HANDBOOK OF EMOTIONS

HANDBOOK OF EMOTIONS

Third Edition

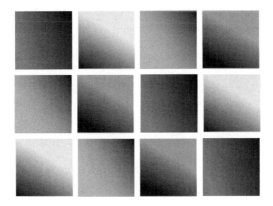

EDITED BY MICHAEL LEWIS,
JEANNETTE M. HAVILAND-JONES,
AND LISA FELDMAN BARRETT

THE GUILFORD PRESS
New York   London

© 2008 The Guilford Press
A Division of Guilford Publications, Inc.
72 Spring Street, New York, NY 10012
www.guilford.com

Printed in the United States of America

This book is printed on acid-free paper.

Last digit is print number: 9 8 7 6 5 4 3 2 1

Library of Congress Cataloging-in-Publication Data

Handbook of emotions / edited by Michael Lewis, Jeannette M. Haviland-Jones,
Lisa Feldman Barrett. — 3rd ed.
    p. cm.
  Includes bibliographical references and index.
  ISBN 978-1-59385-650-2 (cloth : alk. paper)
  1. Emotions. 2. Emotions—Sociological aspects. I. Lewis, Michael, 1937 Jan. 10–
II. Haviland-Jones, Jeannette M.   III. Barrett, Lisa Feldman.
  BF561.H35 2008
  152.4—dc22

                                                          2007042332

About the Editors

Michael Lewis, PhD, is the University Distinguished Professor of Pediatrics and Psychiatry and Director of the Institute for the Study of Child Development at Robert Wood Johnson Medical School, University of Medicine and Dentistry of New Jersey. Dr. Lewis has written or edited more than 30 books on developmental psychology, and he was rated as number one in scholarly impact in the field of developmental psychology in a survey published in *Developmental Review* in 1995. He is coeditor of *The Handbook of Developmental Psychopathology*. His book *Altering Fate: Why the Past Does Not Predict the Future* (1998) was a finalist for the Maccoby Book Award. He recently coedited a new text, *Introduction to Infant Development, Second Edition.*

Jeannette M. Haviland-Jones, PhD, is Professor of Psychology and Director of the Human Emotions Lab at Rutgers, The State University of New Jersey. She has written extensively about emotional development for over 25 years and coauthored *The Hidden Genius of Emotion* with Carol Magai. Her long-time research interests have included lifespan changes in displays of emotion, gender differences in emotions, and the organizing effects of emotion on cognition and on personality. Recently she has initiated research on the chemosensory aspects of emotion communication, including studies on the emotional environment.

Lisa Feldman Barrett, PhD, is Professor of Psychology and Director of the Interdisciplinary Affective Science Laboratory at Boston College, with appointments at Harvard Medical School and Massachusetts General Hospital. Her major research focus is on the nature of emotion from social-psychological, psychophysiological, cognitive science, and neuroscience perspectives. Dr. Barrett has published over 80 papers and book chapters. She has edited, with Peter Salovey, *The Wisdom in Feeling: Psychological Processes in Emotional Intelligence*, and, with Paula Niedenthal and Piotr Winkielman, *Emotion and Consciousness*. She is the recipient of the Career Trajectory Award from the Society for Experimental Social Psychology; the James McKeen Cattell Award from the James McKeen Cattell Fund and the Association for Psychological Science; the NIH Director's Pioneer Award; and a fellowship from the American Philosophical Society. She delivered an APS William James Distinguished Lecture in Psychological Science in 2006 and is currently Co-Editor in Chief of the journal *Emotion Review.*

Contributors

Jo-Anne Bachorowski, PhD, Department of Psychology, Vanderbilt University, Nashville, Tennessee

Lisa Feldman Barrett, PhD, Department of Psychology, Boston College, Chestnut Hill, Massachusetts

John E. Bates, PhD, Department of Psychological and Brain Sciences, Indiana University, Bloomington, Indiana

Gary G. Berntson, PhD, Department of Psychology, Ohio State University, Columbus, Ohio

Eliza Bliss-Moreau, BA, Department of Psychology, Boston College, Chestnut Hill, Massachusetts

George A. Bonanno, PhD, Department of Counseling and Clinical Psychology, Teachers College, Columbia University, New York, New York

Leslie R. Brody, PhD, Department of Psychology, Boston University, Boston, Massachusetts

John T. Cacioppo, PhD, Department of Psychology and Center for Cognitive and Social Neuroscience, University of Chicago, Chicago, Illinois

Linda A. Camras, PhD, Department of Psychology, DePaul University, Chicago, Illinois

Gerald L. Clore, PhD, Department of Psychology, University of Virginia, Charlottesville, Virginia

Michael A. Cohn, BA, Department of Psychology, University of Michigan, Ann Arbor, Michigan

Karin G. Coifman, MA, Department of Counseling and Clinical Psychology, Teachers College, Columbia University, New York, New York

Nathan S. Consedine, PhD, Department of Psychology and Intercultural Institute on Human Development and Aging, Long Island University, Brooklyn, New York

Leda Cosmides, PhD, Department of Psychology and Center for Evolutionary Psychology, University of California at Santa Barbara, Santa Barbara, California

A. D. (Bud) Craig, PhD, Atkinson Research Laboratory, Barrow Neurological Institute, Phoenix, Arizona

Matthew Davidson, BA, Department of Psychology, Columbia University, New York, New York

Brian T. Detweiler-Bedell, PhD, Department of Psychology, Lewis and Clark College, Portland, Oregon

Jerusha B. Detweiler-Bedell, PhD, Department of Psychology, Lewis and Clark College, Portland, Oregon

Michael A. Diefenbach, PhD, Department of Urology and Department of Oncological Sciences, Mount Sinai School of Medicine, New York, New York

Ed Diener, PhD, Department of Psychology, University of Illinois at Urbana–Champaign, Champaign, Illinois

Kenneth A. Dodge, PhD, Department of Public Policy Studies, Duke University, Durham, North Carolina

Seth Duncan, MA, Department of Psychology, Boston College, Chestnut Hill, Massachusetts

Serah S. Fatani, MA, Department of Psychology, DePaul University, Chicago, Illinois

Agneta H. Fischer, PhD, Department of Social Psychology, University of Amsterdam, Amsterdam, The Netherlands

Jennifer E. Fite, MA, Department of Psychological and Brain Sciences, Indiana University, Bloomington, Indiana

Mark Frank, PhD, Department of Communication, University at Buffalo, State University of New York, Buffalo, New York

Barbara L. Fredrickson, PhD, Department of Psychology, University of North Carolina at Chapel Hill, Chapel Hill, North Carolina

Nico H. Frijda, PhD, Department of Psychology, University of Amsterdam, Amsterdam, The Netherlands

Jackson A. Goodnight, BS, Department of Psychological and Brain Sciences, Indiana University, Bloomington, Indiana

Laura Goorin, MA, Department of Counseling and Clinical Psychology, Teachers College, Columbia University, New York, New York

Leslie S. Greenberg, PhD, Department of Psychology, York University, Toronto, Ontario, Canada

James J. Gross, PhD, Department of Psychology, Stanford University, Stanford, California

Jonathan Haidt, PhD, Department of Psychology, University of Virginia, Charlottesville, Virginia

Judith A. Hall, PhD, Department of Psychology, Northeastern University, Boston, Massachusetts

Paul L. Harris, DPhil, Graduate School of Education, Harvard University, Cambridge, Massachusetts

Jeannette M. Haviland-Jones, PhD, Human Emotions Lab, Department of Psychology, Rutgers, The State University of New Jersey, New Brunswick, New Jersey

Marc W. Hernandez, PhD, Department of Psychology, University of Chicago, Chicago, Chicago Illinois

Martin L. Hoffman, PhD, Department of Psychology, New York University, New York, New York

Randall Horton, PhD, Department of Comparative Human Development, University of Chicago, Chicago, Illinois

Alice M. Isen, PhD, Department of Psychology and Johnson Graduate School of Management, Cornell University, Ithaca, New York

Tiffany A. Ito, PhD, Department of Psychology, University of Colorado, Boulder, Colorado

P. N. Johnson-Laird, PhD, Department of Psychology, Princeton University, Princeton, New Jersey

Craig Joseph, PhD, Department of Comparative Human Development, University of Chicago, Chicago, Illinois; Department of Psychology, Northwestern University, Evanston, Illinois

Josh Joseph, BA, BS, Department of Psychology, Columbia University, New York, New York

Dacher Keltner, PhD, Department of Psychology, University of California at Berkeley, Berkeley, California

Margaret E. Kemeny, PhD, Department of Psychiatry, University of California at San Francisco, San Francisco, California

Elizabeth A. Kensinger, PhD, Department of Psychology, Boston College, Chestnut Hill, Massachusetts

Hedy Kober, BS, Department of Psychology, Columbia University, New York, New York

Ann M. Kring, PhD, Department of Psychology, University of California at Berkeley, Berkeley, California

Jeff T. Larsen, PhD, Department of Psychology, Texas Tech University, Lubbock, Texas

Joseph E. LeDoux, PhD, Center for Neural Science, New York University, New York, New York

Elizabeth A. Lemerise, PhD, Department of Psychology, Western Kentucky University, Bowling Green, Kentucky

Howard Leventhal, PhD, Institute for Health, Health Care Policy, and Aging Research, Department of Psychology, Rutgers-The State University of New Jersey, New Brunswick, New Jersey

Michael Lewis, PhD, Institute for the Study of Child Development, Department of Pediatrics, Robert Wood Johnson Medical School, University of Medicine and Dentistry of New Jersey, New Brunswick, New Jersey

Kristen A. Lindquist, BA, Department of Psychology, Boston College, Chestnut Hill, Massachusetts

George Loewenstein, PhD, Department of Social and Decision Sciences, Carnegie Mellon University, Pittsburgh, Pennsylvania

Richard E. Lucas, PhD, Department of Psychology, Michigan State University, East Lansing, Michigan

Diane M. Mackie, PhD, Department of Psychology, University of California at Santa Barbara, Santa Barbara, California

Carol Magai, PhD, Department of Psychology and Intercultural Institute on Human Development and Aging, Long Island University, Brooklyn, New York

Antony S. R. Manstead, DPhil, School of Psychology, Cardiff University, Cardiff, Wales, United Kingdom

David Matsumoto, PhD, Department of Psychology, San Francisco State University, San Francisco, California

John D. Mayer, PhD, Department of Psychology, University of New Hampshire, Durham, New Hampshire

Clark R. McCauley, PhD, Department of Psychology, Bryn Mawr College, Bryn Mawr, Pennsylvania

Suzanne M. Miller, PhD, Division of Population Science, Psychosocial and Behavioral Medicine Program, Behavioral Research Core Facility, and Behavioral Center of Excellence in Breast Cancer, Fox Chase Cancer Center, Philadelphia, Pennsylvania

Marvin Minsky, PhD, Department of Electrical Engineering and Computer Science, and MIT Media Laboratory, Massachusetts Institute of Technology, Cambridge, Massachusetts

Jennifer Mize, BA, Department of Psychology, Boston College, Chestnut Hill, Massachusetts

Paula M. Niedenthal, PhD, Laboratory for Social and Cognitive Psychology, National Center for Scientific Research and University of Clermont-Ferrand, Clermont-Ferrand, France

Keith Oatley, PhD, Cognitive Science Program, University College, University of Toronto, Toronto, Ontario, Canada

Arne Öhman, PhD, Psychology Section, Department of Clinical Neuroscience, Karolinska Institute, Stockholm, Sweden

Andrew Ortony, PhD, Department of Psychology, Northwestern University, Evanston, Illinois

Maureen O'Sullivan, PhD, Department of Psychology, University of San Francisco, San Francisco, California

Michael J. Owren, PhD, Department of Psychology and Center for Behavioral Neuroscience, Georgia State University, Atlanta, Georgia

Jaak Panksepp, PhD, Department of Veterinary and Comparative Anatomy, Pharmacology, and Physiology, College of Veterinary Medicine, Washington State University, Pullman, Washington

Ellen Peters, PhD, Decision Research, Eugene, Oregon

Elizabeth A. Phelps, PhD, Department of Psychology, New York University, New York, New York

Kirsten M. Poehlmann, PhD, Department of Neurosciences, University of California at San Diego, San Diego, California

Matthew Porter, PhD, Department of Oncological Sciences, Mount Sinai School of Medicine, New York, New York

Scott Rick, PhD, Operations and Information Management Department, The Wharton School, University of Pennsylvania, Philadelphia, Pennsylvania

Paul Rozin, PhD, Department of Psychology, University of Pennsylvania, Philadelphia, Pennsylvania

James A. Russell, PhD, Department of Psychology, Boston College, Chestnut Hill, Massachusetts

Carolyn Saarni, PhD, Department of Counseling, Sonoma State University, Rohnert Park, California

Peter Salovey, PhD, Department of Psychology, Yale University, New Haven, Connecticut

Daniel L. Schacter, PhD, Department of Psychology, Harvard University, Cambridge, Massachusetts

Avgusta Shestyuk, PhD, Helen Wills Neuroscience Institute, University of California at Berkeley, Berkeley, California

Michelle N. Shiota, PhD, Department of Psychology, Arizona State University, Tempe, Arizona

Richard A. Shweder, PhD, Department of Comparative Human Development, University of Chicago, Chicago, Illinois

Eliot R. Smith, PhD, Department of Psychological and Brain Sciences, Indiana University, Bloomington, Indiana

Robert C. Solomon, PhD (deceased), Department of Philosophy, University of Texas at Austin, Austin, Texas

Peter N. Stearns, PhD, Department of History and Office of the Provost, George Mason University, Fairfax, Virginia

Michael Stefanek, PhD, Behavioral Research Center, American Cancer Society, Atlanta, Georgia

Nancy L. Stein, PhD, Department of Psychology and Department of Comparative Human Development, University of Chicago, Chicago, Illinois

Jan E. Stets, PhD, Department of Sociology, University of California at Riverside, Riverside, California

John Tooby, PhD, Department of Anthropology and Center for Evolutionary Psychology, University of California at Santa Barbara, Santa Barbara, California

Tom Trabasso, PhD (deceased), Department of Psychology, University of Chicago, Chicago, Illinois

Jonathan H. Turner, PhD, Department of Sociology, University of California at Riverside, Riverside, California

Tor D. Wager, PhD, Department of Psychology, Columbia University, New York, New York

Arlene S. Walker-Andrews, PhD, Department of Psychology and Office of the Provost, University of Montana, Missoula, Montana

Sherri C. Widen, PhD, Department of Psychology, Boston College, Chestnut Hill, Massachusetts

Patricia J. Wilson, PhD, Department of Psychology, La Salle University, Philadelphia, Pennsylvania

Preface

When we published the first edition of the *Handbook of Emotions* in 1993, research in emotions was beginning to blossom. Since then, its study has been recognized as an essential aspect of any study of humankind. At the beginning of the new century, the value of studying emotions—as they interface with cognition, with personality, and with social and health issues—has become obvious to all. The second edition of the *Handbook* was an attempt to meet this new challenge by allowing us to consider the work already accomplished and to begin exploring the new work that lies ahead.

The first edition was rated by *Choice* as an "Outstanding Academic Book" in 1995. The third edition continues this tradition, as it seeks to be both a compendium of what we have learned and an introduction to new areas that have caught our imagination. For those who are just beginning to take an interest in the field of emotion research, this volume should propel their interest further, with new areas to investigate and old questions to be viewed in new ways. For those of us who continue to work in the field and who once labored as isolated scientists, this third edition demonstrates the strength and vitality of the field as new areas open up and new investigators make notable contributions. Such a development reflects the large community of scholars who are now invested in research and conceptual questions about emotions. These research activities are only enhanced when such a gathering of scholars reaches the mass it has now attained.

This edition contains new chapters by authors who made different contributions to the first two editions, updates to chapters in the first and second editions that reflect the research of the last 15 years, and chapters by new contributors that reflect the expanding understanding of how emotions interface with other aspects of behavior. Thus this edition includes work by pioneers of the field who are continuing to expand their original ideas, as well as efforts by new investigators whose contributions to the study of emotion are well documented. In this third edition, we have maintained our interest in "Interdisciplinary Foundations," adding revised chapters on several topics and a new chapter on economics to this first part of the book. Part II, "Biological and Neurophysiological Approaches," now includes new chapters on neuroimaging and olfaction. Whereas in the second edition "Social and Personality Issues" was considered in a single part of the book, we have now divided this section into two separate parts, reflecting how emotions have increasingly become a part of the study of the social world as well as personality. Part III, "Developmental Changes," now includes a new chapter on life course in emotional development. Both the "Cognitive Factors" and "Health and

Emotions" parts have been expanded, including new chapters on artificial intelligence and the role of emotions in the neuroendocrine and immune systems. The final part, "Select Emotions," also now reflects the interest in positive emotions. Our efforts to look at emotions from a broad as well as a more focused perspective allow the reader access not only to the role of emotion in diverse fields, but also to more focused views of work in specific emotions.

Although this edition of the *Handbook* follows the same basic organization of the first edition, there has been such an increase in the possible topics that could have been included that we greatly regret having to omit some areas. We have chosen some areas because we believe that they will emerge as significant; others because they have already been enormously productive; and still others simply to provide balance to the various perspectives. Bringing together the broadening content of the *Handbook* and working with this large, diverse group of scholars were great challenges and privileges. It is to our contributors that the volume owes its strength.

We continue to hope that scholars, clinicians, and students from a variety of disciplines will find our efforts helpful. Finally, we would like to express our appreciation to Stacey Napoli, without whom this edition would not have been possible.

MICHAEL LEWIS
JEANNETTE M. HAVILAND-JONES
LISA FELDMAN BARRETT

Contents

PART I. INTERDISCIPLINARY FOUNDATIONS

PART II. BIOLOGICAL AND NEUROPHYSIOLOGICAL APPROACHES

PART III. DEVELOPMENTAL CHANGES

PART IV. SOCIAL PERSPECTIVES

PART V. PERSONALITY ISSUES

PART VI. COGNITIVE FACTORS

PART I

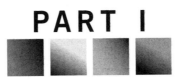

INTERDISCIPLINARY
FOUNDATIONS

CHAPTER 1

The Philosophy of Emotions

ROBERT C. SOLOMON

"What is an emotion?" That question was asked in precisely that form by William James, as the title of an essay he wrote for *Mind* well over 100 years ago (James, 1884). But philosophers have been concerned about the nature of emotion since Socrates and the "pre-Socratics" who preceded him, and although the discipline has grown up (largely because of Socrates and his student Plato) as the pursuit of reason, the emotions have always lurked in the background—often as a threat to reason and a danger to philosophy and philosophers. One of the most enduring metaphors of reason and emotion has been the metaphor of master and slave, with the wisdom of reason firmly in control and the dangerous impulses of emotion safely suppressed, channeled, or (ideally) in harmony with reason. But the question "What is an emotion?" has proved to be as difficult to resolve as the emotions have been to master. Just when it seems that an adequate definition is in place, some new theory rears its unwelcome head and challenges our understanding.

The master–slave metaphor displays two features that still determine much of the philosophical view of emotion today. First there is the inferior role of emotion—the idea that emotion is as such more primitive, less intelligent, more bestial, less dependable, and more dangerous than reason, and thus needs to be controlled by reason (an argument that Aristotle and other enlightened Athenians used to justify the political institution of slavery, as well). Second, and more profoundly, there is the reason–emotion distinction itself—as if we were dealing with two different natural kinds, two conflicting and antagonistic aspects of the soul. Even those philosophers who sought to integrate them and reduce one to the other (typically reducing emotion to an inferior genus of reason, a "confused perception" or "distorted judgment") maintained the distinction and continued to insist on the superiority of reason. It was thus a mark of his considerable iconoclasm that the Scottish skeptic David Hume (1739/1888), in the 18th century, famously declared that "reason is, and ought to be, the slave of the passions." But even Hume, despite an ingenious analysis of the structure of emotions, ultimately fell back on the old models and metaphors. His work remains an exemplary celebration of reason, even while challenging its limits.

Philosophy is a historical discipline. It is constrained and defined as much by its past as by any particular field of phenomena. Philosophical theories and debates today cannot be understood or appreciated without some understanding of philosophy's rich and convoluted past. Even when a philosopher pretends to understand the phenomenon of emotion "in itself," or to analyze the language of emotion without reference to history or to any earlier attempts at analysis, both the wisdom and the folly of generations of accumulated reflection and argument are nevertheless inescapable. Although one might impatiently demand from the outset that one "define the terms" before the current discussion commences, the truth is that a definition emerges only at the end of a long discussion, and even then it is always tentative and appropriate only within a limited context and certain models of culture and personal character.

In what follows, I have tried to sketch a somewhat selective history of philosophical attempts to understand emotion, followed by a brief summary of questions still central to philosophical debate. Given the nature of philosophy and its emphasis on reason, however, we would expect that the focus of most philosophical analysis has been and remains the more cognitive aspects of emotion, with the physiological and to a certain extent the social and behavioral dimensions of emotion diminished or even denied. The dialectic in philosophy, accordingly, tends to go back and forth in its rediscovery of these often neglected dimensions. Sometimes emotions are dismissed as mere feelings and physiology, utterly unintelligent, even subhuman. In reaction, emotions are then ascribed the virtues of true wisdom; they are defended as the proper masters of reason and even the very foundation of our being-in-the-world. Most philosophers, however, try to find some more moderate, multidimensional position.

One might object that philosophical theories of emotion tend to be "armchair" speculation, devoid of the empirical support supplied by social scientists. However, this objection ignores the fact that philosophers, contrary to their own self-styled reputations as men and women of pure reason, have emotions themselves, and in most (but not all) cases a sufficiently rich repertoire of emotions to fund and support a dozen theories of emotion. As Descartes (1649/1989) said in his introduction to the subject, "everyone has experience of the passions within himself, and there is no necessity to borrow one's observations from elsewhere in order to discover their nature." Ultimately, there is no justification for the century-old feud between philosophy and psychology. Their history is in fact the same, and the phenomenon of emotion lies equally open to both of them.

THE HISTORY OF THE PHILOSOPHY OF EMOTION

Although the history of philosophy has often been described as the history of the development of reason—for example, by the great 19th-century German philosopher G. W. F. Hegel—philosophers have never entirely neglected emotion, even if they have almost always denied it center stage. It would be a mistake, however, to put too much emphasis on the term "emotion," for its range and meaning have altered significantly over the years, due in part to changes in theories about emotion. So too, the word "passion" has a long and varied history, and we should beware of the misleading assumption that there is a single, orderly, natural class of phenomena that is simply designated by different labels in different languages at different times. The language of "passion" and "emotion" has a history into which various feelings, desires, sentiments, moods, attitudes, and more explosive responses enter and from which they exit, depending not on arbitrary philosophical stipulation but on an extensive network of social, moral, cultural, and psychological factors. Thus we will often find that the focus is not emotion as such, but rather some particular class of emotions or particular emotion and its role in the manners or morals of the time.

The emotions as such, accordingly, do not form one of the three aspects of Plato's (ca. 428–347 B.C.) tripartite soul as defined in *The Republic* (1974). There are reason, spirit, and appetite; not only does what we call emotion seem divided between spirit and appetite, but, considering Plato's discussion of *eros* as the love of the Good in his dialogue *The Symposium* (1989), there are emotions involved in reason as well. Aristotle (384–322 B.C.), by contrast, did seem to have a view of emotion as such, but although he had a mania for taxonomies, he spent relatively little time listing or analyzing the emotions—as he did, for example, the virtues and the various kinds of birds. In his *Rhetoric* (1941), however, he defined emotion "as that which leads one's condition to become so transformed that his judgment is affected, and which is accompanied by pleasure and pain. Examples of emotion include anger, fear, pity, and the like, as well as the opposites of these."[1] (He did not tell us what these "opposites" might be.) Aristotle discussed certain emotions at length, notably anger, which he described in remarkably modern terms. In the *Rhetoric* he defined anger as "a distressed desire for conspicuous vengeance in return for a conspicuous and unjustifiable contempt of one's person or friends." He added that "anger is always directed toward someone in particular, for example, Cleon, and not toward all of humanity," and mentioned (if only in passing) the physical distress that virtually always accompanies such emotion.

The key to Aristotle's analysis, however, is the notion of a "slight." This is the cause of anger, and it may be an instance of "scorn, spite, or insolence." Aristotle made allowances for only imagined slights (in other words, unwarranted anger is nevertheless anger), and he gave a central place to the desire for revenge, thus introducing a behavioral component at the heart of the emotion. We might note that Aristotle, who was so precocious in so many disciplines, seems to have anticipated most of the main contemporary theories. His analysis of anger includes a distinctive cognitive component, a specified social context, a behavioral tendency, and a recognition of physical arousal. He even noted that physical or psychological discomfort—sickness, poverty, love, war, breached expectations, or ingratitude—yields a predisposition for anger. It is worth noting that Aristotle had little to say of "feeling," presumably not because the Greeks were anesthetic, but rather because what we (inconsistently) call "affect" and inner sensation generally held little interest for them and played no significant role in their language or their psychology.

Perhaps the most important single point to make about Aristotle's view of emotion is the fact that his analyses make sense only in the context of a broader ethical concern. Anger was of interest to him because it is a natural reaction to offense and a moral force, which can be cultivated and provoked by reason and rhetoric. (Thus its inclusion in a book on that topic.) Anger (and several other emotions, notably pride) is also prominent in Aristotle's classical list of virtues in his *Nicomachean Ethics* (1941), where he discussed in some detail those circumstances in which it is appropriate to get angry, those in which it is not, and what amount or intensity of anger is justified. He suggested that forgiveness may be a virtue, but only sometimes. He also insisted that only fools don't get angry, and that although overly angry people may be "unbearable," the absence of anger (aimed at the right offenses) is a vice rather than a virtue. In this as in all else, Aristotle defended moderation, the "mean between the extremes." So too, he discussed fear at length in the *Ethics* with regard to courage, which is not fearlessness or "overcoming" fear so much as it is having just the right amount of fear—not being either foolhardy or cowardly. The emotions, in other words, are central and essential to the good life, and the analysis of their nature is part and parcel of an ethical analysis.

So too, in Roman times, we find the conjunction of ethics and emotion in the philosophy of the Stoics (see Sorabji, 2003, and Nussbaum, 1994). But whereas Aristotle took emotion to be essential to the good life, the Stoics analyzed emotions as conceptual errors, conducive to misery. In modern terms, the Stoics Seneca and Chrysippus developed a full-blooded cognitive theory of the emotions two millennia ago (see especially Seneca, 1963). Emotions, in a word, are judgments—judgments about the world and one's place in it. But the world of Roman society was not a happy or a particularly rational place. (Seneca served under the Emperor Nero, and ultimately committed suicide at his behest.) And as the Stoics saw the world they lived in as out of control and beyond any reasonable expectations, they saw the emotions, which impose such expectations on the world, as misguided judgments about life and our place in the world. The emotions consequently make us miserable and frustrated. Accordingly, the Stoics made a careful study of the component judgments that compose the emotions—the presumptuousness of moral judgment in anger, the vulnerability of love, the self-absorption of security in fear. The alternative was seen as "psychic indifference," or *apatheia* (apathy). The Stoics believed in a "higher" reason, one transcending the vanities of the social world. But they felt that the best life in that world could be achieved only by getting straight about the ultimate pointlessness of emotional attachments and involvement.

Throughout the Middle Ages, the study of emotion was again typically attached to ethics, and it was central to Christian psychology and the theories of human nature in terms of which the medievals understood themselves (see Hyman & Walsh, 1973). There were elaborate, quasi-medical studies of the effects of the various "humours" (gall, spleen, choler, and blood itself) on emotional temperament, but there were (as there were among the Stoics) especially rich studies of the cognitive and "conative" aspects of the emotions. Emotions were essentially linked with desires, particularly self-interested, self-absorbed desires. And so the Christian preoccupation with sin led to elaborate analyses of those emotions, passions, and desires designated as sins (notably greed, gluttony, lust, anger, envy, and pride; sloth, perhaps, is a special case). The tight linkage between the study of emotion and ethics is particularly evident in the curious observation that the highest virtues, such as love, hope, and faith, were not classified as emotions as such, but were rather elevated to a higher status and often (e.g., by Thomas Aquinas) equated with reason. The old master–slave metaphor remained alive and well, and as some emotions were seen as sins, the highest virtues could hardly be counted among the mere emotions.

Reviewing the ancient and medieval literature on emotion, René Descartes (1596–1650) was provoked to write that what they taught was "so slight, and for the most part so far from credible, that I am unable to entertain any hope of approximating the truth excepting by shunning the paths they followed" (1649/ 1989). Descartes is typically recognized as the "father" of modern philosophy, and, in a more scholarly vein, as the bridge between the scholastic world of the Middle Ages and our own. But Descartes was fundamentally a scientist and a mathematician, awed by "the natural light of reason" and fascinated by the unique autonomy of the human mind. Accordingly, he disdained the bodily and the bestial, insisting that the mind is a separate "substance" from the body (and that beasts therefore do not have minds). The separation of mind and body proved to be a famously difficult problem for Descartes and his successors, however, and nowhere was that problem more evident than in his attempt to deal with the emotions.

Thoughts about mathematics may be clearly "in" the mind, as stomach contractions are in the body, but an emotion seems to require the interaction of mind and body in an undeniable way. Accordingly, Descartes defended a theory in his treatise *On the Passions of the Soul* (1649/1989), in which the mind and body "meet" in a small gland at the base of the brain (now known as the pineal gland), and the latter affects the former by means of the agitation of "animal spirits" (minute particles of blood), which bring about the emotions and their physical effects in various parts of the body. But the emotions also involve not only sensations caused by this physical agitation, but perceptions, desires, and beliefs as well. Thus over and above the physical agitation and familiar sensations, the emotion of hatred ultimately arises from the perception of an object's potential harmfulness and involves a desire to avoid it. Accordingly, it is not as if an emotion is merely a perception of the body; it may also be, as Descartes put it, a perception of the soul (e.g., a perception of desire), and some perceptions (as in dreams) may in fact be of things that do not exist at all.

An emotion is one type of "passion," for Descartes defined the passions in general as "the perceptions, feelings or emotions of the soul which we relate specifically to it, and which are caused, maintained, and fortified by some movement of the [animal] spirits." The passions in general are distinguished from "clear cognition," and render judgment "confused and obscure." Emotions are particularly disturbing passions. And yet emotions can be influenced by reason. For example, writing of courage, Descartes stated:

> To excite courage in oneself and remove fear, it is not sufficient to have the will to do so, but we must also apply ourselves to consider the reasons, the objects or examples which persuade us that the peril is not great; that there is always more security in defense than in flight, that we should have the glory and joy of having vanquished, while we should expect nothing but regret and shame for having fled, and so on.

And so the physiological account gives way to a cognitive account, and the emotions move from being merely bodily to becoming an essential ingredient in wisdom: "The utility of the passions consists alone in their fortifying and perpetuating in the soul thoughts which it is good that it should preserve, and which without that might easily be effaced from it." How then can there be "bad" emotions? "The harm is that they fortify these thoughts more than necessary, or they conserve others on which it is not good to dwell." Somewhat bewildered by the physiology (though he was at the cutting edge of the science of his times), Descartes ultimately tended to a value-oriented analysis of emotion. His six "primitive" passions—wonder, love, hatred, desire, joy, and sadness—are not meaningless agitations of the animal spirits, but ingredients in the good life.

Baruch (Benedict) Spinoza (1632–1677) might well be considered to be a latter-day Stoic, like Chrysippus and Seneca in ancient Rome. Just as the Stoics saw the emotions as misguided judgments about life and our place in the world, Spinoza too saw the emotions as a form of "thoughts" that, for the most part, misunderstand the world and consequently make us miserable and frustrated. But unlike the Stoics, Spinoza did not aspire to that "psychic indifference" known as *apatheia*; rather, in his *Ethics* (1677/1982), he urged the attainment of a certain sort of "bliss," which can be achieved only once we get straight our thinking about the world. In particular, we have to give up the idea that we are or can be in control of our own lives, and adopt instead the all-embracing idea of ourselves and our minds as part of God. Most of the emotions, which are passive reactions to our unwarranted expectations of the world, will leave us hurt, frustrated, and enervated.

The active emotions, by contrast, emanate from our own true natures and heighten our sense of activity and awareness. Spinoza, like the Stoics, developed an early version of the cognitive theory of emotion. But Spinoza also defended a grand and complex metaphysics, in which all substance is one, and mind and body are but dual "aspects" of one and the same being. Accordingly, he did not face Descartes's formidable "mind–body" problem; although he himself would not have predicted this, he anticipated some of the subtle emotion–brain research that is being carried out today.

David Hume (1711–1776) was one of the most outspoken defenders of the Enlightenment, that very vocal and often rebellious intellectual movement that challenged old orthodoxies, elevated science and put religion on the defensive, attacked superstition and irrationality in all quarters, practiced and encouraged vigorous debate and discussion, and put a pre-mium on the virtues of reason. But Hume, in carrying out the directives of reason to challenge, debate, and question, came to question the role and capacities of reason itself, and in particular the power of reason to motivate even the most basic minimum of moral behavior. "It is not against reason," he declared in one of his most outrageous proclamations, "to prefer the destruction of half the world to the scratching of my finger" (1739/1888). What motivates us to right (and wrong) behavior, Hume insisted, were our passions, and rather than being relegated to the margins of ethics and philosophy, the passions deserve central respect and consideration.

Accordingly, he gave the passions the large middle portion of his great first book, *A Treatise of Human Nature* (1739/1888). Unfortunately, however, most philosophers then and since have preferred to read the first and third parts, on knowledge and ethics, and to ignore the central position of the passions.

Hume's theory is especially important not only because he challenged the inferior place of passion in philosophy and questioned the role of reason. He also advanced a theory of the passions that, although limited and encumbered by his general theory of mind, displayed dazzling insight and a precocious attempt to grapple with problems that would only be formulated generations later. Hume, like many of his contemporaries and predecessors, defined an emotion as a certain kind of sensation, or what he called an "impression," which (as in Descartes) is physically stimulated by the movement of the "animal spirits" in the blood. Such impressions are either pleasant or unpleasant, but the differentiation of the many emotions is not to be found in the nature of these impressions as such. Rather, the impressions that constitute our emotions are always to be located within a causal network of other impressions and, importantly, ideas. Ideas cause our emotional impressions, and ideas are caused in turn by them. The pleasant impression of pride, for example, is caused by the idea that one has achieved or accomplished something significant, and the impression in turn causes another idea, which Hume described as an idea of the self, *simpliciter*.

The emotion, in other words, cannot be identified with the impression or sensation alone, but can only be identified by the whole complex of impressions and ideas. What Hume acknowledged with his emphasis on the essential place of ideas in emotion is what we now call the cognitive dimension of emotion, in addition to the physiological ("animal spirits") and merely sensational ("impression") aspects of emotion. Moreover, his inclusion of the second idea of the self in his analysis of pride indicates his grappling with the notion of intentionality (the "aboutness" of emotions)—an effort further reinforced by his somewhat obscure insistence that the connection between an emotion (the impression) and this consequent idea is "original" or "natural," or something more than the merely causal associations that form the usual bonds between ideas and impressions.

The emotions, for Hume, form an essential part of ethics. There are good emotions and bad emotions. Pride, he declared, is a good emotion. Humility, its opposite (an unpleasant feeling brought about by the idea that we are inadequate or deeply flawed beings), is a bad emotion, a "monkish" emotion. Here we can see again the extent to which, as so often, a theory of emotion serves to grind some larger philosophical ax—in this case, Hume's Enlightenment attack on religion. In this regard too, we might mention another aspect of Hume's moral philosophy, followed in kind by his illustrious Edinburgh friend and colleague Adam Smith (1723–1790, also the author of *The Wealth of Nations* [1776/1976], the bible of modern capitalism).

Hume and Smith both defended the importance of what they called "the moral sentiments" (see Smith, 1759/1976), the foremost of which is sympathy, our ability to "feel with" other people and appreciate (if not suffer with) their misfortunes. Sympathy, they argued, is a universal feature of human nature (countering and mitigating the self-interest that Smith in particular famously championed in *The Wealth of Nations*), and it is the bedrock foundation of society and morality. Emotion, in other words, is not an embarrassment or part of the refuse of the human psyche, but rather the very essence of human social existence and morality. It is not to be unfavorably contrasted and opposed to reason, but, on the contrary, is to be celebrated and defended along with it.

Immanuel Kant (1724–1804) was also a champion of the Enlightenment, but although he too questioned the capacities and limits of reason, he was uncompromising in its defense—against Hume's skepticism, against any attempt to replace reason by irrational faith, and against any attempt to ground ethics in fleeting human feeling instead of the univer-

sal and necessary dictates of reason. Thus Kant reinforced the crucial distinction between reason and what he called "the inclinations" (emotions, moods, and desires) and dismissed the latter (including the moral sentiments) as inessential to morals at best and intrusive and disruptive at worst. And yet, although Kant felt no need to develop a theory of emotion to accompany his elaborate and brilliant "critiques" of reason, his position on the "inclinations" is more ambiguous than is usually supposed, and his respect for "feeling" more significant. It was Kant, a quarter-century before Hegel (who is credited with it), who insisted that "nothing great is ever done without passion," and it was Kant, in his *Critique of Judgment* (1793/1953, concerned in part with art and aesthetics), who celebrated the importance of shared ("intersubjective") feeling in the appreciation of beauty and the awe with which we try to comprehend the wonder of God's creation. Indeed, even Kant's central notions of respect and human dignity—the very heart of his rationalist ethics—are sometimes suggested to be matters of feeling as well as reason, thus calling into question the harshness of his ruthlessly divided self. When his successor Hegel took over the reins of German philosophy in the early 19th century, the overstated distinction between reason and passion was again called into question, and Hegel's own odyssey of reason (in an epochal book called *The Phenomenology of Spirit* [1807/1977]) has rightly been called a "logic of passion" as well.

Friedrich Nietzsche (1844–1900) was a philosopher for whom passion was the watchword and reason a source of suspicion. He was the culmination of a long line of "Romantics," beginning with the *Sturm und Drang* poets of the previous century and continuing through the philosophy of Nietzsche's own favorite influence, the neo-Kantian pessimist Arthur Schopenhauer. Nietzsche anticipated the global skepticism and conceptual chaos of the 20th century; like Freud, who admired him, he described (and celebrated) the darker, more instinctual, and less rational motives of the human mind. Accordingly, in his *On the Genealogy of Morals* (1887/1967), he praised the passions and, in an ironic twist, described the passions as themselves having more reason than Reason. But this was not to say that all passions are wise; some, he declares, "drag us down with their stupidity," and others, notably the "slave morality" emotion of resentment, are devious and clever but to a disastrous end—the "leveling" of the virtuous passions and the defense of mediocrity. Nietzsche never developed a "theory" of emotions, but his distinctions were remarkable in their insight and subtlety. His celebration of passion scared the wits out of a great many philosophers in Europe, however, who saw more than enough passion and irrationality in World War I and then the rise of National Socialism in Germany. Accordingly, the ancient celebration of reason would once more rule philosophy, and emotion was again relegated to the sidelines.

In the 20th century, one can trace the fate of emotion in Western philosophy through two very different tracks. In North America and in England, the emotions were given short shrift, in large part because of the newly exaggerated emphasis on logic and science. The great British philosopher Bertrand Russell gave elaborate praise to love and passion in the opening pages of his autobiography (1967), but in his philosophy he said virtually nothing about them. Of course, the nature of emotion was a major concern of William James and the young John Dewey in the early years of the century, but with James's emphasis on the physiological nature of emotion (he argued [1884] that an emotion is a sensation or set of sensations caused by a physiological disturbance, which in turn is prompted by some "perception" or other), coupled with the subsequent and quite unfortunate split between philosophy and psychology as academic disciplines, questions about emotion were relegated to the realm of psychology (where they were also treated with less than the full respect due them). Indeed, the first major attention to emotion in Anglo-American philosophy came in midcentury, when an ethical theory named "emotivism" came to dominate both the English and the North American scene. But emotivism, which was part and parcel of an across-the-board philosophical purgative known as "logical positivism," was essentially a dismissal of ethical (and many other) questions in philosophy as "meaningless" (i.e., unscientific and without verifiable solutions). Emotion came back onto the stage of philosophy, but only as the butt of the argument: Ethical statements were viewed as meaningless because they were seen as nothing but expressions of emotion.

During the same period in Europe, however, the emotions enjoyed more attention. Franz Brentano (1874/1971) succeeded the British "moral sentiment" theorists in attempting to found an ethics on a foundation of emotions.

(Sigmund Freud was one of his students.) Following the "phenomenology" of Edmund Husserl (1838/1960), Max Scheler (1916/1970), Martin Heidegger (1927/1962), and more recently, Paul Ricoeur (1950/1966) developed ambitious philosophies in which emotions were given a central place in human existence and accorded with considerable respect. Heidegger, in particular, defended what he generally called "moods" as our way of "being tuned" to the world. In the shadow of World War II, Jean-Paul Sartre offered the slim but important *The Emotions: Sketch of a Theory* (1939/1948), followed by his magnificent tome *Being and Nothingness* (1943/1956), which includes embedded within its many pages a number of detailed "phenomenological" analyses of emotion. Sartre's conception of emotions as "magical transformations of the world"— willful strategems for coping with a difficult world—added a new "existential" dimension to the investigation of emotion. But, predictably, philosophy in both France and Germany turned again to other interests, although the study of emotion continued despite the perennial shift in fashions.

In Anglo-American philosophy, however, the fortunes of emotion were also to change. In an article simply entitled "Emotion" (indicating how rarely the topic had even been broached), Errol Bedford (1956/1964) addressed the Aristotelean Society in London on the nature of emotion and the errors of thinking of emotions as "feelings." The essay might have sat on the shelves gathering dust except for the fact that the then dean of Oxford philosophers, J. L. Austin (1956–1957/1964), took it upon himself to remark on one of Bedford's claims. (Austin's own essay was not about emotions at all.) Austin's attention kept the article alive and occasionally anthologized until the 1960s, when the subject seemed to come to life again.

Today, one finds a rich variety of arguments about emotions on both sides of the Atlantic Ocean and the English Channel. Given the nature of philosophy and its current concern with epistemological matters, it is again not surprising that the focus is on the conceptual structures of emotion, rather than the sensory, social, or physiological aspects of emotion. But there has been a reaction even within philosophy to the "hypercognizing" of emotion; consequently, there has been a serious effort to join forces with psychologists, neurologists, anthropologists, and moral philosophers to obtain a more holistic theory of emotion.

SOME PHILOSOPHICAL QUESTIONS ABOUT EMOTION

What is an emotion? Because philosophy is a discipline concerned with the essential nature and the "definition" of things, the basic question facing theories of emotion in philosophy is still the question posed by James and answered, in a fashion, by Aristotle. It is, on the face of it, a quest for a definition, a conceptual analysis. But it is also a much larger quest for an orientation: How should we think about emotion—as intrusive, as essential to our rationality, as constitutive of meaning, as dangerous, as dispensable, as an excuse for irresponsibility, or as a mode of responsibility? Which of the evident aspects of emotion—that is, the various sensory, physiological, behavioral, cognitive, and social phenomena that typically correspond with an emotion—should we take to be essential? Many philosophers hold onto the old "Cartesian" view that an emotion cannot lack its "subjective" or "introspective" aspect, although what this means (and how accessible or articulate an emotion must be on inspection) is itself a subject of considerable dispute, for instance, in Freud (1915/1935), Sartre (1943/1956), Lyons (1980), and de Sousa (1987). But many philosophers have become skeptical about such subjective essentialism and, like their associates in the sciences, have pushed the analysis of emotion toward more public, observable criteria. Accordingly, philosophers have formulated their own versions of behaviorism, physiologism, and social construction theory, for example, although they have not always been mutually aware of their counterparts in the social sciences, especially.

The seemingly self-evident Cartesian demand that first-person experience is ineliminable is evident, nevertheless, even among the most radical philosophical behaviorists. For instance, Gilbert Ryle (1951) chastised philosophers for their "myth of the ghost in the machine" and suggested that many emotions are mere "agitations" (much as Descartes had insisted) and dispositions to behave in certain ways. But Ryle did not give up the idea that some of the symptoms of emotion consist of "tingles and itches" or some such "feeling." Can one have an emotion without feeling? What is a "feeling"? According to William James (1884), it is a specifiable sort of sensation, the sensation of one or more "visceral disturbances"—changes in the body due, for instance, to the stimulation of the autonomic nervous system. The great virtue of the Jamesian theory is that it ties down the nature of emotional "feelings" to quite particular and therefore verifiable bodily responses. Unfortunately, the Jamesian theory has often been shown to be wrong, at least in its details (e.g., Cannon, 1929/2003; Dewey, 1894/2003; Schachter & Singer, 1962). How specifically are emotional feelings tied to physiological processes? To be sure, whatever goes on in the mind must now be supposed to have some correlate and cause in the brain, but can we not and should we not describe the "phenomenology" of those feelings quite apart from their brain correlations and causes? Some theorists have tried to save feeling theory by employing the vague, general (and technical) notion of "affect" and its cognates ("affective tone") (Stocker, 1996). But do such terms do anything more than cover up the problem with another word, whose meaning can only be explained by "the kind of feeling you get when you have emotion X"? It is a heuristic mistake to suppose that such feelings are indescribable or "ineffable," whether out of excessive romanticism (as if understanding undermines passion) or dismissive scientism (why talk about feelings if we can't experimentally test them?)

Most feelings have at least an "as if" familiarity ("It feels as if I'd known her for years" or "It felt as if he had shot me through the heart, it was so sudden and so traumatizing"). Many feelings have a distinctive structure, which (not surprisingly) emerges in the thoughts (and then in the verbal expressions) of the emotions. Thus we should identify the *experience* of having an emotion (as opposed to just a simple "feeling") as embodying thoughts, judgments, and other cognitive elements. In general, one should ask how much cognition and learning are presupposed in the feelings that we identify as emotions. It may well be that at least some "basic" emotions are largely to be explained by reference to one or another neurophysiological "affect programs," but even the most basic emotions involve or come to involve "intentionality"—an engagement with the world. And this involves perception and some knowledge, as well as the abilities to act in the world. Thus an emotional experience is not just a Jamesian sensation, but a complex awareness of one's engagements in the world and one's tendencies to act in it. (There may be, however, a kind of "borrowed intentionality" peculiar to emotional sensations; Goldie, 2000.) Whether or not there are Jamesian sensations that accompany such engagements and action tendencies (and no doubt usually there are), the emotion is first of all a mode of engagement. But it should be said that we are not always fully aware of our engagements in the world, nor are we usually fully cognizant of our feelings.

Thus there is room for "unconscious" emotions—a grab-bag concept that embraces everything from the Freudian "Unconscious," to the fact that we misidentify and fail to recognize our own emotions, to the more bracing claims of some neuroscientists that an emotion is essentially not conscious and that awareness (if it happens at all) comes late in the neurological game. As for the feelings (the sensations) themselves, Freud was right in wondering whether it makes any sense to claim that they can be unconscious, given that their whole existence seems *to be to be experienced*. But this embodies just the confusion that one would expect with such a grab-bag concept of the unconscious: On the one hand, an unfelt feeling or sensation makes no sense, but the observation that we are not always aware *that* we have a certain feeling or sensation is quite evident. And because the experience of an emotion is so complex (engaging one's beliefs about the world, oneself, and other people, as well as any number of preferred scenarios and outcomes), it is obvious how and why we may not recognize an emotion when we have it. But what does seem essential to all emotions, including those that are most "basic," is some sense of what is going on in the world, some "cognition," whether or not one is or even can be (reflectively) aware of it. Thus no neurological syndrome or "affect program" can be an emotion if it does not engage the world in some way, perhaps by virtue of a more or less automatic "appraisal" or some possibly subliminal stimulus. The affect programs typical of, say, fear and anger do not actually constitute fear and anger if there are no appropriate appraisals, beliefs, or judgments accompanying them. A person may well feel flushed, uncomfortable, and "as if " he or she wants to flee or start a fight with someone—but if there is no fearful object (more precisely, if the person has no sense of a fearful object), or if there is nothing objectionable, frustrating, or offensive (to the person), then those feelings do not count as fear and anger (or even as "feeling afraid" or "feeling angry").

Recent advances in neurology have disclosed illuminating structural and functional patterns in the central nervous system that are correlated with, and that under experimental conditions bring about, certain emotional reactions. Do these patterns dictate the structure of an adequate theory of emotion, or are those findings but one more set of (contingent) considerations for inclusion in an all-embracing theory? Whatever the case, it is now clear that philosophers cannot ignore or neglect the rich neurophysiological literature on emotions. Indeed, there is now a interdisciplinary subfield in philosophy called "neurophilosophy," which makes the new neurology central to any adequate analysis of emotion and "the mind" (Churchland, 1986). Philosophers may continue to argue that Aristotle knew all about emotions even though he did not know anything about the brain, but they do so at their peril—and in the face of the obvious fact that among the factors that have altered the history of philosophy and its concepts most radically have been new advances in previously unknown or undeveloped sciences.

Virtually all emotions get expressed (however minimally) in behavior. Should behavioral tendencies or sequences of actions or certain basic gestures be taken as essential? A great deal of detailed work in psychology has shown the enormous subtlety and the seemingly "hard-wired" nature of basic patterns of facial expression. And yet philosophers remain skeptical about the implied shift in conception from the emotion to a symptom of emotion. The emotion would seem to be the experience, the perception, the awareness—what is expressed, not the expression itself. On the other hand, many philosophers of a somewhat behaviorist bent (following Wittgenstein's later *Philosophical Investigations* [1953] and Gilbert Ryle's *The Concept of Mind* [1951]) have suggested that an emotion is *nothing but* its behavioral expression, though certainly not a single gesture but an open-ended sequence of actions. An emotion is not a "ghostly inner event," according to Ryle, but a "multitrack disposition" to behave in any number of recognizable ways. So too, philosophers have tried to understand emotion not as an inner feeling but as a value-laden description of a social situation. Thus Errol Bedford (1956/1964) suggested in his pioneering article that the difference between shame and embarrassment, for example, is not some shade of difference between internal *qualia*, but the difference between two contrasting descriptions of the situation.

What remains at the core of all such theories, however, is an awareness that all emotions presuppose or have as their preconditions certain sorts of cognitions—an awareness of danger in fear, recognition of an offense in anger, appreciation of someone or something lovable in love. Even the most hard-headed neurological or behavioral theory must take account of the fact that no matter what the neurology or the behavior, if a person is totally unaware (and not just "consciously unaware") of a certain state of affairs or facts, he or she cannot have certain emotions. If neurologically induced rage does not include some object of anger, that reaction (whatever else it may be) cannot be anger. So too, Freud's "free-floating anxiety" would count as an emotion only insofar as it does indeed (as Freud [1915/1935] argued) have an object, albeit "unconscious." Philosophers (following Aristotle and the scholastics of the Middle Ages) have come to call this the "formal object" of emotion, and one might well think of this as the minimum essential set of "beliefs" defining an emotion type and a more or less specific kind of emotional experience. The formal object of fear, to take an obvious case, is a fearful object, together with the at least minimal beliefs constituting the awareness of the presence or threat of such an object.

Other emotions are more complicated and, accordingly, are more often topics of philosophical debate and disagreement. Anger would seem to require a formal object involving an offense, but some authors would allow frustration alone to count as anger (Gordon, 1987). Still others would argue that anger is to a large extent "socially constructed," and its manifestation in any given culture will therefore be more or less specific (though probably not unique) to that culture (Averill, 1985). Jealousy is more difficult still, for its object seems to involve not only a threatened loss but a perpetrator as well (perhaps the threatened object as a perpetrator too), and possibly the larger social situation in which jealousy involves not only loss but humiliation as well (Neu, 1980). But although the exact natures of the formal objects and requisite beliefs of various emotions are matters of lively debate (and there is even more doubt and debate over the very idea of a generalized formal object for emotions as such), the presumption is that every emotion must have a cognitive basis and an object (intentionality). There is some corollary debate concerning the status of moods and mood-like emotions (e.g., joy), which do not have a determinate object, but it can be argued that moods do have an object—namely, the world as a whole. "A depressed man lives in a depressed world," wrote Wittgenstein (1953).

There is also considerable debate over the nature of cognition itself. Beliefs seem to be established states and therefore lack the spontaneity that characterizes many emotions. Beliefs also seem to be too fully articulate for the unreflective reaction that characterizes most emotions. For that reason, some theorists prefer the concept of "judgment" or "evaluative judgment" (e.g., the ancient Stoics; Solomon, 1976, 2003; Nussbaum, 2003), while others prefer the term "thought" (e.g., Spinoza, 1677/1982; Neu, 1977, 1999). Psychologists seem to prefer "appraisal," although it should be said that the social sciences have been much more keen to understand "appraisal" in a multilevel fashion than philosophers, at least until recently (Prinz, 2004). Others have preferred the less cognitively committal notion of a way of seeing ("seeing as")—sometimes as a rejection of the cognitive view, but more appropriately, perhaps, as a refinement of it (Calhoun, 1984, Roberts, 2003). The nature of an emotional cognition, and whether it must be fully conscious or capable of articulation, remain matters for considerable debate. Indeed, if certain holistic suggestions can be worked out, it may be that the very distinctions that philosophers have so long presupposed among cognition, behavior, physiology, and feeling are themselves inadequate and ought to be integrated into a single picture (Damasio, 1994).

One point of general agreement among philosophers is that emotions have intentionality. "Intentionality" is a technical notion, but its common-sense meaning can be captured by the idea that emotions are always "about" something or other. One is always angry about something; one is always in love with someone or something (even if one is also "in love with love"); one is always afraid of something (even if one doesn't know what it is). Thus we can understand the "formal object" of an emotion as its essential intentionality—the kind of object (event, person, state of affairs) to which it must be directed if it is to be that emotion. But intentionality has also been the object of philosophical consternation for over a century now, because despite its appeal as a way of understanding the nature of perception and other mental "acts" (which gets us away from the image of images or representations "in" the mind), intentionality has its own peculiar complications (Kenny, 1963; Searle, 1983). Some philosophers have argued for a more dynamic and action-laden concept than "aboutness," perhaps "motility" or "engagement" (as above) (Merleau-Ponty, 1962/1994; Solomon, 2003). Many philosophers accept the idea of intentionality, but try to integrate it into a neo-Jamesian analysis of emotions as physiology plus sensation, by way of an intricate causal theory of perception (Prinz, 2004). It could be argued that in so doing, they are denying intentionality with the right hand while endorsing it with the left.

Most troubling for philosophers is the obvious fact that an emotion may be "about" some nonexistent, merely imagined object. The object of fear may be nowhere around. The imagined threat in jealousy may not exist. The person one still loves may be dead. (Indeed, the problem seems to remain whether the lover knows of the death or not. In either case, the emotion is directed at a person who is in no position to receive it.) Moreover, the object of an emotion would seem to be one and the same object, whether it exists or not. (It is one and the same devil that is the object of a child's fear, whether the devil exists or not.) Thus the ontological status of the intentional object of emotion causes considerable commotion, particularly in the area of aesthetics and "make-believe" (Walton, 1990). In recent decades, many Anglo-American language-oriented or "analytic" philosophers have reduced the seemingly mysterious notion of intentionality to the supposedly more manageable notion of "intensionality," a precisely defined feature of certain sorts of sentences (Dennett, 1978, 1991). But whether intensionality does in fact capture the necessary features of intentionality is itself a topic of considerable debate; at least it seems to confuse the language in which we describe emotions with the nature of the emotions themselves (Searle, 1983).

Philosophers have also become concerned with the "why?" of emotions—their function and their explanation. Most of the work here has been done on the explanation of particular instances of emotion, although a few investigators have recently tackled the much larger question of the evolution and function of emotions as such (de Sousa, 1987; Gibbard, 1990). Particular instances of emotion seem to be subject to two different sorts of explanations. On the one hand, because they are intentional and essentially involve beliefs (as well as desires, needs, attitudes, and values), emotions seem to require an explanation that invokes a person's belief and attitudes toward the world. A person is angry because he believes that so-and-so wronged him, or someone is saddened because she has found out that she has just lost a loved one, and so on. But this cannot be a complete account of emotional explanation. We also explain emotions by citing the fact that a person has been sleepless all week, or is ill, or has been given some medication. In other words, explanation of emotion may cite an underlying cause that may or may not make mention of the object of emotion. The cause may be physiological—for example, an underlying state of irritability, an ingested drug, or a direct surgical stimulation of the brain. The cause may be some state of affairs or incident that "triggered" the person's emotion, but this may not be the object of the person's emotion, nor need he or she have any memory or awareness of it. (Again, "subliminal" messages presumably work this way.)

How is causal explanation to be reconciled with an explanation in terms of beliefs and attitudes? Many philosophers have tended to emphasize the importance of one form of explanation over the other, or to reduce all explanations to either causal explanations or belief-and-desire, "reason"-type explanations. The latter sort of explanation provides a fuller account of the intentionality of an emotion by describing not only its formal object ("He's angry because he's been offended") but the specific details of the situation, as well as the person's beliefs and various attitudes. The former sort of explanation invokes an underlying cause that may or may not make mention of the object of emotion. Very often, however, the citation of a cause of emotion (its initiating stimulus or "trigger") and the account of the object of the emotion will be nominally the same ("He got mad because she stepped on his toe"). The problem that has been addressed by many philosophers and in recent years has become the subject of intense debate between those who prefer some version of the intentionality model of emotion and those who demonstrate a strong preference for a more biological model of emotion (Rorty, 1980;

Nissenbaum, 1985; Griffiths, 1997; Prinz, 2004).

The cognitive basis of emotions also raises another question, one that was often a matter of deep concern for earlier philosophers: the question of the rationality of emotions. Many thinkers have written as if the emotions were not only irrational but also nonrational—not even candidates for cognition. Accounts of emotions as mere feelings or physiological processes would make them nonrational (one cannot have a "stupid" headache, except by way of a roundabout complaint about its inconvenience). Aristotle, on the other hand, simply assumed that an emotion can be appropriate or inappropriate, foolish or prudent, not just on the basis of whether or not it is acceptable in the circumstance in question (though that social dimension is certainly essential), but on the basis of the perceptions, beliefs, desires, and situation of the individual. The fact that emotions consist at least in part of cognitions means that they can be evaluated in terms of the same epistemic, social, and even ethical criteria that we use to evaluate beliefs and intentions: Are they appropriate to the context? Do they consider the facts of the matter? Are their perceptions fair and their evaluations reasonable? Indeed, the argument is now prevalent and persuasive that emotions cannot be understood without grasping their reasons, and these reasons in turn give us a basis for evaluation (de Sousa, 1987; Greenspan, 1988). The current debate, however, concerns how these reasons are to be understood, and whether the rationality of emotions can indeed be fairly compared to the evaluation of more fully deliberative, articulate activities.

The rationality of emotions also moves to center stage the question of emotions and ethics that we have been following through the history of philosophy. How does emotion enter into ethical understanding, and how do our ethics affect our emotions? One thing is clear: The commingling of emotions and ethics is not grounds for dismissing either ethics or emotion, as the midcentury "emotivists" suggested. But it is worth noting that a new conception of the emotional foundations of ethics has taken root in the Anglo-American tradition and, in an appropriate irony, has taken the name "emotivism" (Gibbard, 1990). Of course, one of the questions that remains, left over from the charge that emotions are "subjective," is that emotions vary too much from culture to culture to provide a firm basis for ethics; in other words, they are "relative." But though philosophers alone cannot answer the empirical question of the universality or relativity of emotions, they can and should clear away the dogmatic assumptions and mistaken conceptions that have often occupied philosophy in the past. There is nothing in the nature of emotion (including the human brain, which changes significantly with experience and varies considerably from person to person) that assures universality, but neither is it so obvious that emotions differ so much from place to place either. (This is indicated not only by studies of facial expression, but by the logic of the "human condition" and its more general features.) Indeed, the whole question of "human nature" is once again up for grabs.

One of the most critical questions about human nature is the extent to which we can transcend our own biology. In one sense, of course, this is absurd, but in another it is perfectly plausible. Human beings did not evolve to fly, but through technology we now have "frequent flyer" programs. Human beings did evolve with anger and jealousy as putatively universal emotions, but the question remains whether we can overcome our anger and jealousy, or perhaps even eliminate them from our emotional repertoires. This raises the question of emotions and choice, and challenges the supposition that we are passive regarding our emotions. Sartre (1939/1948, 1943/1956) suggested that the emotions are both choices and strategies, but many philosophers who do not share Sartre's extreme voluntarism would agree that emotions are indeed ways of coping, whether inherited through natural selection or cultivated in the less articulate practices of a society. But are we at the mercy of our emotions? Do we simply "have" them, or do we perhaps to some extent cultivate them and "do" them ourselves? Obviously, a good deal of ethics and our attitudes toward ourselves depend on this. The study of emotion in philosophy is, accordingly, not a detached and marginal discipline, but the very core of our inquiry into ourselves and our own natures. It was Socrates, the great champion of reason, who took as his mottos the slogan at Delphi ("Know thyself") and the rather extreme injunction that "The unexamined life is not worth living." But part of that knowledge, surely, is our understanding and appreciation of our emotions, which are, after all, much of what makes life worth living.

NOTE

1. This and other quotations from Aristotle in this chapter have been translated by Jon Solomon.

REFERENCES AND FURTHER READING

Aristotle. (1941). *The basic works of Aristotle* (R. McKeon, Ed.). New York: Random House. See also W. Fortenbaugh (1975). *Aristotle on emotion.* London: Duckworth.

Austin, J. L. (1964). Pretending. In D. Gustafson (Ed.), *Essays in philosophical psychology.* Garden City, NY: Doubleday/Anchor. (Original work published 1956–1957)

Averill, J. R. (1985). The social construction of emotion, with special reference to love. In K. Gergen & K. Davis (Eds.), *The social construction of the person* (pp. 89–109). New York: Springer-Verlag.

Barbalet, J. (1999). William James' theory of emotions. *Journal for the Theory of Social Behavior, 29,* 251–256.

Bedford, E. (1964). Emotion. In D. Gustafson (Ed.), *Essays in philosophical psychology.* Garden City, NY: Doubleday/Anchor. (Original work published 1956)

Ben-Zeev, A. (2000). *The subtlety of emotions.* Cambridge, MA: MIT Press.

Brentano, F. (1971). *Psychology from the empirical standpoint.* London: Routledge. (Original work published 1874)

Calhoun, C. (1984). Cognitive emotions? In C. Calhoun & R. C. Solomon (Eds.), *What is an emotion?* New York: Oxford University Press.

Cannon, W. B. (2003). Bodily changes in pain, hunger, fear and rage [Excerpt]. In R. Solomon (Ed.), *What is an emotion?* (2nd ed.). New York: Oxford University Press. (Original work published 1929)

Charland, L. (2002). The natural kind status of emotion. *British Journal for the Philosophy of Science, 53,* 511–537.

Churchland, P. S. (1986). *Neurophilosophy.* Cambridge, MA: MIT Press.

Damasio, A. (1994). *Descartes' error.* New York: Putnam.

Dennett, D. (1978). *Brainstorms.* Cambridge, MA: MIT Press.

Dennett, D. (1991). *Consciousness explained.* Boston: Little, Brown.

Descartes, R. (1989). *On the passions of the soul* (S. Voss, Trans.). Indianapolis, IN: Hackett. (Original work published 1649)

de Sousa, R. (1987). *The rationality of emotion.* Cambridge, MA: MIT Press.

Dewey, J. (2003). The theory of emotion [Excerpt]. In R. Solomon (Ed.), *What is an emotion?* (2nd ed.). New York: Oxford University Press. (Original work published 1894)

Ekman, P. (1973). *Darwin and facial expression.* New York: Academic Press.

Ekman, P. (2003). *Emotions revealed.* New York: Times Books.

Ekman, P., & Davidson, R. J. (Eds.). (1994). *The nature of emotion.* New York: Oxford University Press.

Ellsworth, P. (1994). William James and emotion: Is a century of fame worth a century of misunderstanding? *Psychological Review, 101,* 222–229.

Elster, J. (2000). *Alchemies of the mind.* Cambridge, UK: Cambridge University Press.

Freud, S. (1935). The unconscious (C. M. Baines, Trans.). In *Essays in metapsychology.* London: Liveright. (Original work published 1915)

Frijda, N. (1986). *The emotions.* Cambridge, UK: Cambridge University Press.

Gibbard, A. (1990). *Wise choices, apt feelings: A theory of normative judgment.* Cambridge, MA: Harvard University Press.

Goldie, P. (2000). *The emotions: A philosophical exploration.* Oxford: Clarendon Press.

Gordon, R. M. (1987). *The structure of emotion.* Cambridge, UK: Cambridge University Press.

Greenspan, P. (1988). *Emotions and reasons.* New York: Routledge.

Griffiths, P. (1997). *What emotions really are.* Chicago: University of Chicago Press.

Hamlyn, D. W. (1978). The phenomenon of love and hate. *Philosophy, 53,* 5–20. Includes a discussion of Brentano's theory.

Hegel, G. W. F. (1977). *The phenomenology of spirit* (A. N. Miller, Trans.). Oxford: Oxford University Press. (Original work published 1807)

Heidegger, M. (1962). *Being and time.* New York: Harper & Row. (Original work published 1927) See also the following explications of Heidegger: C. Guignon (1984). Moods in Heidegger's *Being and time;* H. Dreyfus, (1991). *Being-in-the-world: A commentary on Heidegger's Being and time.* Cambridge, MA: MIT Press.

Hobbes, T. (1994). *Leviathan.* Indianapolis, IN: Hackett. (Original work published 1651)

Hume, D. (1888). *A treatise of human nature* (L. A. Selby-Bigge, Ed.). Oxford: Oxford University Press. (Original work published 1739) See also A. Baier (1991). *A progress of sentiments: Reflections on Hume's treatise.* Cambridge, MA: Harvard University Press. And see also D. Davidson (1976). Hume's cognitive theory of pride. *Journal of Philosophy, 73,* 733–757.

Husserl, E. (1960). *Cartesian meditations* (D. Cairns, Trans.). The Hague: Nijhoff. (Original work published 1938)

Hyman, A., & Walsh, J. (1973). *Philosophy in the Middle Ages.* Indianapolis, IN: Hackett.

James, W. (1884). What is an emotion? *Mind, 9,* 188–205.

James, W. (1950). *Principles of psychology.* New York: Dover. (Original work published 1890)

Kant, I. (1953). *Critique of judgment* (J. H. Bernard, Trans.). New York: Hafner. (Original work published 1793)

Kenny, A. (1963). *Action, emotion and will*. London: Routledge & Kegan Paul.

Lane, R. (1999). *The cognitive neuroscience of emotion*. New York: Oxford University Press.

Lazarus, R. S. (1994). *Emotion and adaptation*. New York: Oxford University Press.

LeDoux J. (1996). *The emotional brain*. New York: Simon & Schuster.

Lyons, D. (1980). Emotion. Cambridge, UK: Cambridge University Press.

Merleau-Ponty, M. (1994). *The phenomenology of perception*. (C. Smith, Trans.). New York: Routledge. (Original work published 1962)

Neu, J. (1977). *Emotion, thought and therapy*. Berkeley: University of California Press.

Neu, J. (1980). Jealous thoughts. In A. Rorty (Ed.), *Explaining emotions*. Berkeley: University of California Press.

Neu, J. (1999). *A tear is an intellectual thing*. New York: Oxford University Press.

Nietzsche, F. (1967). *On the genealogy of morals* (W. Kaufmann, Trans.). New York: Random House. (Original work published 1887)

Nissenbaum, H. (1985). *Emotions and focus*. Stanford, CA: CSLI.

Nussbaum, M. (1994). *The therapy of desire*. Princeton, NJ: Princeton University Press. A sympathetic and detailed discussion of the Stoics on the place of emotion in life.

Nussbaum, M. (2003). *Upheavals of thought*. Cambridge, UK: Cambridge University Press.

Ortony, A., Clore, G., & Collins, A. (1988). *The cognitive structure of emotions*. New York: Cambridge University Press.

Plato. (1974). *The republic* (E. M. A. Grube, Trans.). Indianapolis, IN: Hackett.

Plato. (1989). *The symposium* (A. Nehamas & P. Woodruff, Trans.). Indianapolis, IN: Hackett.

Prinz, J. (2004). *Gut reactions*. New York: Oxford University Press.

Ricoeur, P. (1966). *The voluntary and the involuntary* (E. Kohak, Trans.). Evanston, IL: Northwestern University Press. (Original work published 1950)

Roberts, R. (2003). *Emotions*. New York: Cambridge University Press.

Robinson, J. (1995). Startle. *Journal of Philosophy*, 92(2), 53–74.

Robinson, J. (2005). *Deeper than reason*. New York: Oxford University Press.

Rorty, A. (1980). Explaining emotions. In A. Rorty (Ed.), *Explaining emotions*. Berkeley: University of California Press.

Russell, B. (1967). *The autobiography of Bertrand Russell* (Vol. 1). Boston: Little, Brown.

Ryle, G. (1951). *The concept of mind*. New York: Barnes & Noble.

Sartre, J.-P. (1948). *The emotions: Sketch of a theory* (B. Frechtman, Trans.). New York: Philosophical Library. (Original work published 1939) See the commentary in R. C. Solomon (1988). *From Hegel to existentialism*. Oxford: Oxford University Press.

Sartre, J.-P. (1956). *Being and nothingness* (H. Barnes, Trans.). New York: Washington Square Press. (Original work published 1943) See also J. Fell (1965). *Sartre's theory of the passions*. New York: Columbia University Press.

Schachter, S., & Singer, J. (1962). Cognitive, social and physiological determinants of emotional state. *Psychological Review*, 69(5), 379–399. For a good philosophical rejoinder, see R. M. Gordon (above), Ch. 5.

Scheler, M. (1970). *The nature of sympathy*. New York: Archon. (Original work published 1916)

Searle, J. (1983). *Intentionality: An essay in the philosophy of mind*. Cambridge, UK: Cambridge University Press.

Seneca. (1963). *De ira*. Oxford: Loeb Classical Library, Oxford University Press.

Smith, A. (1976). *Theory of the moral sentiments*. Oxford: Oxford University Press. (Original work published 1759)

Smith, A. (1976). *An inquiry into the nature and causes of the wealth of nations*. Indianapolis, IN: Liberty Classics. (Original work published 1776) For a good study of the relation between Smith's ethics and his economic theory, see P. Werhane (1991). *Ethics and economics: The legacy of Adam Smith for contemporary capitalism*. Oxford: Oxford University Press.

Solomon, R. (1976). *The passions*. Notre Dame, IN: University of Notre Dame Press. See also R. Solomon (1988). *About love*. New York: Simon & Schuster; R. C. Solomon & K. Higgins (Eds.). (1991). *The philosophy of (erotic) love*. Lawrence: University of Kansas Press.

Solomon, R. (Ed.). (2003). *What is an emotion?* (2nd ed.). New York: Oxford University Press.

Solomon, R. (2004). *Not passion's slave*. New York: Oxford University Press.

Sorabji, R. (2003). *Emotion and peace of mind*. New York: Oxford University Press.

Spinoza, B. (1982). *Ethics*. (S. Shirley, Trans.). Indianapolis, IN: Hackett. (Original work published 1677) See also A. Rorty (1991). Spinoza on the pathos of love. In R. C. Solomon & K. Higgins (Eds.), *The philosophy of (erotic) love*. Lawrence: University of Kansas Press.

Stocker, M. (1996). *Valuing emotions*. Cambridge, UK: Cambridge University Press.

Thalberg, I. (1977). *Perception, emotion and action*. New Haven, CT: Yale University Press.

Walton, K. (1990). *Mimesis as make-believe*. Cambridge, MA: Harvard University Press.

Williams, B. (1973). Morality and the emotions. In *Problems of the self*. Cambridge, UK: Cambridge University Press.

Wittgenstein, L. (1953). *Philosophical investigations*. London: Routledge & Kegan Paul.

CHAPTER 2

History of Emotions
Issues of Change and Impact

PETER N. STEARNS

Charting changes in emotion raises an intriguing set of analytical challenges, and at the same time yields vital understandings of emotion itself. Here is the core of the history of emotions as a field, as increasingly widely practiced by historians and kindred sociologists and anthropologists. A specific example will illustrate the claim, highlighting the main features of the analytical strategy, which can then be explored in a more generalized fashion.

Studies of emotional emphases in Western Europe in the wake of the Protestant Reformation have highlighted the pervasiveness of an atmosphere of melancholy—held to be an appropriate religious demeanor, given the snares of this world and the ravages of sin. Paintings frequently seized on melancholy, and diary entries characteristically portrayed dolefulness and grief. This tone began to change, however, with the 18th century, when what can now be seen as a dominant modern Western insistence on cheerfulness emerged. Christian values were gradually recast, with a smiling demeanor held to be an appropriate tribute to a beneficent God. Commercial signals gained new strength, with material goods seen as producing happiness, and a cheerful disposition as most suitable for successful business transactions. As one historian has noted, even improved dentistry entered in, with people more willing to smile openly as the quality of their teeth improved during the century of the Enlightenment (Jones, 1996).

Once launched, the new insistence on cheerfulness gained ground steadily, particularly (as many European observers noted) in the United States. By the late 20th century it affected labor relations as well as commercial interactions, with workers expected to display a sunny disposition as proof of their employability. Media extended the emphasis on cheer, and operations like Disney World—where trams from the parking lots still pipe in messages about how happy everyone is—showed the ubiquity of the norm. Cheerfulness also affected cross-cultural contacts: Franklin Roosevelt, at Yalta, was disconcerted when he could not make the dour Stalin smile, but later, when McDonald's began to penetrate the former Soviet Union, American standards of grinning service pervaded the

17

training standards, imposed, against local custom, on Russian sales personnel. Pervasive American cheerfulness had its obvious downside, however, imposing constraints that undoubtedly helped explain comparatively high rates of depression in the population as a whole (Kotchemidova, 2005).

Here, in a thumbnail sketch, is the historical contribution to emotions research at its best: capable of identifying a significant new trend and tracing its evolution; working to determine the relationship between cultural standards (where change can be readily charted) and actual personal emotional experience; providing at least strong indications of causation, in this case associated with cultural shifts (the Enlightenment) and the emergence of consumerism; and demonstrating impact, both in public spheres such as politics or labor relations (where emotional standards have obvious consequences) and in more private life (where some of the limitations of insistent cheerfulness may be particularly clear). In this instance—and there are several different historical scenarios, depending on the emotion in question—origins of novel emotional standards go well back in time, but historical analysis shows the intensification and widening ramifications of these standards as they continue to shape contemporary emotional life. Arguably—and this is the key point in relation to emotions research more generally—the contemporary American emphasis on cheerfulness simply cannot be adequately understood without the historical contribution.

Historical work on emotions as an explicit subfield is now two decades old as and continues to expand rapidly, dealing with processes of change in emotional standards and emotional experience, or, somewhat more complexly, with emotional continuities amid changing contexts. Historians may also be interested in a third focus: seeking to grasp the characteristic emotional styles of a particular period, in and of themselves, as a means of both enriching the portrayal of that past time and launching the process of comparing one previous period to another. Ultimately, however, the analytical goals center on change, either in emotions themselves or in the environments in which they operate. Here, correspondingly, is the central justification for adding history to the list of disciplines seriously engaged in emotions research. For if emotions change in significant ways—and historians and others have conclu-

sively demonstrated that they do, as in the case of modern cheerfulness—then the process must be grappled with as part of evaluating emotional expressions even in the present time. Adding change to the variables involved in emotions research means adding complexity, but it is empirically inescapable and provides an essential perspective for assessing the results of other social science research on emotion, such as the findings emanating from sociology and anthropology.

Examining change involves establishing baselines, so that new trends can be carefully evaluated against real, rather than assumed or imagined, past standards—a task that historians at their best handle quite well. It involves assessing the causes of change and also its results, in personal emotional lives but also in larger institutions (such as law, education, the media, or the political process).

THE DEVELOPMENT OF EMOTIONS HISTORY

Explicit historical research is still a relative newcomer. Theorists from other social science disciplines provided frameworks for historical assessment that were long ignored by most historians themselves. Thus Norbert Elias's (1938/1982) classic work on how new levels of "civilization" began to constrain more spontaneous emotional expressions, beginning with the Western European aristocracy by the 17th century, focused attention on a key turning point now being widely explored. More generally, the constructivist theory of emotion, generated by several social psychologists as well as sociologists, argues that emotions should be interpreted primarily in terms of the social functions they serve; constructivists also correctly note that as social functions frequently change, emotions will shift substantially as well (Averill, 1980, 1982). Some emotions may disappear as part of this process, and others may newly emerge. Here is a richly suggestive historical framework—only rarely, however, fleshed out by detailed historical research, and until recently largely ignored by professional historians. The constructivist approach, including the common attention to cultural context as a functional area or as an intermediary between function and emotion, independently affecting ideas about emotional experiences and the vocabularies used to phrase them (Gordon,

1989), in fact tallies closely with recent historical work.

Historians themselves moved into research on emotion hesitantly. The great French social historian Lucien Febvre called over 70 years ago for a "historical psychology" that would "give up psychological anachronism" and "especially detailed inventory of the mental equipment of the time" (Febvre, 1933/1973). His appeal was not quickly heeded. A number of cultural historians dealt with past styles and rituals that had strong emotional components. Johann Huizinga's (1927) masterful portrayal of the late Middle Ages contained a wealth of data relevant to emotions history, and even more limited studies of popular protest or religious life offered important emotional insight into the past periods involved (Stearns with Stearns, 1985). Explicit focus on emotion, however, was lacking. Most historians continued to emphasize the conscious actions and rational decisions of their subjects. Even the advent of social history, bent on detailing the activities and interests of groups of ordinary people, did not quickly break this mold. Indeed, it could confirm it, as social historians insisted on rescuing ordinary people from accusations of mob impulsiveness and so stressed their transcendent rationality (e.g., in protest situations). Ordinary people may have mental worlds different from those of elites, according to the pioneer social historians, but they are no less careful choosing methods appropriate to their goals. Emotion, in this formulation, was not a significant variable.

The advent of psychohistory in the 1960s brought attention to the role of emotions in the past, but on a very limited scale. Most psychohistorians, from the great Erik Erikson (1958) to more recent practitioners, have concentrated on biography and have utilized a largely Freudian theoretical framework. They have linked emotional characteristics to historical developments—thus Erikson translates Luther's tense relationship with his harsh father into Lutheranism's preoccupation with an angry and omnipotent God—but they have not dealt with emotional change, and they have tended to enmesh emotional factors in a rigid and unchanging psychodynamic. Furthermore, while psychohistorians generated interesting work, their approach never won wide acceptance within the historical discipline, and (because of pervasive Freudianism) had a limited reception in other fields as well. (See, however,

Gay, 1984–1986, for a more ambitious psycho-historical treatment of the emotional lives and standards of the Victorian bourgeoisie.)

The direct antecedents of historical research on emotion, however, awaited a final ingredient, provided by the 1970s through the maturation of social history as the leading branch of historical inquiry. By this point, historians throughout the United States and Western Europe increasingly focused not only on the activities and value systems of ordinary people, but also on institutions and behaviors in addition to formal politics, as the central stuff of the past. New topics meant new materials, and also promoted the analysis of change as the dominant mode of historical presentation, displacing the mere narration of political and military events.

From social history, in turn, the issues emerged that led a number of historians to consider emotional patterns as central to their task and that produced increasing confluence with other disciplines dealing with the social contexts of emotional life. Social historians inevitably developed a strong interest in family history. Initially they focused on "objective" features of family organization—size, household composition, marriage age, and the like—where indeed important changes could be traced. Quickly, however, concern about the emotional quality of family relationships began to shape research agendas. Discussion of affective parental ties with children followed, for example, from analysis of the impact of changes in family size. A general linkage emerged between reductions in birth rate and greater affectionate intensity between parents and individual children, although which came first was (and is) not always easy to discern. Other aspects of household composition related to emotional factors. When the property power of older family members began to decline, in a more commercial economy in which independent jobs for younger adults became more abundant, affective links between young adults and older parents might well improve. Finally, efforts to explain changes in marriage patterns—in rates of marriage, ages at marriage, and age ratios between partners—generated attention to the emotional implications of courtship behaviors and subsequent spousal relationships. (For a solid survey of the family history field, see Mintz & Kellogg, 1989; see also Gillis, 1995.) The social history of emotion—the effort to trace emotional norms in groups of relatively ordinary people and their impact on key institutions of daily life—was born above all from the progressive extension of family history.

By the late 1970s, various studies were directly confronting the emotional aspects of family history. Historians working on France, Britain, Germany, and colonial North America uncovered a pronounced increase in familial affection in the late 17th and 18th centuries, contrasting with the more restrained emotional tone seemingly characteristic of families in earlier centuries. John Demos (1970), a historian dealing with colonial New England, noted an effort in 17th-century Plymouth to keep families free from the angry bickering still tolerated among neighbors; this effort to control anger was accompanied by the encouragement of conjugal love. European families may have tolerated outbursts of anger as part of appropriate family hierarchy for a slightly longer time—it is possible that in the unsettled conditions of the colonies, preservation of family harmony proved particularly important in North America—but a similar evolution set in throughout much of Western Europe by the 18th century (Stone, 1977; Flandrin, 1979; Trumbach, 1978; Shorter, 1975). Child-rearing methods that had focused on breaking children's wills, reflecting parental anger at animal-like offspring and generating intense if necessarily repressed anger in turn, yielded to greater reliance on affectionate persuasion, although the change was gradual and uneven. Mothers began to be defined as central ingredients of the network of familial affection. Romantic love began to influence courtship and marital expectations; the absence of love even served, by the 18th century, as a valid reason for the dissolution of engagements. On the eve of its decline as an economic unit, the family began taking on important new emotional functions and began to generate new expectations (Leites, 1986). Although the rise of various kinds of love headed the innovation list (Stone, 1977), other emotions entered in. Here was the context in which 18th-century family manuals began to urge repression of anger within the family, particularly enjoining men to treat their wives, children, and servants with appropriate decorum.

While the expansion of family history began to introduce emotional change as an explicit historical topic—indeed, a central issue in dealing with the rise of new kinds of family relationships in the 17th and 18th centuries—another kind of social history promoted attention to other emotional issues. Here French historians led the way, in contrast to Anglo-Saxon dominance in the pioneering family history studies. A field of "mentalities" research emerged, focusing on deeply held popular beliefs about self, environment, and society, which were expressed more frequently in ritual behavior than in formal declarations of principle. Historians of mentalities probed what ordinary people really meant by their religious observances, often discovering that beneath a Christian veneer a variety of magical ingredients still held sway. Emotional beliefs, or emotional components of other beliefs, increasingly engaged this field of inquiry. Robert Muchembled (1985) and Jean Delumeau (1978, 1989) emphasized the high level of fear characteristic of French peasants from the Middle Ages to the 18th century, expressed in various religious and magical practices and in festival rituals. Anxiety about death, about crop failure, and about violence generated intense community practices that might relieve fears of the outside world. Delumeau, in particular, painted a picture of popular religion dominated by the need to control constantly overspilling fear. Delumeau also argued, however, that as with family emotion, the 18th century saw a pronounced change in popular emotional life: Growing confidence about measures that could control the natural and social environment reduced the need for fear-managing rituals, leading to a shift in religious emphasis and a redefinition of fear that (in a process Delumeau did not himself trace) would ultimately to the 20th-century formulation of fear as an interior emotion focused on inward demons. Mentalities historians also dealt with relationships between elite and popular belief systems. Here too they emphasized a significant change opening up in the 17th and 18th centuries. Elite Europeans began to look askance at a leisure tradition in which they had once willingly shared. A key focus of their dismay was emotional spontaneity—those occasions when emotion generated physical behaviors, such as crowd frenzy, ribald dances, or exuberant sports, that now seemed both vulgar and disorderly. Correspondingly, the elite launched a variety of disciplinary and legal measures designed to curb spontaneity, and won some success in denting the traditional festivals of European peasants and artisans

(Burke, 1978; Mitzman, 1987). A historian dealing with colonial Virginia has subsequently traced a somewhat similar process of elite–mass divergence over emotional spontaneity in leisure, taking shape in the later 18th century in parts of North America (Isaac, 1982).

In various ways, in sum, analysis of emotional change and its impact had become inescapable by the late 1970s. Without launching a specific subfield concentrating on the history of emotions, social historians were vigorously engaged in dealing with several facets of emotional change, with familial emotions, fear, and spontaneity heading the list. A number of topical inquiries, initially directed toward other issues (e.g., family life or leisure), pointed conclusively both to the existence of substantial emotional change in the past and to the importance of this change in grasping key passages in social history. Attention centered particularly on the early modern period, with analyses of the several different ways Europeans and North Americans were changing their emotional rules or seeing these rules changed during the 17th and 18th centuries. The link between these findings and Elias's earlier model of increasing civilized restraint was not immediately drawn, but it soon added a theoretical ingredient to the emerging picture.

A MATURING FIELD

The history of emotions emerged as an explicit and increasingly polished research area during the 1980s. Earlier findings continued to vivify the field, but a number of features were added or redrawn. In the first place, growing numbers of social historians began dealing with the history of emotions in and of itself, rather than as an adjunct to family or mentalities study. Changes in a particular emotion, and the relationship between these changes and other aspects of a historical period, began to constitute respectable (if still clearly innovative) historical topics. Social historians also expanded the list of emotions that could be subjected to historical scrutiny. Along with love and fear, anger, envy, jealousy, shame, guilt, grief, disgust, and sadness began to receive significant historical attention, and interest in augmenting the range of emotions considered as part of research on historical change continues strong. Significant work more recently has addressed not only cheerfulness but also nostalgia.

The contexts in which emotional change can be explored have also been elaborated. Predominant attention, particularly in Anglo-American research, continues to go to family settings and related emotional socialization, but studies of emotional change have now dealt with workplace relations, religion, leisure and its emotional symbolism, and legal standards and uses of the law to reflect new emotional norms. A growing body of work also deals with the intriguing relationships between emotions and modern consumerism.

In addition, the maturation of emotions history has involved growing recognition of a need to modify some of the impulses toward reifying stark contrasts that characterized much of the initial work. Premodern families, for example, are no longer seen as emotionally cold. Affection for children is not a modern invention, nor—despite the fascinating argument of a feminist French historian (Badinter, 1980)—is mother love. Recognition of some biological constants in emotional expressions, and simply more extensive data probes, has modified the earlier picture or sharp premodern–modern emotional dichotomies. Better use of theory has come into play. Historians using Jerome Kagan's (1979) findings on child rearing can understand that evidence of severe physical discipline in the past, once taken as a sign of emotional distancing, is in fact compatible with real affection. Change has continued to organize historical research on emotion, but change is now seen as more subtle than it was previously regarded as being. For example, one study intriguingly complicates the emotional history of the European Middle Ages, contesting undue emphasis on unrestrained anger, and in the process challenging key assumptions of the Elias school (Rosenwein, 2006).

The process of reassessing initial overstatements generated some interesting byways. Some revisionists began to argue that certain emotional relationships do not change; Linda Pollock (1983), most notably, tried to demonstrate that European parents manifested consistent love for their children from the 16th century onward, though in fact her evidence clustered around 1700. In another important variant, Philip Greven (1977; see also the later extension of the argument, Greven, 1991) posited three basic emotional socialization styles in colonial North America, which have since persisted; change was involved in establishing the initial variety, but thenceforward continuity has prevailed. Angry parents in the 1990s have been trapped in the same culture that generated their predecessors in 1750. These approaches have not captured dominant historical attention, but they have compelled more sophisticated treatment of change.

Love offers a clear illustration of the current approach. Historians now realize that their initial impulse to contrast economically arranged marriages with modern romance was overly simple. Economics remains a factor in modern love, and love entered into premodern courtship. The nature and experience of love were different, however. Love in 17th-century Western Europe was less intense and less individually focused than would become the norm in the 18th and 19th centuries. The system of arranged marriage led to groups of young men and women stimulating each other emotionally, for an individual could not be singled out prior to final arrangement. The 18th-century decline of arranged marriages cut into the group-oriented experience of premarital excitement; this shift soon led to an unprecedented association of love with privacy and with one-on-one intensity. (For an intriguing study of changes and in emotional expectations in 18th-century courtships, see Eustace, 2001.) Finally, expressions of love pulled away from a traditional range of vigorous bodily manifestations. Suitors in Wales stopped urinating on their fiancées' robes as a sign of affection; kissing became gentler, biting far less common. The relationship of love and the body, in other words, changed substantially (Gillis, 1985; Leites, 1986; Stearns & Stearns, 1988). This means that a new definition of love—a modern kind of romantic love—did indeed emerge in the late 17th and 18th centuries. The significance of the change is, if anything, enhanced by its fuller definition, even if the complexity increases as well. Similar modifications of initial generalizations about grief (e.g., over infant death) and parent–child affection have generated more subtle, but also richer, definitions of what emotional change entails (Lofland, 1985; Rosenblatt, 1983). A crucial part of this increased sophistication has resulted from historians' growing recognition of distinctions between emotional standards—the "feeling rules" or emotionology that describes socially prescribed emotional values, and often the criteria individuals themselves use to evaluate their emotional experience—and emotional experience itself. Both topics are important, but they are not the same. The rise of official approval of love in courtship and marriage is genuinely significant—it began to influence legal reactions to marital distress, for example (Griswold, 1986)—but it is not the same thing as a rise of the experience of love. The actual experience may have changed less, or at least differently, than the new standards imply. Historians of emotion still try to deal with both aspects of their subject, but in distinguishing between culture and experience they greatly improve their precision.

Finally, maturation of emotions history has involved increasing interaction between historians and other scholars working on the social context of emotion. The revival of attention to emotions research in sociology brought new interest in the issue of emotional change from this camp. North American sociologists and social psychologists dealt with a number of changes in emotional standards in the 20th century, using many of the same materials historians themselves relied upon (Cancian, 1987; Shields & Koster, 1989; Cancian & Gordon, 1988). More recent additions to the list of sociologists' contributions to emotional history include the work on cheerfulness, and also an important study of gender, shyness, and change (McDaniel, 2003). European sociologists, particularly in the Netherlands, have taken a somewhat longer view. Relying heavily on the Elias (1938/1982) framework, they have dealt with new forms of emotional control in earlier centuries and particularly have tried to place 20th-century patterns of emotional management, including a new informality, in the context of earlier shifts (de Swaan, 1981; Wouters, 2004). Systematic interaction between emotions historians and psychologists remains limited, but the rise of a minority school, deeply committed to exploring the cultural construction of mental states, provides one vigorous connection. Interdisciplinary concern for the relationship between language and emotion, including linguistic change, is another connection that involves psychology, though also cultural studies and other social sciences (Harré & Stearns, 1995; Gergen, 1998). Finally, although most anthropologists dealing with emotions continued to focus on durable cultural traditions, several major studies, such as Robert Levy's (1973) work on Tahiti, also treated alterations in emotional expression under the impact of such changes as missionary contact.

Historians, for their part, have become more aware of relevant work in other fields.

ISSUES OF RANGE AND OF THEORY

Growing interest in the history of emotions has generated research in a variety of historical areas, though from a disciplinary point of view important imbalance remains both chronologically and geographically. A handful of classical historians have dealt with emotion in antiquity. The medieval field is richer. A substantial literature exists on the rise and subsequent impact of chivalric love. A 1997 presidential address to the American Historical Association, by a leading medievalist, specifically invoked the importance of changes in emotional forms between medieval and early modern Europe (Bynum, 1997). The study of medieval anger opens this period to new complexities, from the standpoint of emotions history (Rosenwein, 2006). But further work on earlier periods remains highly desirable, if only to provide fuller perspective on modern trajectories.

Geographic gaps remain even more troubling, and (in contrast to some purely contemporary work, such as Salovey's [1991] volume on jealousy) there is almost no explicitly comparative historical analysis where emotions are concerned. Mark Elvin and others have examined emotions history in China (Elvin, 1989, 1991). A history of Maoism notes the Chairman's appeal for emotional reconfiguration on the part of peasants, toward releasing the anger necessary to fuel revolution (Solomon, 1971). Advances in the history of childhood, particularly in China and Latin America, also have implications for emotions history, and there is promise of further gains in the future. But the challenge of extending explicit work on emotional change to non-Western areas and to comparative treatment remains compelling.

Theoretical work may also have lagged somewhat, aside from continuing utilization of the Elias framework or ideas about informalization. There are theoretical challenges in abundance, but with a few exceptions historical advances from the 1990s onward have emphasized empirical case studies. Only William Reddy's (2001) ambitious work stands out, seeking to apply psychological and social science theory to his own framework, applied in turn to emotional changes and their political and legal consequences during the French revolutionary period. Various American historians have also speculated about the special role of psychology in shaping national emotional life (Pfister & Schnog, 1997)—an inquiry that has both theoretical and comparative implications. Finally, the increasing clustering of studies of consumerism and emotions sets the basis for more extensive theoretical statements. Here too, however, opportunities have not been fully realized, and the gaps also affect the relationship between historical findings and work in other fields such as psychology.

KEY CHANGES OF WESTERN SOCIETY

Significant historical findings do already exist, providing both basis and model for additional work and for interdisciplinary collaborations. The richest literature, steadily expanding, applies to modern Western history (Western Europe and the United States), beginning about 1500 and extending to the present. Three periods command primary attention and generate the most extensive findings, for significant emotional change emerges in sporadic bursts, not consistently in every decade.

Historical research continues to embellish the picture of a fundamental transformation in emotional standards during the early modern centuries, and particularly the 17th and 18th centuries. Imaginative research on the German peasantry has even discerned some symptoms of emotional change, toward fuller identification of an emotional self, in the century after 1500 (Sabean, 1984). In addition to refinements in the understanding of changes in parental and marital love, and to the ongoing work on fear and spontaneity, historians have made a number of other changes to the early modern transformation model. John Demos (1988), looking at New England in the colonial and early national periods, traces a shift from pervasive use of shame in dealing with children and miscreant adults to guilt, from the 18th to the early 19th century. As community cohesion declined, parents had to find new ways to internalize behavioral guidelines; they were able to use newly intense love as the basis for instilling a greatly heightened level of guilt. A comparable shift, toward guilt rather than public shaming, describes innovations in the principles of social discipline and criminal justice in the same period. The work on the balance between cheerfulness and acceptable sadness adds another important dimension. On yet another front, Alain Corbin (1986) describes a vast transformation in the emotion of disgust: As Frenchmen from the 18th century onward began to manifest intense disgust at a new range of objects, they began using the emotion to motivate a variety of new sanitary and cosmetic behaviors and to justify new social distinctions between the washed and the unwashed. Here emotional change is directly linked to altered experience of the senses. This kind of emotions research, linked to the mentalities approach, has expanded into historical inquiries about changes in gestures and humor (Bremmer & Roodenburg, 1997).

Research on 19th-century emotions history has become increasingly active, though it lacks the focus of the early modern framework. To some extent, the very notion of a great transformation in the 17th and 18th centuries overshadows findings on the 19th century, as many developments served to amplify and disseminate to new social groups the basic trajectories established earlier. Yet amplification can carry important new messages. North American studies on the apotheosis of mother love go well beyond 18th-century findings concerning new expectations for parental affection (Lewis, 1989), and the standards applied to children, in terms of anticipated emotional reward, escalated as well (Zelizer, 1985). Several important studies on the 19th-century version of romantic love similarly point to novel and distinctive features (Stearns, 1989; Lystra, 1989). Love became for many in the American middle classes virtually a religious ideal, involving self-abnegation and worshipful devotion to the other; 18th-century standards had not sought so much. Jealousy was redefined in this process, as a largely female emotion and a contradiction of proper selflessness in love; older ideas of jealousy in defense of honor fell by the wayside. Grief gained new attention and vast new symbolic expression in Victorian funeral practices (Houlbrooke, 1989). Anger received more explicit condemnation, particularly in the family setting. Gender distinctions urged total suppression of anger in women, but an ability to channel anger toward competition and righteous indignation in men (Stearns & Stearns, 1986).

Victorian emotional patterns thus provided no overall new direction, but they did adjust prior trends to the new sanctity of the family in an industrial world; to new social class divisions; and to the new need to define emotional distinctions between boys and girls, men and women. Whereas love was seen as uniting men and women in common emotional goals, negative emotions became highly gender-linked; in addition to jealousy and anger, the conquest of fear was redefined to serve purposes of gender identity (Stearns, 2006). Although the primary focus has been on the new standards urged in 19th-century Western society and within the middle class, spelled out in a surge of new kinds of prescriptive literature, various evidence suggests considerable behavioral impact. Men and women did have, with some frequency, the kind of love experiences now recommended, while adjusting their premarital sexuality accordingly; they did work toward appropriate training of children concerning anger and fear. Still not entirely defined, the 19th century stands as a rich source of materials on emotional history and as the scene of a number of significant modifications in norms and experience.

The 20th century, finally, has received sharper definition from the historical perspective. Several emotions historians, to be sure, trace a variety of oscillations in 20th-century standards without an overarching theme. Some analysis concentrates on the need to refute facile modernization ideas that urge (against virtually all available findings) that the 20th century should be seen simply in terms of increasing openness of emotional expression, as older repressions have gradually fallen away. Significant work also stresses continuities from the 19th century, particularly in the gender-linked quality of certain emotional standards; women, for example, continue to be held to a particularly self-sacrificing image of love, even as male standards may have changed (Cancian, 1987). A few historians have argued for continuity pure and simple, from the 19th or even the 18th century (Kasson, 1990; Flandrin, 1979).

Two related approaches focus a number of the most important current findings about the 20th century. The first, emanating particularly from several Dutch sociologists, grapples with the problem of growing emotional informality and apparent liberalization, in a context that continues to insist on a great deal of self-control. Spontaneity has revived, but within strict (if unacknowledged) limits. The general argument is that most Westerners have learned so well the lessons of restraint of violence and of unwanted sexuality that they can be allowed a good bit of informal emotional idiosyncrasy as part of personal style. Rules of emotional expression have become more complex, and judgments are made about appropriate emotional personalities on the basis of various individual interactions rather than rigid and hierarchical codes (de Swann, 1981; Wouters, 1992; Gerhards, 1989). Increasing democratization is also part of this shift, as emotional standards used in the 19th century to separate respectable and unrespectable classes are now more widely enjoined (Wouters, 2004). The second approach similarly urges that the 20th century constitutes a period of considerable and reasonably coherent change in emotional standards. It focuses on implicit attacks on 19th-century emotional formulas, beginning in the 1920s and extending over a transition period of several decades (Stearns, 1994). Hostility to negative emotions has increased. Gender linkages, though by no means absent, have been muted in favor of more uniform standards of emotional control. The importance of managing emotions through talking out rather than active expression has become a dominant theme. Reference to embarrassment in front of others has come to supplement guilt and shame as enforcement for emotional normality (Stearns & Stearns, 1986; Stearns, 1989). Amid a host of specific changes, including new emphasis on avoiding rather than mastering fear as part of building character, the dominant theme is a new aversion to undue emotional intensity (Shields & Koster, 1989; Stearns & Haggerty, 1991). The decline of the acceptability of open grief is a key index to the new emotional regime. Even good emotions have dangers; earlier icons of intense emotion, such as the idealized Victorian mother or fervid romantic love, have come in for substantial criticism. In this context, Arlie Hochschild (1997) has noted how work sometimes provides an easier emotional climate than home life. Also vital is the relationship between increasingly overt sexuality and emotional formulations; sexual prowess may compete with emotional links. Growing approval of envy has adjusted 19th-century standards to the needs of a consumer economy (White, 1993; Shumway, 1998; Seidman, 1991; Matt, 1998; Hochschild, 1997).

PROBLEMS AND RESPONSES

None of the three chronological focal points of historical research on emotion is entirely worked out. Gaps, disagreements, and issues of synthesis persist. One of the obvious current challenges involves pulling together diverse findings on emotional transformation, even for the early modern period, toward a fuller understanding of relationships among different facets of change. Historians also grapple with indications of change in the most recent decade or two, where their perspective needs to be combined with data emanating from the social and behavioral sciences: How fast, and how fundamentally, are emotional formulations changing now in a society such as the United States? Do trends mainly launched in the second quarter of the 20th century continue to shape a predominant American Western emotional framework?

Positioning historical work in interdisciplinary context remains an issue, as historians themselves oscillate between interesting their disciplinary colleagues in the relevance of emotions research to more standard topics, such as the consequences of the French Revolution, and working across boundaries. Active collaboration with sociology is gaining ground, despite the continued impulse of some American sociologists to treat the pre-20th-century past in terms of undifferentiated traditionalism. And there is also friendly overlap with anthropology and with some work on the philosophy of emotion.

Contacts with psychology, in contrast, are less well developed, despite their mutual importance in terms of theory. The maverick "discursive" or constructionist school uses historical data readily, and contributes in turn; moreover, work by some individuals, such as Stephanie Shields, directly enriches emotions history. In principle, additional case studies could be developed that examine cultural context and change along with more durable emotional expressions and functions (comparative work could be revealing here), to determine more precisely where the boundary lines are and to improve the statement of what changes in emotions and emotional standards involve. But the dominant cultures and funding sources of history and its disciplinary allies (such as anthropology and much sociology) on the one hand, and psychology on the other, so far inhibit the desirable interactions. What should be a knowledge frontier awaits additional settlers.

Furthermore, some obvious problems are endemic to the history field itself. Finding data appropriate for dealing with the emotional standards, and even more the emotional experience, of dead people is no easy task. The distinction between professed values and actual emotions helps. Historical research has become progressively more inventive in finding materials on emotional standards and in interpreting them through nuances of language and choices of metaphor, as well as through explicit message. Changes in word meanings ("temper," "lover") and outright neologisms ("sissy," "tantrum") provide direct testimony. Absence of comment may sometimes prove revealing, as in the avoidance of elaborate jealousy discussions in Victorian culture. Utilization of diary evidence, available in Western society from the 17th century and also in 19th-century Japan (Walthall, 1990), provides insight into internalization standards and self-evaluations, though there are problems of representativeness. (For an instance of work using diaries and letters to calculate the role of love in 18th-century American courtship, see Eustace, 2001.) A growing number of historians utilize rituals and various ethnographic evidence to get at emotional expressions in the past (Gillis, 1988). History adds greatly to the cases available for assessing the social contours of emotion, and while its service as laboratory has some undeniable empirical complexities, major strides in data sources continue.

Emotions history also enters researchers into versions of debates important in other social science fields. The results complicate the field, but also allow historical work to contribute to larger issues. Research on emotional change obviously provides yet another confrontation between definitions of basic emotions—biologically predetermined, though perhaps variable in target and expression—and emphasis on the cultural preconditions of emotional experience. Like other emotions researchers, historians, as they have gained in theoretical sophistication, participate in these discussions from various vantage points; the fact of significant change in aspects of emotional perception adds a vital dimension to the larger debates, challenging excessive focus on inherent basic responses.

In addition, emotions history generates some theoretical issues of its own, associated with the focus on tracing change. These issues merit further exploration, not only in history but in other areas of emotions research as historical findings are increasingly taken into account. Problems of timing constitute one example. When emotional standards begin to change in a society, how long does it take for key groups to internalize the changes, at least to some significant extent? Are there generalizable factors that speed or delay the response? For example, advice givers in the United States began early in the 19th century to urge that parents not use fear as a disciplinary tool with children. But manualists were still arguing against the "bogeyman" style a century later, implying that many parents still held out; and studies of rural areas in the 1930s reveal explicit and only mildly embarrassed use of the ploy. Yet change did come: By the 1950s, most prescriptive literature no longer judged the warnings necessary. The issue is not whether change occurred, but at what pace, and what factors determined the timing. Another instance involves implementation of standards in the public sphere: Available findings in the 19th and 20th centuries, again in the United States, suggest a three- to five-decade lag between significant middle-class acceptance of standards (about marital love, jealousy, or grief) and translation of these standards into relevant laws about divorce, jealousy-provoked crime, or grief-related damage suits (Stearns, 1994). Again, can we devise more general models to describe the probable speed of change, at least in modern societies, or will we be confined (as is currently inescapable) to case-by-case judgments? A similar problem arises in dealing with the interaction of dominant prescriptions, issued by leading religious (or, in modern cases, scientific) popularizers, and the effective emotional standards of subcultures (ethnic or socioeconomic). Historians have done much better with middle- and upper-class emotions history than with immigrant or lower-class.

A final set of historically generated theoretical issues involves the relationship between recreations and emotions. Historical work makes it increasingly clear that cultural expressions—in theater, or reading matter, or ritual, or sports—sometimes serve to train individuals in dominant emotional norms. Middle-class parents in the United States about 1900 believed that boxing was a good way to teach boys to retain and express anger (Stearns & Stearns, 1986), while confining its intensity to appropriate targets. In other instances, however, culture can be used in reverse fashion, as an outlet for emotions that are proscribed in daily life. Chinese love poems issued from a society highly intolerant of love in actual youth relationships (Goode, 1959). Spectator sports allow 20th- and 21st-century men to vent emotions that they know are normally inappropriate, despite greater acceptability in the past. Historians of leisure talk about "compensations" for the daily restrictions of contemporary life, but their approach needs further integration with emotions history. The historical perspective is not the only means of entry into these issues of cultural–emotional relationships, but it provides a growing list of significant and diverse examples.

THE STRENGTHS OF THE HISTORICAL APPROACH

Emotions history, despite its various limitations, has already generated a number of important findings about changes in standards and their relationship to aspects of emotional experience. The direction of changes in three major periods in modem Western history, although by no means fully captured, is becoming increasingly clear. The results in turn add evidence and issues to a number of basic discussions in emotions research, highlighting the phenomenon of change as an essential analytical factor.

In this context, historical analysis permits deeper exploration of the causation operating in the social context of emotions—an area suggested by constructivist theory, but not systematically probed. Historical research deals with the factors that induce new emotional formulations, permitting a kind of causation analysis that differs from and is more extensive than that possible in cross-cultural comparisons of relevant variables. In the major cases explored thus far, historians have picked up on the role of shifts in larger beliefs in inducing new emotional standards. For example, the Protestant Reformation encouraged reevaluation of emotions within the family, while new elite culture prompted reassessment of popular spontaneity. The role of changing expertise in the 20th and 21st centuries provides an opportunity to assess cultural causation of another sort. Economic and organization systems provide the second major strand of causation. Increased commercialization prompted new attention to family emotionality in the early modern period, as relationships among other adults became more competitive (Nelson, 1969). The separation of home and work prompted emotional reevaluations in the 19th century. Most of the leading judgments on basic shifts in the 20th century point to the impact of new organizational experiences and styles, attendant on the rise of a service economy, corporate management hierarchies, and mass consumerism. A causation topic of growing importance, where the historical approach to change over time is essential, involves the role of modern media in both shaping and reflecting public and even private emotion—helping to organize, for example, grief or fear reactions. Definitive statements of causation remain elusive, particularly in terms of assigning priority and precedence to one set of variables over another, but the analytical task has been engaged. It involves evaluations that, though rooted in history, inevitably apply to other social research on emotion as well.

Historical research also encourages renewed attention to the impact of emotion and emotional standards, again in a context of change. Emotions research in other disciplines sometimes assumes that further understanding of emotions themselves constitutes a sufficient end result. The growing group of researchers interested in emotions history certainly seeks to add to this understanding, and accepts it as a major goal. Historians, however, are typically interested in relating one facet of the human experience to others, so it is natural that they seek to discuss the effects of emotional change on other aspects of society, whatever the time period involved. The effort to distinguish between emotional standards and outright experience adds to this inclination, for new standards often have measurable impact—on the law, for example—even when basic emotional experience may remain more obdurate.

Historians of emotion have consistently commented on the interaction between emotional change and other facets of family life, such as marriage choice or birth rate decisions. History is proving to be a crucial means of improving the articulation between gender and

emotion. Because gender is in large measure a
cultural construct and varies greatly over time,
historical research is central to the determination of the origins and results of particular gender formulas for emotional expression. One of
the key findings of researchers dealing with the
19th and 20th centuries thus involves recognizing the central importance of gender distinctions in Victorian emotional prescriptions, and
then their reconfiguration beginning in the
1920s. Emotional standards also intertwine
with power relationships, even aside from gender. Emotions are used regularly to enforce,
and sometimes to conceal, such relationships.
Research on emotion in the early modern period deals extensively with the interrelationship
between changes in this area and revision of
family hierarchies. Research on differences in
rates and directions of emotional change, even
in the 21st century, provides new insight into
the often hidden hierarchies of contemporary
social and economic life. It also explains the
changing emotional bases for collective protest
within the configuration of power—including
the decline of emotionally charged protest, the
late 1960s excepted, from the 1950s to the
present in Western society (Moore, 1978).

Dealing with emotions through change also
facilitates evaluation of shifting emotional
problems—another kind of consequence
broadly construed. Seeing the disadvantages of
intensifying pressures for cheerfulness, for example, is easier when cheerfulness itself is
grasped as an evolving emotional goal. Emotions history can clearly be linked with analysis
of changing disease patterns and categories.

Historical research on emotion generates important new data, evaluative tools, and theoretical perspectives for emotions research more
generally. It provides prior examples of emotional reassessments and an explicit historical
vantage point for evaluating current directions
of change. Emotions history, increasingly en-
sconced in the broader field of social history
despite its newcomer status, thus becomes part
of an interdisciplinary inquiry into the constituents of emotional experience and the role of
emotion in social life. The history of emotions
adds challenge and complexity to the study of
emotion by introducing the factor of change as
a central ingredient. Emotions history also provides many of the tools necessary to deal with
the issue of change and to use its analysis to
move toward fuller understanding of the ways
in which emotions develop and function.

GROWING MOMENTUM

Work in emotions history from the 1990s onward suggests how the field is gaining ground,
beginning to tackle some of the major items on
the research agenda. Use of findings by historians not explicitly concerned with emotion also
suggests important cross-fertilization—for example, in work on changing patterns of spousal
abuse (Del Mar, 1996). Although the break-
through in interdisciplinary collaboration with
psychologists has not yet occurred, particularly
in real collaborative research, the discussions
with social psychologists as well as avowed
constructionists are encouraging. Newer research also provides sophisticated treatment of
changes in scientific paradigms of emotion and
their impact on wider emotional expectations
(Dror, 1998).

Equally important are the extensions within
history itself, including the coverage of additional emotions such as envy, the increased attention to medieval history, and the fuller explorations of the complexities of 20th-century
change. Some big tasks still await attention,
such as comparison and wider exploration of
emotions history in Asian, African, and Latin
American contexts. But emotions historians in
the United States are beginning to grapple with
one vital task: the evaluation of the relations of
subgroups to dominant European American
middle-class standards. Emergence of a distinctive African American religious–emotional sub-
culture took on new significance about 1900,
for example, because its trajectory contrasted
so markedly with changing patterns in middle-
class emotionology (Phillips, 1998). Differences in timing between Catholic emotional
culture and its Protestant counterpart provide
important insights into uses of fear (Kelly &
Kelly, 1998; Griffith, 1998).

Another growth area involves extending the
inquiry in the consequences of emotional culture and emotional change. Here, as in exploring change itself, historians offer considerable
experience in dealing with causation and with
interlocking factors. Corbin's (1986) work has
shown the impact of emotional reactions in
helping to shape social class relations, but
also sanitary policies, in 19th-century France.
Research on changing patterns of friendship
suggests another vital impact area (Rotundo,
1989; Rosenwein, 2006). Fuller understanding
of 20th-century change in emotional expectations is being applied to parent–child relations,

as well as to wider phenomena such as consumerism (Stearns, 1998). American work has extended the idea of changes in emotional culture as links between large structural shifts—the rise of a corporate, service-based economy, for example—and alterations in law, political behavior, and even military policy (Stearns, 1997, 1999; Wouters, 1992). Connections between changes in emotional style (Wouters, 1996) and shifts in the crime rate are being explored. Clearly, this diverse use of emotional patterns as cause, though still tentative, is a major new frontier in the field.

A number of historians and kindred sociologists are attempting to further the contributions of emotions history by defining topics based explicitly on contemporary patterns, and moving backward toward historical explanation and assessment, in a movement currently labeled "behavioral history" (Stearns, 2005). Thus novel preferences for house size and furniture purchases in the United States are evaluated in terms of changes in nostalgia (explained in turn through emotional reactions to shifting residential patterns). A challenging opportunity for behavioral history emerges concerning public, and in some cases private, experiences of fear in the contemporary United States. Several sociologists have posited counterproductive levels of fear (Glassner, 1999), but they encounter difficulties in explaining the emotions—their primary focus is on irresponsible media—and in locating them in terms of change. Emotions history, applied to current fear behaviors, can do a better job in measuring public fears over time (e.g., comparing reactions to Pearl Harbor to those roused by the terrorist attacks of 9/11), and also in assessing causation; the media role thus makes no sense if it is not juxtaposed with broader shifts in the socialization of fear. Emotions history can also join in evaluating the consequences of current American fear and—tentatively—in exploring remediation (Stearns, 2006). Here is a significant new frontier for interdisciplinary inquiry.

Emotions history has carved a noticeable (though hardly dominant) niche in the larger history discipline, and a measurably increasing role in interdisciplinary work. It has considerably expanded available knowledge about the range of emotional cultures and behaviors. It has fed important theories about processes of change and, increasingly, the consequences of change. Its interactions with other relevant disciplines have produced mutually significant results. Real challenges remain, however—in societies, periods, and topics still unexplored, as well as in the pressing need for comparative work and for fuller cross-disciplinary collaboration. The vitality of the subfield suggests the possibility of addressing these broader research needs.

REFERENCES

Averill, J. R. (1980). A constructivist view of emotion. In R. Plutchik & H. Kellerman (Eds.), *Emotion: Theory, research, and experience: Vol. 1. Theories of emotion* (pp. 305–339). New York: Academic Press.

Averill, J. R. (1982). *Anger and aggression: An essay on emotion.* New York: Springer-Verlag.

Badinter, E. (1980). *L'amour en plus: Histoire de l'amour maternel.* Paris: Flammarion.

Bremmer, J., & Roodenburg, H. (Eds.). (1997). *A cultural history of humor.* Cambridge, MA: Polity Press.

Burke, P. (1978). *Popular culture in early modern Europe.* New York: New York University Press.

Bynum, C. (1997). Wonder. *American Historical Review, 102,* 1–26.

Cancian, F. M. (1987). *Love in America: Gender and self development.* Cambridge, UK: Cambridge University Press.

Cancian, F. M., & Gordon, S. (1988). Changing emotion norms in marriage: Love and anger in U.S. women's magazines since 1900. *Gender and Society, 2*(3), 303–342.

Corbin, A. (1986). *The foul and the fragrant: Odor and the French imagination.* Cambridge, MA: Harvard University Press.

Del Mar, D. (1996). *What trouble I have seen: A history of violence against wives.* Cambridge, MA: Harvard University Press.

Delumeau, J. (1978). *La peur en Occident, XIVe–XVIIe siecles: Uné cite assiégée.* Paris: Fayard.

Delumeau, J. (1989). *Rassurer et proteger: Le sentiment de sécurité dans l'Occident d'autrefois.* Paris: Fayard.

Demos, J. (1970). *A little commonwealth: Family life in Plymouth Colony.* New York: Oxford University Press.

Demos, J. (1988). Shame and guilt in early New England. In C. Z. Stearns & P. N. Stearns (Eds.), *Emotion and social change: Toward a new psychohistory* (pp. 69–86). New York: Holmes & Meier.

de Swaan, A. (1981). The politics of agoraphobia: On changes in emotional and relational management. *Theory and Society, 10*(3), 359–385.

Dror, O. E. (1998). Creating the emotional body: Confusion, possibilities, and knowledge. In P. N. Stearns & J. Lewis (Eds.), *Emotional history of the United States* (pp. 173–196). New York: New York University Press.

Elias, N. (1982). *The history of manners* (E. Jephcott,

Trans.). New York: Pantheon Books. (Original work published 1938)

Elvin, M. (1989). Tales of the Shen and Xien: Body-personal and heart-mind in China during the last 150 years. *Zone, 4,* 266–349.

Elvin, M. (1991). The inner world of 1830. *Daedalus, 120*(2), 33–61.

Erikson, E. (1958). *Young man Luther.* New York: Norton.

Eustace, N. (2001). The cornerstone of a copious work: Love and power in eighteenth-century courtship. *Journal of Social History, 34*(3), 517–546.

Febvre, L. (1973). *A new kind of history.* New York. Harper & Row. (Original work published 1933)

Flandrin, J. L. (1979). *Families in former times* (R. Southern, Trans.). Cambridge, UK: Cambridge University Press.

Gay, P. (1984–1986). *The bourgeois experience: Victoria to Freud* (2 vols.). New York: Oxford University Press.

Gergen, K. J. (1998). History and psychology: Three weddings and a future. In P. N. Stearns & J. Lewis (Eds.), *Emotional history of the United States* (pp. 15–32). New York: New York University Press.

Gerhards, J. (1989). The changing culture of emotions in modern society. *Social Science Information, 28,* 737–754.

Gillis, J. R. (1985). *For better for worse: British marriages, 1600 to the present.* New York: Oxford University Press.

Gillis, J. R. (1988). From ritual to romance: Toward an alternate history of love. In C. Z. Stearns & P. N. Stearns (Eds.), *Emotion and social change: Toward a new psychohistory* (pp. 87–122). New York: Holmes & Meier.

Glassner, B. (1999). *The culture of fear: Why Americans are afraid of the wrong things.* New York: Basic Books.

Goode, W. J. (1959). The theoretical importance of love. *American Sociological Review, 24*(1), 38–47.

Gordon, S. L. (1989). The socialization of children's emotion: Emotional culture, competence, and exposure. In C. Saarni & P. Harris (Eds.), *Children's understanding of emotion* (pp. 319–349). Cambridge, UK: Cambridge University Press.

Greven, P. J., Jr. (1977). *The Protestant temperament: Patterns of child-rearing, religious experience and the self in early America.* New York: Knopf.

Greven, P. J., Jr. (1991). *Spare the child: The religious roots of punishment and the psychological impact of physical abuse.* New York: Knopf.

Griffith, R. M. (1998). "Joy unspeakable and full of glory": The vocabulary of pious emotion in the narratives of American Pentecostal women, 1910—1945. In P. N. Stearns & J. Lewis (Eds.), *Emotional history of the United States* (pp. 218–240). New York: New York University Press.

Griswold, R. L. (1986). The evolution of the doctrine of mental cruelty in Victorian American divorce, 1790–1900. *Journal of Social History, 20,* 127–148.

Harré, R., & Stearns, P. N. (Eds.). (1995). *Discursive psychology in practice.* London: Sage.

Hochschild, A. R. (1997, April 20). There's no place like work. *The New York Times Magazine,* pp. 50—55, 81–84.

Houlbrooke, R. (Ed.). (1989). *Death, ritual and bereavement.* New York: Routledge/Chapman & Hall.

Huizinga, J. (1927). *The waning of the Middle Ages.* London: Arnold.

Isaac, R. (1982). *The transformation of Virginia, 1740–1790.* Chapel Hill: University of North Carolina Press.

Jones, C. (1996). The great chain of buying: Medical advertisement, the bourgeois public sphere, and the origins of the French Revolution. *The American Historical Review, 10*(1), 13–40.

Kagan, J. (1979). *The growth of the child: Reflections on human development.* New York: Norton.

Kasson, J. F. (1990). *Rudeness and civility: Manners in nineteenth-century urban America.* New York: Hill & Wang.

Kelly, T., & Kelly, J. (1998). American Catholics and discourse of fear. In P. N. Stearns & J. Lewis (Eds.), *Emotional history of the United States* (pp. 259–282). New York: New York University Press.

Kotchemidova, C. (2005). From good cheer to "drive-by smiling." *Journal of Social History, 39,* 5–38.

Leites, E. (1986). *The Puritan conscience and modern sexuality.* New Haven, CT: Yale University Press.

Levy, R. I. (1973). *Tahitians: Mind and experience in the Society Islands.* Chicago: University of Chicago Press.

Lewis, J. (1989). Mother's love: The construction of an emotion in nineteenth-century America. In A. E. Barnes & P. N. Stearns (Eds.), *Social history and issues in human consciousness* (pp. 209–229). New York: New York University Press.

Lofland, L. (1985). The social shaping of emotion: The case of grief. *Symbolic Interaction, 8*(2), 171–190.

Lystra, K. (1989). *Searching the heart: Women, men, and romantic love in nineteenth-century America.* New York: Oxford University Press.

Matt, S. J. (1998). Frocks, finery, and feelings: Rural and urban women's envy, 1890–1930. In P. N. Stearns & J. Lewis (Eds.), *Emotional history of the United States* (pp. 377–395). New York: New York University Press.

McDaniel, P. A. (2003). *Shrinking violets and Caspar Milquetoasts: Shyness, power, and intimacy in the United States, 1950–1995.* New York: New York University Press.

Mintz, S., & Kellogg, S. (1989). *Domestic revolutions: A social history of American family life.* New York: Free Press.

Mitzman, A. (1987). The civilizing offensive: Mentalities, high culture and individual psyches. *Journal of Social History, 20,* 663–688.

Moore, B. F. (1978). *Injustice: The social basis of obedience and revolt.* White Plains, NY: Sharpe.

Muchembled, R. (1985). *Popular culture and elite culture in France, 1400–1750* (L. Cochrane, Trans.). Baton Rouge: Louisiana State University Press.

Nelson, B. (1969). *The idea of usury: From tribal brotherhood to universal brotherhood.* Princeton, NJ: Princeton University Press.

Pfister, J., & Schnog, N. (Eds.). (1997). *Inventing the psychological: Toward a cultural history of emotional life in America.* New Haven, CT: Yale University Press.

Phillips, K. L. (1998). "Stand by me": Sacred quartet music and emotionology of African American audiences, 1900–1930. In P. N. Stearns & J. Lewis (Eds.), *Emotional history of the United States* (pp. 241–258). New York: New York University Press.

Pollock, L. A. (1983). *Forgotten children: Parent–child relations from 1500 to 1900.* Cambridge, UK: Cambridge University Press.

Reddy, W. (2001). *Navigation of feeling: A framework for the history of emotions.* Cambridge, UK: Cambridge University Press.

Rosenblatt, P. (1983). *Bitter, bitter tears: Nineteenth-century diarists and twentieth-century grief theories.* Minneapolis: University of Minnesota Press.

Rosenwein, B. H. (2006). *Emotional communities in the early middle ages.* Ithaca, NY: Cornell University Press.

Rotundo, A. (1989). Romantic friendship: Male intimacy and middle-class youth in the northern United States, 1800–1900. *Journal of Social History, 23,* 1–25.

Sabean, D. (1984). *Power in the blood: Popular culture and village discourse in early modern Germany.* Cambridge, UK: Cambridge University Press.

Salovey, P. (Ed.). (1991). *The psychology of jealousy and envy.* New York: Guilford Press.

Seidman, S. (1991). *Romantic longings: Love in America, 1830–1980.* New York: Routledge.

Shields, S. A., & Koster, B. A. (1989). Emotional stereotyping of parent in child rearing manuals, 1915–1980. *Social Psychology Quarterly, 52*(1), 44–55.

Shorter, E. (1975). *The making of the modern family.* New York: Basic Books.

Shumway, D. R. (1998). Something old, something new: Romance and marital advice in the 1920s. In P. N. Stearns & J. Lewis (Eds.), *Emotional history of the United States* (pp. 305–318). New York: New York University Press.

Solomon, R. H. (1971). *Mao's revolution and Chinese political culture.* Berkeley: University of California Press.

Stearns, C. Z., & Stearns, P. N. (1986). *Anger: The struggle for emotional control in America's history.* Chicago: University of Chicago Press.

Stearns, C. Z., & Stearns, P. N. (Eds.). (1988). *Emotion and social change: Toward a new psychohistory.* New York: Holmes & Meier.

Stearns, P. N. (1989). *Jealousy: The evolution of an emotion in American history.* New York: New York University Press.

Stearns, P. N. (1994). *American cool: Constructing a twentieth century emotional style.* New York: New York University Press.

Stearns, P. N. (1997). Emotional change and political disengagement in the 20th-century United States. *Innovation—The European Journal of Social Sciences, 10*(4), 361–380.

Stearns, P. N. (1998). Consumerism and childhood: New targets for American emotions. In P. N. Stearns & J. Lewis (Eds.), *Emotional history of the United States* (pp. 396–416). New York: New York University Press.

Stearns, P. N. (1999). Perceptions of death in the Korean War. *War in History, 6,* 72–87.

Stearns, P. N. (2005). *American behavioral history: An introduction.* New York: New York University Press.

Stearns, P. N. (2006). *American fear: The causes and consequences of high anxiety.* New York: Routledge.

Stearns, P. N., with Stearns, C. Z. (1985). Emotionology: Clarifying the history of emotions and emotional standards. *American Historical Review, 90*(4), 813–836.

Stone, L. (1977). *The family, sex and marriage in England, 1500–1800.* New York: Harper & Row.

Trumbach, R. (1978). *The rise of the egalitarian family: Aristocratic kinship and domestic relations in eighteenth century England.* New York: Academic Press.

Walthall, A. (1990). The family ideology of the rural entrepreneurs in nineteenth-century Japan. *Journal of Social History, 23,* 463–484.

White, K. (1993). *The first sexual revolution: The emergence of male heterosexuality in modern America.* New York: New York University Press.

Wouters, C. (1991). On status competition and emotion management. *Journal of Social History, 24*(4), 690–717.

Wouters, C. (1992). On status competition and emotion management: The study of emotions as a new field. *Theory Culture and Society, 9,* 229–252.

Wouters, C. (1995). Etiquette books and emotion management in the 20th century. *Journal of Social History, 29,* 107–124, 325–340.

Wouters, C. (1996). *Changing patterns of social controls and self-controls: On the rise of crime since the 1950s.* Paper presented at the "Causes of Crisis" symposium, Edinburgh, Scotland.

Wouters, C. (2004). *Sex and manners: Female emancipation in the west.* London: Sage.

Zelizer, V. (1985). *Pricing the priceless child.* New York: Basic Books.

CHAPTER 3

The Sociology of Emotions

JAN E. STETS and JONATHAN H. TURNER

Within sociology, the study of emotions is a comparatively recent field of specialization, first emerging in its modern form in the 1970s (Heise, 1979; Hochschild, 1979; Kemper, 1978). This late arrival of a field so essential to understanding human interaction and social organization is partly the result of weak foundational statements by the first sociologists, who, with few exceptions, did not offer detailed analyses of human emotional arousal. For example Karl Marx (1867/1990) emphasized the negative arousal of alienation and anger that would push the proletariat to revolutionary class conflict; Emile Durkheim (1912/1965) identified the negative emotions of egoism and anomie while detailing the positive emotions that come with the copresence of individuals and rituals directed at totems symbolizing the group; and Charles Horton Cooley (1902/1964) recognized that pride and shame are the background emotions for self-appraisals in the "looking glass" provided by others' responses to a person's behaviors. However, none of these early theorists' analyses of emotions provided a strong program for sociological work. Even George Herbert Mead

(1934), whose ideas formed the foundation for sociological analysis of micro-level social processes for the entire 20th century, failed to conceptualize emotions. Consequently, the sociology of emotions remained a recessive mode of inquiry until its resurgence in the 1970s. Since then, the study of emotions has become one of the leading edges of theory and research in sociology, particularly sociological social psychology.

A sociological analysis of emotions begins with the view that human behavior and interaction are constrained by individuals' location in social structures guided by culture. Individuals are seen as incumbents in positions within a set of positions (i.e., social structures) that are regulated by systems of cultural symbols. Both cognitive appraisal (people's internal representation of themselves, others, and situations) and emotional arousal are constrained in interaction by culture and social structure. Figure 3.1 outlines the essential elements of a sociological analysis of emotions.

"Culture" is defined as systems of symbols that humans create and use to regulate their behaviors and interactions, with the key elements

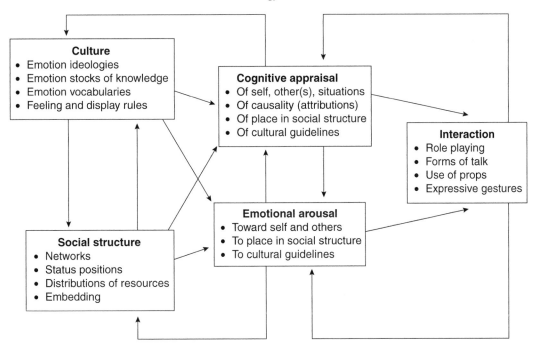

FIGURE 3.1. A sociological analysis of emotions.

of culture including emotion ideologies (appropriate feelings and emotional responses in different situations), emotion stocks of knowledge (emotional experiences that build up over time and become available for use in interaction), emotion vocabularies, and feeling and display rules (Turner & Stets, 2005). These elements are invoked and used to guide social structure and individuals' cognitions.

"Social structure" is conceptualized as either a node in a network revealing varying properties such as density, centrality, and power, or as a set of status positions carrying varying levels of prestige and other resources (Turner & Stets, 2005). Structures distribute resources, often unequally, while being embedded inside of each other. For example, encounters are inside of groups, which are inside organizations, communities, and social categories, which are inside institutional domains and stratification systems (Turner, 2002).

"Cognitive appraisals" revolve around the following: general definitions of self, other(s), and situations; attributions for the causes behind situational outcomes; awareness of one's place in the social structure; and recognition of cultural guidelines. "Emotional arousal" is generally conceived to flow along a positive–negative polarity, with specific emotions

emerging as a result of the responses to self and others, a cognitive assessment of one's place in social structure, and knowledge of the relevant cultural guidelines (Turner & Stets, 2005). "Interaction" is the process whereby the behaviors of one or more persons influence the behaviors of one or more others. For sociologists, behavior is only relevant to the extent that it takes into consideration the actual or anticipated responses of others. Interaction involves role playing and the presentation of self through forms of talk, the use of props, and expressive gestures.

As is evident from the reverse causal arrows connecting elements in Figure 3.1 (i.e., the arrows going from right to left), sociological analysis always emphasizes the recursive nature of interaction, which always feeds back to and affects emotional arousal, cognitions, social structure, and culture. Culture and social structure are reproduced or potentially changed by the cognitions and emotions that emerge during the course of interactions among individuals.

As we review in this chapter, there are now at least five theoretical research traditions in the sociology of emotions, which correspond to the essential elements of a sociological analysis of emotions outlined in Figure 3.1. Moving from left to right in the model, we review the dramaturgical (culture), structural (social structure), symbolic-interactionist (cognitive appraisal), and ritual and exchange (interaction) perspectives on emotion. Each tradition examines only some of the causal connections portrayed in the figure, but together the theories develop concepts, propositions, and empirical assessments for all of the direct, indirect, and recursive causal relations outlined in the figure. As we will review at the end of this chapter, there are several critical issues beyond varying points of emphasis that divide sociological theorizing and research. However, before exploring these contentious issues, we review each of the traditions that have emerged in the sociology of emotions over the last 30 years.

DRAMATURGICAL APPROACHES

Dramaturgical approaches to the sociology of emotions emphasize the importance of culture in providing emotion ideologies, stocks of knowledge, vocabularies, and feeling rules. These elements of culture operate as cognitive guidelines to what emotions should be experienced and expressed in a situation, as well as to what vocabularies are to be used in adjusting emotional responses to the situation (Gordon, 1981; Peterson, 2006). Some good examples of research focusing on the role of culture on emotions include work on grief (Charmaz & Milligan, 2006) and sympathy (Clark, 1997; Schmitt & Clark, 2006). These studies show how emotions are culturally scripted as to "when" to feel and "how" to express these feelings. Through the socialization process, individuals learn how to associate particular emotion vocabularies with specific eliciting situations, internal sensations, and expressive displays. For example, a study by Pollak and Thoits (1989) of a therapeutic nursery reveals how adult caretakers teach children how to identify and express their emotions.

What makes this approach dramaturgical is that individuals are viewed as acting on a stage configured by social structure in front of an audience (of others). Actors not only use the cultural script to orchestrate their presentations of self to an audience; they also use staging props provided by social structure. However, individuals are more than dramatic actors manipulating emotions through expressive control in accordance with the feeling and display rules

of culture. They are also strategists who present themselves to others, manipulating their forms of talk, role cues, bodies, staging props, and expressive display to their audience to realize their goals (Goffman, 1967). Individuals often use their emotional displays strategically to con and/or to gain favor, power, or status over others (Clark, 1997).

When individuals violate the cultural script, however, they experience embarrassment and perhaps shame, which leads them to engage in repair rituals that restore the normal order, while signaling to others that the breach of this order was only temporary (Goffman, 1967). Recent work in dramaturgy has emphasized that social structures and cultural rules often demand that individuals display emotions that they do not feel, and that in fact are systematically generated by social structures. Under these conditions, individuals must engage in "emotion work" or "emotion management" to control their emotional display so that it is in accordance with the feeling rules of the situation (Hochschild, 1983; Rosenberg, 1990; Thoits, 1990).

Hochschild's (1983) classic research on airline attendants and bill collectors is one of the best illustrations of how dramaturgy can be incorporated into the study of emotions. She adopts elements of Goffman's analysis to show how individuals engage in emotion management to maintain a presentation of self that conforms to emotion ideologies, cultural feeling rules, and cultural display rules of a society. When such emotion management is done at work, for a wage, it constitutes emotional labor. Another classic piece in this genre is Pierce's (1995) study of lawyers and paralegals in law firms. Her analysis highlights how emotional labor is gendered either because of the different positions men and women hold in law firms (men are chiefly the lawyers and are expected to be aggressive, while women are typically the paralegals and are expected to be nurturing), or because of the double standard on the emotion norms for the same job (men can be aggressive lawyers, but aggressive women lawyers are considered unfeminine and domineering).

Various cognitive and behavioral strategies are available for managing emotions (Gross, Richards, & John, 2006; Hochschild, 1983; Rosenberg, 1990; Thoits, 1990). Cognitive strategies include invoking thoughts associated with the emotions demanded in the situation to shore up the emotions, using meditation to arouse the emotions dictated by the culture, or psychologically withdrawing from the situation to mask the incongruence between actual feelings and feelings expected in the situation. Behavioral strategies include evoking expressive gestures consistent with the emotion norms of the situation to arouse the culturally appropriate emotions, seeking help and advice from others on how to manage one's emotions, or physically leaving the situation that generates the discrepancy between actual and expected feelings.

Using a national sample of respondents, Stets and Tsushima (2001) have examined how individuals use these cognitive and behavioral strategies to cope with anger at work and at home. Indeed, to remain in a continual state of anger is too disruptive for relationships; anger management is needed. They find that individuals have a tendency to use behavioral coping strategies, such as seeking social support from others to help them manage their anger, to deal with work-related problems. In contrast, persons have a tendency to use cognitive strategies, such as praying to God, for family-related problems. Other researchers have more closely examined emotion management among select groups of individuals, such as wheelchair users (Cahill & Eggleston, 1994), medical students (Smith & Kleinman, 1989), and animal shelter workers (Arluke, 1994).

The emphasis on culture and self-presentation in dramaturgical approaches helps inform us how emotional responses are learned and managed in situations. To advance this approach further, however, several issues should be examined. There needs to be a more precise conceptualization of the elements of emotion cultures, a clearer description of how they are learned, and a better explanation of how they are used strategically in interaction. The concept of emotion work also needs more development, including the conditions under which it is facilitated or impeded, its positive and negative consequences for the self and others in interaction, and the impact of these consequences on social-structural arrangements and social change.

STRUCTURAL APPROACHES

All sociological approaches to the study of emotions include social structure as part of the analysis. Indeed, emphasis on the effects of social structure and culture on behavior and interaction, and vice versa, is the defining characteristic of sociology. It is not the analysis of structure per se, but the relative emphasis on the properties of social structure, that is important. In the sociology of emotions, theorizing and research tend to emphasize a relatively small range of social-structural properties. The most prominent set of approaches, working from diverse theoretical traditions, examine micro-level power (authority) and status (prestige) differences among individuals as these affect their cognitive assessments and emotions during the course of interaction, which in turn either reproduce or change the power and status order. In contrast, relatively few approaches focus on macro-level processes, including institutional spheres and stratification systems as they determine the distribution of resources, and in turn the power and status order at the micro level.

Microstructural Analysis of Emotions

One set of approaches conceptualize the micro-level order of interaction as revealing differences in the relative power and status among individuals or among the positions occupied by individuals. Sometimes these differences are imposed by an existing social structure, and at other times they emerge during the course of interaction. Once in place, status differences establish expectation states for the relative competence and performances of those who are high and low in the status order (Berger, Fisek, Norman, & Zelditch, 1977; Berger & Webster, 2006). Moreover, these differences can become codified into cultural beliefs about the relative qualities of those in high and low positions. Such beliefs are most likely to emerge for diffuse status characteristics, such as gender, ethnicity, age, and other status differences that are widely known in a society and that generate expectation states for competence and performances. In general, when individuals act in accordance with expectation states and cultural beliefs, those in higher-ranking positions experience positive emotions such as happiness and pride, while those in lower-ranking positions experience negative emotions like anger and fear.

Attribution processes are brought into most of these power and status theories, because the valence and direction of emotional arousal depends on the attributions made by actors for confirmation or disconfirmation of their relative status (Houser & Lovaglia, 2002; Lovaglia

& Houser, 1996). Typically, higher-ranking individuals will make self-attributions for their rank, and thus experience satisfaction, happiness, and pride when their performances confirm their rank. At times, however, higher-ranking individuals make external attributions, seeing their rank as due to broader structural conditions rather than their performances. As a result, they will experience status insecurity and will be vulnerable to negative emotional arousal, particularly variants of fear and anxiety.

Lower-ranking persons' emotional arousal will also be influenced by attribution dynamics. If individuals perceive that their low rank is their own fault (i.e., that it is due to lack of ability and/or performance), they will experience low levels of positive emotions such as satisfaction. If they have difficulty accepting their low rank as their own fault, they will experience mild negative emotions such as sadness and alienation. If lower-ranking persons do not accept their situation as the result of their own lack of ability, but rather as a consequence of structural arrangements that work unfairly against them, they will experience anger—and, if possible, will direct this anger outward toward higher-ranking persons and the larger social structure.

Different theories stress varying facets of the general approach summarized above. In Kemper's interactional theory (Kemper, 1978; Kemper & Collins, 1990) or power–status theory of emotions (Kemper, 2006), emotions are related to individuals' relative power (what he labels "involuntary compliance") and status ("voluntary compliance"), changes in relative power and status, and expectations for gains or losses of power and status. Thus Kemper considers both dimensions of social relations—power and status—in his theory, rather than just status.

According to Kemper, when individuals gain power, they will experience satisfaction, confidence, and security; when they lose power and when they do not experience an expected gain in power, they will experience fear, anxiety, and loss of confidence. When they possess status or gain expected status, they will experience satisfaction and well-being, and they will express positive sentiments to others. When individuals lose prestige, the emotional dynamics are influenced by attributions. When individuals blame themselves for a loss of status, they will experience shame and embarrassment, and if the loss is great, they will also feel sad and depressed.

If, however, they blame others for their loss of status, they will experience anger and seek to force others to honor their status claims.

In a direct test of the power–status approach, Kemper (1991) analyzed data gathered from an eight-nation study (Scherer, Wallbott, & Summerfield, 1986). Of particular interest to him were respondents' reports of fear, joy, sadness, and anger. He investigated whether the power–status antecedents could be found in respondents' accounts of the situational circumstances leading to the four emotions. For example, would fear emerge from power loss by the self or power gain by another? Would joy emerge from status gain by the self? Coders' evaluated respondents' open-ended responses regarding the events leading up to emotions as instances of power gain or loss and status gain or loss. The results indicated that the power–status conditions did lead to the expected emotions at a rate higher than would be expected by chance.

Many sociological social psychologists work within the expectation states theory research program, which, as its name suggests, emphasizes the effects of expectations on emotional arousal. The focus is on the expectations associated with status. Unlike Kemper's theory, power is not considered. Furthermore, in expectation states theory, emotion is only one outcome of the status process in interaction, so emotion does not play a major role in the theory as it does in Kemper's power–status theory.

In expectation states theory, when individuals meet performance expectations associated with their status (e.g., when high-status actors outperform low-status actors), positive emotions will be felt by both sets of actors. In this way, status expectations shape emotion. However, emotions may themselves shape the development of a status hierarchy (Ridgeway, 2006). They may act as an additional factor that shapes performance expectations (e.g., if we like a person, we will evaluate his or her performance more positively, thereby giving that person higher status). Alternatively, it may be an additional factor that influences performance expectations only in certain situations, when there is not much at stake in a group decision—as opposed to a crisis situation, where performance is important rather than sentiments about each other. To date, the results are not definite as to which emotions may influence the status hierarchy.

Ridgeway (1994, 2006; Ridgeway & Johnson, 1990) has shown how the evaluation of task suggestions in a group (either agreeing or disagreeing with the task suggestions) not only is important in the establishment of a status hierarchy in the group, but also is an elicitor of positive and negative emotions, thereby setting into motion affective dynamics in a group. Ridgeway has emphasized the emotions that ensue when there are disagreements between higher- and lower-status individuals in task groups. If a person is at the same rank as, or at a higher rank than, another with whom a disagreement occurs, this person will experience mild anger or annoyance toward the other; if this individual is at a lower rank, he or she will experience sadness and potentially, depression. Moreover, lower-status members of the group will often negatively sanction a lower-ranking individual who disagrees with a higher-status person, thus increasing the negative emotional arousal. In contrast, agreements work to increase the flow of positive emotions in the group. With agreements between higher- and lower-status persons, the higher-status individual will experience satisfaction, and as a consequence will be disposed to give off positive emotions to lower-status persons, who will experience satisfaction and potentially happiness. Similarly, agreements among persons at the same status will produce pleasure and even gratitude. Because positive emotional arousal leads individuals to positively sanction each other, thus ratcheting up the flow of positive emotions, groups tend to develop biases for behaviors that maintain the status order. To challenge the order works to arouse negative emotions, which lead to negative sanctioning and negative emotional arousal.

Macrostructural Analysis of Emotions

Relatively few researchers in the sociology of emotions examine social structure from a more macro-level perspective. Particular subfields within sociology, such as the study of collective behavior, social movements, political legitimization, terrorism, or revolutions, employ implicit conceptions of collective emotional arousal, but these approaches typically do not develop a robust analysis of emotions. One exception to this conclusion is work by Barbalet (1998). Although Barbalet does not develop a systematic theory of emotions, he does explore the relationship among certain aspects of social structure—especially those having to do with inequality, power, and specific emotions (namely, resentment, fear, confidence, vengeful-

ness, and shame)—from a more macro-level perspective.

For Barbalet, emotions are distributed differentially across segments of a society, most typically corresponding to each segment's socioeconomic status. Individuals react emotionally to their respective shares of money, power, and prestige in ways that cannot be fully captured in small-group experiments. Resentment is an emotion that arises when subpopulations perceive that others gain power and prestige that is not deserved or that violates cultural rules of justice. For example, in his conceptual reexamination of Sennett and Cobb's (1972) classic study of the hidden injuries of class, Barbalet maintains that much of the resentment of working-class males against welfare recipients is sublimated resentment about their lack of rewards for their hard work. Rather than resent the class system and the forces that have pushed them at the lower rungs of the system, working-class males sublimate their resentment and transfer it to those who are perceived to gain without doing the work.

Fear is another emotion that Barbalet conceptualizes to be differentially distributed across a society. Fear comes from a lack of power, and if individuals attribute this fear to their own shortcomings, then fear leads to withdrawal and flight responses; if individuals make external attributions, fear turns into anger, aggression, and fight responses. Confidence, another emotion Barbalet discusses, arises among those members of a society who perceive that their future is under their control and is predictable. Vengefulness occurs among subpopulations, usually the less powerful, who often see the powerful as denying them the right to occupy high-status positions and play roles in society that allow them to form meaningful and cooperative social relationships. Finally, shame emerges among individuals who claim or are given status that they do not deserve.

Thus Barbalet's preliminary and speculative analysis points to a form of social-structural analysis: the view that emotions are like most resources, and are thereby distributed unequally. Specific kinds of emotion states emerge among subpopulations under predictable conditions, and sociological theory will need to specify these conditions and their potential effects on collective action in societies.

Most structural theories on emotions are decidedly micro-level in focus, examining processes in face-to-face interaction such as power and status. However, micro-level processes occur within a larger macrostructure in which power and resources are unequally distributed. For a structural theory of emotions to develop, it needs to make connections between micro- and macrostructures. Whole categories of individuals based on gender, class, or race, for example, can experience similar emotions because they stand in the same place in the stratification system. They are structurally equivalent; they are likely to have the same experiences; and hence they are likely to have similar emotional reactions. Barbalet's work comes closet to linking macrostructural processes to emotions at the micro level, but much more of such inquiry is needed.

SYMBOLIC INTERACTIONIST APPROACHES

All symbolic interactionist theories and research programs emphasize the central place of self and identities in the arousal of emotions. Two types of cognitive appraisals revolve around individuals: (1) *transsituational* and general conceptions of themselves as particular kinds of individuals, and (2) *situational* identities about themselves in particular roles in the social structure. Individuals formulate self-meanings/identity standards, obtain self-perceptions of who they are in situations, assess the degree of congruence between self-meanings and situational self-meanings, and experience emotional reactions (Stets, 2006). The emotional responses will be positive when situational self-meanings are congruent with one's own self-meanings/identity standards, and negative when they are incongruent. In the latter case, individuals are motivated to bring into congruence the self-meanings and situational self-meanings. When individuals habitually cannot confirm an identity, they will engage in cognitive or behavioral strategies or both (discussed below) to derive positive emotions.

The gestalt-like processes described above lead toward consistency among cognitions about the self, others, and (by extension) one's place in the social structure and in reference to cultural standards. There are also more psychoanalytic versions of symbolic interactionist theory and research, which emphasize that negative emotions like shame and guilt are painful and hence are likely to activate defense mechanisms revolving around repression, thus disrupting the control system that seeks to sustain

consistency among cognitions about self, other, social structure, and culture (Turner, 2006). Below we examine representative approaches in both the gestalt and psychoanalytic variants of symbolic interactionism.

Control Theoretical Variants of Symbolic Interactionism

Symbolic interactionist approaches to emotions generally view the emotional reactions to either verification or nonverification of self or identity as part of a perceptual control system (Burke, 1991; Heise, 1979). Negative emotional arousal signals to a person that a general self-conception or more situational identity is not confirmed, and this distress, anxiety, or sadness motivates individuals to employ a number of cognitive and behavioral strategies. For example, cognitive strategies might include selectively perceiving or interpreting the gestures of others so as to verify one's identity or making external attributions that blame others, the situation, or the social structure for failing to verify the self. Behavioral strategies might involve changing one's behavior to obtain verification or leaving the situation.

In several symbolic interactionist theories, a hierarchy of identities is conceptualized, with those high in the hierarchy of "salience" (Stryker, 1980/2002, 2004) or "prominence" (McCall & Simmons, 1978) more likely to be presented in situations than those low in the hierarchy. When a highly salient identity is disconfirmed, individuals will feel negative emotions, and the identity may move down the hierarchy. Research appears to support this idea. For example, Ellestad and Stets (1998) have found that when the mother identity is more prominent for women, they are more likely to report the negative emotion of jealousy when fathers intrude into caretaking activities traditionally reserved for mothers. Unless the women reassert their nurturing role in the situation, such as spending more time with their children and not allowing their spouses to intrude, the mother identity may not be maintained and thus may move down the hierarchy of identities. Indeed, Stryker theorizes that when an identity is not being confirmed in a situation, an alternative identity that is being confirmed and that produces positive emotions such as satisfaction and happiness may move up the identity hierarchy and guide behavior.

In the perceptual control system of identities, particularly identity control theory, there is an "identity standard," which is the stored set of self-meanings attached to an identity that guides behavior in situations. Individuals compare the self-meanings of who they are in a situation, which are based on reflected appraisals (feedback from others) and self-appraisals (their own assessment), with their identity standard (Burke, 1991, 1996). When self-meanings in the situation correspond with identity standard meanings, positive emotions will be experienced. A lack of correspondence in meanings will lead to negative emotions, and in response, the cognitive and behavioral strategies mentioned previously will be used to generate congruency in meanings.

In a series of laboratory experiments, Stets (2003, 2005) has found that a lack of correspondence between self-meanings in a situation and identity standard meanings does not always lead to negative emotions; in fact, it leads to positive emotions when the identity nonverification is in a positive direction (receiving feedback that is more positive or higher than one's identity standard), compared to a negative direction. Stets argues that this unexpected finding may have been obtained because participants in her studies were not given sufficient time to compare the positive feedback with their self-views, as well as because participants were not invested in the identity that was invoked in the laboratory. Having the mental resources to access one's self-views, and being invested in one's self-views, are both important conditions in the verification process (Swann, Rentfrow, & Guinn, 2003); when they are absent, the emotional response following feedback from others may be different from what is expected. Indeed, other research reveals that when, for example, investment in one's self-views is present in a situation, nonverification in a positive direction does produce negative emotions (Burke & Harrod, 2005).

Another perceptual control theory of identities is affect control theory (Heise, 1979). Affect control theorists array emotions along lines of "evaluation" (goodness–badness), "potency" (powerful–powerless), and "activity" (active–passive). This is known as the EPA dimension. The theorists emphasize cognitions about the identities of self and others, the behaviors of others, and the situation in which identities emerge. The key idea is that individuals seek to keep their fundamental sentiments (culturally established affective meanings [along the EPA dimension] about identities and behaviors that transcend particular situations)

in line with their transient impressions (feelings about what is actually occurring in a particular situation in terms of people's identities and behaviors) (Robinson, Smith-Lovin, & Wisecup, 2006). For example, if the mother identity is on average evaluated as good, somewhat powerful, and somewhat active, but in a particular situation one finds a mother scolding a child, this person will view the mother identity more negatively because she is evaluated as bad rather than good (for scolding) and as somewhat less powerful (for losing control of her child). There would be no change in the degree of activity of the mother identity. When a discrepancy between fundamental sentiments and transient impressions occurs, emotions will emerge, but their valence will depend upon the transient meaning and its direction of change from the original fundamental sentiments. For example, if transient meanings are more positive than fundamental meanings, one will feel more positive, while transient meanings that are more negative than fundamental meanings will lead to negative emotions. Empirical tests have supported the role of emotions in affect control theory (Heise & Weir, 1999; Robinson, Smith-Lovin, & Tsoudis, 1994).

Psychoanalytic Variants of Symbolic Interactionism

Psychoanalytic approaches in the sociology of emotions try to bring the Freudian legacy, particularly as it was incorporated into the seminal analysis of Helen Block Lewis (1971), into the perceptual control models presented by mainstream symbolic interactionism (Scheff, 1988, 1990; Turner, 1999, 2002, 2006). Individuals will often engage in defensive strategies to protect the self from negative emotions. Specifically, when individuals behave incompetently in front of others and/or breach the micro-level social order, they experience shame; when they act in ways violating cultural values, they experience guilt (Turner, 2002).

For shame in particular, persons will repress this negative feeling to varying degrees (Turner, 2006), because shame attacks the self and makes a person feel small and unworthy (Tangney & Dearing, 2002). Turner (2006) argues that once negative emotions are repressed, they will often intensify and be transmuted into new emotions. For example, he maintains that shame often emerges from the cortical sensors as periodic spikes of anger, which, ironically, lead to more shame that is repressed. This is consistent with Lewis's (1971) idea that individuals can become locked into shame–anger–shame cycles, with the successive repression of the shame intensifying the mix of unconscious emotions that periodically erupt as anger.

For psychoanalytic versions of symbolic interactionism, individuals are often unaware of the disjuncture between meanings given off by their self-presentations and meanings as to how others see them in a particular situation, because repression has pushed below the level of consciousness the negative emotions that result and that are important to the perceptual control system posited by mainstream symbolic interactionism. Psychoanalytic theories thus add a corrective to the gestalt dynamics of symbolic interactionism, arguing that when negative emotions are intense, defense mechanisms may change the dynamics of the control system, sometimes with severe consequences for the individual.

Such consequences can extend to more macro-level social structures. For example, Scheff and Retzinger (1991) have argued that the repression of shame in societies can lead to collective violence at the societal and even intersocietal levels when the repressed shame is transmuted into anger and, through mobilization by leaders and the mass media, is directed at "enemies" within a society. In their analysis of the origins of World War II, they contend that the unacknowledged shame experienced by Germans as a result of their blame and humiliation as the sole instigators of World War I, coupled with Hitler's repression of shame and rage toward his father and obsession with Jews, provided a lethal combination: The shame and anger of both the German people and Hitler spiraled out of control and caused the murder of millions of people.

The strength of the symbolic interactionist approach is its emphasis on self and identity in understanding emotions. However, future work on integrating the perceptual control and psychoanalytic views of self is required. Whereas the former emphasizes the self-verification process, the latter emphasizes repression and defense mechanisms that may emerge when the self is not verified. The conditions under which repression and defensive strategies emerge in the perceptual control system, as well as the consequences of this emergence for future self-verification and one's emotional experiences, need to be studied.

RITUAL APPROACHES

Interaction ritual theories borrow from Durkheim's (1912/1965) secondary analysis of "collective effervescence" among Australian aboriginals. When aboriginals would periodically gather, their copresence would lead to animated interaction, which in turn would generate a collective effervescence of positive emotions. This effervescence led individuals to perceive that there was a power or *mana* external to their actions and, indeed, guiding their actions. As a result, they would begin to represent this power with totems. When rituals were directed to these totems to symbolize the power of the gods, they would rekindle the sense of effervescence and *mana*. Durkheim concluded that the aboriginals' religion was nothing more than the personification of their group solidarity, which they saw as all-powerful and in need of representation with totems and reverence through rituals.

This ritual approach has recently been expanded by Collins (2004) and Summers-Effler (2004b, 2006) into a general theory of micro-dynamic processes that operate as the underpinnings of more macro-level social structures. Social structures bring individuals into copresence, often allocating varying degrees of symbolic, material, and power resources to persons occupying different positions in the structure. Individuals are seen as motivated to augment their positive emotional energy (initiative and enthusiasm) and cultural capital in all situations. Those with high levels of resources and power (higher-status persons) will give orders in situations, and they will generally act in ways that allow them to increase their emotional energy and cultural capital. By contrast, lower-status persons will have more difficulty augmenting their emotional energy and cultural capital, because they must take orders.

These more recent versions of the theory emphasize that interaction rituals are of two kinds (Collins, 2004). One kind consists of the transient rituals that open and close interactions and that arouse mild positive emotions (e.g., handshakes, greetings). Another kind of ritual, such as a church service, is more inclusive and incorporates the larger sequence of interaction whereby individuals become copresent, reveal a common focus of attention, and develop a shared mood, which in turn causes a rhythmic synchronization of talk and body alignment, leading to a collective effervescence and increased level of emotional energy.

In general, the escalation of positive emotional energy in interaction rituals of the second kind increases group solidarity, which leads individuals to symbolize the group with words, emblems, phrases, and other "totems." The more the group is symbolized in these terms, the more likely it is that iterated interactions will reinforce the symbols of the group. And as symbols circulate among members, they develop particularized cultural capital unique to the group. Even individuals' internal conversations or thoughts about the symbols of the group have the capacity to arouse positive emotions, all of which increase group solidarity while enhancing cultural capital. Similarly, iterations of this more inclusive interaction ritual will charge up group symbols and, in so doing, enhance not only particularized cultural capital but also social structure. Thus such interaction rituals provide a firm micro-level basis for macrostructures. When initial ritual openings do not cause even mild transient emotions, or when any other element of the early phases of the encounter (such as mutual focus of attention, shared mood, and rhythmic synchronization) do not ensue, then emotional effervescence and positive emotional energy will be low and perhaps even become negative, thereby reducing group solidarity. In turn, cultural capital will not be produced and solidarity will be low, thus undermining macro-level social structures.

Empirical work that uses concepts from Collins's theory includes Summers-Effler's (2004a) analysis of two altruistic social movement organizations: a Catholic Worker house seeking to establish a communal lifestyle, and an anti-death-penalty organization. She shows how interactions among group members generate high degrees of group solidarity through the arousal of positive emotional energy and the circulation of particularized cultural capital.

The reconceptualization of Durkheim's work into a more robust conception of the dynamics of interaction and emotions provided by current ritual theories confronts several problems. One is the portrayal of emotions in terms only of negative and positive valence states. There is a rich array of complex specific emotions that needs to be investigated beyond their positive or negative valences. Another problem is that ritual approaches posit a need for people to maximize emotional energy, and with the exception of Summers-Effler's (2004c) recent work, more research on instances where individuals stay in relationships arousing negative emotional energy needs to be conducted. While Summers-Effler discusses how individuals develop strategies that minimize the loss of emotional energy when they cannot leave interactions that produce negative emotional energy, the ways in which individuals defend themselves from situations in which negative emotional energy prevails have not been adequately conceptualized by ritual theories. Part of the problem is that unlike symbolic interactionism, ritual theories do not include an adequate conceptualization of self, which is needed in understanding the strategies for managing negative emotional arousal.

EXCHANGE APPROACHES

Exchange theories view individuals as motivated to seek valued resources/rewards in excess of their costs (alternative sources of rewards forgone) and investments (accumulated costs over time). Actors give resources to others with the expectation that they will receive more valuable resources in return, thereby making a profit. Payoffs are assessed not only in terms of the level of profit, but also against normative standards of justice and fair exchange. Cognitive calculations of justice and fairness also involve a comparison process of assessing one's own payoffs relative to the payoffs (including costs and investments) of others.

In general, individuals experience positive emotions such as happiness when they receive a profit that is defined as "just," and when others' profits are proportionate to their costs and investments as compared to the costs and investments of the persons making the comparisons. When payoffs are not proportionate to individuals' own costs and investments, when others receive higher payoffs disproportionate to their costs and investments, and when norms of fair exchange and justice are violated, individuals will experience negative emotions (primarily anger). The nature of intensity of emotional arousal is, however, governed by several additional considerations: the type of exchange, the relative power and dependence of individuals on each other for valued resources, the expectations for payoffs, the particular standards of justice invoked, and the attributions that individuals make for profits and loses.

With respect to the nature of exchanges, there are four basic types (Lawler, 2001): "productive," where close coordination of activities occurs and where each person's relative contribution to payoffs is difficult to separate from that of others; "negotiated," where individuals bargain, making offers and counteroffers, in seeking resources from each other; "reciprocal," where a person provides resources to another with assurances of receiving resources in return at a later point in time; and "generalized," where an individual gives resources to another who in turn gives them to another who does the same, in a chain that eventually circles back to the original individual. Conceptually, productive exchanges will generate the most intense emotions, whether positive or negative, followed by negotiated, reciprocal, and generalized (Lawler, 2001). Molm's (1997) research reveals how negotiated exchanges often introduce conflict into interaction, and hence arouse anger and other conflict-oriented emotions. Reciprocal exchanges generate trust and positive emotions revolving around the expectation that the giving of resources will be reciprocated.

The relative power of individuals in an exchange influences payoffs. The power of actor A over actor B is a function of the dependence of B on A for valued resources (Emerson, 1962). Power-advantaged actors will typically impose additional costs on dependent actors for resources, thus increasing the negative emotions (such as anger) among dependent actors. In a series of experimental studies, Lawler and Yoon have shown how actors who are equally dependent on each other for resources (high total power) and who thus possess equal levels of power will have a high rate of exchange among themselves, and how this high rate of exchange will in turn generate more positive emotions (pleasure, satisfaction, interest, excitement), more relational cohesion, and more commitment behaviors during exchanges (Lawler & Yoon, 1996, 1998; Thye, Yoon, & Lawler, 2002). Lawler and Yoon's work, known as the theory of "relational cohesion," operates much like the interaction ritual theories discussed above. In the theory of relational cohesion, new resources—positive emotions, cohesion, and commitments—are introduced into the exchange and generate a kind of mild "collective effervescence" reminiscent of ritual theories.

Moreover, commitments to exchanges operate to produce positive emotional arousal, because they reduce the fear and anxiety that comes with uncertainty over exchange payoffs from others (Kollock, 1994).

The greater the expectations for payoffs at a given level, the more intense the negative emotional arousal (anger, fear, frustration) when they are not forthcoming—and, conversely, the greater the satisfaction and happiness when these payoffs are forthcoming (Jasso, 2006). Moreover, it takes much less underreward below expectations to generate anger than it does overreward to cause a person to feel guilty (Hegtvedt, 1990). In fact, individuals will typically feel guilty only when their overreward is perceived to cause underreward to others (Hegtvedt & Killian, 1999).

The nature of the rules of justice invoked will also influence emotional arousal. In general, violation of any rule of justice causes a person to experience and express anger. Norms of equity (payoffs are to be proportionate to relative costs and investments of individuals) will typically trump those of procedures (fairness of the procedures used in determining payoffs). When payoffs are equitable but procedures are perceived as unfair, individuals will still experience positive emotions, whereas when norms of equity are violated, individuals will almost always see procedures as unfair and experience anger.

Emotional arousal is further influenced by the attributions that individuals make for their payoffs. Receipt of a profit in exchanges reveals a proximal bias (Lawler, 2001), causing individuals to experience positive emotions toward self, such as pride and self-satisfaction; failure to make a profit will arouse negative emotions that reveal a distal bias, whereby the individual blames others or the social structure. When others are blamed, the dominant emotion is anger, while when social structure is blamed, alienation is the more likely emotion. When others are seen to facilitate profitable exchange payoffs, gratitude will be experienced and expressed, whereas when social structure is seen to facilitate profitable payoffs, individuals will experience commitments and attachment to this structure.

The strength of exchange approaches to emotions is the link between the arousal of specific emotions to the structure of the situation and to the dynamics of attribution. However, like ritual theories, exchange theories do not include a conceptualization of self; thus we do not know how actors protect the self when they experience negative outcomes in a situation beyond the notion of external attributions. Another problem with exchange theories is that they are based on experimental research where the level of emotional arousal is low. Although it is remarkable that simple tasks and contrived exchanges can generate emotions, thus indicating that the dynamics under study are important for generating emotions, more intense emotions need to be examined, and these are likely to take us out of the experimental setting.

CONCLUSION: REMAINING PROBLEMS AND FUTURE PROSPECTS

Despite the late start, the sociology of emotions has made considerable progress over the last 30 years, as this cursory review of approaches documents (for more comprehensive reviews, see Stets & Turner, 2006; Turner & Stets, 2005). There are now many difference theories and research programs testing these theories; as a consequence, considerable accumulation of knowledge is now evident. There are, however, several issues that need to be addressed if the sociology of emotions is to continue making progress.

The Number and Types of Emotions

Sociologists view happiness, fear, anger, sadness, disgust, and surprise as the primary emotions, with the presumption that these emotions are hard-wired in the human neuroanatomy (Turner, 2000). Even the most extreme social constructivist in sociology would generally admit this, although they would also emphasize that the expression of these emotions is socially constructed. Within sociology, several efforts to classify emotions have been made (Kemper, 1987; Thamm, 2006; Turner, 2000). Beyond the classification of a few emotions as primary, there is no consensus over the various classifications; nor do researchers agree on which are hard-wired and which are purely social constructions. In the future, sociology will need to make some decisions on those emotions that are basic to human organization, and, if possible, to resolve the debate over those emotions that are hardwired and those that are wholly cultural constructions.

The Relative Neglect of Biology

For many decades, sociologists have been highly suspicious of *any* view of human behavior, interaction, or social organization as biologically based. Fears of "reductionism"—and, more implausibly, of a return to forms of racism that accompanied early 20th-century efforts at incorporating biology—still haunt the discipline. The study of emotions provides an opportunity to reject these unfounded fears about biology, because there can be little doubt that many emotions have a strong neurological basis that evolved among our hominid ancestors. Sociologists need not buy into all of the assumptions of sociobiology or evolutionary psychology to study the selection pressures that worked on human neuroanatomy (Franks, 2006). Indeed, sociologists are well positioned to provide insights into the biology of emotions, because the discipline is sensitive to the sociocultural forces that constrain emotional arousal and that no doubt guided selection of hominid neuroanatomy. With a better understanding of the biology of emotions, it will be possible to connect biology, cognition, emotions, behavior, interaction, social structure, and culture into more robust models of emotional dynamics.

Cognition and Emotions

Like psychology, the sociology of emotions reveals a cognitive bias. Emotions are seen by many approaches as signals to the self that there is incongruence among some set of cognitions (about the self, behavior, other[s], culture, and social-structural location). In response to this incongruence, individuals become motivated to bring their cognitions into line. With the exception of a few who work with psychoanalytic theory, the dynamics of repression and other defense mechanisms are not emphasized in sociological approaches to emotions. But it is now clear that humans store unconscious memories and unconsciously activate subcortical emotion centers of the brain. People often display emotions to others that they do not feel. In the future, it will be necessary to incorporate unconscious emotions into theories and research programs.

The Study of Weak Emotions

A consideration related to the one just discussed is that much research on emotions in sociology is conducted in experimental laboratories and typically focuses on task behaviors. There are, of course, strengths to this approach, because measurements can be more precise and controls can be imposed. Emotions are generally measured by pencil-and-paper tests, reactions to vignettes, and interactions with real persons (or, more often, unreal persons, through computer-mediated interaction with "virtual others"). As a result, the emotions studied generally evidence rather weak valences.

Though clear findings emerge from studies arousing weak emotional valences, the intensity of emotions *does* matter in most human affairs, if only because intense negative emotional arousal increases the likelihood of activation of defense mechanisms or because it mobilizes people to collective action. When emotions are intense, they have greater effects that cannot be adequately mapped in the laboratory. Thus it will be necessary in the future to conduct careful studies of highly valenced emotions in more naturalistic settings—using, for example, the experience-sampling method (Hektner, Schmidt, & Csikszentmihalyi, 2007) —to better understand the dynamics of strong emotional arousal.

The Micro-Level Bias in Conceptions of Social Structure

By virtue of experimental designs in most research on emotions, the conception of social structure reveals a micro-level bias. Small numbers of individuals in small social structures with just a few positions or nodes in a network exist in most experiments. Differences in relative power or prestige in small groups dominate the research. But human societies reveal macro-level domains, such as society-wide distributions of power and wealth, that have large effects on people's emotions. Though these often come into focus in micro-level encounters as status differences, the more macro-level distribution of resources and the structure of institutional domains have large effects that make large differences in how emotions are collectively experienced. And, from collective experiences, we obtain some sense as to how macro-level social structures are sustained or changed. With a few exceptions (Barbalet, 1998; Scheff, 1994; Scheff & Retzinger, 1991), the more macro-level consequences of emotional arousal among subpopulations in a society have not

been studied by those in the sociology of emotions. They need to be.

The Emphasis on Culture

Along with the bias toward the micro level in conceptions of social structure, there is a cultural bias. Considerable emphasis is placed on emotion ideologies, vocabularies, and rules as these influence social structure, cognitions, emotional arousal, and interaction. This emphasis on culture often supports a social-constructionist view, because sociologists tend to view culture as a purely human creation that is independent of biology (except for the recognition that big brains allow humans to create culture, thus obviating human biology as a major force in human behavior, interaction, and social organization). Despite this emphasis on culture, there is surprisingly little in the way of detailed analysis of *specific* emotion ideologies, vocabularies, and rules. These ideas are used in a highly metaphorical way without specifying the exact substantive content of these systems of culture and their effects on the arousal of emotions, or vice versa. If there is an emotion culture, its components need to be conceptualized in more precise terms—and the reciprocal effects among biology, behavior, interaction, and social structure on the one side, and culture on the other, need to be more adequately conceptualized.

Despite the problems described above, the sociology of emotions has made remarkable progress over the last 30 years. With more theoretical integration and more robust data, the field will continue to be a leading edge of theorizing and research in sociology.

REFERENCES

Arluke, A. (1994). Managing emotions in an animal shelter. In A. Manning & J. Serpell (Eds.), *Animals in human society: Changing perspectives* (pp. 145–165). New York: Routledge.

Barbalet, J. M. (1998). *Emotion, social theory, and social structure: A macrosociological approach.* Cambridge, UK: Cambridge University Press.

Berger, J., Fisek, M. H., Norman, R. Z., & Zelditch, M., Jr. (1977). *Status characteristics and social interaction: An expectation–states approach.* New York: Elsevier.

Berger, J., & Webster, M., Jr. (2006). Expectations, status, and behavior. In P. J. Burke (Ed.), *Contemporary social psychological theories* (pp. 268–300). Stanford, CA: Stanford University Press.

Burke, P. J. (1991). Identity processes and social stress. *American Sociological Review, 56,* 836–849.

Burke, P. J. (1996). Social identities and psychosocial stress. In H. B. Kaplan (Ed.), *Psychosocial stress: Perspectives on structure, theory, life course, and methods* (pp. 141–174). San Diego: Academic Press.

Burke, P. J., & Harrod, M. M. (2005). Too much of a good thing? *Social Psychology Quarterly, 68,* 359–374.

Cahill, S. E., & Eggleston, R. (1994). Managing emotions in public: The case of wheelchair users. *Social Psychology Quarterly, 57,* 300–312.

Charmaz, K., & Milligan, M. J. (2006). Grief. In J. E. Stets & J. H. Turner (Eds.), *Handbook of the sociology of emotions* (pp. 516–543). New York: Springer.

Clark, C. (1997). *Misery and company: Sympathy in everyday life.* Chicago: University of Chicago Press.

Collins, R. (2004). *Interaction rituals.* Princeton, NJ: Princeton University Press.

Cooley, C. H. (1964). *Human nature and the social order.* New York: Schocken Books. (Original work published 1902)

Durkheim, E. (1965). *The elementary forms of the religious life.* New York: Free Press. (Original work published 1912)

Ellestad, J., & Stets, J. E. (1998). Jealousy and parenting: Predicting emotions from identity theory. *Sociological Perspectives, 41,* 639–668.

Emerson, R. M. (1962). Power–dependence relations. *American Sociological Review, 27,* 31–40.

Franks, D. (2006). The neuroscience of emotions. In J. E. Stets & J. H. Turner (Eds.), *Handbook of the sociology of emotions* (pp. 38–62). New York: Springer.

Goffman, E. (1967). *Interaction ritual: Essays on face-to-face behavior.* Garden City, NY: Anchor Books.

Gordon, S. L. (1981). The sociology of sentiments and emotion. In M. Rosenberg & R. H. Turner (Eds.), *Social psychology: Sociological perspectives* (pp. 562–592). New York: Basic Books.

Gross, J. J., Richards, J. M., & John, O. P. (2006). Emotional regulation in everyday life. In D. K. Snyder, J. A. Simpson, & J. N. Hughes (Eds.), *Emotion regulation in couples and families: Pathways to dysfunction and health* (pp. 13–35). Washington, DC: American Psychological Association.

Hegtvedt, K. A. (1990). The effects of relationship structure on emotional responses to inequity. *Social Psychology Quarterly, 53,* 214–228.

Hegtvedt, K. A., & Killian, C. (1999). Fairness and emotions: Reactions to the process and outcomes of negotiations. *Social Forces, 78,* 269–303.

Heise, D. R. (1979). *Understanding events: Affect and the construction of social action.* Cambridge, UK: Cambridge University Press.

Heise, D. R., & Weir, B. (1999). A test of symbolic interactionist predictions about emotions in imagined situations. *Symbolic Interaction, 22,* 139–161.

Hektner, J. M., Schmidt, J. A., & Csikszentmihalyi, M. (2007). *Experience sampling method: Measuring the quality of everyday life.* Thousand Oaks, CA: Sage.

Hochschild, A. R. (1979). Emotion work, feeling rules, and social structure. *American Journal of Sociology, 85,* 551–575.

Hochschild, A. R. (1983). *The managed heart: Commercialization of human feeling.* Berkeley: University of California Press.

Houser, J. A., & Lovaglia, M. J. (2002). Status, emotion, and the development of solidarity in stratified task groups. *Advances in Group Processes, 19,* 109–137.

Jasso, G. (2006). Emotion in justice processes. In J. E. Stets & J. H. Turner (Eds.), *Handbook of the sociology of emotions* (pp. 321–346). New York: Springer.

Kemper, T. D. (1978). *A social interactional theory of emotions.* New York: Wiley.

Kemper, T. D. (1987). How many emotions are there?: Wedding the social and autonomic components. *American Journal of Sociology, 93,* 263–289.

Kemper, T. D. (1991). Predicting emotions from social relations. *Social Psychology Quarterly, 54,* 330–342.

Kemper, T. D. (2006). Power and status and the power-status theory of emotions. In J. E. Stets & J. H. Turner (Eds.), *Handbook of the sociology of emotions* (pp. 87–113). New York: Springer.

Kemper, T. D., & Collins, R. (1990). Dimensions of microinteraction. *American Journal of Sociology, 96,* 32–68.

Kollock, P. (1994). The emergence of exchange structures: An experimental study of uncertainty, commitment, and trust. *American Journal of Sociology, 100,* 313–345.

Lawler, E. J. (2001). An affect theory of social exchange. *American Journal of Sociology, 107,* 321–352.

Lawler, E. J., & Yoon, J. (1996). Commitment in exchange relations: A test of a theory of relational cohesion. *American Sociological Review, 61,* 89–108.

Lawler, E. J., & Yoon, J. (1998). Network structure and emotion in exchange relations. *American Sociological Review, 63,* 871–894.

Lewis, H. B. (1971). *Shame and guilt in neurosis.* New York: International Universities Press.

Lovaglia, M. J., & Houser, J. A. (1996). Emotional reactions and status in groups. *American Sociological Review, 61,* 867–883.

Marx, K. (1990). *Capital.* New York: Penguin. (Original work published 1867)

McCall, G. J., & Simmons, J. L. (1978). *Identities and interactions.* New York: Free Press.

Mead, G. H. (1934). *Mind, self, and society.* Chicago: University of Chicago Press.

Molm, L. D. (1997). *Coercive power in exchange.* Cambridge, UK: Cambridge University Press.

Peterson, G. (2006). Cultural theory and emotions. In J. E. Stets & J. H. Turner (Eds.), *Handbook of the sociology of emotions* (pp. 114–134). New York: Springer.

Pierce, J. L. (1995). *Gender trials: Emotional lives in contemporary law firms.* Berkeley: University of California Press.

Pollak, L. H., & Thoits, P. A. (1989). Processes in emotional socialization. *Social Psychology Quarterly, 52,* 22–34.

Ridgeway, C. L. (1994). Affect. In M. Foschi & E. J. Lawler (Eds.), *Group processes: Sociological analyses* (pp. 205–230). Chicago: Nelson-Hall.

Ridgeway, C. L. (2006). Expectation states theory and emotions. In J. E. Stets & J. H. Turner (Eds.), *Handbook of the sociology of emotions* (pp. 347–367). New York: Springer.

Ridgeway, C. L., & Johnson, C. (1990). What is the relationship between socioemotional behavior and status in task groups? *American Journal of Sociology, 95,* 1189–1212.

Robinson, D. T., Smith-Lovin, L., & Tsoudis, O. (1994). Heinous crime or unfortunate accident?: The effects of remorse on responses to mock criminal confessions. *Social Forces, 73,* 175–190.

Robinson, D. T., Smith-Lovin, L., & Wisecup, A. K. (2006). Affect control theory. In J. E. Stets & J. H. Turner (Eds.), *Handbook of the sociology of emotions* (pp. 179–202). New York: Springer.

Rosenberg, M. (1990). Reflexivity and emotions. *Social Psychology Quarterly, 53,* 3–12.

Scheff, T. J. (1988). Shame and conformity: The deference–emotion system. *American Sociological Review, 53,* 395–406.

Scheff, T. J. (1990). Socialization of emotion: Pride and shame as causal agents. In T. D. Kemper (Ed.), *Research agendas in the sociology of emotions* (pp. 281–304). Albany: State University of New York Press.

Scheff, T. J. (1994). *Bloody revenge: Emotions, nationalism, and war.* Boulder, CO: Westview Press.

Scheff, T. J., & Retzinger, S. M. (1991). *Emotions and violence: Shame and rage in destructive conflicts.* Lexington, MA: Lexington Books.

Scherer, K. R., Wallbott, H. G., & Summerfield, A. B. (Eds.). (1986). *Experiencing emotion: A cross-cultural study.* Cambridge, UK: Cambridge University Press.

Schmitt, C. S., & Clark, C. (2006). Sympathy. In J. E. Stets & J. H. Turner (Eds.), *Handbook of the sociology of emotions* (pp. 467–492). New York: Springer.

Sennett, R., & Cobb, J. (1972). *The hidden injuries of class.* New York: Knopf.

Smith, A. C., & Kleinman, S. (1989). Managing emotions in medical school: Students' contacts with the living and the dead. *Social Psychology Quarterly, 52,* 56–69.

Stets, J. E. (2003). Justice, emotion, and identity theory. In P. J. Burke, T. J. Owens, R. T. Serpe, & P. A. Thoits (Eds.), *Advances in identity theory and research* (pp. 105–122). New York: Kluwer Academic/Plenum.

Stets, J. E. (2005). Examining emotions in identity theory. *Social Psychology Quarterly, 68,* 39–56.

Stets, J. E. (2006). Identity theory and emotions. In J. E. Stets & J. H. Turner (Eds.), *Handbook of the sociology of emotions* (pp. 203–223). New York: Springer.

Stets, J. E., & Tsushima, T. (2001). Negative emotion and coping responses within identity control theory. *Social Psychology Quarterly, 64,* 283–295.

Stets, J. E., & Turner, J. H. (Eds.). (2006). *Handbook of the sociology of emotions.* New York: Springer.

Stryker, S. (2002). *Symbolic interactionism: A social structural version.* Caldwell, NJ: Blackburn Press. (Original work published 1980)

Stryker, S. (2004). Integrating emotion into identity theory. *Advances in Group Processes, 21,* 1–23.

Summers-Effler, E. (2004a). *Radical saints and reformer heroes: Culture, interaction, and emotional intensity in altruistic social movement organizations.* Unpublished doctoral dissertation, University of Pennsylvania.

Summers-Effler, E. (2004b). A theory of the self, emotion, and culture. *Advances in Group Processes, 21,* 273–308.

Summers-Effler, E. (2004c). Defensive strategies: The formation and social interactions of patterned self-destructive behavior. *Advances in Group Processes, 21,* 309–325.

Summers-Effler, E. (2006). Ritual theory. In J. E. Stets & J. H. Turner (Eds.), *Handbook of the sociology of emotions* (pp. 135–154). New York: Springer.

Swann, W. B., Jr., Rentfrow, P. J., & Guinn, J. S. (2003). Self-verification: The search for coherence. In M. R. Leary & J. P. Tangney (Eds.), *Handbook of self and identity* (pp. 367–383). New York: Guilford Press.

Tangney, J. P., & Dearing, R. L. (2002). *Shame and guilt.* New York: Guilford Press.

Thamm, R. A. (2006). The classification of emotions. In J. E. Stets & J. H. Turner (Eds.), *Handbook of the sociology of emotions* (pp. 11–37). New York: Springer.

Thoits, P. A. (1990). Emotional deviance: Research agendas. In T. D. Kemper (Ed.), *Research agendas in the sociology of emotions* (pp. 180–203). Albany: State University of New York Press.

Thye, S. R., Yoon, J., & Lawler, E. J. (2002). The theory of relational cohesion: Review of a research program. *Advances in Group Processes, 19,* 139–166.

Turner, J. H. (1999). Toward a general sociological theory of emotions. *Journal for the Theory of Social Behavior, 29,* 132–162.

Turner, J. H. (2000). *On the origins of human emotions: A sociological inquiry into the evolution of human affect.* Stanford, CA: Stanford University Press.

Turner, J. H. (2002). *Face-to-face: Towards a sociological theory of interpersonal behavior.* Stanford, CA: Stanford University Press.

Turner, J. H. (2006). Psychoanalytic sociological theories and emotions. In J. E. Stets & J. H. Turner (Eds.), *Handbook of the sociology of emotions* (pp. 276–294). New York: Springer.

Turner, J. H., & Stets, J. E. (2005). *The sociology of emotions.* New York: Cambridge University Press.

CHAPTER 4

The Affective Brain and Core Consciousness
How Does Neural Activity Generate Emotional Feelings?

JAAK PANKSEPP

Joy & Woe are woven fine,
A Clothing for the Soul divine;
Under every grief & pine
Runs a joy with silken twine.
—WILLIAM BLAKE,
"Auguries of Innocence"

How does neural activity create affective experience? How feelings are created may be the most important question in basic emotion research; although it has barely been addressed empirically, it is the source of heated philosophical and psychological debate. Without affect, we might not feel alive. Without positive affect, there are few reasons for living, and people in depressive despair often choose death over life. Without affect, there is neither fun nor pain. Affect is the source of all intimacy—the profound interpersonal giving of oneself exhibited by people who are in love with life and others. Affect encourages people to dig deeply into their biological "souls"—to find empathy, to communicate their major concerns sincerely, and to hope that their depth of feeling is reciprocated.

Without affect, we humans would have little to talk about and no special reason to reach out to others. Affect motivates our urge to play and to speak: When one of the highest brain regions that encodes sadness, grief, and social bonding, the anterior cingulate, is damaged, people fall into akinetic mutism. Such unfortunates retain the physical capacity to speak, but they have no urge or wish to communicate (Devinsky, Morrell, & Vogt, 1995).

Although affect and cognition are completely blended in mature psychological experience, brain research and great art provide unique ways to distinguish cognition from primary-process affect. All artistic creations require great cognitive skills, but works that do not stir our affects communicate little. In art as in life, affect motivates cognitive flow much as flames (now batteries) allow torches to illuminate the darkness. But we must differentiate neuroscientifically between cognition and affect, since they reflect substantially different, albeit interactive, aspects of brain organization (Ciompi & Panksepp, 2004; Panksepp, 2003b). Cognition involves the neocortical processing of information gleaned largely from environmental inputs via exteroceptive senses. Affects are not encoded as information. They are diffuse global *states* generated by deep subcortical brain structures, interacting with primitive viscerosomatic body (core self) representations that remain poorly mapped (Panksepp, 1998a, 1998b). There is presently more scientific work on the cognitive aspects than on the affective nature of emotions, even though, down through history, various scholars have noted that cognitions are handmaidens to the passions. Cognitions also resolve raw affects into higher emotions.

Many questions about emotions remain empirically unanswered, but also some remain largely unasked in this modern era, as psychology remains timid of engaging with the power and importance of cross-species neuroscience (Panksepp, 2005b, 2007a). The manner in which the brain generates emotional feelings is the biggest of them all. Frijda states in Chapter 5 of this volume: "As far as I know . . . there exist no detailed hypotheses at the functional level of how innate affective stimuli evoke affect" (p. 84). How then might we understand affects in a way that is scientifically credible? Presumably through psychologically guided brain research.

TOWARD A TAXONOMY AND NEUROBIOLOGY OF AFFECTS

Affects fill the mind with a large variety of desirable and undesirable experienced states that are hard to define objectively or to talk about clearly. Partly this is because raw affects are pre-propositional forms of consciousness comprising brain and bodily processes of kaleidoscopic complexity. But there seem to be several distinct types. Some accompany major bodily disturbances (e.g., pain and fatigue); some reflect sensory pleasures and displeasures (ranging from tasty delights to disgust); still others gauge bodily need states (e.g., hunger and thirst); and perhaps most mysteriously, certain intrinsic brain–body arousal states are strongly valenced—the emotional affects.

We do not yet agree upon a generally accepted taxonomy of primary-process affects,[1] but the preceding description contains at least three distinct types: (1) sensory affects, (2) bodily-homeostatic ones, and (3) brain emotional ones. Each is initially expressed at primary-process levels, but during development they come to include learned object relations (secondary-process affects) and get linked to thoughts and other cognitive activities (tertiary-process affects). Until some international congress cobbles together an agreement, there are bound to be conceptual disagreements concerning where certain entities belong. For instance, in a recent commentary I have argued that disgust should not be considered a primary-process *emotion*; it fits better in other categories, and only through learning might it be deemed a secondary- or tertiary-process emotion (see Panksepp, 2007a, discussing Toronchuk & Ellis, 2007b). In other words, when the affective power of primary *sensory* or *homeostatic* disgust/nausea is cognitively resymbolized, social disgust may emerge as a socially constructed emotion.

The basic emotional affects are primary brain/mind processes, similar to seeing a color. One can use a word, like "red," as a label for a color, but this word does not explain the experience of seeing red. If someone is blind, the word "red" is meaningless. In order to explain seeing red, one must discover the neurophysiological and neurochemical causes of visual experience. Similarly, one cannot use words to *explain* primary-process raw emotions. Words can only be used as second-order symbols to discuss affective experiences, but they do not adequately capture the fundamental causes of feelings. Like first-order sensory experiences, primary-process affects are best understood if we clarify the attending brain functions. Thus neural criteria are needed to define core emotional processes, as summarized in Figure 4.1 (adapted from Panksepp, 1998a).

The aim of this chapter is to address how subjectively experienced emotional feelings may arise from the activities of neural circuits. As we begin to understand the neurology of affect, we can avoid the circularity that usually attends verbal descriptions of basic processes. If we understand the neurology of affect, we are beginning to define primary-process experiential concepts, even when dealing with nonhu-

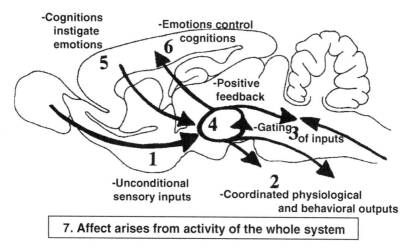

FIGURE 4.1. Proposed neural definition of an emotional system. These seven neural interactions are postulated to be characteristics of all major primary-process emotional systems of the brain. (1) A few sensory stimuli can unconditionally access emotional systems, but most inputs are developmentally learned. (2) Emotional systems can promote coherent instinctual action outputs, as well as (3) modulate sensory inputs. (4) Emotional systems have positive-feedback components that can sustain emotional arousal after precipitating events have passed. Also, (5) these systems can be modulated by cognitive inputs and (6) can modify and channel cognitive activities. The important criterion that emotional systems create affective states is not included, but it is assumed that arousal of the whole executive circuitry for each emotion is essential for elaborating emotional feelings within the brain, perhaps by interacting with other subneocortical brain circuits for organismic visceral self-representation. Adapted from Panksepp (1998a). Copyright 1998 by Oxford University Press. Adapted by permission.

man species that have homologous brain systems (Panksepp, 1982, 1998a). When such basic phenomenal experiences are defined in terms of brain "mechanisms," we can use affective concepts noncircularly in our explanatory endeavors—something we cannot do *scientifically* as long as affects are defined only verbally.

EVIDENCE FOR EMOTIONAL AFFECTS IN OTHER ANIMALS

There is substantial experimental evidence to indicate that other mammals are affective creatures. Probably all vertebrates that exhibit strong instinctual emotional behaviors experience affects (Panksepp, 1990a, 2005b, 2007c). The issue of affects among invertebrates remains a more open question, but preliminary evidence for evaluative processes exists for a few species (Panksepp & Huber, 2004).

What is the best neural evidence for affect? First, one can elicit powerful emotional responses by localized electrical stimulations of specific neural systems (LESSNS). Indeed,

across all mammalian species, specific subcortical brain regions are where LESSNS can evoke the most powerful emotional reactions (Hess, 1957). Second, these subcortical structures are homologous throughout the mammalian kingdom. So if one stimulates FEAR[2] circuits in rats, cats, or primates, all exhibit similar fear responses with differences in species-typical details (Panksepp, 1990a). Third, comparably localized stimulations of the human brain yield congruent affective experiences—felt emotional arousals that typically appear without reason (Heath, 1996). Fourth, human beings report basic emotional feelings that are commensurate with animal emotional behaviors (Panksepp, 1985); this, along with the accruing evidence that both the feeling and behavioral responses emanate from homologous areas of the brain, strongly suggests that other animals also experience primary-process emotions, even though they obviously cannot talk about them. Fifth, by all measures imaginable, one can demonstrate that animals like and dislike stimulation of brain regions that evoke instinctual emotional behaviors (Panksepp, 1998a, 2005a). Their affective preferences are well indexed by conditioned place preferences and place aversions, as well as by the tendency to voluntarily turn LESSNS on and off. Sixth, basic instinctual emotional urges, even ones as complex as social play, remain intact after radical neodecortication early in life (Panksepp, Normansell, Cox, & Siviy, 1994); thus the neocortex is not essential for the generation of primary-process emotionality.

Abundant evidence now supports the medial subneocortical locus of control for instinctual emotional behaviors that are accompanied by raw affective experiences in all mammals that have been studied with LESSNS. Modern brain imaging of self-referential processes in humans (including affective ownership) also highlights higher medial limbic regions of the brain (Northoff, Heinzel, de Greck, Bermpohl, & Panksepp, 2006), long implicated in the regulation of emotional feelings in humans (MacLean, 1990). Thus the weight of evidence indicates not only that all other mammals have affective lives, but also that their basic emotions are homologous across mammalian species. Many still disagree, but this debate typically continues, because discussants fail to consider all the evidence and fear even evolutionarily justified anthropomorphism. Concerned scientists need to situate themselves in a truth diagram (see Figure 4.2) based on their reading of the evidence (e.g., Panksepp, 2005a), as opposed to clinging to belief systems passed down through generations. I encourage cultivation of the upper left quadrant, which is more empirically defensible than situating oneself in the traditionally mandated lower right quadrant.

FROM LOGICAL POSITIVISM TO MODERN REDUCTIONISM: THE SCIENTIFIC DEATH OF AFFECT IN BEHAVIORAL NEUROSCIENCE

In spite of robust evidence, many behavioral neuroscientists do not acknowledge the affective lives of other animals. This bias has deep roots in Judeo-Christian and other dualistic philosophies, as well as in the 19th-century battle between vitalism and materialism. Vitalism, a prevailing mode of thought prior to the middle of the 19th century, postulated nonmaterial "vital principles"—life forces such as *élan vital*. Such beliefs had long prevented powerful materialistic scientific modes of thought from gaining the influence they deserved. In particular, physiologists who sought to study the body as a biophysical entity, and to base the medical curriculum on solid anatomy, physiology, and biochemistry, wished to discard spooky "life forces" from their science. Descendants of these wise revolutionaries eventually decided to dualistically conflate emotional feelings with other nonmaterial "life forces," and the neuroaffective baby was tossed out with the vitalistic bathwater. In fact, affects are thoroughly biological.

The transition to hard-core materialism was effected when influential continental scientists joined forces to form what is now called the Berlin Biophysics Club, led by "heavy hitters" such as Carl Ludwig (1816–1895), Emil du Bois-Reymond (1818–1896), Hermann von Helmholtz (1821–1894), and Ernst Brücke (1819–1892). These scholars erased nonobjective entities from the landscape of physiology and medicine (see Greenspan & Baars, 2005).

	The True Nature of the World	
Our Judgments about the World	Animals Experience Emotional Feelings	Animals Have No Emotional Feelings
Animals Experience Emotional Feelings	Valid Anthropomorphism	Type I Error
Animals Have No Emotional Feelings	Type II Error	Valid Anthropodenial

FIGURE 4.2. Truth diagram concerning the validity of anthropomorphism in the study of emotional feelings in animals. Perhaps the appropriate project for the 20th century was to avoid Type I errors. With the advent of neuroscience, and our search for the actual mechanisms of emotional feelings, we should be equally careful to avoid Type II errors. The weight of evidence currently indicates that the quadrant that is most concordant with research evidence is the upper left quadrant. Surprisingly, most behavioral neuroscientists seem happy to reside in the lower right quadrant, as they were trained as students.

They succeeded in establishing a rigorous medical curriculum on a solid scientific base. Their victory led to an evidence-based medicine that remains the foundation of modern medical education. Members of this coterie were not concerned with emotional matters, but some of their followers were. Pavlov studied under Ludwig, and Freud under Brücke. Pavlov never marginalized affect in his studies of autonomic reflexes in dogs, and even discovered neurotic behaviors in his animals after Neva River floods destroyed his lab. Freud eventually developed an emotion-based "metapsychology," but psychoanalysis eventually lacked the hard stamp of science that exists when one is concerned with the evolved mechanisms of the brain.

Our current, lingering problems arose when excessive antivitalistic forces spilled over into experimental psychology, where mental constructs were eventually deemed too spooky to be accepted as scientific. The physiologist Jacques Loeb, a peripheral member of the Berlin Biophysics movement, brought antimentalistic biases to the United States. At the University of Chicago, he enthralled John B. Watson, the eventual "father of behaviorism." At Harvard, B. F. Skinner came under the spell of another Loeb protégé, William Crozier. Together, Watson and Skinner inaugurated a methodologically rigorous, and eventually doctrinaire, radical behaviorism. As they brought a new level of sophistication to the environmentally controlled analysis of learning, they actively discouraged instinct- and brain-based psychologies. Through their influence, radical behaviorism, with no room for emotionality, became the focus of inquiry.

Watson (1919) was initially interested in emotions. Skinner (1953) famously claimed "The 'emotions' are excellent examples of the fictional causes to which we commonly attribute behavior" (p. 160). Their important contributions to methodologically rigorous behavioral analysis resulted in narrow, nonaffective views of animal behavior (Panksepp, 1990b). As they marginalized instincts (inbuilt tools for behaving and feeling) in preference to learning, they impoverished our understanding of the evolved emotional and motivational underpinnings of mind.

Watson and Skinner's radical "black box" of behaviorism overwhelmed academic psychology until the 1970s, whereupon an oversimplified computer-inspired mentality—information processing that could be rigorously monitored by reaction times and other objective measures—moved to center stage as cognitive science. This transition did not happen in animal research, where behaviorism continued to rule. In the 1970s dramatic shifts in funding (partly resulting from Vietnam War expenditures) coaxed many American behaviorists to become neuroscientists, with little interest in emotional processes that control animal behavior.

To this day, neurobehaviorists are generally unwilling to discuss affective processes within animal brains. This inhibits linkages between biological psychiatry and neuroscientific psychology. Most behavioral neuroscientists consider it unrealistic to consider that affective feelings actually exist in animal brains; thus they position themselves in the lower right quadrant of Figure 4.2. Most subscribe to ruthless neural reductionism, where psychological processes play no role in the control of behavior.

In this context, it is noteworthy that the first "law" of behavior—Thorndike's (1911) "law of effect"—envisioned how "satisfying" and "annoying" events could mediate learning. These affective concepts were eventually transformed by behaviorists into "positive reinforcements" and "punishments," more by self-appointed decisions than through evidence-based discussions. Thus the diverse affective aspects of the "law of effect" were discarded because they raised the specter of scientifically unobservable internal processes—apparent nonmaterial principles—within the brain.

Now that we can link affects to observable brain events (Berridge, 2000; Panksepp, 1998a, 2005a; Peciña, Smith, & Berridge, 2006), we must reconsider that a "law of affect" does control behavior: Animals do seek brain/mind affective comfort zones and avoid discomforts. Such visions of animal minds could nourish the current affective revolution in human psychology. Primary brain/mind processes can only be well studied in animal models. Indeed, the *process* of "reinforcement" may arise from fluctuations of affective states. Reinforcers may only be potent to the degree to which they arouse or diminish affective processes (Panksepp, 2005b).

Modern cognitive science has become fascinated, even enchanted, with the topic of affects, and some researchers recognize that such processes are prereflective (Lambie & Marcel,

2002). Some social constructivists are beginning to postulate that raw positive and negative affect may be birthrights of the human brain (Barrett, 2006; Russell, 2003). Despite this turn toward nativism, they rarely consider the possibility that many positive and negative affective birthrights exist in mammalian brains (Panksepp, in press-b).

Thus cognitive scientists have difficulty generating realistic psychobiological hypotheses of how emotional feelings arise from brain networks, above and beyond highlighting brain regions revealed by modern brain imaging—which are correlative, not causal, approaches (Panksepp, 2007c). The potentially misleading use of correlative data to generate causal conclusions also remains common in behavioral neuroscience. For instance, recording of activity from brain dopamine neurons (namely, listening to what these cells are listening to) has been used to generate causal "reward error prediction"/teaching-signal hypotheses for what dopamine neurons do in the brain (Schultz, 2006). In fact, such neurophysiological studies tell us much about what dopamine neurons are listening to, but little about what dopamine release is doing upstream within the brain. Abundant evidence that dopamine arousal of brain "reward" circuits actually promote affective SEEKING urges, based on many causal experiments (Alcaro, Huber, & Panksepp, 2007; Ikemoto & Panksepp, 1999; Panksepp, 1998a), is commonly ignored—because such views imply that neuroaffective processes lie at the heart of animal foraging behaviors.

A "dual-aspect monism" approach suggests that certain complex neurodynamics create emotional feelings. Accordingly, instinctual behaviors may provide public evidence for internal affective states.[3] This yields many testable neurochemical hypotheses, derived from animal research, for the underpinning of primary-process emotional feelings in humans (Panksepp, 1999; Panksepp & Harro, 2004).

THE ABC's OF AFFECT: AFFECTIVE, BEHAVIORAL, AND COGNITIVE NEUROSCIENCE VIEWS OF AFFECTIVE CONTROL

Many modern brain researchers (e.g., Berridge & Robinson, 2003; Craig, 2003; Damasio, 2003; Dolan, 2002) have asserted that human

beings experience affects, whereas animals display only emotional behaviors. They suggest various "readout" hypotheses of how higher brain functions in humans create emotional feelings from presumably unconscious emotional processes of animal brains.

There currently exist three major neurally based schools of thought regarding how affective experience emerges from neural activities. First, an ultrareductionistic *behavioral neuroscience* view denies that affective capacities exist as inherent aspects of mammalian life; such scholars exhibit little tolerance for discussions of affective control in the governance of animal behaviors. Affects, if they exist, are assumed to be epiphenomenal aspects of higher cognitive activities in human brains. In contrast, *cognitive neuroscience* envisions affects as inherently coupled to higher human cognitive functions; hence other animals, because of their comparatively modest cognitive abilities, may not be capable of experiencing affects. Along with neurobehaviorists, cognitive neuroscientists often assert that the emotional behaviors of other animals are unconscious. Finally, *affective neuroscience* proposes that affects emanate from deep subcortical structures found in the brains of all mammals. Let us consider these views in more detail.

The Behavioral Neuroscience View

Just as traditional black-box behaviorism marginalized the study of feelings, for neurobehaviorists affects remain scientific nonstarters, because they cannot be *directly* monitored with objective neurophysiological measures. Also, animals cannot provide verbal feedback about their feelings. The worrisome fact that most aspects of nature are as invisible to direct observation as subatomic particles has not convinced behaviorists to utilize indirect measures. Still, two behavioral neuroscientists, Gray and Rolls, have envisioned how emotional feelings are created by reinforcement contingencies.

I have critiqued Gray's (1990) debatable assertion that emotional feelings are created, rather than just triggered, by reinforcement contingencies; alternatively, I have suggested that the *process* of reinforcement is mediated by affective change within the brain (Panksepp, 1990c). Rolls (2005) has further advanced a position similar to Gray's, suggesting that reinforcement is a more fundamental neurobiological construct than emotional feelings. Rolls proposes that our human affective experience emerges from the capacity of our cognitive cortex to re-represent various unconscious processes, shared by animals, in linguistic terms. It is merely a concept, not a process. This makes affect phlogiston-like in our attempts to understand animal behavior.

The Cognitive Neuroscience View

Damasio (1994, 1999), and LeDoux (1996) have offered two well-resolved cognitive neuroscience views. Damasio discovered that cognitive decision making is impaired when the affective structures of orbito-frontal cortex are damaged. LeDoux helped refine our understanding of how classical conditioning of fear is elaborated within the amygdala. Both propose modernized James–Lange "cortical readout" views of affective experience.

Damasio's "somatic marker" hypothesis, although neuroscientifically more sophisticated than the classic James–Lange view, essentially envisions affect as the emotional turmoil of bodily states within the somatosensory representation areas of the neocortex. As originally highlighted by MacLean (1990), most investigators, including Damasio, are recognizing the importance of insular cortex in the genesis of various affective experiences, ranging from disgust (Toronchuk & Ellis, 2007) to nicotine craving (Naqvi, Rudrauf, Damasio, & Bechara, 2007).

Damasio's superb neuroimaging of the primal affective states of anger, fear, sadness, and joy (Damasio et al., 2000) has led him to incorporate animalian subcortical emotional systems as contributors to emotional behaviors (Damasio, 1999), but not, apparently, to emotional feelings; he repeatedly states that animals exhibit emotional behaviors, while humans have emotional feelings (Damasio, 2003; critiqued by Panksepp, 2003a). Few cognitivists believe that subneocortical systems can generate affective mentality on their own, but only the physiological and behavioral emotional turmoil that gets translated into psychological experience by the higher brain systems mediating reflective awareness. This view does not seem to distinguish adequately between raw phenomenal experience and reflective awareness, and, like the behavioral neuroscience view, it envisions feelings as arising from cognitive *readout* of the unconscious emotional commotions of the body. Such views discour-

age effective utilization of abundant animal data on the functions of subcortical emotional systems for understanding primary-process homeostatic and emotional affects in humans (Denton, 2006; Panksepp, 2003b, 2003c).

Some investigators also make the assumption that emotional experience is irrelevant for understanding animal emotions. For instance, LeDoux (1996) has suggested that human emotional feelings arise when subcortical information about emotional bodily changes reaches higher working memory and cognitive consciousness generators in the dorsolateral frontal cortex.

Compounding misplaced confidence in modern cortical readout theories of emotions are the prevailing claims about the overriding importance of the amygdala in emotional feelings. The central nuclei of amygdala are clearly part of the unconditional FEAR circuit (Panksepp, 1991), but their capacity to promote fearful feelings probably relies on intact hypothalamic and midbrain FEAR circuitry (Panksepp, 1998a, Fig. 10.4).

The Affective Neuroscience View

Abundant animal emotion research indicates that emotional feelings arise from long swaths of subcortical tissues that control visceral processes, long known as the "limbic system." The emotional–visceral brain extends from medial frontal regions throughout the core of midbrain, and all brain areas in between. Evidence for medial subcortical emotional behavioral circuits in the generation of emotional feelings remains robust for humans (Heath, 1996; Panksepp, 1985) and other animals (Panksepp, 1998a, 2005a). To the best of our knowledge, raw emotional feelings arise from ancient prepropositional subneocortical substrates that are homologous in all mammals. If so, animal brain research becomes a critically important strategy for deriving detailed causal knowledge about the *major* sources of the emotional affects within the human brain. The major representatives of this school of thought are MacLean (1990) and myself (Panksepp, 1982, 1998a).

Denton (2006) has also highlighted how the basic motivations, such as thirst, air, hunger, and various other needs of the body, are represented deep in the brain. Even though he calls such homeostatic feelings "emotions" (perhaps a category error), clearly these affective states correspond to arousals of the primitive brain areas that animal research has revealed as critically important for generating the instinctual behaviors associated with those bodily *drives*—a principle central to the affective neuroscience view of basic feelings (Panksepp, 1998a). If one images brain arousals during intense affective feelings such as orgasms (Holstege et al., 2003a), as well as feelings like anger, sadness, and fear (Damasio et al., 2000), animalian subcortical circuits light up. If anything, higher neocortical systems exhibit diminished arousal (Liotti & Panksepp, 2004; Panksepp, 2003b).

As already noted, we can evoke a variety of specific instinctual emotional action tendencies by activating very specific brain regions in all mammals. Animals clearly enjoy some of these types of stimulation and dislike others. Comparable LESSNS of human brains yield commensurate affective experiences that people can verbalize. Also, decorticate animals display the same basic emotions as neurologically intact animals (Kolb & Tees, 2000), even ones as complex as play (Panksepp et al., 1994). Comparable evidence is available for human children (Shewmon, Holmse, & Byrne, 1999).

Solid evidence exists for at least seven basic emotional operating systems in mammalian brains (Panksepp, 1998a, 2005a). There is insufficient space to cover all these systems here, so I discuss two of special importance for social neuroscience—PANICky separation distress and PLAYful joy. These systems had not received neuroscientific attention before our work in the 1970s.

THE BRAIN SUBSTRATES OF SADNESS AND PANIC

Our research into the nature of separation distress was initiated in 1972 when the first neurotransmitter receptor, for brain opioids, was discovered. We suspected that separation distress had evolved from ancient pain mechanisms of the brain, and thus evaluated whether brain opioids mediate social bonding. We predicted that endogenous opioids released during positive social interactions would facilitate social bonding by alleviating psychic pain in the same way that exogenous opiates can reduce physical pain. This idea provided an evolutionary rationale for why opiates are habit-forming: Social bonding is a naturally addictive process. Social attachments and addictive de-

pendencies share three key attributes: (1) an initial intense positive affect ("loving") phase, followed by (2) a tolerance phase with diminished positive feelings, which sets up (3) a powerful separation distress phase of opiate withdrawal in drug addiction and physiologies of grief following social loss (Panksepp, 1998a, Fig. 13.5). Such hypotheses have been extended to other high-incentive rewards, including food treats (Colantuoni et al., 2002).

Such causal relations between drug addictions and social rewards clarify why lonely, disenfranchised individuals are powerfully attracted to opiate drugs. Addicts commonly lack enough positive human contact to sustain happiness and satisfaction, and opiate intake is partly self-medication (Khantzian, 2003 with five commentaries). Indeed, the pleasure of touch is partly opioid-mediated (Keverne, Nevison, & Martel, 1997; Panksepp, Bean, Bishop, Vilberg, & Sahley, 1980; Panksepp & Bishop, 1981; Roth & Sullivan, 2006).

The social implications of such ideas are far-reaching. Why waste money putting more and more people in jails and fighting perpetual wars on drugs, rather than seeking to build social structures that support human connections?

Now we know that the affective qualities of early social bonds leave lasting marks on human and animal development (Champagne, Francis, Mar, & Meaney, 2003; Meaney, 2001; Panksepp, 2001). Early attachment failures promote depression (Heim & Nemeroff, 1999), and opiates can exert strong antidepressant effects. Indeed, relatively nonaddictive opiates such as buprenorphine are excellent antidepressants (Bodkin, Zornberg, Lukas, & Cole, 1995).

When we initiated this work, discrete brain systems for social affect were not being entertained in neuroscience, although behavioral evidence had long been suggestive (Bowlby, 1969). The prevailing behaviorist assumption was that social attachments arise indirectly from the learned association of social "objects" with primary rewards, especially nourishment and warmth. Our approach revealed the first lawful psychobiological relationship in social neuroscience—namely, that brain opioids regulate the intensity of separation distress. This effect was evident in puppies (Panksepp, Herman, Conner, Bishop, & Scott, 1978), young guinea pigs (Herman & Panksepp, 1978), chicks (Panksepp, Vilberg, Bean, Coy, & Kastin, 1978), and subsequently all other mammals tested. Hence human sadness and grief were envisioned in part as opioid withdrawal states—a proposition affirmed in humans a quarter of a century later (Zubieta et al., 2003).

Many others have confirmed and extended our animal findings (e.g., Kalin, Shelton, & Barksdale, 1988; Kehoe & Blass, 1986; Keverne et al., 1997; Moles, Kieffer, & D'Amato, 2004). It is now certain that social-emotional processes are regulated by opioid and oxytocinergic dynamics (Nelson & Panksepp, 1998), but in recent years the oxytocinergic extensions of the work to adult bonding have garnered more popular attention (Carter, Lederhendler, & Kirkpatrick, 1999; Insel, 2003; Young & Wang, 2004). Still, mother–infant attachments may be more closely related to dynamics of PANIC/separation distress and CARE/maternal-nurturance systems than any other primary social system, while those of older animals have strong contributions from LUST/sexuality and PLAY systems.

Accordingly, in early work we used localized LESSNS to map out the separation distress systems in guinea pigs and chicks (Bishop, 1984;

Herman, 1979). We were pleased that the trajectories of these systems were remarkably similar in these divergent species, as well as in primates (for summaries, see Newman, in press; Panksepp, Normansell, Herman, Bishop, & Crepeau, 1988). Functional brain imaging with positron emission tomography (PET) has highlighted these same brain regions during human sadness (Damasio et al., 2000; see Figure 4.3).

During our initial work, no other psychoactive drugs commonly used in psychiatry, except clonidine, had effects as robust as those of opioids (Rossi, Sahley, & Panksepp, 1983). Of the many other neuropeptides we evaluated across the years (a total of more than 30, each injected into brain ventricles, since neuropeptides do not penetrate the brain readily following peripheral administration), we found that only oxytocin and prolactin had equally robust calming effects. Conversely, other peptides, especially corticotropin-releasing factor (CRF) and the excitatory amino acid glutamate, could robustly promote separation calls (Panksepp, 1998a). Along the way we found how many other social behaviors, from simple

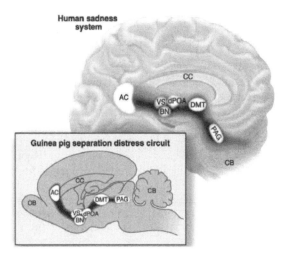

FIGURE 4.3. There are remarkable similarities between regions of the guinea pig brain where LESSNS provoke separation distress calls (data from Herman, 1979; Panksepp et al., 1988) and areas of the human brain that are activated during feelings of sadness (data from Damasio et al., 2000). Areas of subhuman mammalian brains where separation calls are evoked are the anterior cingulate (AC), the ventral septal (VS) and dorsal preoptic areas (dPOA), the bed nucleus of the stria terminalis (BN), the dorsomedial thalamus (DMT), and the periaqueductal central gray area of the brainstem (PAG). Both human sadness and separation distress are low-brain-opioid states (Panksepp, 1998a; Zubieta et al., 2003). The correspondence between the brain regions activated during human sadness and those activated during animal separation distress suggests that human feelings may arise from the instinctual emotional action systems of ancient regions of the mammalian brain. OB, olfactory bulb; CC, corpus callosum; CB, cerebellum. Adapted from Panksepp (2003c). Copyright 2003 by the Association for the Advancement of Science. Adapted by permission.

gregariousness to playfulness, are regulated by brain opioids, confirming and extending the opioid theory of social affect (Panksepp, Bean, Bishop, Vilbers, & Sahlberg, 1980; also see application to autism, Panksepp, Lensing, Leboyer, & Pouvard, 1991).

Although many details remain to be worked out, these animal findings have provided the first entry points for understanding the neurochemical and evolutionary bases of pro-social feelings in humans. When the PANIC (separation distress) system is quiescent, individuals experience a "secure emotional base" for their life activities. Other animal studies have indicated that high opioid tone makes animals more confident and dominant (Panksepp, Jalowiec, DeEskinazi, & Bishop, 1985), and oxytocin facilitates feelings of trust and social sensitivity (Kosfeld, Heinrichs, Zak, Fischbacher, & Fehr, 2005). It is important to note that some of the effects of oxytocin may be indirectly mediated by opioids, since oxytocin can strongly reduce accruing tolerance to endogenous opioids (Kovacs, Sarnyai, & Szabo, 1998). In contrast, diminished chemistries of bonding are expected to promote sadness, grief, and ultimately chronic feelings of emotional emptiness and depressive despair (Panksepp, Yates, Ikemoto, & Nelson, 1991). Indeed, depression may be rapidly reversed with nonaddictive opioids (Bodkin et al., 1995).

In summary, those areas of the brain where we can evoke separation calls with LESSNS (e.g., Herman & Panksepp, 1981; Panksepp et al., 1988) may contain emotional "command" circuitry that generates feelings of social loss in humans—from sadness to panic, depending on the intensity of arousal. Opioids, along with oxytocin and prolactin, are brain neurochemistries that powerfully promote feelings of confidence and the social comfort-enhancing effects of friendly companionship. However, because of habituation processes (perhaps reflecting decreased receptor sensitivity), such feelings may typically recede into the background of consciousness.

Only when there is a loss of an attachment "object" (a loved one) do feelings of emotional dependency reemerge as the separation distress/PANIC system becomes aroused, perhaps by rapidly escalating glutamatergic and CRF tone, along with diminished activity of neuropeptides that engender feelings of social comfort. Thus the power of companionate love to promote happy minds arises in part from these neurochemistries of social attachment.

THE BRAIN SUBSTRATES OF PLAYFUL JOY AND LAUGHTER

To gain a further understanding of positive social-emotional systems, we initiated a parallel research program on social play in the late 1970s. It provided the first working hypothesis of how social joy is created in the brain. When one asks young children what they like to do more than anything else, the universal reply is "To play!" This urge is widespread throughout the animal kingdom (Burghardt, 2005). Three decades of research on the nature of rough-and-tumble play in juvenile rats has clarified that PLAY urges arise from primary-process emotional systems of the mammalian brain. This PLAY system probably evolved in mammalian brains to help young animals learn about the social structures into which they are born, and to provide them with a host of experience-expectant social-emotional skills that, through the power of positive affect, allow them to become well-integrated members of their communities. We think that the implications for child rearing practices are profound (Panksepp, 2001; Sunderland, 2006).

The available evidence (see Panksepp, Siviy, & Normansell, 1984; Panksepp, 1998a; Pellis & Pellis, 1998; Siviy, 1998; Vanderschuren, Niesink, & Van Ree, 1997) indicates that rough-and-tumble play circuitry, like all primary-process emotional systems, is concentrated in subcortical regions of the brain (Panksepp et al., 1994), especially diencephalic regions. In particular, dorsomedial parafascicular regions of the thalamus are important for processing the somatosensory stimuli (Siviy & Panksepp, 1987). Within the hypothalamus, play-induced brain dopamine release (Panksepp, 1993) certainly facilitates the good feelings of play (Burgdorf & Panksepp, 2006). However, if one simply pushes this system pharmacologically into chronic overactivity, play invariably diminishes (Beatty, Dodge, Doge, Whike, & Panksepp, 1982). This may indicate that dopamine must operate in a state of dynamic, as opposed to static, facilitation in order for play to occur. Furthermore, play vocalizations in rats, 50-kHz ultrasonic chirps, are strongly controlled by brain dopamine (Burgdorf, Knutson, Panksepp, & Shippenberg, 2001; Burgdorf, wood, Kroes, Moskal, & Panksepp, in press).

Many other neurochemical modulators of play have been identified (Panksepp, Normansell, Cox, Crepeau, & Sacks, 1987; Vanderschuren et al., 1997), but nothing as clear-cut as the neuropeptides that regulate separation distress. Small doses of opiates can consistently elevate play (Panksepp, Jalowiec, et al., 1985). We have also obtained modest facilitations of play with peripheral injections of the nicotinic acetylcholine receptor antagonist mecamylamine (Panksepp et al., 1984) and with intracerebral neurotensin and thyrotropin release hormone (Panksepp, 1998). Developmentally, it is likely that access to play has positive effects, such as facilitating the construction of a fully social brain through the experience-dependent maturation of prosocial brain circuits, perhaps in part through the genetic activation of neuronal growth factors (Gordon, Burke, Akil, Watson, & Panksepp, 2003) and many other gene expressions (Kroes, Panksepp, Burgdorf, Otto, & Moskal, 2006).

We believe that the relative lack of real play among children of our culture has implications for understanding childhood problems such as attention-deficit/hyperactivity disorder, which are routinely treated with dopamine-promoting psychostimulants that may have long-term effects on brain maturation (Panksepp, 2001). Such drugs may sensitize the brain, thereby chronically amplifying SEEKING urges that may provide fertile breeding grounds for addictive tendencies (Nocjar & Panksepp, 2002). With both "pro" and "con" data on this, we question the wisdom of substituting play-inhibiting drug treatment for the natural, neurochemically mediated brain benefits and joys of physical play (Panksepp, 1998a, 1998b, 2007d).

After many years of research, we encountered an intriguing sound, a ~50-kHz ultrasonic play vocalization, that had previously been heard primarily in the context of sexual solicitation in adult rats. To a lesser extent, this sound is emitted during the anticipation of all major rewards, and we focused on the idea that this might be a way to monitor appetitive motivational intensity (Knutson, Burgdorf, & Panksepp, 2002). Indeed, this response may be the first easily conditioned, natural measure of drug desire (Burgdorf et al., 2001; Panksepp, Knutson, & Burgdorf, 2002). However, more

than anything, the sound is a superb indicator of social joy that accompanies rough-and-tumble play.

Juvenile play arouses this vocalization more than any other social activity. We now believe that it may be evolutionarily related to the instinctual fixed-action patterns of laughter, which is so common during human play (Scott & Panksepp, 2003). Accordingly, we started to tickle juvenile rats, and the 50-kHz play chirps rose dramatically (Panksepp & Burgdorf, 1999, 2003). After years of focused work, we know much about the underlying circuitry. It courses along the ascending mesolimbic dopamine systems that innervate the nucleus accumbens and medial frontal cortex (Burgdorf et al., 2001, 2007).

Perhaps primordial forms of joyful laughter are more prevalent among the playful juveniles of our fellow animals than scientists ever suspected. Traditionally, laughter has been deemed a unique trait of humans and perhaps chimpanzees (Provine, 2000). Our work brings that anthropocentric supposition into question. Tickling (or, more formally, heterospecific hand play) robustly promotes 50-kHz ultrasonic chirping, with characteristics suggestive of ancestral laughter (Panksepp & Burgdorf, 2003; Panksepp, 2007d). We have evaluated this idea abundantly without disconfirmations. Accordingly, we propose that this is a neuroscientifically workable model for understanding the neural details of social joy in mammalian brains.

Here are a dozen reasons to consider relations between childhood laughter in our species and play chirping in young rats (more fully discussed in Panksepp & Burgdorf, 2003; Burgdorf & Panksepp, 2006):

1. The 50-kHz ultrasonic chirping is provoked robustly by positive social interchange (namely, play), and even more powerfully by tickling.
2. All negative affective stimuli, including fearful foot shock, cat smell, scary places, bright lights, and unpleasant handling, reduce the chirping response.
3. Juvenile rats chirp more than mature rats.
4. Rats that chirp most abundantly during tickling also play the most with each other.
5. Animals approach hands that have tickled them more than those that have only petted them.
6. Young rats readily learn to run down alleys

and to press levers to get tickled, but not to be picked up and petted.

7. Rats show conditioned place preferences for tickling and seek out stimuli that have been associated with tickling (e.g., if tickled by a hand that smelled of coffee grounds, they are attracted to that smell in other situations).

8. The tickling response classically conditions rapidly to cues that predict tickling.

9. Children are more ticklish in certain bodily regions (e.g., ribs), and young rats have "tickle skin" concentrated at the nape of the neck, where they typically direct their own play activities.

10. Juvenile rats prefer to spend more time with adults that still chirp a lot than those that do not.

11. Tickle-induced chirping is hard-wired in the brain and is a temperamental characteristic of rats, for it can be successfully increased or decreased within four generations of selective breeding (Burgdorf, Panksepp, Brudzynski, Kroes, & Moskal, 2005).

12. Tickling circuitry courses along the dopamine-modulated self-stimulation circuitry, and such brain regions are aroused when humans laugh. (For a more detailed summary of evidence relevant for understanding the sources of human and rat laughter, see Panksepp, in press-d).

This model system offers a simplified way to understand the primary-process social joy systems of the mammalian brain. We are currently in the 17th generation of selectively breeding animals for high and low chirping in response to tickling. Behavioral phenotyping of these lines has been initiated (see Burgdorf & Panksepp, 2006; Burgdorf et al., 2007; Harmon et al., in press). Our microarray-based screening of how play modifies gene expression patterns in the brain is already indicating that the genetic "orchestra" is dramatically modified by play (a third of 1,200 brain genes significantly changed activity).

We anticipate that a fuller understanding of the neurochemistries of joy will yield new insights and new molecular targets for treating human depression. Comparable possibilities exist for all the other basic emotional systems, and some relevant clinical issues are discussed elsewhere (Panksepp, 2004, 2006).

AFFECTIVE NEUROSCIENCE ONTOLOGY

All basic psychological processes are thoroughly dependent on brain biophysical processes, working in concert with body, environment, and culture. Within our current scientific understanding of mind, there are no emotional feelings that are independent of neuronal activities, operating in the complexities of bodies within environments. In spite of abundant evidence, however, the neuroscientific and psychological communities remain unconvinced that other animals experience affects of great relevance for understanding primary-process human feelings. Many in behavioral neuroscience consider affects to be epiphenomenal—conceptual flotsam of idle anthropomorphism (Figure 4.2).

Much philosophical ink has been spilled concerning the existence and causal efficacy of mental processes. Besides battalions of reductionist neuroscientists, some philosophers do not accept mentality as "really" doing any causal work in our physiochemical universe. Others advocate a foundational "panpsychic" or "panexperiential" view of the physical universe. For example, they appear to accept the so-far empirically inconsequential "mind-dust" as a property of matter—a possibility that William James (1890) entertained, tongue in cheek, in his *Principles of Psychology*. Within our dust-to-dust existence, no "seeds" of mentality have yet been detected in brute matter. Still, some brilliant people are willing to argue that if no fundamental panpsychic "mind-dust" stuff exists in the physical universe—if no kind of protoconsciousness exists at the quantum level—then surely our own experiences of mentality must be epiphenomenal. Such arguments hold little water. Emergence is a pervasive aspect of nature, and new functions do arise from interacting levels of organization.

Even if the physical universe has no intrinsic qualities of mentality, no intrinsic values, evolved brains most certainly do. Affective experience is an emergent function of complex network-level neurodynamics, intimately connected to body and world. Primary-process affects arise from complex neuronal network interactions (see Figure 4.1), yielding intrinsic brain/mind tools that help animals survive.

ON THE EVOLUTION OF AFFECTIVE ADAPTATIONS

Organisms have competed for resources since the beginning of life. Initially the competition may have been largely reflexive, with no mentality. However, experiential specializations presumably led to increasingly successful competition in unpredictable environments. Without interanimal competition, neural networks for generating affects probably would not have evolved; reflexive zombie-like behavioral controls might have sufficed. With ever-increasing levels of competition, there were new choices to be made, and affects may have been ideal heuristics for effective decision making. Affects present survival "compass" bearings for the cognitive apparatus. The most competitive brains developed affective heuristics—which are completely biological, largely neuronal, but with strong bodily and cultural connections—to facilitate rapid decision making for individual benefits, as well as empathy and group sharing of survival-related resources. In short, affects are real brain functions. Their most important infrastructure is neuronal.

Accordingly, a great deal of cognitive activity may be less conscious than the affects. Consider the dispersion of dopamine cells at the mesodiencephalic junction. The more medial ventral tegmental area (VTA) neurons projecting to nucleus accumbens mediate urges to seek resources, and thereby to learn about the contingencies of the world (Ikemoto & Panksepp, 1999; Panksepp, 1998a). The more lateral neurons in substantia nigra (SN) have similar electrophysiological properties during learning (Schultz, 2006), but they are more important in laying down habitual ways of behaving as learning is consolidated into well-worn paths (habit learning), especially within the dorsal striatum (in the caudate–putamen complex). We may ask this question: Which of these two regions sustains experienced feelings more? By the measure of self-stimulation, animals show vigorous self-stimulation of the medial VTA regions, and little of SN regions. Thus arousal of medial, more ancient brain regions is valued more than that of evolutionarily more recent lateral regions.

Instinctual feelings (basic tools for living) presumably present survival knowledge to the cognitive apparatus. Increasing positive feelings, of diverse kinds, inform the cognitive apparatus that organisms are behaving with a high probability of facilitating survival. Various bad feelings inform the cognitive apparatus that ongoing actions may harm survival (Cabanac, 1992). For instance, disgust is an affective response that helps prevent severe nausea once sickness has taken hold. Both feelings guard against death.

Affects, although genetically ingrained, are largely intrinsic anticipatory states that facilitate learning by interacting with information-processing abilities of the cognitive apparatus. Perhaps the primal feeling is pain. For instance, when I feel excruciating, throbbing pain in my occasionally gouty toe, it controls my behavior unambiguously. When I take pain-dissolving medicines, I can again walk with relative ease. Pain rarely informs the rest of our brain that we are at death's door. It typically tells us to protect an injured body part, optimizing healing. Without painful feelings, all humans would die prematurely.

Evolutionarily, the primal capacity to experience pain may have promoted the possibility of generating other negative feelings (such as separation distress), which promote grief and loneliness (Panksepp, 2005c, 2005d). After the emergence of maternal nurturance, the oxytocin-driven sexual affects of females may have been recrafted to generate the pleasures of maternal interactions (Panksepp, 1998a).

Affects control behavior because they are part and parcel of brain *network* functions, which are increasingly accepted in psychiatry and psychoanalysis (Panksepp, 1999, 2004, 2006). The discarding of affective concepts in behavioral neuroscience may be tantamount to crippling our ability to discuss the nature of large-scale adaptive network functions of the brain, and aborting our ability to envision how an understanding of affective mentality provides many avenues to reconceptualizing psychiatric disorders (Johnson-Laird, Mancini, & Gangemi, 2006; Panksepp, 2006). If so, a better neural understanding of affect is a foundational issue for all of psychology and psychiatry, as well as for anyone interested in the functional organization of the mammalian brain. This is not to deny that an enormous amount of autonomic and cognitive brain activity can proceed unconsciously and habitually (Wegner, 2002), but to assert, in agreement with Freud, that affects are quintessentially experienced and real, even in dreams.

Although discussions about affect are becoming more common in psychology (e.g., Lambie & Marcel, 2002; Russell, 2003), relevant fact finding remains sparse. That awaits more intellectual commerce (joint *causal* research) between psychologists and neuroscientists. Indeed, understanding the nature of affect neuroscientifically may become a major gateway for understanding consciousness (Watt & Pincus, 2004). To do that well, we need new neurophilosophical perspectives.

DUAL-ASPECT MONISM

We have identified emotional systems through LESSNS that arouse distinct emotional behaviors in animals. People experience affects when these same brain networks are stimulated, and animals are never neutral about such arousals. They either seek to avoid such states or to reexperience them. Because these affective and emotional responses emerge from homologous brain areas, and because the choice behaviors of animals are commensurate with the affects that human beings verbalize, the underlying circuits may be envisioned in terms of a Spinozan "dual-aspect monism." The "dual-aspect" refers to the fact that certain emotional arousals concurrently generate instinctual emotional urges as well as complementary emotional feelings. The "monism" rejects Cartesian dualism by asserting that both behavior and experience are manifestations of the physical brain. This view coaxes psychology to accept neuroscience as an essential partner for clarifying primary-process affective issues (Panksepp, 2005a). This view also restores many other animals back into the circle of affective mental life, from which they were excluded by the radical behaviorists of the 20th century.

If we share homologous instinctual circuits with our animal cousins, as subcortical anatomical, neurochemical, and functional studies suggest, we mammals should have similar primary-process affective feelings—albeit not secondary- and tertiary-process cognitive abilities, which arise from our differential neocortical complexities. We humans have much more random-access-type neocortical information-processing and memory space for re-representing primary-process experiences. These capacities can parse affective space into complex conceptual structures, many of which may never be illuminated by research on other animals. Our cortical abilities can construct cultural differences and subtleties that exist in no other species. Many emotional complexities emerge from these epigenetic cortical re-representations of raw experience.

Dual-aspect monism is a robust working strategy for understanding primary-process affective experience, but not necessarily associated cognitive processes. Dual-aspect monism maintains, as did William James, that a substantial part of the affectively experienced side of life is completely entwined with neuronal processes that generate certain instinctual behavior patterns. For example, a cat that appears angry because of LESSNS-induced instinctual displays of rage actually experiences anger within the brain. Such large-scale network activities do their work well because they are experienced. Thus classical behavioral *reinforcers* may need to promote affective-experiential states within the brain. According to this approach, the instinctual behavioral neurodynamics are isomorphic with the primary-process affective dynamics, but are only preconditions for associated cognitive moldings of experience that ultimately serve affective needs. In this view, there is no logical problem in asserting that affects, because they are completely neuronal, do regulate behavior.

In summary, affects can be conceived of as a primordial form of consciousness that arose as a way for the brain to represent biological survival values to the evolutionarily emergent cognitive deliberations of the brain (Denton, 2006; Panksepp, 1998a, 2005a; Merker, 2007). How cognitive activities reciprocally mold and parse affective experience remains an open empirical question. If the model described above is on the right track, then the facilitation of learned behavioral change may be dependent in part on the emergence of brain affective changes when animals are rewarded and punished. How might this be tested?

If affective change is pharmacologically prevented, the progression of learning should be changed. The likelihood that the reinforcement is fundamentally affective helped us interpret a strange behavior we discovered almost 30 years ago—the inhibition of extinction by low doses of morphine in juvenile rats trained to run for social rewards (Panksepp & DeEskinazi, 1980). Since social reward is partly due to brain opioid release (Panksepp,

1981), it was reasonable that a reduced brain capacity to experience affective change during extinction would drastically retard extinction of learned habits. Indeed, low doses of morphine that dramatically diminish separation distress blocked extinction almost completely. In similar work with food reward, antiextinction effects were half the size as seen with social reward (Panksepp & DeEskinazi, 1980).

AFFECTIVE FOUNDATIONS OF CORE CONSCIOUSNESS AND CORE SELF

The foundation of phenomenal experience, including primordial affective mentality, is called "core consciousness" (Panksepp, 2007). The understanding of conscious *awareness*—a reflective higher brain function—may require the prior clarification of the neural mechanisms of phenomenal consciousness, which may come in two primal varieties: (1) the here-and-now perceptual fields (the movie in the head, so to speak) and (2) affective experiences (the many nonpropositional valenced ways we feel alive). Our fledgling attempts to understand phenomenal affective experience may require some kind of a "core self" conceptualization—a coherent organismic representation of the organism within the brain, to provide a body-feeling foundation for affective states (Damasio, 1999; Panksepp, 1998a, 1998b, 2005a).

My preferred theoretical vision is that the visceral nervous system has a coherent representation of the inside of the body laid out in primitive action coordinates of the somatic musculoskeletal system. In contrast to Damasio's view of the core self as closely linked to the somatosensory cortex, I envision a considerably more ancient neurosymbolic representation of organisms within the ancient medial subcortical regions that abound in visceral organ representations (Hess, 1957). Both approaches seek to specify the brain circuits, neurochemistries, and neurodynamics that help construct core feelings, but I see the visceral homunculus as highly coordinated with instinctual emotional action coordinates (Panksepp, 1998b, 2000a).

The neurodynamics of such a core SELF may vary as a function of basic emotional and motivational homeostatic and sensory states, all generating distinct affective feelings (see above). Such a vision needs to be given substance with a huge amount of research, but existing electrophysiological approaches may be currently beset by seemingly insurmountable challenges (Panksepp, 2000b). At present, the easiest way to untangle this Gordian knot is to focus on the likelihood that there exists some kind of neurochemical, especially neuropeptide, coding of emotional affects (Panksepp & Harro, 2004), as well as of certain sensory affects that have clear behavioral indicators (Peciña et al., 2006; Steiner, Glaser, Hawilo, & Berridge, 2001), within this complex homuncular representation of the SELF.

The neurochemical aspects are presently comparatively easy to address empirically, because of the discovery of hundreds of neuropeptides concentrated within visceral, subcortical brain regions (Panksepp, 1993; Tohyama & Takatsuji, 1998). Many of these neuropeptides may establish distinct neurodynamics, which are psychologically experienced as distinct affective states, within the subcortical trajectory of the core SELF (Panksepp & Harro, 2004). The concurrent abundances of neuropeptides in peripheral visceral organs and in visceral parts of the brain suggest continuities between the neurochemical regulation of certain bodily functions and brain emotional functions. A striking example is the fact that both oxytocin and prolactin, which regulate the metabolic nourishment of infants by regulating the production and dispensation of milk, are important for the infant's social-emotional nourishment. Both neuropeptides are powerful inhibitors of separation distress (Panksepp, 1998a) and facilitators of a variety of maternal, sexual, and other prosocial behaviors (Carter, 2003; Insel, 2003; Young & Wang, 2004). As already noted, maternal circuits may be evolutionary outgrowths of brain systems that promote female sexuality, helping explain their shared neurochemical controls. Separation distress may be an outgrowth of pain systems (Panksepp, 2003c)

Similar theoretical linkages could be made with many other central and peripheral neuropeptides, allowing us to envision harmonious evolutionary continuities between peripheral bodily and central affective functions (Panksepp, 1993). Thus the regional localizations of brain neuropeptide systems—their abilities to regulate specific classes of emotional behaviors—again affirm that many varieties of positive and negative affects are critically linked to the dynamics of ancient subcortical regions of the brain (Panksepp, 1998a, 2005a). The recent social-constructivist idea that primal positive and negative affects are brain substrates from which the complexity of emotional life is created (Barrett, 2006; Russell, 2003) awaits neurobiological support. No causal tests have been proposed, while abundant predictions are available for a more resolved vision of primary-process emotional systems (Panksepp, 2005a, 2007). Why is it not good news for social constructivists that at the primary-process level there are various core affective tools from which the complexities of individual lives and cultures could be constructed?

The possibility that core emotional affects reflect the neurodynamics of various brain systems that control instinctual emotional actions is eminently testable in humans via psychopharmacological approaches (Depue & Collins, 1999; Panksepp, 1999; Panksepp & Harro, 2004). The core SELF hypothesis is not as easily evaluated, and may first require abundant research characterizing the primitive viscerosomatic homuncular topography that exists in subcortical regions of the brain (Hess, 1957). Because of modern functional magnetic resonance imaging (fMRI) techniques, this feat is already achievable for higher reaches of self-representation (Northoff et al., 2006)—in brain regions where neural firing rates are much higher than in the depths of the visceral nervous system. However, PET studies have had some success in monitoring brain dynamics during diverse forms of emotional and motivational arousal (Damasio et al., 2000; Denton, 2006).

CONCLUDING REMARKS

Can we ever scientifically understand how affective feelings are generated by neural activities? Given the wealth of supportive data, it is evident that mammals and many other vertebrates do experience emotional, sensory, and homeostatic affects, and hence provide workable model systems via which the infrastructure can be objectively characterized. Past LESSNS demonstrate that powerful emotional responses emanate from specific subcortical brain systems that are homologous across species. Arousals of homologous sites in the hu-

man brain evoke affective feelings that are commensurate with the instinctual emotional actions evoked in other animals (Heath, 1996; Panksepp, 1985). Also, animals that have been surgically deprived of their neocortices continue to display spontaneous primary-process emotional behaviors with apparent affective contents, whether they are rats (Kolb & Tees, 2000; Panksepp et al., 1994), cats (Villablanca & Marcus, 1972), or human beings (Shewmon et al., 1999).

I have summarized historical issues that persuaded psychologists to reject affective considerations in favor of behavior-only and eventually cognition-only research strategies. In contrast, affective neuroscience approaches can now envision how subcortical networks constitute the affective crucible of the brain (Panksepp, 1998a, 2005a). I have focused on two emotional systems, SADNESS/PANIC and PLAY/JOY, that highlight how social isolation/ loss and the urge to enjoy positive social interactions are fundamental needs of the mammalian brain.

At birth, the basic emotional systems, and accompanying raw affects, have few intrinsic "object relations." However, life experiences rapidly promote development linkage to world events and objects. Such cognitivized affects enhance behavioral guidance, allowing animals to compete and cooperate with each other successfully in order to survive. All raw affects interpenetrate the cognitive apparatus in the higher reaches of the limbic system—cortices such as cingulate, insula, temporal, and hippocampal paleocortices—allowing animals to generate more flexible adaptive responses to previously neutral stimuli. The neocortex comes to reflect on such experiences, providing ultimately conscious *awareness*.

Finally, I have considered the hypothesis that affective feelings arise when primary-process emotional systems interact with a shared core SELF that is laid out in primitive visceral and somatic coordinates. Clarification of such ancient neural networks may help illuminate the biological nature of the "soul."

Even if this core affective SELF model remains imprecise, it does not diminish the persuasive power of the evidence supporting various basic emotional systems in the mammalian brain. These systems are homologous across species; they are aroused by homologous neurochemicals, and they produce homologous behaviors and commensurate affects. These data, coupled with the abundance of converging positive evidence suggesting that animals are affective creatures (from Darwin, 1872/1998, to Panksepp, 1998a, 2005a), highlight the great value that animal research can provide to the science of mind and its emotional disorders.

ACKNOWLEDGMENTS

I appreciate comments on an earlier draft of this chapter by Luce Bivins and Terry McGuire. This work was partially supported by the Hope for Depression Research Foundation.

NOTES

1. "Primary processes" reflect brain/mind functions that are intrinsic in the normal biological organization of the brain. These are contrasted with "secondary processes," which reflect learned resymbolizations and other developmental landscapes of each organism (such as thoughts about the world), and higher "tertiary processes," which may be uniquely human, constituting thoughts about thoughts and emotions. As basic affects come to be molded by learned individual and cultural influences, the shades and subtlety of emotions become enormous. An understanding of primary-process emotions, best studied in animal models where the necessary neuroscientific work can be done, is essential for making sense of higher-order derivative processes, which can only be well studied through the analysis of human experience. This chapter focuses on primary-process emotions.
2. To highlight the fact that we are talking about the necessary neural substrates for various emotional constructs rather than any comprehensive sets of attributes of such systems operating in the real world, the labels for the various systems are given in small capital letters. In other words, the labels refer to specific neural systems that remain poorly understood.
3. It is noteworthy that John Dewey held the view that emotional feelings occur prior to instinctual actions, and dissipate as a consequence of instinctual discharge. This conjecture may reflect the fact that humans often actively inhibit their instinctual displays, and that this inhibition leaves the instinctual urge within the brain active. It may be the inhibited activity of such urges, which is commonly evident in enculturated humans, that prolongs emotional affect in the absence of overt instinctual displays during which covert instinctual arousal may still be present. At the same time, each emotion is indeed self-limiting, and hence the display gradually does dissipate the underlying, neurochemically based emotional "energy." In this way, Dewey's view can be seen to be a harmonious variant of the present view.

REFERENCES

Alcaro, A., Huber, R., & Panksepp, J. (2007). Behavioral functions of the mesolimbic dopaminergic system: An affective neuroethological perspective. *Brain Research Reviews, 56,* 283–321.
Barrett, L. F. (2006). Are emotions natural kinds? *Perspectives on Psychological Science, 1,* 28–58.
Beatty, W. W., Dodge, A. M., Dodge, L. J., Whike, K., & Panksepp, J. (1982). Psychomotor stimulants, social deprivation and play in juvenile rats. *Pharmacology, Biochemistry and Behavior, 16,* 417–422.
Berridge, K. C. (2000). Measuring hedonic impact in animals and infants: Microstructure of affective taste reactivity patterns. *Neuroscience and Biobehavioral Reviews, 24,* 173–198.
Berridge, K. C., & Robinson, T. E. (2003). *Parsing reward.* Trends in Neurosciences, 9, 507–513.
Bishop, P. (1984). *Brain and opiate modulation of avian affective vocalizations.* Unpublished doctoral dissertation, Bowling Green State University.
Bodkin, J. A., Zornberg, C. L., Lukas, S. E., & Cole, J. O. (1995). Buprenorphine treatment of refractory depression. *Journal of Clinical Psychopharmacology, 15,* 49–57.
Bowlby, J. (1969). *Attachment: Vol. 1. Attachment and loss* (2nd ed.). New York: Basic Books.
Burgdorf, J., Knutson, B., Panksepp, J., & Shippenberg, T. (2001). Evaluation of rat ultrasonic vocalizations as predictors of the conditioned aversive effects of drugs. *Psychopharmacology, 155,* 35–42.
Burgdorf, J., & Panksepp, J. (2006). The neurobiology of positive emotions. *Neuroscience and Biobehavioral Reviews, 30,* 173–187.
Burgdorf, J., Wood, P. L., Kroes, R. A., Moskal, J. R., & Panksepp, J. (2007). Neurobiology of 50-kHz ultrasonic vocalizations in rats: Electrode mapping, lesion, and pharmacological studies. *Behavioural Brain Research, 182,* 274–283.
Burghardt, G. M. (2005). *The genesis of animal play.* Cambridge, MA: MIT Press.
Cabanac, M. (1992). Pleasure: The common currency. *Journal of Theoretical Biology, 155,* 173–200.
Carter, C. S. (2003). Developmental consequences of oxytocin. *Physiology and Behavior, 79,* 383–397.
Carter, C. S., Lederhendler, I., & Kirkpatrick, B. (Eds.). (1999). *The integrative neurobiology of affiliation.* Cambridge, MA: MIT Press.
Champagne, F. A., Francis, D. D., Mar, A., & Meaney, M. J. (2003). Variations in maternal care in the rat as a mediating influence for the effects of environment on development. *Physiology and Behavior, 79,* 359–371.
Ciompi, L., & Panksepp, J. (2004). Energetic effects of emotions on cognitions: Complementary psychobiological and psychosocial finding. In R. Ellis & N. Newton (Eds.), *Consciousness and emotions* (Vol. 1, pp. 23–55). Amsterdam: Benjamins.
Colantuoni, C., Rada, P., McCarthy, J., Patten, C., Avena, N. M., Chadeayne, A., et al. (2002). Evidence

that intermittent, excessive sugar intake causes endogenous opioid dependence. *Obesity Research 10*, 478–488.

Craig, A. D. (2003). How do you feel? Interoception: The sense of the physiological condition of the body. *Nature Reviews Neuroscience, 3*, 655–666.

Damasio, A. R. (1994). *Descartes' error.* New York: Putnam.

Damasio, A. R. (1999). *The feeling of what happens.* New York: Harcourt, Brace.

Damasio, A. R. (2003). *Looking for Spinoza.* Orlando, FL: Harcourt, Brace.

Damasio, A. R., Grabowski, T. J., Bechara, A., Damasio, H., Ponto, L. L. B., Parvizi, J., et al. (2000). Subcortical and cortical brain activity during the feeling of self-generated emotions. *Nature Neuroscience, 3*, 1049–1056.

Darwin, C. (1998). *The expression of the emotions in man and animals* (3rd ed.). New York: Oxford University Press. (Original work published 1872)

Denton, D. (2006). *The primordial emotions: The dawning of consciousness.* New York: Oxford University Press.

Depue, R. A., & Collins, P. F. (1999). Neurobiology of the structure of personality: Dopamine, facilitation of incentive motivation, and extraversion. *Behavioral and Brain Sciences, 22*, 491–517.

Devinsky, O., Morrell, M. J., & Vogt, B. A. (1995). Contributions of anterior cingulate cortex to behavior. *Brain, 118*, 279–306.

Dolan, R. J. (2002). Emotion, cognition, and behavior. *Science, 298*, 1191–1194.

Gordon, N. S., Burke, S., Akil, H., Watson, J., & Panksepp, J. (2003). Socially induced brain fertilization: Play promotes brain derived neurotrophic factor expression. *Neuroscience Letters, 341*, 17–20.

Gray, J. A. (1990). Brain systems that medicate both emotion and cognition. *Cognition and Emotion, 4*, 269–288.

Greenspan, R. J., & Baars, B. J. (2005). Consciousness eclipsed: Jacques Loeb, Ivan P. Pavlov and the rise of reductionistic biology after 1900. *Consciousness and Cognition, 14*, 219–230.

Harmon, K. M., Cromwell, H. C., Burgdorf, J., Moskal, J. R., Brudzynski, S. M., Kroes, R. A., & Panksepp, J. (in press). Rats selectively bred for low levels of 50 kHz ultrasonic vocalizations exhibit alterations in early social motivation. *Developmental Psychobiology.*

Heath, R. G. (1996). *Exploring the mind–body relationship.* Baton Rouge, LA: Moran.

Heim, C., & Nemeroff, C. B. (1999). The impact of early adverse experiences on brain systems involved in the pathophysiology of anxiety and affective disorders. *Biological Psychiatry, 46*, 1509–1522.

Herman, B. H. (1979). *An exploration of brain social attachment substrates in guinea pigs.* Unpublished doctoral dissertation, Bowling Green State University.

Herman, B. H., & Panksepp, J. (1978). Effects of morphine and naloxone on separation distress and approach attachment: Evidence for opiate mediation of social affect. *Pharmacology, Biochemistry and Behavior, 9*, 213–220.

Herman, B. H., & Panksepp, J. (1981). Ascending endorphinergic inhibition of distress vocalization. *Science, 211*, 1060–1062.

Hess, W. R. (1957). *The functional organization of the diencephalon.* New York: Grune & Stratton.

Holstege, G., Georgiadis, J. R., Paans, A. M., Meiners, L. C., van der Graaf, F. H., & Reinders, A. A. (2003). Brain activation during human male ejaculation. *Journal of Neuroscience, 23*, 9185–9193.

Ikemoto, S., & Panksepp, J. (1999). The role of nucleus accumbens DA in motivated behavior: A unifying interpretation with special reference to reward-seeking. *Brain Research Reviews, 31*, 6–41.

Insel, T. R. (2003). Is social attachment an addictive disorder? *Physiology and Behavior, 79*, 351–357.

James, W. (1890). *Principles of psychology.* New York: Holt.

Johnson-Laird, P. N., Mancini, F., & Gangemi, A. (2006). A hyper-emotion theory of psychological illnesses. *Psychological Review, 113*, 822–841.

Kalin, N. H., Shelton, S. E., & Barksdale, C. M. (1988). Opiate modulation of separation-induced distress in non-human primates. *Brain Research, 440*, 285–292.

Kehoe, P., & Blass, E. M. (1986). Opioid-mediation of separation distress in 10-day-old rats: Reversal of stress with maternal stimuli. *Developmental Psychobiology, 19*, 385–398.

Keverne, E. B., Nevison, C. M., & Martel, F. L. (1997). Early learning and the social bond. *Annals of the New York Academy of Sciences, 807*, 329–339.

Khantzian, E. J. (2003). Understanding addictive vulnerability: An evolving psychodynamic perspective. *Neuro-Psychoanalysis, 5*, 5–56.

Knutson, B., Burgdorf, J., & Panksepp, J. (2002). Ultrasonic vocalizations as indices of affective states in rat. *Psychological Bulletin, 128*, 961–977.

Kolb, B., & Tees, C. (Eds.). (2000). *The cerebral cortex of the rat.* Cambridge, MA: MIT Press.

Kosfeld, M., Heinrichs, M., Zak, P. J., Fischbacher, U., & Fehr, E. (2005). Oxytocin increases trust in humans. *Nature, 435*, 673–676.

Kovacs, G. L., Sarnyai, Z., & Szabo, G. (1998). Oxytocin and addiction: A review. *Psychoneuroendicronol, 23*, 945–962.

Kroes, R. A., Panksepp, J., Burgdorf, J., Otto, N. J., & Moskal, J. R. (2006). Social dominance–submission gene expression patterns in rat neocortex. *Neuroscience, 137*, 37–49.

Lambie, J. A., & Marcel, A. J. (2002). Consciousness and the varieties of emotion experience: A theoretical framework. *Psychological Review, 109*, 219–259.

LeDoux, J. E. (1996). *The emotional brain.* New York: Simon & Schuster.

Liotti, M., & Panksepp, J. (2004). On the neural nature

of human emotions and implications for biological psychiatry. In J. Panksepp (Ed.), *Textbook of biological psychiatry* (pp. 33–74). Hoboken, NJ: Wiley-Liss.

MacLean, P. (1990). *The triune brain.* New York: Plenum Press.

Meaney, M. J. (2001). Maternal care, gene expression, and the transmission of individual differences in stress reactivity across generations. *Annual Review of Neuroscience, 24,* 1161–1192.

Merker, B. (2007). Consciousness without a cerebral cortex: A challenge for neuroscience and medicine. *Behavioral and Brain Sciences, 30,* 63–134.

Moles, A., Kieffer, B. L., & D'Amato, F. R. (2004). Deficit in attachment behavior in mice lacking the mu-opioid receptor gene. *Science, 304,* 1983–1986.

Naqvi, N. H., Rudrauf, D., Damasio, H., & Bechara, A. (2007). Damage to the insula disrupts addiction to cigarette smoking. *Science, 315,* 531–534.

Nelson, E. E., & Panksepp, J. (1998). Brain substrates of infant–mother attachment: Contributions of opioids, oxytocin, and norepinephrine. *Neuroscience and Biobehavioral Reviews, 22,* 437–452.

Newman, J. D. (2007). Neural circuits underlying crying and cry responding in mammals. *Behavioural Brain Research, 182,* 155–165.

Nocjar, C., & Panksepp, J. (2002). Chronic intermittent amphetamine pretreatment enhances future appetitive behavior for drug- and natural-reward: Interaction with environmental variables. *Behavioural Brain Research, 128,* 189–203.

Northoff, G., Heinzel, A., de Greck, M., Bermpohl, F., & Panksepp, J. (2006). Our brain and its self: The central role of cortical midline structures. *NeuroImage, 15,* 440–457.

Panksepp, J. (1981). Brain opioids: A neurochemical substrate for narcotic and social dependence. In S. Cooper (Ed.), *Progress in theory in psychopharmacology* (pp. 149–175). London: Academic Press.

Panksepp, J. (1982). Toward a general psychobiological theory of emotions. *Behavioral and Brain Sciences, 5,* 407–467.

Panksepp, J. (1985). Mood changes. In P. Vinken, G. Bruyn, & H. Klawans (Eds.), *Handbook of clinical neurology* (pp. 271–285). Amsterdam: Elsevier.

Panksepp, J. (1990a). The psychoneurology of fear: Evolutionary perspectives and the role of animal models in understanding human anxiety. In G. D. Burrows, M. Roth, & R. Noyes, Jr. (Eds.), *Handbook of anxiety* (pp. 3–58). Amsterdam: Elsevier/North-Holland.

Panksepp, J. (1990b). Can "mind" and behavior be understood without understanding the brain?: A response to Bunge. *New Ideas in Psychology, 8,* 139–149.

Panksepp, J. (1990c). Gray zones at the emotion–cognition interface: A commentary. *Cognition and Emotion, 4,* 289–302.

Panksepp, J. (1991). Affective neuroscience: A conceptual framework for the neurobiological study of emotions. In K. T. Strongman (Ed.), *International review of emotion* (Vol. 1, pp. 59–99). Chichester, UK: Wiley.

Panksepp, J. (1993). Neurochemical control of moods and neuropeptides. In M. Lewis & J. Haviland (Eds.), *Handbook of emotions* (pp. 87–107). New York: Guilford Press.

Panksepp, J. (1998a). *Affective neuroscience: The foundations of human and animal emotions.* New York: Oxford University Press.

Panksepp, J. (1998b). The periconscious substrates of consciousness: Affective states and the evolutionary origins of the SELF. *Journal of Consciousness Studies, 5,* 566–582.

Panksepp, J. (1999). Emotions as viewed by psychoanalysis and neuroscience, An exercise in consilience. *Neuro-Psychoanalysis, 1,* 15–38.

Panksepp, J. (2000a). Affective consciousness and the instinctual motor system: The neural sources of sadness and joy. In R. Ellis, & N. Newton (Eds.), *The caldron of consciousness: Motivation, affect and self-organization* (pp. 27–54). Amsterdam: Benjamins.

Panksepp, J. (2000b). The neurodynamics of emotions: An evolutionary–neurodevelopmental view. In M. D. Lewis & I. Granic (Eds.), *Emotion, self-organization, and development* (pp. 236–264). New York: Cambridge University Press.

Panksepp, J. (2001). The long-term psychobiological consequences of infant emotions: Prescriptions for the 21st century. *Infant Mental Health Journal, 22,* 132–173.

Panksepp, J. (2003a). Damasio's error. *Consciousness and Emotion, 4,* 111–134.

Panksepp, J. (2003b). At the interface of affective, behavioral and cognitive neurosciences: Decoding the emotional feelings of the brain. *Brain and Cognition, 52,* 4–14.

Panksepp, J. (2003c). Feeling the pain of social loss. *Science, 302,* 237–239.

Panksepp, J. (Ed.). (2004). *Textbook of biological psychiatry.* Hoboken, NJ: Wiley-Liss.

Panksepp, J. (2005a). Affective consciousness: Core emotional feelings in animals and humans. *Consciousness and Cognition, 14,* 30–80.

Panksepp, J. (2005b). On the embodied neural nature of the core emotional affects. *Journal of Consciousness Studies, 5,* 158–184.

Panksepp, J. (2005c). Social support and pain: How does the brain feel the ache of a broke heart? *Journal of Cancer Pain and Symptom Palliation, 1,* 59–65.

Panksepp, J. (2005d). Feelings of social loss: The evolution of pain and the ache of a broken heart. In R. Ellis & N. Newton (Eds.), *Consciousness and emotions* (Vol. 1, pp. 23–55). Amsterdam: Benjamins.

Panksepp, J. (2006). Emotional endophenotypes in evolutionary psychiatry. *Progress in Neuro-Psychopharmacology and Biological Psychiatry, 30,* 774–784.

Panksepp, J. (2007a). The neuroevolutionary and

neuroaffective psychobiology of the prosocial brain. In C. Crawford & D. Krebs (Eds.), *Handbook of evolutionary psychology* (pp. 145–162). New York: Erlbaum/Taylor & Francis.

Panksepp, J. (2007b). Criteria for basic emotions: Is DISGUST a primary "emotion"? *Cognition and Emotion, 21*, 1819–1828.

Panksepp, J. (2007c). Neurologizing the psychology of affects: How appraisal-based constructivism and basic emotion theory can co-exist. *Perspectives on Psychological Science, 2*, 281–296.

Panksepp, J. (2007d). Neuroevolutionary sources of laughter and social joy: Modeling primal human laughter in laboratory rats. *Behavioural Brain Research, 182*, 231–244.

Panksepp, J., Bean, N. J., Bishop, P., Vilberg, T., & Sahley, T. L. (1980). Opioid blockade and social comfort in chicks. *Pharmacology, Biochemistry and Behavior, 13*, 673–683.

Panksepp, J., & Bishop, P. (1981). An autoradiographic map of ^{3}H diprenorphine binding in the rat brain: Effects of social interaction. *Brain Research Bulletin, 7*, 405–410.

Panksepp, J., & Burgdorf, J. (1999). Laughing rats?: Playful tickling arouses high frequency ultrasonic chirping in young rodents. In S. Hameroff, D. Chalmers, & A. Kazniak (Eds.), *Toward a science of consciousness III* (pp. 231–244). Cambridge, MA: MIT Press.

Panksepp, J., & Burgdorf, J. (2003). "Laughing" rats and the evolutionary antecedents of human joy? *Physiology and Behavior, 79*, 533–547.

Panksepp, J., & DeEskinazi, F. G. (1980). Opiates and homing. *Journal of Comparative and Physiological Psychology, 94*, 650–663.

Panksepp, J., & Harro, J. (2004). The future of neuropeptides in biological psychiatry and emotional psychopharmacology: Goals and strategies. In J. Panksepp (Ed.), *Textbook of biological psychiatry* (pp. 627–660). Hoboken, NJ: Wiley-Liss.

Panksepp, J., Herman, B., Conner, R., Bishop, P., & Scott, J. P. (1978). The biology of social attachments: Opiates alleviate separation distress. *Biological Psychiatry, 9*, 213–220.

Panksepp, J., Herman, B. H., Vilberg, T., Bishop, P., & DeEskinazi, F. G. (1980). Endogenous opioids and social behavior. *Neuroscience and Biobehavioral Reviews, 4*, 473–487.

Panksepp, J., & Huber, R. (2004). Ethological analyses of crayfish behavior: A new invertebrate system for measuring the rewarding properties of psychostimulants. *Behavioural Brain Research, 153*, 171–180.

Panksepp, J., Jalowiec, J., DeEskinazi, F. G., & Bishop, P. (1985). Opiates and play dominance in juvenile rats. *Behavioral Neuroscience, 99*, 441–453.

Panksepp, J., Knutson, B., & Burgdorf, J. (2002). The role of emotional brain systems in addictions: A neuro-evolutionary perspective. *Addiction, 97*, 459–469.

Panksepp, J., Lensing, P., Leboyer, M., & Bouvard, M. P. (1991). Naltrexone and other potential new pharmacological treatments of autism. *Brain Dysfunction, 4*, 281–300.

Panksepp, J., Normansell, L. A., Cox, J. F., Crepeau, L., & Sacks, D. S. (1987). Psychopharmacology of social play. In B. Olivier, J. Mos, & B. F. Brain (Eds.), *Ethnopharmacology of social behavior* (pp. 132–144). Dordrecht, The Netherlands: Nijhoff.

Panksepp, J., Normansell, L. A., Cox, J. F., & Siviy, S. (1994). Effects of neonatal decortication on the social play of juvenile rats. *Physiology and Behavior, 56*, 429–443.

Panksepp, J., Normansell, L. A., Herman, B., Bishop, P., & Crepeau, L. (1988). Neural and neurochemical control of the separation distress call. In J. D. Newman (Ed.), *The physiological control of mammalian vocalizations* (pp. 263–300). New York: Plenum Press.

Panksepp, J., Siviy, S., & Normansell, L. A. (1984). The psychobiology of play: Theoretical and methodological perspectives. *Neuroscience and Biobehavioral Reviews, 8*, 465–492.

Panksepp, J., Vilberg, T., Bean, N. J., Coy, D. H., & Kastin, A. J. (1978). Reduction of distress vocalization in chicks by opiate-like peptides. *Brain Research Bulletin, 3*, 663–667.

Panksepp, J., Yates, G., Ikemoto, S., & Nelson, E. (1991). Simple ethological models of depression: Social-isolation induced "despair" in chicks and mice. In B. Olivier, J. Mos, & J. L. Slangen (Eds.), *Animal models in psychopharmacology* (pp. 161–181). Basel: Birkhauser-Verlag.

Peciña, S., Smith, K., & Berridge, K. C. (2006). Hedonic hot spots in the brain. *The Neuroscientist, 12*, 500–511.

Pellis, S. M., & Pellis, V. C. (1998). Structure–function interface in the analysis of play fighting. In M. Bekoff & J. A. Byers (Eds.), *Animal play: Evolutionary, comparative, and ecological perspectives* (pp. 115–140). Cambridge, UK: Cambridge University Press.

Provine, R. R. (2000). *Laughter: A scientific investigation.* New York: Viking.

Rolls, E. T. (2005). *Emotions explained.* Oxford: Oxford University Press.

Rossi, J., III, Sahley, T. L., & Panksepp, J. (1983). The role of brain norepinephrine in clonidine suppression of isolation-induced distress in the domestic chick. *Psychopharmacology, 79*, 338–342.

Roth, T. L., & Sullivan, R. M. (2006). Examining the role of endogenous opioids in learned odor-stroke associations in infant rats. *Developmental Psychobiology, 48*, 71–78.

Russell, J. A. (2003). Core affect and the psychological construction of emotion. *Psychological Review, 110*, 145–173.

Schultz, W. (2006). Behavioral theories and the neurophysiology of reward. *Annual Review of Psychology, 57*, 87–115.

Scott, E., & Panksepp, J. (2003). Rough-and-tumble play in human children. *Aggressive Behaviour, 29,* 539–551.

Shewmon, D. A., Holmse, D. A., & Byrne, P. A. (1999). Consciousness in congenitally decorticate children: Developmental vegetative state as self-fulfilling prophecy. *Developmental Medicine and Child Neurology, 41,* 364–374.

Siviy, S. M., & Panksepp, J. (1987). Juvenile play in the rat: Thalamic and brain stem involvement. *Physiology and Behavior, 41,* 39–55.

Skinner, B. F. (1953). *Science and human behavior.* New York: Macmillan.

Steiner, J. E., Glaser, D., Hawilo, M. E., & Berridge, K. C. (2001). Comparative expression of hedonic impact: Affective reactions to taste by human infants and other primates. *Neuroscience and Biobehavioral Reviews, 25,* 53–74.

Sunderland, M. (2006). *Science of parenting.* London, UK: Doring Kindersley Books.

Thorndike, E. L. (1911). *Animal intelligence.* New York: Macmillan.

Tohyama, M., & Takatsuji, K. (Eds.). (1998). *Atlas of neuroactive substances and their receptors.* New York: Oxford University Press.

Toronchuk, J. A., & Ellis, G. F. R. (2007). Disgust: Sensory affect or primary emotional system? *Cognition and Emotion, 21,* 1799–1818.

Vanderschuren, L. J., Niesink, R. J., & Van Ree, J. M. (1997). The neurobiology of social play behavior in rats. *Neuroscience and Biobehavioral Reviews, 21,* 309–326.

Villablanca, J., & Marcus, R. (1972). Sleep-wakefulness, EEG and behavioral studies of chronic cats without neocortex and striatum: The 'diencephalic' cat. *Archives Italiennes de Biologie, 110,* 348–382.

Watson, J. B. (1919). A schematic outline of the emotions. *Psychological Review, 26,* 165–196.

Watt, D. F., & Pincus, D. I. (2004). Neural substrates of consciousness: Implications for clinical psychiatry. In J. Panksepp (Ed.), *Textbook of biological psychiatry* (pp. 627–660). Hoboken, NJ: Wiley-Liss.

Wegner, D. M. (2002). *The illusion of conscious will.* Cambridge, MA: MIT Press.

Young, L. J., & Wang, Z. (2004). The neurobiology of pair bonding. *Nature Neuroscience, 7,* 1048–1054.

Zubieta, J. K., Ketter, T. A., Bueller, J. A., Xu, Y., Kilbourn, M. R., Young, E. A., et al. (2003). Regulation of human affective responses by anterior cingulate and limbic mu-opioid neurotransmission. *Archives of General Psychiatry, 60,* 1145–1153.

CHAPTER 5

The Psychologists' Point of View

NICO H. FRIJDA

The psychological point of view is that "emotion" represents a meaningful and necessary concept. This statement is not a truism. One can hold that "emotion" is no more than a chapter heading (Bentley, 1928), or a folk conception based on preconceptions rather than facts. As Magda Arnold wrote in 1970, there are a number of "perennial problems in the field of emotion." The definition of emotion is one of them, and so is the question of whether it represents a coherent domain of study.

Indeed, the word "emotion" itself may give reasons for doubt. It may not represent a natural class of phenomena. It also is of relatively recent origin. In its present sense, it dates from about 1649, the publication date of Descartes's *Passions de l'Âme*. Not all languages possess a more or less equivalent concept (Wierzbicka, 1995). Nevertheless, most languages do, and for good reason. The word fills a need in pointing to particular phenomena of feeling and behavior. Which phenomena these are transpires from the term itself, and from its equivalents in other languages. Around the time that Descartes (1649/1970) first used "emotions"

for *les emotions de l'âme*, it meant "uproar" or "social unrest," with implications of unruliness and vehemence (Cayrou, 1924). Ancient Greek used the term *pathèma*, and early French and English used *passion*—that is, mental events involving passivity. "Passions" differ from "actions," in that the individual feels the actions or inclinations for them passively coming over him or her, rather than flowing from their initiative. The Latin near-equivalent, *affectus*, had a similar connotation: an event or experience that one is affected by. Sanskrit employed *bhava*, meaning something like a "state of mind that becomes"—that is, one that movements flow from (Shweder & Haidt, 2000). The notions of passivity, being affected, and uproar all refer to the phenomenon that certain feelings and behavioral inclinations tend to intrude upon ongoing thought and behavior. They seek to assume control, tend to persist over time, and may do so even when prevailing conditions make it advisable for them not to do so.

These control shifts appear largely due to feelings. *Pathèma*, *affectus*, emotion, and *bhava* all are felt. People profess to feelings, and perhaps do so everywhere. Feelings indeed loom large in definitions of emotion (see Kleinginna & Kleinginna, 1981). Humans appear to "express" them in movements and sounds that do not appear to serve instrumental purposes, but still function in communicating states of mind to others. Both feelings and behavior pivot around acceptance and rejection of people (including oneself), objects, or events. They pivot around inclinations and disinclinations to deal with them, around professed feelings of like and dislike or of pleasure and pain, and around judgments of good and bad (Nussbaum, 2001). The distinction between good and bad appears to be a universal component of language (Wierzbicka, 1995).

People, objects, and events, and the feelings they evoke, moreover, do not leave one cold. They affect one's body and one's cognitive functioning. One may tremble, become confused, or believe what one knows to be untrue.

The psychologists' point of view thus points to a domain of phenomena of feelings, behaviors, and bodily reactions. These phenomena require explanations different from those required for explaining habit, voluntary action, and sensory impressions and thought as such. They appear to demand explanatory concepts such as pleasure and pain, evaluation, control priorities, preferences, and desires.

This psychological perspective has two interconnected implications. First, its focus is on phenomena manifested or felt by individuals. Second, the explanations for these phenomena require hypotheses about intrapersonal causal processes. "Emotion," first of all, serves as a shorthand for, or pointer to, intrapersonal processes and mechanisms. It thereby also points to a human and animal system architecture that enables such mechanisms (Sloman, 1987).

The notion of emotion thereby serves to resolve discrepancies between what people do or feel and the events surrounding them; between the immediate cues for why they do what they do and what they actually do; between what they do and what they say; between what they do and what seems most appropriate, most useful, most reasonable, and best organized; and between what they do and what they profess to know they should do. It serves to help our understanding that different people may react in different ways to the same situations, and that one given person may react differently to one given situation on different occasions.

THE TASK OF THE PSYCHOLOGY OF EMOTION

The psychology of emotion has the task of describing features and patterns of phenomena that qualify as "emotional," and of explaining them in terms of underlying processes and the species' and individuals' process repertoires. Explanations include operating characteristics such as sensitivities and thresholds, processing and response repertoires, and attentional and energetic resources. They also include analysis of the various kinds of information that these processes have to work with. Some of that information is received from the environment; some is generated by an individual's bodily processes; and some comes from the individual's store of representations of facts, cognitive schemas, and behavioral skills. The psychological point of view focuses on intraindividual processes, even if these may represent convergence points for influences of sociocultural origin.

Explanations can be formulated at different levels of description. Dennett (1987) has distinguished an intentional or phenomenological level (description in terms of feelings, aims, desires, and expectations), a functional or properly psychological level (description in terms of habits, programs, information-processing procedures, and memory stores), and a hardware or neural and neurohumoral level. Within each level, there are gradations of integration of elements, and corresponding levels of description. There are neurons, neuron circuits, and neurohumoral systems. There are muscle twitches, movements, and actions at many scales of hierarchical complexity. There are momentary feelings of discontent, and feelings that the world is heading toward its ruin. The descriptions may not immediately reflect the underlying integration and complexity. Suffering from foreseeing the world's doom is not necessarily a more complex feeling than suffering from pain in one's toe. Only the foundational processes differ in complexity and, of course, so do the explications of the feelings and their implications for behavior.

These relationships complicate the task of psychology. Operation, properties, and effects of more integrative phenomena usually cannot be meaningfully reduced to some combination of those of the founding elements, or be predicted from these. They may possess emergent properties, such as a sense of agency or of being affected (Metzinger, 2003). Founding elements may change their operation within the integrated whole, in what has been called "circular causation" (Lewis, 1996). For instance, the effects of emotional feelings on thought may drastically differ from the mere effects of somatic feelings, even if the latter are among the foundations of the former.

Among its explanatory tools, the psychology of emotion includes the dynamic interactions of the individual with his or her environment. These interactions bring sensory stimuli in from environment and body, produce effects on how smoothly the individual's faculties and processes function, and produce effects on the environment as well as feedback from that environment.

Psychological explanations of emotion phenomena thus are composed of three terms: the structure (properties, capacities, propensities) of the individual; incoming and stored information; and online dynamic interaction with the environment. How the emotional phenomena emerge from what corresponds to those three terms raises several of the other perennial problems that Arnold (1970) alluded to.

The three terms can be combined in an indefinite number of ways. Theoretical orientations differ in emphasizing one or another of them. Classical behaviorism favored structural simplicity, together with simple rules of information acquisition; McDougall's (1923) innate instincts theory formed a contrast. In emotion theory proper, Mandler's (1984) view explains emotions with few structural provisions: Emotions are viewed as arousal responses triggered by goal interruption. Russell's (2003) core affect theory likewise requires only pleasure–pain and activation provisions as basic elements. Both theories contrast with Ekman's (1992) highly structured neurocultural theory of basic emotions, and with that of Öhman and Mineka (2001)—which, for instance, posits an evolved fear module, innately sensitive to particular sets of stimuli. Striving for structural simplicity is reductionist. It seeks to follow the principle of Occam's razor: Be as stingy with structure as possible. Complexity is motivated by the effort to account as fully as possible for phenomenal variety. Dynamic interaction seeks to combine structural simplicity and richness of phenomena.

All efforts at description and explanation aim to find regularities among responses, and in the links among antecedents, responses, and further outcomes. Ideally, the regularities indicate causal laws, such as "All emotional reactions are instigated by appraisal processes," or "Anger is the inevitable consequence of frustration." However, it may well be that true laws cannot be found at any integrative level of description. Elster (1999a) has argued that at such levels, explanatory rules must and do have a limited scope, and are subject to unspecified restrictions. They are rules, not laws; Elster calls them "mental mechanisms." Their limitations are due to the fact that the conditions under which each rule applies cannot be strictly specified because of the chaotic nature of psychological causation. Elster illustrates the argument with the following pair of rules: Rule 1, "Tyranny decreases the likelihood of rebellion," and Rule 2, "Tyranny increases the likelihood of rebellion." Both are true; however, their respective conditions cannot be exhaustively specified because of their unbounded context dependence, which can reverse the balances.

WHAT ARE EMOTIONS?

Emotions thus do exist. This does not imply, however, that these phenomena justify a single concept or form a natural class. The underlying processes or provisions may not possess sufficient unity and specificity. In that sense, one may repeat the question: Do emotions exist? Do the phenomena justify assuming a distinct function of "Emotion," separate from "Cognition" and "Conation," as an older psychology would have it?

Specificity and unity of emotions are commonly assumed; the assumptions are not necessarily correct, however. Nor are they universally held. James (1884) did not adhere to the one about specificity. Emotional behavior, in his view, does not differ from other behavior called forth by key stimuli. James supposed it to originate in the cerebral cortex, just like all other behavior; it took Cannon's work on subcortical mechanisms to prove him wrong. Neither did he give emotional feeling any special status; he viewed it as just consisting of body sensations resulting from feedback from movements and other bodily responses. Other investigators also argued that there is nothing specific in emotion experience. For instance, "emotional experience is a highly variable state [and] often partakes of the complicated nature of a judgment" (Landis & Hunt, 1932, quoted by Hebb, 1949, p. 237). Duffy (1941) took a different nonspecificity position. In her view, what are called "emotions" are just the high and low levels of activation, with no qualitative property separating them from the emotionally neutral middle range.

One may also deny the unity assumption. Dumas (1948) and Hebb (1949) denied that goal-directed reactions such as angry attack or fearful flight have anything in common with the diffuse ones of mere upset or excitement, or of emotional shock and behavioral disorganization. More recently, LeDoux (1996) has suggested that the various emotions may not involve shared mechanisms.

There are good reasons to raise the unity and specificity issues. The central problem is the modest agreement between investigators about which features so-called emotions might share. Bentley (1928), in the paper mentioned earlier, concluded: "Well, emotion is at least a topic! It is something to talk about and to disagree upon" (p. 21). The main problem is that the features mentioned in my first section (passivity, feeling, driving force, etc.), as well as the various behavioral, experiential, and physiological response aspects, do not strongly covary. They each define overlapping but nonidentical sets of responses. Theorists select different features for their definitions, and as a consequence, these definitions are numerous and may diverge widely (Kleinginna & Kleinginna, 1981).

In some definitions, the essence of emotions is feeling, notably that of pleasure or pain. Affective valence is commonly regarded as a criterial aspect. Emotions, say Ortony, Clore, and Collins (1988), are valenced reactions, or conscious experiences of events with valenced meanings (e.g., Elster, 1999a). Affects, pleasure and pain, certainly set the experiences in which they occur apart from all other kinds of experience—if only because, as feelings, they cannot be readily reduced to something else, such as cognitions or body sensations (Frijda, 1986, 2007a). Yet, conversely, many valenced reactions are not usually classed as emotions. Tasting sweet substances merely produces a pleasant sensation that usually is not regarded as an emotion. By contrast, some reactions are often considered emotions even though they do not involve pleasure or pain. Surprise and wonder are among them. But, precisely for that reason, Spinoza (1677/1989) did not include them among the emotions; he saw them as merely cognitive reactions.

Even feelings may not be considered criterial for emotions, though. Emotions occur even in lower animals, according to behavioral criteria. Valenced reactions—acceptance and rejection, pursuit and avoidance—occur without awareness. They occur in insects and fish. They occur in humans in response to pleasant and unpleasant stimuli that are not consciously perceived. Backward masking of such stimuli may lead to subsequent affect ratings (e.g., Zajonc, 1980), or even to enhanced consumption of liked drinks (Berridge, 2004).

But the latter findings point to a level of analysis that might enlarge the domain of responses that share pleasure or pain: viewing the feelings as but one kind of expression of the underlying processes that Berridge (2004) has called "core pleasure" and "core pain." These processes are also expressed in readiness for event acceptance or rejection.

Pleasure and pain, in turn, result from a still larger process domain: that of "appraisal." Appraisal processes are defined as intrasubjective processes that turn incoming stimulus events into ones with affective value and further meaning for well-being and motive satisfaction (Lazarus, 1991). Event appraisal can be considered one of the basic abilities of human and animal systems; emotions can therefore be defined as processes that involve appraisal. Appraisal processes vary in kind and complexity, ranging from immediate, automatic affect arousal (stimuli may directly evoke pleasure or pain because one has innate or acquired dispositions for them to do so; LeDoux, 1996) to complex integration of cues for promotion or obstruction in achieving goals and safeguarding concerns. The latter are often designated as "cognitive appraisals" (e.g., Lazarus, 1991; Oatley, 1992; Scherer, 2001; Stein & Trabasso, 1992). Because of the role of appraisals in emotional feelings and action instigations (Elster, 1999a; Scherer, 2001), emotions haven been defined as kinds of judgments (e.g., Nussbaum, 2001). However, regardless of complexity, appraisal processes mostly proceed automatically and nonconsciously, even if one is often aware of their outcomes (Bargh, 1997; Zajonc, 1980). Obviously, the extent to which felt and overt responses are taken to share the processes of appraisal depends on one's level of analysis and theoretical interpretation.

Another domain that looms large in efforts to define emotions is that of motivation. Emotional behavior as well as felt emotions strongly suggest a certain prominence of urges to act, desires, or motive states (including those of loss or decay of motivation, as observed in emotional confusion and depressive apathy). Motivation was central in older emotion theories, such as those of Thomas Aquinas, McDougall (1923), Tomkins (1962), and Wallon (1942), and more recently that of Magda Arnold (1960). The motivational side of emotions has been lost from view in more recent theoretical attempts.

Yet motive states as occurring in what we call emotions are rather specific for them. They are triggered by events as appraised. They are felt as urges and lead to impulsive actions, which means that they do not result from planning and are little controlled by foresight. They command actions that are not premeditated. Impulses to act represent a mode of action instigation and control differing from that of automatic and habitual behavior, as well as from that of planned behavior. Impulsive control of action was indeed prominent among the phenomena that gave rise to the emotion-like notions.

Emotions can therefore be regarded as passions—as defined as event-instigated or object-instigated states of action readiness with control precedence. "States of action readiness" are states of readiness for actions to maintain or modify one's relationship with the world or oneself, including loss or decay of motivation to relate (Frijda, 1986, 2007a). "Readiness" implies being set for action if and when appropriate conditions arise, and if relevant actions are available in one's action repertoire. Some states of action readiness are diffuse and have no aim other than to relate or not to relate in general; they are called "activation states." Besides apathy, diffuse excitement and unfocused receptivity, as in some states of meditation, are examples. Other states of action readiness have the aim of achieving, maintaining, or modifying one's relationship to a particular object or event in a particular way—by seeking proximity, by moving away or protecting oneself, or by moving against and blocking interference. They are called "action tendencies," and command actions that can fulfill their aim.

Action readiness is conspicuous in event-triggered actions that a definition of emotions in terms of only pleasure and pain would leave out. Desire is the clearest instance, since many desires are not guided by foresight of pleasure, or by a wish to escape from pain other than that of unfulfilled desire. Surprise and wonder are further instances that I have already mentioned. Conversely, emotions defined by action readiness do include instances of pleasure and pain that produce some change in action readiness: hunger that leads to restlessness and the urge to find food, and craving for something irresistibly attractive.

Many reactions that are considered "emotional" do not include much overt action. States of action readiness may remain just that: states of readiness. However, the actions for which action readiness is readiness include cognitive actions: changes in beliefs. Emotions have been defined by Aristotle as well as by Spinoza as inclinations to think one way rather than another.

Such cognitive actions share with overt actions one of the defining aspects of passion and action readiness: They are not initiated by voluntary planning, nor can they be readily modified at will. By contrast, they possess the feature that I have termed "control precedence" (Frijda, 1986, 2007). They tend to take control and overrule other actions or action instigations—the passivity aspect of passion. They not only command actions to fulfill their aim, but also are set toward achieving that aim in the face of delays, obstacles, and other difficulties, turning action into persistent striving. They seek precedence over ongoing behavior or interference from other sources.

Perhaps the major feature of passions, their emotionally driven actions, and their belief changes is their being reward-insensitive (Elster, 1999b). One tends to do certain things—in love, in hate, in greed, and in addiction—even when one knows that only bad things will come from it. One shrugs one's shoulders over such things. By contrast, passions are stimulus-governed; one feels irresistibly drawn to good-smelling food, or to unattainable but attractive sexual targets, in proportion to their perceptual salience (Frijda, 2007a). The smell of alcohol, the cues for a heroin shot, and the sight of a syringe may fill an addicted individual with frenzy (Berridge, 2004). This aspect of impulsive action control is lawful: Feeling and action instigation are inverse hyperbolic functions of temporal distance to the target in time. Ainslie's (2001) law of time discounting describes the "breakdown of will" when a person is facing temptations, and the null effects of mere warnings of future misery. Hume said that reason is emotion's slave. That may not be entirely true (Solomon, 2004): One can to some extent control one's emotions; one can even to some extent choose them. But even if one is not truly passion's slave, one certainly is not their master.

Viewing the role of motive states as central in emotion resembles the view that defines emotions by activation of largely innate action systems, each with a particular adaptive function (e.g., Bradley, Codispoti, Cuthbert, & Lang, 2001; Buck, 1999; Damasio, 2003; Öhman, Chapter 44, this volume; Plutchik, 2003). Both views presumably cover many of the same behavioral phenomena, except that the action system view is silent on the behavioral and motivational dynamics, and the action readiness view is silent on the provenance of modes of action readiness and the action repertoires.

So far, these are various possible bases for defining emotions. What specifies and unifies the reactions with the phenomena discussed may not, however, be one or the other of the various components, or even a particular combination of them. "Emotion" can perhaps best be taken to designate any process in which the various components are intimately connected. The concept properly fits states of synchronization of several components (Scherer, 2000, 2007). "Synchronization" here does not mean that fixed linkages exist between particular components, but rather that the various components flexibly influence each other. In this flexible fashion, they represent a unitary reaction of the entire system. Synchronization in this sense is involved whenever appraisal and action readiness are evoked, and when control precedence is operative. The three tend to be coupled and to involve a number of further components, such as autonomic arousal and cognitive orientation (Frijda, 2007b).

THE EMOTION CONCEPT

Just as there are arguments to restrict the domain of emotion (smaller than all impulsive motor reactions, such as startle; smaller than all affective responses), there also are arguments to enlarge it.

There is a large class of emotional phenomena called "emotional attitudes" or "sentiments" (Arnold, 1960; Shand, 1920). They are usually treated as distinct from emotions. Being frightened by a nearby dog and afraid of dogs are not the same sort of thing. The distinction is that between an occurrent state and a disposition. Emotions have a limited duration; sentiments may persist over a lifetime. But nevertheless, occurrent emotions and sentiments are not totally separate. Emotions and sentiments have the same structure. They can both be characterized by an object, its appraisal, and a particular propensity to act in relation to the object—a latent, dispositional propensity in the case of sentiments, and an acute, occurrent propensity in the case of emotions proper. Also, sentiments are not all that dispositional. One can feel that one fears dogs and that one loves one's beloved. One can know these sentiments and act accordingly—by avoiding places where one knows a dog to live, or by going upstairs to embrace the beloved. One can also know that the sentiment may turn into an emotion at the slightest provocation. One may, in other words, join sentiments and occurrent emotions together in one emotion category, contrary to what Kenny (1963) proposed. Some authors in fact do this.

The preceding section has been mainly concerned with the definition of emotions. So is much debate in emotion theory. Such debate can be considered an unprofitable undertaking. Natural processes of any complexity are not tailored into discrete categories. The question of whether or not someone has an emotion nevertheless is sometimes meaningful. It comes up when wondering whether a given reaction is a "false" or faked emotion. This has a moral or legal side: Has some act been committed "coolly" or "with emotion"? There also exist imagined and empathic emotions, as well as anticipated emotions (e.g., anticipated guilt, shame, or regret), which exert powerful social control (Harré & Parrott, 1996) and which may be absent in some individuals like psychopaths.

However, the multicomponent nature of emotions entails a looseness of structure that leads to considering a discrete category labeled "emotion" as only a shorthand. The same may be true of the distinctions between emotions and sentiments and between feelings and moods. Distinguishing categories reflects the general problem of using "substance concepts" (Cassirer, 1908) instead of function concepts, when organizing continuous and continuously varying phenomena. Emotions indeed are often treated as thing-like states. Language sustains this; emotions are usually referred to by nouns. This may be useful in social communication. For psychological analysis, however, it might be better to treat emotions as the observable results of processes that are better denoted by verbs. "She is angering" might not be a bad expression, which neatly matches "She has been angered," as well as "She is loving."

Instead of talking about emotions, one might instead describe streams of concurrent and interacting ongoing processes: appraisals that last and change, that activate processes of action readiness that generate action preparations and overt actions, which in turn act back upon appraisals, and that all vary in degree of activation, each having different time courses and different moments at which they die down. This is the picture sketched by multicomponential emotion theory (e.g., Scherer, 2000), according to which matching categories to ongoing processes—"an emotion," "a mood," and even "anger!" or "excitement!"—can only be sloppy, often a bit arbitrary, and not very consequential except for verbal communication.

The usefulness of category labels for verbal interaction does not imply, incidentally, that they are needed for nonverbal communication. States of action readiness, degrees of activation, and degrees of control precedence of feelings and action urges can be grasped directly by an observer, and can probably be copied directly in motor empathy (Gallese, 2005). In psychological analysis, too, the various phenomena can be described directly in terms of the ongoing processes. All these processes are graded in strength, and making cutoffs at certain levels of strength is arbitrary; that, of course, was the point of Duffy's (1941) attack on the emotion concept. Her analysis was limited by its focus on activation. The same applies to other emotional processes, such as action readiness, appraisals, and control precedence. Degree of articulation of an intentional object, for instance, can be considered a parameter. Its introduction would turn the distinction between emotions and moods into a continuum of "emotionness" versus "moodness."

EMOTION INSTANCES

So far, I have referred to emotions as modes of acting and reacting, or as modes of feeling and doing. This is decidedly vaguer than calling them "responses" or "reactions." There is, however, good reason to do so. What we use words like "emotion" for are usually complex response patterns spread out over time. Their components show variations in duration and time course. Brief facial expressions occur alongside longer-lasting changes in heart rate or respiration, interspersed with flashes of strong feeling against a background of feeling that waxes and wanes.

These observable and experienced phenomena can in fact be described at very different levels of analysis and integration. One can describe single response components, such as a smile or an angry facial expression. One can describe more or less coherent expressive and behavioral sequences, such as a series of fearful movements when a person is facing an ongoing frightening event, or of various angry expressions (a scowl, a glare, a deep frown, a clenching of fists) during a hostile interchange. One can observe a sequence of behavior and feeling modes that all center around dealing with a particular event, such as viewing something with apprehension that grows into alarm and turns into anger, then calms down to mere watchfulness. Such sequences form "emotion episodes."

Emotion episodes are in fact what subjects usually recount when asked to recall some instance of an emotion (Frijda, Mesquita, Sonnemans, & Van Goozen, 1991). Episodes usually include several emotions (Oatley & Duncan, 1994). All this is obviously relevant for the question of what represents an emotion instance, and how long emotions last. The duration depends on what one focuses on. It may be 5 seconds at most, for an individual facial response. It may be an hour for a hostile or fearful interchange. It is up to days or longer for emotion episodes that continue over restless dream-ridden sleep. It is up to a lifetime when the notion of emotions is extended to sentiments and their latent readiness for emotions in the acute, occurrent sense (Frijda, 2007a).

How long one considers an emotion to last is to some extent, as emotions of any personal importance tend to entail extensions. They may instigate the individual to ruminate, to walk around pondering revenge or ways of restoring self-esteem, or to engage in social sharing of one's emotion (Rimé, 2005). It is not immediately transparent when an emotion terminates, since all components may do so at different moments; lowered thresholds (e.g., irritability, rapid tears) may outlast all more manifest components. It is also a matter of taste which of the phenomena discussed are considered as belonging to the emotion itself, and which to its antecedents or consequents (e.g., Dumas, 1948). Conscious appraisal is as much a part of the emotion as an antecedent for action impulse. These questions clearly lose much of their sense when "emotion" is understood to refer to a collection of interacting processes, and not to a single or a solidly integrated entity.

Emotion instances thus can be viewed at very different levels. That is why "response" or "reaction" is not the best designation for an emotion instance. Most instances are complex. Actions and feelings in a particular emotion form part of interactions and interchanges. An emotion thus can thus be viewed as an intrapersonal state of feeling, arousal, activation, and so forth, but also as the individual's share in an interactive occurrence that involves dealing with another person and one's mutual relationship. Which level of analysis is selected can have appreciable consequences. A focus on feelings, for instance, readily loses sight of the intentional nature of emotion—its being, and being experienced as, an event between the individual and the other (Lambie & Marcel, 2002). A focus on motor responses may, in experience and in analysis, turn an action into a mere movement.

Analyses at different levels are compatible; they coexist. However, incompatibilities may arise when emotions are categorized on different levels. One cannot, as a rule, reduce descriptions at some higher, more integrative level to a combination of more elementary constituents without loss. Jealousy, as pain caused by rivalry, is not just pain, nor is it just anger, nor is it just despair; it is an interpersonal pain that can change its face at any moment. Likewise, higher-level categorizations cannot always be built up from the lower-level phenomena. Higher-level categorizations often (or perhaps usually) include more phenomena, as well as more interactions between the lower-level phenomena, or feedback from them. Indignation is more than anger with a moral overtone, since it is felt as carried by one's moral values rather than by one's personal interests.

Noticing that emotions are streams of independent but interacting processes raises questions about the nature of these interactions. Process analyses suggest that processes that logically follow from certain other processes may still, by their feedback, influence those latter. Facial expressions that respond to appraisals in turn influence appraisals. The expected effect of one's emotion on others influences the actual occurrence of that emotion. Processes may produce a higher-order outcome (say, a categorization of one's state) that then controls and modifies logically prior processes (say, appraisal). Such processes have been called "processes of vertical causality." Emotion processes thus are not linearly organized. A nonlinear, dynamic model is called for (Lewis, 1996, 2005); such a model accounts better for how emotions actually proceed and how they obtain and modify their shape.

The interactions suggest that given subprocesses do not follow each other in a very regular manner, even if the links are lawful. The actual linkages are sensitive to a host of feedback influences, and to influences from various levels. Whether certain stimuli actually elicit certain responses, or certain appraisals elicit certain emotions, may strongly depend on secondary conditions such as personality, mood, the state of the organism, and coincidences in the physical and social situation. These secondary conditions may be so important that a model involving chaotic determination may be more satisfactory than the usual linear model. It also is what makes Elster's (1999a) mental mechanisms better explanatory tools than "laws" in a strict sense.

HOW ARE WE TO DISTINGUISH DIFFERENT EMOTIONS?

How are we to distinguish different emotions properly or profitably? Verbal categories have been used as the starting point, since some of them suggest elementary entities. Some emotion labels have indeed been interpreted as reflecting elementary, irreducible feelings or *qualia*, with other labels representing their blends or subspecies (Izard, 1977; Oatley, 1992). The feelings may reflect (or be part of) basic organized component structures, including motivational states (e.g., Oatley, 1992), action and expression patterns (e.g., Ekman, 1992; Izard, 1977; Tomkins, 1962), and patterns of physiological reactions (e.g., James, 1884). The feelings may not be irreducible *qualia*, but themselves patterns of values on two feeling dimensions of hedonic tone and activation—variants of "core affect" (Barrett, 2005; Russell, 2003).

There is no a priori reason why verbal labels should offer a good clue to distinct emotions. Languages differ in their taxonomies, and verbal labels may reflect eliciting contingencies rather than modes of feeling and doing (e.g., likelihood of certain social sanctions or particular rewards).

Several hypotheses on how the various components are related and organized have oriented research. In one major hypothesis, the various components form solidly coherent packets, each based on a common neural and neurohumoral disposition. Activation of the dispositions by events jointly activates the various components. This basic-emotions hypothesis exists in several variants (Buck, 1999; Ekman, 1992; Izard, 1977; Öhman, Chapter 44, this volume; Panksepp, Chapter 4, this volume; Tomkins, 1962). Such a hypothesis finds support in indications for the existence of dedicated brain circuits and neurohumors (Panksepp, Chapter 4, this volume), apart from the unstable evidence for label-specific facial and other expressions (Ekman, 1992; Izard, 1977); however, correlations in the occurrence of various components tend to be moderate or weak (Scherer, 2005).

A second hypothesis starts from this last finding. The "multicomponential view" (Scherer, 2000) views emotions as more or less unordered collections of components, jointly activated by how an emotional event is appraised and by individual component propensities. Emotions can occupy almost any position in a multidimensional space, with as many dimensions as there exist components. Each component is activated by separate external conditions or aspects of the event–subject interaction as appraised (Ortony & Turner, 1990; Scherer, 2001).

This second hypothesis leads to abandoning the very notion of distinct emotion types. Each emotion instance stands on is own. Emotions are just bundles of component processes. Emotion labels just loosely and fuzzily cover subregions of the multicomponential space, or delimit such subregions themselves by culturally, linguistically, or ecologically determined prototypes or scripts linked to them (Russell, 1991).

Several theorists have taken this second option. Emotion labels are viewed as arbitrary distinctions in a more or less unstructured domain (Mandler, 1984), reflecting ecologically frequent or socially important patterns of components (as in Scherer's [1992] conception of "modal emotions"), or reflecting cultural concerns and values that give emphasis to some, and not to other, sets of feelings and modes of behavior (as in social-constructivist theory; see, e.g., Harré & Parrott, 1996).

The multicomponential view appears better able to deal with cultural differences in emotion taxonomies (e.g., Lutz, 1988), as well as with differences in the precise semantic content of similar categories in different languages (such as "anger" in English and *ikari* in Japanese, or "shame" in English and *hassam* in Arabic). On the other hand, a basic-emotions view more readily handles evidence suggesting that certain emotion categories are very common (Mesquita, Frijda, & Scherer, 1997) and may even occur in most or all languages (Hupka, Lenton, & Hutchinson, 1999; Shaver, Wu, & Schwartz, 1992; but see Russell, 1991).

The two hypotheses may not be as dissimilar as they seem, though. The basic-emotions view has ample room for cultural differences. Basic emotions can be considered to represent functionally defined classes (Ekman, 1992). Within each class, the precise antecedents, nature of the objects, full gamut of appraisal components, precise type of action goal or action to deal with the appraised contingency, and significance of the emotion (see below) all may vary. They all provide the leeway that cultural and individual differences require. More pertinent still is the fact that any component— facial expression, autonomic reaction, action tendency—is the joint outcome of the emotion disposition as such, and of facilitation by situational and other momentary factors. Respiration rate is influenced by excitement as well as by moving fast. Smiling flows from pleasure and from desire to please. The moderate correlations between components can be readily accommodated within the basic-emotions view.

Conversely, even within the multicomponential hypothesis, the componential space is not at all fully unstructured. Many components mutually constrain or entrain each other. There exist coordinate structures. Vigorous action requires sympathetic energy arousal, and readiness for it prepares it; feeling consists in part of feedback from autonomic and skeletal responses and from states of action readiness; motor relaxation and high autonomic arousal are incompatible; and so forth.

In a third, hierarchical approach, components differ in their organizational power. Some are more central than others. Pleasantness and unpleasantness may each cascade into collections of separate subsystems and component streams (Bradley et al., 2001). Action tendency may well organize all other components for implementing its aim. This third approach would fit the functional interpretation of different emotions as different, specifically focused adaptive provisions (Damasio, 2003; Frijda, 1986, 2007; Plutchik, 2003).

The multicomponential and hierarchical approaches follow the shift from categorical to process conceptualizations. This shift extends from the phenomena of emotions as such to the emotion components themselves. Many components are best broken down into smaller components and their variable conjunctions. This has appeared necessary for "autonomic arousal"; no valid, consistent index has been found, because indices do not strongly covary (Levenson, 2003; Stemmler, 2003). The same has been argued for facial expressions. Most patterns, even those presumably typical for particular emotions, are best understood as built up from individual facial action units that each can be considered functional units, such as serving protective, attentional, or force-assembling functions (e.g., eye narrowing, eye widening, or vertical frowning, respectively, in these three examples) (Camras, 2000; Ortony & Turner, 1990; Smith & Scott, 1997; Scherer, 1992). In any case, shifting from category to process approaches turns the relationships between components into a subject for unprejudiced research on several basic questions. Which processes are linked to which other processes, and to what degree? Which linkages are due to joint response to the same antecedent contingencies, and which to their forming coordinative motor structures? Which linkages represent functional dependence? Which represent the effects of a shared command system (Lewis, 2005)?

THE RELATIONS BETWEEN EMOTION AND MOTIVATION

The relations between motivation and emotion constitute another of the perennial problems. Many emotions form motivational states, but many motivational states (e.g., need for food) are not emotions. This has led some investigators (e.g., Bindra, 1959) to abandon the emotion–motivation distinction. This does not appear justified, however, because there is a real distinction that counts.

The term "motivation" suffers from a polysemy that is similar to that for "emotion." It, too, has an occurrent reading (referring to emotions proper) as well as a dispositional one (referring to sentiments). When saying that one's social motivation causes one to be unhappy when alone, a dispositional reading is meant. Saying that felt loneliness motivates one to seek company implies an occurrent reading; loneliness is an emotion. "Motivation" thus can label a cause, a consequence, or an aspect of an emotion. It is a cause in its dispositional sense, and a consequence and/or aspect in the occurrent one.

This type of distinction can generally be considered fruitful. McDougall (1923) distinguished dispositional "instincts" from emotions as their actualizations. Buck (1999) calls emotions the "readouts" of motivation. Oatley (1992) distinguishes "goals" from emotions, with the latter identified as the responses to contingencies in achieving or not achieving goals. Goals, in this context, function as dispositions that drive the occurrent emotional motivations to reach them.

Such a distinction is important. Dispositional motives (I call them "concerns"; "interests" is a useful alternative) belong to the major explanatory notions for emotions (with "action tendencies" as the latter's occurrent motivational component). Concerns are what render events and objects emotionally relevant in the first place. The psychology of motivation forms the cornerstone of emotion analysis. Why do we seek and enjoy company, and why does loneliness makes us sad? Because being with and interacting with others are our concerns. Concerns of course also form the cornerstone of dynamic exploration of emotional conflict: Conflict flows from incompatible concerns, such as desiring wealth and estimating personal decency.

The two senses of "motivation" are not always easy to tease apart, though. Is "love" a dispositional or an occurrent motivation, a concern or an emotion? And what about being in love? Both obviously can be both—the former more continuously, the latter more intermittently.

EMOTION ELICITATION

What elicits emotions? The simplest type of answer is that different emotions are evoked by different kinds of events—each emotion by a different one. In behaviorist parlance, emotions are different reflex-like response patterns to different unconditioned stimuli. The range of elicitors then is augmented by the usual conditioning constellations. This was Watson's (1929) answer. It is still dominant in emotion explanations from evolutionary psychology and evolutionary orientation generally (e.g., Bradley et al., 2001; Tooby & Cosmides, Chapter 8, this volume; Öhman, Chapter 44, this volume).

Later behaviorism and more recent analyses have refined the type of explanation a bit. Stimulus events are pleasant or unpleasant, or represent rewards or punishments. They may have come to do so by evolutionary selection or by actual need or concern satisfaction or frustration. But different emotions are aroused when rewards are embedded in constellations involving the temporal context: their advent, decrease, or omission (Bouton, 2005; Gray, 1987; Mowrer, 1960; Rolls, 2005). This refinement has been extended to include further context aspects, such as previous reinforcement or nonreinforcement of particular responses to deal with the event (Gray, 1987). In appraisal approaches, the context variables are formulated in cognitive rather than contingency terms. They are designated as "appraisal components" (e.g., Ellsworth & Scherer, 2003). "Appraisal of coping resources," as a component of emotion antecedents, thus is largely equivalent to previous reinforcement or nonreinforcement of coping responses. What differs between behaviorist and cognitive approaches is the process by which one or the other emotion is supposedly evoked: It is linked more strongly to environmental events in behaviorist theory, but more strongly to subject-bound processing variables in appraisal theory.

A major, somewhat different conceptualization starts from the previously mentioned central place of dispositional motivation in behavior, rather than that of stimulus–response connections. This conceptualization posits processes of appraisal of the goal or concern relevance of events—or, for short, of events' relevance to well-being (Lazarus, 1991; Oatley, 1992; Stein & Trabasso, 1992). Those events elicit emotions that are appraised as beneficial or harmful for achieving the individual's well-being. This conceptualization seeks to account for positive and negative reward values, or pleasantness and unpleasantness of events, from a general perspective. It implies a different account of the basic mode of operation of human and animal systems. In the end, this approach and the behavioral approach may turn out not to be as different as they seem, since the definitions of "unconditioned stimuli" and "states of satisfaction of concerns" may not always be so drastically different, as evidenced by Hull's (1953) notion of "drive reduction." On the other hand, their emphasis differs. Sensitivities for the various concerns are, by their nature, more general than can be formulated as sensitivities for sets of discrete stimuli. "Novel" stimuli (that trigger curiosity) present a case in point: Novelty is not a stimulus attribute. The same is true of interpersonal warmth and of relevance to self-esteem.

The emotional efficacy of eliciting events cannot always be meaningfully reduced to "unconditioned" stimuli contained in or signaled by them. Reduction is often problematic. Several elementary event types may converge on a given higher-order sensitivity. Personal loss elicits sadness because it implies loss of personal warmth, of protection, or of soothing stimuli. It may elicit sadness by any mixture of those. The stimuli may have nothing more in common than that they all engage an interpersonal intimacy-achieving system.

Moreover, events are not always emotionally efficacious because of the stimuli they contain or signal. Some are efficacious by enabling or obstructing exerting particular skills and competences. Novel stimuli may be pleasurable (when they are) because and when they enable cognitive assimilation skills (Frijda, 2007).

Emotion elicitors can be more profitably understood at some intermediary level between specific stimuli such as painful stimuli, mutilated bodies, snakes, or spiders, and the general level of negative and positive rewards. "Concern relevance" points at emergent properties that reside not in the positive or negative stimuli as such, but in a more involved interaction. Exploring why certain stimuli or actions are rewarding or aversive—receiving a gift or giving one (Mauss, 1914/1957), being sensitive to a magic curse, shrinking back from seeing mutilated bodies—forms a challenging task for emotion psychology.

THE ORIGINS OF EMOTIONS

Nature or nurture? Here is another of the perennial problems in emotion. Specifically, how much, and what, in the phenomena that suggest "emotion"—and in the precise sets of phenomena that are labeled as "joy" or "fear"—are due to provisions and constraints laid down in the mechanisms with which humans are by nature equipped? How much, and what, are the results of individual learning, social shaping, and social pressure?

Nobody, I think, contests that emotions have biological bases. There is compelling evidence of neural and neurochemical mechanisms (see LeDoux & Phelps, Chapter 10, this volume; Panksepp, Chapter 4, this volume). Basic phenomena and underlying processes—unlearned action systems, appraisal processes, pleasure and pain, control shift provisions—extend beyond the human species over many other animal species. Some may extend over invertebrates.

Indications for several different emotions are shared by most or all birds and mammals. The indications include evidence for dedicated neural and neurohumoral circuits (Buck, 1999; Panksepp, Chapter 4, this volume), and for action systems with particular functions: for approach, for establishing close nonhostile interaction, for hostility, for escape and avoidance, for active rejection, for behavioral inhibition. As I have mentioned, verbal emotion labels that imply references to these occur in almost all languages.

Cross-species and intrahuman generalities offer strong support for arguments that some or most of the preceding phenomena and processes have an evolutionary basis (e.g., Ekman, 1994). These arguments are strengthened by the adaptive utility of the behavior systems linked to the emotions: protecting oneself from intruders, predators, and rivals; warding these off and threatening them; obtaining food and drink; detecting and contacting mates; seeking shelter; protecting the young; submitting to the more powerful. For all of them, utility in promoting reproductive fitness is obvious or can be readily constructed (Buss, 1994; Tooby & Cosmides, Chapter 8, this volume).

Nevertheless, reservations are in order. So far, it is rather unclear what precisely the various neural circuits do in functional terms. Do extended amygdala circuits link affective appraisal to particular stimuli or contingencies, or to sets of prewired motor programs, or to motivational reactions activating motor programs that have been shaped in other than specific emotional contexts? The last of these is not unlikely.

By itself, universality in fact does not prove biological origin. Major emotions correspond to sensitivities to universal contingencies or core relational themes, such as threat, loss, competition, or success (Lazarus, 1991). Universal contingencies themselves present universal occasions for learning, and for universally similar modes of problem solving and dynamic compilation of action patterns. Take anger, for example. Its behavior repertoire could be explained by the facts that harm is universally painful, and that one is equipped with several sorts of actions that can produce external changes in general and social changes in particular. Kicking, scratching, throwing objects, and shouting are useful within emotional contexts (e.g., when chasing intruders), as well as outside such contexts (e.g., when cracking nuts, breaking branches, and throwing over one's companions in play). Instrumental behaviors have an applicability range. The efficacy of such actions can be discovered in the dynamic contexts of hostile, playful, and instrumental interactions, in the same way that a baby discovers the possibility of walking when body weight and muscle strength have reached the right relationship (Thelen, 1985). In other words, universality can be explained in more than one way. Biological roots are still involved, but may well exist at deeper or more elementary levels than being roots of emotional response patterns as such.

And then, even if biological roots are involved, it may not be easy to assess what they are. Mother–child and child–mother attachment no doubt have such roots, but which are they, and what is their role? Western attachment theory and findings, on close scrutiny, may reflect more cultural influences than prima facie likelihood suggests. Independence may not be a general component of the attachment system, but one more characteristic of the Western world (Rothbaum, Weisz, Pott, Miyake, & Morelli, 2000).

Biological dispositions, moreover, need inner and outer environments to take behavioral and experiential shape. It may be useful to stress that the role of cultural differences in emotional phenomena depends to an important degree upon one's level of analysis: The deeper the level, the larger the generality (Mesquita et al., 1997). What is usually translated into English as "shame" differs strongly in social role and behavioral implications between Western and Arab cultures; yet both flow from a similar sensitivity to being socially accepted and involve a similar motivation to correct one's deviations from acceptance. But again, they strongly diverge in what represents such deviations and how to correct for them. Cultural prescriptions and models provide such shaping, and it may even shape the motivation to such an extent that the emotions are not recognizably similar (Mesquita, 2003). Both symbolic capacities and social interactions penetrate every phenomenon, its occasions for appearing, and its duration. It largely remains to explore how far these penetrations can go, and what the implications of cultural differences are.

THE FUNCTIONS OF EMOTIONS

The negative aspects of emotions dominated earlier theorizing in both philosophy and psychology. For Aquinas, most emotions belonged to the capital sins. For Kant, emotions represented illnesses of the mind ("*Krankheiten des Gemüts*"). Several early 20th-century authors considered emotions to be "states of functional decortication" or of neural disorganization (e.g., Claparède, 1928; Hebb, 1949).

In contemporary theorizing, the tides have turned, mainly under the influence of evolutionary interpretations. Emotions are largely viewed as adaptively useful, or at least as having been so in the evolutionary past. The functional perspective now dominates.

Considering the evidence for phylogenetic origin and continuity, this functional perspective on emotions is plausible. It is also plausible because of the wide range of likely functions of emotions—wider than dealing very directly with individual or species survival or reproductive fitness. Joy can be understood as motivating readiness for novel exploits and expanding competences (Fredrickson & Cohn, Chapter 48, this volume). Anger, shame, guilt-feeling, and sympathy are powerful regulators of social interaction (Hoffman, Chapter 27, this volume; Fischer & Manstead, Chapter 28, this volume). Sadness may serve disengagement from attachments after personal loss. Irrational-seeming emotions like compassion

and desire for revenge serve adaptive purposes: They represent one's commitment, and signal others that one may act upon them; they thereby outweigh occasional costs in short-term interaction (Frank, 1988).

Evolutionary origins may mean that emotions are now mere obsolete remnants, since the original adaptive problems have waned (e.g., nonhuman predators) or rationally devised methods for dealing with such problems are now available (e.g., precision bombing). Energy mobilization by sympathetic arousal may be wasteful, now that rationally guided mental actions can be instigated. However, by and large, emotions and emotional actions are still generally adaptive in about the original sense. Love still drives sexual reproduction; intimacy is still profitable for child care and social support; fear still motivates prudence; anger still promotes our interests and may discourage rivals. Expressive behaviors, it can likewise be argued, still serve to strengthen relations (e.g., smiling), to discourage offenses (e.g., bracing, shouting, readying for a fight), and to protect one's body (e.g., ducking and closing one's eyes). Considerable amounts of work have gone into generating plausible functional hypotheses and assembling evidence (Frijda & Tcherkassof, 1997; Scherer, 1992; Keltner & Busswell, 1997).

Many emotions and emotional behaviors are, moreover, functional in a somewhat different sense. They may not be adaptive in promoting survival, and this may not have been what made them come into existence—but they do have effects on oneself and on others that keep them going. Joy is an obvious example; it may not help, but it is nice. Similarly, positive excitement and curiosity keep boredom at bay and keep one's competences active. Grief may not have any direct advantage, but its anticipation keeps people together. It helps to know that one will be missed when the time has come.

One needs to be cautious with functional interpretations, though. They are easily found, and the evolutionary perspective almost forces searching for them. Anger? Small wonder if it is innate, since it helps in protecting one's territory and offspring. Grief? It may well serve to detach oneself from lost attachments. Apathy in grief? Small wonder again; it saves expending energy that would be useless after the loss. Heart rate increase in fear? It was obviously useful when the emotion developed under threat of rivals and predators, and when one had to be always ready to climb a tree; although its net profit even then can be doubted (Arnold, 1960). Aversion to pictures of blood and mutilation? It obviously serves prudence, and thus survival (Bradley et al., 2001). But does it? It might hinder the process of keeping one's enemies off.

In fact, in the ancient adaptational environment, no observer was around to gauge the various benefits against the costs that anger, apathy, the wear caused by heart rate increase, and fear of the sight of blood might have entailed. Evolutionary emotion hypotheses rarely examine such implications or possible alternative, more dynamic explanations. Emotional phenomena may indeed have originated as mere "spandrels"—chance offshoots of quite different potentials (Gould & Lewontin, 1979). Anger, as I have indicated, might largely have emerged as a by-product of provisions for power deployment that developed for cracking nuts; moral disgust may stem from a pre-adaptation for ejecting foul substances (Rozin, 1999).

Functional advantages of emotions can readily be thought of; that does not make these advantages actually occur, nor do they actually explain the emotions' origins. Grief may not help anything at all. Grief of loss may be similar to pain in a phantom limb: Pain generally is useful, but not all pain is. Depression may be an offshoot when all objects worth striving for have dropped away, and exhaustion has set in because of fruitless efforts to regain them; Weiss, Glazer, and Poherecky (1976) opposed this hypothesis to Seligman's learned helplessness hypothesis. Emotional shock may just represent disorganization due to sudden impact that cannot be managed; that is how Dumas (1984) and Hebb (1949) interpreted it. There is no doubt that emotions, by and large, fulfill profitable functions, but one should not fall prey to the Panglossian fallacy (Gould & Lewontin, 1979). Pangloss, as readers may recall, was the philosopher in Voltaire's *Candide* who, upon every misfortune, echoed Leibniz's dictum that we live in the best of all possible worlds. By now we know that we do not. Many emotional events are simply beyond human and animal coping resources. Such resources are of necessity limited in an 80-kilogram organism that has to be operational after only a 9-month gestation. Disturbance of optimal functioning can just be dysfunctional.

And, as noted, emotions that in principle represent functional provisions are often disadvantageous or outright harmful. Emotions can cause suboptimal action. In panic, people press through narrow exits; stage fright spoils performance; nervousness spoils precision of movement; rage may lead to childish behavior and destroy social harmony (De Waal, 1996). Parrott (2001) has convincingly shown that whether or not emotions are functional depends critically on the adequacy of the appraisals that led to these emotions, on the choice and control of behavior that is motivated by the emotions, and on adequately evaluating the impact on others of both the behaviors and one's feelings.

In short, a functional perspective on emotions should not lose sight of the limits within which this perspective holds.

EMOTION AND COGNITION

Traditionally, emotion and cognition have been considered different faculties. They have been put in opposition; so have feeling and thinking. Pondering and raging would seem to constitute opposite ends of a continuum.

Contemporary psychology tends to consider these oppositions problematic. The contrasts tend to dissolve upon analysis of how intimately information processing and acting, reacting emotionally and appraising emotional meanings, and goal setting and pursuing impulsive aims and desires are intertwined. Oppositions dissolve at lower levels of analysis, when scrutiny of processes replaces categorical distinctions.

The emotion–cognition distinction has frequently been confounded with that between conscious and nonconscious information processing. The distinctions are, however, orthogonal (Clore, Storbeck, Robinson, & Centerbar, 2005); I return to the latter one below. But the problems in giving an account of information processing in emotion are considerable, because most of this processing cannot be analyzed in the way that the processing of propositional, discursive information can. Cognitive psychology has invented representational tools such as schemas, cognitive networks, and symbolic representations, and ultimately abstract representations in "mentalese." These tools do not appear appropriate for information that operates in emotion processes. The term "intuition" is often used (Arnold, 1960). "Appraisal" is contrasted with "knowledge" (Lazarus, 1991)—a distinction needed because of the central problem that so much information that is in principle relevant to emotional arousal often fails to arouse, and knowledge that shows events to be neutral still does not prevent emotional arousal. Tools for understanding the processes involved in rendering information emotionally efficacious have begun emerging only slowly and recently. One consists of recourse to concrete and mode-specific representations and their networks (Barsalou, 1999). Another is recognizing the important role of motor representations, both as underlying identification of emotional meanings in the behavior of other individuals, and as underlying action programs, action representations, and action foresight (e.g., Gallese, 2005; Meltzoff, 2002). This is one of the areas that gave rise to extensive recognition of what has been termed "embodied cognition" (Niedenthal, Barsalou, Ric, & Krauth-Gruber, 2005). Still another tool, not used yet in understanding emotions, is representation of processes over time, as is being developed in the description and analysis of human movement.

Besides the problems of representing emotional processes and information are those that concern the structures of the involved information. These structures range from simple stimulus–response transductions (which imply representations of stimulus "keys" that fit representations of particular response "locks"), to elaborate multimodal networks of associations, and on to abstract meanings and inferences. Massive research over the last two or three decades has demonstrated how very elementary information can on occasion be emotionally effective (e.g., Zajonc, 1980). Research has also shown how complex emotional information often is (Barsalou, 1999), even when it does not immediately appear to be so because it operates nonconsciously (Clore et al., 2005).

Close to the contrast between emotion and thinking has been that between emotion and reason. "Reason" has at least two different meanings: that of using complex thought processes such as logical inference, and that of using means–end relationships to reach optimal problem solutions. The first meaning contrasts

reason with the intuitive and impulsive processes; the second contrasts it with the often harmful and disorganizing aspects of emotions, and their command of primitive responses. Both contrasts have been attenuated in modern theory. The first is weakened by recognition of the complex appraisals that underlie most emotions. These appraisals derive from standards of comparison, cultural values, and thwarting or fulfillment of expectancies and concerns. All are involved in elicitation of social emotions such as shame and regret. The second contrast is weakened by recognition of the "rationality of emotions" (de Sousa, 1987): recognition of emotions as in principle reasonable and functionally appropriate responses to events as appraised. Emotions also appear as conditions for rational choice (Damasio, 1994; de Sousa, 1987; Frank, 1988; Solomon, 1993, 2004), because they respond to a wider array of relevant variables.

And nevertheless, both contrasts between emotion and rationality remain. The emotions aroused by simple stimuli may override further cognitions, notably those relevant to consequences that are more remote in time. Emotionally effective beliefs may disagree with simultaneously held, more solidly founded beliefs. People with spider phobias often recognize that spiders are harmless, and still fear them. Dysfunctional emotions have been discussed previously. As de Sousa (1987) has argued, emotions possess only "local rationality." But the contrast is perhaps not really between emotions and rationality, but between what does elicit emotions and what could elicit emotions if and when "rational" information were to acquire emotional appeal.

EMOTION EXPERIENCE

One major problem has hovered over the field of emotion study, and it still does: that of conscious feelings. What are they, and what role do they play with regard to emotional behavior and the conduct of life?

It was not too long ago that "emotions" were defined as particular states of consciousness that causally determine bodily and behavioral responses. That time has changed. In the current literature, one frequently comes across the view that feelings are mere epiphenomena of neural and bodily processes. Neural and bodily processes come first, and can proceed entirely or largely without the intervention of feelings. This view has solid support in the conviction that all conscious phenomena find their roots in neural processes, reflect neural processes, and depend on neural processes. Also, there is the fairly general conviction that physical causal sequences are closed. Neural processes may give rise to conscious experience, but it is hard to conceive that conscious experience might influence neural processes in turn.

Yet this view contradicts everyday experience. It does so outside the domain of emotions. Although there is appreciable "blindsight"—the name given to perception without conscious awareness—the blind-sighted person is severely handicapped (Weiskrantz, 1997). It also contradicts experience within the emotion domain. One refuses to enter some dark alleyway because it looks threatening, breaks off a friendship with someone who has made one very angry, and goes to great lengths to please someone who provides warmth and joy. One decides to go to the movies because that spells fun.

Much of such everyday experience may well be illusionary. One often acts for other reasons than the feelings one is aware of or constructs. Psychoanalytic exploration found evidence that this is so; contemporary experiments have confirmed it. So, everyday experience notwithstanding, feelings might still be useless. The general theoretical argument for this conclusion has been mentioned: How could feelings possibly influence neurons? One can state this as a problem, rather than as an argument. It has been called "the" hard problem of consciousness (Chalmers, 1996): how to conceive of the relationship between body and consciousness. It is the problem that comes clearest to the fore in emotions, where feelings, but also cognitions, appear to influence the body and get information back from the latter. It is the problem that Descartes was the first to truly recognize, in his *Passions de l'Âme*. It is still entirely unsolved, recourse to Spinoza (Damasio, 2003) notwithstanding.

There is good reason, other than everyday experience, not to be satisfied with considering feelings epiphenomenal and irrelevant for behavior. That view makes feeling into an evolutionary oddity. It came about—when? with the advent of humans? with the advent of primates? with the advent of vertebrates?—with-

out any adaptive advantage. It is unlikely. This means that research has to continue on the possible effects of conscious feelings, and on how such effects can occur if they exist.

What created the doubts about the function of feelings has been twofold. First, there has been the force of James's argument that feelings are the "readouts" from bodily emotional reactions, which therefore must have been present before the feelings. Second, there is the massive evidence that affective reactions can occur without the subject's being aware of their objects, of the emotionally relevant attributes, or even of the reactions' having taken place (Bargh, 1997; Berridge, 2004; Moors & De Houwer, 2006; Zajonc, 1980).

Yet the range of emotional reactions shown to occur nonconsciously is as yet limited. It includes nonconsciously induced liking for neutral stimuli, enhanced preferences for liked substances or stimulus objects, nonconscious imitation of behaviors, and delayed extinction of conditioned physiological arousal. To what extent affective influences may unwittingly determine strivings, goal-directed behavior, and the conduct of life remains to be demonstrated.

Examining the role of conscious feelings in emotions is rendered difficult because of the various ways in which feelings can occur. Conscious experience occurs in various modes: reportable or not reportable, diffuse and global or articulate and amenable to verbal description. The several modes have given rise to sharp disagreements about the nature of emotional feelings: irreducible *qualia*, sensory body sensations, central body state and position representations, action representations, or perceptions of external events with emotional meanings (Frijda, 2005, 2007a; Lambie & Marcel, 2003). It can be argued that all can occur, depending on circumstances and attentional attitude; if so, this has perhaps given rise to needless disagreements.

CONCLUDING REMARKS

Will the perennial problems in the psychology of emotion remain? Such problems in various fields often cannot be resolved, since they reflect either different world views or our limited human capacity for conceptualization. The wave–particle dilemma in physics would seem to be something of the latter sort; the contrast between social constructivism and explanation by laws and mechanisms something of the former. But perhaps the scope of the problems in emotion psychology can be narrowed somewhat by insight into the relationships between proposed solutions for the various problems.

As I have remarked, psychological explanations of emotional phenomena are being sought at different levels. Answers to several questions may seem incompatible when they are answers to questions being sought at different levels of explanation or at different levels of the phenomena.

The study of emotion may advance, I think, when Dennett's (1987) level distinctions are better heeded, and when his functional or psychological level receives more attention. In current analyses of emotion antecedents, little is being said about what constitutes a reinforcement and why; Schroeder (2004) has courageously presented a single effort. Only preliminary endeavors are being made at constructing models of appraisal processes and of the inner structure of concerns, both of which play such a pivotal role in explaining emotions. As far as I know, for instance, there exist no detailed hypotheses at the functional level of how innate affective stimuli evoke affect. I have no idea how sugar evokes not only the sensation of sweetness but also the experience of pleasantness, even granted that somehow opoids may become active. Ultimately, intentional phenomena such as experiences, desires, and goals should be clarified in terms of subpersonal, functionally defined processes. But such clarifications are scarce (however, see Metzinger, 2003). As a consequence, jumps are being made from the intentional level to the hardware or neurophysiological level, and vice versa. Fear arousal is mediated by the amygdalae, but how exactly do the amygdalae do that? We sure like certain things, but how does that proceed?

All this is important for advances in emotion research, because there is no guarantee that categories of analysis at one level will project onto coherent categories at another level. There is no guarantee that emotions as defined experientially or behaviorally will all involve one mechanism, or one coherent set of mechanisms. The mechanisms of fear of failure may have little in common with the mechanisms of fear of the unknown or of spiders, except that they all share the final common pathways of ef-

forts to escape or behavioral inhibition. That all stimuli evoking emotions are in some way appraised does not imply the existence of one single coherent appraisal mechanism. And so on.

How explanations at different levels are related depends on the findings at different levels, of course. It would be profitable if researchers in different areas and on different levels talked and listened more to each other. It would be profitable if they knew better what is happening at other areas and levels. Experimental investigators of emotions often know little of the social and cultural psychology of emotions, and vice versa. Such limitations of knowledge painfully restrict the range of emotion elicitors considered in the explanatory hypotheses. Students of the neuropsychology of emotion often know little of the contemporary psychology of emotion. They sometimes write as if the paradigm of what causes emotions is an electric shock, and as if the paradigm of motivation is thirst or hunger, or something weird like "survival." To most psychological researchers, the limbic area is merely somewhere in the brain, and the amygdala is an amorphous blob of tissue. There is no real reason why all of this should remain so. To facilitate communication across disciplines, of course, is one of the main purposes of this handbook.

REFERENCES

Ainslie, G. (2001). *Breakdown of will*. Cambridge, UK: Cambridge University Press.

Arnold, M. B. (1960). *Emotion and personality* (Vol. I). New York: Columbia University Press.

Arnold, M. B. (1970). Perennial problems in the field of emotion. In M. B. Arnold (Ed.), *Feelings and emotions: The Loyola Symposium* (pp. 169–186). New York: Academic Press.

Bargh, J. A. (1997). The automaticity of everyday life. In R. S. Wyer (Ed.), *Advances in social cognition* (Vol. 10, pp. 1–61). Mahwah, NJ: Erlbaum.

Barrett, L. F. (2005). Feeling is perceiving: Core affect and conceptualization in the experience of emotion. In L. F. Barrett, P. M. Niedenthal, & P. Winkielman (Eds.), *Emotion and consciousness* (pp. 255–286). New York: Guilford Press.

Barsalou, L. W. (1999). Perceptual symbol systems. *Behavioral and Brain Sciences, 22,* 577–660.

Bentley, M. (1928). Is "emotion" more than a chapter heading? In M. L. Reymert (Ed.), *Feelings and emotions: The Wittenberg Symposium* (pp. 17–23). Worcester, MA: Clark University Press.

Berridge, K. C. (2004). Unfelt affect and irrational desire: A view from the brain. In A. R. S. Manstead, N. H. Frijda, & A. Fischer (Eds.), *Feelings and emotions: The Amsterdam Symposium* (pp. 243–262). Cambridge, UK: Cambridge University Press.

Bindra, D. (1959). *Motivation: A systematic reinterpretation.* New York: Ronald Press.

Bouton, M. E. (2005). Behavior systems and the contextual control of anxiety, fear, and panic. In L. F. Barrett, P. M. Niedenthal, & P. Winkielman (Eds.), *Emotion and consciousness* (pp. 205–230). New York: Guilford Press.

Bradley, M. M., Codispoti, M., Cuthbert, B. N., & Lang, P. J. (2001). Emotion and motivation I: Defensive and appetitive reactions in picture processing. *Emotion, 1,* 276–298.

Buck, R. (1999). Biological affects: A typology. *Psychological Review, 106,* 301–336.

Buss, D. M. (1994). *The evolution of desire.* New York: Basic Books.

Camras, L. A. (2000). Surprise!: Facial expressions can be coordinative motor structures. In M. D. Lewis & I. Granic (Eds.), *Emotion, development, and self-organization* (pp. 100–124). New York: Cambridge University Press.

Cassirer, E. (1908). *Substanzbegriff und funcktionsbegriff* [Substance concepts and function concepts]. Leipzig, Germany: B. Cassirer.

Cayrou, G. (1924). *Le français classique. Lexique de la langue française du dix-septième siècle* (2nd ed.). Paris: Dedier.

Chalmers, D. (1996). *The conscious mind: In search of a fundamental theory.* New York: Oxford University Press.

Claparède, E. (1928). Emotions and feelings. In M. L. Reymert (Ed.), *Feelings and emotions: The Wittenberg Symposium* (pp. 124–139). Worcester, MA: Clark University Press.

Clore, G. L., Storbeck, J., Robinson, M. D., & Centerbar, D. (2005). The seven deadly sins of research on affect. In L. F. Barrett, P. M. Niedenthal, & P. Winkielman (Eds.), *Emotion and consciousness* (pp. 384–408). New York: Guilford Press.

Damasio, A. (1994). *Descartes' error: Emotion, reason, and the human brain.* New York: Putnam.

Damasio, A. (2003). *Looking for Spinoza: Joy, sorrow, and the feeling brain.* London: Heinemann.

Dennett, D. C. (1987). *The intentional stance.* Cambridge, MA: MIT Press.

de Sousa, R. (1987). *The rationality of emotion.* Cambridge, MA: MIT Press.

Descartes, R. (1970). *Les passions de l'âme* [*The passions of the soul*]. Paris: Vrin. (Original work published 1649)

De Waal, F. B. M. (1996). *Good natured.* Cambridge, MA: Harvard University Press.

Duffy, E. (1941). An explanation of "emotional" phenomena without the use of the concept "emotion." *Journal of General Psychology, 25,* 283–293.

Dumas, G. (1948). *La vie affective.* Paris: Presses Universitaires de France.

Ekman, P. (1992). An argument for basic emotions. *Cognition and Emotion, 6,* 169–200.

Ekman, P. (1994). Strong evidence for universals in facial expression: A reply to Russell's mistaken critique. *Psychological Bulletin, 115,* 268–287.

Ellsworth, P. C., & Scherer, K. R. (2003). Appraisal processes in emotion. In R. Davidson, K. R. Scherer, & H. H. Goldsmith (Eds.), *Handbook of the affective sciences* (pp. 572–596). Mahwah, NJ: Erlbaum.

Elster, J. (1999a). *Alchemies of the mind.* Cambridge, UK: Cambridge University Press.

Elster, J. (1999b). *Strong feelings.* Cambridge, MA: MIT Press.

Frank, R. H. (1988). *Passions within reason: The strategic role of the emotions.* New York: Norton.

Frijda, N. H. (1986). *The emotions.* Cambridge, UK: Cambridge University Press.

Frijda, N. H. (2005). Emotion experience. *Cognition and Emotion, 19,* 473–498.

Frijda, N. H. (2007a). *The laws of emotion.* Mahwah, NJ: Erlbaum.

Frijda, N. H. (Ed.). (2007b). Klaus Scherer's article on "What are emotions?": Comments. *Social Science Information, 46,* 381–443.

Frijda, N. H., Mesquita, B., Sonnemans, J., & Van Goozen, S. (1991). The duration of affective phenomena, or emotions, sentiments and passions. In K. T. Strongman (Ed.), *International review of studies on emotion* (Vol. 1, pp. 187–225). Chichester, UK: Wiley.

Frijda, N. H., & Tcherkassof, A. (1997). Facial expressions as modes of action readiness. In J. A. Russell & J. M. Fernández-Dols (Eds.), *The psychology of facial expression* (pp. 78–102). Cambridge, UK: Cambridge University Press.

Gallese, V. (2005). Embodied simulation: From neurons to phenomenal experience. *Phenomenology and the Cognitive Sciences, 4,* 23–48.

Gould, S. J., & Lewontin, R. C. (1979). The spandrels of San Marco and the Panglossian paradigm: A critique of the adaptationist programme. *Proceedings of the Royal Society of London, 205,* 581–598.

Gray, J. A. (1987). *The psychology of fear and stress* (2nd ed.). Cambridge, UK: Cambridge University Press.

Harré, R., & Parrott, W. G. (Eds.). (1996). *The emotions: Social, cultural and biological dimensions.* Thousand Oaks, CA: Sage.

Hebb, D. O. (1949). *The organization of behavior.* New York, Wiley.

Hull, C. L. (1953). *A behavior system: An introduction to behavior theory concerning the individual organism.* New Haven, CT: Yale University Press.

Hupka, R. B., Lenton, A. P., & Hutchison, K. A. (1999). Universal development of emotion categories in natural language. *Journal of Personality and Social Psychology, 77,* 247–278.

Izard, C. E. (1977). *Human emotions*. New York: Plenum Press.

James, W. (1884). What is an emotion? *Mind*, 9, 188–205.

Keltner, D., & Buswell, B. N. (1997). Embarrassment: Its distinct form and appeasement functions. *Psychological Bulletin*, 122, 250–270.

Kenny, A. (1963). *Action, emotion and will*. London: Routledge & Kegan Paul.

Kleinginna, P. R., & Kleinginna, A. M. (1981). A categorized list of emotion definitions, with suggestions for a consensual definition. *Motivation and Emotion*, 5, 345–379.

Lambie, J., & Marcel, A. (2002). Consciousness and emotion experience: A theoretical framework. *Psychological Review*, 109, 219–259.

Landis, C., & Hunt, W. A. (1932). Adrenalin and emotion. *Psychological Review*, 39, 467–485.

Lazarus, R. S. (1991). *Emotion and adaptation*. New York: Oxford University Press.

LeDoux, J. (1996). *The emotional brain*. New York: Simon & Schuster.

Levenson, R. W. (2003). Autonomic specificity and emotion. In R. J. Davidson, K. R. Scherer, & H. H. Goldsmith (Eds.), *Handbook of affective sciences* (pp. 212–224). New York: Oxford University Press.

Lewis, M. (1996). Self-organizing cognitive appraisals. *Cognition and Emotion*, 10, 1–26.

Lewis, M. D. (2005). Bridging emotion theory and neurobiology through dynamic system modeling. *Behavioral and Brain Sciences*, 28, 105–131.

Lutz, C. (1988). *Unnatural emotions: Everyday sentiments on a Micronesian atoll and their challenge to Western theory*. Chicago: University of Chicago Press.

Mandler, G. (1984). *Mind and body: The psychology of emotion and stress*. New York: Norton.

Mauss, M. (1957). *Essai sur le don* [*The gift*]. London: Routledge & Kegan Paul. (Original work published 1914)

McDougall, W. (1923). *Outline of psychology*. New York: Scribner.

Meltzoff, A. N. (2002). Imitation as a mechanism of social cognition: Origins of empathy, theory of mind, and the representation of action. In U. Goswami (Ed.), *Handbook of childhood cognitive development* (pp. 6–25). Oxford: Blackwell.

Mesquita, B. (2003). Emotions as dynamic cultural phenomena. In R. J. Davidson, K. R. Scherer, & H. Goldsmith (Eds.), *Handbook of affective sciences* (pp. 871–890). New York: Oxford University Press.

Mesquita, B., Frijda, N. H., & Scherer, K. R. (1997). Culture and emotion. In P. R. Dasen & T. S. Saraswathi (Eds.), *Handbook of cross-cultural psychology* (Vol. 2, pp. 255–298). Boston: Allyn & Bacon.

Metzinger, T. (2003). *Being no one: The self-model theory of subjectivity*. Cambridge, MA: MIT Press.

Moors, A., & De Houwer, J. (2006). Automaticity: A theoretical and conceptual analysis. *Psychological Bulletin*, 132, 297–326.

Mowrer, O. H. (1960). *Learning theory and behavior*. New York: Wiley.

Niedenthal, P. M., Barsalou, L. W., Ric, F., & Krauth-Gruber, S. (2005). Embodiment in the acquisition and use of emotion knowledge. In L. F. Barrett, P. M. Niedenthal, & P. Winkielman (Eds.), *Emotion and consciousness* (pp. 21–50). New York: Guilford Press.

Nussbaum, M. C. (2001). *Upheavals of thought: The intelligence of emotions*. New York: Cambridge University Press.

Oatley, K. (1992). *Best laid schemes: The psychology of emotions*. Cambridge, UK: Cambridge University Press.

Oatley, K., & Duncan, E. (1994). The experience of emotions in daily life. *Cognition and Emotion*, 8, 369–382.

Öhman, A., & Mineka, S. (2001). Fears, phobias, and preparedness: Toward an evolved module of fear and fear learning. *Psychological Review*, 108, 483–522.

Ortony, A., Clore, G., & Collins, A. (1988). *The cognitive structure of emotions*. Cambridge, UK: Cambridge University Press.

Ortony, A., & Turner, T. (1990). What's basic about basic emotions? *Psychological Review*, 97, 315–331.

Parrott, W. G. (2001). Implications of dysfunctional emotions for understanding how emotions function. *Review of General Psychology*, 5, 180–186.

Plutchik, R. (2003). *Emotions and life*. Washington, DC: American Psychological Association.

Rimé, B. (2005). *Emotion et expression*. Paris: Presses Universitaires de France.

Rolls, E. T. (2005). *Emotion explained*. Oxford: Oxford University Press.

Rothbaum, F. M., Weisz, J. R., Pott, M., Miyake, K., & Morelli, G. (2000). Attachment and culture: Security in the United States and Japan. *American Psychologist*, 55, 1093–1104.

Rozin, P. (1999). Preadaptation and the puzzles and properties of pleasure. In D. Kahneman, E. Diener, & N. Schwarz (Eds.), *Well-being: The foundations of hedonic psychology. Scientific perspectives on enjoyment and suffering* (pp. 109–133). New York: Russell Sage Foundation.

Russell, J. A. (1991). Culture and the categorization of emotions. *Psychological Bulletin*, 110, 426–450.

Russell, J. A. (2003). Core affect and the psychological construction of emotion. *Psychological Review*, 110, 145–172.

Scherer, K. R. (1992). What does facial expression express? In K. T. Strongman (Ed.), *International review of studies on emotion* (Vol. 2, pp. 139–165). Chichester, UK: Wiley.

Scherer, K. R. (2000). Emotions as episodes of subsystem synchronization driven by nonlinear appraisal processes. In M. D. Lewis & I. Granic (Eds.), *Emotion, development, and self-organization* (pp. 70–99). New York: Cambridge University Press.

Scherer, K. R. (2001). Appraisal considered as a process of multilevel sequential checking In K. R. Scherer, A. Schorr, & T. Johnstone (Eds.), *Appraisal processes in emotion: Theory, methods, research* (pp. 92–120). New York: Oxford University Press.

Scherer, K. R. (2005). What are emotions? And how can they be measured? *Social Science Information, 44,* 695–729.

Schroeder, T. (2004). *Three faces of desire.* Oxford: Oxford University Press.

Shand, A. F. (1920). *The foundations of character: A study of the emotions and sentiments.* London: Macmillan.

Shaver, P., Wu, S., & Schwartz, J. C. (1992). Cross-cultural similarities and differences in emotion and its representation: A prototype approach. In M. Clark (Ed.), *Review of personality and social psychology* (Vol. 13, pp. 175–212). Newbury Park, CA: Sage.

Shweder, R. A., & Haidt, J. (2000). The cultural psychology of the emotions: Ancient and new. In M. Lewis & J. M. Haviland-Jones (Eds.), *Handbook of emotions* (2nd ed., pp. 397–416). New York: Guilford Press.

Sloman, A. (1987). Motives, mechanisms and emotions. *Cognition and Emotion, 1,* 217–234.

Smith, C. A., & Scott, H. H. (1997). A componential approach to the meaning of facial expressions. In J. A. Russell & J.-M. Fernández-Dols (Eds.), *The psychology of facial expression* (pp. 229–254). Cambridge, UK: Cambridge University Press.

Solomon, R. C. (1993). *The passions* (2nd ed.). Indianapolis, IN: Hackett.

Solomon, R. C. (2004). *Not passion's slave.* New York: Oxford University Press.

Spinoza, B. (1989). *Ethics.* (G. H. R. Parkinson, Trans.). London: Dent. (Original work published 1677)

Stein, N., & Trabasso, T. (1992). The organization of emotional experience: Creating links between emotion, thinking, and intentional action. *Cognition and Emotion, 6,* 225–244.

Stemmler, G. (2003). Methodological considerations in the psychophysiological study of emotion. In R. J. Davidson, K. R. Scherer, & H. H. Goldsmith (Eds.), *Handbook of affective sciences* (pp. 225–255). New York: Oxford University Press.

Thelen, E. (1995). Motor development: A new synthesis. *American Psychologist, 50,* 79–95.

Tomkins, S. S. (1962). *Affect, imagery and consciousness: Vol. 1. The positive affects.* New York: Springer.

Wallon, H. (1942). *De l'acte à la pensée.* Paris: Flammarion.

Watson, J. B. (1929). *Psychology from the standpoint of a behaviorist* (3rd ed.). Philadelphia: Lippincott.

Weiskrantz, L. (1997). *Consciousness lost and found: A neuropsychological exploration.* Oxford: Oxford University Press.

Weiss, J. M., Glazer, H. I., & Poherecky, L. A. (1976). Coping behavior and neurochemical changes: An alternative explanation for the original "learned helplessness" experiments. In A. Serban & A. Kling (Eds.), *Animal models in human psychobiology* (pp. 141–173). New York: Plenum Press.

Wierzbicka, A. (1995). Everyday conceptions of emotion: A semantic perspective. In J. A. Russell, J.-M. Fernández-Dols, A. S. R. Manstead, & J. Wellenkamp (Eds.), *Everyday conceptions of emotion* (pp. 17–48). Dordrecht, The Netherlands: Kluwer.

Zajonc, R. B. (1980). Thinking and feeling: Preferences need no inferences. *American Psychologist, 35,* 151–175.

CHAPTER 6

The Clinical Application of Emotion in Psychotherapy

LESLIE S. GREENBERG

This chapter addresses the emerging focus on emotion in psychotherapy. Given that emotion is seen as information (i.e., as signaling the significance of a situation to a person's well-being), and that affect regulation is seen as a key human motivation, it has become clear that emotion needs to be focused on, validated, and worked with directly in therapy to promote emotional change (Greenberg, 2002; Samoilov & Goldfried, 2000; Fosha, 2000). The idea that accessing and exploring painful emotions, within the context of a secure therapeutic relationship, makes one feel better has been widely held by several schools of psychotherapy (Freud, 1915/1957; Rogers, 1951; Perls, 1969), but it has been difficult to prove. However, over the last decade, newer therapeutic approaches that treat affect as a primary target of intervention within the context of an empathic relationship have been developed and tested. In this chapter, results of evidence-based treatment studies that show evidence for effectiveness of emotion-focused treatment of mood disorders, personality disorders, and trauma are reviewed briefly. Principles of emotion assessment and emotional change are then discussed. These provide a map for differential intervention with emotion by showing that different classes of emotions in therapy benefit from different types of interventions—ranging from awareness of adaptive emotions, through regulation of dysregulated emotions, to transformation of maladaptive emotions. The chapter concludes with a discussion of different methods of activating new emotional responses to change habitual problematic emotional responses.

EVIDENCE-BASED TREATMENT

A number of treatment approaches that focus on painful emotions have been demonstrated in randomized clinical trials to be effective (Elliott, Greenberg, & Lietaer, 2004; Greenberg & Pascual-Leone, 2006; Whelton, 2004). A manualized form of emotion-focused therapy (EFT) for depression has been found to be highly effective in treating depression in three separate studies (Greenberg & Watson, 1998;

Goldman, Greenberg, & Angus, 2006; Watson, Gordon, Stermac, Kalogerakos, & Steckley, 2003). In these studies, EFT was found to be as effective as or more effective than either a purely relational empathic treatment or a form of cognitive-behavioral therapy (CBT). Both the treatments with which it was compared were themselves also found to be highly effective in reducing depression, but EFT was found to be more effective in both reducing interpersonal problems and promoting change in symptoms than the purely relational treatment. It also was found to be highly effective in preventing relapse.

The objective of EFT is to access and restructure the habitual maladaptive emotional states that are seen as the source of the depression. This involves accessing feelings of shame-based worthlessness, anxious dependence, powerlessness, abandonment, and invalidation, and transforming these through accessing adaptive emotions (such as healthy grief and empowering anger), as well as reflecting on emotional experience to create new meaning and develop new narratives. This process of emotional change is aided by the use of specific therapeutic techniques that help stimulate both the arousal and processing of emotion. Various experiential interventions—such as two-chair dialogue in response to in-session statements of self-critical conflicts, empty-chair dialogue in response to in-session statements of unresolved feelings toward a significant other, and focusing on bodily felt meaning in response to an unclear felt sense—are used to engage patients in emotion processing in session.

Short-term dynamic therapy, which works on overcoming defenses and treats affect phobia by exposure to dreaded emotion, has been found to be effective in treating personality disorders in two studies (Winston et al., 1994; Svartberg, Stiles, & Seltzer, 2004). EFT for adult survivors of childhood abuse, which uses empathy plus empty-chair work and involves the arousal and processing of painful emotions, has been found effective in treating abuse (Paivio & Nieuwenhuis, 2001). Emotionally focused couple therapy (Greenberg & Johnson, 1988; Johnson, 1996), which involves partners' revealing their underlying attachment- and identity-related vulnerable feelings to each other, has been found to be effective in treating couples' distress (Johnson, Hunsley, Greenberg, & Schindler, 1999). In addition, versions of CBT based on exposure to imaginal

stimuli have been shown to be effective for posttraumatic stress disorder (PTSD) and other anxiety disorders (Borkovec, Alcaine, & Behar, 2004; Shapiro, 1999). Finally, therapy based on an avoidance theory in which worry is understood as a cognitive response that orients individuals to a threat, while insulating them from the immediacy of their emotional experience, has recently gained support (Borkovec et al., 2004).

A recent study examining the therapists' stance in interpersonal therapy (IPT) and CBT for depression showed the importance of focusing on emotion, regardless of orientation. This study (Coombs, Coleman, & Jones, 2002) found that collaborative emotional exploration (which occurred significantly more frequently in IPT) was found to relate positively to outcome in both forms of therapy, whereas educative/directive process (which was more frequent in CBT) had no relationship to outcome. Helping people overcome their avoidance of emotions, focusing collaboratively on emotions, and exploring them in therapy thus appears to be important in therapeutic change, whichever therapeutic orientation is employed. What is needed now is a more differentiated understanding of how to work with emotion. A differential approach to assessment and intervention has recently emerged.

DIFFERENTIAL EMOTION ASSESSMENT AND INTERVENTION

In assessing and working with emotion in therapy, it is helpful to make certain distinctions between different types of emotional experiences and expressions, which require different types of in-session interventions. This involves differentiating between "primary" emotions and "secondary" or "reactive" emotions, and between "adaptive" and "maladaptive" emotional experiences (Greenberg, 2002). Primary emotions are people's first, gut-level emotional responses to situations. These responses need to be accessed and assessed for whether they provide adaptive information and the capacity to organize action, or whether they are maladaptive. Maladaptive emotions are learned responses that are not appropriate to current situations and thus are no longer adaptive; these emotions need to be regulated and transformed. Secondary emotions are those responses that are secondary to other, more primary internal processes and may be defenses against these, such as feeling ashamed of one's sadness or hopeless when angry. Secondary maladaptive emotions need to be explored to access their more primary cognitive or emotional generators. These distinctions between different types of emotions thus provide clinicians with a map for differential intervention with emotions.

PRINCIPLES OF WORKING WITH EMOTION

Outcome and process research findings point toward emotional processing as centrally important to good therapy, but what good processing is actually remains to be elucidated. Emotional insight, catharsis, awareness, and exposure have all been put forward as explanations of the role of emotion in change, but there is still not a comprehensive, empirically based understanding of how emotion and its processing lead to change. The following five principles provide an empirically based understanding of emotional change processes in clinical change: (1) increasing awareness of emotion, (2) expressing emotion, (3) enhancing emotion regulation, (4) reflecting on emotion, and (5) transforming emotion (Greenberg, 2002; Greenberg & Watson, 2006).

Emotion Awareness

The first and most general goal of emotional change is for clients to become aware of their emotions in general and their primary adaptive emotions in particular. Increased emotion awareness is therapeutic in a variety of ways. Becoming aware of core emotional experience and symbolizing it in words provide access to both the adaptive information and action tendency in the emotion. Labeling emotions is often a first step in problem definition. It is important to note that emotion awareness is not thinking about feeling; it involves feeling the feeling in awareness. Only once an emotion is felt does its articulation in language become an important component of its awareness.

The therapist thus needs to help clients approach, tolerate, and accept their emotions. Acceptance of emotional experience as opposed to its avoidance is the first step in awareness work. Once clients have accepted their emotions rather than avoided them, the thera-

pist then helps the clients in the utilization of emotion to improve coping. That is, clients are helped to make sense of what each emotion is telling them and to identify the goal/need/concern that it is organizing them to attain. Emotion is thus used both to inform and to move.

A measure of levels of emotion awareness has been developed by Lane and Schwartz (1992). Five such levels can be measured. In ascending order, these are physical sensations, action tendencies, single emotions, blends of emotions, and blends of blends of emotional experience (the capacity to appreciate complexity in the experiences of self and other). The dynamic interactions among phenomenal experience, establishing a representation of it, elaborating that representation (e.g., identifying the source of the emotional response), and integrating it with other cognitive processes are the fundamental processes involved in the cognitive elaboration of emotion and addressed by the levels of this measure. Scores on the measure have been found to correlate significantly with self-reported self-restraint and impulse control. Individual differences in emotion awareness have also been found to predict recovery of positive mood and decrements in ruminative thoughts following a distressing stimulus (Salovey, Mayer, Golman, Turvey, & Palfai, 1995).

Awareness of emotion also involves overcoming the avoidance of emotional experience. There is a strong human tendency to avoid or interrupt painful emotions. Normal cognitive processes often deny, distort, or interrupt emotion and transform adaptive but unpleasant emotions into dysfunctional behaviors designed to avoid feeling. Leahy (2002) has defined "emotional schemas" as cognitive structures that frame the interpretation of emotional experience and guide the strategies used in coping with emotion. He has noted that there are two fundamental coping pathways for dealing with emotion. One involves attending to and labeling emotions in a manner that accepts and normalizes them; the other pathway pathologizes some emotional experiences, and this leads to attempts to distort or avoid them (initiating guilt, frantic efforts at control, obsessive rumination, etc.). To overcome emotion avoidance, clients must first be helped to approach emotions by attending to their emotional experience. This often involves changing the cognitions governing their avoidance. Then clients must allow and tolerate being in live contact with their emotions. These two steps are consistent with notions of exposure.

Emotional Arousal and Expression

Emotional expression has recently been shown to be a unique aspect of emotional processing that predicts adjustment to breast cancer (Stanton et al., 2000). Women who coped with cancer through expressing emotion had fewer medical appointments, enhanced physical health and vigor, and decreased distress than those low in emotional expression did. Expressive coping was also related to increased quality of life for those who perceived their social environment to be highly receptive. Analyses further suggested that expressive coping enhanced the pursuit of goals, perhaps by helping clients attend to and clarify central concerns, but that this relationship was mediated by hope. Emotional arousal and its expression in therapeutic contexts thus appear to constitute a therapeutic aspect of emotional processing. Expressing emotion in therapy does not involve simply venting emotion, but rather overcoming avoidance of, strongly experiencing, and expressing previously constricted emotions.

There is a long line of evidence on the effectiveness of arousal of and exposure to previously avoided feelings as a mechanism of change. Results from a variety of studies indicate that emotional engagement (fear expression) with trauma memories during exposure in early sessions, and habituation (reduced distress) during exposure over the course of therapy, predict better outcome (Foa & Jaycox, 1999; Jaycox, Foa, & Morral, 1998). Emotional engagement with trauma memories early in therapy appears to be important in overcoming trauma. However, only a subgroup of individuals are able to engage in the exposure technique and therefore maximally benefit from therapy (Jaycox et al., 1998). Pretreatment severity of PTSD symptoms is also associated with engagement difficulties and poorer outcome. Foa, Zoellner, Feeny, Hembree, and Alvarez-Conrad (2002) have shown that although imaginal exposure, which arouses strong emotion, can exacerbate symptoms in some clients, it does this in relatively few cases, and even then this does not impede a long-term positive outcome. Overall, a chain of factors beginning with trauma symptom severity, through initial engagement in imaginal exposure, activation of the fear structure, and re-peated exposure while providing new information, appears to predict outcome (Jaycox et al., 1998).

However, studies on exposure and arousal do not take into account the importance to client change of the therapeutic relationship. In a process–outcome study evaluating EFT for adult survivors of childhood abuse (Paivio, Hall, Holowaty, Jellis, & Tran, 2001), the therapeutic alliance, initial engagement in the primary imaginal confrontation intervention, the overall dosage of this intervention (quality × frequency), and client predisposing variables all contributed to reduced global and trauma-specific symptomatology and interpersonal problems. The effect of emotional arousal in therapy also depends on the quality of the working alliance. Beutler, Clarkin, and Bongar (2000) studied several therapies, in an attempt to match patient variables with treatments. Across modalities, emotional intensity of sessions was a strong predictor of outcome, but this effect was mediated by the working alliance. Likewise, Iwakabe, Rogan, and Stalikas (2000) documented that high arousal predicted good session outcome only when there was a strong alliance.

Learning to contain and regulate strong emotions is central to adaptive emotional arousal and expression, and these skills are often lacking in people seeking therapy. The ability to regulate emotion is believed to emerge from early attachment experiences of validation, soothing, and safety, and involves attending to emotions and dampening or expressing them as appropriate. The emotional validation and empathy of the therapist seem to be particularly important in allowing clients with dysregulated emotions to learn to self-soothe and restore emotional equilibrium (Greenberg, 2002).

It is clear is that emotional arousal and expression are not always helpful or appropriate in therapy or in life, and that for some clients, training in the capacity for emotion regulation (see next section) must precede or accompany it (Greenberg, 2002). Any benefits believed to accrue from the intense expression of emotion are generally predicated on the client's overregulation (overcontrol) or suppression of emotion (Gross, 1999), but it is apparent that for some individuals with certain psychological disorders or in particular situations, emotions are under- or dysregulated (Linehan, 1993; Gross, 1999). Some support has been found for the cathartic expression of feeling in therapy, but only with certain people under specified circumstantial conditions (Pierce, Nichols, & DuBrin, 1983). Catharsis is not helpful all the time for all people. Process–outcome research on EFT for depression, however, has shown that higher expressed emotional arousal at midtreatment predicted positive treatment outcomes (Warwar, 2003). This supports the importance of expressed arousal as a key change process in these treatments. It is important also to note that this study measured *expressed* as opposed to *experienced* emotion. A follow-up study examining in-session client reports of *experienced* emotional intensity (Warwar, Greenberg, & Perepeluk, 2003) found that client reports of in-session experienced emotion were not related to positive therapeutic change. A discrepancy was observed between clients' reports of in-session *experienced* emotions and the emotions that were actually *expressed*, based on arousal ratings of videotaped therapy segments. For example, one client reported that she had experienced intense emotional pain and anger in a session. Her level of expressed emotional arousal, however, was judged to be very low by observers who rated emotional arousal from videotaped therapy segments.

Exposure methods have established a basis for understanding the emotional processing required for therapeutic change in the treatment of fear and anxiety. Hunt (1998), however, looked at emotional processing of depressive events and found that although greater short-term attention to negative feelings induced short-term emotional pain, those who went through this pain felt better in the long run than individuals who engaged in problem solving or avoided processing their feelings after the depressive event. This benefit was mediated by degree of emotional arousal, suggesting again that emotions must be "up and running" and must be experienced for beneficial emotional processing to occur. Evidence also has been found supporting the specific effectiveness of arousing and expressing *anger* in the treatment of depression and traumatic sexual abuse (Beutler et al., 1991; Van Velsor & Cox, 2001). Anger can be a means for survivors of sexual abuse to develop self-efficacy, heal memories, and correctly attribute blame. In these studies, arousal and expression of anger was related to the development of agency, self-efficacy, and self-assertion. In a review of research literature related to the benefits and dangers of reexperiencing painful emotion in therapy, Littrell (1998) concluded that when therapy is designed so as to allow for the planned restructuring of painful memories, the reexperience of pain in therapy has been demonstrated to be beneficial and therapeutic.

Pierce et al. (1983) found that catharsis was therapeutically useful only under very specific circumstances and only for certain people. There can be no universal rule about the effectiveness of arousing emotion or evoking emotional expression. The role of arousal and the degree to which it may be useful in therapy depend on what emotion is expressed and about what issue; how it is expressed, by whom, to whom, when, and under what conditions; and in what way the emotional expression is followed by other experiences of affect and meaning (Whelton, 2004). Nonetheless, the evidence suggests that emotional processing is mediated by arousal, so that for emotion processing to occur, the distressing affective experience must be activated and viscerally experienced by the client. Arousal is necessary but not sufficient for therapeutic progress. Recently we (Greenberg, Auszra, & Herrmann, 2007) found that the productivity of processing of aroused emotions, rather than arousal alone, distinguished good from poor outcomes.

Emotion Regulation

The third principle of emotional processing involves the regulation of emotion. Important issues in any treatment are what emotions are to be regulated and how. Undercontrolled secondary emotions and maladaptive emotions are what need to be regulated. Clients with these types of underregulated affect have been shown to benefit both from validation and from the learning of specific emotion regulation and distress tolerance skills (Linehan, 1993).

The provision of a safe, validating, supportive, and empathic environment is the first level of intervention for automatically generated underregulated distress (Bohart & Greenberg, 1997). Linehan et al. (2002) found evidence for the effectiveness of emotional validation and soothing as part of the treatment for borderline personality disorder. Empathy from another person seems to be particularly important in learning to self-soothe, restore emotional equilibrium, and strengthen the self.

Emotion regulation skills—including such things as identifying and labeling emotions, allowing and tolerating emotions, establishing a working distance, increasing positive emotions, reducing vulnerability to negative emotions, self-soothing, breathing, and distraction—also have been found to help with high distress (Linehan, 1993). Particularly important among these skills are getting some distance from overwhelming shame, despair, hopelessness, and/or shaky vulnerability, and developing self-soothing capacities to calm and comfort core anxieties and humiliation. Forms of meditative practice and self-acceptance are often most helpful in achieving a working distance from overwhelming core emotions. The ability to regulate breathing, and to observe one's emotions and let them come and go, are important processes to help regulate emotional distress. Mindfulness treatments have been shown to be effective in treating generalized anxiety disorder and panic (Kabat-Zinn et al., 1992), treating chronic pain (Kabat-Zinn, Lipworth, Burney, & Sellers, 1986), and preventing relapse in depression (Teasdale et al., 2000).

Another important aspect of regulation, however, is developing clients' abilities to tolerate emotion and to self-soothe *automatically*. Such abilities can be developed at various levels of processing. Physiological soothing involves teaching clients to activate the parasympathetic nervous system to regulate heart rate, breathing, and other sympathetic functions that speed up under stress. At the more deliberate behavioral and cognitive levels, promoting clients' abilities to receive and be compassionate to their emerging painful emotional experience is the first step toward helping them develop automatic emotion tolerance and self-soothing. This form of self-soothing involves, among other things, diaphragmatic breathing, relaxation, and the development of self-empathy and self-compassion.

Soothing also comes interpersonally in the form of another's empathic attunement to one's affect and through acceptance and validation by another person. Internal security develops from feeling that one exists in the mind and heart of another, and the security of being able to soothe the self develops through internalizing the soothing functions of the protective other (Sroufe, 1996). It is also important to make a distinction in emotion work between intensity of emotion per se and the depth of processing of the emotion. It is the latter that is the aim in EFT, not the former, and the regulation of overwhelming emotional intensity is vi-

tal in promoting the required depth of processing of emotion.

Reflection on Emotion

The fourth principle of emotional change is related to the first principle, emotion awareness, in that it involves making meaning of emotion. Reflection on emotion helps people make sense of their experience and promotes its assimilation into their ongoing self-narratives. What we make of our emotional experience makes us all who we are. In addition to the informational value of emotion awareness, symbolizing emotion in awareness promotes reflection on experience to create new meaning, and this helps people develop new narratives to explain their experience (Pennebaker, 1995; Greenberg & Angus, 2004). Understanding an emotional experience always involves putting it into narrative form. In therapy as well as in literature, all emotions occur in the context of significant stories, and all stories involve significant emotions (Greenberg & Angus, 2004). Therapy thus involves both change in emotional experiences and change in the narratives in which they are embedded.

In particular, symbolizing traumatic emotion memories in words helps promote their assimilation into people's ongoing self-narratives (van der Kolk, 1995). This process of verbalization allows *previously unsymbolized* experience in emotion memory to be assimilated into people's conscious, conceptual understandings of self and world, where it can be organized into a coherent story. Once such emotions are in words, they allow people to reflect on what they are feeling, create new meanings, and evaluate their own emotional experience. For example, reflecting on interpersonal difficulties and understanding that one is prone to get angry at one's partner because one is feeling abandoned, and that this relates to one's own history of abandonment rather than to the withholding nature of the partner, can be most therapeutic.

Pennebaker and colleagues have shown the positive effects of writing about emotional experience on autonomic nervous system activity, immune functioning, and physical and emotional health. Pennebaker (1995) concludes that through language, individuals are able to organize, structure, and ultimately assimilate both their emotional experiences and the events that may have provoked the emotions.

Both insight and reframing of emotional experience have long been viewed as ways to change emotion. The role in psychotherapy of humans' capacity for conscious awareness of the processes and contents of their own minds, and for reason and insight to shed light on unconscious motivations, has been substantial—from the beginnings of psychoanalysis right up to the present day. In addition, many therapists have written on the importance of changing people's assumptive frameworks in therapy (see, e.g., Frank, 1961).

In a study of events in which problematic issues were resolved in session, Watson (1996) found that vivid descriptions, emotional arousal, and cognitive meaning making interacted in complex yet orderly stages to produce therapeutic change. Theses stages allowed for clients to reflect on the emotions they were experiencing. Similarly, Stalikas and Fitzpatrick (1995) did an intensive analysis of "good client moments" and showed that in-session change was related to the combination of strength of feeling and higher-order levels of reflection. In addition, computer-assisted studies of verbal patterns in psychodynamic and other therapies have shown that in the key moments in therapy in which substantial shifts happened, there was a frequent co-occurrence of high emotion tone (emotional arousal) and high abstraction (a reflection on this emotional process)—a beneficial co-occurrence that was called "making a connection" (Mergenthaler, 1996). It seems to be the timely conjunction of emotional arousal and a thoughtful exploration of the emotion's meaning that generates change.

Thus, as well as having emotions, we also live in a constant process of making sense of our emotions. A dialectical-constructivist view of human functioning has been offered to explain this process (Greenberg & Pascual-Leone, 1995, 2001; Neimeyer & Mahoney, 1995). In this view, personal meaning emerges from the self-organization and explication of one's own emotional experience, and optimal adaptation involves an integration of reason and emotion. This integration is achieved by an ongoing circular process of making sense of experience by symbolizing bodily felt sensations in awareness and articulating them in language, thereby constructing new ones.

In this dialectical-constructivist view, symbol and bodily felt referents are viewed as interacting to carry meaning forward, and newly symbolized experience is organized in different ways to construct new views. Attending to and discovering preconceptual elements of emotional experience influence the process of meaning construction. New experiential elements from many sources from within, and sometimes from without, can be integrated into this process. People are then viewed as constantly striving toward making sense of their preconceptual emotional experience by symbolizing it, explaining it, and putting it into narrative form. Preconceptual tacit meaning carries implications and acts to constrain, but does not fully determine, meaning. Rather, it is synthesized with conceptual, explicit meaning to form explanations constrained by experiencing (Greenberg & Pascual-Leone, 1995, 2001). This provides the ongoing narrative of a person's life.

Thus, although the recipe for emotional processing from the perspective of behavioral therapies and CBT is that arousal plus habituation to the distressing stimulus produces change, approach, arousal, acceptance, and tolerance of emotional experience are necessary but not sufficient from an EFT perspective. Optimum emotional processing involves in addition the integration of cognition and affect and the creation of new meaning (Greenberg, 2002; Greenberg & Pascual-Leone, 1995; Pos, Greenberg, Goldman, & Korman, 2003). Once contact with emotional experience is achieved, clients must also cognitively orient to that experience as information, and explore, reflect on, and make sense of it.

EFT appears to work by enhancing emotional processing, and this involves helping people both accept their emotions and make sense of them (Pos et al., 2003; Goldman, Greenberg, & Pos, 2005). Deepening of experience over therapy as measured by the Experiencing Scales (Klein, Mathieu-Coughlan, & Kiesler, 1986), which measure clients' ability to focus on feelings and use them to solve problems and create new meaning, has been shown to be a specific change process that predicts outcome over and above the change predicted by the therapeutic alliance. Past studies also show a strong relationship between in-session emotional experiencing and therapeutic gain in dynamic, cognitive, and experiential therapies (Castonguay, Goldfried, Wiser, Raue, & Hayes, 1996; Silberschatz, Fretter, & Curtis, 1986). This suggests that this variable may be a common factor that helps explain change across approaches.

In addition, it has been shown that therapists' depth of experiential focus influenced clients' depth of experiencing in the next moment, and that this predicted outcome. Moreover, the effect of early emotional processing on outcome was found to be mediated by late emotional processing, where "emotional processing" was defined as depth of experiencing emotion episodes (Pos et al., 2003). Early capacity for emotional processing alone thus did not guarantee good outcome. Nor did entering therapy without this capacity guarantee poor outcome. Therefore, although early emotional processing skill was probably an advantage, it appeared not as critical as the ability to acquire and/or increase depth of experiencing throughout therapy. In this study, late emotional processing independently added 21% to the explained variance in reduction in symptoms over and above early alliance and early emotional processing level.

In another study (Warwar, 2003), not only did midtherapy expressed emotional arousal predict outcome; a client's ability to use internal experience to make meaning and solve problems as measured by the Experiencing Scales, particularly in the late phase of treatment, added to the outcome variance over and above middle-phase emotional arousal. This study thus showed that a combination of emotional arousal and reflection was a better predictor of outcome than either index alone. Reflection on aroused emotion thus appears to be an important change process (Missirlian, Toukmanian, Warwar, & Greenberg, 2005).

Emotion Transformation

The final and probably most fundamental principle of emotional change is the transformation of one emotion into another. This applies most specifically to transforming primary maladaptive emotions—those old familiar bad feelings that occur repeatedly but do not change by contact with more adaptive emotions. Although the more traditional ways of transforming emotions (either exposure through experience, expression, and completion, or reflection on them) can occur with primary maladaptive emotions, another process appears to be more important. This is a process of *changing emotion with emotion* (Greenberg, 2002). In other words, a maladaptive emotional state can be transformed best by undoing it with another, more adaptive emotion. In time, the activation of the more adaptive emotion along with or in response to the maladaptive emotion helps transform the maladaptive emotion. While thinking usually changes thoughts, only feeling can change emotions.

Spinoza was the first to note that emotion is needed to change emotion; he proposed that "an emotion cannot be restrained nor removed unless by an opposed and stronger emotion" (1677/1967, p. 195). Reason clearly is seldom sufficient to change automatic emergency-based emotional responses. Darwin (1872/1998), on jumping back from the strike of a glassed-in snake, noted that despite his having approached it with the determination not to start back, his will and reason were powerless against the imagination of a danger that he had never even experienced. Rather than reasoning with an emotion, one needs to transform the emotion by accessing another emotion.

In an interesting line of investigation, positive emotions have been found to undo lingering negative emotions (Frederickson, 2001). The basic observation is that key components of positive emotions are incompatible with negative emotions. Frederickson (2001) suggests that by broadening a person's momentary thought–action repertoire, a positive emotion may loosen the hold that a negative emotion has on the person's mind. The experiences of joy and contentment were found to produce faster cardiovascular recovery from negative emotions than a neutral experience. Frederickson, Mancuso, Branigan, and Tugade (2000) also found that resilient individuals coped by recruiting positive emotions to regulate negative emotional experiences. They found that these individuals manifested a physiological "bounce-back" that helped them to return to cardiovascular baseline more quickly.

It thus seems possible to replace bad feelings with happy feelings—not in a simple manner, by trying to look on the bright side, but by evoking meaningfully embodied alternative experiences to undo the negative feelings. For example, in grief, laughter has been found to be a predictor of recovery; thus being able to remember the happy times, to experience joy, serves as an antidote to sadness (Bonanno & Keltner, 1997). Similarly, warmth and affection are often antidotes to anxiety. In depression, a protest-filled, submissive sense of worthlessness can be transformed therapeutically by guiding people to the desire that drives their protest—a desire to be free of their cages and to access their feelings of joy and excitement for life. Isen (1999) notes that at least some of the positive effects of happy feelings have been hypothesized to depend on the effects of the neurotransmitters involved in the emotion of joy on specific parts of the brain that influence purposive thinking. Mild positive affect has been found to facilitate problem solving.

In a study of self-criticism, Whelton and Greenberg (2004) found that people who were more vulnerable to depression showed more contempt but also less resilience in response to self-criticism than people less vulnerable to depression. The less vulnerable people were able to recruit positive emotional resources, such as self-assertive pride and anger, to combat the depressogenic contempt and negative cognitions. In other words after a distressing experience, resilient people appear to generate a positive feeling (often through imagery or memory) in order to soothe themselves, and they can combat negative feelings and views of self in this more resilient state. Accessing a positive emotional state therefore helps them counteract the effect of a negative emotional state. These studies together indicate that positive affect can be used to regulate negative feelings.

Davidson (2000) suggests that the right-hemispheric, withdrawal-related negative affect system can be transformed by activation of the approach-related system in the left prefrontal cortex. He defines "resilience" as the maintenance of high levels of positive affect and well-being in the face of adversity; he highlights that it is not that resilient people do not feel negative affect, but that their negative affect does not persist. Levenson (1992) has reviewed research indicating that specific emotions are associated with specific patterns of autonomic nervous system activity, providing evidence that different emotions change one's physiology differentially. Emotion also has been shown to be differentially transformed by people's differing capacity to self-generate imagery to replace unwanted, automatically generated emotions with more desirable imagery scripts (Derryberry & Reed, 1996); this finding suggests the importance of individual differences in this domain.

It is important to note that the process of changing emotion with emotion goes beyond ideas of catharsis, completion, exposure, extinction, or habituation, in that the maladaptive feeling is not purged, nor is it simply attenuated by the person feeling it. Rather, another feeling is used to transform or undo it. Although exposure to emotion at times may be helpful to overcome affect phobia in many situations in therapy, change also occurs because one emotion is transformed by another emotion rather than simply attenuated. In these instances emotional change occurs by the activation of an incompatible, more adaptive experience that undoes or reverses the old response.

Clinical observation and research suggest that emotional transformation occurs through a process of dialectical synthesis of opposing schemes. When opposing schemes are coactivated, they synthesize compatible elements from the coactivated schemes to form new higher-level schemes, just as in development when schemes for standing and falling, in a toddler, are dynamically synthesized into a higher-level scheme for walking (Greenberg & Pascual-Leone, 1995; Pascual-Leone, 1991). Schemes of different emotional states are similarly synthesized to form new higher-level states. Thus, in therapy, maladaptive fear, once aroused, can be transformed into security by evoking the more boundary-establishing emotions of adaptive anger or disgust, or the softer feelings of compassion or forgiveness. Similarly, maladaptive anger can be undone by adaptive sadness. Maladaptive shame can be transformed by accessing anger at violation, self-comforting feelings, and pride and self-worth. For example, the tendency to shrink into the ground in shame is transformed by the thrusting-forward tendency in newly accessed anger at violation. Withdrawal emotions from one side of the brain are replaced with approach emotions from another part of the brain, or vice versa (Davidson, 2000). Once the alternative emotion has been accessed, it transforms or undoes the original state, and a new state is forged.

Given the importance of accessing new, more adaptive emotions to transform old maladaptive emotions, this question arises: "How then are new emotions accessed?" How does a therapist help people in the midst of maladaptive experiences access emotions that will help them transform their maladaptive feelings and beliefs? Some different ways are listed below (Greenberg, 2002; Greenberg & Watson, 2006).

1. *The therapeutic relationship.* A good therapeutic relationship provides an ongoing source of new emotions by providing a secure empathic environment that soothes and calms.

2. *Shifting attention.* Shifting people's focus of attention so that they pay attention to a background feeling is a key method of helping them change their emotional states. On the edge of awareness or in the background, behind their current dominant emotion, often lies a subdominant emotion that can be found if attended to or searched for. Another feeling is there, but not yet in focal awareness. Behind anger is sadness, love, or forgiveness; at the edge of sadness is anger; within hurt or fear is anger; behind shame are pride and self-esteem. The subdominant emotion is often present in the room nonverbally, in tone of voice or manner of expression.

3. *Accessing needs/goals.* A more process-directive way in which a therapist can help clients access their healthy healing emotions and internal resources is by asking them when they are in a maladaptive state, such as shame, what they *need* to resolve their pain. People usually know what they need when they are suffering their pain. Once they know what they need in a situation, they often begin to feel as if they have some control over it. Raising a need or a goal to a self-organizing system has a number of effects. At the conscious, intentional level, it opens a problem space to search for a solution. At an affective level, it conjures up a feeling of what it is like to reach the goal, and opens up neural pathways to both the feeling and the goal. Most important, raising a need that is unmet helps a new feeling such as anger or sadness to emerge.

4. *Positive imagery.* Another way to activate alternative feelings is to use imagery. Imagination is a means of bringing about an emotional response. This involves helping clients use their conscious capacities to generate new experience. People can use their imaginations to create scenes that they know will help them feel an emotion, and can use this emotion as an antidote to a maladaptive feeling they want to change. They can change what they feel, not by changing feelings with reason, but by using imagination to evoke new emotions. With practice, people can learn how to generate opposing emotions through imagery and use these as antidotes to negative emotions.

5. *Expressive enactment of the emotion.* Yet another way to access alternate emotions is to have people enact a feeling that is not currently being experienced. This goes back to William James's idea that we feel afraid because we run. The therapist asks clients to adopt certain emotional stances, and helps

them to deliberately assume the expressive posture of that feeling and then to intensify it. Thus a therapist might use a psychodramatic enactment and instruct a client, "Try telling him, 'I'm angry.' Say it again—yes, louder. Can you put your feet on the floor and sit up straight? Yes, do it some more." Here the therapist coaches the person in expressing an emotion until the emotion actually begins to be experienced. This is not encouraging phony expression, but trying to facilitate access to a suppressed, disallowed experience. Instructions to take on expressive postures are always balanced by asking people what they experience after doing this.

6. *Remembering another emotion.* Remembering a situation in which an emotion occurred can bring the emotion memory alive in the present. This technique is related to the imaging process described above. Remembering past emotional scenes clearly produces emotion. To help people change what they feel, a therapist has to help them access and restructure their emotion memories. One important way of changing emotion memories involves accessing the emotion memory to be changed and then transforming it with another emotion memory. Once another emotion memory is evoked, either the new memory dominates and the old one recedes into the background and becomes less accessible, or the new one eventually transforms the old memory.

7. *Cognitive change.* A therapist can also help people access a new emotion by talking with them about the more desirable emotion. This is using cognitive meaning to generate new feelings. Talking about an emotional episode helps people reexperience the feelings they had in that episode.

8. *Expressing the emotion for the client.* A therapist might express outrage or sadness for a client that the client is not yet able to express. This gives the client permission to begin experiencing this emotion. We all often see ourselves in the reflections of ourselves that we get back from others. Seeing that our stories have an impact on others and that they are moved can also move us.

9. *Using the therapy relationship to generate a new emotion.* A new emotion can be evoked in response to a new interaction with a therapist. The therapist can evoke a particular emotion in a client by taking a particular position in the interaction. For example, a therapist who is comforting will evoke soft feelings; one who is confrontive will evoke anger.

EMOTION COACHING

A view of the therapist as an "emotion coach"—a view that encompasses the importance of both the therapeutic relationship and emotional processing—has been proposed as a model of the therapist's role and function in working with emotion. Emotion coaching (Gottman, 1997; Greenberg, 2002) is essentially aimed at helping people become aware of and make sense of their emotional experience. The effects of a good therapeutic relationship on outcome is widely recognized (Norcross, 2002), and there is good reason to believe that a good alliance is also a prerequisite to productive emotional processing, as noted throughout this chapter. An accepting, empathic relational environment provides people with the experience of emotional soothing and support they need to pay attention to their bodily felt experience. This type of relational environment helps people to sort out their feelings, develop self-empathy, and find alternative inner resources from which new responses can be constructed. Within this relational context, emotion coaching aims to help clients be informed by their emotions, regulate them, transform them, and use them intelligently to solve problems in living.

In addition to following where the client is moment by moment, the therapist acting as an emotion coach guides the client in new ways of processing experiential information. Emotion coaching thus involves a style that combines leading and following, and embodies the idea that it is possible to influence the construction of people's subjective experience. Change and novelty can be introduced in the emotional domain by training people to become aware of their emotional processes, and by guiding their attention and meaning construction processes.

Based on a major principle that one cannot leave an emotional place until one has arrived, two phases of emotion coaching—the "arriving" phase and the "leaving" phase—have been proposed. Each phase includes four steps designed to help people experience their emotions more skillfully. The first phase, focused on awareness of emotion, is designed to help people arrive at what they feel and involves the following steps:

1. The coach helps people attend to their emotions.
2. The coach encourages people to welcome their emotional experience and allow it (this does not necessarily mean they must express everything they feel to other people; rather, they must acknowledge it themselves). People also need to be coached in skills of emotion regulation if these are needed.
3. The coach helps people to describe their feelings in words, in order to aid them in solving problems.
4. The coach guides people to become aware of whether their emotional reactions are their primary feelings in this situation. If not, they need help in discovering what their primary feelings are.

The second phase focuses on emotion utilization or transformation and is designed to help clients leave the place where they have arrived. This stage involves moving on and transforming core feelings when necessary. It is here that the coaching aspect is more central.

5. When a person has been helped to experience a primary emotion, the coach and person together need to evaluate whether the emotion is a healthy, adaptive emotion or an unhealthy, maladaptive response to the current situation. If it is healthy, it should be used as a guide to action. If it is unhealthy, it needs to be changed.
6. If the accessed primary emotion is unhealthy, the person has to be helped to identify the negative cognition associated with this emotion.
7. Alternative, adaptive emotional responses and needs are now processed and developed.
8. People are coached to challenge the destructive thoughts in their maladaptive emotions from their new inner voice, based on their adaptive primary emotions and needs, and to regulate maladaptive emotions when necessary.

Coaching in the emotional domain thus involves helping clients verbally label each emotion they are feeling, accept the emotion, talk about what it is like to experience the emotion, develop new ways of processing the emotion, and learn ways of soothing or regulating the emotion. It is important to note that people often cannot simply be explicitly taught new strategies for dealing with difficult emotions; they have to be assisted to engage in the new process experientially, and only later explicitly taught what to do. For example, accessing a need or goal may be very helpful in overcoming a sense of passivity or defeat or to help a painful feeling. However, explicitly teaching people that this is what they should do is not nearly as helpful as interpersonally facilitating this by asking them at the right time what it is they need. For example, it is through experiencing a process of shifting from negative to more positive emotional states that the experiential links between states are best forged. This then is consolidated only later by explicit knowledge of the process.

CONCLUSION

EFT emphasizes becoming aware of and reflecting on primary emotions, as well as regulating and transforming maladaptive emotions. Both the utilization and the transformation of emotion are seen as therapeutic. A two-step therapeutic process is recommended when the core emotion accessed is adaptive. First, the symptomatic secondary emotion (such as feeling upset, despairing, or hopeless) is evoked in therapy; then the core primary adaptive emotion that is being interrupted (such as sadness, grief, or empowering anger) is accessed and validated and utilized to promote adaptive action. A three-step sequence is required to transform a core maladaptive emotion. In this sequence, the secondary emotion is first evoked; then the core maladaptive emotion being avoided (such as shame, fear, or anger) is accessed. This latter emotion is then transformed by accessing a more adaptive emotion (such as anger, sadness, or compassion). When adaptive emotions finally are evoked, they are incorporated into new views of self and used to transform personal narratives.

REFERENCES

Beutler, L. E., Clarkin, J. F., & Bongar, B. (2000). *Guidelines for the systematic treatment of the depressed patient*. New York: Oxford University Press.

Beutler, L., Engle, D., Mohr, D., Daldrup, R., Bergan, M., & Merry, W. (1991). Predictors of differential response to cognitive, experiential, and self-directed psychotherapeutic procedures. *Journal of Consulting and Clinical Psychology, 59*, 333–340.

Bohart, A. C., & Greenberg, L. S. (Eds.). (1997). *Empathy reconsidered: New directions in psychotherapy*. Washington, DC: American Psychological Association.

Bonanno, G. A., & Keltner, D. (1997). Facial expressions of emotion and the course of conjugal bereavement. *Journal of Abnormal Psychology, 106*, 126–137.

Borkovec, T. D., Alcaine, O., & Behar, E. (2004). Avoidance theory of worry and generalized anxiety disorder. In R. G. Heimberg, C. L. Turk, & D. S. Mennin (Eds.), *Generalized anxiety disorder: Advances in research and practice* (pp. 77–108). New York: Guilford Press.

Castonguay, L. G., Goldfried, M. R., Wiser, S., Raue, P. J., & Hayes, A. M. (1996). Predicting the effect of cognitive therapy for depression: A study of unique and common factors. *Journal of Consulting and Clinical Psychology, 64*, 497–504.

Coombs, M. M., Coleman, D., & Jones, E. E. (2002). Working with feelings: The importance of emotion in both cognitive-behavioral and interpersonal therapy in the NIMH Treatment of Depression Collaborative Research Program. *Psychotherapy: Theory, Research, Practice, Training, 39*, 233–244.

Darwin, C. (1998). *Expression of the emotions in man and animals* (3rd ed.). London: HarperCollins.

Davidson, R. J. (2000). Affective style, psychopathology, and resilience: Brain mechanisms and plasticity. *American Psychologist, 5*(11), 1193–1196.

Derryberry, D., & Reed, M. A. (1996). Regulatory processes and the development of cognitive representations. *Development and Psychopathology, 8*, 215–234.

Elliott, R., Greenberg, L., & Lietaer, G. (2004). Research on experiential psychotherapy. In M. Lambert (Ed.), *Bergin and Garfield's handbook of psychotherapy and behavior change* (pp. 493–539). New York: Wiley.

Foa, E. B., & Jaycox, L. H. (1999). Cognitive-behavioral theory and treatment of posttraumatic stress disorder. In D. Spiegel (Ed.), *Efficacy and cost-effectiveness of psychotherapy* (pp. 23–61). Washington, DC: American Psychiatric Press.

Foa, E. B., Zoellner, L. A., Feeny, N. C., Hembree, E. A., & Alvarez-Conrad, J. (2002). Does imaginal exposure exacerbate PTSD symptoms? *Journal of Consulting and Clinical Psychology, 70*, 1022–1028.

Fosha, D. (2000). *The transforming power of affect: A model of accelerated change*. New York: Basic Books.

Frank, J. (1961). *Persuasion and healing*. Baltimore: Johns Hopkins University Press.

Frederickson, B. (2001). The role of positive emotions in positive psychology: The broaden-and-build theory of positive emotions. *American Psychologist, 56*(3), 218–226.

Frederickson, B., Mancuso, R., Branigan, C., & Tugade, M. (2000). The undoing effects of positive emotion. *Motivation and Emotion, 24*, 237–258.

Freud, S. (1957). Instincts and their vicissitudes. In J. Strachey (Ed. & Trans.), *The standard edition of the complete psychological works of Sigmund Freud* (Vol. 14, pp. 109–140). London: Hogarth Press. (Original work published 1915)

Goldman, R., Greenberg, L. S., & Angus, L. (2006).

The effects of adding emotion-focused interventions to the therapeutic relationship in the treatment of depression. *Psychotherapy Research, 16,* 537–549.

Goldman, R., Greenberg, L., & Pos, A. (2005). Depth of emotional experience and outcome. *Psychotherapy Research, 15,* 248–260.

Gottman, J. (1997). *The heart of parenting: How to raise an emotionally intelligent child.* New York: Simon & Schuster.

Greenberg, L. S. (2002). *Emotion-focused therapy: Coaching clients to work through their feelings.* Washington, DC: American Psychological Association.

Greenberg, L. S., & Angus, L. (2004). The contributions of emotion processes to narrative change in psychotherapy: A dialectical constructivist approach. In L. Angus & J. McLeod (Eds.), *Handbook of narrative psychotherapy* (pp. 331–352). Thousand Oaks, CA: Sage.

Greenberg, L. S., Auszra, L., & Herrmann, I. (2007). The relationship between emotional productivity, emotional arousal and outcome in experiential therapy of depression. *Psychotherapy Research, 2,* 57–66.

Greenberg, L. S., & Johnson, S. M. (1988). *Emotionally focused therapy for couples.* New York: Guilford Press.

Greenberg, L. S., & Pascual-Leone, A. (2006). Emotion in psychotherapy: A practice-friendly research review. *In Session: Psychotherapy in Practice, 62,* 611–630.

Greenberg, L. S., & Pascual-Leone, J. (1995). A dialectical constructivist approach to experiential change. In R. A. Neimeyer & M. Mahoney (Eds.), *Constructivism in psychotherapy* (pp. 169–191). Washington, DC: American Psychological Association.

Greenberg, L. S., & Pascual-Leone, J. (2001). A dialectical constructivist view of the creation of personal meaning. *Journal of Constructivist Psychology, 14*(3), 165–186.

Greenberg, L. S., & Watson, J. (1998). Experiential therapy of depression: Differential effects of client-centered relationship conditions and process experiential interventions. *Psychotherapy Research, 8,* 210–224.

Greenberg, L. S., & Watson, J. C. (2006). *Emotion-focused therapy for depression.* Washington, DC: American Psychological Association.

Gross, J. J. (1999). Emotion and emotion regulation. In L. A. Pervin & O. P. John (Eds.), *Handbook of personality: Theory and research* (2nd ed., pp. 525–552). New York: Guilford Press.

Hunt, M. G. (1998). The only way out is through: Emotional processing and recovery after a depressing life event. *Behaviour Research and Therapy, 36,* 361–384.

Isen, A. (1999). Positive affect. In T. Dalgleish & M. Power (Eds.), *Handbook of cognition and emotion.* Chichester, UK: Wiley.

Iwakabe, S., Rogan, K., & Stalikas, A. (2000). The relationship between client emotional expressions, therapist interventions, and the working alliance: An exploration of eight emotional expression events. *Journal of Psychotherapy Integration, 10,* 375–402.

Jaycox, L. H., Foa, E. B., & Morral, A. R. (1998). Influence of emotional engagement and habituation on exposure therapy for PTSD. *Journal of Consulting and Clinical Psychology, 66,* 185–192.

Johnson, S. (1996). *The practice of emotionally focused couples therapy: Creating connections.* New York: Brunner-Routledge.

Johnson, S., Hunsley, J., Greenberg, L., & Schlindler, D. (1999). Emotionally focused couples therapy: Status and challenges. *Clinical Psychology: Science and Practice, 6,* 67–79.

Kabat-Zinn, J., Lipworth, L., Burney, R., & Sellers, W. (1986). Four year follow-up of a meditation-based program for the self-regulation of chronic pain: Treatment outcomes and compliance. *Clinical Journal of Pain, 2,* 159–173.

Kabat-Zinn, J., Massion, A. O., Kristeller, J., Peterson, L. G., Fletcher, K. E., Pbert, L., et al. (1992). Effectiveness of a meditation-based stress reduction program in the treatment of anxiety disorders. *American Journal of Psychiatry, 149,* 936–943.

Klein, M. H., Mathieu-Coughlan, P., & Kiesler, D. J. (1986). The Experiencing Scales. In L. S. Greenberg & W. M. Pinsof (Eds.), *The psychotherapeutic process: A research handbook* (pp. 21–71). New York: Guilford Press.

Lane, R. D., & Schwartz, G. E. (1992). Levels of emotional awareness: Implications for psychotherapeutic integration. *Journal of Psychotherapy Integration, 2,* 1–18.

Leahy, R. L. (2002). A model of emotional schemas. *Cognitive and Behavioral Practice, 9,* 177–191.

Levenson, R. W. (1992). Autonomic nervous system differences among emotions. *Psychological Science, 3,* 23–27.

Linehan, M. M. (1993). *Cognitive-behavioral treatment of borderline personality disorder.* New York: Guilford Press.

Linehan, M. M., Dimeff, L. A., Reynolds, S. K., Comtois, K. A., Shaw Welch, S., Heagerty, P., et al. (2002). Dialectical behavior therapy versus comprehensive validation plus 12 step for the treatment of opioid dependent women meeting criteria for borderline personality disorder. *Drug and Alcohol Dependence, 67,* 13–26.

Littrell, J. (1998). Is the reexperience of painful emotion therapeutic? *Clinical Psychology Review, 18,* 71–102.

Mergenthaler, E. (1996). Emotion–abstraction patterns in verbatim protocols: A new way of describing psychotherapeutic processes. *Journal of Consulting and Clinical Psychology, 64,* 1306–1315.

Missirlian, T., Toukmanian, S., Warwar, S., & Greenberg, L. (2005). Emotional arousal, client perpetual processing, and the working alliance in experiential psychotherapy for depression. *Journal of Consulting and Clinical Psychology, 73*(5), 861–871.

Neimeyer, R. A., & Mahoney, M. (1995). *Constructivism in psychotherapy*. Washington, DC: American Psychological Association.

Norcross, J. C. (2002). Empirically supported therapy relationships. In J. C. Norcross (Ed.), *Psychotherapy relationships that work: Therapist contributions and responsiveness to patients* (pp. 3–16). London: Oxford University Press.

Paivio, S. C., Hall, I. E., Holowaty, K. A. M., Jellis, & Tran, (2001). Imaginal confrontation for resolving child abuse issues. *Psychotherapy Research, 11*, 56–68.

Paivio, S. C., & Nieuwenhuis, J. A. (2001). Efficacy of emotionally focused therapy for adult survivors of child abuse: A preliminary study. *Journal of Traumatic Stress, 14*, 115–134.

Pascual-Leone, J. (1991). Emotions, development and psychotherapy: A dialectical constructivist perspective. In J. Safran & L. S. Greenberg (Eds.), *Emotion, psychotherapy, and change* (pp. 302–335). New York: Guilford Press.

Pennebaker, J. W. (Ed.). (1995). *Emotion, disclosure, and health*. Washington, DC: American Psychological Association.

Perls, F. S. (1969). *Gestalt therapy verbatim*. Lafayette, CA: Real People Press.

Pierce, R. A., Nichols, M. P., & DuBrin, J. R. (1983). *Emotional expression in psychotherapy*. New York: Gardner Press.

Pos, A. E., Greenberg, L. S., Goldman, R. N., & Korman, L. M. (2003). Emotional processing during experiential treatment of depression. *Journal of Consulting and Clinical Psychology, 71*, 1007–1016.

Rogers, C. R. (1951). *Client-centered therapy*. Boston: Houghton Mifflin.

Salovey, P., Mayer, J. D., Golman, S. L., Turvey, C., & Palfai, T. P. (1995). Emotional attention, clarity, and repair: Exploring emotional intelligence using the Trait Meta-Mood Scale. In J. W. Pennebaker (Ed.), *Emotion, disclosure, and health* (pp. 125–154). Washington, DC: American Psychological Association.

Samoilov, A., & Goldfried, M. (2000). Role of emotion in cognitive behavior therapy. *Clinical Psychology: Science and Practice, 7*, 373–385.

Shapiro, F. (1999). Eye-movement desensitization and reprocessing (EMDR) and the anxiety disorders: Clinical and research implications of an integrated psychotherapy treatment. *Journal of Anxiety Disorders, 13*, 35–67.

Silberschatz, G., Fretter, P. B., & Curtis, J. T. (1986). How do interpretations influence the process of psychotherapy? *Journal of Consulting and Clinical Psychology, 54*, 646–652.

Spinoza, B. (1967). *Ethics (Part IV)*. New York: Hafner. (Original work published 1677)

Sroufe, L. A. (1996). *Emotional development: The organization of emotional life in the early years*. New York: Cambridge University Press.

Stalikas, A., & Fitzpatrick, M. (1995). Client good moments: An intensive analysis of a single session. *Canadian Journal of Counselling, 29*, 160–175.

Stanton, A., Danoff-Burg, S., Cameron, C., Bishop, M., Collins, C., Kirk, S. B., et al. (2000). Emotionally expressive coping predicts psychological and physical adjustment to breast cancer. *Journal of Consulting and Clinical Psychology, 68*, 875–882.

Svartberg, M., Stiles, T. C., & Seltzer, M. H. (2004). Randomized, controlled trial of the effectiveness of short-term dynamic psychotherapy and cognitive therapy for Cluster C personality disorders. *American Journal of Psychiatry, 161*, 810–817.

Teasdale, J. D., Segal, Z. V., Williams, J. M. G., Ridgeway, V. A., Soulsby, J. M., & Lau, M. A. (2000). Prevention of relapse/recurrence in major depression by mindfulness-based cognitive therapy. *Journal of Consulting and Clinical Psychology, 68*, 615–623.

van der Kolk, B. A. (1995). The body, memory, and the psychobiology of trauma. In J. L. Alpert (Ed.). *Sexual abuse recalled: Treating trauma in the era of the recovered memory debate* (pp. 29–60). Northvale, NJ: Aronson.

Van Velsor, P., & Cox, D. L. (2001). Anger as a vehicle in the treatment of women who are sexual abuse survivors: Reattributing responsibility and accessing personal power. *Professional Psychology: Research and Practice, 32*, 618–625.

Warwar, N. (2003). *Relating emotional processes to outcome in experiential psychotherapy of depression.* Unpublished doctoral dissertation, York University, Toronto.

Warwar, N., Greenberg, L. S., & Perepeluk, (2003, June). *Reported in-session emotional experience in therapy*. Paper presented at the annual meeting of the International Society for Psychotherapy Research, Weimar, Germany.

Watson, J. C. (1996). The relationship between vivid description, emotional arousal, and in-session resolution of problematic reactions. *Journal of Consulting and Clinical Psychology, 64*, 459–464.

Watson, J. C., Gordon, L. B., Stermac, L., Kalogerakos, F., & Steckley, P. (2003). Comparing the effectiveness of process-experiential with cognitive-behavioral psychotherapy in the treatment of depression. *Journal of Consulting and Clinical Psychology, 71*, 773–781.

Whelton, W. J. (2004). Emotional processing in psychotherapy: Evidence across therapeutic modalities. *Clinical Psychology and Psychotherapy, 11*, 58–71.

Whelton, W., & Greenberg, L. (2005). Emotion in self-criticism. *Personality and Individual Differences, 38*, 1583–1595.

Winston, A., Laikin, M., Pollack, J., Samstag, L., McCullough, L., & Muran, C. (1994). Short-term psychotherapy of personality disorders: 2 year follow-up. *American Journal of Psychiatry, 151*, 190–194.

CHAPTER 7

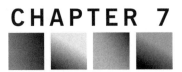

Emotions, Music, and Literature

P. N. JOHNSON-LAIRD and KEITH OATLEY

Most human activities have emotional consequences. And what we humans do in our leisure is often designed to elicit emotions. The enjoyment of works of art is no exception. Novels, plays, and movies can all prompt real emotions about unreal events. The mechanisms we use to understand fiction are the same as those we use to understand the everyday world (Gerrig, 1993); part of the result is that we may laugh or weep about what we know is imaginary. Music is still more mysterious. Why should a piece of pure music—Beethoven's late piano sonata, the "Hammerklavier," say— have any emotional impact on us? It can move us even though it refers to nothing at all. If we feel sad as a result of listening to a piece of music, then the music isn't the object of our emotion, but its cause. Usually we cannot say why this piece of music makes us happy, whereas that piece makes us sad. Philosophers have struggled with these problems, but they have reached no consensus (see, e.g., Budd, 1985; Robinson, 1997; Nussbaum, 2001). Psychologists and others have addressed emotions and the arts (see, e.g., Hjort & Laver, 1997). But no one appears to have a complete explanation of the causal link between the perception of a work of art and the ensuing emotional experience. Our goal in the present chapter is both to review the psychology of emotions in relation to music and literature, as befits a chapter in a handbook, and at the same time to take some steps toward a solution to this mystery.

Music is older than writing: The earliest musical instrument, a flute found in Slovenia, is more than 43,000 years old (Huron, 2003), whereas the invention of writing is only about 5,000 years old (Coulmas, 1996). Painting and sculpture started with the creation of objects that are models or metaphors for something else—marks on a cave wall that depict a bison. They survive from 30,000 years ago (Mithen, 1996), about the same time as the start of burial practices, and presumably of myths about the afterlife. Coming at the beginning and end of this sequence of emergence, music and literature are our topics.

Pure music is without propositional content. By "pure" music, we mean music that is not a setting for words—that does not follow a program such as Richard Strauss's *Til Eulenspiegel's Merry Pranks*, or that does not depict a series of events such as Claude Debussy's *La Mer*, with its three movements entitled, "From dawn till noon on the ocean," "Play of the waves," and "Dialogue of wind and sea."

In contrast, literature does have propositional content. It relies on understanding the propositions that the writer expresses. If you cannot understand "It is a truth universally acknowledged, that a single man in possession of a good fortune, must be in want of a wife," then you will not make much of Jane Austen's novel *Pride and Prejudice* (1813/1906), of which it is the opening sentence. The appeal of Austen's novel occurs because many of us are moved by the love that develops between Elizabeth Bennet and Mr. Darcy. The propositional content of the novel, and the ways in which Austen expresses it, lead us to experience a sequence of emotional states, even though we know that the characters and their actions are fictitious. Other arts—plays, movies, operas, and representational paintings and sculptures—can also convey propositional contents that have an emotional impact on us. Before children learn to read, these sorts of art can affect them. Hence written literature is an ideal case study, because it depends more than any other art on the mental work that we put into its interpretation.

Our plan for this chapter is to begin with a representative cognitive theory of emotions, which makes the contrasts that we need to solve our puzzle. We then consider the nature of music, and as we review the area, we propose a theory of how music evokes emotions in listeners. We next describe relevant aspects of literature, and extend our theory to cope with the effects of propositional content on emotions. Finally, we draw some conclusions about relations between the arts in general and human emotions.

A COMMUNICATIVE THEORY OF EMOTIONS

The vital problems that social mammals, such as human beings, must solve are those created in their internal environment, such as fatigue and pain; those created in their physical environment, such as the need for shelter; and those created in their social environment, such as the desire for a mate and for offspring. According to a "communicative" theory of emotions (Oatley & Johnson-Laird, 1987, 1996), emotions are communications, in which a small set of signals conveys an individual's emotional states to others. Although the idea of basic emotions and their expressions remains somewhat controversial (see, e.g., Oatley, Keltner, & Jenkins, 2006; Russell, Bachorowski, & Fernandez-Dols, 2003) it is scarcely controversial that a smile is recognized in all cultures as a signal of happiness and social welcome, whereas weeping is a signal of sadness that often elicits sympathy. Such nonverbal signals are human universals (see, e.g., Keltner, Ekman, Gonzaga, & Beer, 2003) although the cognitive appraisals that elicit them may differ among cultures (Johnson-Laird & Oatley, 2000). The way in which such signals are recognized is very different from the interpretation of propositions expressed in language. Human facial expressions, gestures, and vocal tone can all contribute to distinctive signals of emotions, akin to signals of enjoyment, alarm, threat, or submission made by other species of social mammals. Their interpretation is carried out in specialized regions of the brain. In contrast, the meaning of a sentence is composed from the meanings of its parts according to the grammatical relations among them. It depends on working memory, because grammatical structures are often recursive (Fitch, Hauser, & Chomsky, 2005), and because the interpretation of discourse calls for readers to determine the referents of expressions.

Many messages that travel through the brain carry specific information of a propositional nature. The communicative theory, however, postulates an evolutionarily older, and cruder, form of internal communication by means of simple signals that are the internal equivalent of the nonverbal expressions we have just discussed. They do not require working memory for their interpretation, because their meanings are not composed grammatically from the meanings of their parts. One set of these signals concerns bodily feelings such as hunger and thirst, which arise from the monitoring of the internal environment. Another set of signals concerns *basic* emotions, which direct attention, mobilize innate bodily resources, and prepare appropriate suites of behaviors. They don't carry propositional information, but set the brain into specific states to coordinate our multiple goals and plans, given the constraints of time pressure and of our limited intellectual resources.

An emotional signal begins with an appraisal, which may or may not be conscious. But, the transition from the appraisal to the emotion is always unconscious. We cannot switch the emotion on or off. As Aristotle (1984, *Nichomachean Ethics*, line 1106a3) wrote, we cannot choose to feel anger or fear. Hence our emotions are a primitive sort of unconscious reasoning that manifests itself not in propositions, but in simple signals. Typically, we are aware of both the signal and of the appraisal. Introspection can tell us that we are angry because someone insulted us, but it cannot reveal the transition from the appraisal (that an insult has occurred) to the emotion.

The communicative theory postulates *basic* emotions and *complex* emotions (Oatley & Johnson-Laird, 1987, 1996). Basic emotions are innate and have their own distinctive signals in the brain (see, e.g., Panksepp, 1998, 2005) and in universal nonverbal expressions. They include happiness, sadness, anger, and fear. Basic emotions can arise as a result of rudimentary appraisals, and they can be experienced for no known reason (Oatley & Johnson-Laird, 1996). Basic emotions are the biological foundation of the *complex* emotions that appear to be unique to humans. Complex emotions depend on conscious appraisals that relate to our models of ourselves, and often to comparisons between alternative possibilities or between actual events and possibilities that we imagine in alternative histories. They therefore can be experienced only for known reasons. They include such emotions as empathy, jealousy, pride, and embarrassment. We feel empathy when we imagine ourselves in someone else's position and feel that person's sadness. Thus complex emotions integrate a basic emotional signal and a conscious cognitive appraisal. Complex emotions appear to depend on a region in the prefrontal lobes of the brain. If this region is damaged, individuals suffer impairments in their experience of these emotions, and cease to be able to plan their lives or to make sensible decisions (see, e.g., Damasio, 1994).

MUSIC AND EMOTIONS

Music appears to be universal to all cultures. Some evolutionary psychologists have argued that it serves no useful purpose (e.g., Pinker, 1997); others have suggested to the contrary that it may serve an adaptive role in sexual selection (e.g., Miller, 2000)—an idea that goes back to Darwin (1872/1965). The issue does not appear amenable to empirical testing. Nevertheless, music does depend on some innate predispositions. For example, 2-day-old hearing infants of congenitally deaf parents prefer singing that is intended for infants, which is more emotional, than singing that is intended for adults (Masataka, 1999). Likewise, infants recognize melodies that are transposed to a new key or played at a different tempo (Trehub, 2003). At 2 months of age, they prefer consonance to dissonance (Trainor, Tsang, & Cheung, 2002); at 4 months, they prefer a consonant melody to a dissonant one (Zentner & Kagan, 1998). So why is music universal? What is its appeal?

Most of us respond to this question with the answer that music stirs our emotions. But not everyone agrees. The great 19th-century music critic Eduard Hanslick argued that the appreciation of music does not depend on the emotions that it creates. He wrote (Hanslick, 1854/ 1957, p. 11): "An art aims, above all, at producing something beautiful which affects not our feelings but the organ of pure contemplation, our *imagination*" (italics Hanslick's). And the great 20th-century composer Igor Stravinsky (1936, p. 91) wrote: "I consider that music is, by its very nature, powerless to express anything at all, whether a feeling, an attitude of mind, a psychological mood, etc." A common argument in defense of this position is that emotions are *about* something, but pure music does not have any propositional content that enables it to be about anything (see, e.g., Nussbaum, 2001, and Sloboda & Juslin, 2001, for discussion). According to the communicative theory, however, basic emotions can be experienced in the absence of propositional content. They needn't be about anything. Indeed, from the 1890s onward, many experiments have shown that individuals *are* emotionally moved by music (Gilman, 1891, 1892; Downey, 1897), that it is a reliable way to induce moods, and that it elicits activity in regions of the brain known to mediate emotions. (For reviews of these three topics, see, respectively, Gabrielsson & Lindström, 2001; Västfjäll, 2002; and Peretz & Zatorre, 2003.)

A subtle distinction occurs between the emotions that listeners experience from listening to a piece of music and their judgments about what emotion the music expresses. Listeners can tell that a piece is intended to convey happiness, though they themselves are irritated by it. The same distinction occurs for readers of imaginative literature. As Oscar Wilde remarked about Charles Dickens's *The Old Curiosity Shop*, "One would have to have a heart of stone to read the death of Little Nell without laughing." Granted this distinction, studies that evoke emotions by way of music are essentially over when the experimenter has selected the materials. That is, their selection shows that at least one individual—the experimenter—is affected by the music.

Anecdotal evidence also supports the idea that music evokes emotions. In the 46th minute of Alfred Hitchcock's 47th movie, *Psycho*, the director did something shocking: He killed off his leading lady, Janet Leigh. He had planned to have no music during her murder in the shower, just sounds of the shower and her struggle with her assailant. Unbeknownst to him, the composer of the film's music, Bernard Herrmann, had put together a sequence of scary music—high-pitched shrieks on the violins, which anyone who has seen the movie is likely to recall. Hitchcock viewed both versions of the movie, one with natural sounds and the other with Herrmann's music, and declared that he had been wrong. The montage was much more frightening with the music (see also Oatley, 2004).

The standard answer is therefore correct: Music moves us. But it raises a mystery: How does it do so? It also raises another mystery: Why do we like to have our emotions stirred by music and other forms of art? We have only a little to say about this second mystery in our conclusions, and so we turn to the fundamentals of music pertinent to emotion.

Music is a social activity in most cultures. In the West, the single most popular piece of music is "Happy Birthday to You," which serves a social function. Readers may be surprised to learn that it is not a folk tune, but was composed by Mildred and Patti Hill and published in 1893. Most music in Western culture consists of a melody and an accompaniment, where the accompaniment is a simultaneous performance of other pitches in the form of chords.

A "melody" is a rhythmical sequence of pitches in a metrical framework. "Meter" is a regular pulse that provides the framework for rhythm (see, e.g., Lerdahl & Jackendoff, 1983; Longuet-Higgins & Lee, 1984; Johnson-Laird, 2002). It makes prediction easier, especially for musicians who have to synchronize their per-

formances. But meter is more than the number of beats in the measure: Beats and their subdivisions can be grouped in different ways. A good example is the contrast between two beats to the measure that are each subdivided into three, and waltz time, with three beats to the measure each subdivided into two. One measure in these two meters contains the same number of units, but their structures differ: One has two main pulses, and the other has three main pulses. Even individuals who are not musicians perceive meter, as shown in an unpublished experiment that Johnson-Laird carried out with Jung-Min Lee and Malcolm Bauer. The experimenter counts, "1, 2, 3, 4," in a regular way to establish a meter, and then claps the following rhythm in the same tempo:

$$\left| \ \flat \ \flat \ \flat \ \flat \ \right|$$

Listeners judge all four notes to be of the same duration. If, instead, the experimenter claps:

$$\left| \ \flat \ \flat \ \flat \ \natural \ \flat \ \right|$$

then the listeners judge the last note to be shorter than the others. Of course, the claps are all of the same brief duration. So why is the last note in the first case judged to be longer than the last note in the second case? The answer must be that listeners perceive both rhythms as having a meter of four beats to the measure, and that they tacitly infer that there will be a note on the first beat of the next measure. The interval from the onset of the last clap to the onset of this imagined clap is indeed longer in the first case than in the second. Hence listeners infer unconsciously that the onset of the next clap, even though it is imaginary, will occur on the first beat of the next measure. These judgments demonstrate the cognitive reality of metrical structure even for nonmusicians.

As many theorists have pointed out (e.g., Povel, 1984), the critical feature of a rhythm is the sequence of onsets of its notes. Hence if you clap the rhythm of a familiar piece, then listeners will be able to identify it. Clapping, of course, provides information only about onset times. If you play the sequence of pitches in a melody with each pitch having the same duration, it is hard for listeners to identify the melody. You might therefore suppose that more information is conveyed by the rhythm than by the sequence of pitches. The conclusion is unwarranted. The problem is that the equal duration of the pitches produces a new, albeit uniform, rhythm, which masks the real rhythm of the melody.

A simple demonstration showing that a sequence of pitches can identify a melody is Parsons's (1975) *Directory of Tunes and Musical Themes*. This directory represents any melody merely by its contour. It represents, for example, the famous opening of Beethoven's Fifth Symphony as follows:

> *R R D U R R D . . .

where * denotes the first note, R a repeat of the previous note, U an upward step, and D a downward step. As the directory shows, these eight symbols are common to five other themes, including one from Gilbert and Sullivan's *HMS Pinafore*. But once the first 15 notes of any theme in the classical repertory have been encoded in the notation, it is almost always identified uniquely.

In the Western tradition, melodies are "tonal" from the earliest music that survives through the great classical composers, the Romantics, and most 20th-century music (including popular songs, jazz, and rock and roll). Tonal melodies are made up from a subset of the possible pitches in the Western scale, and in this subset one note, the "tonic," is more important than the others. This note also gives its name to the key of the piece. For example, a melody in the key of C major is made up from the following 7 notes (from the standard scale of 12 notes): C D E F G A B. The chorus of The Beatles's "Yellow Submarine" starts with the following sequence of pitches, which we've transposed to the key of C major:

> I G G G G A I D D D D D D I D D D D D I C C C C C I

The vertical lines demarcate the measures. The key of C minor, which is slightly more dissonant, is made up from the following notes: C D E♭ F G A B C. Only one note makes the key a minor one, E♭ (i.e., E flat).

Western music has a number of global variables, whose values are normally held constant for some length of time during a piece. The seven most important of these variables are as follows:

1. Tempo, which varies from slow to fast.
2. Volume, which varies from soft to loud.
3. Register, which may be high or low (e.g., a melody may be a sequence of low pitches).
4. Dissonance, which includes whether the key is major or minor.
5. Timbre, which depends on the particular instrument that is played.
6. Range of melody, which may include only notes close to each other or may include large jumps in pitch.
7. Meter, which is the number of beats per measure.

Our theory of how music creates emotions is, like Aristotle's (1984, *Politics*, line 1340a11 et seq.), a mimetic one. Its first hypothesis is that music in itself creates only the basic emotions of happiness, sadness, anxiety, and anger. Music can also manipulate our level of arousal, and thus our general level of excitement. Of course, factors outside music, such as lyrics or a drama that it accompanies, can elicit complex emotions. Similarly, individuals can acquire associations between certain sorts of music and emotions, such as the association between waltzes and dancing, and these too can color the emotions that music creates. But what the present hypothesis rules out is that music alone can create object-oriented emotions of love or hate, or complex emotions. Evidence corroborates this account. Children of ages 4–6 are able to discriminate music expressing basic emotions (Cunningham & Sterling, 1988). Adults can recognize these emotions in music (Krumhansl, 1997). Music therapists can improvise music to convey these emotions to others (Bunt & Pavlicevic, 2001).

Meyer (1956), in one of the earliest and best-known theories of emotion and music, argued that music sets up expectations, which may be delayed in fulfillment: "Emotion or affect is aroused when a tendency to respond is arrested or inhibited" (p. 14). The longer resolution is postponed, the greater the affect. Hence emotion depends on the structure of music. This account is not incompatible with our hypothesis, and it may explain how music affects arousal. But it has little to say about the different emotions, such as happiness or sadness, that music evokes (Budd, 1985).

Arguments to the contrary of our hypothesis also exist. The music critic Deryck Cooke (1959) argued that music can express attitudes; that is, it does have propositional content. Hence he allocated to the different notes of the scale complex emotions, such as "pleasurable longing in the context of flux." And he assigned different emotions to various sequences of pitches in melodies. Gabriel (1978) failed to corroborate their occurrence in an experimental investigation (cf. Sloboda, 1985, p. 63). Scherer (2004) also argues that basic emotions are far too impoverished to do justice to our experiences of listening to music. One aspect of the perception of music, however, is that it is easy to "project" a program onto pure music—a propensity that musicians, critics, and nonmusicians all possess (see, e.g., Downey, 1897). This propensity can in turn lead us to ascribe emotions other than basic ones to a piece of music. Ives (1962, p. 36), for example, does so when he describes the opening of Beethoven's Fifth Symphony as "the soul of humanity at the door of divine mysteries, radiant in the faith that it will be opened—and the human become divine." McClary (1991, p. 128) goes a step further but in the opposite direction when she writes about Beethoven's Ninth Symphony, "The point of recapitulation in the first movement in the *Ninth* is one of the most horrifying moments in music, as the carefully prepared cadence is frustrated, damming up energy which finally explodes in the throttling, murderous rage of a rapist incapable of attaining release." When listeners indulge in this practice, they are imagining a program for which the music might make a suitable accompaniment, rather than responding to the music in itself. Pure music has no propositional content, and so it cannot express anything other than basic emotions. One person's program is another person's parody.

The second hypothesis of our theory is that music creates emotions in a mimetic way. It mimics the main characteristics of emotional behavior, speech, and thought (Scherer, 1986; Davies, 1994; Juslin & Laukka, 2003). It does so, in part, with settings of global parameters that create basic emotions. A simple illustration is that when people are sad, they move slowly and speak softly, with an intonation contour that does not make great leaps. When people are happy, however, they move more rapidly and speak loudly, with an intonation contour that can make great leaps for emphasis. The theory accordingly postulates the following sorts of settings:

Happiness—medium tempo, loud, concordant
Sadness—slow, muted, slightly discordant
Anxiety—scurrying, low pitch, discordant
Anger—fast, loud, high pitch, discordant

Bunt and Pavlicevic (2001) report a similar list of settings in the music that therapists improvise to convey emotions. Juslin (2001) also describes such a list, which he relates to innate programs for the vocal expression of emotions.

The third hypothesis of our theory is that music creates basic emotions because they depend on rudimentary cognitive appraisals calling for only minimal computational power. "Computational power" concerns what a system can compute, and minimal computational power depends on a system that has only a finite number of states; it makes no use of working memory for the results of intermediate computations (Hopcroft & Ullman, 1979). One corroboration of this hypothesis is the speed with which music conveys emotions. Individuals need less than a quarter of a second—a chord or a few notes of melody—to identify whether a musical excerpt is happy or sad (Peretz, Gagnon, & Bouchard, 1998).

Another corroboration comes from a computer program that Johnson-Laird devised to create melodies. A common view among composers is that melodies are a result of unconscious inspiration. Aaron Copland (1957, p. 102) wrote: "The composer starts with his theme; and the theme is a gift from heaven. He doesn't know where it comes from—has no control over it. It comes almost like automatic writing." The process of creating a melody is indeed akin to improvisation. Beethoven was a great improviser, and had no time for musicians who could not improvise:

> It has always been known that the greatest pianoforte players were also the greatest composers; but how did they play? Not like the pianists of to-day, who prance up and down the keyboard with passages that they have practised—putsch, putsch, putsch; what does that mean? Nothing! (Beethoven, quoted in Kinderman, 2000, p. 106)

Melodies are often the results of unconscious processes, and so they too are created—at least in their initial form—using minimal computational power, because unconscious processes have no access to working memory. But the creation of melodies can rely on long-term memories of other melodies, and of musical structures such as chord sequences. A minimal-finite-state system that is capable of infinitely many different outputs is one based on a matrix of transitions. Many theorists have analyzed the transition probabilities from one pitch to another in a set of melodies (e.g., Simonton, 2001). But a melody also has a rhythm, which needs to be taken into account. One solution, which the computer makes possible, is to construct an array of transitions from one pitch *and* its duration to the interval of the next pitch and its duration. The program takes as input a corpus of melodies and constructs such an array from them. The user then provides a chord sequence and specifies the number of beats in the bar. The program uses the probabilities in its array of transitions to generate a novel melody. Each call to the program generates a new melody, and the chances of its creating the same melody twice are negligible. Johnson-Laird used the program to construct arrays of transitions from corpora of happy, sad, and anxiety-provoking melodies, and then to generate melodies from these arrays. Figure 7.1 presents examples of each sort of melody. Audiences to whom they were played concurred that they conveyed the appropriate emotion, even though the melodies exploited only some of the relevant global variables.

Melodies may have an improvisational quality, at least when they first come to a composer's mind, but the process of composition may lead to modifications. Even though Beethoven was a great improviser, his process of composition was laborious; at least 8,000 pages of his notebooks survive. Composed music has a large-scale structure, and Beethoven began his career by using "models" of these structures from Haydn and Mozart (Sisman, 2000). Such structures, and the sequences of chords, call for more computational power than unconscious processes can muster. They need a working memory for the results of intermediate computations (see Johnson-Laird, 2002), and musical notation can act as a substitute for such a memory. Musical structure, however, is what Hanslick (1854/1957) considered as crucial for beauty. Our perception of this structure may in turn lead to an "esthetic" emotion (Scherer, 2004)—an emotion that we regard as akin to awe, a complex emotion rooted in anxiety.

LITERATURE AND EMOTIONS

Just as pure music is nonpropositional, fictional literature is propositional. When we read fiction, we expect to experience emotions. The question is this: How can such propositional content prompt these emotions?

As with music, we distinguish the esthetic emotion that occurs in response to literature from the emotions of involvement in a story (Oatley, 1994). The esthetic emotion depends on an appreciation of beauty in the use of language. It calls for readers to achieve an esthetic distance from the work (Cupchik, 2002) and for them to have had a sufficient experience with literature to develop an appreciation of its skillful use. Consider, for instance, the first stanza of Coleridge's "Kubla Khan," published in 1816 (Coleridge, 1977):

> In Xanadu did Kubla Khan
> A stately pleasure dome decree:
> Where Alph, the sacred river, ran
> Through caverns measureless to man
> Down to a sunless sea.

The iambic rhythm, the assonance on the sound of "ah," the alliterations (e.g., "Kubla Khan"), the rhymes (e.g., "Khan, ran, man"),

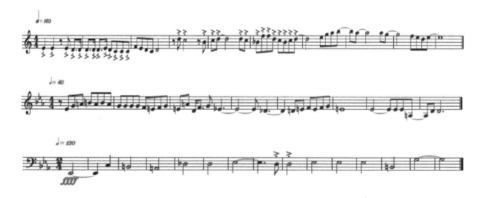

FIGURE 7.1. Three melodies (happy in the key of C major, sad in the key of C minor, and anxious in the key of C minor) created by a computer program using a finite-state system of transitions derived from corpora of real melodies.

and the exoticism ("Xanadu") may all move us in a way akin to music. However, our understanding of the propositional content of literature also elicits emotions. In "Kubla Khan," the content is difficult. We come to understand it either from several readings and much contemplation, or from knowing some of Coleridge's preoccupations, or from having someone knowledgeable explain it to us (e.g., Paglia, 2005). The poem is a metaphor for the place of art and the artist in society. Hence the pleasure dome is a metonymic figure (a "synecdoche") for art in general. The sacred river is a metaphor for the stream of artistic creativity that flows through society. The poem evokes further images as it continues: the source of creativity in nature and sexuality ("as if this earth in fast thick pants were breathing"), the potential enmity between the artist and society ("ancestral voices prophesying war"), an image of the artist ("A damsel with a dulcimer"), and the status of the artist as demigod ("for he on honey dew hath fed / and drunk the milk of paradise"). Some poetry, such as Mallarmé's, makes its emotional effect almost entirely in terms of its music rather than its propositional content. It was Mallarmé who reminded his painter friend, Degas, that poetry was made from words, not ideas.

Certain novelists, notably Flaubert, have insisted that the arrangements of words in their works should be as delicate and precise as those of poetry (see, e.g., Williams, 2004). Yet, in prose, the emphasis shifts toward a primacy of the propositional. Consider the opening line of L. P. Hartley's (1953) novel *The Go-Between*: "The past is another country: they do things differently there." "Another country" is a wonderful metaphor, but it does not have the rhythmic and alliterative music of "A damsel with a dulcimer." Above all in literature, propositional content prompts our emotions. These emotions can be basic, but they can be complex emotions too, depending on appraisals of the self in relation to others. Consider jealousy. It springs from our suspicion that a third person might displace us in a relationship with someone we love. The basic emotion may be fear or anger, but jealousy depends on inferences about the relations among three individuals, and these inferences in turn hinge on propositional content. A beautiful depiction of jealousy occurs in Frank O'Connor's short story "My Oedipus Complex" (O'Connor, 1963). The protagonist is a young boy, and the story follows his growing understanding of the impact of his father's return from the war and his own displacement from the center of his mother's affections. We enter his world and empathize with his anger and distress as he realizes that he has been displaced. The emotional effect on us is powerful and fascinating, because it resonates with emotions that we have experienced too. But something mysterious and ambiguous remains: The boy has not quite understood his own emotion.

T. S. Eliot (1919/1953) argued that artists do not describe emotions subjectively, but offer instead an external, objective pattern of events, which he referred to as the "objective correlative." Our appraisal of these events leads us to experience emotions. This view foreshadows those theories of emotions that hinge on our cognitive appraisals. We use our knowledge of the language to assemble the meanings of sentences from the meanings of the words and the grammatical relations among them. And, as experiments have shown, we use these meanings to construct a mental model of the individuals and events to which the discourse refers (see, e.g., Johnson-Laird, 1983, Ch. 14; Garnham, 2001). But how does such a model—the objective correlative—suggest emotions?

We propose three hypotheses intended to answer this question (see Oatley, 1994). The first hypothesis is that literature can suggest emotions because we identify with the protagonist and resist antagonists. The propositional content of a story affects us most powerfully when, like Alice through the looking glass, we enter through its surface into its interior. The typical mode of narrative, as Bruner (1986) has pointed out, concerns human plans and their vicissitudes. The author provides us with the content that allows us to construct a dynamic model that simulates such a world, its characters, and their interactions (Oatley, 1999). And we enter the simulation when we identify with a character in the story (see Freud, 1905–1906/ 1985). Flaubert is supposed to have said, "Madame Bovary, c'est moi." But we too can become Madame Bovary as we read the novel. We are caught up in her experience (see also Miall & Kuiken, 2002; Zillmann, 1994). We run her plans on our own planning processors. When these plans meet vicissitudes, we experience emotions. They occur within our simulation, and they are our emotions. Identification is empathy, as shown in the emotions elicited from movies (Trabasso & Chung, 2004). But the empathy is not quite as it is in real life, because we empathize with a fiction—a nonexistent individual whom we have created in our simulation of the story (see also Lipps, 1962; Kreitler & Kreitler, 1962). Although the effects are familiar, they remain surprising. As Hamlet says, after witnessing an actor affected by emotion as he plays a part, "What's Hecuba to him, or he to Hecuba?" (Shakespeare, c. 1600/ 1981). It may be that actors, during rehearsal though not necessarily during performance (Konijn, 2000), use Stanislavski's (1936) method of drawing on their own autobiographies to reexperience certain emotions.

Our second hypothesis is that literature can prompt us to feel an emotion about a character. Tan and Frijda have proposed a theory that is a version of this idea, but intended to cover the same ground as our first hypothesis about identification with characters (Tan, 1996; Tan & Frijda, 1999). They argue that an author provides appraisal patterns and that we pick up these patterns as they apply to characters. As a result, we may feel sympathetic emotions toward these characters. Tan (1996) calls these "witness emotions." We argue that when we analyze events in our simulation, we infer how they would strike a character in it so that we can feel sympathy for the character, but in our view the process coexists with identification. Indeed, we may like or admire a protagonist, or fear or loathe a villain. When Dorothea, the heroine of George Eliot's novel *Middlemarch* (1872/1991), agrees to marry the aged scholar Casaubon, she is full of enthusiasm to help him with his work, and we share some of her enthusiasm. At the same time, our hearts sink. We respond this way in part because Eliot has conveyed Casaubon's character to us in a way that goes beyond Dorothea's understanding of him. One of the skills of great writers is to make us feel the emotions of a character with whom we identify, and quite different emotions toward the same character.

This distinction was important for medieval Indian literary theorists such as Abhinavagupta (see, e.g., Ingalls, Massson, & Patwardhan, 1990). They described the emotions depicted by an actor in a play, using facial expressions, gestures, tone of voice, and the content of utterances, and the corresponding emotions (*rasas* in Sanskrit) that occur in audiences (see Oatley et al., 2006, p. 112). For example, when an actor depicts amusement or anger, the audience identifies and feels amusement or anger. But when an actor depicts sorrow, the audience feels compassion for the character; when an actor depicts something disgusting, the audience feels loathing. According to these theorists, *rasas* are literary emotions and subtly distinct from the emotions of daily life. Each well-constructed work should be based on a single *rasa*, which is the basis for a genre (e.g., a love story, a comedy, a tragedy). Within a story, other *rasas* may also occur, but in a supporting and transient way. Hogan (2003) has reviewed stories worldwide and reports that the two most common genres are the love story and the story of an angry conflict.

The third hypothesis of our theory is that emotions can also depend on personal memories (Larsen & Seilman, 1998). Events in a simulation may elicit only our memory of an emotion, while the events themselves remain implicit. Hence, according to Scheff (1979), we may cry at the fate of the protagonists in *Romeo and Juliet* because we are reexperiencing earlier losses of our own, which are reactivated, though not necessarily consciously, by the play's events.

Following these hypotheses we can propose a generalization. Along with the cues in a text that enable the reader or audience member to construct a simulation, any literary work has also what Oatley (1999) has called a "suggestion structure." It is principally this structure that prompts emotions in the ways indicated by our three hypotheses: by suggesting (1) empathetic identifications, (2) sympathies and antagonisms, and (3) scenes that might prompt memories. Although figurative language is not necessary to this structure (see, e.g., Oatley, 2004), tropes such as metaphor and metonymy (see Lodge, 1977) prompt emotions principally by suggestion. An individual may read Hartley's (1953) metaphor, "The past is another country," and think of a visit to another country, Kashmir—which triggers thoughts of being in a 450-year-old painting by Bruegel, with chickens walking in the road, and people carrying bundles of firewood. This thought adds emotional potency to the metaphor. Western theories of poetics neglect the role of suggestion, but in Eastern poetics it is stressed, and there is a Sanskrit word for it, *dhvani*. Abhinavagupta argued that *dhvani* is the heart of poetry (see Ingalls et al., 1990).

Experiments have shown that stories do elicit emotions in people who read them (Miall & Kuiken, 2002; Oatley, 2002). Furthermore, a study by Nundy (1996) has corroborated the role of personal suggestion. The participants read a short story by Russell Banks in which a man cruelly severs his relationship with a woman. The participants experienced strong emotions as a result, but their nature differed from one person to another: Some readers were angry, others were sad, and a few were disgusted. Another corroboration of suggestion is that readers of a narrative piece had more memories that were personal (as compared with generic memories) than readers of a nonnarrative piece of the same length, propositional content, and reading difficulty (Mar, Oatley, & Eng, 2003).

CONCLUSIONS

Emotions arise from unconscious transitions, and so we are often puzzled by our emotional reactions. Sometimes they are so aberrant in intensity and so prolonged in their effects that they create a psychological illness (Johnson-Laird, Mancini, & Gangemi, 2006). Art may help us to understand them better. One of the principal theories of emotion's relation to art is that of Collingwood (1938): Art is the expression of an emotion in a particular language—words, sculpture, paintings—so that we come to understood the emotion better (Oatley, 2003). Music is mystifying in its emotional effects, but we enjoy the emotions it creates. In contrast, literature helps us to understand the relation between propositional content and subjective feelings—to understand the causes of an emotion, and why a particular individual in a particular circumstance feels a particular emotion. The Indian theorists said that we fail to understand our emotions because a thick crust of egotism obscures our vision. *Rasas*, however, allow us to see more deeply into their nature, because of their literary context. Nussbaum (1986) similarly translates Aristotle's *katharsis* as "clarification" or "illumination." In literary fiction, it becomes possible to understand emotions as they occur in a wider set of circumstances than we would encounter in our ordinary lives.

REFERENCES

Aristotle. (1984). *The complete works of Aristotle* (Vols. 1 and 2, rev. Oxford trans., J. Barnes, Ed.). Princeton, NJ: Princeton University Press.

Austen, J. (1906). *Pride and prejudice*. London: Dent. (Original work published 1813)

Bruner, J. (1986). *Actual minds, possible worlds*. Cambridge, MA: Harvard University Press.

Budd, M. (1985). *Music and the emotions: The philosophical theories*. London: Routledge.

Bunt, L., & Pavlicevic, M. (2001). Music and emotion: Perspectives from music therapy. In P. N. Juslin & J. A. Sloboda (Eds.), *Music and emotion: Theory and research* (pp. 181–201). Oxford: Oxford University Press.

Coleridge, S. T. (1977). *The portable Coleridge*. Harmondsworth, UK: Penguin.

Collingwood, R. G. (1938). *The principles of art*. Oxford: Oxford University Press.

Cooke, D. (1959). *The language of music*. Oxford: Oxford University Press.

Copland, A. (1957). *What to listen for in music*. New York: McGraw-Hill.

Coulmas, F. (1996). *The Blackwell encyclopedia of writing systems*. Oxford, UK: Blackwell.

Cunningham, J. G., & Sterling, R. S. (1988). Developmental change in the understanding of affective meaning in music. *Motivation and Emotion, 12*, 399–413.

Cupchik, G. C. (2002). The evolution of psychical distance as an aesthetic concept. *Culture and Psychology, 8*, 155–187.

Damasio, A. R. (1994). *Descartes' error: Emotion, reason, and the human brain*. New York: Putnam.

Darwin, C. (1965). *The expression of the emotions in man and animals*. Chicago: University of Chicago Press. (Original work published 1872)

Davies, S. (1994). *Musical meaning and expression*. Ithaca, NY: Cornell University Press.

Downey, J. E. (1897). A musical experiment. *American Journal of Psychology, 9*, 63–69.

Eliot, G. (1991). *Middlemarch*. New York: Knopf. (Original work published 1872)

Eliot, T. S. (1953). Hamlet. In J. Hayward (Ed.), *T. S. Eliot: Selected prose* (pp. 104–110). Harmondsworth, UK: Penguin. (Original work published 1919)

Fitch, W. T., Hauser, M., & Chomsky, N. (2005). The evolution of the language faculty: Clarifications and implications. *Cognition, 97*, 179–210.

Freud, S. (1985). Psychopathic characters on the stage. In A. Dickson (Ed.), *Pelican Freud library: Vol. 14: Art and literature* (pp. 119–127). London: Penguin. (Original work published 1905–1906)

Gabriel, C. (1978). An experimental study of Deryck Cooke's theory of music and meaning. *Psychology of Music, 6*, 13–20.

Gabrielsson, A., & Lindström, E. (2001). The influence of musical structure on emotional expression. In P. N. Juslin & J. A. Sloboda (Eds.), *Music and emotion: Theory and research* (pp. 223–248). Oxford: Oxford University Press.

Garnham, A. (2001). *Mental models and the representation of anaphora*. Hove, UK: Psychology Press.

Gerrig, R. J. (1993). *Experiencing narrative worlds: On*

the psychological activities of reading. New Haven, CT: Yale University Press.

Gilman, B. I. (1891). Report of an experimental test of musical expressiveness. *American Journal of Psychology, 4,* 558–576.

Gilman, B. I. (1892). Report of an experimental test of musical expressiveness (continued). *American Journal of Psychology, 5,* 42–73.

Hanslick, E. (1957). *The beautiful in music* (7th ed., G. Cohen, Trans.). New York: Liberal Arts Press. (Original work published 1854; this ed. originally published 1885)

Hartley, L. P. (1953). *The go-between.* London: Hamilton.

Hjort, M., & Laver, S. (Eds.). (1997). *Emotion and the arts.* Oxford: Oxford University Press.

Hogan, P. C. (2003). *The mind and its stories: Narrative universals and human emotion.* Cambridge, UK: Cambridge University Press.

Hopcroft, J. E., & Ullman, J. D. (1979). *Formal languages and their relation to automata.* Reading, MA: Addison-Wesley.

Huron, D. (2003). Is music an evolutionary adaptation? In I. Peretz & R. Zatorre (Eds.), *The cognitive neuroscience of music* (pp. 57–75). Oxford: Oxford University Press.

Ingalls, D. H., Masson, J. M., & Patwardhan, M. V. (1990). *The Dhvanyaloka of Anandavardana with the Locana of Abhinavagupta.* Cambridge, MA: Harvard University Press.

Ives, C. (1962). *Essays before a sonata and other writings.* (H. Boatwright, Ed.). New York: Norton.

Johnson-Laird, P. N. (1983). *Mental models: Towards a cognitive science of language, inference, and consciousness.* Cambridge, MA: Harvard University Press.

Johnson-Laird, P. N. (2002). How jazz musicians improvise. *Music Perception, 19,* 415–442.

Johnson-Laird, P. N., Mancini, F., & Gangemi, A. (2006). A hyper-emotion theory of psychological illnesses. *Psychological Review, 113,* 822–841.

Johnson-Laird, P. N., & Oatley, K. (2000). The cognitive and social construction of emotions. In M. Lewis & J. M. Haviland-Jones (Eds.), *Handbook of emotions* (2nd ed., pp. 458–475). New York: Guilford Press.

Juslin, P. N. (2001). Communicating emotion in music performance: A review and theoretical framework. In P. N. Juslin & J. A. Sloboda (Eds.), *Music and emotion: Theory and research* (pp. 309–337). Oxford: Oxford University Press.

Juslin, P. N., & Laukka, P. (2003). Communication of emotions in vocal expression and music performance: Different channels, same code? *Psychological Bulletin, 129,* 770–814.

Keltner, D., Ekman, P., Gonzaga, G. C., & Beer, J. (2003). Facial expression of emotion. In R. J. Davidson, K. R. Scherer, & H. H. Goldsmith (Eds.), *Handbook of affective sciences* (pp. 415–432). New York: Oxford University Press.

Kinderman, W. (2000). The piano music: Concertos, sonatas, variations, small forms. In G. Stanley (Ed.), *The Cambridge companion to Beethoven* (pp. 105–126). Cambridge, UK: Cambridge University Press.

Konijn, E. (2000). *Acting emotions: Shaping emotions on stage.* Amsterdam: Amsterdam University Press.

Kreitler, H., & Kreitler, S. (1972). *Psychology and the arts.* Durham, NC: Duke University Press.

Krumhansl, C. L. (1997). An exploratory study of musical emotions and psychophysiology. *Canadian Journal of Experimental Psychology, 51,* 336–352.

Larsen, S. F., & Seilman, U. (1988). Personal meanings while reading literature. *Text, 8,* 411–429.

Lerdahl, F., & Jackendoff, R. (1983). *A generative theory of tonal music.* Cambridge, MA: MIT Press.

Lipps, T. (1962). Empathy, inner imitation, and sense feeling. In M. Rader (Ed.), *A modern book on esthetics: An anthology* (3rd ed., pp. 374–382). New York: Holt, Rinehart & Winston.

Lodge, D. (1977). *The modes of modern writing: Metaphor, metonymy, and the typology of modern fiction.* Ithaca, NY: Cornell University Press.

Longuet-Higgins, H. C., & Lee, C. S. (1984). The rhythmic interpretation of monophonic music. *Music Perception, 1,* 424–441.

Mar, R., Oatley, K., & Eng, A. (2003, August). *Abstraction and the vividness of details in fiction.* Paper presented at the annual convention of the American Psychological Association, Toronto.

Masataka, N. (1999). Preference for infant-directed singing in 2-day-old hearing infants of deaf parents. *Developmental Psychology, 35,* 1001–1005.

McClary, S. (1991). *Feminine endings: Music, gender, and sexuality.* Minneapolis: University of Minneapolis Press.

Meyer, L. B. (1956). *Emotion and meaning in music.* Chicago: University of Chicago Press.

Miall, D. S., & Kuiken, D. (2002). A feeling for fiction: Becoming what we behold. *Poetics, 30,* 221–241.

Miller, G. (2000). Evolution of human music through sexual selection. In N. L. Wallis, B. Merker, & S. Brown (Eds.), *The origins of music* (pp. 319–360). Cambridge, MA: MIT Press.

Mithen, S. (1996). *The prehistory of the mind: The cognitive origins of art and science.* London: Thames & Hudson.

Nundy, S. (1996). *The effects of emotion on human inference: Towards a computational model.* Unpublished doctoral dissertation, University of Toronto.

Nussbaum, M. C. (1986). *The fragility of goodness: Luck and ethics in Greek tragedy and philosophy.* Cambridge, UK: Cambridge University Press.

Nussbaum, M. C. (2001). *Upheavals of thought: The intelligence of emotions.* Cambridge, UK: Cambridge University Press.

Oatley, K. (1994). A taxonomy of the emotions of literary response and a theory of identification in fictional narrative. *Poetics, 23,* 53–74.

Oatley, K. (1999). Why fiction may be twice as true as fact: Fiction as cognitive and emotional simulation. *Review of General Psychology, 3,* 101–117.

Oatley, K. (2002). Emotions and the story worlds of fiction. In M. C. Green, J. J. Strange, & T. C. Brock (Eds.), *Narrative impact: Social and cognitive foundations* (pp. 39–69). Mahwah, NJ: Erlbaum.

Oatley, K. (2003). Creative expression and communication of emotion in the visual and narrative arts. In R. J. Davidson, K. R. Scherer, & H. H. Goldsmith (Eds.), *Handbook of affective sciences* (pp. 481–502). New York: Oxford University Press.

Oatley, K. (2004). Scripts, transformations, and suggestiveness, of emotions in Shakespeare and Chekhov. *Review of General Psychology, 8,* 323–340.

Oatley, K., & Johnson-Laird, P. N. (1987). Towards a cognitive theory of emotion. *Cognition and Emotion, 1,* 29–50.

Oatley, K., & Johnson-Laird, P. N. (1996). The communicative theory of emotions: Empirical tests, mental models, and implications for social interaction. In L. L. Martin & A. Tesser (Eds.), *Striving and feeling: Interactions among goals, affect, and self-regulation* (pp. 363–393). Mahwah, NJ: Erlbaum.

Oatley, K., Keltner, D., & Jenkins, J. M. (2006). *Understanding emotions* (2nd ed.). Malden, MA: Blackwell.

O'Connor, F. (1963). *My Oedipus complex, and other stories.* Harmondsworth, UK: Penguin.

Paglia, C. (2005). *Break, blow, burn.* New York: Pantheon.

Panksepp, J. (1998). *Affective neuroscience: The foundations of human and animal emotions.* Oxford: Oxford University Press.

Panksepp, J. (2005). Affective consciousness: Core emotional feelings in animals and humans. *Consciousness and Cognition, 14,* 30–80.

Parsons, D. (1975). *The directory of tunes and musical themes.* Cambridge, UK: Brown.

Peretz, I., Gagnon, L., & Bouchard, B. (1998). Music and emotion: Perceptual determinants, immediacy, and isolation after brain damage. *Cognition, 68,* 111–141.

Peretz, I., & Zattore, R. J. (Eds.). (2003). *The cognitive neuroscience of music.* New York: Oxford University Press.

Pinker, S. (1997). *How the mind works.* New York: Norton.

Povel, D.-J. (1984). A theoretical framework for rhythm perception. *Psychological Research, 45,* 315–337.

Robinson, J. (Ed.). (1997). *Music and meaning.* Ithaca, NY: Cornell University Press.

Russell, J. A., Bachorowski, J. A., & Fernandez-Dols, J. M. (2003). Facial and vocal expression of emotion. *Annual Review of Psychology, 54,* 329–349.

Scheff, T. J. (1979). *Catharsis in healing, ritual, and drama.* Berkeley: University of California Press.

Scherer, K. R. (1986). Vocal affect expression: A review and a model for future research. *Psychological Bulletin, 99,* 143–165.

Scherer, K. R. (2004). Which emotions can be induced by music? What are the underlying mechanisms? And how can we measure them? *Journal of New Music Research, 33,* 239–251.

Shakespeare, W. (1981). *Hamlet* (H. Jenkins, Ed.). London: Methuen. (Original work performed c. 1600)

Simonton, D. K. (2001). Emotion and composition in classical music: Historiometric perspectives. In P. N. Juslin & J. A. Sloboda (Eds.), *Music and emotion: Theory and research* (pp. 205–222). Oxford: Oxford University Press.

Sisman, E. (2000). "The spirit of Mozart from Haydn's hands": Beethoven's musical inheritance. In G. Stanley (Ed.), *The Cambridge companion to Beethoven* (pp. 45–63). Cambridge, UK: Cambridge University Press.

Sloboda, J. A. (1985). *The musical mind: The cognitive psychology of music.* Oxford: Clarendon Press.

Sloboda, J. A., & Juslin, P. N. (2001). Music and emotion: Commentary. In P. N. Juslin & J. A. Sloboda (Eds.), *Music and emotion: Theory and research* (pp. 453–462). Oxford: Oxford University Press.

Stanislavski, C. (1936). *An actor prepares* (E. R. Habgood, Trans.). New York: Routledge.

Stravinsky, I. (1936). *Chronicles of my life.* New York: Simon & Schuster.

Tan, E. S. (1996). *Emotion and the structure of film: Film as an emotion machine.* Mahwah, NJ: Erlbaum.

Tan, E. S., & Frijda, N. H. (1999). Sentiment in film viewing. In C. Plantinga & G. M. Smith (Eds.), *Passionate views: Film, cognition, and emotion* (pp. 48–64). Baltimore: Johns Hopkins University Press.

Trabasso, T., & Chung, J. (2004, January). *Empathy: Tracking characters and monitoring their concerns in film.* Paper presented at the Winter Text Conference, Jackson Hole, WY.

Trainor, L. J., Tsang, C. D., & Cheung, V. H. W. (2002). Preference for consonance in 2- and 4-month-old infants. *Music Perception, 20,* 187–194.

Trehub, S. E. (2003). Musical predispositions in infancy: An update. In I. Peretz & R. Zatorre (Eds.), *The cognitive neuroscience of music* (pp. 3–20). Oxford: Oxford University Press.

Västfjäll, D. (2002). Emotion induction through music: A review of the musical mood induction procedure. *Musicae Scientiae,* 173–211.

Williams, T. (2004). The writing process: Scenarios, sketches and rough drafts. In T. Unwin (Ed.), *The Cambridge companion to Flaubert* (pp. 165–179). Cambridge, UK: Cambridge University Press.

Zentner, M. R., & Kagan, J. (1998). Infants' perception of consonance and dissonance in music. *Infant Behavior and Development, 21,* 483–492.

Zillmann, D. (1994). Mechanisms of emotional involvement with drama. *Poetics, 23,* 33–51.

CHAPTER 8

The Evolutionary Psychology of the Emotions and Their Relationship to Internal Regulatory Variables

JOHN TOOBY and LEDA COSMIDES

Evolutionary psychology is an attempt to unify the psychological, social, and behavioral sciences theoretically and empirically within a single, mutually consistent, seamless scientific framework. The core of this enterprise is the integration of principles and findings drawn from evolutionary biology, cognitive science, anthropology, economics, and neuroscience with psychology in order to produce high-resolution maps of human nature. By "human nature," evolutionary psychologists mean the evolved, reliably developing, species-typical computational architecture of the human mind, together with the physical structures and processes (in the brain, in development, and in genetics) that give rise to this information-processing architecture. For evolutionary psychologists, all forms of knowledge about brains and behavior are relevant, but the pivotal step is using these facts to form accurate models of the information-processing structure of psychological mechanisms.

The discovery of a correct information-processing description of a psychological mechanism is the fundamental clarifying scientific step, because each mechanism came into existence and was organized by natural selection in order to carry out its particular set of information-processing functions. It is not a metaphor but a reality that the brain is a computer—a physical system that came into existence to carry out computations. The computations were needed to solve the adaptive problem of regulating behavior successfully. Hence the brain (and its subsystems) evolved to carry out specific varieties of computation in order to regulate behavior so that it was biologically successful—that is, to assemble the individual somatically and neurally, to prevent prereproductive death, to increase the probability of achieving conditions (social and physical) that would have led to successful reproduction in the ancestral world, to reproduce successfully, and to assist genetic relatives (including children) to achieve and maintain conditions for their own successful reproduction.

In short, the functional subcomponents (programs) that constitute our psychological architecture were designed by natural selection to solve adaptive problems faced by our hunter–gatherer ancestors by regulating behavior in ways that increased genetic propagation—what biologists call "fitness." Against the otherwise disordering forces of entropy that pervade all of physical reality, natural selection is the only process that introduces functional organization into the designs of organisms (Tooby, Cosmides, & Barrett, 2003). So, to the extent that there is functional organization in the human psychological architecture, it was created by, reflects, and is explained by the operation of natural selection among our ancestors. This is why evolutionary psychology is not a specific subfield of psychology, such as the study of vision, reasoning, or social behavior. It is a way of approaching the science of psychology that produces (or is intended to produce) stable functional descriptions of the elements of the mind. (Detailed arguments for these positions can be found in Tooby & Cosmides, 1990a, 1990b, 1992a, 2005, and in Cosmides & Tooby, 1987, 1992, 1997.)

Researchers less familiar with evolutionary psychology often equate adaptive problems exclusively with short-run threats to physical survival. However, survival per se is not central to evolution: All individual organisms die sooner or later. In contrast, genes—which can be thought of as particles of design—are potentially immortal, and design features spread by promoting the reproduction of the genes that participate in building them. Survival is significant only insofar as it promotes the reproduction of design features into subsequent generations. Survival is no more significant than anything else that promotes reproduction, and is often advantageously risked or sacrificed in the process of promoting reproduction in self, children, or other relatives. Nearly every kind of event or condition has the potential to have some impact on the prospect of reproduction for individuals, their children, and their relatives. Consequently, selection on neural designs for functional behavior reaches out to encompass, in a network of cause and effect linkages, virtually all of human life, from the subtleties of facial expression to attributions of responsibility to the intrinsic rewards of play. The realm of adaptive information-processing problems is

not limited to one area of human life, such as sex, violence, or resource acquisition. Instead, it is a dimension cross-cutting all areas of human life, as weighted by the strange, nonintuitive metric of their cross-generational statistical effects on direct and kin reproduction.

By "computation," evolutionary psychologists simply mean the organized causation of patterned information input–output relations. Natural selection poses adaptive problems of behavior regulation, and the mechanisms of the brain evolved to engineer solutions in the form of these regulatory input–output relations. Of course, these computational relations must be embodied physically in neural tissue, and must be designed to develop reliably. Adaptations are not just the products of the genes, but are the products of the coordinated interaction of a stable genetic inheritance and the evolutionarily long-enduring features of the environment.

A model of an evolved neurocomputational mechanism or program would answer questions such as these: What information does the program take as input? How is this information encoded, formatted, and represented as data structures? What operations are performed on these data structures to transform them into new representations or regulatory elements? And how do these procedures and data structures interact to generate and regulate behavior? In short, how does each program work in cause-and-effect terms?

AN EVOLUTIONARY-PSYCHOLOGICAL APPROACH TO THE EMOTIONS

Although an evolutionary-psychological approach can be applied to any topic in psychology, it is especially illuminating when applied to the emotions. To the extent that there is functional order to be found in the mechanisms responsible for the emotions, it was forged over evolutionary time by natural selection acting on our ancestors. The analysis of adaptive problems that arose ancestrally has led evolutionary psychologists to apply the concepts and methods of the evolutionary sciences to scores of topics that are relevant to the study of emotion. These include anger, cooperation, sexual attraction, jealousy, aggression, parental love, friendship, romantic love, the aesthetics of landscape preferences, coalitional aggression, incest avoidance, disgust, predator avoidance, kinship, and family relations (for reviews, see Barkow, Cosmides, & Tooby, 1992; Buss, 2005; Crawford & Krebs, 1998; Daly & Wilson, 1988; Pinker, 1997).

Indeed, a rich theory of the emotions naturally emerges out of the core principles of evolutionary psychology (Tooby, 1985; Tooby & Cosmides, 1990a; Cosmides & Tooby, 2000; see also Nesse, 1991). In this chapter, we (1) briefly state what we think emotions are and what adaptive problem they were designed to solve; (2) explain the evolutionary and computational principles that led us to this view; (3) identify how the emotions relate to motivational and other underlying regulatory variables the human brain is designed to generate and access; and (4) using this background, explicate in a more detailed way the design of emotion programs and the states they create.

It may strike some as odd to speak about love, jealousy, or disgust in computational terms. "Computation" has an affectless, flavorless connotation. But if the brain evolved as a system of information-processing relations, then emotions are, in an evolutionary sense, best understood as information-processing relations—that is, programs—with naturally selected functions. Initially, the commitment to exploring the underlying computational architecture of the emotions may seem infelicitous, but viewing them as programs leads to a large number of scientific payoffs. In particular, the claim that emotion is computational does not mean that an evolutionary-psychological approach misconstrues human experience as bloodless, affectless, disembodied ratiocination. It is simply the claim that one can describe the underlying set of informational relationships that explain emotional phenomena, including the nature of emotional experience. Every mechanism in the brain—whether it does something categorizable as "cold cognition" (such as reasoning, inducing a rule of grammar, or judging a probability) or as "hot cognition" (such as computing the intensity of parental fear, the imperative to strike an adversary, or an escalation in infatuation)—depends on an underlying computational organization to give its operation its patterned structure, as well as a set of neural circuits to implement it physically. In these terms, an evolutionary and computational view of emotion can open up for

exploration new empirical and theoretical possibilities obscured by other frameworks.

AN EVOLUTIONARY-PSYCHOLOGICAL THEORY OF THE EMOTIONS

Both deductions from theoretical evolutionary psychology and a large supporting body of empirical findings in psychology, biology, and neuroscience support the view that the human mental architecture is crowded with evolved, functionally specialized programs. Each is tailored to solve a different adaptive problem that arose during human evolutionary history (or before), such as face recognition, foraging, mate choice, heart rate regulation, sleep management, or predator vigilance, and each is activated by a different set of cues from the environment.

But the existence of all these diverse programs itself creates an adaptive problem: Programs that are individually designed to solve specific adaptive problems could, if simultaneously activated, deliver outputs that conflict with one another, interfering with or nullifying each other's functional products. For example, sleep and flight from a predator require mutually inconsistent actions, computations, and physiological states. It is difficult to sleep when your heart and mind are racing with fear, and this is no accident: Disastrous consequences would ensue if proprioceptive cues were activating sleep programs at the same time that the sight of a stalking lion was activating ones designed for predator evasion. To avoid such consequences, the mind must be equipped with superordinate programs that override and deactivate some programs when others are activated (e.g., a program that deactivates sleep programs when predator evasion subroutines are activated). Reciprocally, many adaptive problems are best solved by the coordinated activation of a specific subset of programs, with each program being entrained into the computational settings most appropriate for the particular adaptive problem being faced. For example, predator avoidance may require simultaneous shifts in both heart rate and auditory acuity (see below). To do this, a special type of program is required that manages and harmonizes other programs, aligning each of them into the proper configuration at the right time.

In general, to behave functionally according to evolutionary standards, the mind's many subprograms need to be orchestrated so that their joint product at any given time is coordinated to deal with the adaptive challenge being faced, rather than operating in a self-defeating, discoordinated, and cacophonous fashion. We argue that such coordination is accomplished by a special class of programs: the emotions that evolved to solve these superordinate demands. In this view, the best way to understand what the emotions are, what they do, and how they operate is to recognize that mechanism orchestration is the function that defines the emotions, and explains in detail their design features. They are the neurocomputational adaptations that have evolved in response to the adaptive problem of matching arrays of mechanism activation to the specific adaptive demands imposed by alternative situations (Tooby & Cosmides, 1990a; Tooby, 1985; Cosmides & Tooby, 2000; Nesse, 1991).

Thus each emotion evolved to deal with a particular, evolutionarily recurrent situation type. The design features of the emotion program, when the emotion is activated, presume the presence of an ancestrally structured situation type (regardless of the actual structure of the modern world). Hence the exploration of the statistical structure of ancestral situations and their relationship to the mind's battery of functionally specialized programs is central to mapping the emotions. This is because the most useful (or least harmful) deployment of programs at any given time will depend critically on the exact nature of the situation being encountered. The abstract, distilled, recurrent characteristics of the situation are reflected in the architecture of the emotion. For example, because sexual rivals could be advantageously driven off by violence or its threat in a substantial fraction of the trillions of ancestral cases of mate competition, sexual jealousy is engineered to prepare the body physiologically for combat, and (when the rival is weak or unwary) motivates the individual to behave violently. In modern situations of potential or actual infidelity, police and prisons create additional consequences, and so violence against a sexual rival is likely to lead to maladaptive outcomes now. However, the design features of jealousy were designed to mesh with the long-enduring structure of the ancestral world, and not the modern world—so the emotion program continues to execute its own ancestral functional logic even under modern conditions.

How did emotions arise and assume their distinctive structures? Fighting, falling in love, escaping predators, confronting sexual infidelity, experiencing a failure-driven loss in status, responding to the death of a family member, and so on each involved conditions, contingencies, situations, or event types that recurred innumerable times in hominid evolutionary history. Repeated encounters with each kind of situation selected for adaptations that guided information processing, behavior, and the body adaptively through the clusters of conditions, demands, and contingencies characterizing that particular class of situation.

The payoffs accruing to alternative mutant designs for program activation, in interaction with recurrent classes of situations, engineered programs each of which jointly mobilizes a subset of the psychological architecture's other programs in a particular configuration. Each configuration was selected to deploy computational and physiological mechanisms in a way that, when *averaged* over individuals and generations, would have led to the most fitness-promoting subsequent lifetime outcome, given that ancestral situation type. Thus an emotion is a bet placed under conditions of uncertainty: It is the evolved mind's bet about what internal deployment is likely to lead to the best average long-term set of payoffs, given the structure and statistical contingencies present in the ancestral world when a particular situation was encountered. Running away in terror, vomiting in disgust, or attacking in rage are bets that are placed because these responses had the highest average payoffs for our ancestors, given the eliciting conditions.

This coordinated adjustment and entrainment of mechanisms constitutes a mode of operation for the entire psychological architecture, and serves as the basis for a precise computational and functional definition of each emotion state (Tooby & Cosmides, 1990a; Tooby, 1985; Cosmides & Tooby, 2000). Each emotion entrains various other adaptive programs—deactivating some, activating others, and adjusting the modifiable parameters of still others—so that the whole system operates in a particularly harmonious and efficacious way when the individual is confronting certain kinds of triggering conditions or situations. The conditions or situations relevant to the emotions are those that (1) recurred ances-trally; (2) could not be negotiated successfully unless there was a superordinate level of pro-gram coordination (i.e., circumstances in which the independent operation of programs caused no conflicts would not have selected for an emotion program, and would lead to emo-tionally neutral states of mind); (3) had a rich and reliable repeated structure; (4) had recog-nizable cues signaling their presence; and (5) would have resulted in large fitness costs if an error had occurred (Tooby & Cosmides, 1990a; Tooby, 1985; Cosmides & Tooby, 2000). When a condition or situation of an evolutionarily recognizable kind is detected, a signal is sent out from the emotion program that activates the specific constellation of subprograms appropriate to solving the type of adaptive problems that were regularly embed-ded in that situation, and deactivates programs whose operation might interfere with solving those types of adaptive problems. Programs di-rected to remain active may be cued to enter subroutines that are specific to that emotion mode, and that were tailored by natural selec-tion to solve the problems inherent in the trig-gering situation with special efficiency. (Where there was no repeated structure, or there were no cues to signal the presence of a repeated structure, then selection could not build an ad-aptation to address the situation.)

According to this theoretical framework, an emotion is a superordinate program whose function is to direct the activities and interac-tions of the subprograms governing perception; attention; inference; learning; memory; goal choice; motivational priorities; categorization and conceptual frameworks; physiological re-actions (such as heart rate, endocrine function, immune function, gamete release); reflexes; behavioral decision rules; motor systems; com-munication processes; energy level and effort allocation; affective coloration of events and stimuli; recalibration of probability estimates, situation assessments, values, and regulatory variables (e.g., self-esteem, estimations of rela-tive formidability, relative value of alternative goal states, efficacy discount rate); and so on. An emotion is not reducible to any one cate-gory of effects, such as effects on physiology, behavioral inclinations, cognitive appraisals, or feeling states, because it involves evolved in-structions for all of them together, as well as other mechanisms distributed throughout the human mental and physical architecture.

FEAR AS A MODE OF OPERATION

Consider the following example. The ances-trally recurrent situation is being alone at night, and a situation detector circuit perceives cues that indicate the possible presence of a hu-man or animal predator. The emotion mode is a fear of being stalked. (In this conceptualiza-tion of emotion, there might be several distinct emotion modes that are lumped together under the folk category "fear," but that are at least partially distinguishable, computationally and empirically, by the overlapping but nonidenti-cal constellation of programs each entrains.) When the situation detector signals that one has entered the situation of "possible stalking and ambush," the following kinds of mental programs are entrained or modified:

1. There are shifts in perception and atten-tion. You may suddenly hear with far greater clarity sounds that bear on the hypothesis that you are being stalked, but that ordinarily you would not perceive or attend to, such as creaks or rustling. Are the creaks footsteps? Is the rus-tling caused by something moving stealthily through the bushes? Signal detection thresh-olds shift: Less evidence is required before you respond as if there were a threat, and more true positives will be perceived at the cost of a higher rate of false alarms.

2. Goals and motivational weightings change. Safety becomes a far higher priority. Other goals and the computational systems that subserve them are deactivated: You are no longer hungry; you cease to think about how to charm a potential mate; practicing a new skill no longer seems rewarding. Your planning fo-cus narrows to the present; worries about yes-terday and tomorrow temporarily vanish. Hunger, thirst, and pain are suppressed.

3. Information-gathering programs are redi-rected: Where is my child? Where are others who can protect me? Is there somewhere I can go where I can see and hear what is going on better?

4. Conceptual frames shift, with the auto-matic imposition of categories such as "danger-ous" or "safe." Walking a familiar and usually comfortable route may now be mentally tagged as "dangerous." Odd places that you normally would not occupy—a hallway closet, the branches of a tree—suddenly may become sa-lient as instances of the category "safe" or "hiding place."

5. Memory processes are directed to new retrieval tasks: Where was that tree I climbed before? Did my adversary and his friend look at me furtively the last time I saw them?

6. Communication processes change. Depending on the circumstances, decision rules may cause you to emit an alarm cry, or be paralyzed and unable to speak. Your face may automatically assume a species-typical fear expression.

7. Specialized inference systems are activated. Information about a lion's trajectory or eye direction may be fed into systems for inferring whether the lion saw you. If the inference is yes, then a program automatically infers that the lion knows where you are; if no, then the lion does not know where you are (the "seeing-is-knowing" circuit identified by Baron-Cohen, 1995, as impaired in persons with autism). This variable may automatically govern whether you freeze in terror or bolt. Are there cues in the lion's behavior that indicate whether it has eaten recently, and so is unlikely to be predatory in the near future? (Savanna-dwelling ungulates, such as zebras and wildebeests, commonly make this kind of judgment; Marks, 1987.)

8. Specialized learning systems are activated, as the large literature on fear conditioning indicates (e.g., LeDoux, 1995; Mineka & Cook, 1993; Pitman & Orr, 1995). If the threat is real, and the ambush occurs, you may experience an amygdala-mediated recalibration (as in posttraumatic stress disorder) that can last for the remainder of your life (Pitman & Orr, 1995).

9. Physiology changes. Gastric mucosa turn white as blood leaves the digestive tract (another concomitant of motivational priorities changing from feeding to emergency motor activity in pursuit of safety); adrenalin spikes; heart rate may go up or down (depending on whether the situation calls for flight or immobility), blood rushes to the periphery, and so on (Cannon, 1929; Tomaka, Blascovich, Kibler, & Ernst, 1997); instructions to the musculature (face and elsewhere) are sent (Ekman, 1982). Indeed, the nature of the physiological response can depend in detailed ways on the nature of the threat and the best response option (see, e.g., Marks, 1987).

10. Behavioral decision rules are activated: Depending on the nature of the potential threat, different courses of action will be potentiated: hiding, flight, self-defense, or even tonic immobility (the last of these is a common response to actual attacks, both in other animals and in humans[1]). Some of these responses may be experienced as automatic or involuntary.

From the point of view of avoiding danger, these computational changes are crucial: They are what allowed the adaptive problem to be solved with high probability, on average over evolutionary time. Of course, in any single case they may fail, because they are only the evolutionarily computed best bet, based on ancestrally summed outcomes; they are not a sure bet, based on an unattainable perfect knowledge of the present.

Whether individuals report consciously experiencing fear is a separate question from whether their mechanisms assumed the characteristic configuration that, according to this theoretical approach, defines the fear emotion state. Individuals often behave as if they are in the grip of an emotion, while denying they are feeling that emotion. We think it is perfectly possible that individuals sometimes remain unaware of (or lose conscious access to) their emotion states, which is one reason we do not use subjective experience as the *sine qua non* of emotion. At present, both the function of conscious awareness, and the principles that regulate conscious access to emotion states and other mental programs, are complex and unresolved questions (but see Tooby, Cosmides, Sell, Lieberman, & Sznycer, in press). Mapping the design features of emotion programs can proceed independently of their resolution, at least for the present.

ADAPTATIONIST FOUNDATIONS

Adaptations, By-Products, and Noise

Because of the different roles played by chance and selection, the evolutionary process builds three different types of outcomes into organisms: (1) adaptations—that is, functional machinery built by selection, and usually species-typical (see Tooby & Cosmides, 1990b, for details and exceptions); (2) by-products of adaptations, which are present in the design of organisms because they are causally coupled to traits that were selected for (usually species-typical); and (3) random noise, injected by mutation and other random processes (often not species-typical) (Tooby & Cosmides, 1990a, 1990b, 1992a; Williams, 1966). The emotion of sexual jealousy is an adaptation (Daly, Wilson, & Weghorst, 1982; Buss, 1994); stress-induced physical deterioration is arguably a by-product of the flight–fight system; and heritable personality variation in emotional functioning (e.g., extreme shyness, morbid jealousy, bipolar disorder) is probably noise (Tooby & Cosmides, 1990b). Evidence of the presence (or absence) of high degrees of coordination between adaptive problems and the design features of putative adaptations allows researchers to distinguish adaptations, by-products, and noise from one another (Williams, 1966; Cosmides & Tooby, 1997).

The emotions are often thought of as crude, but we expect emotions to be very well-designed computational adaptations. Biologists have found that selection has routinely produced exquisitely engineered biological machines of the highest order at all scales, from genetic error correction and quality control in protein assembly to photosynthetic pigments, the immune system, efficient bee foraging algorithms, echolocation, and color constancy systems. Indeed, the best-studied psychological adaptation—the eye and visual system—has been held up for centuries as the apotheosis of engineering excellence, as yet unrivaled by any human engineer. There is no principled reason to expect other neurocomputational (i.e., psychological) adaptations to be less well engineered than the eye. Although Stephen Jay Gould (1997) and his followers have energetically argued in the popular science literature that natural selection is a weak evolutionary force, evolutionary biologists, familiar with the primary literature, have found it difficult to take these arguments seriously (Tooby & Cosmides, 1997). So although adaptations are in some abstract sense undoubtedly far from optimal (and there is genetic noise in all systems), the empirical evidence falsifies the claim that evolved computational adaptations tend to be crude or primitive in design, and instead supports the opposite view: that our mental machinery—including the emotions—is likely to be very well designed to carry out evolved functions. For emotion researchers, this means that their working hypotheses (which are always open to empirical revision) should begin with the expectation of high levels of evolutionary functionality, and their research methods should be sensitive enough to detect such organization. This does not mean that emotions are well designed for the modern world—

only that their functional logic is likely to be sophisticated and well engineered to solve ancestral adaptive problems.

The Environment of Evolutionary Adaptedness

Behavior in the present is generated by evolved information-processing mechanisms that were constructed in the past. They were constructed in the past because they solved adaptive problems that were recurrently present in the ancestral environments in which the human line evolved. For this reason, evolutionary psychology is both environment-oriented and past-oriented in its functionalist orientation. Adaptations become increasingly effective as selection makes their design features more and more complementary to the long-enduring structure of the world. The articulated features of the adaptation are designed to mesh with the features of the environment that were stable during the adaptation's evolution, so that their interaction produced functional outcomes. The regulation of breathing assumes the presence of certain long-enduring properties of the atmosphere and the respiratory system. Vision assumes the presence of certain evolutionarily stable properties of surfaces, objects, and terrestrial spectral distributions. The digestive enzyme lactase presupposes an infant diet of milk with lactose. Fear presupposes dangers in the environment, and even presupposes higher probabilities of specific kinds of dangers, given certain cues: darkness, spiders, snakes, heights, predators, open spaces, and so on (Marks, 1987). That is, each emotion program presupposes that certain cues signal the presence of a structure of events and conditions that held true during the evolution of that emotion. Disgust circuits presume a world in which rotten smells signal toxins or microbial contamination, for example.

Accordingly, to understand an adaptation as a problem solver, one needs to model the enduring properties of the task environment that constituted the problem and provided materials that could be exploited for its solution: the "environment of evolutionary adaptedness," or (EEA). Although the human line is thought to have first differentiated itself from the chimpanzee lineage on the African savannahs and woodlands, the EEA is not a place or time. It is the statistical composite of selection pressures that caused the genes underlying the design of an adaptation to increase in frequency until they became species-typical or stably persistent (Tooby & Cosmides, 1990a). Thus statistical regularities define the EEA for any given adaptation. The conditions that characterize the EEA are usefully decomposed into a constellation of specific environmental regularities that had a systematic (though not necessarily unvarying) impact on reproduction, and that endured long enough to work evolutionary change on the design of an adaptation. Some of these regularities are extremely simple: Distance from a predator is protection from the predator. Sex with an opposite-sex adult is more likely to produce offspring than sex with a child or a nonhuman. These regularities can equally well include complex conditionals (e.g., if one is a male hunter–gatherer *and* one is having a sexual liaison with someone else's mate *and* that liaison is discovered, then one is the target of lethal retributory violence 14% of the time). Descriptions of these regularities are essential parts of the construction of a task analysis of the adaptive problem a hypothesized adaptation evolved to solve (Tooby & Cosmides, 1990a). Conceptualizing the EEA in probabilistic terms is fundamental to the functional definition of emotion that we have presented above and will elucidate below.

Each adaptive problem recurred billions or trillions of times in the EEA, and so manifested a statistical and causal structure whose elements were available for specialized exploitation by design features of the evolving adaptation. For example, predators use darkness and cover to ambush (Marks, 1987). Physical appearance varies with fertility and health (Symons, 1979). Among hunter–gatherers, infants that a mother primarily cares for are almost invariably genetic siblings (Lieberman, Tooby, & Cosmides, 2007). Specialized programs—for predator fear, sexual attraction, and kin detection, respectively—could evolve whose configuration of design features embodied and/or exploited these statistical regularities, allowing these adaptive problems to be solved economically, reliably, and effectively. Such specializations, by embodying "innate knowledge" about the problem space, operate better than any general learning strategy could. Children did not have to wait to experience being ambushed and killed in the dark to prudently modulate their activities. Adults did not need to observe the negative effects of incest, because the human kin detection system mobilizes disgust toward having sex with individu-

als the mind has tagged as siblings (Lieberman et al., 2007).

The Functional Structure of an Emotion Program Evolved to Match the Evolutionarily Summed Structure of Its Target Situation

Each emotion program was constructed by a selective regimen consisting of repeated encounters with a particular kind of evolutionarily recurrent situation. By an "evolutionarily recurrent situation," we mean a cluster of repeated probabilistic relationships among events, conditions, actions, and choice consequences that endured over a sufficient stretch of evolutionary time to have favored some variant designs over others. Many of these relationships were probabilistically associated with cues detectable by humans, allowing psychophysical triggers to activate the task-appropriate program.

For example, the condition of having a mate plus the condition of the mate's copulating with someone else constitutes a situation of sexual infidelity—a situation that has recurred over evolutionary time, even though it has not happened to every individual. Associated with this situation were cues reliable enough to allow the evolution of a "situation detector" (e.g., observing a sexual act, flirtation, or even the repeated simultaneous absence of the suspected lovers were cues that could trigger the categorization of a situation as one of infidelity). Even more importantly, there were many necessarily or probabilistically associated elements that tended to be present in the situation of infidelity as encountered among our hunter–gatherer ancestors. These additional elements included (1) a sexual rival with a capacity for social action and violence, as well as allies of the rival; (2) a discrete probability that one's mate had conceived with the sexual rival; (3) changes in the net lifetime reproductive returns of investing further in the mating relationship; (4) a probable decrease in the degree to which the unfaithful mate's mechanisms would value the victim of infidelity (the presence of an alternative mate would lower replacement costs); (5) a cue that the victim of the infidelity was likely to have been deceived about a range of past events, leading the victim to confront the likelihood that his or her memory was permeated with false information; and (6) a likelihood that the victim's status and reputation for being effective at defending his or her interests in general would plummet, inviting challenges in other arenas. These are just a few of the many factors that would constitute a list of elements associated in a probabilistic cluster, and that would constitute the evolutionary recurrent structure of a situation of sexual infidelity. The emotion of sexual jealousy evolved in response to these properties of the world, and there should be evidence of this in its computational design.

Emotion programs have evolved to take such elements into account, whether they can be perceived or not. Thus not only do cues of a situation trigger an emotion mode, but embedded in that emotion mode is a way of seeing the world and feeling about the world related to the ancestral cluster of associated elements. Depending on the intensity of the jealousy evoked, less and less evidence will be required for individuals to believe that these conditions apply to their personal situation. Individuals with morbid jealousy, for example, may hallucinate counterfactual but evolutionarily thematic contents, such as seeing their mates having sex with someone else (Mowat, 1966; Shepherd, 1961). This leads many to consider emotions "irrational," but this property was selected for because it allows emotional computation to go beyond the evidence given, producing correct responses (when averaged over evolutionary time).

To the extent that situations exhibited a structure repeated over evolutionary time, their statistical properties would be used as the basis for natural selection to build an emotion program whose detailed design features were tailored for that situation. This would be accomplished by selection acting over evolutionary time, differentially incorporating program components that dovetailed with individual items on the list of properties probabilistically associated with the situation.

For example, ancestrally a male's ability to inflict costs through violence (his "formidability") was associated with his status and reputation for defending his interests. Moreover, the fitness consequences of being cuckolded are great, and males have become motivated by design to resist this outcome. If a male's mate is sexually unfaithful and this infidelity becomes public, this advertises a weakness previously unappreciated by those who know him best. This decrease in perceived formidability decreases his value to his male allies and increases the probability that he will be challenged by competitors in other domains of life. The sexual jealousy, anger, and shame systems have been shaped by the distillation of these (and other) payoff probabilities. Each of these recurrent subelements in a situation of sexual infidelity, and the adaptive circuits they require, can be added together to form a general theory of sexual jealousy, as well as a theory of the functional coactivation of linked programs (such as anger and shame).

Hence the emotion of sexual jealousy constitutes an organized mode of operation specifically designed to deploy the programs governing each psychological mechanism, so that each is poised to deal with the exposed infidelity. Physiological processes are prepared for such things as violence, sperm competition, and the withdrawal of investment; the goal of deterring, injuring, or murdering the rival emerges; the goal of punishing, deterring, or deserting the mate appears; the desire to make oneself more competitively attractive to alternative mates emerges; memory is activated to reanalyze the past; confident assessments of the past are transformed into doubts; the general estimate of the reliability and trustworthiness of the opposite sex (or indeed everyone) may decline; associated shame programs may be triggered to search for situations in which the individual can publicly demonstrate acts of violence or punishment that work to counteract an (imagined or real) social perception of weakness; and so on.

It is the relationship between the summed details of the ancestral condition and the detailed structure of the resulting emotion program that makes this approach so useful for emotion researchers. Each functionally distinct emotion state—fear of predators, guilt, sexual jealousy, rage, grief, and so on—will correspond to an integrated mode of operation that functions as a solution designed to take advantage of the particular structure of the recurrent situation or triggering condition to which that emotion corresponds. This approach can be used to create theories of each individual emotion, through four steps: (1) Reconstruct the clusters of properties of ancestral situations; (2) analyze what behavioral and somatic alterations would solve the adaptive problem posed by the recurrent situation (or minimize the damage it causes); (3) construct a provisional model of the program architecture of the emotion that could generate the necessary mechanism-, body-, and behavior-regulating outputs, including the cues used, the regulatory variables the emotion needs to track, and so on; and (4) design and conduct experiments and other investigations to test each hypothesized design feature of the proposed emotion program, revising them as necessary.

It is also important to understand that evolutionarily recurrent situations can be arrayed along a spectrum in terms of how rich or skeletal the set of probabilistically associated elements defining the recurrent situation is. Richly structured situations—such as sexual infidelity, exposure to potential disease vectors, or predator ambush—will support a richly substructured emotion program in response to the numerous ancestrally correlated features each manifests: Many detailed adjustments will be made to many psychological mechanisms as instructions for the mode of operation. In contrast, some recurrent situations have less structure (i.e., they share fewer properties), and so the emotion mode makes fewer highly specialized adjustments, imposes fewer specialized and compelling interpretations and behavioral inclinations, and so on. For example, surges of happiness or joy are an emotion program that evolved to respond to the recurrent situation of encountering unexpected positive events. The class of events captured by "unexpectedly positive" is extremely broad and general, and such events have only a few additional properties in common. Emotion programs at the most general and skeletal end of this spectrum correspond to what some call "mood" (happiness, sadness, excitement, anxiety, playfulness, homesickness, etc.).

HOW TO CHARACTERIZE AN EMOTION

To characterize an emotion adaptation, one must identify the following properties of environments and of mechanisms.

1. *An evolutionarily recurrent situation or condition.* A "situation" is a repeated structure of environmental and organismic properties, characterized as a complex statistical composite of how such properties covaried in the environment of evolutionary adaptedness. Examples of these situations are being in a depleted nutritional state, competing for maternal attention, being chased by a predator, being about to

ambush an enemy, having few friends, experiencing the death of a spouse, being sick, having experienced a public success, having others act in a way that damages you without regard for your welfare, having injured a valued other through insufficient consideration of self–other behavioral tradeoffs, and having a baby.

2. *The adaptive problem.* Identifying the adaptive problem means identifying which organismic states and behavioral sequences will lead to the best average functional outcome for the remainder of the lifespan, given the situation or condition. For example, what is the best course of action when others take the products of your labor without your consent? What is the best course of action when you are in a depleted nutritional state? What is the best course of action when a sibling makes a sexual approach?

3. *Cues that signal the presence of the situation.* For example, low blood sugar signals a depleted nutritional state; the looming approach of a large, fanged animal signals the presence of a predator; seeing your mate having sex with another signals sexual infidelity; finding yourself often alone, rarely the recipient of beneficent acts, or actively avoided by others signals that you have few friends.

4. *Situation-detecting algorithms.* A multimodular mind must be full of "demons"—algorithms that detect situations. *The New Hacker's Dictionary* defines a "demon" as a "portion of a program that is not invoked explicitly, but that lies dormant waiting for some condition(s) to occur" (Raymond, 1991, p. 124). Situation-detecting subprograms lie dormant until they are activated by a specific constellation of cues that precipitates the analysis of whether a particular ancestral situation has arisen. If the assessment is positive, it sends the signal that activates the associated emotion program. Emotion demons need two kinds of subroutines:

a. *Algorithms that monitor for situation-defining cues.* These programs include perceptual mechanisms, proprioceptive mechanisms, and situation-representing mechanisms. They take the cues in point 3 above as input.

b. *Algorithms that detect situations.* These programs take the output of the monitoring algorithms and targeted memory registers in point a as input, and through integration, probabilistic weighting, and other decision criteria, identify situations as absent or present with some probability and with some index of the magnitude of the fitness consequences inherent in the situation.

The assignment of a situation interpretation to present circumstances involves a problem in signal detection theory (Tooby & Cosmides, 1990a; Swets, Tanner, & Birdsall, 1961; see also Gigerenzer & Murray, 1987). Animals should be designed to detect what situation they are in on the basis of cues, stored regulatory variables, and specialized interpretation algorithms. Selection will not shape decision rules so that they act solely on the basis of what is most likely to be true, but rather on the basis of the weighted consequences of acts, given that something is held to be true. Should you walk under a tree that might conceal a predator? Even if the algorithms assign a 51% (or even 98%) probability to the tree's being leopard-free, under most circumstances an evolutionarily well-engineered decision rule should cause you to avoid the tree—to act as if the leopard were in it. The benefits of calories saved via a shortcut, scaled by the probability that there is no leopard in the tree, must be weighed against the benefits of avoiding becoming catfood, scaled by the probability that there is a leopard in the tree. Because the costs and benefits of false alarms, misses, hits, and correct rejections are often unequal, the decision rules may still treat as true situations that are unlikely to be true. In the modern world, this behavior may look "irrational" (as is the case with many phobias), but we do it because such decision biases were adaptive under ancestral conditions, given ancestral payoff asymmetries. That is, they were "ecologically rational" (Tooby & Cosmides, 1990a; Haselton & Buss, 2003).

Situation-detecting algorithms can be of any degree of complexity, from demons that monitor single cues (e.g., "snake present") to algorithms that carry out more complex cognitive assessments of situations and conditions (LeDoux, 1995; Lazarus & Lazarus, 1994; Tooby & Cosmides, 1990a). Inherent in this approach is the expectation that the human mind has a series of evolved subsystems designed to represent events in terms of evolutionarily recurrent situations and situational subcomponents. The operations of these representational systems are not necessarily consciously accessible. By their structure, they impose an evolutionary organization on representational spaces that are updated by data inputs. When the representational space assumes certain configurations, an interpretation is triggered that activates the associated emotion program—corresponding approximately to what others have called a "cognitive appraisal" (see, e.g., Lazarus & Lazarus, 1994). It is important to recognize that the evolutionary past frames the experienced present, because these situation-detecting algorithms provide the dimensions and core elements out of which many cross-culturally recurring representations of the world are built. To some extent, the world we inhabit is shaped by the continuous interpretive background commentary provided by these mechanisms.

5. *Algorithms that assign priorities.* A given world state may correspond to more than one situation at a time; for example, you may be nutritionally depleted *and* in the presence of a predator. The prioritizing algorithms define which emotion modes are compatible (e.g., hunger[2] and boredom) and which are mutually exclusive (e.g., feeding and predator escape). Depending on the relative importance of the situations and the reliability of the cues, the prioritizing algorithms decide which emotion modes to activate and deactivate, and to what degree. Selection, through ancestral mutant experiments, would have sorted emotions based on the average importance of the consequences stemming from each, and the extent to which joint activation was mutually incompatible or facilitating. (Prioritizing algorithms can be thought of as a supervisory system operating over all of the emotions.)

6. *An internal communication system.* Given that a situation has been detected, the internal communication system sends a situation-specific signal to all relevant programs and mechanisms; the signal switches them into the appropriate adaptive emotion mode. In addition, information is fed back into the emotion program from other programs and systems that assess body states and other regulatory variables, which may govern the intensity, trajectory, supplantation, or termination of the emotion. Along with the sensorium and motivational systems, the emotions are embedded in and partly responsible for what might be called "feeling computation." In this view, the richly textured representations we experience as feeling constitute our conscious access to a high-bandwidth system of computational devices and program interfaces that amalgamate

valuation information with other representations to guide decision making and to recalibrate decisions in an ongoing way (see, e.g., Tooby et al., 2003).

Some modes of activation of the psychological architecture are accompanied by a characteristic feeling state, a certain quality of experience. The fact that we are capable of becoming aware of certain physiological states—our hearts thumping, bowels evacuating, stomachs tightening—is surely responsible for some of the *qualia* evoked by emotion states that entrain such responses. The fact that we are capable of becoming aware of certain mental states—such as the magnitude of certain regulatory variables or the retrieved memories of past events—is probably responsible for other *qualia*. In our view, the characteristic feeling state that accompanies an emotion mode results (in part) from mechanisms that allow us to sense the signal activating and deactivating the relevant programs, as well as signals communicating necessary parameters and variable magnitudes to the various programs. Such internal sensory mechanisms—analogous to proprioception—can be selected for if there are mechanisms requiring as input the information that a particular emotion mode has been activated. (This might be true, for example, of mechanisms designed to inhibit certain stimulus-driven actions when the conditions are not auspicious.)

7. *Each program and physiological mechanism entrained by an emotion program must have associated algorithms that regulate how it responds to each emotion signal.* These algorithms determine whether the mechanism should switch on or switch off, and if on, what emotion-specialized performance it will implement. For example, there should be algorithms in the auditory system that, upon detecting the fear signal (see point 6), reset signal detection thresholds, increasing acuity for predator-relevant sounds.

WHAT KINDS OF PROGRAMS CAN EMOTIONS MOBILIZE?

Any controllable biological or neurocomputational process that, by shifting its performance in a specifiable way, would lead to enhanced average fitness outcomes should have come to be partially governed by emotional state (see

point 7 above). Some such processes are discussed in this section.

Goals

The cognitive mechanisms that define goal states and choose among goals in a planning process should be influenced by emotions. For example, vindictiveness—a specialized subcategory of anger—may define "injuring the offending party" as a goal state to be achieved. (Although the evolved functional logic of this process is deterrence, this function need not be represented, either consciously or unconsciously, by the mechanisms that generate the vindictive behavior.)

Motivational Priorities

Mechanisms involved in hierarchically ranking goals or calibrating other kinds of motivational and reward systems should be emotion-dependent. What may be extremely unpleasant in one state, such as harming another, may seem satisfying in another state (e.g., aggressive competition may facilitate counterempathy). Different evolutionarily recurrent situations predict the presence—visible or invisible—of different opportunities, risks, and payoffs, so motivational thresholds and valences should be entrained. For example, a loss of face should increase the motivation to take advantage of opportunities for status advancement, and should decrease attention to attendant costs.

Information-Gathering Motivations

Because establishing which situation one is in has enormous consequences for the appropriateness of behavior, the process of detection should in fact involve specialized inference procedures and specialized motivations to discover whether certain suspected facts are true or false. What one is curious about, what one finds interesting, and what one is obsessed with discovering should all be emotion-specific.

Imposed Conceptual Frameworks

Emotions should prompt construals of the world in terms of concepts that are appropriate to the decisions that must be made. When one is angry, domain-specific concepts such as social agency, fault, responsibility, and punishment will be assigned to elements in the situation. When one is hungry, the food–nonfood distinction will seem salient. When one is endangered, safety categorization frames will appear. The world will be carved up into categories based partly on what emotional state an individual is in.

Perceptual Mechanisms

Perceptual systems may enter emotion-specific modes of operation. When one is fearful, acuity of hearing may increase. Specialized perceptual inference systems may be mobilized as well: If you've heard rustling in the bushes at night, human and predator figure detection may be particularly boosted, and not simply visual acuity in general. In fact, nonthreat interpretations may be depressed, and the same set of shadows will "look threatening"—that is, given a specific threatening interpretation such as "a man with a knife"—or not, depending on emotion state.

Memory

The ability to call up particularly appropriate kinds of information out of long-term memory ought to be influenced. A woman who has just found strong evidence that her husband has been unfaithful may find herself flooded by a torrent of memories about small details that seemed meaningless at the time but that now fit into an interpretation of covert activity. We also expect that what is stored about present experience will also be differentially regulated. Important or shocking events, for example, may be stored in great detail (as has been claimed about "flashbulb memories"), but other, more moderate emotion-specific effects may occur as well.

Attention

The entire structure of attention, from perceptual systems to the contents of high-level reasoning processes, should be regulated by emotional state. If you are worried that your spouse is late and might have been injured, it is hard to concentrate on other ongoing tasks (Derryberry & Tucker, 1994), but easy to concentrate on danger scenarios. Positive emotions may broaden attentional focus (Fredrickson, 1998).

Physiology

Each organ system, tissue, or process is a potential candidate for emotion-specific regulation, and "arousal" is insufficiently specific to capture the detailed coordination involved. Each emotion program should send out a different pattern of instructions (to the face and limb muscles, the autonomic system, etc.), to the extent that the problems embedded in the associated situations differ. This leads to an expectation that different constellations of effects will be diagnostic of different emotion states (Ekman, Levenson, & Friesen, 1983). Changes in circulatory, respiratory, and gastrointestinal functioning are well known and documented, as are changes in endocrinological function. We expect thresholds regulating the contraction of various muscle groups to change with certain emotion states, reflecting the probability that they will need to be employed. Similarly, immune allocation and targeting may vary with disgust, with the potential for injury, or with the demands of extreme physical exertion.

Communication and Emotional Expressions

Emotion programs are expected to mobilize many emotion-specific effects on the subcomponents of the human psychological architecture relevant to communication. Most notably, many emotion programs produce characteristic species-typical displays that broadcast to others the emotion state of an individual (Ekman, 1982). Ekman and his colleagues have established in a careful series of landmark studies that many emotional expressions are human universals, both generated and recognized reliably by humans everywhere they have been tested (Ekman, 1994). Indeed, many emotional expressions appear to be designed to be informative, and these have been so reliably informative that humans have coevolved automated interpreters of facial displays of emotion, which decode these public displays into knowledge of others' mental states.

Two things are communicated by an authentic emotional expression:[3] (1) that the associated emotion program has been activated in an individual, providing observers with information about the state of that individual's mental programs and physiology (e.g., "I am afraid"); and (2) the identity of the evolutionarily recurrent situation being faced, in the estimation of the signaler (e.g., the local world holds a danger). Both are highly informative, and emotional expressions provide a continuous commentary on the underlying meaning of things to companions. This provokes the question: Why did selection build facial, vocal, and postural expressions at all? More puzzlingly, why are they often experienced as automatic and involuntary? The apparent selective disadvantages of honestly and automatically broadcasting one's emotional state have led Fridlund (1994), for example, to argue that expressions must be voluntary and intentional communications largely unconnected to emotion state. But even when people deliberately lie, microexpressions of face and voice often leak out (Ekman, 1985), suggesting that certain emotion programs do in fact create involuntarily emitted signals that reliably broadcast the person's emotion state and that are difficult to override. Why?

First, natural selection has shaped emotion programs to signal their activation, or not, on an emotion-by-emotion basis. For each emotion program considered by itself (jealousy, loneliness, disgust, predatoriness, parental love, sexual attraction, gratitude, fear), there was a net benefit or cost to having others know that mental state, averaged across individuals over evolutionary time. For those recurrent situations in which, on average, it was beneficial to share one's emotion state (and hence assessment of the situation) with those one was with, species-typical facial and other expressions of emotion were constructed by selection. For example, fear was plausibly beneficial to signal, because it signaled the presence of a danger that might menace one's kin and cooperators as well, and it also informed others in a way that might recruit assistance. Guilt was not selected to cause a presentation with an unambiguous, distinctive signal.

Nevertheless, averaged over evolutionary time, it was functional for the organism to signal the activation of only *some* emotion states. The conditions favoring signaling an emotion are hard to meet (for conditions and discussion, see Tooby & Cosmides, 1996b; Cosmides & Tooby, 2000a). Consequently, only some emotions out of the total species-typical set are associated with distinctive, species-typical facial expressions. There should be a larger set of emotions that have no automatic display. Moreover, emotions that lack a display are not necessarily less fundamental or less anchored in the evolved architecture of the human mind.

For this reason, the existence of a distinctive expression is not a necessary aspect of an emotion, nor should it be part of its definition. Jealousy and guilt are both genuine emotions lacking distinctive signals.

Precisely because we are designed to monitor broadcast emotions, our attention goes disproportionately to the subset of emotions that do come equipped with emotional expressions. We think it likely that this has had an impact on the history of emotion research—specifically, that the emotions associated with distinctive expressions have been unnecessarily considered "primary" or "fundamental."

Finally, many features of facial expressions may not just be arbitrary, but may be reliable indicators of an emotion state. Many seem to be functional concomitants of the activity associated with the emotion (such as eyes widening or hyperventilation). Others may be signals that are nonarbitrary; that is, they remove barriers to the correct assessment of aspects of the phenotype that the organism benefits by demonstrating. For example, the anger expression may be designed to maximize the perception of strength—an advertisement of a property relevant to the negotiation, and not just an arbitrary signal to others that one is angry (Sell, Tooby, & Cosmides, in press-b). That is, there may be functional reasons why the anger face has the characteristics it does, rather than consisting of ear flapping or nose twitching. Similarly, the baring of teeth may be combat preparation and advertisement (Archer, 1988); the narrowing of the pupil may be preparation for the detection of fast motion; and so on.

Behavior

All psychological mechanisms are involved in the generation and regulation of behavior, so obviously behavior will be regulated by emotion state. More specifically, however, mechanisms proximately involved in the generation of actions (as opposed to such processes as face recognition, which are only distally regulatory) should be very sensitive to emotion state. Not only may highly stereotyped behaviors of certain kinds be released (as during sexual arousal or rage, or as with species-typical facial expressions and body language), but more complex action generation mechanisms should be regulated as well. Specific acts and courses of action will be more available as responses in some states than in others, and more likely to be implemented. Emotion mode should govern the construction of organized behavioral sequences that solve adaptive problems.

Biologists, psychologists, and economists who adopt an evolutionary perspective have recognized that game theory can be used to model many forms of social interactions (Maynard Smith, 1982). If the EEA imposes certain evolutionarily repeated games, then the "strategies" (the evolved cognitive programs that govern behavior in those contexts) should evolve in the direction of choices that lead to the best expected fitness payoffs. The strategy activated in the individual should match the game (e.g., exchange) and the state of play in the game (e.g., having just been cheated)—a process that requires the system of cues, situation detection, and so on, already discussed. So different emotion and inference programs or subprograms may have evolved to correspond to various evolved games, including zero-sum competitive games, positive-sum exchange games, coalitional lottery games, games of aggressive competition corresponding to "chicken," and so on (for exchange, see Cosmides, 1989; Cosmides & Tooby, 1992). Corresponding emotion programs guide the individual into the appropriate interactive strategy for the social "game" being played, given the state of play. Surprisingly, for some games, rigid obligatory adherence to a prior strategy throughout the game is better than the ability to revise and change strategies ("voluntarily") in the light of events. If an individual contemplating a course of action detrimental to you knows you will take revenge, regardless of the magnitude of the punishment to you that this might unleash, then that individual will be less likely to take such harmful action. This may translate into emotion programs in which the desire to attempt certain actions should be overwhelming, to the point where the actions are experienced as compulsory. In the grip of such programs, competing programs, including the normal integration of prudential concerns and social consequences, are muted or terminated. For example, the desire to avenge a murder or an infidelity is often experienced in this way, and crimes resulting from this desire are even culturally recognized as "crimes of passion" (Daly & Wilson, 1988). In modern state societies, where there are police who are paid to punish and otherwise enforce agreements, it is easy to underestimate the importance that deterrence based on the actions of oneself and

one's coalition had in the Pleistocene (Chagnon, 1983). Hirshleifer (1987) and Frank (1988) are evolutionary economists who have pursued this logic the furthest, arguing that many social behaviors are the result of such "commitment problems."

Specialized Inference

Research in evolutionary psychology has shown that "thinking" or reasoning is not a unitary category, but is carried out by a variety of specialized mechanisms. So, instead of emotion's activating or depressing "thinking" in general, the specific emotion program activated should *selectively* activate appropriate specialized inferential systems, such as cheater detection (Cosmides, 1989; Cosmides & Tooby, 1989, 1992), bluff detection (Tooby & Cosmides, 1989), precaution detection (Fiddick, Cosmides, & Tooby, 2000), attributions of blame and responsibility, and so on. For example, fear could influence precautionary reasoning (Boyer & Liénard, 2006), competitive loss could regulate bluff detection, and so on.

Reflexes

Muscular coordination, tendency to blink, threshold for vomiting, shaking, and many other reflexes are expected to be regulated by emotion programs to reflect the demands of the evolved situation.

Learning

Emotion mode is expected to regulate learning mechanisms. What someone learns from stimuli will be greatly altered by emotion mode, because of attentional allocation, motivation, situation-specific inferential algorithms, and a host of other factors. Emotion mode will cause the present context to be divided up into situation-specific, functionally appropriate categories so that the same stimuli and the same environment may be interpreted in radically different ways, depending on emotion state. For example, which stimuli are considered similar should be different in different emotion states, distorting the shape of the individual's psychological "similarity space" (Shepard, 1987). Highly specialized learning mechanisms may be activated, such as those that control food aversions (Garcia, 1990), predator learning (Mineka & Cook, 1993), or fear conditioning (LeDoux, 1995). Happiness is expected to signal the energetic opportunity for play, and to allow other exploratory agendas to be expressed (Frederickson, 1998).

Mood, Energy Level, Effort Allocation, and Depression

Overall metabolic budget will be regulated by emotion programs, as will specific allocations to various processes and facilitation or inhibition of specific activities. The effort that it takes to perform given tasks will shift accordingly, with things being easier or more effortful, depending on how appropriate they are to the situation reflected by the emotion (Tooby & Cosmides, 1990a). Thus fear will make it more difficult to attack an antagonist, whereas anger will make it easier. The confidence with which a situation has been identified (i.e., emotional clarity) should itself regulate the effortfulness of situation-appropriate activities. Confusion (itself an emotional state) should inhibit the expenditure of energy on costly behavioral responses and should motivate more information gathering and information analysis. Nesse (1991) has suggested that the function of mood is to reflect the propitiousness of the present environment for action—a hypothesis with many merits. We have hypothesized (Tooby & Cosmides, 1990a) a similar function of mood, based on recognizing that the action–reward ratio of the environment is not a function of the environment alone, but an interaction between the structure of the environment and the individual's present understanding of it. (By "understanding," we mean the correspondence between the structure of the environment, the structure of the algorithms, and the weightings and other information they use as parameters.) The phenomenon that should regulate this aspect of mood is a perceived discrepancy between expected and actual payoff. The suspension of behavioral activity accompanied by very intense cognitive activity in depressed people looks like an effort to reconstruct models of the world so that future action can lead to payoffs, in part through stripping away previous valuations that led to unwelcome outcomes. Depression should be precipitated by (1) a heavy investment in a behavioral enterprise that was expected to lead to large payoffs that either failed to materialize or were not large enough to justify the investment; or (2) insufficient investment in maintaining a highly valued

person or condition that was subsequently lost (possibly as a consequence); or (3) gradual recognition by situation detectors that one's long-term pattern of effort and time expenditure has not led to a sufficient level of evolutionarily meaningful reward, when implicitly compared to alternative life paths (the condition of Dickens's Scrooge). Discrepancies between expected and actual payoff can occur in the other direction as well: Joy, or a precipitated surge of happiness, is an emotion program that evolved to respond to the condition of an unexpectedly good outcome. It functions to recalibrate previous value states that led to underinvestment in or underexpectation for the successful activities or choices. Moreover, energy reserves that were being sequestered under one assumption about future prospects can be released, given new, more accurate expectations about a more plentiful or advantageous future. Similarly, one can be informed of bad outcomes to choices not made: For example, one may find out that a company one almost invested in went bankrupt, or that the highway one almost took was snowed in. Information of this kind leads to a strengthening of the decision variables used (experienced as pleasure), which is sometimes mistaken for pleasure in the misfortune of others. Reciprocally, one can be informed of good outcomes to choices not made, which will be experienced as unpleasant.

Moreover, the functional definition of emotion given here invites the possibility that many well-known mental states should be recognized as emotion states—such as the malaise engendered by infectious illness, coma, shock, the appreciation of beauty, homesickness, sexual arousal, confusion, nausea, and so on. For example, when you are sick, initiating actions and going about your daily activities is more effortful than usual; your impulse is to stay home and lie still. Although you feel as if your energy reserves are depleted, at a physical level the same fat reserves and digestively delivered glucose are available. Malaise is a computational state, not a physical one, and is designed to cope with the adaptive problem of illness: It shunts energy from behavior to the immune system, and possibly signals the need for aid. Similarly, when situation-detecting algorithms detect the presence of a very grave internal injury, or the potential for one as indicated by a major blow, these may trigger a mode of operation of the psychological architecture that is designed to prevent *any* discretionary movement:

coma. The function of coma, in a world before hospitals, was to prevent further injury from being done, minimize blood loss and internal hemorrhaging, and allow the mobilization of the body's resources toward repair of immediate threats to life. Note that a coma is not a physically mandated state of paralysis; it is a computational state—technically, "a state of unconsciousness from which the patient cannot be roused" (Miller, 1976, p. 46), or "unarousable unresponsiveness" (Berkow, 1992, p. 1398). It can occur even when there has been no damage to the motor system.

INTERNAL REGULATORY VARIABLES AND FEELING COMPUTATION

We expect that the architecture of the human mind, by design, is full of registers for evolved variables whose function is to store summary magnitudes that are useful for regulating behavior and making inferences involving valuation. These are not explicit concepts, representations, goal states, beliefs, or desires, but rather indices that acquire their meaning via the evolved behavior-controlling and computation-controlling procedures that access them. That is, each has a location embedded in the input–output relations of our evolved programs, and their function inheres in the role they play in the decision flow of these the programs.

For example, in our recent mapping of the architecture of the human kin detection system, we have identified a series of regulatory variables needed to make the system work functionally and to explain the data (Lieberman et al., 2007). For example, for each familiar individual i, the system computes and updates a continuous variable, the "kinship index" (K_i), which corresponds to the system's pairwise estimate of genetic relatedness between self and i. When the kinship index is computed or updated for a given individual, the magnitude is taken as input to procedures that are designed to regulate kin-relevant behaviors in a fitness-promoting way. For the case of altruism, the kinship index is fed as one of many inputs to the "welfare tradeoff ratio estimator," whose function is to compute a magnitude, the "intrinsic welfare tradeoff ratio" ($_{int}WTR_i$), which regulates the extent to which the actor is intrinsically disposed to trade off his or her own welfare against that of individual i. A high kinship index up-regulates the weight put on i's welfare, while a low kinship index has little effect on the disposition to treat i altruistically. This is one element that up-regulates the emotion of love, attachment, or caring. Independently, the kinship index is fed as one of many inputs into the "sexual value estimator." Its function is to compute a magnitude, "sexual value" (SV_i), which regulates the extent to which the actor is motivated to value or disvalue sexual contact with individual i. As with altruism, many factors (e.g., health, age, symmetry) affect sexual value, but a high kinship index renders sexual valuation strongly negative, while a low kinship index is expected to have little effect on sexual valuation. The system takes as input two cues, whose values must themselves be stored and updated as regulatory variables. The first is maternal perinatal association (i.e., whether an older sibling observes his or her mother caring for a younger sibling as an infant), and the second is duration of coresidence between birth and the end of the period of parental investment. These two cues are processed to set the value of the kinship index for each familiar childhood companion. This system was designed by natural selection to detect which familiar others were close genetic relatives; to create a magnitude corresponding to the degree of genetic relatedness; and then to deploy this information to motivate both a sexual aversion between brothers and sisters, and a disposition to behave altruistically toward siblings.

An internal regulatory variable like the kinship index or the welfare tradeoff ratio acquires its meaning and functional properties from its relationship to the programs that compute it, and from the downstream decisions or processes that it regulates. The claim is not that such computations and their embedded variables are deliberate or consciously accessible. We think that they are usually nonconscious or implicit. Outputs of processes that access these variables may be consciously experienced—as disgust (at the prospect of sex with a sibling), affection for them, fear (on their behalf), grief (at their loss), and so on. Indeed, we think that it may be possible eventually to arrive at a precise description of computational understructure subserving the world of feeling, by considering feeling to be a special form of computation that evolved to deal with the world of valuation.

Because the computational mapping of motivational systems and emotion programs is a new enterprise, at present it is difficult to know the full range of internal regulatory variables that our psychological architecture is designed to compute and access. On adaptationist grounds, we suspect that the full set may include a surprising variety of registers for specialized magnitudes, corresponding to such things as these: how valuable a mate is, a child is, one's own life is, and so on; how stable or variable the food supply is over the long term; the distribution of condition-independent mortality in the habitat; one's expected future lifespan or period of efficacy; how good a friend someone has been to you; the extent of one's social support; the aggressive formidability for self or others (i.e., the ability to inflict costs); the sexual value of self and others; one's status, as well as the status of the coalition one belongs to; present energy stores; one's present health; the degree to which subsistence requires collective action; and so on. However, even focusing on one small set of internal regulatory variables, welfare tradeoff ratios, offers to clarify the functional architecture of several emotions, including anger, guilt, and gratitude.

ANGER AS AN EVOLVED REGULATORY PROGRAM

Consistent with the views of many other researchers, we have hypothesized that anger is an evolved emotion program with a special relationship to aggression. However, we think that it has an equal relationship to cooperation. In the evolutionary-psychological approach to the emotions, anger (in addition to being an experienced psychological state) is the expression of a functionally structured neurocomputational system whose design features and subcomponents evolved to regulate thinking, motivation, and behavior in the context of resolving conflicts of interest in favor of the angry individual (Sell, 2005; Sell, Tooby, & Cosmides, in press-a, in press-b). Two negotiating tools regulated by this system are the threat of inflicting costs (aggression) and the threat of withdrawing benefits (the down-regulation of cooperation). Humans differ from most other species in the number, intensity, and duration of close cooperative relationships, so traditional models of animal conflict must be modified to integrate the cooperative dimension more fully. Given its apparent functional logic, its universality across individuals and cultures

(Ekman, 1973; Brown, 1991), and its early ontogenetic development (Stenberg, Campos, & Emde, 1983; Stenberg & Campos, 1990), it seems likely that anger is an adaptation designed by natural selection. If so, then its computational structure (i.e., what variables cause anger, what behavioral patterns are enacted by it, and what variables cause it to subside) might be usefully illuminated by testing predictions derived by reference to the selection pressures that designed them.

Humans evolved embedded in small-scale social networks involving both cooperation and conflict. In many situations, each individual has open to him or her a range of alternative behaviors that embody—as one dimension—a spectrum of possible tradeoffs between the individual's own welfare and the welfare of one or more others. By choosing one course of conduct, the individual is intentionally or unintentionally expressing what can be termed a welfare tradeoff ratio with respect to the affected party or parties. For example, an individual might act in a way that weights the welfare of another person slightly or not at all (e.g., being late, theft, marital abandonment, rape, burning down someone's house for the fun of it), in a way that balances the two, or in a way that minimizes one's own welfare by sacrificing one's life for the other party. In this view, humans have a system that, in each individual, computes the welfare tradeoff ratio expressed in the actions of one person toward another (individual i to j), and stores it as a summary characterization of i's disposition toward j in the form of a regulatory variable—the welfare tradeoff ratio of i to j (WTR_{ij}). Indeed, there are at least two parallel, independent welfare tradeoff ratios: the intrinsic one ($_{int}WTR$), which guides an individual's behavior toward another, regardless of whether his or her actions are being observed; and the public one ($_{public}WTR$), which guides an individual's behavior when the recipient (or others) can observe the behavior. Some altruism is motivated through love, and some through fear, shame, or hope of reward—and the mechanisms involved are different.

If the human mind really contains welfare tradeoff ratios as regulatory variables that control how well one individual treats another, then evolution can build emotions whose function is to alter welfare tradeoff ratios in others toward oneself. Anger is conceptualized as a mechanism whose functional product is the recalibration in the mind of another of this other person's welfare tradeoff ratio with respect to oneself. That is, the goal of the system (rather than a conscious intention) is to change the targeted person's disposition to make welfare tradeoffs so that he or she more strongly favors the angered individual in the present and the future. As in animal contests, the target of anger may relinquish a contested resource, or may simply in the future be more careful to help or to avoid harming the angered individual. In cooperative relationships, where there is the expectation that the cooperative partner will spontaneously take the welfare of the individual into account, the primary threat from the angered person that potentially induces recalibration in the targeted individual is the signaled possibility of the withdrawal of future help and cooperation if the welfare tradeoff ratio is not modified. If the withdrawal of this cooperation would be more costly to the target of the anger than the burden of placing greater weight on the welfare of the angry individual, then the target should increase his or her welfare tradeoff ratio toward the angry individual, and so treat him or her better in the future.

Reciprocally, the program is designed to recalibrate the angry individual's own welfare tradeoff ratio toward the target of the anger for two functional reasons. This first is that it curtails the wasteful investment of cooperative effort in individuals who do not respond with a sufficient level of cooperation in return. The second is that the potential for this downward recalibration functions as leverage to increase the welfare tradeoff ratio of the target toward the angry individual. In the absence of cooperation, the primary threat is the infliction of damage. In the presence of cooperation, the primary threat is the withdrawal of cooperation. Concepts that are anchored in the internal regulatory variable $_{public}WTR$ include respect, consideration, deference, status, rank, and so on.

For example, ancestrally, one major cue that an individual would have been able to inflict costs to enforce welfare tradeoff ratios in his or her favor was the individual's physical strength (as noted earlier, we call the ability to inflict costs "formidability"). Consistent with this, in many species the degree to which an organism values a nonrelative is determined primarily by the relative strength of the two; thus animals with higher relative strength will, when other factors are held constant, fight more effectively for resources and have a higher expectation of gaining a larger share of disputed resources or social rank. Because strength was consistently one factor (out of several) relevant under ancestral conditions, and the nervous system had reliable access to the body, it seems plausible and worth investigating that the mind is designed to compute a strength self-assessment automatically and nonconsciously, and to use this self-assessment as an input regulating behavior. Thus the human brain should have evolved a set of programs that (1) evaluates one's own and others' formidabilities; (2) transforms each of these evaluations into a magnitude (a "formidability index") associated with each person; and, in situations where cooperation is not presumed, (3) implicitly expects or accords some level of deference based on relative formidability.

The approach briefly sketched above can be unpacked into a large number of empirical predictions derived from this analysis of the design features of the program regulating anger. For example, it is predicted that in humans, physical strength should be a partial cause of individual differences in the likelihood of experiencing and expressing anger. Other things being equal, stronger individuals are predicted to be more likely to experience anger and express anger; they should feel more entitled; they should expect others to give greater weight to their welfare, and become angrier when they do not. Although physical strength by no means exhausts the set of relevant variables, it offers an easily operationalizable and measurable gateway into a series of tests of this general model of the logic underlying the regulation of anger. Arguments precipitated by anger should reflect the underlying logic of the welfare tradeoff ratio: The complainant will emphasize the cost of the other's transgression to him or her, as well as the value of the complainant's cooperation to the transgressor, and will feel more aggrieved if the benefit the transgressor received (the justification) is small compared to the cost inflicted. A series of empirical studies supports both sets of predictions of this theory about the design of anger (Sell, 2005; Sell et al., in press-a, in press-b).

RECALIBRATIONAL EMOTIONS SUCH AS GUILT AND GRATITUDE

The EEA was full of event relationships (e.g., "Mother is dead") and psychophysical regularities (e.g., "Blood indicates injury") that cued reliable information about the functional meanings and properties of things, events, persons, and regulatory variables to the psychological architecture. For example, certain body proportions and motions indicated immaturity and need, activating the emotion program of experiencing cuteness (see Eibl-Ebesfeldt, 1970). Others indicated sexual attractiveness (Symons, 1979; Buss, 1994). To be moved with gratitude, to be glad to be home, to see someone desperately pleading, to hold one's newborn baby in one's arms for the first time, to see a family member leave on a long trip, to encounter someone desperate with hunger, to hear one's baby cry with distress, to be warm while it is storming outside—these all *mean* something to us. How does this happen? In addition to the situation-detecting algorithms associated with major emotion programs such as fear, anger, or jealousy, we believe that humans have a far larger set of evolved specializations, which we call "recalibrational releasing engines." These are activated by situation-detecting algorithms, and their function is to trigger appropriate recalibrations, including affective recalibrations, when certain evolutionarily recognizable situations are encountered.

We believe that the psychophysical or interpretive "front ends" of emotion programs use these cues not only to trigger the appropriate emotion, but to alter the weightings of regulatory variables embedded in decision rules. (For example, if you experience someone treating you disrespectfully, it makes you angry.) Indeed, most evolutionarily recurrent situations that selected for corresponding emotion programs bristle with information that allows the recomputation of one or more variables. Recalibration (which, when consciously accessible, appears to produce rich and distinct feeling states) is therefore a major functional component of most emotion programs. Jealousy, for example, involves several sets of recalibrations (e.g., diminution in estimate of one's own mate value, diminution of trust, lowering of the welfare tradeoff ratio toward the mate).

Indeed, from an evolutionary-psychological perspective, recalibrational emotion programs appear to be the dominant (but not the only) components of such emotions as guilt, grief, depression, shame, and gratitude. Their primary function is not to orchestrate any short-run behavioral response (as fear or anger do), but instead to carry out valuation recomputations in the light of the new information relevant to evolved regulatory variables that is provided by external or internal environments (Tooby & Cosmides, 1990a). An evolutionary viewpoint is a utilitarian one, which suggests that the time humans spend simply feeling—attending inwardly not to factual representations, but to something else—is doing something useful that will be reflected eventually in behavior. The hypothesis is that feeling is a form of computational activity that takes time and attention, that can compete with or preempt motivation to engage in other activities, and whose function is to recalculate and reweight the regulatory variables implicated by the newly encountered information. This approach has the potential to provide an account of the characteristics of emotions such as guilt or depression, which appear otherwise puzzling from a functional perspective. The feelings these emotion programs engender interfere with short-term utilitarian action that an active organism might be expected to engage in. If they were not useful, the capacity to feel them would have been selected out.

Consider guilt: We believe that guilt functions as an emotion mode specialized for recalibration of regulatory variables that control tradeoffs in welfare between self and other (Tooby & Cosmides, 1990a). Three important reasons why humans evolved to take the welfare of others into account are genetic relatedness toward relatives (Hamilton, 1964), the positive externalities others emit (Tooby & Cosmides, 1996a), and the maintenance of cooperative relationships (Trivers, 1971; Tooby & Cosmides, 1996a). The regulatory variable approach provides a clear framework for understanding why guilt evolved and what its underlying logic is. In this view, guilt involves the recalibration of regulatory variables considered when one is making decisions about tradeoffs in welfare between the self and others, based on new information about actual or potential harm arising from having placed too little weight on the other person's welfare in past actions. Kin selection would favor a mechanism designed to effect such recalibration toward those the kin detection mechanism identifies as close genetic relatives. Similarly, individuals have an intrinsic interest in the welfare of those whose existence benefits them, and with whom they share deep engagement relationships

(Tooby & Cosmides, 1996a). Third, reciprocal, exchange, or cooperative relationships need to be proximately motivated, so that benefit flows are appropriately titrated. Individuals who experienced guilt (and the associated modification of decision rules) would have been less likely to injure relationship partners repeatedly, and they would have had more success in maintaining beneficial cooperative relationships.

In the case of kin selection, we now have an empirical map of the architecture of the neurocomputational program that detects genetic relatedness and passes this information to the welfare tradeoff system (Lieberman et al., 2007). The theory of kin selection says nothing, however, about the procedures by which a mechanism could estimate the value of, say, a particular piece of food to oneself and one's kin. The fitness payoffs of such acts of assistance vary with circumstances. Consequently, each decision about where to allocate assistance depends on inferences about the relative weights of these variables. These nonconscious computations (however they are carried out) must be subject to error, selecting for feedback systems of correction.

Imagine a hunter–gatherer woman with a sister. The mechanisms in the woman's brain have been using the best information available to her to weight the relative values of the meat she has been acquiring to herself and her sister, leaving her reassured that it is safe to leave her sister for a while without provisioning her. The sudden discovery that her sister, since she was last contacted, has been starving and has become desperately sick functions as an information-dense situation allowing the recalibration of the algorithms weighting the relative values of the meat to self and sister (among other things). The sister's sickness functions as a cue that the previous allocation weighting was in error and that the variables need to be reweighted—including all of the weightings embedded in habitual action sequences that might be relevant to the sister's welfare. Guilt should be triggered when the individual receives (1) unanticipated information about the welfare of a valued other (or the increased value of the other), indicating that (2) the actor's actions or omissions caused or allowed the welfare of the valued individual to be damaged in a way that is inconsistent with the actor's ideal welfare tradeoff ratio, given (3) the actor's resources and potential for action.

When guilt is triggered, the welfare tradeoff ratio is adjusted, as well as a variety of subsidiary variables expressing this ratio in action. As a result of this recalibration, the guilty individual's behavior should reflect this higher valuation. In cases where the effects were intentional and anticipated, there should be little recalibration.

Existing findings substantiate these predictions and explain some of their otherwise puzzling features. Unsurprisingly, when the valued other is negatively affected unexpectedly, subjects feel guiltier (Baumeister, Stillwell, & Heatherton, 1995, Kubany & Watson, 2003). More surprisingly, individuals feel guiltier when the harm was caused accidentally rather than anticipated, even though individuals are usually considered less responsible and culpable for the harm when it occurs accidentally (McGraw, 1987; Baumeister et al., 1995). If the function of guilt is, however, to recalibrate an improperly set welfare tradeoff ratio, then information that merely confirms the evaluation present in the decision requires no recalibration. If the effect was foreseen and chosen anyway in the light of the existing ratio, then no adjustment is necessary.

Gratitude is a recalibrational emotion program that is complementary to guilt. Guilt turns up the welfare tradeoff ratio toward an individual when one has evidence that one's own actions have expressed too low a valuation of the other. Gratitude is triggered by new information indicating that another places a higher value on one's welfare than one's system had previously estimated—again leading to an up-regulation of the WTR toward that person. Anger, guilt, and gratitude all play different roles in cooperation, and their computational structure reflects their recalibrational functions with respect to welfare tradeoff ratios and the choice points they involve.

The evolutionary-psychological stance motivating the investigation of the program architecture of the emotions suggests that the emotions are intricate, functionally organized, and sensitively related to the detailed structure of ancestral problems. In this view, the emotions are likely to be far more sophisticated engineering achievements than previously appreciated, and there are many decades of work ahead for emotion researchers before they are comprehensively mapped.

NOTES

1. Marks (1987, pp. 68–69) vividly conveys how many aspects of behavior and physiology may be entrained by certain kinds of fear:

> During extreme fear humans may be "scared stiff" or "frozen with fear." A paralyzed conscious state with abrupt onset and termination is reported by survivors of attacks by wild animals, by shell-shocked soldiers, and by more than 50% of rape victims (Suarez & Gallup, 1979). Similarities between tonic immobility and rape-induced paralysis were listed by Suarez & Gallup (features noted by rape victims are in parentheses): (1) profound motor inhibition (inability to move); (2) Parkinsonian-like tremors (body-shaking); (3) silence (inability to call out or scream); (4) no loss of consciousness testified by retention of conditioned reactions acquired during the immobility (recall of details of the attack); (5) apparent analgesia (numbness and insensitivity to pain); (6) reduced core temperature (sensation of feeling cold); (7) abrupt onset and termination (sudden onset and remission of paralysis); (8) aggressive reactions at termination (attack of the rapist after recovery); (9) frequent inhibition of attack by a predator . . .

2. We think that some emotion programs evolved in response to the situation cue provided by a strong drive state, such as hunger, when the motivational intensity reached a point that other mechanisms became dominated and entrained by the magnitude of the motivation. We see no principled reason for distinguishing strong drive states from other emotion programs, and suspect that this practice originated from outdated notions of natural selection that separated "survival-related" functions (hunger, thirst) from other functions, such as mate acquisition or reciprocity. Thus we propose that it is useful to model specialized motivational states as emotion programs, just as one would disgust, anger, or fear.

3. The evolutionary purpose of deceitful emotional expressions is to (falsely) communicate the same two things.

REFERENCES

Archer, J. (1988). *The behavioural biology of aggression*. Cambridge, UK: Cambridge University Press.

Barkow, J., Cosmides, L., & Tooby, J. (Eds.). (1992). *The adapted mind: Evolutionary psychology and the generation of culture*. New York: Oxford University Press.

Baron-Cohen, S. (1995). *Mindblindness: An essay on autism and theory of mind*. Cambridge, MA: MIT Press.

Baumeister, R., Stillwell, A., & Heatherton, T. (1995). Personal narratives about guilt. *Basic and Applied Social Psychology*, 17(1–2), 173–198.

Berkow, R. (Ed.). (1992). *The Merck manual of diagnosis and therapy* (16th ed.). Rahway, NJ: Merck.

Brown, D. (1991). *Human universals*. New York: McGraw-Hill.

Boyer, P., & Liénard, P. (2006). Why ritualized behavior? Precaution systems and action parsing in developmental, pathological, and cultural rituals. *Behavioral and Brain Sciences*, 12(6), 595–613.

Buss, D. M. (1994). *The evolution of desire*. New York: Basic Books.

Buss, D. M. (Ed.). (2005). *The handbook of evolutionary psychology*. Hoboken, NJ: Wiley.

Cannon, W. (1929). *Bodily changes in pain, hunger, fear and rage: Researches into the function of emotional excitement*. New York: Harper & Row.

Chagnon, N. (1983). *Yanomamo: The fierce people* (3rd ed.). New York: Holt, Rinehart & Winston.

Cosmides, L. (1989). The logic of social exchange: Has natural selection shaped how humans reason? Studies with the Wason selection task. *Cognition, 31*, 187–276.

Cosmides, L., & Tooby, J. (1987). From evolution to behavior: Evolutionary psychology as the missing link. In J. Dupre (Ed.), *The latest on the best: Essays on evolution and optimality* (pp. 276–306). Cambridge, MA: MIT Press.

Cosmides, L., & Tooby, J. (1989). Evolutionary psychology and the generation of culture: Part II. Case study: A computational theory of social exchange. *Ethology and Sociobiology, 10*, 51–97.

Cosmides, L., & Tooby, J. (1992). Cognitive adaptations for social exchange. In J. Barkow, L. Cosmides, & J. Tooby (Eds.), *The adapted mind: Evolutionary psychology and the generation of culture* (pp. 163–228). New York: Oxford University Press.

Cosmides, L., & Tooby, J. (1997). Dissecting the computational architecture of social inference mechanisms. In G. Bock & G. Cardeco (Eds.), *Characterizing human psychological adaptations* (Ciba Symposium No. 208, pp. 132–156). Chichester, UK: Wiley.

Cosmides, L., & Tooby, J. (2000). Evolutionary psychology and the emotions. In M. Lewis & J. M. Haviland-Jones (Eds.), *Handbook of emotions* (2nd ed., pp. 91–115). New York: Guilford Press.

Crawford, C., & Krebs, D. (Eds.). (1998). *Handbook of evolutionary psychology*. Mahwah, NJ: Erlbaum.

Daly, M., & Wilson, M. (1988). *Homicide*. New York: Aldine.

Daly, M., Wilson, M., & Weghorst, S. J. (1982). Male sexual jealousy. *Ethology and Sociobiology, 3*, 11–27.

Derryberry, D., & Tucker, D. (1994). Motivating the focus of attention. In P. M. Neidenthal & S. Kitayama (Eds.), *The heart's eye: Emotional influences in perception and attention* (pp. 167–196). San Diego, CA: Academic Press.

Eibl-Ebesfeldt, I. (1970). *Ethology: The biology of behavior*. New York: Holt, Rinehart & Winston.

Ekman, P. (1973). Cross-cultural studies of facial expression. In P. Ekman (Ed.), *Darwin and facial ex-

pression: A century of research in review (pp. 169–222). New York: Academic Press.

Ekman, P. (Ed.). (1982). *Emotion in the human face* (2nd ed.). Cambridge, UK: Cambridge University Press.

Ekman, P. (1985). *Telling lies*. New York: Norton.

Ekman, P. (1994). Strong evidence for universals in facial expressions. *Psychological Bulletin, 115,* 268–287.

Ekman, P., Levenson, R., & Friesen, W. (1983). Autonomic nervous system activities distinguishes between emotions. *Science, 221,* 1208–1210.

Fiddick, L., Cosmides, L., & Tooby, J. (2000). No interpretation without representation: The role of domain-specific representations and inferences in the Wason selection task. *Cognition, 77,* 1–79.

Frank, R. (1988). *Passions within reason: The strategic role of the emotions.* New York: Norton.

Fredrickson, B. (1998). What good are positive emotions? *Review of General Psychology, 2,* 300–319.

Fridlund, A. (1994). *Human facial expression: An evolutionary view.* San Diego, CA: Academic Press.

Garcia, J. (1990). Learning without memory. *Journal of Cognitive Neuroscience, 2,* 287–305.

Gigerenzer, G., & Murray, D. (1987). *Cognition as intuitive statistics.* Hillsdale, NJ: Erlbaum.

Gould, S. J. (1997, June 12). Darwinian fundamentalism. *New York Review of Books,* pp. 34–38.

Hamilton, W. D. (1964). The genetical evolution of social behaviour. *Journal of Theoretical Biology, 7,* 1–52.

Haselton, M. G., & Buss, D. M. (2003). Biases in social judgment: Design flaws or design features? In J. Forgas, K. Williams, & B. von Hippel (Eds.), *Responding to the social world: Implicit and explicit processes in social judgments and decisions* (pp. 23–43). New York: Cambridge University Press.

Hirshleifer, J. (1987). On the emotions as guarantors of threats and promises. In J. Dupre (Ed.), *The latest on the best: Essays on evolution and optimality* (pp. 307–326). Cambridge, MA: MIT Press.

Kubany, E., & Watson, S. (2003). Guilt: Elaboration of a multidimensional model. *Psychological Record, 53,* 51–90.

Lazarus, R., & Lazarus, B. (1994). *Passion and reason.* New York: Oxford University Press.

LeDoux, J. (1995). In search of an emotional system in the brain: Leaping from fear to emotion to consciousness. In M. S. Gazzaniga (Ed.), *The cognitive neurosciences* (pp. 1049–1061). Cambridge, MA: MIT Press.

Lieberman, D., Tooby, J., & Cosmides, L. (2007). The architecture of human kin detection. *Nature, 445,* 727–731.

Marks, I. (1987). *Fears, phobias, and rituals.* New York: Oxford University Press.

Maynard Smith, J. (1982). *Evolution and the theory of games.* Cambridge, UK: Cambridge University Press.

McGraw, K. (1987). Guilt following transgression: an attribution of responsibility approach. *Journal of Personality and Social Psychology, 53*(2), 247–256.

Miller, S. (Ed.). (1976). *Symptoms: The complete home medical encyclopedia.* New York: Crowell.

Mineka, S., & Cook, M. (1993). Mechanisms involved in the observational conditioning of fear. *Journal of Experimental Psychology: General, 122,* 23–38.

Mowat, R. R. (1966). *Morbid jealousy and murder: A psychiatric study of morbidly jealous murders at Broadmoor.* London: Tavistock.

Nesse, R. (1991). Evolutionary explanations of emotions. *Human Nature, 1,* 261–289.

Pinker, S. (1997). *How the mind works.* New York: Norton.

Pitman, R., & Orr, S. (1995). Psychophysiology of emotional and memory networks in posttraumatic stress disorder. In J. McGaugh, N. Weinberger, & G. Lynch (Eds.), *Brain and memory: Modulation and mediation of neuroplasticity* (pp. 75–83). New York: Oxford University Press.

Raymond, E. S. (1991). *The new hacker's dictionary.* Cambridge, MA: MIT Press.

Sell, A. (2005). *Regulating welfare trade-off ratios: Three tests of an evolutionary–computational model of human anger.* Doctoral dissertation, Department of Psychology, University of California, Santa Barbara.

Sell, A., Tooby, J., & Cosmides, L. (in press-a). *The logic of anger: Formidability regulates human conflict.*

Sell, A., Tooby, J., & Cosmides, L. (in press-b). *Computation and the logic of anger.*

Shepard, R. N. (1987). Evolution of a mesh between principles of the mind and regularities of the world. In J. Dupre (Ed.), *The latest on the best: Essays on evolution and optimality* (pp. 251–275). Cambridge, MA: MIT Press.

Shepherd, M. (1961). Morbid jealousy: Some clinical and social aspects of a psychiatric symptom. *Journal of Mental Science, 107,* 687–753.

Stenberg, C. R., & Campos, J. J. (1990). The development of anger expression in infancy. In N. Stein, B. Leventhal, & T. Trabasso (Eds.), *Psychological and biological approaches to emotion* (pp. 247–282). Hillsdale, NJ: Erlbaum.

Stenberg, C. R, Campos, J. J., & Emde, R. N. (1983). The facial expression of anger in seven-month-old infants. *Child Development, 54*(1), 178–184.

Suarez, S. D., & Gallup, G. G. (1979). Tonic immobility as a response to rage in humans: A theoretical note. *Psychological Record, 29,* 315–320.

Swets, J. A., Tanner, W. D., & Birdsall, T. G. (1961). Decision processes in perception. *Psychological Review, 68,* 301–340.

Symons, D. (1979). *The evolution of human sexuality.* Oxford: Oxford University Press.

Tomaka, J., Blascovich, J., Kibler, J., & Ernst, J. (1997). Cognitive and physiological antecedents of threat and challenge appraisal. *Journal of Personality and Social Psychology, 73,* 63–72.

Tooby, J. (1985). The emergence of evolutionary psychology. In D. Pines (Ed.), *Emerging syntheses in science: Proceedings of the founding workshops of the Santa Fe Institute* (pp. 1–6). Santa Fe, NM: Santa Fe Institute.

Tooby, J., & Cosmides, L. (1989, August). *The logic of threat.* Paper presented at the meeting of the Human Behavior and Evolution Society, Evanston, IL.

Tooby, J., & Cosmides, L. (1990a). The past explains the present: emotional adaptations and the structure of ancestral environments. *Ethology and Sociobiology, 11,* 375–424.

Tooby, J., & Cosmides, L. (1990b). On the universality of human nature and the uniqueness of the individual: The role of genetics and adaptation. *Journal of Personality, 58,* 17–67.

Tooby, J., & Cosmides, L. (1992). The psychological foundations of culture. In J. Barkow, L. Cosmides, & J. Tooby (Eds.), *The adapted mind: Evolutionary psychology and the generation of culture* (pp. 19–136). New York: Oxford University Press.

Tooby, J., & Cosmides, L. (1996a). Friendship and the banker's paradox: Other pathways to the evolution of adaptations for altruism. In W. G. Runciman, J. M. Smith, & R. I. M. Dunbar (Eds.), *Evolution of Social Behaviour Patterns in Primates and Man. Proceedings of the British Academy, 88,* 119–143.

Tooby, J., & Cosmides, L. (1996b). *The computationalist theory of communication.* Paper presented at the meeting of the Human Behavior and Evolu-

tion Society Meetings, University of Arizona, Tucson.

Tooby, J., & Cosmides, L. (1997). On evolutionary psychology and modern adaptationism: A reply to Stephen Jay Gould. Available online at *www.psych.ucsb.edu/research/cep/critical_eye.htm*

Tooby, J., & Cosmides, L. (2005). Conceptual foundations of evolutionary psychology. In D. M. Buss (Ed.), *The handbook of evolutionary psychology* (pp. 5–67). Hoboken, NJ: Wiley.

Tooby, J., & Cosmides, L. (in press). Internal regulatory variables and the design of human motivation: An evolutionary and computational approach. In A. Elliot (Ed.), *Handbook of approach and avoidance motivation.* Mahwah, NJ: Erlbaum.

Tooby, J., Cosmides, L., & Barrett, H. C. (2003). The second law of thermodynamics is the first law of psychology: Evolutionary developmental psychology and the theory of tandem, coordinated inheritances. *Psychological Bulletin, 129*(6), 858–865.

Tooby, J., Cosmides, L., Sell, A., Lieberman, D., & Sznycer, D. (in press). Internal regulatory variables and the design of human motivation: An evolutionary and computational approach. In A. Elliot (Ed.), *Handbook of approach and avoidance motivation.* Mahwah, NJ: Erlbaum.

Trivers, R. L. (1971). The evolution of reciprocal altruism. *The Quarterly Review of Biology, 46,* 35–37.

Williams, G. C. (1966). *Adaptation and natural selection: A critique of some current evolutionary thought.* Princeton, NJ: Princeton University Press.

CHAPTER 9

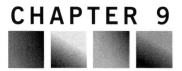

The Role of Emotion in Economic Behavior

SCOTT RICK and GEORGE LOEWENSTEIN

IMMEDIATE AND EXPECTED EMOTIONS

Consequentialist Models of Decision Making

Economic models of decision making are consequentialist in nature; they assume that decision makers choose between alternative courses of action by assessing the desirability and likelihood of their consequences, and integrating this information through some type of expectation-based calculus. Economists refer to the desirability of an outcome as its "utility," and decision making is depicted as a matter of maximizing utility.

This does not, however, imply that consequentialist decision makers are devoid of emotion or immune to its influence. To see why, it is useful to draw a distinction between "expected" and "immediate" emotions (Loewenstein, Weber, Hsee, & Welch, 2001; Loewenstein & Lerner, 2003). Expected emotions are those that are anticipated to occur as a result of the outcomes associated with different possible courses of action. For example, if Laura, a potential investor, were deciding whether to purchase a stock, she might imagine the disappointment she would feel if she bought it and it declined in price, the elation she would experience if it increased in price, and possibly emotions such as regret and relief that she might experience if she did not purchase the stock and its price either rose or fell. The key feature of expected emotions is that they are experienced when the outcomes of a decision materialize, but not at the moment of choice, at the moment of choice they are only cognitions about future emotions.

Immediate emotions, by contrast, are experienced at the moment of choice and fall into one of two categories. "Integral" emotions, like expected emotions, arise from thinking about the consequences of one's decision, but integral emotions, unlike expected emotions, are experienced at the moment of choice. For example, in the process of deciding whether to purchase the stock, Laura might experience immediate fear at the thought of the stock's losing value. "Incidental" emotions are also experienced at the moment of choice, but arise from dispositional or situational sources objectively unrelated to the task at hand (e.g., the TV program playing in the background as Laura called her brokerage house).[1]

The notion of expected emotions is perfectly consistent with the consequentialist perspective of economics. Nothing in the notion of utility maximization rules out the idea that the utility an individual associates with an outcome might arise from a prediction of emotions; for example, one might assign higher utility to an Italian restaurant dinner than a French restaurant dinner because one anticipates being happier at the former. While not explicitly denying the idea that utilities might depend on expected emotions, however, most economists until recently viewed detailed accounts of such emotions as outside the purview of their discipline.

Integral immediate emotions can also be incorporated into a consequentialist framework, although it takes one farther afield from conventional economics. Integral emotions, it can and in fact has been argued, might provide decision makers with information about their own tastes—for instance, to help inform Laura of how she would actually feel if she purchased the stock and it rose or declined in value. However, this assumes, contrary to the usual assumption in economics, that people have an imperfect understanding of their own tastes.

An influence of incidental immediate emotions on decision making would pose a much more fundamental challenge to the consequentialist perspective, because such emotions, by definition, are irrelevant to the decision at hand. Any influence of incidental emotions would suggest that decisions are influenced by factors unrelated to the utility of their consequences.

Figure 9.1 presents a schematic representation of the traditional perspective of economics. Although immediate emotions are represented in the figure, they would not be part of any traditional economist's representation of their framework, because they play no role in decision making; they are "epiphenomenal" by-products of, but not determinants of, decisions.

However, a great deal of market activity can be understood in terms of *both* expected and immediate emotions. Much advertising attempts to inform consumers, whether accurately or not, about emotions that they can expect to feel if they do or do not buy a particular good. "One-day-only" sales, for example, are probably effective because they make consumers think that they will regret not seizing the

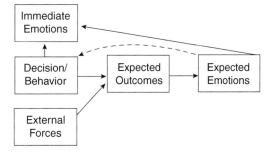

FIGURE 9.1. Consequentialist model of decision making.

opportunity. Marketers also attempt to capitalize on immediate emotions—for example, charitable organizations that make potential donors feel guilty about what they squander their money on while less fortunate people starve.

The food industry is particularly motivated to capitalize on immediate emotions. Mrs. Field's Cookies, for example, has been known to pump enticing cookie smells into the atmosphere of shopping malls to stimulate hunger (Hoch & Loewenstein, 1991). A company named "ScentAir" sells similar odors (e.g., "Glazed Donut," "Iced Cinnamon Pretzel," "Blue Cotton Candy") to businesses looking to stimulate hunger.[2] By contrast, the dieting industry often attempts to market its services by focusing people on the positive emotions they can anticipate experiencing once they are finally able to fit into the perfect pair of jeans.

Enter Behavioral Economics

Fortunately, many economists would view the snapshot of their discipline presented above as outdated. This is largely attributable to the advent of "behavioral economics," a subdiscipline of economics that incorporates more psychologically realistic assumptions to increase the explanatory and predictive power of economic theory. The field first achieved prominence in the 1980s and has been gaining influence since then. And much of the thrust of behavioral economics has involved, or at least could be construed as involving, an enhanced understanding of emotions.

The first, and less controversial, interaction of behavioral economics with emotions was to question the neglect of the topic and to begin to examine exactly how utility depended on outcomes. For example, whereas conventional economics assumes that the utility of an outcome depends only on the outcome itself, some economists showed how counterfactual emotions (e.g., regret), which arise from considering alternative outcomes that could have occurred, can influence decision making. Note that these analyses focus on expected emotions and hence help to elaborate the connection among outcomes, emotions, and utility, but do not challenge the consequentialist perspective.

More recently, economists as well as psychologists who are specifically interested in decision making have begun to take greater account of immediate emotions. Some of the research has shown that immediate integral emotions play a critical role in decision making. However, other research has shown that immediate emotions, and especially but not exclusively incidental emotions, often propel decisions in different directions from expected emotions—that is, in directions that run contrary to the predictions of a consequentialist perspective. The new research thus suggests that the consequentialist perspective is much too simple to be a descriptively valid account of actual behavior.

In this chapter, we review some of the critical (consequentialist) assumptions and predictions of the dominant economic models of risky decision making, intertemporal choice, and social preferences. For each of these areas, we first discuss behavioral phenomena that are anomalous from the consequentialist perspective, but that are rectified once the role of expected emotions is taken into account. Next, we discuss phenomena that can potentially be illuminated by taking account of immediate emotions, both integral and incidental. We conclude by proposing directions for future research on the role of emotion in decision making.

DECISION MAKING UNDER RISK

Most decisions, including decisions of economic importance, entail an element of risk, because the consequences of alternative courses of action are rarely known with certainty. Thus decision making under risk is a central topic in economics.

Since first proposed by Daniel Bernoulli (1738/1954), the "expected utility" (EU) model has served as the normative benchmark for decision making under risk in economics.

EU assumes that people choose between alternative courses of action by assessing the desirability or "utility" of each action's possible outcomes and linearly weighting those utilities by their probability of occurring. The normative status of the EU model was enhanced by von Neumann and Morgenstern's (1944) demonstration that it could be derived from a primitive, intuitively appealing set of axioms—for example, that preferences are transitive (if A is preferred to B, and B is preferred to C, then A should be preferred to C). In addition to its normative appeal, this model's assumption that decisions are based on EU, rather than expected value, gives it descriptive appeal as well. For instance, it assumes that the difference in happiness (i.e., utility) between winning $1 and winning $2 is not necessarily equal to the difference in happiness between winning $101 and winning $102 (though the difference in *value* is equal).

However, empirical research has documented many behavioral phenomena that are inconsistent with the basic axioms, and thus inconsistent with the predictions of the EU model, and many of these anomalies can be attributed to unrealistic assumptions about the determinants of expected emotions and the influence of immediate emotions. Several models have accounted for some of these anomalies by making more realistic assumptions about the determinants of expected emotions. We next review some of these theoretical innovations. We then discuss anomalies that can potentially be explained by taking account of the influence of immediate emotions.

Innovations to the EU Model Involving Expected Emotions

Relaxing the Asset Integration Assumption

In its original form, the EU model assumes that people do not narrowly focus on potential outcomes when making a decision, but rather on how those outcomes affect their overall wealth. Thus the utility of a particular outcome is not simply based on that outcome, but instead on the integration of that outcome with all assets accumulated to that point. However, as originally noted by Markowitz (1952) and developed more fully by Kahneman and Tversky (1979), people typically make decisions with a narrower focus. When evaluating the potential outcomes of a decision, people tend to think in terms of incremental gains and losses, rather than in terms of changes in overall welfare.

Suppose, for example, that Bob must decide whether to accept or reject a gamble that offers a 50% chance of winning $20 and a 50% chance of losing $10. If Bob currently possesses $1 million in wealth, then the EU model assumes that he views the gamble as offering a 50% chance of experiencing the utility of $1,000,020 and a 50% chance of experiencing the utility of $999,990. Markowitz (1952) argued, however, that most people would instead process the gamble as it was presented, namely as offering a 50% chance of experiencing the utility of winning $20 and a 50% chance of experiencing the disutility of losing $10.[3]

Relaxing the Assumption That Utility Is Strictly Defined over Realized Outcomes

Another problematic assumption of the EU model is that unrealized outcomes do not influence how we feel about realized outcomes. For example, suppose you anticipate a pay raise of $10,000 and subsequently receive a $5,000 raise. Although the raise is a gain relative to the status quo, you will likely code it as a loss, since it fails to meet expectations. Indeed, Koszegi and Rabin (2006) have recently proposed a model assuming that gains and losses are defined relative to expectations, rather than the status quo.

Additionally, several modifications of the EU model incorporate the tendency to compare what happens to what was expected to happen (e.g., Loomes & Sugden, 1986; Mellers, Schwartz, Ho, & Ritov, 1997). Other theories attempt to account for regret, a counterfactual emotion that arises from a comparison between the outcome one experiences as a consequence of one's decision and the outcome one could have experienced as a consequence of making a different choice. Early versions of regret theory (e.g., Loomes & Sugden, 1982) predicted that regret aversion could lead to violations of fundamental axioms of the EU model, such as monotonicity (i.e., stochastically dominating gambles are preferred to the gambles they dominate).

Regret can also lead to violations of transitivity. Consider, for example, the three gambles below. Assume that there are three equally likely states of nature; the table lists what each gamble pays if a particular state of nature is realized. If people care more about one big regret

than they do about two smaller ones, as assumed in Loomes and Sugden (1982), then Gamble A will be preferred to Gamble B. Similarly, B is likely to be preferable to C. Since A is preferred to B, and B is preferred to C, then transitivity requires that A is preferred to C. However, in fact C is preferred to A, since choosing A over C exposes one to the risk of one large regret instead of two small ones.

	State 1	State 2	State 3
Gamble A	$10	$20	$30
Gamble B	$20	$30	$10
Gamble C	$30	$10	$20

Disappointment aversion and regret aversion theories have only met with modest empirical support. One problem with the predictive validity of regret aversion theories may be that anticipated regret only influences decision making when the possibility of regret is salient (Zeelenberg & Beattie, 1997; Zeelenberg, Beattie, van der Plight, & De Vries, 1996). Consider, for example, the following gambles, in which one of four colors can be drawn with varying probability:

Gamble A

90% chance of White, which pays $0
6% chance of Red, which pays $45
1% chance of Green, which pays $30
3% chance of Yellow, which pays -$15

Gamble B

90% chance of White, which pays $0
7% chance of Red, which pays $45
1% chance of Green, which pays –$10
2% chance of Yellow, which pays –$15

Since Green wins $30 in Gamble A and loses $10 in Gamble B, choosing B could produce regret if Green is drawn. This very salient potential for regret could lead to a preference for A over B, even though such a preference violates monotonicity. However, the gambles can be rewritten to make the possibility of regret less salient:

Gamble A′

90% chance of White, which pays $0
6% chance of Red, which pays $45
1% chance of Green, which pays $30
1% chance of Blue, which pays –$15
2% chance of Yellow, which pays –$15

Gamble B′

90% chance of White, which pays $0
6% chance of Red, which pays $45
1% chance of Green, which pays $45
1% chance of Blue, which pays –$10
2% chance of Yellow, which pays –$15

Note that Gambles A' and B' are equivalent to Gambles A and B, respectively; A and A' both have an expected value of $2.55, and B and B' both have an expected value of $2.75. However, the potential for regret is no longer salient. Rather, B' pays at least as much as A' for each possible color. Thus, even though A and A' are equivalent, A' is likely to be less attractive than A, only because the way A' and B' are framed obfuscates the potential for regret.[4]

However, note that regret is often more salient in prospect than in retrospect.[5] Consider, for example, a study by Gilbert, Morewedge, Risen, and Wilson (2004) that examined the extent to which subway passengers regretted missing their train. Passengers who entered a subway station within 6 minutes of missing the train (experiencers) were told that they missed their train by either 1 minute or 5 minutes. They were then asked to report how much regret they felt. These ratings were compared to the ratings of passengers leaving the station (forecasters), who were asked to imagine how much regret they would feel if they missed their train by 1 or 5 minutes. Forecasters anticipated feeling greater regret if they missed their train by 1 minute than by 5 minutes, though actual regret did not depend on how close experiencers came to catching the train. A subsequent study suggested that the effect was driven by forecasters' inability to realize how quickly they would absolve themselves of responsibility for the disappointing outcome.

Although work remains to be done to incorporate more determinants of expected emotions into consequentialist models of decision making under risk, great progress has been made. We now discuss risky choice phenomena driven by immediate emotions.

Innovations to the EU Model Involving Immediate Emotions

Integral Emotions Influence Risky Decision Making

When sufficiently strong, immediate emotions can directly influence behavior, completely precluding cognitive decision making (Loewenstein, 1996). Ariely and Loewenstein (2005) experimentally examined the influence of sexual arousal on (hypothetical) risky decision making (see also Loewenstein, Nagin, & Paternoster, 1997). Male participants were given a laptop computer and asked to answer a

series of questions. In the control treatment, participants answered the questions while in their natural (presumably not highly aroused) state. In the arousal treatment, participants were first asked to self-stimulate (masturbate) while viewing erotic photographs, and were presented with the same questions only after they had achieved a high but suborgasmic level of arousal. When asked about their intention to use birth control in the future, aroused participants were less likely to report intending to use a condom. Although arousal affected participants' risk *attitudes*, it did not affect their risk *perception*. For example, aroused participants were no less likely to endorse this statement: "If you pull out before you ejaculate, a woman can still get pregnant." Although the authors did not ask questions that would permit mediational analyses, the preliminary results suggest that immediate emotions had a direct effect on (predicted) behavior.

When experienced at more moderate levels, however, affect can mediate the relationship between cognition and behavior. Antonio Damasio and his colleagues (Damasio, 1994; Bechara, Damasio, Tranel, & Damasio, 1997) have argued that decision makers encode the consequences of alternative courses of action affectively, and that such "somatic markers" critically influence decision making. Damasio and colleagues have further argued that the ventromedial prefrontal cortex (VMPFC) plays a critical role in this affective encoding process. Bechara et al. (1997) investigated the proposed role of the VMPFC in an experiment in which patients suffering damage to the VMPFC and non-brain-damaged individuals played a game in which the objective was to win as much money as possible. Players earned hypothetical money by turning over cards that yielded either monetary gains or losses. On any given turn, players could draw from one of four decks, two of which included $100 gains and two of which contained $50 gains. The high-paying decks also included a small number of substantial losses, resulting in a net negative expected value for these decks. Bechara et al. (1997) found that both nonpatients and those with VMPFC damage avoided the high-paying decks immediately after incurring substantial losses. However, individuals with VMPFC damage resumed sampling from the high-paying decks more quickly than nonpatients did after encountering a substantial loss. Thus, even though patients understood the game and wanted to win, they often went "bankrupt." Bechara et al. (1997) reasoned that patients "knew" the high-paying decks were risky, but that their failure to experience fear when contemplating sampling from these decks made risky draws more palatable.[6] While the Bechara et al. (1997) study has not been immune to criticism (see Maia & McClelland, 2004, for a particularly compelling critique, and Dunn, Dalgleish, and Lawrence, 2005, for a review of several critiques), the somatic marker hypothesis remains intuitively appealing.

Other evidence suggesting that integral emotion influences decision making comes from studies of consumers' willingness to insure against a variety of risks. Johnson, Hershey, Meszaros, and Kunreuther (1993), for example, asked participants how much they would be willing to pay for flight insurance that protected against death due to "any act of terrorism" or "any reason." Since terrorism is only one of many reasons why a plane might crash, consequentialist models of decision making predict that participants will pay more for insurance covering all types of crashes than for insurance just covering terrorism. However, Johnson et al. (1993) found that participants were willing to pay slightly more for insurance protecting against terrorism.[7]

Additional evidence of integral emotions' impact on risky decision making comes from studies of probability weighting. The EU model assumes that the weight an outcome's probability receives in decision making is independent of the outcome; in fact, the model assumes linear probability weighting (i.e., that outcomes are weighted in exact proportion to their likelihood of occurring). However, more recent models of decision making under risk have challenged this assumption, suggesting instead that probabilities are weighted nonlinearly, as in Figure 9.2 (Kahneman & Tversky, 1979). Kahneman and Tversky's (1979) proposed "probability-weighting function" suggests that small probabilities are overweighted and large probabilities are underweighted.

Despite the innovation, models such as Kahneman and Tversky's (1979) still assume that probability weights are independent of outcomes. This suggests, for example, that a 1% chance of losing $1 has the same psychological impact as a 1% chance of losing your life. Rottenstreich and Hsee (2001) suggest that the probability-weighting function is flatter for affect-rich outcomes than for affect-poor out-

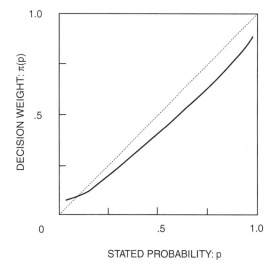

FIGURE 9.2. Kahneman and Tversky's probability-weighting function. From Kahneman and Tversky (1979). Copyright 1979 by the Econometric Society. Reprinted by permission.

comes. They speculate that affect-rich prizes elicit greater degrees of hope and fear, and thus an extreme overweighting of small probabilities and an extreme underweighting of large probabilities. Indeed, Rottenstreich and Hsee (2001) found that participants' willingness to pay to avoid an electric shock was insensitive to the probability of the shock, whereas willingness to pay to avoid losing $20 was extremely sensitive to the probability of the loss.[8]

Incidental Emotion Influences Risky Decision Making

In a study of market index returns across 26 countries from 1982 to 1997, Hirshleifer and Shumway (2003) found that the amount of sunshine (relative to expected amount of sunshine for a given time of year) was positively and significantly correlated with market returns. The authors speculate that the phenomenon may be driven by incorrect attributions of good mood to positive economic prospects rather than correct attributions to the sunshine (cf. Schwarz & Clore, 1983). Similarly, Edmans, García, and Norli (2007) have found that stock market returns plummet when a country's soccer team is eliminated from an important tournament (e.g., the World Cup). They also document a dip in market returns following important losses in other sports (e.g., cricket, rugby, and hockey) in countries where those sports are popular.[9]

INTERTEMPORAL CHOICE

Models of intertemporal choice address how decision makers choose between alternatives involving costs and benefits that are distributed over time. The "discounted utility" (DU) model is the dominant model of intertemporal choice in economics (Samuelson, 1937). Structurally, this model is closely parallel to the EU model—and, like the EU model, has been derived from a series of intuitively compelling axioms (Koopmans, 1960). However, a number of anomalies have been identified that call into question the descriptive validity of these axioms, and thus the predictions of the DU model (Loewenstein & Prelec, 1992). We next review anomalies that can be reconciled with this model once more realistic assumptions are made about the determinants of expected emotions; we then discuss anomalies that can be explained by taking account of immediate emotions.

Innovations to the DU Model Involving Expected Emotions

Relaxing the Assumption That Utility Is Strictly Defined over Realized Outcomes

Like the EU model, the DU model assumes that utility (and thus expected emotion) is only a function of realized outcomes. If people devalue future emotions, they should want to experience pleasurable outcomes immediately and postpone painful outcomes whenever possible. However, contrary to this basic assumption, in many situations people prefer to get unpleasant outcomes over with quickly, or to "leave the best for last." In an early study documenting this phenomenon, Loewenstein (1987) asked 30 undergraduates how much they would be willing to pay immediately to obtain a kiss from the movie star of their choice and to avoid receiving a (nonlethal) 110-volt shock, after several time delays. Contrary to the predictions of the DU model, respondents were willing to pay more to experience a kiss delayed by 3 days than an immediate kiss or one delayed by 3 hours or 1 day, and were also willing to pay more to avoid a shock that was delayed for 1 year

or 10 years than to avoid a shock experienced within the next 3 days.

These anomalies can be reconciled with the DU model if one takes account of the observation that utility is not strictly a function of realized outcomes, but also of emotions experienced while waiting for those outcomes to occur. Loewenstein (1987) proposes that people derive utility from "savoring" future good outcomes and disutility from dreading bad outcomes.[10] Indeed, in a brain imaging study in which participants were confronted with the prospect of a *real* impending shock, Berns et al. (2006) found that components of the brain's "pain matrix" (a cluster of regions that are activated during the experience of pain) are also active in anticipation of shock. Furthermore, providing support for the idea that utility from anticipation plays a causal role in the desire to expedite negative outcomes, individual differences in activation in response to anticipatory pain predict individual tendencies to expedite shocks.[11]

Incorporating Affective Forecasting Errors

For the DU model to be descriptively valid, people must be able to forecast accurately how they will react emotionally to future outcomes. However, there is by now substantial evidence that people have difficulty making such forecasts. Consider, for instance, a study by Brickman, Coates, and Janoff-Bulman (1978) in which lottery winners, persons with paraplegia or quadriplegia, and a control group were asked to report their current happiness on a 5-point scale. The lottery group ($n = 22$) consisted of people who had recently won at least $50,000 in the Illinois state lottery. The paraplegic and quadriplegic participants ($n = 29$) had become paralyzed within the past year. Lottery winners reported a mean level of happiness virtually identical to that of the control group (4.00 vs. 3.82), whose happiness was significantly different from, but surprisingly close to, the mean happiness level among paraplegic and quadriplegic participants (2.96). Although the lottery winners and the paraplegic and quadriplegic participants were not prospectively asked to predict their future happiness (since they could not be identified beforehand), it seems likely that both groups would have overestimated the hedonic impact of their future circumstances.[12]

Loewenstein and Adler (1995) examined whether people could predict falling subject to the "endowment effect" (Thaler, 1980), which refers to the tendency for people to value an object more highly if they possess it than they would value the same object if they did not. In the typical demonstration of the effect (see, e.g., Kahneman, Knetsch, & Thaler, 1990), some participants (sellers) are endowed with an object and given the option of trading it for various amounts of cash; other participants (choosers) are not given the object, but are given a series of choices between receiving the object and receiving various amounts of cash. Although the objective wealth position of the two groups is identical, as are the choices they face, endowed participants hold out for significantly more money than those who are not endowed. Loewenstein and Adler (1995) informed some participants that they would be endowed with an object (a mug engraved with their school logo) and asked them to predict the price at which they would sell the object back to the experimenter once they were endowed. These participants, and others who did not make a prediction, were then endowed with the object and given the opportunity to sell it back to the experimenter. Participants who were not yet endowed substantially underpredicted their own postendowment selling prices. In a second study, selling prices were elicited from participants who were actually endowed with an object and from others who were told they had a 50% chance of getting the object. Selling prices were substantially higher for the former group, and the valuations of participants who were not sure of getting the object were indistinguishable from the buying prices of participants who did not have the object.

Loewenstein and Adler's (1995) results suggest that participants who were not endowed with an object failed to predict how painful it would be to part with the object once they possessed it. That is, non-endowed participants made "affective forecasting" errors when predicting their future attachment to the object. However, a recent study by Kermer, Driver-Linn, Wilson, and Gilbert (2006) suggests that it may be the *sellers* who are making the affective forecasting error (see also Galanter, 1992). Kermer et al. (2006) first asked participants to report their baseline affect. Participants then received a $5 show-up fee and were told that a coin would be flipped to determine whether they would win an additional $3 or lose $2. Next, they predicted how they would feel im-

mediately after the coin toss. The experimenter then flipped a coin and paid participants accordingly. Participants then rated how they felt at that moment. Some participants were also asked to report what they would think after the coin toss, and once the coin had actually been tossed, they were asked to report their actual thoughts. Kermer et al. (2006) found that people expected losing $3 to diminish their happiness (relative to happiness reported at the beginning of the experiment) more than it actually did.[13] This suggests that the predictors in Loewenstein and Adler (1995) may have accurately based their predicted selling prices on how they would actually feel after losing an object. Sellers, by contrast, may have based their selling prices on unrealistically negative forecasts of how they would feel after losing an object.[14]

In a behavioral economic model of intertemporal choice that incorporates affective forecasting errors, Loewenstein, O'Donoghue, and Rabin (2003) propose that people exaggerate the degree to which their future tastes will resemble their current tastes. Conlin, O'Donoghue, and Vogelsang (2007) find evidence of such "projection bias" in catalog orders of cold-weather-related clothing items and sports equipment. People are overinfluenced by the weather at the time they make decisions, as measured by their likelihood of returning the item: A decline of 30° F on the date an item is ordered increases the probability of a return by 3.95%.

Economists have incorporated more realistic assumptions about expected emotions into models of intertemporal choice. However, some phenomena, driven by immediate emotions, remain anomalous from the perspective of such models. We now turn to these phenomena.

Innovations to the DU Model Involving Immediate Emotions

Relaxing the Assumption of Exponential Discounting

The DU model assumes that people discount future flows of utility at a fixed discount rate based on when the utility will be experienced. Discounting at a fixed rate (i.e., "exponential" discounting) means that a given time delay leads to the same amount of discounting regardless of when it occurs. According to the DU model, delaying the delivery of a good by 1 day leads to the same degree of time discounting whether that delay makes the difference between consuming the good tomorrow rather than today or in 101 days rather than 100 days. However, an overwhelming amount of empirical work suggests that people (as well as animals) do not discount the future exponentially (Kirby & Herrnstein, 1995; Rachlin & Raineri, 1992). Rather, people care more about the same time delay if it is proximal rather than distal—a general pattern that has been refereed to as "hyperbolic time discounting" (Ainslie, 1975). For example, delaying consumption of a pleasurable good from today to tomorrow is more distressing than delaying consumption from 100 days from now to 101 days from now. Hyperbolic time discounting predicts that people will behave farsightedly when the consequences of their decision are delayed. In such situations, decision makers will place great weight on long-term costs and benefits. However, when consequences are immediate, hyperbolic time discounting will produce behavior that appears impulsive.[15]

Consider, for example, an experiment by Read, Loewenstein, and Kalyanaraman (1999) in which participants were asked to select 1 of 24 movies to watch. Some of the movies were "highbrow" (e.g., *Schindler's List*), and some were "lowbrow" (e.g., *The Mask*). Some participants were asked to choose a movie to watch that night, whereas others were asked to choose a movie to watch in the future. Consistent with hyperbolic discounting, "lowbrow" movies (ones that are high in short-run benefits, but low in long-run benefits) were most popular among participants selecting a movie for immediate viewing.[16]

Behavioral economists have made great progress in modeling hyperbolic discounting (e.g., Laibson, 1997). Such models implicitly assume that discounting leads to impulsive behavior by diminishing the importance of expected emotions. However, when the timing of consumption is held constant, various other situational factors can also lead to impulsivity. Walter Mischel (1974) and colleagues, for example, have extensively studied the impact of physical proximity of rewards on the impulsivity of children. Children faced with the choice between a small immediate reward (e.g., one marshmallow immediately or two marshmallows in 15 minutes) and a larger delayed reward (two marshmallows) tend to behave more impatiently when the immediate reward is visible.

Thus impulsivity may reflect factors other than a devaluation of expected emotions. Immediate emotions may also produce nonexponential discounting. To examine the influence of immediate emotions on impulsivity, McClure, Laibson, Loewenstein, and Cohen (2004) measured the brain activity of participants with functional magnetic resonance imaging (fMRI) while they made a series of intertemporal choices between small proximal rewards ($R available at delay d) and larger delayed rewards ($R' available at delay d'), where $R < $R' and d < d'. Rewards ranged from $5 to $40 Amazon.com gift certificates, and the delay ranged from the day of the experiment to 6 weeks later. McClure et al. (2004) investigated whether there were brain regions that showed elevated activation (relative to a resting state benchmark) only when immediacy was an option (i.e., activation when d = 0, but no activation when d > 0), and whether there were regions that showed elevated activation when participants were making any intertemporal decision irrespective of delay. McClure et al. (2004) found that time discounting is associated with the engagement of two neural systems. Limbic and paralimbic cortical structures, which are known to be rich in dopaminergic innervation, were preferentially recruited for choices involving immediately available rewards. In contrast, fronto-parietal regions, which support higher cognitive functions, were recruited for all intertemporal choices. Moreover, the authors found that when choices involved an opportunity for immediate reward, thus engaging both systems, greater activity in fronto-parietal regions than in limbic regions was associated with choosing larger delayed rewards.[17] These results suggest that the experience of immediate emotion rather than the devaluation of expected emotion may, at least in some situations, drive impulsivity.[18]

Integral Emotions Influence Intertemporal Choice

Suppose you are deciding whether or not to buy a CD for $10. The DU model predicts that you will buy the CD if the anticipated pleasure of listening to it exceeds its "opportunity cost" (i.e., the forgone pleasure that could have been purchased with the $10). However, Frederick, Novemsky, Wang, Dhar, and Nowlis (2006) suggest that people do not spontaneously consider opportunity costs when deciding whether or not to purchase goods. Frederick et al. (2006) asked participants whether they would (hypothetically) be willing to purchase a desirable video for $14.99. They simply varied whether the decision not to buy it was framed as "not buy this entertaining video" or "keep the $14.99 for other purchases." Although the two phrases described objectively equivalent actions, the latter highlighted the pleasure that would be forgone by purchasing the video. Frederick et al. (2006) found that drawing attention to opportunity costs significantly reduced the proportion of participants willing to purchase the video, suggesting that many participants were not spontaneously considering opportunity costs (cf. Jones, Frisch, Yurak, & Kim, 1998).

If many people do not take opportunity costs into account when deciding whether or not to purchase goods, then how do they make such decisions? In a project wiht Brian Knutson, Elliott Wimmer, and Drazen Prelec (Knutson, Rick, Wimmer, Prelec, & Loewenstein, 2007), we investigated this question in an experiment in which participants chose whether or not to purchase a series of discounted consumer goods while having their brains scanned with fMRI. The goods ranged in retail price from $10 to $80, and were offered at a 75% discount to encourage spending. Participants were given $20 to spend and were told that one of their decisions would be randomly selected to count for real. At the conclusion of the experiment, participants indicated how much they liked each product and how much they would be willing to pay for it.

We found that the extent to which participants reported liking the products correlated positively with activation in nucleus accumbens, a target of dopaminergic projections that has previously been associated with anticipation of gains and self-reported happiness (Knutson, Adams, Fong, & Hommer, 2001). Moreover, consumer surplus (i.e., the difference between self-reported willingness to pay for the good and its price) correlated positively with activation in medial prefrontal cortex, a region previously associated with the receipt of unexpectedly large gains (e.g., Knutson, Fong, Bennett, Adams, & Hommer, 2003). We also found that activation in both regions correlated positively with purchasing decisions. However, we found that activation in insula during the period when subjects first saw the price correlated negatively with pur-

chasing decisions. Insula activation has previously been observed in connection with aversive stimuli such as disgusting odors (Wicker et al., 2003), unfairness (Sanfey, Rilling, Aronson, Nystrom, & Cohen, 2003), and social exclusion (Eisenberger, Lieberman, & Williams, 2003). Thus when the delayed costs of immediage indulgence are not explicitly represented (as in, e.g., McClure et al., 2004), but rather implicitly captured by prices, participants appear to rely on an anticipatory "pain of paying" (Prelec & Loewenstein, 1998) to curtail their spending.

Incidental Emotions Influence Consumer Choice

In other research conducted wiht Cynthia Cryder (Rick, Cryder, & Loewenstein, 2008) investigated whether individuals chronically differed in their tendency to experience anticipatory pain when making purchasing decisions. We hypothesized that individuals who typically experience an intense pain of paying may generally spend less than they would ideally like to spend, whereas individuals who experience minimal pain of paying may typically spend more than they would ideally like to spend. We developed a "Spendthrift–Tightwad" scale to measure individual differences in the pain of paying and found that tightwads outnumbered spendthrifts by a 3:2 ratio in a sample of more than 13,000 people. Rick (2007) hypothesized that incidental sadness could help both tightwads and spendthrifts overcome their prepotent affective responses to spending. The hypothesis was based on previous experimental work suggesting that sadness deepens deliberation (e.g., Tiedens & Linton, 2001) and motivates people to change their circumstances (e.g., Lerner et al., 2004). Rick (2007) tested the hypothesis in an experiment in which tightwads and spendthrifts decided whether or not to purchase a variety of goods while listening to neutral or sad music. As predicted, tightwads spent more when sad than when in a neutral state, and spendthrifts spent less when sad than when in a neutral state.

SOCIAL PREFERENCES

Although there are widely accepted normative benchmarks for risky decision making and intertemporal choice, no such benchmarks exist for how people should behave toward others.

However, many economic models make the simplifying, but unrealistic, assumption that people are strictly self-interested. Below we review behavioral economic models of social preferences that have incorporated more realistic assumptions about the determinants of expected emotions in social interactions. We then review anomalies driven by immediate emotions.

Expected Emotion: Relaxing the Pure Self-Interest Assumption

Economists frequently study social preferences in the context of the "ultimatum game" (Guth, Schmittberger, & Schwarze, 1982). In the typical ultimatum game, a "proposer" offers some portion of an endowment to a "responder," who can either accept the offer or reject it. If the responder accepts the offer, the money is divided according to the proposed split. If the responder rejects the offer, both players leave with nothing. Since purely self-interested responders should accept any positive offer, self-interested proposers should offer no more than the smallest positive amount possible. However, average offers typically exceed 30% of the pie, and offers of less than 20% are frequently rejected (see Camerer, 2003).

Several behavioral economic models have emerged that incorporate a taste for fairness.[19] Rabin (1993) proposes a model in which people derive utility from reciprocating intentional (un)kindness with (un)kindness (see also Dufwenberg & Kirchsteiger, 2004). Blount (1995) conducted an interesting variant of the ultimatum game to investigate the role of intentions in social behavior. Some responders were told that the proposer with whom they were paired would make an offer, as in the standard ultimatum game. Other responders were told that the offer would be randomly generated. Blount (1995) found that responders were willing to accept significantly less when the offer was generated randomly than when it came from the proposer.

Sanfey, Rilling, Aronson, Nystrom, and Cohen (2003) conducted a similar study in which participants played the ultimatum game while having their brains scanned with fMRI. Participants, all responders, were told they would play the ultimatum game with 10 different human proposers (though offers were actually determined by the experimenters). Responders received five "fair" offers ($5 for proposer, $5 for respondent) and five unfair offers. In 10 other

trials, responders received the same offer, but this time from a computer. As in Blount (1995), participants were more willing to accept low offers from computer proposers than from human proposers. Moreover, activation in anterior insula, a region commonly implicated in the experience of pain (e.g., Knutson et al., 2007), was greater for unfair offers from human proposers than for fair offers from human proposers. Insula activation was also significantly greater in response to unfair offers from human proposers than in response to unfair offers from computer proposers. In fact, whether players rejected unfair offers from human proposers could be predicted reliably by the level of their insula activity. Thus it appears that integral emotions influence responders' behavior in the ultimatum game (cf. Pillutla & Murninghan, 1996).

Behavioral economists have created more descriptively valid models of social preferences by relaxing the assumption of pure self-interest. However, some phenomena driven by immediate emotion cannot be explained by such models. We review such anomalies below.

Integral Emotions Influence Social Preferences

Recent work on the "identifiable-victim effect" (Small & Loewenstein, 2003), which refers to the tendency to give more to identifiable victims than to statistical victims, suggests that integral emotions play a role in generosity toward others (see also Schelling, 1968; Kogut & Ritov, 2005). Subsequent research has demonstrated that people are also more punitive toward identifiable wrongdoers than toward equivalent but unidentified wrongdoers, and that anger mediates the effect of identifiability on punishing behavior (Small & Loewenstein, 2005). To capture these phenomena, as well as a variety of experimental findings, Loewenstein and Small (2007) have proposed a dual-process model of helping behavior in which a sympathetic but highly immature emotional system interacts with a more mature but uncaring deliberative system.

Incidental Emotions Influence Social Preferences

Andrade and Ariely (2006) investigated the impact of incidental emotions on behavior in the ultimatum game. They induced either incidental happiness or anger, and then had participants play the role of responder in an ultimatum game in which they were offered $4 of a $20 endowment. After deciding whether to accept or reject the offer, participants then played the role of proposer in a second ultimatum game, with a presumably different partner than in the first game. Andrade and Ariely (2006) found that happy responders were less likely than angry responders to reject unfair offers in the initial ultimatum game. Surprisingly, however, proposers who were initially induced to feel happy made *more* selfish proposals in the second ultimatum game. The authors reasoned that angry individuals, who were more likely to reject unfair offers than happy individuals in the initial ultimatum game, misattributed their behavior to stable preferences rather than to incidental affect. Later, due to a "false-consensus effect" (Ross, Greene, & House, 1977; but see Dawes & Mulford, 1996), the previously angry individuals inferred that others would also be likely to reject unfair offers and therefore, as proposers, made very generous offers. By contrast, the authors reasoned that happy individuals, who were less likely to reject unfair offers than angry individuals in the initial ultimatum game, also misattributed their behavior to stable preferences. Accordingly, previously happy individuals inferred that others would also be unlikely to reject unfair offers and therefore, as proposers, made very selfish offers.[20]

CONCLUSION

As the foregoing review indicates, emotions influence economic behavior in two distinct ways. First, people anticipate, and take into account, how they are likely to feel about the potential consequences of alternative courses of action. As discussed, such a role for *expected* emotions is entirely consistent with consequentialist economic accounts of decision making. Research on the role of expected emotions in decision making has taken a variety of directions. It has assessed the types of emotions that people actually experience when different outcomes are realized, with a special focus on counterfactual emotions. It has examined people's predictions of what emotions they will experience, and the accuracy of such predictions. And, it has sought to determine the degree to which decisions are in fact guided by predicted emotions.

Second, substantial research supports the idea that immediate emotions also play an important role in decision making. Integral immediate emotions arise from contemplating the potential outcomes of a decision. In some cases, these emotions seem to play a beneficial role in decision making, informing decision makers about their own values. But in other cases, such as the disproportionate fear commonly associated with flying as opposed to driving, integral emotions may cause people to act contrary to their own material interests. In contrast to the mixed role played by integral emotions, it is much more difficult to justify the well-documented role of incidental emotions, which by definition are unrelated to the decision at hand.

In general, research on expected emotions is far more advanced than that on immediate emotions. As a result, there is a pressing need for more research to examine the causes and consequences of immediate emotions, and to understand the complex interplay of immediate and expected emotions in the production of behavior. In some cases, immediate and expected emotions seem to complement one another. This is true, for example, when immediate emotions provide decision makers with a better understanding of their own values—an understanding that may help them to better predict their own future feelings. For instance, the experience of anticipatory guilt may help students who are contemplating cheating on an exam to appreciate the guilt they would experience after doing so. In other cases, however, immediate and expected emotions come into conflict. For example, the immediate effect of a positive mood may be to make decision makers more inclined to take risks—but, by a different, consequentialist path, a positive mood might also make decision makers more risk-avoidant, with the goal of not risking a disturbance to the positive feelings (Isen, Nygren, & Ashby, 1988; Kahn & Isen, 1993).

The clash between immediate and expected emotions is also a major cause of self-control problems. For example, people are often driven by immediate emotions to eat, drink, and make merry, but in some of these situations, contemplation of expected emotional consequences may discourage indulgence. Psychologists have for decades been developing "dual-process" models that can be interpreted in such terms (see Evans, 2008, for a review), and in recent years economists have begun to follow their lead. Thaler and Shefrin (1981) were the first economists to do so; their model adopts a principal–agent framework, in which a far-sighted planner (the principal) attempts to reconcile the competing demands of a series of myopic doers (the agents). More recently, many dual-process models have focused on the problem of self-control (Brocas & Carrillo, 2006; Fudenberg & Levine, 2006; Benhabib & Bisin, 2005; Loewenstein & O'Donoghue, 2004; Bernheim & Rangel, 2004).

Although most of the dual-process models proposed by economists have sought to adhere to the standard consequentialist perspective, introducing a role for immediate emotions should raise questions about whether such a perspective is "up to the job" of providing a useful account of human behavior. Behavior under the control of immediate emotions bears little resemblance to the reflective weighing of costs and benefits that is the prototype of rational economic decision making. Instead, it is a much more reflexive process that often drives behavior in exactly the opposite direction from that suggested by a weighing of costs and benefits. Whether behavior driven by immediate emotions even warrants the label of "decision making" seems questionable.

In closing, we note two potential (and, we believe, fruitful) directions for future research on the role of emotion in decision making. The first is the need to study stronger emotions than have generally been examined in the empirical literature. Many vitally important decisions are made "in the heat of the moment," and indeed important economic decisions such as major purchases often evoke powerful emotions. But studying the impact of such emotions is difficult—in part because it is difficult if not impossible to manipulate such strong emotional states experimentally, and in part because people generally do not like to be studied when they are in heightened emotional states. Gaining a better understanding of the role of immediate emotions in economic decision making, therefore, is going to require researchers who are willing to extend themselves into "hot" situations and creative enough to find natural experiments in which people are naturally assigned to different emotional states before they make important decisions.

The second pressing need is for economic research that takes fuller account of the range of insights that psychologists are developing into emotions. Thus, for example, economists studying the impact of weather on the stock market have generally taken a rather simplistic view—that bad weather should lead to negative emotions, which should in turn lead to negative price movements. But psychologists studying the impact of emotions on risk taking find that different specific negative emotions can have very different effects. More relevant to the central theme of this chapter, that they have found negative emotions can exert conflicting effects on risk taking, depending on whether the mechanism is consequentialist or more reflexive.

Economists' understanding of the role of emotions in economic behavior has made enormous strides in recent decades. However, there is still a long distance to go.

NOTES

1. Note that the distinction between expected and immediate emotions closely maps onto other commonly discussed distinctions in economics and psychology, such as the broad distinction between cognition and emotion, or Adam Smith's (1759/1981) distinction between the "impartial spectator" and the "passions."

2. On the surface, it seems somewhat unethical to artificially induce visceral states in order to sell products. However, food companies that failed to prey on the affective vulnerability of consumers would probably be driven out of business by other companies that did. Hence one could argue that food companies that pump artificial smells into the atmosphere to stimulate hunger are not evil, but rather are doing what they must to stay afloat.

3. Note that narrowly focusing on gains and losses rather than on changes in overall welfare suggests that all people, regardless of their current wealth position, view gambles the same way. Indeed, such a narrow focus may explain why some extraordinarily wealthy individuals take big risks to achieve small gains and avoid small losses (e.g., Martha Stewart, worth hundreds of millions of dollars, engaged in insider trading to avoid a loss of less than $50,000).

4. As Sugden (1986) notes, another problem with regret-aversion models may be that it is *recrimination*—regret accompanied by the feeling that one should have behaved differently—rather than regret that one cares about and attempts to avoid. Suppose, for example, you take your car to your regular mechanic, Sue, for an oil change. You have never had a problem with this mechanic's work, but this time she uses the wrong type of oil, which causes the car to break down. In this situation, you surely regret that the mistake was made, but you probably

do not blame yourself for taking it to Sue, since you had no reason to anticipate such a mistake based on her past performance. Now suppose that you instead had decided to change your own oil. You have never done so before, but you decide it is worth trying to save the money. Your inexperience leads you to use the wrong type of oil, causing the car to break down. As in the previous scenario, you regret that the mistake was made. However, now there is likely to be recrimination as well: You think that you should have known better than to try to change your own oil.

5. Interestingly, however, Kivetz and Keinan (2006) show that regret from choosing virtues over vices increases over time, whereas regret from choosing vices over virtues diminishes over time.

6. Note that the extent to which emotional deficits lead to poor decision making depends largely on situational factors. In a similar study in which risky choices had a higher expected value than riskless choices, Shiv, Loewenstein, Bechara, Damasio, and Damasio (2005) found that patients with damage to brain regions associated with processing emotion earned *more* than control participants.

7. One natural explanation for these results is that "unpacking" vivid subsets of a larger set provides a more effective retrieval cue when people are recalling past causes of plane crashes (e.g., Tversky & Koehler, 1994). Such an account would be consistent with a consequentialist model of decision making that allows for errors in judging probabilities. However, other work suggests that this result should not be interpreted in purely cognitive terms. Slovic, Fischhoff, and Lichtenstein (1980), for example, speculated that people's willingness to insure themselves against unlikely losses may be related to how much these potential losses cause worry or concern. Consistent with this view, a number of studies have shown that knowing someone who has been in a flood or earthquake, or having been in one oneself, greatly increases the likelihood of purchasing insurance (Browne & Hoyt, 2000). Although this finding, like that of Johnson et al. (1993), could be explained in consequentialist terms as resulting from an increase in individuals' expectations of experiencing a flood or earthquake in the future, the effect remains significant even after subjective expectations are controlled for (Kunreuther et al., 1978).

8. Similarly, Ditto, Pizarro, Epstein, Jacobson, and MacDonald (2006) conducted an experiment in which participants were given the opportunity to play a game that would either result in winning chocolate chip cookies or being required to work on a boring task for an extra 30 minutes. Half of the participants were only told about the cookies, whereas for the other half the cookies were freshly baked in the lab and placed in front of the participants as they decided whether or not to play the game. Consistent with Rottenstreich and Hsee

(2001), Ditto et al. (2006) found that participants' willingness to play the game was insensitive to the probability of winning cookies when the cookies were baked in the lab, whereas willingness to play was very sensitive to the probability of winning when the cookies were merely described.

9. Also, Lerner and Keltner (2001) find that dispositional (i.e., incidental) anger and fear have opposing effects on risk preferences. Specifically, angry people tend to prefer risk (see also Fessler, Pillsworth, & Flamson, 2004), whereas fearful people tend to avoid it. The authors explain their results in terms of the cognitive appraisals generated by the emotions (Smith & Ellsworth, 1985). Anger is generally associated with appraisals of certainty and individual control, whereas fear is generally associated with appraisals of uncertainty and situational control. These incidental emotions, through their associated appraisals, appear to influence participants' cognitive evaluations of the problem, thus influencing their subsequent decisions.

10. Loewenstein's model applies only to deterministic outcomes (e.g., a guaranteed kiss from a movie star in the future). Caplin and Leahy (2001) note that many anticipatory emotions (e.g., suspense) are driven by uncertainty about the future. They propose a model that modifies the EU model to incorporate such anticipatory emotions, and then show that it can explain a variety of phenomena (e.g., the overwhelming preference for riskless bonds over stocks).

11. In addition to savoring and dread, an entirely different type of anticipation may also drive intertemporal choice: the anticipation of *memories* (Elster & Loewenstein, 1992). For example, people may perform challenging but unpleasant activities (e.g., mountain climbing) partly because they savor the pleasant memories of conquering the challenge (see also Keinan, 2006).

12. Addressing an important limitation of the Brickman et al. (1978) study, Gilbert et al. (1998) conducted a study in which affective forecasts could be elicited prior to an important life event. Specifically, Gilbert et al. (1998) studied assistant professors' forecasts of how they would feel after their tenure decisions; the investigators compared these forecasts to the self-reported well-being of others whose tenure decisions had been made in the past. The sample consisted of all assistant professors who were considered for tenure in the liberal arts college of a major university over a 10-year period, and it was divided into three categories: current assistant professors, those whose decisions were made less than 5 years earlier, and those whose decisions were made more than 5 years earlier. Current assistant professors predicted that they would be much happier during the first 5 years after a positive decision, but that this difference would dissipate during the subsequent 5 years. Thus they expected to adapt much more slowly than others actually did: There was no

significant difference in reported well-being between those who had and had not received tenure in
either the first 5 or the next 5 years afterward.

13. By contrast, participants accurately predicted how
    much winning the coin flip would increase their
    happiness.

14. Why are people often unable to accurately predict
    their affective reactions to negative events? Kermer
    et al. (2006) suggest that people do not realize how
    capable they are of finding "silver linings." For ex-
    ample, participants who were asked to report their
    thoughts before and after losing the coin flip were
    significantly more likely to think about their $2
    profit after losing the coin flip than before the coin
    was flipped. Conversely, participants were more
    likely to think they would focus on the $3 loss be-
    fore the coin was flipped than they actually did after
    losing the coin flip. Other researchers (e.g., Schkade
    & Kahneman, 1998) attribute affective forecasting
    errors to "focusing illusions," whereby people exag-
    gerate the impact of specific narrow changes in their
    circumstances on well-being. Both are plausible ex-
    planations of the affective forecasting errors docu-
    mented in the studies discussed here.

15. However, Kivetz and Simonson (2002) suggest that
    some people have a hard time selecting luxuries
    (items that are presumably high in short-run bene-
    fits, but low in long-run benefits) over cash when ei-
    ther would be received shortly after the decision.
    They demonstrate that choosing luxuries over cash
    is easier when the consequences of the decision are
    delayed.

16. Goldstein and Goldstein (2006) document a similar
    phenomenon among Netflix customers, who watch
    and return low-brow movies right away, but let
    high-brow movies sit around much longer before
    watching them.

17. However, note that since the rewards were gift cer-
    tificates, the consumption they afforded was not im-
    mediate in any conventional sense. To address this
    limitation, McClure, Ericson, Laibson, Loewen-
    stein, and Cohen (2007) ran an experiment in which
    participants were asked not to drink any liquids
    during the 3 hours preceding their session. While
    having their brains scanned with fMRI, participants
    made a series of choices between receiving a small
    amount of juice or water immediately (by having it
    squirted into their mouths) and receiving a larger
    amount of juice or water up to 20 minutes later.
    Like McClure et al. (2004), McClure et al. (2007)
    found that limbic regions were preferentially re-
    cruited for choices involving immediately available
    juice or water, whereas fronto-parietal regions were
    recruited for all choices.

18. The results are consistent with earlier behavioral re-
    search by Shiv and Fedorikhin (1999), who found
    that cognitive load increases the likelihood of
    choosing cake over fruit salad. The McClure et al.
    (2004) results suggest that cognitive load interfered
    more with activation in fronto-parietal regions than

with activation in limbic regions, making participants' visceral attraction to the cake more
influential.

19. But see Dana, Weber, and Kuang (2007) for evidence
    suggesting that some actions that appear to reflect a
    taste for fairness may in fact reflect a desire to ap-
    pear to have a taste for fairness.

20. Incidental emotion also influences prosocial behav-
    ior. Darlington and Macker (1966), for example,
    found that incidental guilt increased participants'
    willingness to donate blood. Alice Isen and her col-
    leagues (e.g., Isen & Levin, 1972; Isen, Horn, &
    Rosenhan, 1973; Isen, Clark, & Schwartz, 1976)
    have found in a variety of settings that incidental
    happiness (induced, e.g., by finding a dime in a
    phone booth or receiving free cookies) increases
    people's willingness to help others (e.g., by picking
    up their dropped papers or by helping the experi-
    menter with a subsequent task; but see Isen &
    Simmonds, 1978). Incidental gratitude also in-
    creases people's willingness to help others (Bartlett
    & DeSteno, 2006). Although the preceding studies
    did not deal directly with money, note that the help-
    ing behavior they documented did involve expendi-
    tures of costly resources (e.g., blood, effort, atten-
    tion).

REFERENCES

Ainslie, G. (1975). Specious reward: A behavioral theory of impulsiveness and impulse control. *Psychological Bulletin, 82*(4), 463–496.

Andrade, E. B., & Ariely, D. (2006). *Short- and long-
term consequences of emotions in decision making.*
Manuscript in preparation, University of California,
Berkeley.

Ariely, D., & Loewenstein, G. (2005). The heat of the
moment: The effect of sexual arousal on sexual decision making. *Journal of Behavioral Decision
Making, 18*(1), 1–12.

Bartlett, M. Y., & DeSteno, D. (2006). Gratitude and
prosocial behavior: Helping when it costs you. *Psychological Science, 17*(4), 319–325.

Benhabib, J., & Bisin, A. (2005). Modeling internal commitment mechanisms and self-control: A neuroeco-
nomics approach to consumption-saving decisions.
Games and Economic Behavior, 52(2), 460–492.

Bechara, A., Damasio, H., Tranel, D., & Damasio, A. R.
(1997). Deciding advantageously before knowing the
advantageous strategy. *Science, 275,* 1293–1295.

Bernheim, B. D., & Rangel, A. (2004). Addiction and
cue-triggered decision processes. *American Economic Review, 94*(5), 1558–1590.

Bernoulli, D. (1954). Specimen theoriae novae de
mensura sortis [Exposition of a new theory on the
measurement of risk]. *Econometrica, 22*(1), 23–36.
(Original work published 1738)

Berns, G. S., Chappelow, J., Cekic, M., Zink, C. F.,
Pagnoni, G., & Martin-Skurski, M. E. (2006). Neu-

robiological substrates of dread. *Science, 312,* 754–758.

Blount, S. (1995). When social outcomes aren't fair: The effect of causal attributions on preferences. *Organizational Behavior and Human Decision Processes, 63*(2), 131–144.

Brickman, P., Coates, D., & Janoff-Bulman, R. (1978). Lottery winners and accident victims: Is happiness relative? *Journal of Personality and Social Psychology, 36*(8), 917–927.

Brocas, I., & Carrillo, J. D. (2006). *The brain as a hierarchical organization.* Manuscript in preparation, University of Southern California.

Browne, M. J., & Hoyt, R. E. (2000). The demand for flood insurance: empirical evidence. *Journal of Risk and Uncertainty, 20*(2), 271–289.

Buchel, C., & Dolan, R. J. (2000). Classical fear conditioning in functional neuroimaging. *Current Opinion in Neurobiology, 10*(2), 219–233.

Camerer, C. (2003). *Behavioral game theory: Experiments in strategic interaction.* Princeton, NJ: Princeton University Press.

Caplin, A., & Leahy, J. (2001). Psychological expected utility theory and anticipatory feelings. *Quarterly Journal of Economics, 116*(1), 55–80.

Conlin, M., O'Donoghue, T., & Vogelsang, T. J. (2007). Projection bias in catalog orders. *American Economic Review, 97*(4), 1217–1249.

Damasio, A. R. (1994). *Descartes' error: Emotion, reason, and the human brain.* New York: Putnam.

Dana, J., Weber, R. A., & Kuang, J. X. (2007). Exploiting moral wiggle room: Experiments demonstrating an illusory preference for fairness. *Economic Theory, 33*(1), 67–80.

Darlington, R. B., & Macker, C. E. (1966). Displacement of guilt-produced altruistic behavior. *Journal of Personality and Social Psychology, 4*(4), 442–443.

Dawes, R. M., & Mulford, M. (1996). The false consensus effect and overconfidence: Flaws in judgment or flaws in how we study judgment? *Organizational Behavior and Human Decision Processes, 65*(3), 201–211.

Ditto, P. H., Pizarro, D. A., Epstein, E. B., Jacobson, J. A., & MacDonald, T. K. (2006). Visceral influences on risk-taking behavior. *Journal of Behavioral Decision Making, 19*(2), 99–113.

Dufwenberg, M., & Kirchsteiger, G. (2004). A theory of sequential reciprocity. *Games and Economic Behavior, 47*(2), 268–298.

Dunn, B. D., Dalgleish, T., & Lawrence, A. D. (2005). The somatic marker hypothesis: A critical evaluation. *Neuroscience and Biobehavioral Reviews, 30*(2), 1–33.

Edmans, A., García, D., & Norli, Ø. (2007). Sports sentiment and stock returns. *Journal of Finance, 62*(4), 1967–1998.

Eisenberger, N. I., Lieberman, M. D., & Williams, K. D. (2003). Does rejection hurt? An fMRI study of social exclusion. *Science, 302,* 290–292.

Elster, J., & Loewenstein, G. (1992). Utility from memory and anticipation. In G. Loewenstein & J. Elster (Eds.), *Choice over time.* New York: Russell Sage Foundation.

Evans, J. St. B. T. (2008). Dual-processing accounts of reasoning, judgment, and social cognition. *Annual Review of Psychology, 59.*[pp tk]

Fessler, D. M. T., Pillsworth, E. G., & Flamson, T. J. (2004). Angry men and disgusted women: An evolutionary approach to the influence of emotions on risk taking. *Organizational Behavior and Human Decision Processes, 95,* 107–123.

Frederick, S., Novemsky, N., Wang, J., Dhar, R., & Nowlis, S. (2006). *Opportunity costs and consumer decisions.* Manuscript in preparation, Massachusetts Institute of Technology.

Fudenberg, D., & Levine, D. K. (2006). A dual-self model of impulse control. *American Economic Review, 96*(5), 1449–1476.

Galanter, E. (1992). Utility functions for nonmonetary events. *American Journal of Psychology, 65,* 45–55.

Gilbert, D. T., Morewedge, C. K., Risen, J. L., & Wilson, T. D. (2004). Looking forward to looking backward: The misprediction of regret. *PsychologicalScience, 15*(5), 346–350.

Gilbert, D. T., Pinel, E. C., Wilson, T. D., Blumberg, S. J., & Wheatley, T. P. (1998). Immune neglect: A source of durability bias in affective forecasting. *Journal of Personality and Social Psychology, 75*(3), 617–638.

Goldstein, D. G., & Goldstein, D. C. (2006). Profiting from the long tail. *Harvard Business Review, 84*(6), 24–28.

Guth, W., Schmittberger, R., & Schwarze, B. (1982). An experimental analysis of ultimatum bargaining. *Journal of Economic Behavior and Organization, 3*(4), 367–388.

Hirshleifer, D., & Shumway, T. (2003). Good day sunshine: Stock returns and the weather. *Journal of Finance, 58*(3), 1009–1032.

Hoch, S. J., & Loewenstein, G. (1991). Time-inconsistent preferences and consumer self-control. *Journal of Consumer Research, 17,* 492–507.

Isen, A. M., Clark, M., & Schwartz, M. F. (1976). Duration of the effect of good mood on helping: Footprints on the sands of time. *Journal of Personality and Social Psychology, 34*(3) 385–393.

Isen, A. M., Horn, N., & Rosenhan, D. L. (1973). Effects of success and failure on children's generosity. *Journal of Personality and Social Psychology, 27*(2), 239–247.

Isen, A. M., & Levin, P. F. (1972). The effect of feeling good on helping: Cookies and kindness. *Journal of Personality and Social Psychology, 15*(4), 294–301.

Isen, A. M., Nygren, T. E., & Ashby, F. G. (1988). Influence of positive affect on social categorization. *Motivation and Emotion, 16*(1), 65–78.

Isen, A. M., & Simmonds, S. F. (1978). The effect of feeling good on a helping task that is incompatible with good mood. *Social Psychology, 41*(4), 346–349.

Johnson, E. J., Hershey, J., Meszaros, J., & Kunreuther,

H. (1993). Framing, probability distortions, and insurance decisions. *Journal of Risk and Uncertainty*, 7(1), 35–51.

Jones, S. K., Frisch, D., Yurak, T. J., & Kim, E. (1998). Choices and opportunities: Another effect of framing on decisions. *Journal of Behavioral Decision Making*, 11(3), 211–226.

Kahn, B. E., & Isen, A. M. (1993). The influence of positive affect on variety seeking among safe, enjoyable products. *Journal of Consumer Research*, 20(2), 257–270.

Kahneman, D., Knetsch, J. L., & Thaler, R. H. (1990). Experimental tests of the endowment effect and the Coase theorem. *Journal of Political Economy*, 98(6), 1325–1348.

Kahneman, D., & Tversky, A. (1979). Prospect theory: An analysis of decision under risk. *Econometrica*, 47(2), 263–291.

Keinan, A. (2006). *Productivity mindset and the consumption of collectible experiences.* Manuscript in preparation, Columbia University.

Kermer, D. A., Driver-Linn, E., Wilson, T. D., & Gilbert, D. T. (2006). Loss aversion is an affective forecasting error. *Psychological Science*, 17(8), 649–653.

Kirby, K. N., & Herrnstein, R. J. (1995). Preference reversals due to myopic discounting of delayed reward. *Psychological Science*, 6(2), 83–89.

Kivetz, R., & Keinan, A. (2006). Repenting hyperopia: An analysis of self-control regrets. *Journal of Consumer Research*, 33, 273–282.

Kivetz, R., & Simonson, I. (2002). Self-control for the righteous: Toward a theory of precommitment to indulgence. *Journal of Consumer Research*, 29, 199–217.

Knutson, B., Adams, C. M., Fong, G. W., & Hommer, D. (2001). Anticipation of increasing monetary reward selectively recruits nucleus accumbens. *Journal of Neuroscience*, 21, RC159.

Knutson, B., Fong, G. W., Bennett, S. M., Adams, C. M., & Hommer, D. (2003). A region of mesial prefrontal cortex tracks monetarily rewarding outcomes: Characterization with rapid event-related fMRI. *NeuroImage*, 18, 263–272.

Knutson, B., Rick, S., Wimmer, G. E., Prelec, D., & Loewenstein, G. (2007). Neural predictors of purchases. *Neuron*, 53, 147–156.

Kogut, T., & Ritov, I. (2005). The "identified victim" effect: An identified group, or just a single individual? *Journal of Behavioral Decision Making*, 18(3), 157–167.

Koopmans, T. C. (1960). Stationary ordinal utility and impatience. *Econometrica*, 28(2), 287–309.

Köszegi, B., & Rabin, M. (2006). A model of reference-dependent preferences. *Quarterly Journal of Economics*, 121(4), 1133–1165.

Kunreuther, H., Ginsberg, R., Miller, L., Sagi, P., Slovic, P., Borkan, B., et al. (1978). *Disaster insurance protection: Public policy lessons.* New York: Wiley.

Laibson, D. I. (1997). Golden eggs and hyperbolic dis-

counting. *Quarterly Journal of Economics*, 112(2), 443–477.

Lerner, J. S., & Keltner, D. (2001). Fear, anger, and risk. *Journal of Personality and Social Psychology*, 81(1), 146–159.

Lerner, J. S., Small, D. A., & Loewenstein, G. (2004). Heart strings and purse strings: Carryover effects of emotions on economic decisions. *Psychological Science*, 15(5), 337–341.

Loewenstein, G. (1987). Anticipation and the valuation of delayed consumption. *The Economic Journal*, 97(387), 666–684.

Loewenstein, G. (1996). Out of control: Visceral influences on behavior. *Organizational Behavior and Human Decision Processes*, 65(3), 272–292.

Loewenstein, G., & Adler, D. (1995). A bias in the prediction of tastes. *The Economic Journal*, 105(431), 929–937.

Loewenstein, G., & Lerner, J. (2003). The role of affect in decision making. In R. J. Dawson, K. R. Scherer, & H. H. Goldsmith (Eds.), *Handbook of affective science* (pp. 619–642). Oxford: Oxford University Pres.

Loewenstein, G., Nagin, D., & Paternoster, R. (1997). The effect of sexual arousal on predictions of sexual forcefulness. *Journal of Crime and Delinquency*, 34(4), 443–473.

Loewenstein, G., & O'Donoghue, T. (2004). *Animal spirits: Affective and deliberative processes in economic behavior.* Manuscript in preparation, Carnegie Mellon University.

Loewenstein, G., O'Donoghue, T., & Rabin, M. (2003). Projection bias in predicting future utility. *Quarterly Journal of Economics*, 118(4), 1209–1248.

Loewenstein, G., & Prelec, D. (1992). Anomalies in intertemporal choice. *Quarterly Journal of Economics*, 107(2), 573–597.

Loewenstein, G., & Small, D. A. (2007). The scarecrow and the tin man: The vicissitudes of human sympathy and caring. *Review of General Psychology*, 11, 112–126.

Loewenstein, G., Weber, E. U., Hsee, C. K., & Welch, N. (2001). Risk as feelings. *Psychological Bulletin*, 127(2), 267–286.

Loomes, G., & Sugden, R. (1982). Regret theory: An alternative theory of rational choice under uncertainty. *The Economic Journal*, 92(368), 805–824.

Loomes, G., & Sugden, R. (1986). Disappointment and dynamic consistency in choice under uncertainty. *Review of Economic Studies*, 53(2), 271–282.

Maia, T. V., & McClelland, J. L. (2004). A reexamination of the evidence for the somatic marker hypothesis: What participants really know in the Iowa gambling task. *Proceedings of the National Academy of Sciences USA*, 101(45), 16075–16080.

Markowitz, H. M. (1952). The utility of wealth. *Journal of Political Economy*, 60(2), 151–158.

McClure, S. M., Ericson, K. M., Laibson, D. I., Loewenstein, G., & Cohen, J. D. (2007). Time discounting for primary rewards. *Journal of Neuroscience*, 27(21), 5796–5804.

McClure, S. M., Laibson, D. I., Loewenstein, G., & Cohen J. D. (2004). Separate neural systems value immediate and delayed monetary rewards. *Science*, 306, 503–507.

Mellers, B. A., Schwartz, A., Ho, K., & Ritov, I. (1997). Decision affect theory: Emotional reactions to the outcomes of risky options. *Psychological Science*, 8(6), 423–429.

Mischel, W. (1974). Processes in delay of gratification. In L. Berkowitz (Ed.), *Advances in experimental social psychology* (Vol. 7). New York: Academic Press.

Pillutla, M. M., & Murnighan, J. K. (1996). Unfairness, anger, and spite: Emotional rejections of ultimatum offers. *Organizational Behavior and Human Decision Processes*, 68(3), 208–224.

Prelec, D., & Loewenstein, G. (1998). The red and the black: Mental accounting of savings and debt. *Marketing Science*, 17, 4–28.

Rabin, M. (1993). Incorporating fairness into game theory and economics. *American Economic Review*, 83, 1281–1302.

Rachlin, H., & Raineri, A. (1992). Irrationality, impulsiveness, and selfishness as discount reversal effects. In G. Loewenstein & J. Elster (Eds.), *Choice over time*. New York: Russell Sage Foundation.

Read, D., Loewenstein, G., & Kalyanaraman, S. (1999). Mixing virtue and vice: Combining the immediacy effect and the diversification heuristic. *Journal of Behavioral Decision Making*, 12(4), 257–273.

Rick, S. (2007). *The influence of anticipatory affect on consumer choice*. Unpublished doctoral dissertation, Department of Social and Decision Sciences, Carnegie Mellon University.

Rick, S., Cryder, C., & Loewenstein, G. (2008). Tightwads and spendthrifts. *Journal of Consumer Research*, 34.

Ross, L., Greene, D., & House, P. (1977). The false consensus effect: An egocentric bias in social perception and attribution processes. *Journal of Experimental Social Psychology*, 13(2), 279–301.

Rottenstreich, Y., & Hsee, C. K. (2001). Money, kisses, and electric shocks: On the affective psychology of risk. *Psychological Science*, 12(3), 185–190.

Samuelson, P. (1937). A note on measurement of utility. *Review of Economic Studies*, 4(2), 155–161.

Sanfey, A. G., Rilling, J. K., Aronson, J. A., Nystrom, L. E., & Cohen, J. D. (2003). The neural basis of economic decision-making in the ultimatum game. *Science*, 300, 1755–1758.

Schelling, T. C. (1968). The life you save may be your own. In S. B. Chase (Ed.), *Problems in public expenditure analysis*. Washington, DC: Brookings Institute.

Schkade, D., & Kahneman, D. (1998). Does living in California make people happy?: A focusing illusion in judgments of life satisfaction. *Psychological Science*, 9(6), 340–346.

Schwarz, N., & Clore, G. (1983). Moods, misattribution, and judgments of well-being: Informative and directive functions of affective states. *Journal of Personality and Social Psychology*, 45(3), 513–523.

Shiv, B., & Fedorikhin, A. (1999). Heart and mind in conflict: The interplay of affect and cognition in consumer decision making. *Journal of Consumer Research*, 26, 278–292.

Shiv, B., Loewenstein, G., Bechara, A., Damasio, H., & Damasio, A. R. (2005). Investment behavior and the negative side of emotion. *Psychological Science*, 16(6), 435–439.

Slovic, P., Fischhoff, B., & Lichtenstein, S. (1980). Facts and fears: Understanding perceived risk. In R. C. Schwing & W. A. Albers, Jr. (Eds.), *Societal risk assessment: How safe is safe enough?* San Francisco: Jossey-Bass.

Small, D. A., & Loewenstein, G. (2003). Helping 'a' victim or helping 'THE' victim: Altruism and identifiability. *Journal of Risk and Uncertainty*, 26(1), 5–16.

Small, D. A., & Loewenstein, G. (2005). The devil you know: The effects of identifiability on punishment. *Journal of Behavioral Decision Making*, 18(5), 311–318.

Smith, A. (1981). *The theory of moral sentiments* (D. D. Raphael & A. L. Macfie, Eds.). Indianapolis, IN: Liberty Fund. (Original work published 1759)

Smith, C. A., & Ellsworth, P. C. (1985). Patterns of cognitive appraisal in emotion. *Journal of Personality and Social Psychology*, 48(4), 813–838.

Sugden, R. (1986). Regret, recrimination, and rationality. In L. Daboni, A. Montesano, & M. Lines (Eds.), *Theory and decision library series: Vol. 47. Recent developments in the foundations of utility and risk theory*. Dordrecht, The Netherlands: Reidel.

Thaler, R. H. (1980). Toward a positive theory of consumer choice. *Journal of Economic Behavior and Organization*, 1(1), 39–60.

Thaler, R. H., & Shefrin, H. M. (1981). An economic theory of self-control. *Journal of Political Economy*, 89(2), 392–410.

Tiedens, L. Z., & Linton, S. (2001). Judgment under emotional certainty and uncertainty: The effects of specific emotions on information processing. *Journal of Personality and Social Psychology*, 81(6), 973–988.

Tversky, A., & Koehler, D. J. (1994). Support theory: A nonextensional representation of subjective probability. *Psychological Review*, 101(4), 547–567.

von Neumann, J., & Morgenstern, O. (1944). *Theory of games and economic behavior*. New York: Wiley.

Wicker, B., Keysers, C., Plailly, J., Royet, J-P., Gallese, V., & Rizzolatti, G. (2003). Both of us disgusted in my insula: The common neural basis of seeing and feeling disgust. *Neuron*, 40, 655–664.

Zeelenberg, M., & Beattie, J. (1997). Consequences of regret aversion: 2. Additional evidence for effects of feedback on decision making. *Organizational*

Behavior and Human Decision Processes, 72(1), 63–78.

Zeelenberg, M., Beattie, J. van der Plight, J., & De Vries, N. K. (1996). Consequences of regret aversion: Effects of expected feedback on risky decision making. *Organizational Behavior and Human Decision Processes*, 65(2), 148–158.

PART II

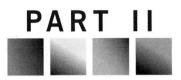

BIOLOGICAL AND NEUROPHYSIOLOGICAL APPROACHES

CHAPTER 10

Emotional Networks in the Brain

JOSEPH E. LEDOUX and ELIZABETH A. PHELPS

Contemporary neuroscientists have available a vast arsenal of tools for understanding brain functions, from the level of anatomical systems to the level of molecules. Localization of function at the anatomical level is the oldest but also the most basic approach. Until the function in question can be localized to a specific set of structures and their connections, application of cellular and molecular approaches is the neurobiological equivalent of a search for a needle in a haystack. Fortunately, considerable progress has been made in understanding the anatomical organization of one emotion, fear, and this chapter focuses on this work. Whereas most of the progress in the past came from studies of experimental animals, recent studies in humans, some capitalizing on new techniques for imaging the human brain, have confirmed and extended the animal work.

IN SEARCH OF
THE EMOTIONAL BRAIN

Our understanding of the brain mechanisms of emotion has changed radically over the past 120 years. In the late 19th century, William James (1884) suggested that emotion is a function of sensory and motor areas of the neocortex, and that the brain does not possess a special system devoted to emotional functions. This idea was laid low by studies showing that emotional reactions require the integrity of the hypothalamus (Cannon, 1929; Bard, 1929). On the basis of such observations, Papez (1937) proposed a circuit theory of emotion involving the hypothalamus, anterior thalamus, cingulate gyrus, and hippocampus. MacLean (1949, 1952) then named the structures of the Papez circuit, together with several additional regions (amygdala, septal nuclei, orbito-frontal cortex, portions of the basal ganglia), the "limbic system"; he viewed the limbic system as a general-purpose system involved in the mediation of functions required for the survival of the individual and the species.

MacLean's writings were very persuasive, and for many years the problem of relating emotion to brain mechanisms seemed solved at the level of anatomical systems. However, the limbic system concept came under fire beginning in the 1980s (see Brodal, 1982; Swanson,

1983; LeDoux, 1987, 1991; Kotter & Meyer, 1992). It is now believed that the concept suffers from imprecision at both the structural and functional levels. For example, it has proven impossible to provide unequivocal criteria for defining which structures and pathways should be included in the limbic system (Brodal, 1982; Swanson, 1983). A standard criterion, connectivity with the hypothalamus, extends the limbic system to include structures at all levels of the central nervous system, from the neocortex to the spinal cord. Furthermore, classic limbic areas, such as the hippocampus and mammillary bodies, have proven to be far more important for cognitive processes (such as declarative memory) than for emotional processes (e.g., Squire & Zola, 1996; Cohen & Eichenbaum, 1993).

Nevertheless, one limbic area that has been consistently implicated in emotional processes in a variety of situations is the amygdala (e.g., Weiskrantz, 1956; Gloor, 1960; Goddard, 1964; Mishkin & Aggleton, 1981; Aggleton & Mishkin, 1986; LeDoux, 1987, 1996; Rolls, 1986, 1992; Halgren, 1992; Aggleton, 1992; Davis, 1992; Kapp, Whalen, Supple, & Pascoe, 1992; Ono & Nishijo, 1992; Damasio, 1994; Everitt & Robbins, 1992; McGaugh et al., 1995). Interestingly, the amygdala was not part of the Papez circuit model and was clearly a second-class citizen, relative to the hippocampus at least, in the limbic system hypothesis. However, the survival of the limbic system hypothesis for so long is in part due to the inclusion of the amygdala (LeDoux, 1992). Otherwise, the relation between emotional functions and classic limbic areas would have been far less prominent over the years.

THE AMYGDALA
AS AN EMOTIONAL COMPUTER

The contribution of the amygdala to emotion emerged from studies of the Kluver–Bucy syndrome, a complex set of behavioral changes brought about by damage to the temporal lobe in primates (Kluver & Bucy, 1937). Following such lesions, animals lose their fear of previously threatening stimuli, attempt to copulate with members of other species, and attempt to eat a variety of things that "normal" primates find unattractive (feces, meat, rocks). Studies by Weiskrantz (1956) then determined that lesions confined to the amygdala and sparing

other temporal lobe structures produce the emotional components of the syndrome. Weiskrantz proposed that amygdala lesions interfere with the ability to determine the motivational significance of stimuli. A host of subsequent studies have shown that the amygdala is a key structure in the assignment of reward value to stimuli (Jones & Mishkin, 1972; Spiegler & Mishkin, 1981; Gaffan & Harrison, 1987; Gaffan, Gaffan, & Harrison, 1988; Everitt & Robbins, 1992; Ono & Nishijo, 1992; Rolls, 1992), in the conditioning of fear to novel stimuli (Blanchard & Blanchard, 1972; Kapp et al., 1992; Davis, 1992, 1994; LeDoux, 1996; Maren & Fanselow, 1996), in the self-administration of rewarding brain stimulation (Kane, Coulombe, & Miliaressis, 1991; Olds, 1977), and in the elicitation by brain stimulation of a host of behavioral and autonomic responses typical of emotional reactions (Hilton & Zbrozyna, 1963; Fernandez de Molina & Hunsperger, 1962; Kapp, Pascoe, & Bixler, 1984; Iwata, Chida, & LeDoux, 1987). These and other findings have led a number of authors to conclude that the amygdala plays an important role in the assignment of affective significance to sensory events. As important as the various studies described above have been in establishing that the amygdala plays a role in emotional processes, most of the studies were done with little appreciation for the anatomical organization of the amygdala. It is generally believed that there are at least a dozen different nuclei, and that each has several subdivisions, each with its own set of unique connections (e.g., Pitkänen, Savander, & LeDoux, 1997). If we are to understand how the amygdala participates in computation of emotional significance, we need to take these distinctions into account.

NEURAL PATHWAYS INVOLVED
IN FEAR PROCESSING

Much of our understanding of the role of different regions of the amygdala in emotional processes has come from studies of fear conditioning, where an auditory stimulus, a conditioned stimulus (CS), is paired with footshock, the unconditioned stimulus (US) (Figure 10.1). The reason this task has been so successful in mapping the pathways is, in large part, the simplicity of the task itself. It involves a discrete, well-defined CS and stereotyped autonomic

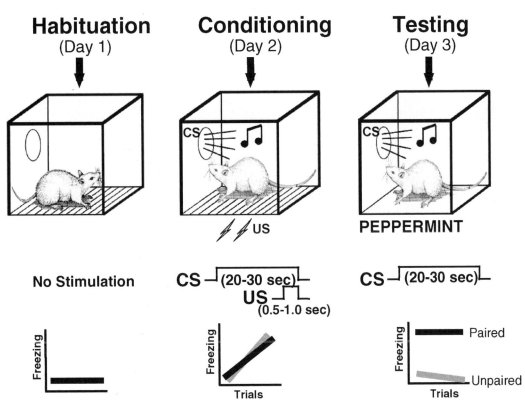

FIGURE 10.1. Fear conditioning. Fear conditioning occurs in three phases. In habituation, the rat is acclimated to the chamber. No stimuli are presented. During conditioning, the tone conditioned stimulus (CS) is paired with the footshock unconditioned stimulus (US). Testing then involves presentation of the CS without the US the next day. Typically, the rat exhibits freezing responses to the CS during the test. If the rat received unpaired presentations of the CS and US during conditioning, it freezes little to the CS, indicating that it did not come to associate the CS with the US.

and behavioral conditioned responses (CRs). These two features—a well-defined stimulus and stereotyped responses—are very helpful when trying to relate brain function to brain structure. Also, fear conditioning can and has been used similarly in animal and human studies, which has allowed the establishment of commonalities in the underlying brain systems. Fear conditioning may not be able to tell us everything we need to know about emotions and the brain, or even about fear and the brain, but it has been an excellent starting point.

Basic Circuits

The pathways involved in conditioning of fear responses to a single-tone CS are shown in Figure 10.2. The CS is transmitted through the auditory system to the auditory thalamus, including the subregions of the medial geniculate body (MGB) and adjacent regions of the posterior thalamus (LeDoux, Sakaguchi, & Reis, 1984; LeDoux, Ruggiero, & Reis, 1985; LeDoux, Farb, & Ruggiero, 1990). The signal is then transmitted from all regions of the auditory thalamus to the auditory cortex, and from a subset of thalamic nuclei to the amygdala. The thalamo-amygdala pathway originates primarily in the medial division of the MGB and the associated posterior intralaminar nucleus (LeDoux, Cicchetti, Xagoraris, & Romanski, 1990). The auditory association cortex also gives rise to a projection to the amygdala (Romanski & LeDoux, 1993; Mascagni, McDonald, & Coleman, 1993). Both the thalamo-amygdala and thalamo-cortico-amygdala pathways terminate in the sensory input region of the amygdala, the lateral nucleus (LA) (see Turner & Herkenham, 1991; LeDoux, Cicchetti, et al., 1990; Romanski & LeDoux,

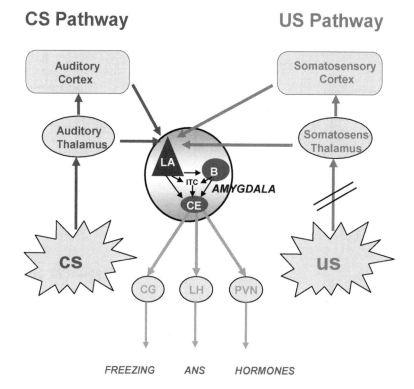

FIGURE 10.2. Neural circuit of fear conditioning. Fear conditioning occurs in the brain via the modification of the processing of the auditory CS by the somatosensory US. As shown, the CS and US converge in the lateral amygdala (LA), which receives CS and US inputs from both thalamic and cortical areas. The LA then communicates with the central amygdala (CE) both directly and by way of other amygdala areas, including the basal nucleus (B) and the intercalated masses (ITC). The CE connects with brainstem and hypothalamic areas that control the expression of fear responses, including freezing behavior (mediated by the central gray, CG), autonomic nervous system (ANS) responses (mediated by the lateral hypothalamus, LH), and hormonal responses (mediated by the paraventricular hypothalamus).

1993; Mascagni et al., 1993). In fact, the two pathways converge onto single neurons in LA (Li, Stutzman, & LeDoux, 1996). Damage to LA interferes with fear conditioning (LeDoux, Cicchetti, et al., 1990), which can be mediated by either the thalamo-amygdala or thalamo-cortico-amygdala pathways (for discussions, see Romanski & LeDoux, 1993; Campeau & Davis, 1995; Corodimas & LeDoux, 1995). Temporary inactivation of LA and the adjacent basal nucleus (Helmstetter & Bellgowan, 1994; Muller, Corodimas, Fridel, & LeDoux, 1997; Wilensky, Schafe, & LeDoux, 1999, 2000), or pharmacological blockade of excitatory amino acid receptors in this region (Miserendino, Sananes, Melia, & Davis, 1990; Kim & Fanselow, 1992; Maren & Fanselow, 1996; Gewirtz & Davis, 1997; Rodrigues, Schafe, & LeDoux, 2004), also disrupts the acquisition of conditioned fear, and facilitation of excitatory amino acid transmission enhances the rate of fear learning (Rogan, Staubli, & LeDoux, 1997). A host of intracellular signaling cascades downstream of excitatory amino acid transmission have been implicated in fear conditioning as well (for a review, see Rodrigues et al., 2004).

Although the auditory cortex is not required for the acquisition of conditioned fear to a simple auditory stimulus (Romanski & LeDoux, 1992; Armony, Servan-Schreiber, Romanski, Cohen, & LeDoux, 1997), processing of the CS by cells in the auditory cortex is modified as a result of its pairing with the US (Weinberger, 1995; Quirk, Armony, & LeDoux, 1997). In situations involving more complex stimuli that must be discriminated, recognized, and/or categorized, the auditory cortex may be critical for aversive learning (e.g., Cranford & Igarashi, 1977; Whitfield, 1980) and may provide an important set of inputs to the amygdala.

What are the advantages of the parallel processing capabilities of this system? First, the existence of a subcortical pathway allows the amygdala to detect threatening stimuli in the environment quickly, in the absence of a complete and time-consuming analysis of the stimulus. This "quick and dirty" processing route may confer an evolutionary advantage to the species. Second, the rapid subcortical pathway may function to "prime" the amygdala to evaluate subsequent information received along the cortical pathway (LeDoux, 1986a, 1986b; Li et al., 1996). For example, a loud noise may be sufficient to alert the amygdala at the cellular level to prepare to respond to a dangerous predator lurking nearby, but defensive reactions may not be fully mobilized until the auditory cortex analyzes the location, frequency, and intensity of the noise, to determine specifically the nature and extent of this potentially threatening auditory signal. The convergence of the subcortical and cortical pathways onto single neurons in the LA (Li et al., 1996) provides a means by which the integration can take place. Third, computational modeling studies show that the subcortical pathway can function as an interrupting device that enables the cortex, by way of amygdalo-cortical projections, to shift attention to dangerous stimuli that occur outside the focus of attention (Armony, Servan-Schreiber, Cohen, & LeDoux, 1996). Modeling studies have also emphasized the evolutionary advantages of the dual-route hypothesis (den Dulk, Heerebout, & Phaf, 2003).

As noted, sensory information from both the thalamus and the cortex enters the amygdala through the LA. Information processed by the LA is then transmitted via intra-amygdala connections (Pitkänen et al., 1997; Pare & Smith, 1998) to the basal and accessory basal nuclei, where it is integrated with other incoming information from other areas and further transmitted to the central nucleus. The central nucleus is the main output system of the amygdala (LeDoux, 1996; Davis, 1992; LeDoux, Iwata, Cicchetti, & Reis, 1988; Carrive, Lee, & Su, 2000; Fendt & Fanselow, 1999; Davis & Whalen, 2001). Damage to the central amygdala or structures that project to it interferes with the acquisition and expression of all CRs, whereas lesions of areas to which

the central amygdala projects interfere with individual responses, such as blood pressure changes, freezing behavior, or hormone release.

With the neural circuits underlying fear conditioning well understood, studies have turned to the molecular mechanisms that make emotional learning possible. These mechanisms (Figure 10.3) are understood in great detail, allowing novel approaches to the treatment of fear-related disorders.

Contextualization of Fear

Whether a stimulus signals danger, and thus elicits fear reactions, often depends on the situation (context) in which it occurs. For example, the sight of a bear in the zoo poses little threat, but the same bear seen while we are on a walk in the woods will probably make us run away in fear. Furthermore, contexts may themselves

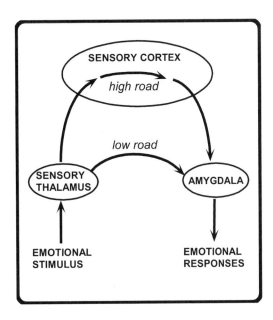

FIGURE 10.3. High road and low road to the amygdala. The amygdala receives inputs from sensory processing regions in the thalamus and cortex. The thalamic pathway, the low road, provides a rapid but crude representation, while the cortical pathway provides slower but more elaborate representation. The low-road inputs are thought to initiate amygdala processing, and the cortical inputs build upon this initial processing. Both pathways in all likelihood process emotional stimuli unconsciously, with conscious awareness of the stimulus requiring prefrontal areas (see Figure 10.4).

acquire aversive value through prior experiences. If we are mugged, we are very likely to feel "uneasy" when we return to the scene of the crime. The relationship between environmental situations and fear responses can been investigated in the laboratory through contextual fear conditioning: When a rat is conditioned to expect a footshock in the presence of a tone CS, it will also exhibit fear reactions to the chamber where the conditioning took place, even in the absence of the CS (Kim & Fanselow, 1992; Phillips & LeDoux, 1992). Several studies have shown that the formation and consolidation of contextual fear associations depend on the hippocampus. Lesions of the hippocampus made prior to training interfere with the acquisition of CRs to the context, without having any effect on the conditioning to the CS (Maren, Anagnostaras, & Fanselow, 1998; Frankland, Cestari, Filipkowski, McDonald, & Silva, 1998; Phillips & LeDoux, 1992, 1994; Selden, Everitt, Jarrard, & Robbins, 1991). Furthermore, hippocampal lesions made after training interfere with the consolidation and retention of contextual fear associations (Kim & Fanselow, 1992). Bidirectional projections between the hippocampal formation and the amygdala (Amaral, Price, Pitkänen, & Carmichael, 1992; Canteras & Swanson, 1992; Ottersen, 1982) provide anatomical channels through which the attachment of emotional value to context may take place. The fibers from the hippocampus to the amygdala terminate extensively in the basal and accessory basal nuclei, and to a much lesser extent in the LA, suggesting why lesions of the LA have little effect on context conditioning, but lesions of the basal nucleus and/or accessory basal nucleus seem to be disruptive (Maren, Aharonov, Stote, & Fanselow, 1996; Majidishad, Pelli, & LeDoux, 1996). The role of the hippocampus in the evaluation of contextual cues in fear conditioning is consistent with current theories of spatial, configural, and/or relational processing in the hippocampus (Cohen & Eichenbaum, 1993; O'Keefe & Nadel, 1978; Sutherland & Rudy, 1989; Rudy, Huff, & Matus-Amat, 2004).

Getting Rid of Fear

Fear responses tend to be very persistent. This has obvious survival advantages, as it allows us to keep a record of previously encountered threatening experiences, and thus allows us to respond quickly to similar situations in the future. Nonetheless, it is also important to be able to learn that a stimulus no longer signals danger. Otherwise, unnecessary fear responses will be elicited by innocuous stimuli and may potentially become liabilities, interfering with other important routine tasks. In humans, the inability to inhibit unwarranted fear responses can have devastating consequences, as observed in phobias, posttraumatic stress disorder, generalized anxiety disorder, and other anxiety disorders. In laboratory experiments, learned fear responses can be reduced (extinguished) by repeatedly presenting the CS without the US. It is important to note, however, that extinction of conditioned fear responses is not a passive forgetting of the CS–US association, but an active process, often involving a new learning (Bouton & Swartzentruber, 1991). In fact, CS-elicited responses can be spontaneously reinstated following an unrelated traumatic experience (Pavlov, 1927/1960; Jacobs & Nadel, 1985; Rescorla & Heth, 1975).

Experimental observations in fear conditioning studies suggest that neocortical areas, particularly areas of the medial prefrontal cortex, are involved in the extinction process. Lesions of the medial prefrontal cortex lead to a potentiation of fear responses and a retardation of the extinction (Morgan, Romanski, & LeDoux, 1993; Morgan & LeDoux, 1995; Quirk, Russo, Barron, & Lebron, 2000; Milad & Quirk, 2002; Quirk, Garcia, & Gonzalez-Lima, 2006; but see Gewirtz & Davis, 1997). These findings complement electrophysiological studies showing that neurons within the orbito-frontal cortex are particularly sensitive to changes in stimulus–reward associations (Thorpe, Rolls, & Maddison, 1983; Rolls, 1999). Lesions of sensory areas of the cortex also retard extinction (LeDoux, Romanski, & Xagoraris, 1989; Teich et al., 1989), and neurons in auditory cortex exhibit extinction resistant changes to an auditory CS (Quirk et al., 1997). Thus the medial prefrontal cortex, possibly in conjunction with other neocortical regions, may be involved in regulating amygdala responses to stimuli based on their current affective value. These findings suggest that fear disorders may be related to a malfunction of the prefrontal cortex that makes it difficult for patients to extinguish fears they have acquired (Morgan et al., 1993; Morgan & LeDoux, 1995; LeDoux, 1996). Imaging studies in humans have confirmed the role of medial prefrontal cortex in extinction and other aspects of fear regulation, as described below.

Stress has deleterious effects on medial prefrontal cortex (Radley et al., 2006; Radley & Morrison, 2005) and also can have effects similar to lesions of the medial prefrontal cortex—that is, potentiation of fear responses (Corodimas, LeDoux, Gold, & Schulkin, 1994; Conrad, Margarinos, LeDoux, & McEwen, 1997; Shors, 2006). Given that stress is a common occurrence in psychiatric patients, and that such patients often have functional changes in the prefrontal cortex (Drevets et al., 1997; Bremner et al., 1995), it is possible that the exaggeration of fear in anxiety disorders results from stress-induced alterations in the medial prefrontal region.

Emotional Action

The defensive responses we have considered so far are hard-wired reactions to danger signals. These are evolution's gifts to us; they provide a first line of defense against danger. Some animals rely mainly on these. But mammals, especially we humans, can do much more. We are able to take charge. Once we find ourselves in a dangerous situation, we can think, plan, and make decisions. We make the transition from reaction to action. Considerably less is understood about the brain mechanisms of emotional action than reaction, due in part to the fact that emotional actions come in many varieties and are limited only by the ingenuity of the actor. For example, once we are freezing and expressing physiological responses to a dangerous stimulus, the rest is up to us. On the basis of our expectations about what is likely to happen next and our past experiences in similar situations, we make a plan about what to do. We become instruments of action. Instrumental responses in situations of danger are often studied by using avoidance conditioning procedures.

Avoidance is a multistage learning process (Mowrer & Lamoreaux, 1946). First, fear CRs are acquired. Then the CS becomes a signal that is used to initiate responses that prevent encounters with the US. Finally, once avoidance responses are learned, animals no longer show the characteristic signs of fear (Rescorla & Solomon, 1967). They know what to do to avoid the danger, and simply perform the response in a habitual way. Consistent with this

is the fact that the amygdala is required for avoidance learning (for the fear conditioning part), but not for the expression of well-trained avoidance responses (the instrumental part) (Parent, Tomaz, & McGaugh, 1992). The involvement of an instrumental component to some aversive learning tasks may explain why these are not dependent on the amygdala for long-term storage (Packard, Williams, Cahill, & McGaugh, 1995; McGaugh et al., 1995). Because avoidance learning involves fear conditioning, at least initially, it will be subject to all the factors that influence fear conditioning and conditioned fear responding. However, because avoidance learning involves more than simple fear conditioning, it is to be expected that avoidance will be subject to influences that have little or no effect on conditioned fear. Much more work is needed to understand how fear and avoidance interact, and thus how emotional actions emerge out of emotional reactions. From what we know so far, it appears that, as in other habit systems (Mishkin, Malamut, & Bachevalier, 1984), interactions among the amygdala, basal ganglia, and neocortex are important in avoidance (Everitt & Robbins, 1992; Gray, 1987; Killcross, Robbins, & Everitt, 1997).

The neural basis of emotional actions has recently been studied using a paradigm called "escape from fear" (Amorapanth, LeDoux, & Nader, 2000). In this paradigm, rats first undergo fear conditioning. They are then placed in a new context and exposed to the CS. Although they initially freeze, at some point they move. When they move, the tone is terminated. Through careful shaping, behaviors that terminate the tone can be established as habits, which are learned because removal of the tone is a negative secondary reinforcer. Damage to the lateral or central amygdala, but not the basal amygdala, prevents learning in the first phase (fear conditioning); damage to the lateral or the basal, but not the central, amygdala prevents learning of the escape-from-fear component. The transition from fear reaction to action thus requires that information processing in the amygdala be diverted from the reaction pathway (lateral to central amygdala) to the action pathway (lateral to basal amygdala) (LeDoux & Gorman, 2001).

The action circuits may be the means through which emotional behaviors that are performed initially as voluntary responses are then converted into habits. Emotional habits can be useful, but can also be quite detrimental. Successful avoidance is known to prevent extinction of conditioned fear, since the opportunity to experience the CS in the absence of the US is eliminated by the avoidance. In real life, this can perpetuate anxiety states. The patient with panic disorder and agoraphobia who never leaves home as a means of avoiding having a panic attack is but one example.

Emotional Influences on Cognition

Emotions influence cognitive processing in a number of ways. The amygdala receives inputs from the sensory processing in the cortex for each modality, and projects to these as well (Amaral et al., 1992; McDonald, 1998). The projections to the amygdala allow it to detect the presence of danger, while the amygdala's projections to the cortex, which are widespread and reach the initial stages of sensory processing, allow the amygdala to influence cortical processing very early in an emotional episode. Thus, once the amygdala is activated by a sensory event, it can begin to regulate the cortical areas that project to it, controlling the kinds of inputs that these areas subsequently send to the amygdala. Through such connections, emotions can have direct influences on attention and perception (see human studies below).

The amygdala also projects (directly or indirectly) to various modulatory networks, including the cholinergic systems in the basal forebrain and brainstem, and the dopaminergic and noradrenergic systems that innervate widespread areas of the cortex. For example, Weinberger and colleagues found that the processing of auditory signals—specifically, the regulation of auditory cortex during fear conditioning—is modulated by cholinergic modulation (see Weinberger, 1995). They proposed that the amygdala plays an important role in activating the cholinergic system, which then modulates cortical arousal and conditioning. Experimental studies have shown that this may occur. Kapp et al. (1992), for example, found that stimulation of the amygdala can change cortical arousal (as measured by electroencephalographic patterns), and that cholinergic blockade prevents this. Furthermore, during the presentation of a CS, cells in the auditory cortex become very active at the time just preceding the occurrence of the US, and lesions of the amygdala prevent this anticipatory response (Quirk et al., 1997; Armony,

Quirk, & LeDoux, 1998). Through projections to the cortex, either directly (see Amaral et al., 1992) or by way of the cholinergic system, the amygdala may direct attentional resources toward environmental stimuli that are eliciting amygdala activity. Thus, once the amygdala detects danger, it can influence sensory and cognitive processing in the cortex by activating these modulatory systems.

The amygdala is also involved in triggering the release of so-called "stress hormones," including epinephrine (adrenaline) and glucocorticoids, from the adrenal gland. The glucocorticoids circulate to the brain, where they bind to specific receptors in the hippocampus, medial prefrontal cortex, other cortical areas, and amygdala. Epinephrine does not enter the brain directly from the bloodstream, but studies by McGaugh and colleagues suggest that it nevertheless influences areas in the brain by changing the activity of the vagus nerve, which then, through several relays in the brain, affects the amygdala and other areas (see McGaugh et al., 1995; Cahill & McGaugh, 1998; McGaugh, 2004). Their work in both animals and humans suggests that peripheral hormones, such as glucocorticoids and epinephrine, can modulate the strength of memories (especially conscious or declarative memories) formed in other brain regions (especially the hippocampus and neocortex), as discussed below when we consider human studies. In brief, intermediate levels of these hormones tend to facilitate declarative memory for events, whereas high levels tend to impair it. This may account for why emotional arousal sometimes leads to an enhancement of memory and sometimes a memory impairment for an event. Glucocorticoids are particularly interesting for their contrasting effects on the amygdala and hippocampus. These hormones are released when the amygdala detects dangerous or otherwise threatening events. When they reach the brain, they inhibit hippocampus-dependent processes (e.g., spatial memory), but enhance amygdala-dependent processes (e.g., fear conditioning) (Corodimas et al., 1994; Conrad, Margarinos, et al., 1997; Conrad, Lupien, Thanosoulis, & McEwen, 1997; Kim & Diamond, 2002). Given that conscious or declarative memory is one of the prime functions of the hippocampus (Squire & Zola, 1996; Cohen & Eichenbaum, 1993), we may conclude that during periods of intense stress the brain's ability to form conscious memories is impaired, but its ability to form unconscious emotional memories is potentiated. This observation has important implications for understanding such processes as memory loss during trauma and stress, and may account for memory disturbances in patients with depression and posttraumatic stress disorder.

EMOTIONAL SYSTEMS IN THE HUMAN BRAIN

Investigations of emotion in the human brain have used animal models of fear learning as a starting point. Findings from studies of amygdala-damaged patients and from functional neuroimaging have demonstrated the importance of the amygdala in fear conditioning (Bechara et al., 1995; LaBar, LeDoux, Spencer, & Phelps, 1995; Buchel, Morris, Dolan, & Friston, 1998; LaBar, Gatenby, Gore, LeDoux, & Phelps, 1998). Furthermore, the hippocampus in humans, as in other animals (see above), plays a key role in the expression of conditioned fear modulated by the learning context (LaBar & Phelps, 2005). In addition, the medial prefrontal cortex has been implicated in fear regulation in both humans and other animals (Phelps, Delgado, Nearing, & LeDoux, 2004). The existing evidence suggests that the neural mechanisms of fear conditioning are preserved across species, although it is difficult to study the unique contribution of different subnuclei of the amygdala in humans.

Fear Acquisition

The similarities in the neural circuitry of fear conditioning among different species provide some assurance when we are speculating about human function on the basis of this animal model. However, fear learning can be significantly more complex than simple fear conditioning. In particular, humans and other primates have developed social means of acquiring fears, which permit learning about the potential aversive properties of stimuli in the environment without necessarily having to experience an aversive event directly.

For example, one can learn that a neutral stimulus, such as a blue square, predicts a potentially painful shock because the blue square was paired with the delivery of a shock. This is an example of simple fear conditioning. However, one could also learn that the blue square predicts a potential shock by being told about this relationship. In this case, the emotional properties of the blue square are communicated symbolically, through language. This type of instructed fear has been shown to lead to fear reactions to a neutral stimulus that predicts a potentially aversive event (i.e., the "threat" stimulus) comparable to those observed with fear conditioning (Hugdahl & Öhman, 1977). In addition, one could learn about the potential aversive properties of stimuli in the environment by watching others. If a conspecific receives a shock that is paired with a blue square, this could lead to a fear response to the blue square when it is presented in a similar context to the observer. This type of observational fear learning has been shown to be effective in producing robust learned fear responses in both human and nonhuman primates (Öhman & Mineka, 2001). These social means of fear learning, instruction and observation, allow us to acquire information about the potential aversive properties of stimuli in the environment without having to undergo physically painful experiences. They can result in fears that are imagined and anticipated, but never experienced; these may account for a significant portion of human fear learning. The questions remains: Do socially acquired fears rely on the same neural circuitry as fear conditioning?

Instructed fear results in a symbolic representation of the emotional properties of a stimulus. The acquisition of this cognitive representation probably does not rely on the amygdala. Patients with amygdala damage, whose hippocampus is intact, can verbally report these types of stimulus contingencies (e.g., a blue square predicts a shock), even when they fail to show physiological evidence of conditioned fear (Bechara et al., 1995; LaBar et al., 1995). On the other hand, patients with hippocampal damage, whose amygdalas are intact, show the opposite pattern—a normal CR, but an inability to report the stimulus contingencies verbally (Bechara et al., 1995). These findings suggest that the retention of an abstract, cognitive representation of fear may depend on the hippocampus. Nevertheless, damage to the left amygdala impairs the physiological expression of instructed fear (Funayama, Grillon, Davis, & Phelps, 2001), and functional magnetic resonance imaging (fMRI) shows enhanced activation in the left amygdala to a "threat" stimulus, relative to one that is instructed to be "safe"

(Phelps et al., 2001). Unlike fear conditioning, where both the right and left amygdala seem to be important (LaBar et al., 1995; LaBar & LeDoux, 1996), instructed fear depends primarily on the left amygdala, perhaps reflecting the linguistic nature of the representation. In instructed fear, it is likely that a symbolic communication system (namely, language) is necessary for acquisition, that the hippocampal memory system underlies the retention of this representation, and that the amygdala mediates the physiological expression of this learning. Although humans and other primates may have developed unique social means of communicating fears, the expression of these fears may take advantage of the phylogenetically shared mechanisms underlying fear conditioning.

Learning through social observation also depends on the amygdala. A recent fMRI study (Olsson & Phelps, 2007) found equally robust activation of the bilateral amygdala both when a participant observed a conspecific receiving a shock paired with a blue square, and when the observer was also presented with a blue square in a similar context. The enhanced blood-oxygenation-level-dependent (BOLD) signal in the amygdala during observation of a conspecific in a fear conditioning paradigm occurred primarily in response to watching the conspecific receive a shock, whereas the amygdala showed an anticipatory BOLD response to the blue square when the observer believed he or she might also receive a shock. In this study, the only knowledge of the contingency between the colored square and shock was through social observation. These results suggest that learning fears by observing others recruits the amygdala to a similar degree as fear conditioning does. It may be that observing others receive an aversive stimulus is aversive to the observer as well, and may act as a US. Participants in this study showed a physiological arousal response both when they watched a conspecific receive a shock and when they believed they might receive a shock themselves. In this way, observational fear learning may be more similar to fear conditioning than learning by instruction. Consistent with this interpretation, observational fear and fear conditioning are both expressed when the CS is presented subliminally without awareness. In contrast, instructed fear learning, which depends on a symbolic representation of the stimulus contingencies, requires awareness for expression

(Olsson & Phelps, 2004). Functional imaging results showing amygdala activation in fear conditioning, instructed fear, and observational fear learning are shown in Pate 10.1 (see color insert).

In summary, the neural mechanisms of fear acquisition and expression are similar across species. Humans and can acquire fears through social means, including instruction and observation. Other primates also have the capacity for observational fear learning. Although the amygdala may only be necessary for the acquisition of some types of socially acquired fears, the amygdala plays a critical role in the physiological expression of fears acquired through fear conditioning, verbal instruction, or social observation. Although social learning in primates may be especially well developed, other species do engage in social learning. For example, rodents use olfactory cues and birds use auditory cues in social learning.

Fear Regulation

Humans also have a range of means to reduce fears once they are established. As in other animals, acquired fears can be diminished through extinction, in which the CS is no longer paired with the aversive US and the expression of the conditioned fear eventually diminishes. As mentioned earlier, animal models of extinction learning indicate that the medial prefrontal cortex, particularly the infralimbic cortex, may be critically involved in extinction. Recent fMRI studies have shown involvement of this region during extinction in humans (Plate 10.2; see color insert). Similar to electrophysiological data from rats (Milad & Quirk, 2002), BOLD responses in the medial prefrontal cortex increase as extinction training progresses (Knight, Smith, Cheng, Stein, & Helmstetter, 2004; Phelps et al., 2004). This increase in BOLD in the medial prefrontal cortex predicts the amount of extinction that has occurred when assessed after a delay and is inversely correlated with the responses in the amygdala (Phelps et al., 2004). A recent anatomical MRI study demonstrated that the relative cortical size of this region predicts the rate of extinction learning across individuals (Milad et al., 2005). Although it is difficult to specify the precise role of the medial prefrontal cortex in extinction learning by using correlational human neuroimaging techniques, the similarities with animal models suggest that this region might be inhibiting the amygdala response. As mentioned earlier, given this importance of the medial prefrontal cortex in extinction, it is possible that dysfunction of this region may underlie some fear-related clinical disorders (Rauch, Shin, & Phelps, 2006).

Of course, we humans do not have to expose ourselves repeatedly to a fear-inducing stimulus to diminish a fear response. We can do the same thing with our minds. Our ability to control and regulate our emotions is critical in normal social behavior and adaptive function. Recent studies of emotion regulation have explored the neural mechanisms underlying the use of cognitive strategies to alter fear responses (e.g., Ochsner, Bunge, Gross, & Gabrieli, 2002; Beauregard, Levesque, & Bourgouin, 2001). These studies, which often use stimuli such as negative, arousing scenes, have shown that the successful use of a strategy to control an emotional response results in a decrease in BOLD signal in the amygdala and an increase in regions of the dorsolateral prefrontal cortex. The dorsolateral prefrontal cortex is a region that is anatomically rather different across species. It may be unique to primates (Preuss & Goldman-Rakic, 1991), and it is thought to underlie higher cognitive functions, such as executive control (Smith & Jonides, 1999). However, this region has few direct projections to the amygdala (McDonald, Mascagni, & Guo, 1996; Stefanacci & Amaral, 2002). As a result, any influence it may have on the amygdala is likely to be mediated by its connections with more ventral and medial regions of the prefrontal cortex. Many studies examining the emotion regulation of scenes also report increased BOLD responses in the medial prefrontal cortex when a negative emotional response is diminished through a cognitive strategy (e.g., Beauregard et al., 2001; Urry et al., 2006)

In order to explore whether the medial prefrontal cortex mediates the influence of the dorsolateral prefrontal cortex on the amygdala when humans are using a cognitive strategy to control fears, a recent study examined the regulation of conditioned fear and its relation to fear extinction (Delgado et al., 2004). Much like extinction training, the use of a cognitive strategy can diminish the physiological expression of conditioned fear. Like extinction training, the regulation of conditioned fear resulted in an increase in BOLD signal in the infralimbic region of the medial prefrontal cortex and a correlated decrease in the amygdala response. Much as in other studies of emotion regulation (e.g., Ochsner et al., 2002), the regulation of conditioned fear resulted in increased BOLD signal in the dorsolateral prefrontal cortex. This increase was more strongly correlated with the responses in the medial prefrontal cortex than the amygdala, indicating that the medial prefrontal cortex may be mediating any influence of the dorsolateral prefrontal cortex and of executive processes on the amygdala and the physiological expression of fear.

These findings suggest that much as in the case of fear acquisition, humans may have developed unique cognitive means for controlling fear responses, but probably did not develop unique neural mechanisms for controlling fears. The use of complex cognitive strategies to control fears may take advantage of phylogenetically shared mechanisms of fear extinction. As mentioned earlier, the medial prefrontal cortex may play a general role in regulating and inhibiting the amygdala response across a range of paradigms and techniques.

Emotional Influence on Perception, Attention, and Memory

Studies of the amygdala in animal models have generally focused on its role in fear conditioning. However, studies in humans have also highlighted a role for the amygdala in mediating emotion's influence on a range of social and cognitive functions.

For example, studies of the perception of facial expression in others have shown that the amygdala is critically involved in the normal perception of fear expressions. Patients with bilateral amygdala damage consistently have difficulty indicating the intensity of fear expressions (Adolphs et al., 1999), and findings from functional neuroimaging demonstrate that fearful faces result in stronger activation of the amygdala than faces with other expressions do (Whalen et al., 1998). Two recent studies have specified the component of fearful faces that may engage the amygdala. Using fMRI, the first study demonstrated that presenting the eyes of fearful versus happy faces results in robust activation of the amygdala (Whalen et al., 2004). Consistent with this correlational evidence suggesting the importance of the eyes in detecting fear expressions, Adolphs et al. (2005) recently demonstrated that patients with amygdala damage fail to focus on the eyes as much as non-brain-damaged control subjects do when viewing fearful faces. Interestingly, if amygdala-damaged patients are instructed to focus on the eyes of a face, their ratings for the intensity of the fear expression are normal. This only occurs, however, when the patients are instructed to focus on the eyes, whereas the control subjects do this spontaneously. This finding suggests that the amygdala may be mediating attentional behaviors that enable the perception of fear from facial expression. In addition to the perception of fear from facial expressions, the amygdala has been shown to be involved in the perception of fear from bodily expressions (de Gelder, Snyder, Greve, Gerard, & Hadjikhani, 2004); the ability to determine trustworthiness from face stimuli (Adolphs, Tranel, & Damasio, 1998; Winston, Strange, O'Doherty, & Dolan, 2002); the response to faces from other races (Phelps et al., 2001); and the ability to attribute social, motivational signals to nonsocial stimuli (Heberlein & Adolphs, 2004). These findings indicate that the amygdala may play a complex role in the perception of a range of social signals.

The amygdala has also been shown be important in mediating emotion's influence on a number of cognitive functions, most notably attention and memory. Emotion influences attention by enhancing the perception of emotional events. This was first described by Cherry (1953) as the "cocktail party effect," in which an emotionally salient stimulus, such as one's name, breaks through a limited attentional bottleneck to reach awareness and receive priority in stimulus processing. More recently, the facilitation of attention with emotion was demonstrated by using the attentional blink paradigm, which examines the temporal limitations of attention (Raymond, Shapiro, & Arnell, 1992). In this task, when two target stimuli are presented in a short temporal window, the ability to identify the second target is diminished. However, if the second target is an arousing stimulus, such as a dirty word, it is much more likely to be correctly identified (Anderson, 2005). Patients with amygdala damage fail to show this attenuation of attentional blink effect with emotion, suggesting that the amygdala is critically mediating emotion's facilitation of attention (Anderson & Phelps, 2001).

Findings from functional neuroimaging suggest that one mechanism by which emotion can influence attention is through the modulation of visual processing regions (Plate 10.3; see color insert). The enhanced amygdala activation observed to fearful versus neutral faces is correlated with a similar enhancement in visual cortex (Morris et al., 1998). This enhanced activation for fearful versus neutral expressions in the visual cortex is diminished if there is damage to the amygdala (Vuilleumier, Richardson, Armony, Driver, & Dolan, 2004). These findings suggest a model by which the amygdala receives information about the emotional significance of a stimulus early in stimulus processing, and then modulates further perceptual processing through its reciprocal connections with visual cortical regions (Amaral, Behniea, & Kelly, 2003). Consistent with the suggestion that the amygdala's influence on attention may be the result of its modulation of the visual cortex (Vuilleumier et al., 2004), it was recently demonstrated that the presentation of a fearful face enhances the detection of early perceptual features known to be coded by early visual cortex—specifically, sensitivity to contrast (Phelps, Ling, & Carrasco, 2006).

The amygdala's influence on attention and perception ensures that stimuli that are arousing and emotionally salient receive priority in initial stimulus processing. The amygdala's influence on memory ensures that emotional events are also more likely to be remembered over time. Most memories for episodic events depend on the hippocampal complex for long-term storage, and are not dependent on the amygdala (Squire & Kandel, 1999). However, when an event is emotional and arousing, the amygdala has a specific role in modulating the hippocampus and enhancing memory consolidation or storage (McGaugh, 2004). In this way, emotional events are more likely to be retained. Animal models indicate that the amygdala's modulation of hippocampal consolidation is dependent on the neurohormonal changes that occur with arousal (McGaugh, 2004). In humans, it has been demonstrated that amygdala activation at encoding for arousing stimuli predicts later memory (Canli, Zhao, Brewer, Gabrieli, & Cahill, 2000; Hamann, Ely, Grafton, & Kilts, 1999). In addition, using a pharmacological agent that blocks the effects of arousal on the amygdala eliminates emotion's influence on later memory (Cahill, Prins, Weber, & McGaugh, 1994). Finally, patients with amygdala damage fail to show the normal enhancement of memory for emotional events (Cahill, Babinsky, Marko-witsch, & McGaugh, 1995), and this failure is more pronounced over time (LaBar & Phelps, 1998), consistent with the suggestion that the amygdala is modulating memory consolidation.

The human amygdala, which is critical for the acquisition and expression of fear conditioning, also appears to modulate a range of social and cognitive functions through its extensive connectivity with cortical regions (Young, Scannell, Burns, & Blakemore, 1994). The amygdala mediates some forms of social perception and has a modulatory effect on a number of cognitive functions, particularly attention and memory. Through this combination of roles, the amygdala helps ensure that stimuli that come to predict potential threat are also more likely to be noticed and remembered.

FEELINGS AND THE BRAIN

How do we become consciously aware that an emotion system in our brains is active? This is the problem that most emotion studies and theories, especially psychological studies of and theories about humans, have focused on (e.g., Lewis & Michalson, 1983). However, we have examined the neural basis of emotion in this chapter without really mentioning feelings. Our hypothesis is that the mechanism of consciousness is the same for emotional and nonemotional subjective states, and that what distinguishes these states is the brain system that consciousness is aware of at the time. This is why we have focused on the nature of the underlying emotion systems throughout the chapter. Now, however, we consider feelings and their relation to consciousness.

Several theorists have proposed that consciousness has something to do with a mental workspace where things can be compared, contrasted, and mentally manipulated (Johnson-Laird, 1988; Kihlstrom, 1984; Schacter, 1989; Shallice, 1988; Baars, 1997, 2005; Dehaene & Naccache, 2001; Dehaene, Kerszberg, & Changeux, 1998; Dehaene, Changeux, Naccache, Sackur, & Sergent, 2006). The operation of this workspace is often described in

terms of working memory (Baddeley, 1986, 1993, 2000), which includes the capacity to integrate information across sensory modalities with long-term memory into unified representations, to maintain the representation temporarily in an active state, and to use the representation in controlling mental activity and behavior.

Various studies of humans and nonhuman primates point to the prefrontal cortex, especially the dorsolateral prefrontal areas, as being involved in working memory processes (Goldman-Rakic, 1987; Fuster, 2000; Smith & Jonides, 1999; D'Esposito et al., 1995; Miller & Cohen, 2001; Ranganath, Johnson, & D'Esposito, 2003; Muller & Knight, 2006). Immediately present stimuli and stored representations are integrated in working memory by way of interactions among prefrontal areas, sensory processing systems (which serve as short-term memory buffers as well as perceptual processors), and the long-term explicit or declarative memory system (involving the hippocampus and related areas of the temporal lobe). Working memory may involve interactions among several prefrontal areas, including the anterior cingulate, insular, and orbital cortical regions, as well as dorsolateral prefrontal cortex (D'Esposito et al., 1995; Gaffan, Murray, & Fabre-Thorpe, 1993; Smith & Jonides, 1999; Muller & Knight, 2006; Ranganath et al., 2003; Rolls, 1999; LeDoux, 2002; Posner & Dehaene, 1994; Pasternak & Greenlee, 2005; Constantinidis & Procyk, 2004; Curtis, 2006). That prefrontal cortex is involved in conscious experiences is strongly suggested by studies in humans showing that sensory stimuli activate sensory cortex and prefrontal areas when the stimulus is consciously perceived, but only sensory cortex when conscious awareness is blocked by masking or other procedures (Rees, Kreiman, & Koch, 2002; Beck, Rees, Frith, & Lavie, 2001; Frith, Perry, & Lumer, 1999; Frith & Dolan, 1996; Cunningham, Raye, & Johnson, 2004; Carter, O'Doherty, Seymour, Koch, & Dolan, 2006; Vuilleumier et al., 2002; Critchley, Mathias, & Dolan, 2002; Critchley, Wiens, Rotshtein, Öhman, & Dolan, 2004).

If a stimulus is affectively charged (say, a trigger of fear), the same sorts of processes will be called upon as for stimuli without emotional implications; in addition, however, working memory will become aware of the fact that the fear system of the brain has been activated. This further information, when added to perceptual and mnemonic information about the object or event, may be the condition for the subjective experience of an emotional state of fear (Figure 10.4).

But what is the further information that is added to working memory when the fear system is activated? As noted, the amygdala projects to many cortical areas, even some from which it does not receive inputs (Amaral et al., 1992). It can thus influence the operation of perceptual and short-term memory processes, as well as processes in higher-order areas. Although the amygdala does not have extensive connections with the dorsolateral prefrontal cortex, it does communicate with the anterior cingulate, insular, and orbital cortex—other components of the working memory network. But in addition, the amygdala projects to brainstem monoaminergic systems involved in the regulation of cortical arousal. And the amygdala controls bodily responses (behavioral, autonomic, endocrine), which then provide feedback that can influence cortical processing indirectly, such as the adrenal hormones mentioned above. Thus working memory receives a greater number of inputs, and receives inputs of a greater variety, in the presence of an emotional stimulus than in the presence of other kinds of stimuli. These extra inputs may just be what are required to add affective charge to working memory representations, and thus to turn subjective experiences into emotional experiences.

An alternative view, the somatic marker hypothesis, proposes that feelings arise when body sensing areas receive feedback about emotional arousal (Damasio, 1994). Somatic feedback and processing by somatosensory areas of the cortex are components of the working memory model as well. However, the working memory model proposes that somatosensory cortex activity is not conscious until it is represented in working memory. The studies described above, showing that prefrontal cortex is active during the conscious processing of external stimuli and not active when the stimuli are not consciously perceived, are consistent with this idea.

Though described in terms of the fear system, the present hypothesis about feelings is a general one that applies to any emotion. That is, an emotional feeling results when working memory is occupied with the fact that an emotion system of the brain is active. The difference between an emotional state and other states of consciousness, then, is not due to different underlying mechanisms that give rise to the qualitatively different subjective experiences. Instead, there is one mechanism of consciousness, and it can be occupied by either mundane events or emotionally charged ones.

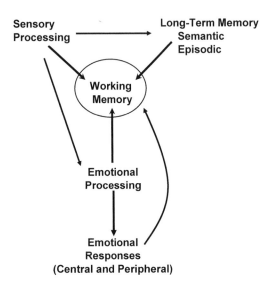

FIGURE 10.4. A model of how the brain consciously experiences emotional stimuli. In this model, the conscious experience of the emotional significance of a stimulus involves the integration in working memory of information about the immediately present stimulus, long-term declarative memories about the stimulus, and the emotional state of the brain and body.

REFERENCES

Adolphs, R., Gosselin, F., Buchanan, T. W., Tranel, D., Schyns, P., & Damasio, A. R. (2005). A mechanism for impaired fear recognition after amygdala damage. *Nature, 433,* 68–72.

Adolphs, R., Tranel, D., & Damasio, A. R. (1998). The human amygdala in social judgment. *Nature, 393,* 470–474.

Adolphs, R., Tranel, D., Hamann, S., Young, A. W., Calder, A. J., Phelps, E. A., et al. (1999). Recognition of facial emotion in nine individuals with bilateral amygdala damage. *Neuropsychologia, 37,* 1111–1117.

Aggleton, J. P. (Ed.). (1992). *The amygdala: Neurobiological aspects of emotion, memory, and mental dysfunction.* New York: Wiley-Liss.

Aggleton, J. P., & Mishkin, M. (1986). The amygdala: Sensory gateway to the emotions. In R. Plutchik & H. Kellerman (Eds.), *Emotion: Theory, research, and experience* (Vol. 3, pp. 281–299). Orlando, FL: Academic Press.

Amaral, D. G., Behniea, H., & Kelly, J. L. (2003). Topographic organization of projections from the amygdala to the visual cortex in the macaque monkey. *Neuroscience, 118,* 1099–1120.

Amaral, D. G., Price, J. L., Pitkänen, A., & Carmichael, S. T. (1992). Anatomical organization of the primate amygdaloid complex. In J. P. Aggleton (Ed.), *The amygdala: Neurobiological aspects of emotion, memory, and mental dysfunction* (pp. 1–66). New York: Wiley-Liss.

Amorapanth, P., LeDoux, J. E., & Nader, K. (2000). Different lateral amygdala outputs mediate reactions and actions elicited by a fear-arousing stimulus. *Nature Neuroscience, 3,* 74–79.

Anderson, A. K. (2005). Affective influences on the attentional dynamics supporting awareness. *Journal of Experimental Psychology: General, 134,* 258–281.

Anderson, A. K., & Phelps, E. A. (2001). Lesions of the human amygdala impair enhanced perception of emotionally salient events. *Nature, 411,* 305–309.

Armony, J. L., Quirk, G. J., & LeDoux, J. E. (1998). Differential effects of amygdala lesions on early and late plastic components of auditory cortex spike trains during fear conditioning. *Journal of Neuroscience, 18,* 2592–2601.

Armony, J. L., Servan-Schreiber, D., Cohen, J. C., & LeDoux, J. E. (1996). Emotion and cognition interactions in the thalamo-cortico-amygdala network: Theory and model. *Cognitive Neuroscience Society Abstracts, 3,* 76.

Armony, J. L., Servan-Schreiber, D., Romanski, L. M., Cohen, J. D., & LeDoux, J. E. (1997). Stimulus generalization of fear responses: Effects of auditory cortex lesions in a computational model and in rats. *Cerebral Cortex, 7,* 157–165.

Baars, B. J. (1997). In the theatre of consciousness. *Journal of Consciousness Studies, 4,* 292–309.

Baars, B. J. (2005). Global workspace theory of consciousness: Toward a cognitive neuroscience of human experience. *Progress in Brain Research, 150,* 45–53.

Baddeley, A. (1986). Modularity, mass-action and memory. *Quarterly Journal of Experimental Psychology A, 38,* 527–533.

Baddeley, A. (1993). Verbal and visual subsystems of working memory. *Current Biology, 3,* 563–565.

Baddeley, A. (2000). The episodic buffer: A new component of working memory? *Trends in Cognitive Sciences, 4,* 417–423.

Bard, P. (1929). The central representation of the sympathetic system: As indicated by certain physiological observations. *Archives of Neurology and Psychiatry, 22,* 230–246.

Beauregard, M., Levesque, J., & Bourgouin, P. (2001). Neural correlates of conscious self-regulation of emotion. *Journal of Neuroscience, 21,* RC165.

Bechara, A., Tranel, D., Damasio, H., Adolphs, R., Rockland, C., & Damasio, A. R. (1995). Double dissociation of conditioning and declarative knowledge relative to the amygdala and hippocampus in humans. *Science, 269,* 1115–1118.

Beck, D. M., Rees, G., Frith, C. D., & Lavie, N. (2001). Neural correlates of change detection and change blindness. *Nature Neuroscience, 4,* 645–650.

Blanchard, C. D., & Blanchard, R. J. (1972). Innate and conditioned reactions to threat in rats with amygdaloid lesions. *Journal of Comparative and Physiological Psychology, 81,* 281–290.

Bouton, M. E., & Swartzentruber, D. (1991). Sources of relapse after extinction in Pavlovian and instrumental learning. *Clinical Psychology Review, 11,* 123–140.

Bremner, J. D., Randall, T., Scott, T. M., Brunen, R. A., Seibyl, J. P., Southwick, S. M., et al. (1995). MRI-based measurement of hippocampal volume in patients with combat-related posttraumatic stress disorder. *American Journal of Psychiatry, 152,* 973–981.

Brodal, A. (1982). *Neurological anatomy.* New York: Oxford University Press.

Buchel, C., Morris, J., Dolan, R. J., & Friston, K. J. (1998). Brain systems mediating aversive conditioning: An event-related fMRI study. *Neuron, 20,* 947–957.

Cahill, L., Babinsky, R., Markowitsch, H. J., & McGaugh, J. L. (1995). The amygdala and emotional memory. *Nature, 377,* 295–296.

Cahill, L., & McGaugh, J. L. (1998). Mechanisms of emotional arousal and lasting declarative memory. *Trends in Neurosciences, 21,* 294–299.

Cahill, L., Prins, B., Weber, M., & McGaugh, J. L. (1994). Beta-adrenergic activation and memory for emotional events. *Nature, 371,* 702–704.

Campeau, S., & Davis, M. (1995). Involvement of subcortical and cortical afferents to the lateral nucleus of the amygdala in fear conditioning measured with fear-potentiated startle in rats trained concurrently with auditory and visual conditioned stimuli. *Journal of Neuroscience, 15,* 2312–2327.

Canli, T., Zhao, Z., Brewer, J., Gabrieli, J. D., & Cahill, L. (2000). Event-related activation in the human amygdala associates with later memory for individual emotional experience. *Journal of Neuroscience, 20,* RC99.

Cannon, W. B. (1929). *Bodily changes in pain, hunger, fear, and rage.* New York: Appleton.

Canteras, N. S., & Swanson, L. W. (1992). Projections of the ventral subiculum to the amygdala, septum, and hypothalamus: A PHAL anterograde tract-tracing study in the rat. *Journal of Comparative Neurology, 324,* 180–194.

Carrive, P., Lee, J., & Su, A. (2000). Lidocaine blockade of amygdala output in fear-conditioned rats reduces Fos expression in the ventrolateral periaqueductal gray. *Neuroscience, 95,* 1071–1080.

Carter, R. M., O'Doherty, J. P., Seymour, B., Koch, C., & Dolan, R. J. (2006). Contingency awareness in human aversive conditioning involves the middle frontal gyrus. *NeuroImage, 29*, 1007–1012.

Cherry, E. C. (1953). Some experiments on the recognition of speech, with one and two ears. *Journal of the Acoustical Society of America, 25*, 975–979.

Cohen, N. J., & Eichenbaum, H. (1993). *Memory, amnesia, and the hippocampal system.* Cambridge, MA: MIT Press.

Conrad, C. D., LeDoux, J. E., Margarinos, A. M., & McEwen, B. S. (1997). Repeated restraint stress fear conditioning independently of causing hippocampal CA3 dendritic atrophyh. *Behavioral Neuroscience, 113*, 902–913.

Conrad, C. D., Lupien, S. J., Thanosoulis, L. C., & McEwen, B. S. (1997). The effects of Type I and Type II corticosteroid receptor agonists on exploratory behavior and spatial memory in the Y-maze. *Brain Research, 759*, 76–83.

Constantinidis, C., & Procyk, E. (2004). The primate working memory networks. *Cognitive, Affective, and Behavioral Neuroscience, 4*, 444–465.

Corodimas, K. P., & LeDoux, J. E. (1995). Disruptive effects of posttraining perirhinal cortex lesions on conditioned fear: Contributions of contextual cues. *Behavioral Neuroscience, 109*, 613–619.

Corodimas, K. P., LeDoux, J. E., Gold, P. W., & Schulkin, J. (1994). Corticosterone potentiation of conditioned fear in rats. *Annals of the New York Academy of Sciences, 746*, 392–393.

Cranford, J. L., & Igarashi, M. (1977). Effects of auditory cortex lesions on temporal summation in cats. *Brain Research, 136*, 559–564.

Critchley, H. D., Mathias, C. J., & Dolan, R. J. (2002). Fear conditioning in humans: The influence of awareness and autonomic arousal on functional neuroanatomy. *Neuron, 33*, 653–663.

Critchley, H. D., Wiens, S., Rotshtein, P., Öhman, A., & Dolan, R. J. (2004). Neural systems supporting interoceptive awareness. *Nature Neuroscience, 7*, 189–195.

Cunningham, W. A., Raye, C. L., & Johnson, M. K. (2004). Implicit and explicit evaluation: FMRI correlates of valence, emotional intensity, and control in the processing of attitudes. *Journal of Cognitive Neuroscience, 16*, 1717–1729.

Curtis, C. E. (2006). Prefrontal and parietal contributions to spatial working memory. *Neuroscience, 139*, 173–180.

Damasio, A. (1994). *Descartes' error: Emotion, reason, and the human brain.* New York: Putnam.

Davis, M. (1992). The role of the amygdala in conditioned fear. In J. P. Aggleton (Ed.), *The amygdala: Neurobiological aspects of emotion, memory, and mental dysfunction* (pp. 255–306). New York: Wiley-Liss.

Davis, M. (1994). The role of the amygdala in emotional learning. *International Review of Neurobiology, 36*, 225–266.

Davis, M., & Whalen, P. J. (2001). The amygdala: Vigilance and emotion. *Molecular Psychiatry, 6*, 13–34.

de Gelder, B., Snyder, J., Greve, D., Gerard, G., & Hadjikhani, N. (2004). Fear fosters flight: A mechanism for fear contagion when perceiving emotion expressed by a whole body. *Proceedings of the National Academy of Sciences of the USA, 101*, 16701–16706.

Dehaene, S., Changeux, J. P., Naccache, L., Sackur, J., & Sergent, C. (2006). Conscious, preconscious, and subliminal processing: A testable taxonomy. *Trends in Cognitive Sciences, 10*, 204–211.

Dehaene, S., Kerszberg, M., & Changeux, J. P. (1998). A neuronal model of a global workspace in effortful cognitive tasks. *Proceedings of the National Academy of Sciences of the USA, 95*, 14529–14534.

Dehaene, S., & Naccache, L. (2001). Towards a cognitive neuroscience of consciousness: Basic evidence and a workspace framework. *Cognition, 79*, 1–37.

Delgado, M. R., Trujillo, J. L., Holmes, B., Nearing, K. I., LeDoux, J. E., & Phelps, E. A. (2004). *Emotion regulation of conditioned fear: The contributions of reappraisal.* Paper presented at the 11th Annual Meeting of the Cognitive Neuroscience Society, San Francisco.

den Dulk P., Heerebout, B. T., & Phaf, R. H. (2003). A computational study into the evolution of dual-route dynamics for affective processing. *Journal of Cognitive Neuroscience, 15*, 194–208.

D'Esposito, M., Detre, J., Alsop, D., Shin, R., Atlas, S., & Grossman, M. (1995). The neural basis of the central executive system of working memory. *Nature, 378*, 279–281.

Drevets, W. C., Price, J. L., Simpson, J. R., Jr., Todd, R. D., Reich, T., Vannier, M., et al. (1997). Subgenual prefrontal cortex abnormalities in mood disorders. *Nature, 386*, 824–827.

Everitt, B. J., & Robbins, T. W. (1992). Amygdala–ventral striatal interactions and reward-related processes. In J. P. Aggleton (Ed.), *The amygdala: Neurobiological aspects of emotion, memory, and mental dysfunction* (pp. 401–429). New York: Wiley-Liss.

Fendt, M., & Fanselow, M. S. (1999). The neuroanatomical and neurochemical basis of conditioned fear. *Neuroscience and Biobehavioral Reviews, 23*, 743–760.

Fernandez de Molina, A., & Hunsperger, R. W. (1962). Organization of the subcortical system governing defense and flight reactions in the cat. *Journal of Physiology, 160*, 200–213.

Frankland, P. W., Cestari, V., Filipkowski, R. K., McDonald, R. J., & Silva, A. J. (1998). The dorsal hippocampus is essential for context discrimination but not for contextual conditioning. *Behavioral Neuroscience, 112*, 863–874.

Frith, C., & Dolan, R. (1996). The role of the prefrontal cortex in higher cognitive functions. *Brain Research: Cognitive Brain Research, 5*, 175–181.

Frith, C., Perry, R., & Lumer, E. (1999). The neural correlates of conscious experience: An experimental framework. *Trends in Cognitive Sciences, 3*, 105–114.

Funayama, E. S., Grillon, C., Davis, M., & Phelps, E. A. (2001). A double dissociation in the affective modulation of startle in humans: Effects of unilateral temporal lobectomy. *Journal of Cognitive Neuroscience*, *13*, 721–729.

Fuster, J. M. (2000). The prefrontal cortex of the primate: A synopsis. *Psychobiology*, *28*, 125–131.

Gaffan, D., & Harrison, S. (1987). Amygdalectomy and disconnection in visual learning for auditory secondary reinforcement by monkeys. *Journal of Neuroscience*, *7*, 2285–2292.

Gaffan, D., Murray, E. A., & Fabre-Thorpe, M. (1993). Interaction of the amygdala with the frontal lobe in reward memory. European *Journal of Neuroscience*, *5*, 968–975.

Gaffan, E. A., Gaffan, D., & Harrison, S. (1988). Disconnection of the amygdala from visual association cortex impairs visual reward-association learning in monkeys. *Journal of Neuroscience*, *8*, 3144–3150.

Gewirtz, J. C., & Davis, M. (1997). Second-order fear conditioning prevented by blocking NMDA receptors in amygdala. *Nature*, *388*, 471–474.

Gloor, P. (1960). Amygdala. In J. Field, H. W. Magoun, & V. E. Hall (Eds.), *Handbook of physiology: Vol. 2. Neurophysiology* (pp. 1395–1420). Washington, DC: American Physiological Society.

Goddard, G. (1964). Functions of the amygdala. *Psychological Review*, *62*, 89–109.

Goldman-Rakic, P. S. (1987). Circuitry of primate prefrontal cortex and regulation of behavior by representational memory. In F. Plum (Ed.), *Handbook of physiology: Section 1. The nervous system. Vol. 5. Higher functions of the brain* (pp. 373–418). Bethesda, MD: American Physiological Society.

Gray, J. A. (1987). *The psychology of fear and stress.* New York: Cambridge University Press.

Halgren, E. (1992). Emotional neurophysiology of the amygdala within the context of human cognition. In J. P. Aggleton (Ed.), *The amygdala: Neurobiological aspects of emotion, memory, and mental dysfunction* (pp. 191–228). New York: Wiley-Liss.

Hamann, S. B., Ely, T. D., Grafton, S. T., & Kilts, C. D. (1999). Amygdala activity related to enhanced memory for pleasant and aversive stimuli. *Nature Neuroscience*, *2*, 289–293.

Heberlein, A. S., & Adolphs, R. (2004). Impaired spontaneous anthropomorphizing despite intact perception and social knowledge. *Proceedings of the National Academy of Sciences of the USA*, *101*, 7487–7491.

Helmstetter, F. J., & Bellgowan, P. S. (1994). Effects of muscimol applied to the basolateral amygdala on acquisition and expression of contextual fear conditioning in rats. *Behavioral Neuroscience*, *108*, 1005–1009.

Hilton, S. M., & Zbrozyna, A.W. (1963). Amygdaloid region for defense reactions and its efferent pathway to the brainstem. *Journal of Physiology*, *165*, 160–173.

Hugdahl, K., & Öhman, A. (1977). Effects of instruction on acquisition and extinction of electrodermal responses to fear-relevant stimuli. *Journal of Experimental Psychology: Human Learning and Memory*, *3*, 608–618.

Iwata, J., Chida, K., & LeDoux, J. E. (1987). Cardiovascular responses elicited by stimulation of neurons in the central amygdaloid nucleus in awake but not anesthetized rats resemble conditioned emotional responses. *Brain Research*, *418*, 183–188.

Jacobs, W. J., & Nadel, L. (1985). Stress-induced recovery of fears and phobias. *Psychological Review*, *92*, 512–531.

James, W. (1884). What is an emotion? *Mind*, *9*, 188–205.

Johnson-Laird, P. N. (1988). *The computer and the mind: An introduction to cognitive science.* Cambridge, MA: Harvard University Press.

Jones, B., & Mishkin, M. (1972). Limbic lesions and the problem of stimulus-reinforcement associations. *Experimental Neurology*, *36*, 362–377.

Kane, F., Coulombe, D., & Miliaressis, E. (1991). Amygdaloid self-stimulation: A movable electrode mapping study. *Behavioral Neuroscience*, *105*, 926–932.

Kapp, B. S., Pascoe, J. P., & Bixler, M. A. (1984). The amygdala: A neuroanatomical systems approach to its contributions to aversive conditioning. In L. R. Squire & N. Butters (Eds.), *Neuropsychology of memory* (pp. 473–488). New York: Guilford Press.

Kapp, B. S., Whalen, P. J., Supple, W. F., & Pascoe, J. P. (1992). Amygdaloid contributions to conditioned arousal and sensory information processing. In J. P. Aggleton (Ed.), *The amygdala: Neurobiological aspects of emotion, memory, and mental dysfunction* (pp. 229–254). New York: Wiley-Liss.

Kihlstrom, J. F. (1984). Conscious, subconscious, unconscious: A cognitive perspective. In K. S. Bowers & D. Meichenbaum (Eds.), *The unconscious reconsidered* (pp. 149–211). New York: Wiley.

Killcross, S., Robbins, T. W., & Everitt, B. J. (1997). Different types of fear-conditioned behaviour mediated by separate nuclei within amygdala. *Nature*, *388*, 377–380.

Kim, J. J., & Diamond, D. M. (2002). The stressed hippocampus, synaptic plasticity and lost memories. *Nature Reviews Neuroscience*, *3*, 453–462.

Kim, J. J., & Fanselow, M. S. (1992). Modality-specific retrograde amnesia of fear. *Science*, *256*, 675–677.

Kluver, H., & Bucy, P. C. (1937). "Psychic blindness" and other symptoms following bilateral temporal lobectomy in rhesus monkeys. *American Journal of Physiology*, *119*, 352–353.

Knight, D. C., Smith, C. N., Cheng, D. T., Stein, E. A., & Helmstetter, F. J. (2004). Amygdala and hippocampal activity during acquisition and extinction of human fear conditioning. *Cognitive, Affective, and Behavioral Neuroscience*, *4*, 317–325.

Kotter, R., & Meyer, N. (1992). The limbic system: A review of its empirical foundation. *Behavioural Brain Research*, *52*, 105–127.

LaBar, K. S., Gatenby, J. C., Gore, J. C., LeDoux, J. E., & Phelps, E. A. (1998). Human amygdala activation during conditioned fear acquisition and extinction: A mixed-trial fMRI study. *Neuron, 20,* 937–945.

LaBar, K. S., & LeDoux, J. E. (1996). Partial disruption of fear conditioning in rats with unilateral amygdala damage: Correspondence with unilateral temporal lobectomy in humans. *Behavioral Neuroscience, 110,* 991–997.

LaBar, K. S., LeDoux, J. E., Spencer, D. D., & Phelps, E. A. (1995). Impaired fear conditioning following unilateral temporal lobectomy in humans. *Journal of Neuroscience, 15,* 6846–6855.

LaBar, K. S., & Phelps, E. A. (1998). Arousal-mediated memory consolidation: Role of the medial temporal lobe in humans. *Psychological Science, 9,* 490–493.

LaBar, K. S., & Phelps, E. A. (2005). Reinstatement of conditioned fear in humans is context dependent and impaired in amnesia. *Behavioral Neuroscience, 119,* 677–686.

LeDoux, J. E. (1986a). Neurobiology of emotion. In J. E. LeDoux & W. Hirst (Eds.), *Mind and brain* (pp. 301–358). New York: Cambridge University Press.

LeDoux, J. E. (1986b). Sensory systems and emotion. *Integrative Psychiatry, 4,* 237–248.

LeDoux, J. E. (1987). Emotion. In F. Plum (Ed.), *Handbook of physiology: Section 1. The nervous system. Vol. 5. Higher functions of the brain* (pp. 419–460). Bethesda, MD: American Physiological Society.

LeDoux, J. E. (1991). Emotion and the limbic system concept. *Concepts in Neuroscience, 2,* 169–199.

LeDoux, J. E. (1992). Emotion and the amygdala. In J. P. Aggleton (Ed.), *The amygdala: Neurobiological aspects of emotion, memory, and mental dysfunction* (pp. 339–351). New York: Wiley-Liss.

LeDoux, J. E. (1996). *The emotional brain.* New York: Simon & Schuster.

LeDoux, J. E. (2002). *Synaptic self: How our brains become who we are.* New York: Viking.

LeDoux, J. E., Cicchetti, P., Xagoraris, A., & Romanski, L. M. (1990). The lateral amygdaloid nucleus: Sensory interface of the amygdala in fear conditioning. *Journal of Neuroscience, 10,* 1062–1069.

LeDoux, J. E., Farb, C., & Ruggiero, D. A. (1990). Topographic organization of neurons in the acoustic thalamus that project to the amygdala. *Journal of Neuroscience, 10,* 1043–1054.

LeDoux, J. E., & Gorman, J. M. (2001). A call to action: Overcoming anxiety through active coping. *American Journal of Psychiatry, 158,* 1953–1955.

LeDoux, J. E., Iwata, J., Cicchetti, P., & Reis, D. J. (1988). Different projections of the central amygdaloid nucleus mediate autonomic and behavioral correlates of conditioned fear. *Journal of Neuroscience, 8,* 2517–2529.

LeDoux, J. E., Romanski, L. M., & Xagoraris, A. E. (1989). Indelibility of subcortical emotional memories. *Journal of Cognitive Neuroscience, 1,* 238–243.

LeDoux, J. E., Ruggiero, D. A., & Reis, D. J. (1985). Projections to the subcortical forebrain from anatomically defined regions of the medial geniculate body in the rat. *Journal of Comparative Neurology, 242,* 182–213.

LeDoux, J. E., Sakaguchi, A., & Reis, D. J. (1984). Subcortical efferent projections of the medial geniculate nucleus mediate emotional responses conditioned to acoustic stimuli. *Journal of Neuroscience, 4,* 683–698.

Lewis, M., & Michalson, L. (1983). *Children's emotions and moods: Developmental theory and measurement.* New York: Plenum Press.

Li, X. F., Stutzmann, G. E., & LeDoux, J. E. (1996). Convergent but temporally separated inputs to lateral amygdala neurons from the auditory thalamus and auditory cortex use different postsynaptic receptors: *In vivo* intracellular and extracellular recordings in fear conditioning pathways. *Learning and Memory, 3,* 229–242.

MacLean, P. D. (1949). Psychosomatic disease and the "visceral brain": Recent developments bearing on the Papez theory of emotion. *Psychosomatic Medicine, 11,* 338–353.

MacLean, P. D. (1952). Some psychiatric implications of physiological studies on frontotemporal portion of limbic system (visceral brain). *Electroencephalography and Clinical Neurophysiology, 4,* 407–418.

Majidishad, P., Pelli, D. G., & LeDoux, J. E. (1996). Disruption of fear conditioning to contextual stimuli but not to a tone by lesions of the accessory basal nucleus of the amygdala. *Society for Neuroscience Abstracts, 22,* 1116.

Maren, S., Aharonov, G., Stote, D. L., & Fanselow, M. S. (1996). N-methyl-D-aspartate receptors in the basolateral amygdala are required for both acquisition and expression of conditional fear in rats. *Behavioral Neuroscience, 110,* 1365–1374.

Maren, S., Anagnostaras, S. G., & Fanselow, M. S. (1998). The startled seahorse: Is the hippocampus necessary for contextual fear conditioning? *Trends in Cognitive Sciences, 2,* 39–41.

Maren, S., & Fanselow, M. S. (1996). The amygdala and fear conditioning: Has the nut been cracked? *Neuron, 16,* 237–240.

Mascagni, F., McDonald, A. J., & Coleman, J. R. (1993). Corticoamygdaloid and corticocortical projections of the rat temporal cortex: A *Phaseolus vulgaris* leucoagglutinin study. *Neuroscience, 57,* 697–715.

McDonald, A. J. (1998). Cortical pathways to the mammalian amygdala. *Progress in Neurobiology, 55,* 257–332.

McDonald, A. J., Mascagni, F., & Guo, L. (1996). Projections of the medial and lateral prefrontal cortices to the amygdala: A *Phaseolus vulgaris* leucoagglutinin study in the rat. *Neuroscience, 71,* 55–75.

McGaugh, J. L. (2004). The amygdala modulates the consolidation of memories of emotionally arousing experiences. *Annual Review of Neuroscience, 27,* 1–28.

McGaugh, J. L., Mesches, M. H., Cahill, L., Parent,

M. B., Coleman-Mesches, K., & Salinas, J. A. (1995). Involvement of the amygdala in the regulation of memory storage. In J. L. McGaugh, F. Bermudez-Rattoni, & R. A. Prado-Alcala (Eds.), *Plasticity in the central nervous system* (pp. 18–39). Mahwah, NJ: Erlbaum.

Milad, M. R., Quinn, B. T., Pitman, R. K., Orr, S. P., Fischl, B., & Rauch, S. L. (2005). Thickness of ventromedial prefrontal cortex in humans is correlated with extinction memory. *Proceedings of the National Academy of Sciences of the USA, 102,* 10706–10711.

Milad, M. R., & Quirk, G. J. (2002). Neurons in medial prefrontal cortex signal memory for fear extinction. *Nature, 420,* 70–74.

Miller, E. K., & Cohen, J. D. (2001). An integrative theory of prefrontal cortex function. *Annual Review of Neuroscience, 24,* 167–202.

Miserendino, M. J., Sananes, C. B., Melia, K. R., & Davis, M. (1990). Blocking of acquisition but not expression of conditioned fear-potentiated startle by NMDA antagonists in the amygdala. *Nature, 345,* 716–718.

Mishkin, M., & Aggleton, J. (1981). Multiple functional contributions of the amygdala in the monkey. In Y. Ben-Ari (Ed.), *The amygdaloid complex* (pp. 409–420). Amsterdam: Elsevier/North-Holland.

Mishkin, M., Malamut, B., & Bachevalier, J. (1984). Memories and habits: Two neural systems. In G. Lynch, J. L. McGaugh, & N. M. Weinberger (Eds.), *Neurobiology of learning and memory* (pp. 65–77). New York: Guilford Press.

Morgan, M. A., & LeDoux, J. E. (1995). Differential contribution of dorsal and ventral medial prefrontal cortex to the acquisition and extinction of conditioned fear in rats. *Behavioral Neuroscience, 109,* 681–688.

Morgan, M. A., Romanski, L. M., & LeDoux, J. E. (1993). Extinction of emotional learning: Contribution of medial prefrontal cortex. *Neuroscience Letters, 163,* 109–113.

Morris, J. S., Friston, K. J., Buchel, C., Frith, C. D., Young, A. W., Calder, A. J., et al. (1998). A neuromodulatory role for the human amygdala in processing emotional facial expressions. *Brain, 121*(Pt. 1), 47–57.

Mowrer, O. H., & Lamoreaux, R. R. (1946). Fear as an intervening variable in avoidance conditioning. *Journal of Comparative Psychology, 39,* 29–50.

Muller, J., Corodimas, K. P., Fridel, Z., & LeDoux, J. E. (1997). Functional inactivation of the lateral and basal nuclei of the amygdala by muscimol infusion prevents fear conditioning to an explicit conditioned stimulus and to contextual stimuli. *Behavioral Neuroscience, 111,* 683–691.

Muller, N. G., & Knight, R. T. (2006). The functional neuroanatomy of working memory: Contributions of human brain lesion studies. *Neuroscience, 139,* 51–58.

Ochsner, K. N., Bunge, S. A., Gross, J. J., & Gabrieli, J. D. (2002). Rethinking feelings: An FMRI study of the cognitive regulation of emotion. *Journal of Cognitive Neuroscience, 14,* 1215–1229.

Öhman, A., & Mineka, S. (2001). Fears, phobias, and preparedness: Toward an evolved module of fear and fear learning. *Psychological Review, 108,* 483–522.

O'Keefe, J., & Nadel, L. (1978). *The hippocampus as a cognitive map.* Oxford: Clarendon Press.

Olds, J. (1977). *Drives and reinforcement.* New York: Raven Press.

Olsson, A., & Phelps, E. A. (2004). Learned fear of "unseen" faces after Pavlovian, observational, and instructed fear. *Psychological Science, 15,* 822–828.

Olsson, A., & Phelps, E. A. (2007). Social learning of fear. *Nature Neuroscience, 10,* 1095–1102.

Ono, T., & Nishijo, H. (1992). Neurophysiological basis of the Kluver–Bucy syndrome: Responses of monkey amygdaloid neurons to biologically significant objects. In J. P. Aggleton (Ed.), *The amygdala: Neurobiological aspects of emotion, memory, and mental dysfunction* (pp. 167–190). New York: Wiley-Liss.

Ottersen, O. P. (1982). Connections of the amygdala of the rat: IV. Corticoamygdaloid and intraamygdaloid connections as studied with axonal transport of horseradish peroxidase. *Journal of Comparative Neurology, 205,* 30–48.

Packard, M. G., Williams, C. L., Cahill, L., & McGaugh, J. L. (1995). The anatomy of a memory modulatory system: From periphery to brain. In N. E. Spear, L. P. Spear, & M. L. Woodruff (Eds.), *Neurobehavioral plasticity: Learning, development, and response to brain insults* (pp. 149–150). Hillsdale, NJ: Erlbaum.

Papez, J. W. (1937). A proposed mechanism of emotion. *Archives of Neurology and Psychiatry, 79,* 217–224.

Pare, D., & Smith, Y. (1998). Intrinsic circuitry of the amygdaloid complex: Common principles of organization in rats and cats. *Trends in Neurosciences, 21,* 240–241.

Parent, M. B., Tomaz, C., & McGaugh, J. L. (1992). Increased training in an aversively motivated task attenuates the memory-impairing effects of posttraining N-methyl-D-aspartate-induced amygdala lesions. *Behavioral Neuroscience, 106,* 789–798.

Pasternak, T., & Greenlee, M. W. (2005). Working memory in primate sensory systems. *Nature Reviews Neuroscience, 6,* 97–107.

Pavlov, I. P. (1960). *Conditioned reflexes* (G. V. Anrep, Trans.) New York: Dover. (Original work published 1927)

Phelps, E. A., Delgado, M. R. Nearing, K. I., & LeDoux, J. E. (2004). Extinction learning in humans: Role of the amygdala and vmPFC. *Neuron, 43,* 897–905.

Phelps, E. A., Ling, S., & Carrasco, M. (2006). Emotion facilitates perception and potentiates the perceptual benefits of attention. *Psychological Science, 17,* 292–299.

Phelps, E. A., O'Connor, K. J., Gatenby, J. C., Gore, J. C., Grillon, C., & Davis, M. (2001). Activation of the left amygdala to a cognitive representation of fear. *Nature Neuroscience, 4,* 437–441.

Phillips, R. G., & LeDoux, J. E. (1992). Differential contribution of amygdala and hippocampus to cued and contextual fear conditioning. *Behavioral Neuroscience, 106,* 274–285.

Phillips, R. G., & LeDoux, J. E. (1994). Lesions of the dorsal hippocampal formation interfere with background but not foreground contextual fear conditioning. *Learning and Memory, 1,* 34–44.

Pitkänen, A., Savander, V., & LeDoux, J. E. (1997). Organization of intra-amygdaloid circuitries in the rat: An emerging framework for understanding functions of the amygdala. *Trends in Neurosciences, 20,* 517–523.

Posner, M. I., & Dehaene, S. (1994). Attentional networks. *Trends in Neurosciences, 17,* 75–79.

Preuss, T. M., & Goldman-Rakic, P. S. (1991). Ipsilateral cortical connections of granular frontal cortex in the strepsirhine primate *Galago,* with comparative comments on anthropoid primates. *Journal of Comparative Neurology, 310,* 507–549.

Quirk, G. J., Armony, J. L., & LeDoux, J. E. (1997). Fear conditioning enhances different temporal components of tone-evoked spike trains in auditory cortex and lateral amygdala. *Neuron, 19,* 613–624.

Quirk, G. J., Garcia, R., & Gonzalez-Lima, F. (2006). Prefrontal mechanisms in extinction of conditioned fear. *Biological Psychiatry, 60,* 337–343.

Quirk, G. J., Russo, G. K., Barron, J. L., & Lebron, K. (2000). The role of ventromedial prefrontal cortex in the recovery of extinguished fear. *Journal of Neuroscience, 20,* 6225–6231.

Radley, J. J., & Morrison, J. H. (2005). Repeated stress and structural plasticity in the brain. *Ageing Research Reviews, 4,* 271–287.

Radley, J. J., Rocher, A. B., Miller, M., Janssen, W. G., Liston, C., Hof, P. R., et al. (2006). Repeated stress induces dendritic spine loss in the rat medial prefrontal cortex. *Cerebral Cortex, 16,* 313–320.

Ranganath, C., Johnson, M. K., & D'Esposito, M. (2003). Prefrontal activity associated with working memory and episodic long-term memory. *Neuropsychologia, 41,* 378–389.

Rauch, S. L., Shin, L. M., & Phelps, E. A. (2006). Neurocircuitry models of posttraumatic stress disorder and extinction: Human neuroimaging research—past, present, and future. *Biological Psychiatry, 60,* 376–382.

Raymond, J. E., Shapiro, K. L., & Arnell, K. M. (1992). Temporary suppression of visual processing in an RSVP task: An attentional blink? *Journal of Experimental Psychology: Human Perception and Performance, 18,* 849–860.

Rees, G., Kreiman, G., & Koch, C. (2002). Neural correlates of consciousness in humans. *Nature Reviews Neuroscience, 3,* 261–270.

Rescorla, R. A., & Heth, C. D. (1975). Reinstatement of fear to an extinguished conditioned stimulus. *Journal of Experimental Psychology: Animal Behavior Processes, 104,* 88–96.

Rescorla, R. A., & Solomon, R. L. (1967). Two process learning theory: Relationships between Pavlovian conditioning and instrumental learning. *Psychological Review, 74,* 151–182.

Rodrigues, S. M., Schafe, G. E., & LeDoux, J. E. (2004). Molecular mechanisms underlying emotional learning and memory in the lateral amygdala. *Neuron, 44,* 75–91.

Rogan, M. T., Staubli, U. V., & LeDoux, J. E. (1997). AMPA receptor facilitation accelerates fear learning without altering the level of conditioned fear acquired. *Journal of Neuroscience, 17,* 5928–5935.

Rolls, E. T. (1986). A theory of emotion, and its application to understanding the neural basis of emotion. In Y. Oomur (Ed.), *Emotions: Neural and chemical control* (pp. 325–344). Tokyo: Japan Scientific Societies Press.

Rolls, E. T. (1992). Neurophysiological mechanisms underlying face processing within and beyond the temporal cortical visual areas. *Philosophical Transactions of the Royal Society of London: Series B. Biological Sciences, 335,* 11–21.

Rolls, E. T. (1999). *The brain and emotion.* Oxford: Oxford University Press.

Romanski, L. M., & LeDoux, J. E. (1992). Bilateral destruction of neocortical and perirhinal projection targets of the acoustic thalamus does not disrupt auditory fear conditioning. *Neuroscience Letters, 142,* 228–232.

Romanski, L. M., & LeDoux, J. E. (1993). Information cascade from primary auditory cortex to the amygdala: Corticocortical and corticoamygdaloid projections of temporal cortex in the rat. *Cerebral Cortex, 3,* 515–532.

Rudy, J. W., Huff, N. C., & Matus-Amat, P. (2004). Understanding contextual fear conditioning: Insights from a two-process model. *Neuroscience and Biobehavioral Reviews, 28,* 675–685.

Schacter, D. L. (1989). On the relation between memory and consciousness: Dissociable interactions and conscious experience. In H. L. I. Roediger & F. I. M. Craik (Eds.), *Varieties of memory and consciousness: Essays in honour of Endel Tulving* (pp. 355–389). Hillsdale, NJ: Erlbaum.

Selden, N. R., Everitt, B. J., Jarrard, L. E., & Robbins, T. W. (1991). Complementary roles for the amygdala and hippocampus in aversive conditioning to explicit and contextual cues. *Neuroscience, 42,* 335–350.

Shallice, T. (1988). Information processing models of consciousness. In A. Marcel & E. Bisiach (Eds.), *Consciousness in contemporary science* (pp. 305–333). Oxford: Oxford University Press.

Shors, T. J. (2006). Stressful experience and learning across the lifespan. *Annual Review of Psychology, 57,* 55–85.

Smith, E. E., & Jonides, J. (1999). Storage and executive processes in the frontal lobes. *Science, 283,* 1657–1661.

Spiegler, B. J., & Mishkin, M. (1981). Evidence for the sequential participation of inferior temporal cortex and amygdala in the acquisition of stimulus–reward associations. *Behavioural Brain Research*, 3, 303–317.

Squire, L. R., & Kandel, E. R. (1999). *Memory: From mind to molecules*. New York: Scientific American Library.

Squire, L. R., & Zola, S. M. (1996). Structure and function of declarative and nondeclarative memory systems. *Proceedings of the National Academy of Sciences of the USA*, 93, 13515–13522.

Stefanacci, L., & Amaral, D. G. (2002). Some observations on cortical inputs to the macaque monkey amygdala: An anterograde tracing study. *Journal of Comparative Neurology*, 451, 301–323.

Sutherland, R. J., & Rudy, J. W. (1989). Configural association theory: The role of the hippocampal formation in learning, memory, and amnesia. *Psychobiology*, 17, 129–144.

Swanson, L. W. (1983). The hippocampus and the concept of the limbic system. In W. Seifert (Ed.), *Neurobiology of the hippocampus* (pp. 3–19). London: Academic Press.

Teich, A. H., McCabe, P. M., Gentile, C. C., Schneiderman, L. S., Winters, R. W., Liskowsky, D. R., et al. (1989). Auditory cortex lesions prevent the extinction of Pavlovian differential heart rate conditioning to tonal stimuli in rabbits. *Brain Research*, 480, 210–218.

Thorpe, S. J., Rolls, E. T., & Maddison, S. (1983). The orbitofrontal cortex: Neuronal activity in the behaving monkey. *Experimental Brain Research*, 49, 93–115.

Turner, B., & Herkenham, M. (1991). Thalamo-amygdaloid projections in the rat: A test of the amygdala's role in sensory processing. *Journal of Comparative Neurology*, 313, 295–325.

Urry, H. L., van Reekum, C. M., Johnstone, T., Kalin, N. H., Thurow, M. E., Schaefer, H. S., et al. (2006). Amygdala and ventromedial prefrontal cortex are inversely coupled during regulation of negative affect and predict the diurnal pattern of cortisol secretion among older adults. *Journal of Neuroscience*, 26, 4415–4425.

Vuilleumier, P., Armony, J. L., Clarke, K., Husain, M., Driver, J., & Dolan, R. J. (2002). Neural response to emotional faces with and without awareness: Event-related fMRI in a parietal patient with visual extinction and spatial neglect. *Neuropsychologia*, 40, 2156–2166.

Vuilleumier, P., Richardson, M. P., Armony, J. L., Driver, J., & Dolan, R. J. (2004). Distant influences of amygdala lesion on visual cortical activation during emotional face processing. *Nature Neuroscience*, 7, 1271–1278.

Weinberger, N. M. (1995). Retuning the brain by fear conditioning. In M. S. Gazzaniga (Ed.), *The cognitive neurosciences* (pp. 1071–1090). Cambridge, MA: MIT Press.

Weiskrantz, L. (1956). Behavioral changes associated with ablation of the amygdaloid complex in monkeys. *Journal of Comparative and Physiological Psychology*, 49, 381–391.

Whalen, P. J., Kagan, J., Cook, R. G., Davis, F. C., Kim, H., Polis, S., et al. (2004). Human amygdala responsivity to masked fearful eye whites. *Science*, 306, 2061.

Whalen, P. J., Rauch, S. L., Etcoff, N. L., McInerney, S. C., Lee, M. B., & Jenike, M. A. (1998). Masked presentations of emotional facial expressions modulate amygdala activity without explicit knowledge. *Journal of Neuroscience*, 18, 411–418.

Whitfield, I. C. (1980). Auditory cortex and the pitch of complex tones. *Journal of the Acoustical Society of America*, 67, 644–647.

Wilensky, A. E., Schafe, G. E., & LeDoux, J. E. (1999). Functional inactivation of the amygdala before but not after auditory fear conditioning prevents memory formation. *Journal of Neuroscience*, 19, RC48.

Wilensky, A. E., Schafe, G. E., & LeDoux, J. E. (2000). The amygdala modulates memory consolidation of fear-motivated inhibitory avoidance learning but not classical fear conditioning. *Journal of Neuroscience*, 20, 7059–7066.

Winston, J. S., Strange, B. A., O'Doherty, J., & Dolan, R. J. (2002). Automatic and intentional brain responses during evaluation of trustworthiness of faces. *Nature Neuroscience*, 5, 277–283.

Young, M. P., Scannell, J. W., Burns, G. A., & Blakemore, C. (1994). Analysis of connectivity: Neural systems in the cerebral cortex. *Reviews in the Neurosciences*, 5, 227–250.

CHAPTER 11

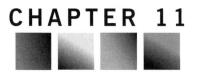

The Psychophysiology of Emotion

JEFF T. LARSEN, GARY G. BERNTSON, KIRSTEN M. POEHLMANN,
TIFFANY A. ITO, and JOHN T. CACIOPPO

> You see me here, you gods, a poor old man,
> As full of grief as age; wretched in both!
> If it be you that stir these daughters' hearts
> Against their father, fool me not so much
> To bear it tamely; touch me with noble anger.
> —SHAKESPEARE, *King Lear*, II.5

Just as Shakespeare used words to give voice to King Lear's outrage at his daughters' betrayal, psychology has often used the words that people use to describe their emotions to understand those emotions (e.g., Green, Salovey, & Truax, 1999; Osgood, Suci, & Tannenbaum, 1957; cf. Cacioppo, Gardner, & Berntson, 1999; LeDoux, 1996). Psychology's reliance on self-reports has been remarkably successful in terms of uncovering functional relationships between different variables. The words people use to describe their current emotions typically show consistent patterns (e.g., Russell, 1980). Those who report feeling happy, for instance, are unlikely to report feeling sad (Russell & Carroll, 1999; but see Larsen, McGraw, & Cacioppo, 2001). In addition, situational manipulations reliably elicit different patterns of self-reported emotional states. People generally report feeling happy when hearing fast music in a major key, and sad when hearing slow music in a minor key (Gagnon & Peretz, 2003). Moreover, children as young as 6 years of age can find words that describe not only their emotions, but the putative causes of their emotions (e.g., Stein & Levine, 1987).

One factor that allows people to use words to convey their emotions is the fact that the world's languages are rich in emotional terms (e.g., Clore, Ortony, & Foss, 1987; Russell, 1978), which are supplemented with even richer metaphors (Fainsilber & Ortony, 1987; Hoffman, Waggoner, & Palermo, 1991). Yet words have their limitations. They are sometimes used to deceive rather than inform (e.g., DePaulo et al., 2003). Even when used in earnest, they are subject to contextual distortions that operate outside of awareness (e.g.,

180

Schwarz & Clore, 1983). One implication is that emotions are not merely cerebral; they are embodied. Indeed, Lear's emotions are most powerfully conveyed not when his lines are read, but when they are portrayed by an actor on the stage. It is perhaps not surprising, then, that many of the metaphors people use to express emotion involve bodily sensations. People express anxiety by remarking that they have butterflies in their stomachs, or anger by remarking that their blood is boiling. Of course, such metaphors are just that. They are not emotions; they merely symbolize emotions—albeit imperfectly.

Dating back to Freud, research from clinical psychology has revealed that some aspects of emotional states can be reported and that others cannot (e.g., Bradley, 2000; Lang, 1971). In addition, research from the neurosciences (e.g., Gazzaniga & LeDoux, 1978; Tranel & Damasio, 2000) and social psychology (e.g., Winkielman, Berridge, & Wilbarger, 2005) has shown that emotional processes can occur in the absence of emotional experience, which is a prerequisite for the verbal expression of emotion. Thus self-reports of emotion tend to be only modestly related to somatovisceral and behavioral aspects of emotion (e.g., Bradley & Lang, 2000a; but see Mauss, Levenson, McCarter, Wilhelm, & Gross, 2005). One goal of the psychophysiology of emotion, then, is to investigate the physiological processes by which emotion is embodied, and thereby to complement and clarify insights gleaned from ratings of emotions that people are willing and able to report. A second goal is to use psychophysiological methods to decompose the component processes that result in an emotional experience or response (Cacioppo & Petty, 1987).

Most contemporary definitions of emotion share several features. Most important is the notion that emotions consist of affective, valenced (i.e., positive and/or negative) reactions to meaningful stimuli (Frijda, 1994). Yet not all valenced reactions constitute emotions. Emotions typically are directed at particular objects, unlike moods, which tend to be more diffuse (Frijda, 1994). Emotions also tend to be short-lived, lasting on the order of seconds to minutes (Ekman, 1994). Other affective reactions, such as moods (Ekman, 1994; Frijda, 1994) and especially attitudes (cf. sentiments; Frijda, 1994), tend to be more enduring (Eagly & Chaiken, 1993). Thus individuals who fear

dogs do not live in a constant state of fear, but the appearance of a dog is likely to elicit fear (Frijda, Chapter 5, this volume).

Fear can be conceptualized as a discrete emotion, along with anger, sadness, happiness, relief, and other states that putatively differ in terms of a variety of factors, including antecedent appraisals (e.g., Scherer, Schorr, & Johnstone, 2001), facial expressions (Ekman, 1994), and action tendencies (Frijda, 1986). Alternatively, emotions can be conceptualized in terms of a small number of dimensions, such as valence and arousal (Russell & Barrett, 1999), positive and negative activation (Watson, Wiese, Vaidya, & Tellegen, 1999), or positivity and negativity (Cacioppo et al., 1999). Though a review of the relative merits of each approach is beyond the scope of this chapter, we have argued that discrete and dimensional approaches are not incommensurable, and that both approaches can be useful (Cacioppo et al., 1999). Indeed, many of the findings reviewed in this chapter indicate that the psychophysiological substrates of emotion are organized in terms of dimensions (e.g., valence), but other findings highlight the utility of postulating the existence of discrete emotions.

OVERVIEW

The nervous system is divided into two broad components. The central nervous system comprises the brain and spinal cord, which send and receive inputs from the peripheral nervous system. In turn, the peripheral nervous system comprises the autonomic and somatic nervous systems. The autonomic nervous system innervates smooth muscles (e.g., the heart) and glands, and is divided into the sympathetic and parasympathetic branches. Whereas the sympathetic branch generally prepares the body for action (e.g., by stimulating heart rate), the parasympathetic branch aids restorative functions (e.g., by stimulating digestion). Finally, the somatic nervous system innervates skeletal muscles, including those of the face.

Common to all definitions of psychophysiology is that it involves the use of physiological signals to understand psychological processes (e.g., Cacioppo, Tassinary, & Berntson, 2007; Coles, Donchin, & Porges, 1986; Stern, Ray, & Quigley, 2001). Cognitive psychophysiology, for instance, is largely concerned with mental processes and has therefore relied heavily on the electroencephalogram (EEG), which reflects electrical activity underlying central nervous system processes (e.g., Coles et al., 1986). So extensive is the embodiment of emotion, however, that surface recordings of both central and peripheral nervous system activity have shed light on the physiological substrates of emotion. Early theory and research on the psychophysiology of emotion focused on the autonomic portion of the peripheral nervous system, so we begin there. We then turn to the somatic nervous system, where research has investigated relationships between emotional states and activation of the facial musculature. Finally, we turn to the central nervous system, where EEG research has helped delineate the neural mechanisms underlying emotion.

THE PERIPHERAL NERVOUS SYSTEM

As mentioned above, many metaphors used to describe emotions involve bodily states. Most of those metaphors make reference to peripheral physiological processes in particular. Though most individuals in Western cultures presumably recognize that the heart is in reality a mere pump, it is often described as the seat of emotion in general and love in particular. Thus our hearts go aflutter when we are in love, but break when our beloved departs. Though intuition about psychological phenomena is often imprecise at best and inaccurate at worst, psychophysiology has demonstrated that peripheral processes in the form of autonomic (i.e., visceral) and somatic (e.g., motor, expressive) events are indeed associated with emotional processes.

The Autonomic Nervous System

The rich connections between the central and peripheral nervous systems have long fueled debates over the precise role of peripheral activity in emotion. These connections are reciprocal, such that the central nervous system both sends and receives input from the viscera. The fact that the brain sends efferents to the periphery raises the possibility that the experience of emotions (i.e., "feelings") cause peripheral changes. On the other hand, the fact that the central nervous receives afferents from the periphery raises the perhaps more counterintuitive possibility that the peripheral changes

contribute to the experience of emotion. The former possibility was set forth by William James (1884, 1890/1950) more than a century ago. By this account, specific somatovisceral patterns can not only precede but also generate the experience of emotion. In an early critique of James's position, however, Cannon (1927) argued that different autonomic patterns do not produce different emotions; rather, different emotions produce different autonomic patterns.

Schachter and Singer (1962) proposed an alternative to both James (1884, 1890/1950) and Cannon (1927). Like James, Schachter and Singer contended that autonomic activity could generate different emotions. Unlike James, however, they also suggested that the same pattern of autonomic activity could result in the experience of different emotions (see also Mandler, 1975). By this account, the perception of neutral, unexplained physiological arousal creates an "evaluative need" that motivates the individual to come up with a cognitive label for the arousal state. Depending on situational cues, the individual may come to experience different emotional states (e.g., anger, euphoria; Schachter & Singer, 1962; cf. Reisenzein, 1983).

Thus theories have proposed three distinct relationships between somatovisceral activity and emotional state. Whereas Cannon (1927) contended that different emotions produce different patterns of somatovisceral activity, James (1884) contended that different patterns of somatovisceral activity can produce different emotions. Finally, Schachter and Singer (1962) contended that even undifferentiated somatovisceral activity can produce distinct and different emotions depending on the situational context. Several subsequent theories of emotion can be seen as falling within each of these camps. Damasio's (1994) somatic marker hypothesis and Barrett's (2006) somatic marker hypothesis and conceptual act model of emotion, for instance, bear resemblance to the conceptualizations of James (1884) and Schachter and Singer (1962), respectively. Researchers have marshaled empirical evidence both for and against each position. Vianna, Weinstock, Elliott, Summers, and Tranel (2006) studied individuals with Crohn's disease, which is associated with excessive visceral outflow from the gut. As both James and Schachter and Singer would expect, individuals with Crohn's disease showed greater gastric myoelectrical activity during emotionally evocative films than did comparison participants, which may help explain why they also experienced more subjective arousal. (For a review of work on interoception and emotion, see Craig, Chapter 16, this volume.) Indirect evidence for James's position comes from Barrett, Quigley, Bliss-Moreau, and Aronson's (2004) recent finding that individuals who are more sensitive to their heartbeats also tend to emphasize the arousal-related meanings of emotion words (see also Critchley, Wiens, Rotshtein, Öhman, & Dolan, 2004).

On the other hand Cannon (1927) provided evidence from animal studies that autonomic events are too slow, insensitive, and undifferentiated to influence emotions. More recently, neuropsychological research with humans suggests that spinal cord injuries have little impact on individuals' experience of emotion (Chwalisz, Diener, & Gallagher, 1988; see also Cobos, Sánchez, Garcia, Vera, & Vila, 2002). Perhaps most problematic for James's hypothesis was that early research failed to demonstrate replicable and generalizable emotion-specific autonomic patterns. Ekman, Levenson, and Friesen (1983; see also Levenson, 1988) attributed such inconsistency to a variety of methodological limitations. For instance, previous investigators made no attempt to equate the intensity of different emotions, and they failed to synchronize physiological recordings with the likely onset and offset of the emotion, or even to collect self-reports or behavioral observations to confirm that the expected emotions had been elicited. Furthermore, Ekman and colleagues argued that differentiation requires simultaneous examination of a number of indices of autonomic nervous system activity.

Ekman et al. (1983) overcame these limitations in a groundbreaking article published in *Science* that provided evidence for emotion-specific autonomic patterns. Ekman et al. measured heart rate, finger temperature, skin resistance, and forearm flexor muscle tension as participants completed two sets of tasks designed to elicit anger, fear, sadness, happiness, surprise, and disgust. In one task participants were asked to remember and relive past emotional episodes. Participants also completed a directed facial action task in which they were asked to contract sets of muscles to produce facial expressions associated with each emotion. During the anger condition, for instance, participants were asked to pull their eyebrows down and together, raise their upper eyelids, push the lower lips up, and press their lips together.

Ekman et al. (1983) found that in addition to differentiating positive from negative emotions, combinations of autonomic measures could differentiate some negative emotions (e.g., fear) from others (e.g., anger). During the facial action task, for instance, happiness was characterized by decreased heart rate, anger by increased heart rate and increased skin temperature, and fear by increased heart rate and decreased skin temperature. Based on such findings, Levenson, Ekman, and Friesen (1990) proposed that each discrete emotion is associated with an innate affect program that coordinates changes in the organism's biological states. They further argued that such changes support the behavioral reactions most often associated with particular emotions (e.g., fleeing, in the case of fear).

Levenson and colleagues' work sparked a flurry of research on emotion-specific autonomic patterning, which has been reviewed by numerous researchers (e.g., Wagner, 1989). Different reviewers, however, have come to strikingly different conclusions (e.g., Levenson, 1992; Zajonc & McIntosh, 1992). Levenson contended that the literature provided compelling evidence for emotion-specific autonomic responding. For instance, he reviewed evidence that sadness is associated with greater heart rate acceleration than anger and fear, which are both associated with greater acceleration than happiness. Disgust, on the other hand, is associated with heart rate decelerations. Zajonc and McIntosh, however, contended that the evidence for emotion-specific autonomic responding was inconsistent at best.

In an attempt to resolve the debate, we (Cacioppo, Berntson, Klein, & Poehlmann, 1997; Cacioppo, Berntson, Larsen, Poehlmann, & Ito, 2000) conducted meta-analyses of all published studies comparing the effects of at least two discrete emotions on at least two autonomic measures. Though meta-analyses allow one to examine statistically the differentiation of discrete emotions by individual measures, it is possible that discrete emotions differ in terms of the patterns of autonomic responses, even if they do not differ in terms of each isolated autonomic response. Nonetheless, the literature contains claims that emotions can be differentiated with individual autonomic measures, and such hypotheses can be rigorously tested with meta-analysis.

The results of our (Cacioppo et al., 2000) meta-analysis were consistent with some of Levenson's (1992) claims. For instance, anger, fear, and sadness were associated with greater heart rate acceleration than disgust. Anger was also associated with higher diastolic blood pressure than fear, and disgust was associated with larger increases in skin conductance level than happiness. Other claims were not supported. For instance, fear was not associated with larger decreases in finger temperature than control conditions, nor was fear associated with larger increases in skin conductance level. Several other reliable results emerged from our (Cacioppo et al., 2000) meta-analyses. In addition to being associated with higher diastolic blood pressure than fear, anger was associated with more nonspecific skin conductance responses, smaller heart rate acceleration, smaller increases in stroke volume and cardiac output, and larger increases in total peripheral resistance, facial temperature, and finger pulse volume than fear. Thus anger appears to be more strongly associated with vascular activity than is fear, but less strongly associated with cardiac activity.

Only a handful of studies were available for many of our (Cacioppo et al., 2000) comparisons, so these results should only be accepted tentatively and may need to be revisited, pending more recent and future research. For instance, we found that anger was associated with greater total peripheral resistance and more nonspecific skin conductance responses than fear, but only a few previous studies had examined these relationships. Thus it is not especially surprising that whereas Pauls and Stemmler (2003) more recently found that anger was associated with greater total peripheral resistance, they also found that anger was associated with *fewer* skin conductance responses than fear. By way of comparison, Pauls and Stemmler's results corroborated our finding that fear was associated with larger increases in heart rate, which was based on 15 studies. Recent and future research will also allow meta-analytic comparisons that Cacioppo et al. (2000) were unable to complete because the necessary data were simply unavailable. Britton, Taylor, Berridge, Mikels, and Iberzon (2006), for instance, measured participants' heart rate and skin conductance as they watched films that elicited happiness, sadness, and disgust. They found that disgust was associated with greater skin conductance than sadness—a comparison that no studies in our database had reported.

As a research literature develops, meta-analysis becomes especially useful for identifying moderator variables. Several narrative reviews (e.g., Zajonc & McIntosh, 1992) have noted that different emotion inductions appear to elicit different autonomic patterns. Skin resistance level, for instance, declines more during sadness than during other negative emotions (e.g., anger) when emotions are induced with imagery tasks; these patterns are not obtained, however, when emotions are induced with facial action tasks (Ekman et al., 1983). Similarly, whereas Cacioppo et al. (2000) found that fear is associated with greater heart rate increases than anger, Labouvie-Vief, Lumley, Jain, and Heinze (2003) found that imagery-induced fear and anger elicited comparably large increases in heart rate. As it turns out, Labouvie-Vief et al.'s null effect is consistent with the results of a more recent meta-analysis by Stemmler (2004) that focused exclusively on the autonomic differentiation of fear and anger. Stemmler's meta-analysis revealed that whereas "real-life" fear inductions (e.g., unanticipated sudden darkness after hearing a frightening short story; Stemmler, 1989) elicited larger heart rate increases than real-life anger inductions (e.g., an experimenter's aggressive demands; Pauls & Stemmler, 2003), fear imagery elicited no larger heart rate increases than anger imagery. Stemmler's (2004) meta-analysis revealed the opposite pattern for diastolic blood pressure: Fear imagery elicited larger increases than anger imagery, but real-life fear elicited no larger increases than real-life anger. Moreover, whereas sadness is typically associated with increased heart rate, sad music seems to decrease heart rate (Etzel, Johnsen, Dickerson, Tranel, & Adolphs, 2006; Krumhansl, 1997). Such intriguing findings are problematic for the notion of *emotion*-specific patterning (e.g., Cacioppo et al., 1997; Zajonc & McIntosh, 1992).

Lang, Bradley, and Cuthbert's (1990; see also Bradley, 2000) distinction between "strategic" and "tactical" aspects of emotions may help explain the limited evidence for emotion-specific patterning. Tactics are the specific, context-bound patterns of action aimed at achieving narrow goals. The same discrete emotion may call for different tactics in different situations. Lang et al. (1990), for instance, note that the behaviors associated with fear can range from freezing to vigilance to flight, all of which pose different metabolic demands. Such tactical variability may account in part for the limited evidence of emotion-specific autonomic patterning (Zajonc & McIntosh, 1992).

In contrast to tactics, strategies direct actions aimed at achieving broad end goals. Securing appetitive stimuli (e.g., food) and avoiding aversive stimuli (e.g., predators), for instance, represent strategic aspects of emotion (Lang et al., 1990). The ability of the autonomic nervous system to mobilize metabolic resources in response to hostile and hospitable stimuli is crucial to survival, so valence-specific patterning may be more pronounced than emotion-specific patterning. Among the ways in which negative and positive affective processes appear to differ, for instance, is the tendency for the change in negative motivational output to be larger than the change in positive motivational output per unit of activation. Though subject to contextual factors (e.g., Smith et al., 2006), this "negativity bias" (Cacioppo & Berntson, 1994; Cacioppo, Larsen, Smith, & Berntson, 2004) has been observed in animal learning (Miller, 1961), risky decision making (Kahneman & Tversky, 1979), human affective judgments (Ito, Cacioppo, & Lang, 1998), and event-related brain potentials to affective stimuli (Ito, Larsen, Smith, & Cacioppo, 1998; Smith, Cacioppo, Larsen, & Chartrand, 2003).

A variety of theoretical and empirical work suggests that, *ceteris paribus*, negative emotions may also elicit greater autonomic activity than positive emotions (e.g., Taylor, 1991). To examine this hypothesis further, we (Cacioppo et al., 2000) conducted additional meta-analyses of autonomic activity in response to all negative emotions combined compared with all positive emotions combined. Diastolic blood pressure, blood volume, cardiac output, left ventricular ejection time, preejection period, pulse transit time, and heart rate all showed significantly greater activation during negative than positive emotions, and no autonomic responses showed the opposite pattern. Thus, whereas Cacioppo et al.'s (2000) meta-analyses indicated that even a limited set of discrete emotions such as happiness, sadness, fear, anger, and disgust could not be fully differentiated by visceral activity alone, they also indicated that negative emotions are associated with stronger autonomic responses than are positive emotions.

Of course, Cacioppo et al.'s (1997, 2000) meta-analyses are mute with respect to the enduring theoretical question of whether autonomic activity contributes to or follows from emotional experience. At first glance, the debate between James (1884) and Cannon (1927) presupposes the existence of a single invariant relationship between emotional experience and peripheral physiological activity. Overlooked is the fact that James actually viewed emotions as being multiply determined. At the outset, James (1884) stated that "the only emotions I propose expressly to consider here are those that have a distinct bodily expression" (p. 189). Thus, in addition to contending that peripheral patterns can produce emotions in a bottom-up fashion, he acknowledged that emotional experiences are sometimes governed by top-down processes that fail to produce somatovisceral activity (Ellsworth, 1994). Along these lines, one neurobiological model delineates the reciprocal relations between ascending and descending systems that may contribute to anxiety (Berntson, Sarter, & Cacioppo, 1998). This model contends that affective states may be primed by top-down processes (e.g., appraisals) or bottom-up processes (e.g., visceral reactivity), and that the top-down and bottom-up mechanisms may mutually reinforce one another (e.g., as in panic disorder).

We (Cacioppo, Berntson, & Klein, 1992) provided a general framework for conceptualizing the multiple pathways by which peripheral activity may shape emotional experience. At one end of the continuum, discrete emotional experiences result from the apperception of distinct somatovisceral patterns (e.g., Ekman et al., 1983; James, 1884; Levenson, 1988; Levenson et al., 1990). At the other end of the continuum, attributional processes instigated by the perception of undifferentiated physiological arousal generate discrete emotional experiences (e.g., Mandler, 1975; Schachter & Singer, 1962). Falling between these extremes is yet another process by which peripheral bodily reactions may contribute to emotional experience. By this account, "somatovisceral illusions" represent the result of an active perceptual process by which ambiguous patterns of somatovisceral afference are immediately and spontaneously disambiguated to produce distinct emotional experiences.

The essential feature of the proposition that discrete emotions may result from somatovisceral illusions can be illustrated by analogy, using the ambiguous visual figure depicted in Figure 11.1 (see Cacioppo, Berntson, et al., 1992, for a more complete description of the model). Even though the figure itself is unchanging, top-down processes allow viewers to perceive two very different images: a young

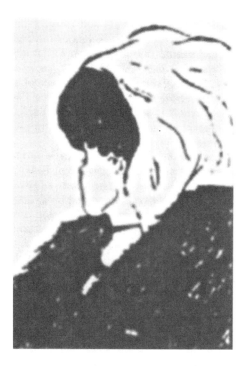

FIGURE 11.1. This ambiguous figure is called "My wife and mother-in-law" and is constructed from overlapping unambiguous elements. The perceptual system tends to group like or related information together. Rather than presenting some odd mixture of the two alternative pictures, partial identification of a young woman or an old woman in this figure supports a stable perception of a single coherent image. The identification of wholes and of parts is reciprocally supportive, contributing further to the locking-in process. A shift in gaze is not necessary for a perceptual change to occur. In what may be analogous to discrete emotional feelings' being spawned by the same ambiguous pattern of somatovisceral information, ambiguous visual figures demonstrate that discrete images can derive from the same ambiguous pattern of visual information. From Boring (1930).

woman facing left or an elderly woman facing right (Leeper, 1935). Thus the same visual afference can lead to two different, discrete, and indubitable perceptual experiences, just as Schachter and Singer (1962) argued that the same physiological afference may lead to two different, discrete, and indubitable emotional experiences. Indeed, the architecture of the somatovisceral apparatus may be better suited to produce ambiguous afference than that of the visual system (Reed, Harver, & Katkin, 1990). For instance, in the perception of ambiguous visual figures, the stimulus is a visual array outside the body. In contrast, the central nervous system serves both to create and to interpret the stimulus and the response to somatovisceral information.

Cacioppo, Berntson, et al.'s (1992) model argues against the tendency to view the psychophysiological mechanisms underlying emotion in terms of a simple central–peripheral dichotomy. It is also in accord with robust findings in the literature that discrete emotional percepts can occur even when the autonomic changes do not fully discriminate the emotions that are experienced, and that autonomic activation can alter the intensity, if not the nature, of emotional experience. From this perspective, the question is not whether emotion-specific autonomic patterns occur, but under what conditions such patterns occur. We have emphasized visceral contributions to emotional experience to this point, but, like Tomkins (1962), Cacioppo, Berntson, et al. (1992) also suggested that somatic processes can also affect emotional experience. In an ingenious test of this hypothesis, Strack, Martin, and Stepper (1988) reported that participants who had unknowingly been induced to smile found comic strips funnier than participants in a control condition. In the next section we examine the relationships between emotion and somatic activity, particularly facial expressions.

The Somatic Nervous System

Scientific studies of the link between facial expressions and emotions originated with Darwin (1890/1989), who noted, for instance, that among grief-stricken individuals, "the eyelids droop; . . . the lips, cheeks, and lower jaw all sink downwards from their own weight. Hence all the features are lengthened; and the face of a person who hears bad news is said to fall" (p. 134). Investigators have since provided provocative evidence that each of at least a subset of discrete emotions is associated with distinct overt facial expressions (Ekman, 1973). Additional evidence suggest that congenitally blind individuals, members of non-Western cultures, and infants make emotional facial expressions similar to those of sighted Western adults, thereby raising the possibility that emotion-specific facial expressions are not merely the product of social learning (e.g., see Ekman, 1973; Ekman & Friesen, 1978; Izard, 1977).

Although facial expressions may often reveal the nature of underlying emotions, many emotional reactions are not accompanied by visible facial actions (Cacioppo & Petty, 1981). Furthermore, although there is evidence that observers across cultures recognize the facial expressions of happiness, sadness, fear, anger, surprise, and disgust (Ekman, 1973), the data are open to alternative interpretations (Russell, 1994). In addition, individuals can invoke display rules to mask or hide the emotion they are feeling, and observers can confuse the meaning of expressions (e.g., fear and surprise; Ekman, 1973; but see Cacioppo, Bush, & Tassinary, 1992). As a result, the coding of overt facial expressions can be a less than perfect measure of emotion. An important complement to visual inspection of facial expression has been the measurement of patterns of electrical activity associated with contraction of the facial muscles. This technique—facial electromyography (EMG)—has made it possible to index muscle activity even in the absence of visible facial expressions (Cacioppo & Petty, 1981; Cacioppo, Tassinary, & Fridlund, 1990).

In pioneering research, Schwartz and colleagues demonstrated that different types of emotional imagery can elicit different patterns of EMG activity over the brow (*corrugator supercilii*), cheek (*zygomaticus major*), and perioral (*depressor anguli oris*) muscle regions. Schwartz, Fair, Salt, Mandel, and Klerman (1976), for instance, asked participants to imagine positive or negative events in their lives. Results revealed that sad imagery elicited more EMG activity over the brow and less activity over the cheek than happy imagery. Thus facial EMG patterns associated with emotional states appeared to represent "miniature representations" of those occurring during overt facial expressions (Schwartz, Fair, Greenberg, Foran, & Klerman, 1975). Subsequent research has examined whether the facial EMG patterns observed by Schwartz et al. (1975, 1976) with

emotional imagery tasks generalize to other types of emotion inductions. Hess, Banse, and Kappas (1995), for instance, found that humorous films elicited greater activity over *zygomaticus major* and *orbicularis oculi*, particularly when participants were accompanied by friends. Patterns similar to those obtained with emotional imagery and films have also been obtained with emotional pictures (Cacioppo, Petty, Losch, & Kim, 1986; Lang, Greenwald, Bradley, & Hamm, 1993; Larsen, Norris, & Cacioppo, 2003) and sounds (Bradley & Lang, 2000b; Larsen et al., 2003).

More recent research also indicates that affective stimuli can automatically elicit facial EMG reactions. Neumann, Hess, Schulz, and Alpers (2005) instructed participants to smile or frown whenever a word appeared on the screen. Facial EMG recordings indicated that participants smiled more quickly when pleasant words appeared and frowned more quickly when unpleasant words appeared. Dimberg, Thunberg, and Elmehed (2000) exposed participants to backwardly masked pictures of angry and happy faces for a mere 30 milliseconds. Results indicated that subliminal happy faces elicited more activity over *zygomaticus major* and less activity over *corrugator supercilii* than did angry faces. Taken together, these results indicate that facial reactions to affective stimuli occur spontaneously (Neumann et al., 2005), even when the eliciting stimulus is presented outside of awareness (Dimberg et al., 2000). An unresolved issue is whether the facial EMG patterns observed by Dimberg et al. (2000) reflect emotional reactions or mere mimicry (cf. Hess, Philippot, & Blairy, 1998). In any event, such mimicry may reflect the operation of circuitry involving mirror neurons in the prefrontal cortex, which fire not only when an individual performs some action (e.g., smiling; Leslie, Johnson-Frey, & Grafton, 2004), but also when the individual observes someone else performing that action.

Though most research has investigated the effects of valence on EMG activity, some research has focused on discrete emotions. Schwartz, Ahern, and Brown (1979) asked subjects to engage in thought and imagery tasks that involved happiness, excitement, sadness, fear, and neutral emotional states. The only significant main effects for discrete emotional states indicated higher EMG activity over the cheek and lower EMG activity over the brow during positive than negative emotions. In a similar study by Brown and Schwartz (1980), fear, anger, and sadness imagery elicited greater activity over the brow than did happiness imagery. Happiness imagery elicited the most activity over the cheek, but fear and anger also elicited elevations over the cheek. Whether these latter elevations reflect "miserable smiles" (Ekman, Friesen, & Ancoli, 1980), cross-talk from other muscles of the middle and lower facial regions, or the putative phylogenetic origin of smiling and laughter in primitive agonistic displays (Andrew, 1963; van Hooff, 1972) is unclear. More recently, Vrana (1993) found that disgust and anger imagery elicited similar levels of activity over the brow and that disgust imagery also elicited greater activity over the *levator labii*, which elevates the upper lip and wrinkles the nose. Thus the literature provides some evidence for distinct covert facial expressions associated with some emotions, but a great deal more evidence for distinct covert facial expressions associated with broad positive and negative affective states (Cacioppo et al., 2000).

THE CENTRAL NERVOUS SYSTEM

EMG activity reflects the end result of central nervous system activity and can therefore shed some light on central processes involved in emotion. Early research by Schwartz et al. (1979) suggested that negative and positive emotional imagery elicited greater activity over the right and left sides of the face, respectively. The facial musculature is to some extent contralaterally innervated, so Schwartz et al.'s findings are consistent with neuropsychological evidence suggesting that the left and right hemispheres are differentially involved in negative and positive emotional processing, respectively (Robinson & Downhill, 1995). Whereas left anterior brain lesions are more likely to produce major depression, for instance, right anterior brain lesions are more likely to produce mania. Subsequent research, however, has provided limited evidence for asymmetries in EMG responses (Hager & Ekman, 1985).

Unlike EMG activity, EEG activity directly reflects central nervous system activity and has therefore been more useful in exploring the hemispheric specialization of emotion. Much of this work has focused on measurement of EEG power in the alpha band (8–13 Hz), which is in-

versely related to hemispheric activity (Lindsley & Wicke, 1974). A variety of EEG evidence has corroborated the neuropsychological evidence that the right hemisphere is more strongly associated with negative affect and the left hemisphere with positive affect. For instance, those with greater relative left frontal activity tend to report higher levels of subjective well-being (Urry et al., 2004) and dispositional behavioral activation (Coan & Allen, 2003; Sutton & Davidson, 1997). Earlier in life, toddlers with greater relative left frontal activity tend to be less behaviorally inhibited (Davidson, 1993).

Davidson (1993, 2003) has integrated these and other findings into a diathesis–stress model linking individual differences in anterior cortical asymmetry to dispositional affective tendencies. According to this model, differences in cerebral asymmetry have greater impact on affective reactions to stressors and other challenges than on baseline affect (e.g., Davidson, 1993; Davidson & Tomarken, 1989). Consistent with the diathesis–stress model, participants with greater relative left frontal asymmetry reported stronger positive affective reactions to pleasant film clips and weaker negative affective reactions to unpleasant film clips, but did not differ from those with greater relative right frontal asymmetry in terms of baseline mood (Tomarken, Davidson, & Henriques, 1990; see also Wheeler, Davidson, & Tomarken, 1993). Similarly, infants who cried when their mother left the room had greater relative right-hemisphere activity prior to the separation (Davidson & Fox, 1989). Some evidence also suggests that those with greater relative left frontal activity experience shorter bouts of negative affect in response to unpleasant pictures (Jackson et al., 2003).

To this point, EEG asymmetry has been related to differences in affective traits, but there is also substantial state-dependent variance in EEG asymmetry (Hagemann, Naumann, Thayer, & Bartussek, 2002), and some of that that variance may be due to differences in affective states. Davidson, Ekman, Saron, Senulis, and Friesen (1990) recorded EEG during a variety of evocative film clips. Participants showed greater relative left frontal activation during those moments when they displayed facial expressions of happiness than when they displayed facial expressions of disgust. Analyses conducted across all artifact-free EEG data (i.e., including those times in which a facial expression was not present) failed to reveal an effect of film valence on EEG asymmetry. Thus it may be that only emotional experiences strong enough to produce overt facial expressions are associated with measurable hemispheric asymmetry.

Recent research has clarified whether frontal activity better reflects approach- and avoidance-related behavioral motivation or positive and negative affective valence. Motivation and valence tend to be correlated, such that positive emotions are associated with approach and negative emotions with avoidance. An interesting exception is anger, which is a negative emotion that is associated with approach motivation. Harmon-Jones and Allen (1998) found that those who tend to experience anger show grater relative left frontal, as opposed to right frontal, activity. Similarly, anger induced with facial action tasks is associated with greater relative left frontal activation (Coan, Allen, & Harmon-Jones, 2001). Such findings indicate that frontal activity reflects approach–withdrawal motivation more than it does positive–negative valence (Harmon-Jones, 2003).

Early conceptualizations of EEG asymmetry focused on the relative difference between activity in the left and right hemispheres. In light of neurophysiological and psychological evidence for separable approach- and avoidance-related motivational systems (e.g., Cacioppo & Berntson, 1994; Larsen et al., 2001), current conceptualizations explicitly link activity in the left hemisphere with approach motivation and activity in the right hemisphere with avoidance motivation. Individuals with depression or a history of depression show less left anterior activity than comparison participants, but do not differ in right anterior activity (Henriques & Davidson, 1990, 1991). These findings suggest that depression reflects hypoactive approach motivation rather than hyperactive avoidance motivation (Henriques & Davidson, 1990, 1991). More recently, Schmidt (1999) extended prior evidence that shyness and sociability are separable by demonstrating that women who report high levels of shyness and sociability show greater right and left frontal activity. Schmidt's findings, in particular, highlight the utility of considering left and right frontal activity separately. Indeed, difference scores would have failed to disambiguate individuals who are both shy and sociable from those who are neither shy nor sociable.

EPILOGUE

As the varied perspectives represented in this volume suggest, a comprehensive understanding of emotions must encompass a wide range of viewpoints. One of the more interesting questions concerning the psychophysiology of emotions in particular is the role of somatovisceral afference in emotional experience. Although it appears that negative emotions are associated with greater autonomic reactivity than positive emotions, the cumulative evidence for emotion-specific patterns remains inconclusive. In addition, facial EMG activity over the cheek (*zygomaticus major*) and periocular (*orbicularis oculi*) muscle regions increase with positivity, whereas EMG activity over the brow (*corrugator supercilii*) muscle region increases with negativity and decreases with positivity; research on EEG asymmetries similarly suggests that anterior brain regions are differentially involved in approach-related versus avoidance-related behavioral processes. Thus EEG activity can differentiate approach- and avoidance-related negative emotions such as anger and fear, respectively.

As detailed above, the patterns of autonomic activity associated with emotion have not been thoroughly delineated. Among the obstacles to identifying emotion-specific autonomic patterns, particularly for dually and antagonistically innervated organs such as the heart, are the multiple causal pathways connecting neural changes and end-organ response (e.g., heart rate). Emotional stimuli do not invariably evoke reciprocal activation of the sympathetic and parasympathetic branches of the autonomic nervous system. For instance, aversive conditioned stimuli can produce coactivation of the sympathetic and parasympathetic branches system, yielding accelerated, decelerated, or even unchanged heart rate, depending on the relative strength of sympathetic versus parasympathetic activation (see Berntson, Cacioppo, & Quigley, 1991). Rainville, Bechara, Naqvi, and Damasio (2006) recently provided initial evidence that measures of sympathetic and parasympathetic activity can differentiate discrete emotions even when end-organ responses cannot. Heart rate increased during both anger and fear imagery in their study, but spectral analyses of heart rate variability indicated that the effect of anger imagery was mediated by sympathetic activation and the effect of fear imagery by parasympathetic deactivation. Whether Rainville et al.'s findings will be replicated with larger samples, different types of emotion inductions (cf. Stemmler, 2004), and different discrete emotions remains to be seen.

Whether or not the conditions for and elements of emotion-specific peripheral patterns of activity can be identified, what does seem clear from the extant research is that discrete emotions can be experienced even in the absence of completely differentiated autonomic patterns. Though Cannon (1927) took this as evidence that somatovisceral afference has no influence on the experience of emotion, we (Cacioppo, Berntson, et al., 1992) outlined three routes by which somatovisceral afferentiation may influence emotional experience: emotion-specific autonomic patterns, somatovisceral illusions, or cognitive labeling of unexplained physiological arousal. From this perspective, the traditional tendency to view the mechanisms underlying emotion in terms of a simple central–peripheral dichotomy is untenable.

Emotions, particularly negative emotions, have also been linked to increases in health problems, including an enhanced susceptibility to infection (e.g., Cohen, Doyle, Turner, Alper, & Skoner, 2003; see review by Herbert & Cohen, 1993), poorer response to an influenza vaccine (Kiecolt-Glaser, Glaser, Gravenstein, Malarkey, & Sheridan, 1996), and impaired wound healing (Kiecolt-Glaser, Marucha, Malarkey, Mercado, & Glaser, 1995). Mediators of the relationship between emotion and health have not yet been fully delineated, but several mechanisms are likely to be involved, some of which imply autonomic differentiation of positive from negative affective states. Health problems increase with aging as well, with negative emotions augmenting age-related declines in health and well-being (e.g., Kiecolt-Glaser, Dura, Speicher, Trask, & Glaser, 1991), and positive emotions having less impact (Ewart, Taylor, Kraemer, & Agras, 1991).

Studies of the psychophysiology of emotion have tended to treat autonomic, somatic, and central nervous system activity in isolation (cf. Davidson et al., 1990; Mauss et al., 2005). Recent work highlights the utility of studying the relationships among these systems and related systems (e.g., the immune system). In a recent study investigating autonomic and immune responses to stress, for instance, individuals who responded to an experimenter's demands with fear, as assessed by facial action coding, showed greater cardiovascular and cortisol reactivity than did those who responded with a combination of anger and disgust (Lerner, Gonzalez, Dahl, Hariri, & Taylor, 2005). In another study Waldstein et al. (2000) found that those who showed greater left frontal EEG activation during anger inductions also showed greater cardiovascular activation. Hagemann, Waldstein, and Thayer (2003) have incorporated such findings into a model that integrates the roles of the central nervous system and autonomic nervous systems in emotion. Hagemann et al.'s (2003) model relied in part on evidence from positron emission tomography (PET) and functional magnetic resonance imaging (fMRI), which now allow psychophysiologists to visualize the human brain during emotional episodes with tremendous spatial resolution (Wager et al., Chapter 15, this volume). One must bear in mind, however, that PET and fMRI have limited temporal resolution, because they rely on relatively gradual changes in blood flow through the brain. Emotional reactions tend to be fleeting (Ekman, 1994), so a useful approach may be to conduct studies combining fMRI data with traditional psychophysiological recordings, many of which offer superior temporal resolution (e.g., Critchley et al., 2003). In the years to come, such integrative approaches promise to yield ever clearer insights into the physiological substrates of emotion.

REFERENCES

Andrew, R. J. (1963). The origin and evolution of the calls and facial expressions of the primates. *Behaviour, 20*, 1–109.

Barrett, L. F. (2006). Solving the emotion paradox: Categorization and the experience of emotion. *Personality and Social Psychology Review, 10*, 20–46.

Barrett, L. F., Quigley, K. S., Bliss-Moreau, E., & Aronson, K. R. (2004). Interoceptive sensitivity and self-reports of emotional experience. *Journal of Personality and Social Psychology, 87*, 684–697.

Berntson, G. G., Cacioppo, J. T., & Quigley, K. S. (1991). Autonomic determinism: The modes of autonomic control, the doctrine of autonomic space, and the laws of autonomic constraint. *Psychological Review, 98*, 459–487.

Berntson, G. G., Sarter, M., & Cacioppo, J. T. (1998).

Anxiety and cardiovascular reactivity: The basal forebrain cholinergic link. *Behavioural Brain Research*, 94, 225–248.

Boring, E. G. (1930). A new ambiguous figure. *American Journal of Psychology*, 42, 444.

Bradley, M. M. (2000). Emotion and motivation. In J. T. Cacioppo, L. G. Tassinary, & G. G. Berntson (Eds.), *Handbook of psychophysiology* (2nd ed., pp. 602–641). New York: Cambridge University Press.

Bradley, M. M., & Lang, P. J. (2000a). Measuring emotion: Behavior, feeling, and physiology. In R. D. Lane & L. Nadel (Eds.), *Cognitive neuroscience of emotion* (pp. 242–276). New York: Oxford University Press.

Bradley, M. M., & Lang, P. J. (2000b). Affective reactions to acoustic stimuli. *Psychophysiology*, 37, 204–215.

Britton, J. C., Taylor, S., F., Berridge, K. C., Mikels, J. A., & Liberzon, I. (2006). Differential subjective and psychophysiological responses to socially and nonsocially generated emotional stimuli. *Emotion*, 6, 150–155.

Brown, S. L., & Schwartz, G. E. (1980). Relationships between facial electromyography and subjective experience during affective imagery. *Biological Psychology*, 11, 49–62.

Cacioppo, J. T., & Berntson, G. G. (1994). Relationship between attitudes and evaluative space: A critical review, with emphasis on the separability of positive and negative substrates. *Psychological Bulletin*, 115, 401–423.

Cacioppo, J. T., Berntson, G. G., & Klein, D. J. (1992). What is an emotion?: The role of somatovisceral afference, with special emphasis on somatovisceral "illusions." *Review of Personality and Social Psychology*, 14, 63–98.

Cacioppo, J. T., Berntson, G. G., Klein, D. J., & Poehlmann, K. M. (1997). The psychophysiology of emotion across the lifespan. *Annual Review of Gerontology and Geriatrics*, 17, 27–74.

Cacioppo, J. T., Berntson, G. G., Larsen, J. T., Poehlmann, K. M., & Ito, T. A. (2000). The psychophysiology of emotion. In M. Lewis & J. M. Haviland-Jones (Eds.), *Handbook of emotions* (2nd ed., pp. 173–191). New York: Guilford Press.

Cacioppo, J. T., Bush, L. K., & Tassinary, L. G. (1992). Microexpressive facial actions as a function of affective stimuli: Replication and extension. *Personality and Social Psychology Bulletin*, 18, 515–526.

Cacioppo, J. T., Gardner, W. L., & Berntson, G. G. (1999). The affect system: Form follows function. *Journal of Personality and Social Psychology*, 76, 839–855.

Cacioppo, J. T., Larsen, J. T., Smith, N. K., & Berntson, G. G. (2004). The affect system: What lurks below the surface of feelings? In A. S. R. Manstead, N. H. Frijda, & A. H. Fischer (Eds.), *Feelings and emotions: The Amsterdam Conference* (pp. 223–242). New York: Cambridge University Press.

Cacioppo, J. T., & Petty, R. E. (1981). Electromyograms as measures of extent and affectivity of information processing. *American Psychologist*, 36, 441–456.

Cacioppo, J. T., & Petty, R. E. (1986). Stalking rudimentary processes of social influence: A psychophysiological approach. In M. P. Zanna, J. M. Olson, & C. P. Herman (Eds.), *Social influence: The Ontario Symposium* (Vol. 5, pp. 41–74). Hillsdale, NJ: Erlbaum.

Cacioppo, J. T., & Petty, R. E. (1987). Stalking rudimentary processes of social influence: A psychophysiological approach. In M. P. Zanna, J. M. Olson, & C. P. Herman (Eds.), *Social influence: The Ontario Symposium* (Vol. 5, pp. 41–74). Hillsdale, NJ: Erlbaum.

Cacioppo, J. T., Petty, R. E., Losch, M. E., & Kim, H. S. (1986). Electromyographic activity over facial muscle regions can differentiate the valence and intensity of affective reactions. *Journal of Personality and Social Psychology*, 50, 260–268.

Cacioppo, J. T., Tassinary, L. G., & Berntson, G. G. (Eds.). (2007). *Handbook of psychophysiology* (3rd ed.). New York: Cambridge University Press.

Cacioppo, J. T., Tassinary, L. G., & Fridlund, A. J. (1990). The skeletomotor system. In J. T. Cacioppo & L. G. Tassinary (Eds.), *Principles of psychophysiology: Physical, social, and inferential elements* (pp. 325–384). New York: Cambridge University Press.

Cannon, W. B. (1927). The James–Lange theory of emotions: A critical examination and an alternative theory. *American Journal of Psychology*, 39, 106–124.

Chwalisz, K., Diener, E., & Gallagher, D. (1988). Autonomic arousal feedback and emotional experience: Evidence from the spinal cord injured. *Journal of Personality and Social Psychology*, 54, 820–828.

Clore, G. L., Ortony, A., & Foss, M. A. (1987). The psychological foundations of the affective lexicon. *Journal of Personality and Social Psychology*, 53, 751–766.

Coan, J. A., & Allen, J. J. B. (2003). Frontal EEG asymmetry and the behavioral activation and inhibition systems. *Psychophysiology*, 40, 106–114.

Coan, J. A., Allen, J. J. B., & Harmon-Jones, E. (2001). Voluntary facial expression and hemispheric asymmetry over the frontal cortex. *Psychophysiology*, 38, 912–925.

Cobos, P., Sánchez, M., Garcia, C., Vera, M. N., & Vila, I. (2002). Revisiting the James versus Cannon debate on emotion: Startle and autonomic modulation in patients with spinal cord injuries. *Biological Psychology*, 61, 251–269.

Cohen, S., Doyle, W. J., Turner, R. B., Alper, C. M., & Skoner, D. P. (2003). Emotional style and susceptibility to the common cold. *Psychosomatic Medicine*, 65, 652–657.

Coles, M. G. H., Donchin, E., & Porges, S. W. (Eds.). (1986). *Psychophysiology: Systems, processes, and applications*. New York: Guilford Press.

Critchley, H. D., Mathias, C. J., Josephs, O., O'Doherty,

J., Zanini, S., Dewar, B., et al. (2003). Human cingulate cortex and autonomic control: Converging neuroimaging and clinical evidence. *Brain*, *126*, 2139–2152.

Critchley, H. D., Wiens, S., Rotshtein, P., Öhman, A., & Dolan, R. J. (2004). Neural systems supporting interoceptive awareness. *Nature Neuroscience*, *3*, 1049–1056.

Damasio, A. R. (1994). *Descartes' error: Emotion, reason, and the human brain.* New York: Putnam.

Darwin, C. (1989). *The expression of emotions in man and animals* (2nd ed.). New York: New York University Press. (Original work published 1890)

Davidson, R. J. (1993). Childhood temperament and cerebral asymmetry: A neurobiological substrate of behavioral inhibition. In K. H. Rubin & J. B. Asendorpf (Eds.), *Social withdrawal, inhibition, and shyness in childhood* (pp. 31–48). Hillsdale, NJ: Erlbaum.

Davidson, R. J. (2003). Affective neuroscience and psychophysiology: Toward a synthesis. *Psychophysiology*, *40*, 655–665.

Davidson, R. J., Ekman, P., Saron, C. D., Senulis, J. A., & Friesen, W. V. (1990). Approach–withdrawal and cerebral asymmetry: Emotional expression and brain physiology I. *Journal of Personality and Social Psychology*, *58*, 330–341.

Davidson, R. J., & Fox, N. A. (1989). Frontal brain asymmetry predicts infants' response to maternal separation. *Journal of Abnormal Psychology*, *98*, 127–131.

Davidson, R. J., & Tomarken, A.J. (1989). Laterality and emotion: An electrophysiological approach. In F. Boller & J. Grafman (Eds.), *Handbook of neuropsychology* (Vol. 3, pp. 419–441). New York: Elsevier.

DePaulo, B. M., Lindsay, J. J., Malone, B. E., Muhlenbruck, L., Charlton, K., & Cooper, H. (2003). Cues to deception. *Psychological Bulletin*, *129*, 74–112.

Dimberg, U., Thunberg, M., & Elmehed, K. (2000). Unconscious facial reactions to emotional facial expressions. *Psychological Science*, *11*, 86–89.

Eagly, A. H., & Chaiken, S. (1993). *The psychology of attitudes.* Orlando, FL: Harcourt Brace Jovanovich.

Ekman, P. (1973). Cross-cultural studies of facial expression. In P. Ekman (Ed.), *Darwin and facial expression: A century of research in review* (pp. 1–83). New York: Academic Press.

Ekman, P. (1994). Moods, emotions, and traits. In P. Ekman & R. J. Davidson (Eds.), *The nature of emotion* (pp. 56–58). New York: Oxford University Press.

Ekman, P., & Friesen, W. V. (1978). *The Facial Action Coding System: A technique for the measurement of facial movement.* Palo Alto, CA: Consulting Psychologists Press.

Ekman, P., Friesen, W. V., & Ancoli, S. (1980). Facial signs of emotional experience. *Journal of Personality and Social Psychology*, *39*, 1125–1134.

Ekman, P., Levenson, R. W., & Friesen, W. V. (1983). Autonomic nervous system activity distinguishes among emotions. *Science*, *221*, 1208–1210.

Ellsworth, P. C. (1994). William James and emotion: Is a century of fame worth a century of misunderstanding? *Psychological Review*, *101*, 222–229.

Etzel, J. A., Johnsen, E. L., Dickerson, J., Tranel, D., & Adolphs, R. (2006). Cardiovascular and respiratory responses during musical mood induction. *International Journal of Psychophysiology*, *61*, 57–69.

Ewart, C. K., Taylor, C. B., Kraemer, H. C., & Agras, W. S. (1991). High blood pressure and marital discord: Not being nasty matters more than being nice. *Health Psychology*, *10*, 155–163.

Fainsilber, L., & Ortony, A. (1987). Metaphorical uses of language in the expression of emotions. *Metaphor and Symbolic Activity*, *2*, 239–250.

Frijda, N. H. (1986). *The emotions.* Cambridge, UK: Cambridge University Press.

Frijda, N. H. (1994). Varieties of affect: Emotions and episodes, moods, and sentiments. In P. Ekman & R. J. Davidson (Eds.), *The nature of emotion* (pp. 59–67). New York: Oxford University Press.

Gagnon, L., & Peretz, I. (2003). Mode and tempo relative contributions to "happy–sad" judgements in equitone mequitone. *Cognition and Emotion*, *17*, 25–40.

Gazzaniga, M. S., & LeDoux, J. E. (1978). *The integrated mind.* New York: Plenum Press.

Green, D. P., Salovey, P., & Truax, K. M. (1999). Static, dynamic, and causative bipolarity of affect. *Journal of Personality and Social Psychology*, *76*, 856–867.

Hagemann, D., Naumann, E., Thayer, J. F., & Bartussek, D. (2002). Does resting electroencephalograph asymmetry reflect a trait?: An application of latent state-trait theory. *Journal of Personality and Social Psychology*, *82*, 619–641.

Hagemann, D., Waldstein, S. R., & Thayer, J. F. (2003). Central and autonomic nervous system integration in emotion. *Brain and Cognition*, *52*, 79–87.

Hager, J. C., & Ekman, P. (1985). The asymmetry of facial actions is inconsistent with models of hemispheric specialization. *Psychophysiology*, *22*, 307–318.

Harmon-Jones, E. (2003). Clarifying the emotive functions of asymmetrical frontal cortical activity. *Psychophysiology*, *40*, 838–848.

Harmon-Jones, E., & Allen, J. J. B. (1998). Anger and frontal brain activity: EEG asymmetry consistent with approach motivation despite negative affective valence. *Journal of Personality and Social Psychology*, *74*, 1310–1316.

Henriques, J. B., & Davidson, R. J. (1990). Regional brain electrical asymmetries discriminate between previously depressed and healthy control subjects. *Journal of Abnormal Psychology*, *99*, 22–31.

Henriques, J. B., & Davidson, R. J. (1991). Left frontal hypoactivation in depression. *Journal of Abnormal Psychology*, *100*, 535–545.

Herbert, T. B., & Cohen, S. (1993). Depression and immunity: A meta-analytic review. *Psychological Bulletin*, *113*, 472–486.

Hess, U., Banse, R., & Kappas, A. (1995). The intensity of facial expression is determined by underlying affective state and social situation. *Journal of Personality and Social Psychology*, *69*, 280–288.

Hess, U., Philippot, P., & Blairy, S. (1998). Facial reactions to emotional facial expressions: Affect or cognition? *Cognition and Emotion*, *12*, 509–531.

Hoffman, R. R., Waggoner, J. E., & Palermo, D. S. (1991). Metaphor and context in the language of emotion. In R. R. Hoffman & D. S. Palermo (Eds.), *Cognition and the symbolic processes: Applied and ecological perspectives* (pp. 163–185). Hillsdale, NJ: Erlbaum.

Ito, T. A., Cacioppo, J. T., & Lang, P. J. (1998). Eliciting affect using the International Affective Picture System: Bivariate evaluation and ambivalence. *Personality and Social Psychology Bulletin*, *24*, 855–879.

Ito, T. A., Larsen, J. T., Smith, N. K., & Cacioppo, J. T. (1998). Negative information weighs more heavily on the brain: The negativity bias in evaluative categorizations. *Journal of Personality and Social Psychology*, *75*, 887–900.

Izard, C. E. (1977). *Human emotions*. New York: Academic Press.

Jackson, D. C., Mueller, C. J., Dolski, I., Dalton, K. M., Nitschke, J. B., Urry, H. L., et al. (2003). Now you feel it, now you don't: Frontal brain electrical asymmetry and individual differences in emotion regulation. *Psychological Science*, *14*, 612–617.

James, W. (1884). What is an emotion? *Mind*, *9*, 188–205.

James, W. (1950). *Principles of psychology* (Vol. 1). New York: Dover. (Original work published 1890)

Kahneman, D., & Tversky, A. (1979). Prospect theory: An analysis of decisions under risk. *Econometrica*, *47*, 263–291.

Kiecolt-Glaser, J. K., Dura, J. R., Speicher, C. E., Trask, O. J., & Glaser, R. G. (1991). Spousal caregivers of dementia victims: Longitudinal changes in immunity and health. *Psychosomatic Medicine*, *53*, 345–362.

Kiecolt-Glaser, J. K., Glaser, R., Gravenstein, S., Malarkey, W. B., & Sheridan, J. (1996). Chronic stress alters the immune response to influenza virus vaccine in older adults. *Proceedings of the National Academy of Sciences of the USA*, *93*, 3043–3047.

Kiecolt-Glaser, J. K., Marucha, P. T., Malarkey, W. B., Mercado, A. M., & Glaser, R. (1995). Slowing of wound healing by psychological stress. *Lancet*, *346*, 1194–1196.

Krumhansl, C. L. (1997). An exploratory study of musical emotions and psychophysiology. *Canadian Journal of Experimental Psychology*, *51*, 336–353.

Labouvie-Vief, G., Lumley, M. A., Jain, E., & Heinze, H. (2003). Age and gender differences in cardiac reactivity and subjective emotion responses to emotional autobiographical memories. *Emotion*, *3*, 115–126.

Lang, P. J. (1971). The application of psychophysiological methods to the study of psychotherapy and behavior change. In A. E. Bergin & S. L. Garfield (Eds.), *Handbook of psychotherapy and behavior change: An empirical analysis* (pp. 75–125). New York: Wiley.

Lang, P. J., Bradley, M. M., & Cuthbert, B. N. (1990). Emotion, attention, and the startle reflex. *Psychological Review*, *97*, 377–395.

Lang, P. J., Greenwald, M. K., Bradley, M. M., & Hamm, A. O. (1993). Looking at pictures: Affective, facial, visceral, and behavioral reactions. *Psychophysiology*, *30*, 261–273.

Larsen, J. T., McGraw, A. P., & Cacioppo, J. T. (2001). Can people feel happy and sad at the same time? *Journal of Personality and Social Psychology*, *81*, 684–696.

Larsen, J. T., Norris, C. J., & Cacioppo, J. T. (2003). Effects of positive affect and negative affect on electromyographic activity over zygomaticus major and corrugator supercilii. *Psychophysiology*, *40*, 776–785.

LeDoux, J. (1996). *The emotional brain*. New York: Simon & Schuster.

Leeper, R. (1935). A study of a neglected portion of the field of learning—the development of sensory organization. *Journal of Genetic Psychology*, *46*, 41–75.

Lerner, J. S., Gonzalez, R. M., Dahl, R. E., Hariri, A. R., & Taylor, S. E. (2005). Facial expressions of emotion reveal neuroendocrine and cardiovascular stress responses. *Biological Psychiatry*, *58*, 743–750.

Leslie, K. R., Johnson-Frey, S. H., & Grafton, S. T. (2004). Functional imaging of the face and hand imitation: Towards a motor theory of empathy. *NeuroImage*, *21*, 601–607.

Levenson, R. W. (1988). Emotion and the autonomic nervous system: A prospectus for research on autonomic specificity. In H. L. Wagner (Eds.), *Social psychophysiology and emotion: Theory and clinical applications* (pp. 17–42). Chichester, UK: Wiley.

Levenson, R. W. (1992). Autonomic nervous system differences among emotions. *Psychological Science*, *3*, 23–27.

Levenson, R. W., Ekman, P., & Friesen, W. V. (1990). Voluntary facial action generates emotion-specific autonomic nervous system activity. *Psychophysiology*, *27*, 363–384.

Lindsley, D. B., & Wicke, J. D. (1974). The electroencephalogram: Autonomous electrical activity in man and animals. In R. Thompson & M. N. Patterson (Eds.), *Bioelectric recording techniques* (pp. 3–79). New York: Academic Press.

Mandler, G. (1975). *Mind and emotion*. New York: Wiley.

Mauss, I. B., Levenson, R. W., McCarter, L., Wilhelm, F. H., & Gross, J. J. (2005). The tie that binds?: Coherence among emotion, experience, behavior, and physiology. *Emotion*, *5*, 175–190.

Miller, N. E. (1961). Some recent studies on conflict behavior and drugs. *American Psychologist*, *16*, 12–24.

Neumann, R., Hess, M., Schulz, S., & Alpers, G. W. (2005). Automatic behavioural responses to valence: Evidence that facial action is facilitated by evaluative processing. *Cognition and Emotion*, *19*, 499–513.

Osgood, C. E., Suci, G. J., & Tannenbaum, P. H. (1957). *The measurement of meaning*. Urbana: University of Illinois Press.

Pauls, C. A., & Stemmler, G. (2003). Repressive and defensive coping during fear and anger. *Emotion*, *3*, 284–302.

Rainville, P., Bechara, A., Naqvi, N., & Damasio, A. R. (2006). Basic emotions are associated with distinct patterns of cardiovascular reactivity. *International Journal of Psychophysiology*, *61*, 5–18.

Reed, S. D., Harver, A., & Katkin, E. S. (1990). Interoception. In J. T. Cacioppo & L. G. Tassinary (Eds.), *Principles of psychophysiology: Physical, social, and inferential elements* (pp. 253–294). New York: Cambridge University Press.

Reisenzein, R. (1983). The Schachter theory of emotion: Two decades later. *Psychological Bulletin*, *94*, 239–264.

Robinson, R. G., & Downhill, J. E. (1995). Lateralization of psychopathology in response to focal brain injury. In R. J. Davidson & K. Hugdahl (Eds.), *Brain asymmetry* (pp. 693–711). Cambridge, MA: MIT Press.

Russell, J. A. (1978). Evidence of convergent validity on the dimensions of affect. *Journal of Personality and Social Psychology*, *36*, 1152–1168.

Russell, J. A. (1980). A circumplex model of affect. *Journal of Personality and Social Psychology*, *39*, 1161–1178.

Russell, J. A. (1994). Is there universal recognition of emotion from facial expressions?: A review of the cross-cultural studies. *Psychological Bulletin*, *115*, 102–141.

Russell, J. A., & Barrett, L. F. (1999). Core affect, prototypical emotional episodes, and other things called emotion: Dissecting the elephant. *Journal of Personality and Social Psychology*, *76*, 805–819.

Russell, J. A., & Carroll, J. M. (1999). On the bipolarity of positive and negative affect. *Psychological Bulletin*, *125*, 3–30.

Schachter, S., & Singer, J. E. (1962). Cognitive, social, and physiological determinants of emotional state. *Psychological Review*, *69*, 379–399.

Scherer, K. R., Schorr, A., & Johnstone, T. (Eds.). (2001). *Appraisal processes in emotion*. New York: Oxford University Press.

Schmidt, L. A. (1999). Frontal brain electrical activity in shyness and sociability. *Psychological Science*, *10*, 316–320.

Schwartz, G. E., Ahern, G. L., & Brown, S.-L. (1979). Lateralized facial muscle response to positive and negative emotional stimuli. *Psychophysiology*, *16*, 561–571.

Schwartz, G. E., Fair, P. L., Greenberg, P. S., Foran, J. M., & Klerman, G. L. (1975). Self-generated affective imagery elicits discrete patterns of facial muscle activity. *Psychophysiology*, *12*, 234. (Abstract)

Schwartz, G. E., Fair, P. L., Salt, P., Mandel, M. R., & Klerman, G. R. (1976). Facial muscle patterning to affective imagery in depressed and nondepressed subjects. *Science*, *192*, 489–491.

Schwarz, N., & Clore, G. L. (1983). Mood, misattribution, and judgments of well-being: Informative and directive functions of affective states. *Journal of Personality and Social Psychology*, *45*, 513–523.

Smith, N. K., Cacioppo, J. T., Larsen, J. T., & Chartrand, T. L. (2003). May I have your attention, please: Electrocortical responses to positive and negative stimuli. *Neuropsychologia*, *41*, 171–183.

Smith, N. K., Larsen, J. T., Chartrand, T. L., Cacioppo, J. T., Katafiasz, H. A., & Moran, K. E. (2006). Being bad isn't always good: Evaluative context moderates the attention bias toward negative information. *Journal of Personality and Social Psychology*, *90*, 210–220.

Stein, N. L., & Levine, L. J. (1987). Thinking about feelings: The development and organization of emotional knowledge. In R. E. Snow & M. Farr (Eds.), *Aptitude, learning, and instruction: Vol. 3. Cognition, conation, and affect* (pp. 165–197). Hillsdale, NJ: Erlbaum.

Stemmler, G. (1989). The autonomic differentiation of emotions revisited: Convergent and discriminant validation. *Psychophysiology*, *26*, 617–632.

Stemmler, G. (2004). Physiological processes during emotion. In P. Phillippot & R. S. Feldman (Eds.), *The regulation of emotion* (pp. 33–70). Mahwah, NJ: Erlbaum.

Stern, R. M., Ray, W. J., & Quigley, K. S. (2001). *Psychophysiological recording*. New York: Oxford University Press.

Strack, F., Martin, L. L., & Stepper, S. (1988). Inhibiting and facilitating conditions of the human smile: A nonobtrusive test of the facial feedback hypothesis. *Journal of Personality and Social Psychology*, *54*, 768–777.

Sutton, S. K., & Davidson, R. J. (1997). Prefrontal brain asymmetry: A biological substrate of the behavioral approach and inhibition systems. *Psychological Science*, *8*, 204–210.

Taylor, S. E. (1991). Asymmetrical effects of positive and negative events: The mobilization-minimization hypothesis. *Psychological Bulletin*, *110*, 67–85.

Tomarken, A. J., Davidson, R. J., & Henriques, J. B. (1990). Resting frontal asymmetry predicts affective responses to films. *Journal of Personality and Social Psychology*, *59*, 791–801.

Tomkins, S. S. (1962). *Affect, imagery, and consciousness: Vol. 1. The positive affects*. New York: Springer.

Tranel, D., & Damasio, A. (2000). Neuropsychology

and behavioral neurology. In J. T. Cacioppo, L. G. Tassinary, & G. G. Berntson (Eds.), *Handbook of psychophysiology* (2nd ed., pp. 119–141). New York: Cambridge University Press.

Urry, H. L., Nitschke, J. B., Dolski, I., Jackson, D. C., Dalton, K. M., Mueller, C. J., et al. (2004). Making a life worth living: Neural correlates of well-being. *Psychological Science, 15*, 367–372.

van Hooff, J. A. R. A. M. (1972). A comparative approach to the phylogeny of laughter and smiling. In R. Hinde (Ed.), *Non-verbal communication* (pp. 129–179). London: Royal Society & Cambridge University Press.

Vianna, E. P. M., Weinstock, J., Elliott, D., Summers, R., & Tranel, D. (2006). Increased feelings with increased body signals. *Scan, 1*, 37–48.

Vrana, S. R. (1993). The psychophysiology of disgust: Differentiating negative emotional contexts with facial EMG. *Psychophysiology, 30*, 279–286.

Wagner, H. (1989). The physiological differentiation of emotions. In H. Wagner & A. Manstead (Eds.), *Handbook of social psychophysiology* (pp. 77–89). New York: Wiley.

Waldstein, S. R., Kop, W. J., Schmidt, L. A., Haufler, A. J., Krantz, D. S., & Fox, N. A. (2000). Frontal electrocortical and cardiovascular reactivity during happiness and anger. *Biological Psychology, 55*, 3–23.

Watson, D., Wiese, D., Vaidya, J., & Tellegen, A. (1999). The two general activation systems of affect: Structural findings, evolutionary considerations, and psychobiological evidence. *Journal of Personality and Social Psychology, 76*, 820–838.

Wheeler, R. E., Davidson, R. J., & Tomarken, A. J. (1993). Frontal brain asymmetry and emotional reactivity: A biological substrate of affective style. *Psychophysiology, 30*, 82–89.

Winkielman, P., Berridge, K. C., & Wilbarger, J. (2005). Unconscious affective reactions to masked happy versus angry faces influence consumption behavior and judgments of value. *Personality and Social Psychology Bulletin, 31*, 121–135.

Zajonc, R. B., & McIntosh, D. N. (1992). Emotions research: Some promising questions and some questionable promises. *Psychological Science, 3*, 70–74.

CHAPTER 12

Vocal Expressions of Emotion

JO-ANNE BACHOROWSKI and MICHAEL J. OWREN

There is now a substantial body of work focused on how emotion is conveyed and perceived from vocal acoustics. Although this research has arguably not enjoyed the same degree of cumulative success as has work on the facial channel, there is nonetheless a solid body of evidence showing that specific vocal acoustic features are reliably associated with affect-related arousal (or activation) on the part of vocalizers, and that listeners in turn can reliably perceive arousal from vocal acoustics. Ongoing debates center on the more pointed question of whether vocal acoustics are routinely associated with either discrete emotional states or affectively valenced experiences. Because reliable associations with either are unconvincing, we suggest a different perspective in which the primary function of vocal signaling is not so much to communicate emotion as to influence listener affect through vocal acoustics, and thereby to influence behavior. In this chapter, we first review the two key theoretical perspectives concerning the expression of affect via the vocal channel, and introduce a third (af-

fect induction) possibility. We then briefly describe the acoustic measures that are most typically examined in empirical work. Next, we consider the results of research concerning the expression and perception of affect via the vocal channel, with particular attention given to the interpretive claims that can reasonably be made in the context of several paradigmatic limitations. We then return to the affect induction perspective, and show how that framework has been useful in understanding results from research on laughter. Finally, we more broadly consider that an affect induction perspective may help shape a more informed understanding of emotion-related signaling via the vocal channel.

THEORETICAL PERSPECTIVES

The notion that vocal acoustics are rich with cues to a vocalizer's emotional state has a long history, with Cicero (55 B.C.E./2001) suggesting that each emotion is associated with a distinctive tone of voice. The first comprehensive account of vocal emotion expression was provided by Darwin (1872/1998), whose detailed comparative descriptions led him to conclude that affective expressions, including those produced via the vocal channel, are veridical. In other words, he presumed that there is a direct correspondence between particular signaler states and the communicative display produced. This position is largely consistent with the best-known contemporary perspective. Exemplified by the ambitious work of Scherer and colleagues (e.g., Scherer, 1986, 1989; Banse & Scherer, 1996; see reviews by Johnstone & Scherer, 2000; Leinonen, Hiltunen, Linnankoski, & Laakso, 1997), this perspective posits that discrete affective states experienced by the vocalizer are reflected in specific patterns of acoustic cues in the speech being produced. Scherer has further proposed that emotion-specific acoustic cues occur subsequent to the outcomes of a vocalizer's affective appraisal processes and associated physiological changes in vocal production anatomy (for details, see Scherer, 1986). The principal contrasting perspective is that emotional cues in speech acoustics instead reflect activation among a small set of continuous dimensions. In this approach, a relatively common suggestion is that emotion-related acoustic effects are specifically traceable to two orthogonal underlying dimensions of arousal and pleasure (Bachorowski, 1999; Cowie, 2000; Frick, 1985; Kappas, Hess, & Scherer, 1991; Pakosz, 1983).

At this juncture, it is worth noting that the discrete-emotion and dimensional perspectives have two important commonalities. First, both expect that affective states will be associated with differentiated acoustics, meaning that specific patterns or configurations of acoustic cues will be reliably associated with affective states. A second commonality is that both perspectives at least implicitly adopt a representational perspective, meaning that information concerning emotional state is encoded in vocal acoustics, and subsequently decoded by listeners in order to make attributions about the vocalizer's state (e.g., Scherer, 1986, 2003; Juslin & Laukka, 2001). We discuss some implications of a representational stance later in this chapter. For now, we note that outcomes from empirical studies suggest that neither the discrete-emotion nor the dimensional approach

is likely to be correct. Data from speech-related research provides only moderate support for a discrete-emotions view, with emotion-related aspects of the acoustics seeming largely to reflect to vocalizer arousal. However, links to a corresponding emotional valence dimension have also been difficult to demonstrate, suggesting a need for alternative interpretations.

One such approach can arguably be traced to the writing of Charles Darwin. Although Darwin (1872/1998) generally emphasized possible veridical associations between vocal acoustics and vocalizer emotional state, he also made two key observations that are central to the position taken here. The first was that vocal signals can induce emotional responses in listeners, and the second was that these vocal signals can elicit learned emotional responses. Thus he recognized that signalers can use sounds to influence listener affect, and that idiosyncratic aspects of these signals can elicit learned emotional responses in recipients who hear them in association with affect-inducing events. These observations form the core of an "affect induction" view of vocal signaling, which began as a functional account of nonhuman primate calling (Owren & Rendall, 1997, 2001; Rendall & Owren, 2002), but may also apply to affect-related vocal signaling in humans (Owren, Rendall, & Bachorowski, 2003).

In the affect induction framework, the primary function of signaling is not to express emotion, but instead to influence listeners' affect and thereby to shape their behavior. Although vocalizations may be triggered by a signaler's emotions, signal function is not to convey information about the nuances of those states, but rather to affect listeners' arousal and affect. In this view, inferences that listeners can make concerning the signaler's affect are a secondary outcome, and reflect attributions that listeners base on their own affective responses to the sounds, their past experience with such sounds, and the context in which signal production is occurring. In sum, the affect induction perspective argues that vocal expressions of emotion are not displays of vocalizer states as much as they are tools of social influence (see also Russell, Bachorowski, & Fernandez-Dols, 2003). We will return to this perspective in the context of describing research outcomes on human laughter.

EMOTION-RELATED VOCAL ACOUSTICS

Speech acoustics are imbued with "indexical" or "personal" cues, which are nonlinguistic aspects of speech production that provide acoustic correlates of the talker's sex, individual identity, age, and emotional state. Indexical cues are also prominent in many nonlinguistic vocalizations, such as laughter. Regardless of the kind of sound produced, the source filter model of speech production (Fant, 1960; Stevens, 2000) has typically guided selection of the acoustic measurements to make (for details, see Owren & Bachorowski, 2007). In this model, vocal acoustics are treated as a linear combination of (1) an underlying energy source, and (2) filtering effects that stem from the resonances of the supralaryngeal vocal tract. Source energy commonly has one of two forms in vocal production, being either "voiced" or "unvoiced." Voicing, also referred to as "phonation," means that the vocal folds are vibrating. Unvoiced sounds, in contrast, are produced without vocal fold vibration, and are typically noisy or breathy. The sounds of particular interest here are those in which vocal fold vibration occurs in a quasi-periodic fashion, producing phonemes such as vowels. The basic rate of that vibration is called the "fundamental frequency" (F_0), and is primary in the perception of pitch. Measures of F_0 and F_0 variability (including both overall range and moment-to-moment perturbations) are the focus of work seeking to identify acoustic correlates of emotional state. However, amplitude or perceived loudness has also been found to be important, particularly when listeners make inferences about a vocalizer's emotional state from speech.

Supralaryngeal resonances (e.g., Johnson, 1997; Lieberman & Blumstein, 1988) can also be measured, with the frequency of these "formants" being of greatest interest. Formant filtering creates a shaping effect on the frequency content of voiced sounds, producing high-amplitude energy bands at resonance locations and attenuating source energy elsewhere in the frequency spectrum. Measuring rapidly occurring formant changes has the potential to reveal the effects of momentary emotional states as they occur, although not much practical attention has yet been paid to this promise. However, global frequency characteristics of emotion-laden voiced speech sounds are readily characterized by calculating a "long-term average spectrum" (LTAS; e.g., Pittam & Scherer, 1993), which usually involves computing mean energy over segments of 30 seconds or more. The LTAS is thus quick and robust, but does not track acoustic cues associated with transient affective experiences.

EXPRESSION OF EMOTION IN SPEECH

Overview of the Research

Although there has been no shortage of debate between those who advocate a discrete-emotions perspective and those who argue instead for a dimensional perspective, few (if any) empirical studies have actually compared the two approaches directly. Direct comparisons are in fact difficult to engineer, with most studies therefore examining smaller sets of predictions derived from one or the other of the two perspectives. Stemming from a discrete-emotions perspective, one prominent example is the work of Banse and Scherer (1996), who analyzed the vocalizations produced by 12 professional actors who each portrayed 14 emotions. This study is notable for both examining a large number of emotions and including very detailed acoustic analyses. A central result was that of 29 acoustic features measured, F_0 and mean amplitude clearly showed the strongest connections to the emotions being portrayed. These findings are particularly important because, regardless of one's theoretical stance, investigators widely agree that these features are more likely to index talker arousal than specifically valenced or differentiated states. Other acoustic measures were also found to be linked with particular emotional portrayals, but these measures accounted for much smaller proportions of the variance. For example, in examinations of the distribution of energy across 18 frequency bands extracted from LTAS analyses, the researchers found that on average, each acted emotion accounted for only 10% of the variance in each band.

Using acoustic outcomes, Banse and Scherer (1996) were able to demonstrate statistical classification accuracies of roughly 40% when using an empirically derived subset of 16 acoustic measures to discriminate among the various emotions that were portrayed (results varied depending on the particular statistical model used, but were generally consistent). On the one hand, these modest classification rates might be expected based on findings from other kinds of indexical cues (e.g., talker identity in speech segments; Bachorowski & Owren, 1999). On the other hand, the recordings had been carefully screened prior to statistical classification; only 224 "high-quality" portrayals from the total of 1,344 recorded samples were used. As a result, classification rates reported in this study were probably inflated relative to those that would have been obtained with an unscreened sample. When Banse and Scherer tested 40 specific hypotheses concerning the links between emotion and vocal acoustics (see Scherer, 1986), 23 predictions were supported; the evidence was tenuous for 6 others; and statistically significant deviations from the expected magnitude and/or direction of effect occurred for 11 predictions. Naturally, any model of such scope will require adjustments in light of empirical findings. The more important point here is that the results were mixed even for a small, carefully selected subsample of the recorded portrayals. Although these results are often cited as evidence of differentiated vocal cues for discrete emotions, we suggest that they cannot be used to substantiate strong claims along these lines.

Other research has produced a similar mix of supportive and contrary outcomes (e.g., Scherer, Banse, Wallbott, & Goldbeck, 1991; Sobin & Alpert, 1999), suggesting a need for further theoretical work or possibly even alternative approaches (e.g., Kappas et al., 1991; Kappas & Hess, 1995; Scherer et al., 1991). In addition, we suggest that the use of acted rather than natural stimuli and carefully screened rather than representative samples may both have important, albeit unintended, consequences in studies of this kind (cf. Scherer, 2003). The obvious problem with relying on acted samples is that these may not necessarily correspond to naturally produced vocalizations. One counterargument is that much of our verbal communication involves making impressions on others, and so having vocalizers act "as if" they were experiencing a particular state is not markedly different from natural communicative circumstances. To resolve this impasse, validation work could be performed, but for the most part has not (cf. Williams & Stevens, 1972). However, when this issue is taken together with evidence from natural emotion-inducing circumstances showing that individual variability in vocalizer acoustics can

be quite substantial (e.g., Streeter, Macdonald, Apple, Krauss, & Galotti, 1983), it may be the case that the careful analysis of acoustic cues to acted emotion is providing more information about emblematic portrayals of affective states than about naturally occurring cueing (cf. Scherer, 2003).

This problem is exacerbated by working with a nonrepresentative subset of the samples in question. In Banse and Scherer's (1996) work, selection was based largely on quality evaluations made by 12 professional acting students, who found that some individual actors (especially females) were much more convincing in their portrayals than others. One result of the selection process, for instance, was that one particular actor contributed a single sample to the final set of 224, while another was represented by 47 utterances. These kinds of sex and talker differences in the "quality" of portrayals have also been found by others (e.g., Leinonen et al., 1997; Pell, 2001; Scherer et al., 1991; Schröder, 2000; Sobin & Alpert, 1999; Walbott & Scherer, 1986). Here again, the issue is whether the results of such studies can be taken at face value when the utterances being classified are not representative of the full range of variation observed in the original dataset.

Comparing the Discrete-Emotions and Dimensional Approaches

Overall, the most reliable empirical outcomes in testing the acoustics of emotional speech have been arousal-related. Numerous studies have shown, for example, that anger and joy are both associated with increased F_0 and higher amplitude in the sounds produced. Even advocates of discrete-emotions perspectives agree that these have been the most prominent effects (e.g., Johnstone & Scherer, 2000; Scherer, 1989). However, associations between valence and vocal acoustics have been less clear-cut (cf. Johnstone, van Reekum, Hird, Kirsner, & Scherer, 2005; Laukka, Juslin, & Bresin, 2005). For instance, we (Bachorowski & Owren, 1995) examined several acoustic features from speech samples produced by 120 naïve participants, who were individually recorded as they performed a lexical-decision task. As part of the task, each participant uttered a stock phrase just after receiving affect-inducing success or failure feedback. The three most prominent acoustic changes from baseline to on-task performance were F_0-related and were taken to reflect increases in vocalizer arousal. Valence-related differences were observed, but only emerged in more complex interactions among such variables as talker sex, the relative proportion of positive and negative feedback each participant received, and trait differences in emotional intensity. Similar findings were obtained when a more exacting comparison was conducted with recordings made of 24 naïve participants who each described the thoughts and feelings evoked by affect-inducing slides (Bachorowski & Owren, 1996). Acoustic outcomes were strongly associated with self-reported arousal and to a much lesser extent with valence. Analyses testing whether acoustic outcomes could be linked to discrete emotional states were largely nonsignificant. The results thus showed that arousal plays a noticeably more important role in shaping speech acoustics than does valence, and that ready links to discrete emotional states are difficult to demonstrate. Similar findings have been reported in other studies in which arousal and valence effects can be at least indirectly compared (Hatfield, Hsee, Costello, Weisman, & Denney, 1995; Leinonen et al., 1997; Millot & Brand, 2001; Paeschke & Sendlmeier, 2000; Pell, 2001; Pereira, 2000; Pittam, Gallois, & Callan, 1990; Protopapas & Lieberman, 1997; Tolkmitt & Scherer, 1986; Trouvain & Barry, 2000).

However, it would be premature to conclude that the acoustics of emotional speech only reflect arousal (see also Johnstone et al., 2005), or that they can be better accounted for by a dimensional than by a discrete-emotions approach. Any such conclusion requires testing predictions from the two perspectives within the same empirical framework, and we are not aware of any such comparisons. Furthermore, as Tassinary and Cacioppo (1992) indicated in the context of facial expressions of emotion, affective intensity may moderate whether discrete or valenced effects are observed. In support of this notion, Juslin and Laukka (2001; see also Banse & Scherer, 1996; Ladd, Silverman, Tolkmitt, Bergmann, & Scherer, 1985; Scherer, Ladd, & Silverman, 1984) showed that the acoustics measured from the vocal portrayals of five emotions were differentially associated with the intensity (i.e., weak or strong) with which each of these emotions were produced.

What is clearest at this point is that the acoustics of emotional speech are influenced by a variety of factors. Arousal and valence effects do not in and of themselves explain the available data concerning vocal emotion effects. Other contributing factors include talker sex, individual talker identity, and emotional traits. Strategic shaping of vocal acoustics that a talker might show in pursuit of social goals, and the particular social context in which the speech is being produced, may well also prove to be important (Bachorowski, 1999; Scherer, 2003).

PERCEPTION OF EMOTION FROM SPEECH

Overview of the Research

Theoretical approaches and empirical outcomes associated with the perception of emotion from speech acoustics generally parallel those noted for production. When listeners are asked to identify the intended emotion in utterances produced by actors, accuracy is significantly better than chance—although at a moderate level overall, typically about 55% (reviewed by Johnstone & Scherer, 2000). Similar identification and misidentification rates are observed across language groups, although error rates increase as vocalizer and listener languages become more dissimilar (Scherer, Banse, & Wallbott, 2001; see also Tickle, 2000).

Identification rates are usually best for anger, fear, and sadness. Performance is quite poor for disgust, perhaps because this state is typically conveyed not through speech, but via vocal emblems or exclamations. Results for positive emotions have varied, but in an informative way. Accuracy is typically quite high when listeners are given only one positive response option, such as "happiness" (e.g., Johnson, Emde, Scherer, & Klinnert, 1986; Scherer et al., 1991). However, correct responses drop significantly when other positively toned options, such as "elation," "contentment," or "interest," are tested (Banse & Scherer, 1996). A similar effect may contribute to the identification of "sadness," which is sometimes the only low-arousal option offered among the negative emotions.

In an elegant set of studies, Laukka (2005) tested for evidence of categorical perception of vocal emotion, using a set of synthetic stimuli derived from four prototypical expressions. These stimuli included expressions of anger, fear, happiness, and sadness produced by a professional actress. Synthesized continua were then created for perceptual testing, using vocal samples that differed by constant physical amounts. Each continuum was anchored at each end by one of two different emotion prototypes, and included five intermediate morphs.

Outcomes from both identification and discrimination paradigms were taken as evidence of categorical perception of vocal emotion—in other words, as supporting a discrete-emotions perspective. Specifically, identification performance produced the distinct category boundaries that are a hallmark feature of categorical perception, and discrimination performance was better for stimulus pairs that crossed category boundaries than for pairs drawn from within a category. However, boundaries were expected to be defined by stimuli representing an equal mix of the two emotions involved. That outcome occurred for only two of the six continua tested. In other cases, a 50–50 blend of emotions could be identified as representing one of the two emotion categories as much as 70% of the time. In a second experiment, listeners were asked to rate each stimulus according to the extent to which each of the four emotions was represented. This more complex task produced fuzzier category boundaries. Moreover, the disparities between the physical 50–50 mix and the listener-perceived 50–50 point were quite large for two of the four continua. For example, the continuum representing an equal mix of anger and fear was identified as being "angry" more than 90% of the time. Thus the categories produced by listeners were not always aligned with the known physical qualities of the stimulus, which suggests at the least that listeners bring important perceptual biases to this task. In addition, the results indicate that categorization can be critically shaped by procedural aspects of the identification task that in theory should have little effect.

As a package, Laukka's (2005) outcomes leave open the possibility of categorical perception of emotion from voice, but with several caveats. As Laukka notes, further work should include stimuli based on more than one talker. We would also add that in testing for categorical perceptual effects, Laukka in effect began

from the assumption that those categories exist and could be represented in prototype form by using single stimuli. In other words, there is a danger of circularity in this design, with the procedures themselves encouraging listeners to confirm categories that were built into the task from the beginning. In emotions research, it is the very existence of the categories themselves that is questioned (Barrett, 2006). Finally, it is questionable whether these results can be used to refute dimensional accounts, because the continua that Laukka tested are not the continua that are proposed in dimensional accounts. Those accounts are typically based on valence- and arousal-based dimensions, and even discrete-emotions theorists who argue for the occurrence of basic-emotion blends might find it hard to imagine speech that is an equal mix of happiness and fear.

The standard strategy for testing emotion perception from speech has not been to use synthetic stimuli as in Laukka's (2005) study, but instead to use acted speech samples in a forced-choice identification paradigm. Stimulus sets usually include only a small number of talkers and emotions, and are often selected so as to include prototypical instances of the emotions in question. As mentioned earlier, Banse and Scherer (1996) used a subset of 224 samples drawn from an original set of 1,344 recordings. Similarly, Leinonen and colleagues (1997) used 120 of their 480 samples to test participants; Scherer et al. (1991, 2001) used either 10 or 30 of 80 samples; and Sobin and Alpert (1999) used 152 of their 620 samples. This overall approach, which relies on acted emotional samples and then tests only a subset selected on the basis of quality (cf. Juslin & Laukka, 2001), should necessarily produce at least some evidence of differentiated perception of emotion. The outcomes described by Scherer et al. (1991) speak directly to this point. These researchers conducted four perception studies, with listeners in the first experiment hearing all the stimuli, but participants in subsequent studies hearing only selected subsets. Not surprisingly, higher performance rates were achieved with the screened samples, regardless of the emotion being tested.

Other factors also affect listener accuracy. Consistent with the literature on facial expressions of emotion, forced-choice procedures produce better performance than free-choice tests (e.g., Johnson et al., 1986; Pakosz, 1983).

Furthermore, Sobin and Alpert (1999) found that participants may be using quite variable criteria when using a particular emotion label, and Scherer et al. (1991) have demonstrated that the particular kind of participant being tested can be important. Their study showed, for example, that college students and community volunteers differed in both accuracy rates and error patterns. A final issue to note is that stimulus duration can play an important role. For instance, Cauldwell (2000) found that words heard as conveying anger when heard in isolation could become less emotion-laden or even neutral when embedded in carrier phrases. This effect occurred even when listeners were exposed to full-length versions before hearing the words individually. Cauldwell's answer to the rhetorical question "Where did the anger go?" was that the emotion was never present in the first place. He suggested instead that the perception of emotion can be an artifact of the particular testing method used.

Comparing the Discrete-Emotions and Dimensional Approaches

There is relatively good agreement among listeners asked to rate the perceived talker arousal of vocal stimuli. Pereira (2000; see also Green & Cliff, 1975; Juslin & Laukka, 2001), for example, had listeners rate acted vocal samples of various discrete emotional states, using dimensional scales. The strongest associations between these ratings and vocal acoustics were clearly arousal-related, with F_0 and amplitude playing crucial roles. The importance of these features in particular was also noted by Streeter et al. (1983), whose listeners rated talker stress levels from speech. Participants reported that vocalizers were stressed when talker F_0 and amplitude were significantly variable, but otherwise usually failed to perceive actually occurring stress.

Paralleling outcomes on the production side, the link between speech acoustics and arousal is generally stronger than the link between acoustics and perceived valence (cf. Laukka et al., 2005). Ladd et al. (1985), for instance, systematically varied several acoustic parameters as participants rated vocalizer affect and attitude. Listeners in this study did not show categorical response patterns in their attributions of emotional states, but rather perceived vocalizer arousal to be varying continuously in accordance with similarly continuous changes in

F_0. Other results have put dimensional and discrete accounts on more equal footing (e.g., Scherer & Oshinsky, 1977; see also Hatfield et al., 1995). Of interest here is the pattern of misidentifications that occurs when participants are asked to identify discrete vocalizer states. Confusion matrices have shown that errors are most likely to occur for emotions that are similar in arousal (e.g., Pakosz, 1983; Pereira, 2000) and between similarly valenced members of emotion "families" (e.g., Banse & Scherer, 1996; see also Breitenstein, Van Lancker, & Daum, 2001; Ladd et al., 1985).

There are thus at least two issues to consider when the discrete-emotions and dimensional approaches are contrasted from perceptual evidence. The first is that listener accuracy is intermediate, averaging about 55% across a number of studies. Some investigators have argued that this result shows that vocalizer emotion is indeed associated with discrete patterns of acoustic cues, and that these effects are perceptible by listeners (e.g., Banse & Scherer, 1996; Johnstone & Scherer, 2000). We take a more cautious stance and argue that even better performance should be expected, given that the samples used have typically been portrayals of emotion produced by trained actors, and have usually been culled for quality or prototypicality by experimenters prior to being tested with listeners. Both aspects may well strongly decrease acoustic variability relative to naturally occurring emotional speech, and thereby artificially inflate listener scores. Given these circumstances, an outcome of 55% correct seems low if emotion-specific acoustics are in fact present, and probably overestimates how listeners would perform under less artificial circumstances.

A second issue to consider is the extent to which emotion-specific cues are actually present in naturally occurring speech, given that attributions about emotion also involve perceptual processes, inferential capabilities, and even simple biases that listeners bring to the situation. For example, listeners tend to place disproportionate weight on particular acoustic cues, whether or not these cues reliably covary with vocalizer state (e.g., Johnstone & Scherer, 2000; Streeter et al., 1983). Given that this sort of "stereotyping" is prominent in many automatic evaluations of personal characteristics in others (Banaji & Hardin, 1996; Kawakami, Young, & Dovidio, 2002), it would not be surprising to find that listener inferences concerning vocalizer affect from acoustics alone are simply not very accurate. Under natural circumstances, a listener would be hearing the speech within a rich social context and often from a familiar vocalizer. Both factors could significantly boost the accuracy of attribution (Bachorowski, 1999; Pakosz, 1983).

From a methodological point of view, it therefore becomes critical to separate these factors explicitly, given that perception of emotion from speech may rely as much or more on active interpretation by a listener as it does on acoustic cues provided by the vocalizer. This possibility is elaborated in the next section, which shifts the focus from hypothesized links between emotional states and vocalizer acoustics to the effects that sounds have on listener affect. Although compatible with various aspects of both discrete and dimensional accounts of emotions and emotional expression, this perspective suggests that emotion-related cueing by vocalizers is actually a secondary outcome of the communication process. The primary function of emotional vocal acoustics is instead proposed to be influencing the listener's state and concomitant behavior.

AN AFFECT INDUCTION ACCOUNT OF VOCAL SIGNALING

Whether from a discrete-emotions or a dimensional perspective, a central theme of work on emotion-related aspects of vocal signals has been that there are veridical links among vocalizer affect, associated vocal acoustics, and listener perception. This perspective assumes that the purpose of emotion-related signaling is for the vocalizer to inform listeners that particular affective states are being experienced. Of course, simply informing listeners about such states is not necessarily beneficial. Instead, the effect that signaling has on subsequent listener behavior must be what has shaped the signaling process over evolutionary time (see Dawkins, 1989; Dawkins & Krebs, 1978; see also Owren & Bachorowski, 2001). It therefore becomes important that there is no guarantee that listeners will behave in ways that benefit vocalizers who are providing veridical cues to their internal states. This observation in turn suggests that the most fundamental selection pressure acting on signalers must be to modulate others' behavior in ways that are beneficial to themselves. This logic leads to a

different way of thinking about affect-related vocal acoustics: From this point of view, their function cannot be to inform as much as to influence. We suggest that such influence can occur either via the direct impact of signal acoustics on listener affective systems or through learned associations between vocalizer acoustics and listener state, thereby shaping the way listeners behave toward the vocalizer. After briefly describing this perspective, we specifically apply it to the case of human laughter—a seemingly ubiquitous, affect-related vocal signal.

Affect Induction through Sound

Anyone who has spent time with a crying infant can well appreciate that auditory stimuli can readily induce emotion-related responses in listeners. Sounds as varied as those of doors opening and closing, sirens wailing, and thunderstorms booming can all elicit attention, arousal, and valenced responses. Laughter and infant crying are two of the more potent, affect-inducing vocal signals, but even speech acoustics can produce emotion in listeners (Neumann & Strack, 2000; Hatfield et al., 1995; Siegman & Boyle, 1993). More broadly, Bradley and Lang (2000) have shown that affective responses occur to an array of environmental and human sounds, and that these responses can be readily organized along arousal and pleasure dimensions.

The fact that sounds can induce affect has played little role in work on production and perception of vocal expression of emotion. Instead, as noted earlier, both the discrete-emotions and dimensional perspectives seemingly approach the problem from a representational standpoint, in the sense that affect-related meaning is "encoded" by vocalizers and subsequently "decoded" by listeners (e.g., Juslin & Laukka, 2001; Scherer, 1988, 2003). Emotional expressions are thus treated as a code that vocalizers use to convey their emotional states—a perspective that at least implicitly draws on a linguistically inspired interpretation.

The "affect induction" model has been proposed as an alternative to representational perspectives. Originally developed in the context of nonhuman primate vocalizations (Owren & Rendall, 1997, 2001; Rendall & Owren, 2002), this approach may also have broad applicability to human affective signaling (Owren et al., 2003). Rather than treating emotional communication as a process of information encoding and decoding, the approach argues that the primary function of emotion-related vocal signals is to influence listeners' affect and thereby also to modulate their behavior. Whereas representational accounts of communication implicitly implicate rather sophisticated but typically undescribed processes of information encoding and decoding, the affect induction approach argues that vocal signals "work" because they have an impact on listeners at comparatively low levels of neural organization by eliciting emotional responses. The effects can be "direct," meaning that signal acoustics themselves have an impact, or "indirect," meaning that listeners experience a learned affective response to sounds as a result of previous experience. For the former, impact depends on the signal energy itself, meaning that such aspects as variability, amplitude, duration, and overall salience are of primary importance. In the latter, learning arises through social interactions, and depends on instances in which individually distinctive sounds produced by a given vocalizer are repeatedly paired with the affect being experienced by a listener.

Differences between the affect induction and representational perspectives can be elucidated in the context of the similarities that exist between them. There are at least two important points of contact, with the first being that both approaches assume some association between the signaler's internal state and the signal produced. The representational approach argues that the function of signaling is to allow the listener to infer that this particular state is occurring in the vocalizer. This view therefore predicts that signals should be strongly associated with differentiated signaler states. The affect induction approach instead proposes that the vocalizer's internal state is important in the mechanistic underpinnings of signal production, but that the function of signaling is to induce emotion in the listener. As a result, signal acoustics need not be strongly linked to vocalizer states, because it may benefit the vocalizer to induce similar responses in the listener across a variety of situations. Conversely, a diverse set of acoustic properties in sounds produced in a given situation may serve a common function in modulating listener arousal and valenced emotion. The affect induction approach therefore expects associations between vocalizer state and physical signal, but maintains that these associations will be probabilistic in nature.

A second point of contact is that listeners are probably able to draw inferences about vocalizer states and/or likely upcoming behaviors. From a representational perspective, such inferences are part and parcel of why communication signals evolve: Signal recipients receive encoded information about a signaler's state and act on that content. The affect induction approach, in contrast, views listener inference as a secondary outcome of vocal behavior, which has evolved first and foremost because it benefits the vocalizer to influence listener affect and behavior. Substantial variability in vocalizing behavior is thus to be expected. However, there will be probabilistic patterning involved, which listeners will inevitably benefit from attending to and learning about, to the extent that they themselves benefit from drawing inferences about vocalizer states and likely behavior.

Although affect-related signals do not have representational value in this view, they are still "meaningful" in the sense that listeners make inferences about their significance based on a host of factors, which can include the acoustic attributes of the sound, the listener's affective state and familiarity with the sound, and the overarching context in which the sound has occurred (see also Bachorowski & Owren, 2002; Hess & Kirouac, 2000; Kappas et al., 1991). A corollary is that affective responses to highly similar sounds may be quite variable. For example, hearing a high-pitched shriek may be pleasurable when one is attending a party, but quite negative when one is walking down a dark, isolated street. In both cases, the acoustics of the shriek are likely to elicit orientation, increase listener arousal, and exacerbate whatever affective state the listener is already experiencing—positive and negative, respectively, in these two situations. In addition, if the sound has distinctive acoustic features that have previously been paired with either positive or negative affect in the listener, the sound will activate corresponding learned responses. Finally, the sound can have a larger and probably more complex inferred significance in a given context—for instance, if the shriek "means" that someone has had too much to drink and should be driven home.

Although it is thus fundamentally different from representational approaches to emotional expression, the affect induction perspective nonetheless has parallels with Scherer's "appeal" and "pull" functions of vocal expression of emotion (Scherer, 1988, 1992; see also Johnstone & Scherer, 2000), as well as with the construct of "emotion contagion." Hatfield, Cacioppo, and Rapson's (1992) notion of "primitive" emotional contagion is particularly relevant, in that this process is described as either unconditioned or conditioned, and as occurring outside the realm of conscious awareness. However, the affect induction perspective takes mechanism a step further than the notions of "appeal," "pull," or "contagion" by specifically emphasizing direct links between the acoustics of affect-related vocalizations and low-level neural responses in listeners.

A larger implication of the affect induction approach is that vocal emotion expressions function most importantly as nonconscious strategies of social influence (see also Bargh & Chartrand, 1999; Zajonc, 1980). Rather than acting as informative beacons to a vocalizer's state, these signals are held to sway or shape perceiver affect and subsequent behavior or attitude toward the vocalizer. Any information value the signal has thus represents a combination of inferences the perceiver may be able to draw, given the context at hand, previous general experience with such signals, and the unique history of interaction shared by the individuals involved (Hess & Kirouac, 2000; Owren & Rendall, 2001).

Applying an Affect Induction Approach to Laughter

There is no shortage of hypotheses concerning the associations between laughter and affect-related states on the part of vocalizers. On the one hand, laughter has obvious links with positive states such as happiness (e.g., Darwin, 1872/1998; Nwokah, Davies, Islam, Hsu, & Fogel, 1993; van Hooff, 1972) and with the enjoyment associated with humor (Deacon, 1989; Edmonson, 1987; Weisfeld, 1993). On the other hand, laughter has also been noted to accompany negative emotions such as guilt, shame, and nervousness (Darwin, 1872/1998; McComas, 1923). Other signaling values have also been suggested, including sexual interest and sexual fitness (Dunbar, 1996; Grammer & Eibl-Eibesfeldt, 1990), self-deprecation (Glenn, 1991–1992), appeasement or submission (Adams & Kirkevold, 1978; Deacon, 1997; Dovidio, Brown, Heltman, Ellyson, & Keating,

1988; Grammer & Eibl-Ebesfeldt, 1990), and denigration (Eibl-Ebesfeldt, 1989).

These approaches to laughter have at least tacitly adopted a representational stance in which laugh acoustics themselves are considered to provide information about vocal state, with listeners being held to make inferences about that state from signal acoustics (and perhaps contextual cues). An implication is therefore that if laughter is to represent vocalizer affect, it should exhibit differentiated acoustic properties that then allow listeners to make inferences about the laugher's corresponding internal states—in other words, that laugh acoustics vary in accordance with affective state. To our knowledge, there are no direct tests of this hypothesis.

As might be expected from the variety of hypothesized functions concerning laughter, the available data in fact show laugh acoustics to be remarkably variable (Bachorowski, Smoski, & Owren, 2001; Grammer & Eibl-Ebesfeldt, 1990; Vettin & Todt, 2004). However, this variability actually poses a challenge for representational perspectives, because it occurs both within and among laughers reporting similar arousal and positive affect states (see Owren & Bachorowski, 2003; Owren et al., 2003). Laughs in the Bachorowski et al. (2001) study were recorded from 97 individuals as they watched humorous film clips either alone or with a same- or other-sex friend or stranger. The results of detailed acoustic analyses revealed that laughs could be reliably grouped into voiced and unvoiced (noisy, breathy) categories, with the latter being further separable into grunt- and snort-like versions. There was striking variability in a number of F_0-related measures in voiced laughs, suggesting that many of these sounds should have significant, direct impact on listener arousal and affect. Specifically, both males and females produced laughs with very high mean and maximum F_0's, as well as considerable variability or F_0 modulation both within single laugh sounds and across bouts of laughter. A number of laughs also had notable acoustic irregularities (i.e., acoustic nonlinearities), which we suspect are especially potent in tweaking listener response systems.

Further analyses (see Bachorowski, Smoski, Tomarken, & Owren, 2008) showed that laugh acoustics were only loosely coupled with self-reported affect—an outcome that is inconsistent with a representational view of these sounds. These acoustics were, however, significantly associated with the social circumstances of the testing situation (see also Devereux & Ginsburg, 2001; Grammer & Eibl-Eibesfeldt, 1990; Vettin & Todt, 2004). So, for example, males laughed the most and produced a high proportion of laughs likely to have potent direct effects on listeners when paired with a friend, especially a male friend. Females, on the other hand, were more likely to produce these kinds of laugh sounds in the company of a male. Although a careful accounting of the interactions between laugher sex and social context is beyond the scope of this chapter, the gist is that both males and females produce more direct-effect laughs when it would benefit them to elicit arousal and affect in listeners, and specifically do not produce such sounds when inducing arousal in listeners might only exacerbate negatively toned (e.g., wary) emotional states in these individuals (Owren & Bachorowski, 2003; Owren et al., 2003).

As on the production side, perceptual responses to laughter have not received much systematic empirical attention. Nevertheless, the available data do show that laugh acoustics elicit affective responses in listeners and can have a modulating effect on a social partner's attitude toward a vocalizer. As a first step toward testing hypotheses about the direct effects that laugh sounds may exert on listener states, we (Bachorowski & Owren, 2001) had listeners rate a sample of voiced and unvoiced laughs. Outcomes were remarkably consistent, regardless of whether listeners rated their own affect in response to hearing a laugh, the likely affective response other listeners would experience, or three affect-related attributes of the laugher. Voiced laughs were given significantly more positive evaluations than were unvoiced laughs, supporting the idea that the acoustic properties of the former (e.g., high mean F_0, marked F_0 modulation, and high amplitude) activate listeners in a direct fashion. More recent work has shown that unvoiced laughs can actually elicit slightly negative affect in listeners (Owren, Trivedi, Schulman, & Bachorowski, 2007). Grammer and Eibl-Eibesfeldt (1990; see also Keltner & Bonanno, 1997) have further shown that the occurrence of voiced laughter is associated with listener interest in the laugher: Males reported being more interested in females they had just met if those females produced a larger number of voiced, but not unvoiced, laughs during a 10-minute interval.

Other research has begun to focus on indirect or learned effects. Here the expectation is that learned emotional responses should accrue in listeners experiencing positive affect, as laughers are able to repeatedly produce individually distinctive sounds in close temporal association with the occurrence of those listener states. We (Bachorowski et al., 2001) achieved moderate success in statistical classification of both the voiced and unvoiced laughs of individual vocalizers, suggesting that laughs are in fact individually distinctive. Initial behavioral support for the notion of indirect effects was obtained by finding that laughter is far more likely to show coincident occurrence between friends than between strangers (Smoski & Bachorowski, 2003a), and that this temporal link is more frequent for voiced than for unvoiced laughs (Smoski & Bachorowski, 2003b).

The studies reviewed here are just the beginning, however, with much remaining to be learned about this affect-related vocal signal. In the current context, the most important point to note is that there are some important connections between the major findings emerging from studies of emotional communication through speech acoustics and laughter.

CONCLUSIONS: VOCAL EXPRESSIONS OF EMOTION AS SOCIAL TOOLS

Laughter resembles speech in being a decidedly social event (Provine & Fischer, 1989) and a critical part of the communicative processes that are central to human social relationships. There also appear to be some telling commonalities in how the acoustic features of both speech and laughter function in emotional aspects of communication. A routine finding for speech is that F_0- and amplitude-related features play a primary role. On the one hand, speech produced while a vocalizer is experiencing salient emotion usually shows significant changes in these particular characteristics, which also clearly have an impact on listener perception and attributions of emotion. On the other hand, there is little indication that these or other acoustic features of speech are tightly coupled with either discrete emotional states or valenced affect, and when listeners are asked to identify vocalizer states, performance based on speech acoustics alone is modest. Although less information is available for laughter, outcomes so far have been similar. For example, the degree of variability occurring in laugh sounds produced during positive states alone argues against the possibility of emotion-specific acoustics. Laugh sounds nonetheless have unambiguous impact on listener emotion, with voicing and F_0-related features playing a central role.

It has thus been difficult to demonstrate clearly differentiated, state-specific acoustic effects for either speech or laughter, but quite easy to show that acoustics nonetheless have general and robust effects on listeners' emotions and evaluation of vocalizers (see also Scherer, 1986). To us, these results raise questions about the adequacy of representational approaches, and are instead more compatible with the view that vocalizers are using relatively undifferentiated acoustics that have potent effects on listener affect. The evidence is far from definitive, particularly as much of the work conducted on human vocal expression of emotion has assumed rather than tested the proposition that representational signaling is involved. However, it is therefore also noteworthy that relevant research has largely failed to support this assumption either for production or for perception. Although listeners readily hear emotional "content," their judgments about a vocalizer's states are constrained and context-dependent. Our interpretation is that these inferences primarily reflect the listeners' own arousal and valenced responses, which are richly interpreted while also taking other information about the vocalizer and context into account. Affective communication in both speech and laughter thus becomes a process of attributing emotion to vocalizers, rather than one of recovering encoded information.

A larger implication of this view is that emotional expressions in general function most importantly as nonconscious strategies of social influence, rather than as veridical representations of internal state (see also Bargh & Chartrand, 1999; Zajonc, 1980). Rather than informing per se, both kinds of signals function to sway or shape the perceiver's affect and attitude, promoting behavioral effects that ultimately benefit the signaler. The information value of a signal is thus critically dependent on a perceiver's previous general experience, particular history with the signaler, and ability to take signaling context into account (Hess & Kirouac, 2000; Owren & Rendall, 2001).

These are difficult distinctions to make, however, and illustrate the need to significantly improve on the data that are currently available concerning vocal emotion expression (Douglas-Cowie, Campbell, Cowie, & Roach, 2003). We suggest that it will be useful to focus on vocalizations acquired under controlled but naturalistic circumstances, where vocalizers are experiencing actual rather than simulated emotions. Furthermore, alternative interpretations should be contrasted as directly as possible, including discrete-emotions versus dimensional approaches and representational versus affect induction perspectives within the same experimental framework. Finally, it will be important to broaden the scope of inquiry, so that the inferential processes used by listeners to make attributions about vocalizer states can be uncovered. With these desiderata as a framework, a deeper understanding of how humans use emotion-related vocal acoustics in their communicative endeavors should be within reach.

ACKNOWLEDGMENTS

During this work, Michael J. Owren was supported in part by National Institute of Mental Health Prime Award No. 1 R01 MH65317-01A2, Subaward No. 8402-15235-X; by the Brains and Behavior Program of Georgia State University; and by the Center for Behavioral Neuroscience, STC Program of the National Science Foundation, under Agreement No. IBN-9876754.

REFERENCES

Adams, R. M., & Kirkevold, B. (1978). Looking, smiling, laughing, and moving in restaurants: Sex and age differences. *Environmental Psychology and Nonverbal Behavior, 3*, 117–121.

Bachorowski, J.-A. (1999). Vocal expression and perception of emotion. *Current Directions in Psychological Science, 8*, 53–57.

Bachorowski, J.-A., & Owren, M. J. (1995). Vocal expression of emotion: Acoustic properties of speech are associated with emotional intensity and context. *Psychological Science, 6*, 219–224.

Bachorowski, J.-A., & Owren, M. J. (1996). Vocal expression of emotion is associated with vocal fold vibration and vocal tract resonance. *Psychophysiology, 33*(Suppl. 1), S20.

Bachorowski, J.-A., & Owren, M. J. (1999). Acoustic correlates of talker sex and individual talker identity are present in a short vowel segment produced in running speech. *Journal of the Acoustical Society of America, 106*, 1054–1063.

Bachorowski, J.-A., & Owren, M. J. (2001). Not all laughs are alike: Voiced but not unvoiced laughter readily elicits positive affect. *Psychological Science, 12,* 252–257.

Bachorowski, J.-A, & Owren, M. J. (2002). The role of vocal acoustics in emotional intelligence. In L. F. Barrett & P. Salovey (Eds.), *The wisdom in feeling: Psychological processes in emotional intelligence* (pp. 11–36). New York: Guilford Press.

Bachorowski, J.-A., Smoski, M. J., & Owren, M. J. (2001). The acoustic features of human laughter. *Journal of the Acoustical Society of America, 110,* 1581–1597.

Bachorowski, J.-A., Smoski, M. J., Tomarken, A. J., & Owren, M. J. (2008). *Laugh rate and acoustics are associated with social context.* Manuscript submitted for publication.

Banaji, M. R., & Hardin, C. D. (1996). Automatic stereotyping. *Psychological Science, 7,* 136–141.

Banse, R., & Scherer, K. R. (1996). Acoustic profiles in vocal emotion expression. *Journal of Personality and Social Psychology, 70,* 614–636.

Bargh, J. A., & Chartrand, T. L. (1999). The unbearable automaticity of being. *American Psychologist, 54,* 462–479.

Barrett, L. F. (2006). Are emotions natural kinds? *Perspectives on Psychological Sciences, 1,* 28–58.

Bradley, M. M., & Lang, P. J. (2000). Affective reactions to acoustic stimuli. *Psychophysiology, 37,* 204–215.

Breitenstein, C., Van Lancker, D., & Daum, I. (2001). The contribution of speech rate and pitch variation to the perception of vocal emotions in a German and an American sample. *Cognition and Emotion, 15,* 57–79.

Cauldwell, R. T. (2000). Where did the anger go?: The role of context in interpreting emotion in speech. In R. Cowie, E. Douglas-Cowie, & M. Schröder (Eds.), *Proceedings of the International Speech Communication Association Workshop on Speech and Emotion* (pp. 127–131). Belfast: Textflow.

Cicero, M. T. (1904). *De oratore* (2nd ed.). Translated and with an introduction by E. N. P. Moor. London: Methuen.

Cowie, R. (2000). Describing the emotional states expressed in speech. In R. Cowie, E. Douglas-Cowie, & M. Schröder (Eds.), *Proceedings of the International Speech Communication Association Workshop on Speech and Emotion* (pp. 11–18). Belfast: Textflow.

Darwin, C. (1998). *The expression of the emotions in man and animals.* New York: Oxford University. (Original work published 1872)

Dawkins, R. (1989). *The selfish gene* (2nd ed.). Oxford: Oxford University Press.

Dawkins, R., & Krebs, J. R. (1978). Animal signals: Information or manipulation? In J. R. Krebs & N. B. Davies (Eds.), *Behavioural ecology: An evolutionary approach* (pp. 282–309). Oxford: Blackwell Scientific.

Deacon, T. W. (1989). The neural circuitry underlying primate calls and human language. *Human Evolution, 4,* 367–401.

Deacon, T. W. (1997). *The symbolic species.* New York: Norton.

Devereux, P. G., & Ginsburg, G. P. (2001). Sociality effects on the production of laughter. *Journal of General Psychology, 128,* 227–240.

Douglas-Cowie, E., Campbell, N., Cowie, R., & Roach, P. (2003). Emotional speech: Towards a new generation of databases. *Speech Communication, 40,* 33–60.

Dovidio, J. F., Brown, C. E., Heltman, K., Ellyson, S. L., & Keating, C. F. (1988). Power displays between women and men in discussions of gender-linked tasks: A multichannel study. *Journal of Personality and Social Psychology, 55,* 580–587.

Dunbar, R. I. M. (1996). *Grooming, gossip, and the evolution of language.* London: Faber &Faber.

Edmonson, M. S. (1987). Notes on laughter. *Anthropological Linguistics, 29,* 23–34.

Eibl-Ebesfeldt, I. (1989). *Human ethology.* New York: Aldine de Gruyler.

Fant, G. (1960). *Acoustic theory of speech production.* S-Gravenhage, The Netherlands: Mouton.

Frick, R. W. (1985). Communicating emotion: The role of prosodic features. *Psychological Bulletin, 97,* 412–429.

Glenn, P. J. (1991–1992). Current speaker initiation of two-party shared laughter. *Research on Language and Social Interaction, 25,* 139–162.

Grammer, K., & Eibl-Eibesfeldt, I. (1990). The ritualization of laughter. In W. Koch (Ed.), *Naturlichkeit der sprache und der kultur: Acta colloquii* (pp. 192–214). Bochum, Germany: Brockmeyer.

Green, R. S., & Cliff, N. (1975). Multidimensional comparisons of structures of vocally and facially expressed emotion. *Perception and Psychophysics, 17,* 429–438.

Hatfield, E., Cacioppo, J. T., & Rapson, R. L. (1992). Primitive emotional contagion. In M. S. Clark (Ed.), *Emotion and social behavior* (pp. 151–177). London: Sage.

Hatfield, E., Hsee, C. K., Costello, J., Weisman, M. S., & Denney, C. (1995). The impact of vocal feedback on emotional experience and expression. *Journal of Social Behavior and Personality, 10,* 293–312.

Hess, U., & Kirouac, G. (2000). Emotion expression in groups. In M. Lewis & J. M. Haviland-Jones (Eds.), *Handbook of emotions* (2nd ed., pp. 368–381). New York: Guilford Press.

Johnson, K. (1997). *Acoustic and auditory phonetics.* Cambridge, MA: Blackwell.

Johnson, W. F., Emde, R. N., Scherer, K. R., & Klinnert, M. D. (1986). Recognition of emotion from vocal cues. *Archives of General Psychiatry, 43,* 280–283.

Johnstone, T., & Scherer, K. R. (2000). Vocal communication of emotion. In M. Lewis & J. M. Haviland-Jones (Eds.), *Handbook of emotions* (2nd ed., pp. 220–235). New York: Guilford Press.

Johnstone, T., van Reekum, C. M., Hird, K., Kirsner, K., & Scherer, K. R. (2005). Affective speech elicited with a computer game. *Emotion, 5,* 513–518.

Juslin, P. N., & Laukka, P. (2001). Impact of intended emotional intensity on cue utilization and decoding accuracy in vocal expression of emotion. *Emotion, 1,* 381–412.

Kappas, A., & Hess, U. (1995). Nonverbal aspects of oral communication. In D. U. M. Quasthoff (Ed.), *Aspects of oral communication* (pp. 169–180). Berlin: De Gruyter.

Kappas, A., Hess, U., & Scherer, K. R. (1991). Voice and emotion. In B. Rime & R. Feldman (Eds.), *Fundamentals of nonverbal behavior* (pp. 200–238). Cambridge, UK: Cambridge University Press.

Kawakami, K., Young, H., & Dovidio, J. F. (2002). Automatic stereotyping: Category, trait, and behavioral activations. *Personality and Social Psychology Bulletin, 28,* 3–15.

Keltner, D., & Bonanno, G. (1997). A study of laughter and dissociation: Distinct correlates of laughter and smiling during bereavement. *Journal of Personality and Social Psychology, 73,* 687–702.

Ladd, D. R., Silverman, K. E. A., Tolkmitt, F., Bergmann, G., & Scherer, K. R. (1985). Evidence for the independence of intonation contour type, voice quality, and F_0 range in signaling speaker affect. *Journal of the Acoustical Society of America, 78,* 435–444.

Laukka, P. (2005). Categorical perception of vocal emotion expressions. *Emotion, 5,* 277–295.

Laukka, P., Juslin, P. N., & Bresin, R. (2005). A dimensional approach to vocal expression of emotion. *Cognition and Emotion, 19,* 633–653.

Leinonen, L., Hiltunen, T., Linnankoski, I., & Laakso, M.-L. (1997). Expression of emotional–motivational connotations with a one-word utterance. *Journal of the Acoustical Society of America, 102,* 1853–1863.

Lieberman, P., & Blumstein, S. E. (1988). *Speech physiology, speech perception, and acoustic phonetics.* Cambridge, UK: Cambridge University Press.

McComas, H. C. (1923). The origin of laughter. *Psychological Review, 30,* 45–56.

Millot, J.-L., & Brand, G. (2001). Effects of pleasant and unpleasant ambient odors on human voice pitch. *Neuroscience Letters, 297,* 61–63.

Neumann, R., & Strack, F. (2000). "Mood contagion": The automatic transfer of mood between persons. *Journal of Personality and Social Psychology, 79,* 211–223.

Nwokah, E. E., Davies, P., Islam, A., Hsu, H. C., & Fogel, A. (1993). Vocal affect in three-year-olds: A quantitative acoustic analysis of child laughter. *Journal of the Acoustical Society of America, 94,* 3076–3090.

Owren, M. J., & Bachorowski, J.-A. (2001). The evolution of emotional expression: A "selfish-gene" account of smiling and laughter in early hominids and humans. In T. Mayne & G. A. Bonanno (Eds.), *Emotions: Current issues and future directions* (pp. 152–191). New York: Guilford Press.

Owren, M. J., & Bachorowski, J.-A. (2003). Reconsidering the evolution of nonlinguistic communication: The case of laughter. *Journal of Nonverbal Behavior, 27,* 183–200.

Owren, M. J., & Bachorowski, J.-A. (2007). Measuring vocal acoustics. In J. A. Coan & J. J. B. Allen (Eds.), *The handbook of emotion elicitation and assessment* (pp. 239–266). New York: Oxford University Press.

Owren, M. J., & Rendall, D. (1997). An affect-conditioning model of nonhuman primate signaling. In D. H. Owings, M. D. Beecher, & N. S. Thompson (Eds.), *Perspectives in ethology: Vol. 12. Communication* (pp. 299–346). New York: Plenum Press.

Owren, M. J., & Rendall, D. (2001). Sound on the rebound: Bringing form and function back to the forefront in understanding nonhuman primate vocal signaling. *Evolutionary Anthropology, 10,* 58–71.

Owren, M. J., Rendall, D., & Bachorowski, J.-A. (2003). Nonlinguistic vocal communication. In D. Maestripieri (Ed.), *Primate psychology* (pp. 359–394). Cambridge, MA: Harvard University Press.

Owren, M. J., Trivedi, N., Schulman, A., & Bachorowski, J.-A. (2007). *An implicit association test (IAT) with nonlinguistic auditory stimuli: Listener evaluations of human laughter.* Manuscript submitted for publication.

Paeschke, A., & Sendlmeier, W. F. (2000). Prosodic characteristics of emotional speech: Measurements of fundamental frequency movements. In R. Cowie, E. Douglas-Cowie, & M. Schröder (Eds.), *Proceedings of the International Speech Communication Association Workshop on Speech and Emotion* (pp. 75–80). Belfast: Textflow.

Pakosz, M. (1983). Attitudinal judgments in intonation: Some evidence for a theory. *Journal of Psycholinguistic Research, 12,* 311–326.

Pell, M. D. (2001). Influence of emotion and focus location on prosody in matched statements and questions. *Journal of the Acoustical Society of America, 109,* 1668–1680.

Pereira, C. (2000). Dimensions of emotional meaning in speech. In R. Cowie, E. Douglas-Cowie, & M. Schröder (Eds.), *Proceedings of the International Speech Communication Association Workshop on Speech and Emotion* (pp. 25–28). Belfast: Textflow.

Pittam, J., Gallois, C., & Callan, V. (1990). The long-term spectrum and perceived emotion. *Speech Communication, 9,* 177–187.

Pittam, J., & Scherer, K. R. (1993). Vocal expression and communication of emotion. In M. Lewis & J. M. Haviland (Eds.), *Handbook of emotions* (pp. 185–197). New York: Guilford Press.

Protopapas, A., & Lieberman, P. (1997). Fundamental frequency of phonation and perceived emotional stress. *Journal of the Acoustical Society of America, 101,* 2267–2277.

Provine, R. R., & Fischer, K. R. (1989). Laughing, smiling, and talking: Relation to sleeping and social context in humans. *Ethology, 83,* 295–305.

Rendall, D., & Owren, M. J. (2002). Animal vocal communication: Say what? In M. Bekoff, C. Allen, & G.

Burghardt (Eds.), *The cognitive animal* (pp. 307–314). Cambridge, MA: MIT Press.

Russell, J. A., Bachorowski, J.-A., & Fernandez-Dols, J.-M. (2003). Facial and vocal expressions of emotion. *Annual Review of Psychology, 54,* 329–349.

Scherer, K. R. (1986). Vocal affect expression: A review and model for future research. *Psychological Bulletin, 99,* 143–165.

Scherer, K. R. (1988). On the symbolic functions of vocal affect expression. *Journal of Language and Social Psychology, 7,* 79–100.

Scherer, K. R. (1989). Vocal measurement of emotion. In R. Plutchik & H. Kellerman (Eds.), *Emotion: Theory, research, and experience Vol. 4. The measurement of emotions* (pp. 233–259). New York: Academic Press.

Scherer, K. R. (1992). Vocal affect expression as symptom, symbol, and appeal. In H. Papoušek, U. Jürgens, & M. Papoušek (Eds.), *Nonverbal vocal communication: Comparative and developmental approaches* (pp. 43–60). Cambridge, UK: Cambridge University Press.

Scherer, K. R. (2003). Vocal communication of emotion: A review of research paradigms. *Speech Communication, 40,* 227–256.

Scherer, K. R., Banse, R., & Wallbott, H. G. (2001). Emotion inferences from vocal expression correlate across languages and cultures. *Journal of Cross-Cultural Psychology, 32,* 76–92.

Scherer, K. R., Banse, R., Wallbott, H. G., & Goldbeck, T. (1991). Vocal cues in emotion encoding and decoding. *Motivation and Emotion, 15,* 123–148.

Scherer, K. R., Ladd, D. R., & Silverman, K. E. A. (1984). Vocal cues to speaker affect: Testing two models. *Journal of the Acoustical Society of America, 76,* 1346–1356.

Scherer, K. R., & Oshinsky, J. S. (1977). Cue utilization in emotion attribution from auditory stimuli. *Motivation and Emotion, 1,* 331–346.

Schröder, M. (2000). Experimental study of affect bursts. In R. Cowie, E. Douglas-Cowie, & M. Schröder (Eds.), *Proceedings of the International Speech Communication Association Workshop on Speech and Emotion* (pp. 132–135). Belfast: Textflow.

Siegman, A. W., & Boyle, S. (1993). Voices of fear and anxiety and sadness and depression: The effects of speech rate and loudness on fear and anxiety and sadness and depression. *Journal of Abnormal Psychology, 102,* 430–437.

Smoski, M. J., & Bachorowski, J.-A. (2003a). Antiphonal laughter between friends and strangers. *Cognition and Emotion, 17,* 327–340.

Smoski, M. J., & Bachorowski, J.-A. (2003b). Antiphonal laughter in developing friendships. *Annals of the New York Academy of Sciences, 1000,* 300–303.

Sobin, C., & Alpert, M. (1999). Emotion in speech: The acoustic attributes of fear, anger, sadness, and joy. *Journal of Psycholinguistic Research, 28,* 347–365.

Stevens, K. N. (2000). *Acoustic phonetics.* Cambridge, MA: MIT Press.

Streeter, L. A., Macdonald, N. H., Apple, W., Krauss, R. M., & Galotti, K. M. (1983). Acoustic and perceptual indicators of emotional stress. *Journal of the Acoustical Society of America, 73,* 1354–1360.

Tassinary, L. G., & Cacioppo, J. T. (1992). Unobservable facial actions and emotion. *Psychological Science, 3,* 28–33.

Tickle, A. (2000). English and Japanese speakers' emotion vocalisation and recognition: A comparison highlighting vowel quality. In R. Cowie, E. Douglas-Cowie, & M. Schröder (Eds.), *Proceedings of the International Speech Communication Association Workshop on Speech and Emotion* (pp. 104–109). Belfast: Textflow.

Tolkmitt, F. J., & Scherer, K. R. (1986). Effects of experimentally induced stress on vocal parameters. *Journal of Experimental Psychology: Human Perception and Performance, 12,* 302–313.

Trouvain, J., & Barry, W. J. (2000). The prosody of excitement in horse race commentaries. In R. Cowie, E. Douglas-Cowie, & M. Schröder (Eds.), *Proceedings of the International Speech Communication Association Workshop on Speech and Emotion* (pp. 86–91). Belfast: Textflow.

van Hooff, J. A. R. A. M. (1972). A comparative approach to the phylogeny of laughter and smiling. In R. A. Hinde (Ed.), *Non-verbal communication* (pp. 209–241). Cambridge, UK: Cambridge University Press.

Vettin, J., & Todt, D. (2004). Laughter in conversation: Features of occurrence and acoustic structure. *Journal of Nonverbal Behavior, 28,* 93–115.

Wallbott, H. G., & Scherer, K. R. (1986). Cues and channels in emotion recognition. *Journal of Personality and Social Psychology, 51,* 690–699.

Weisfeld, G. E. (1993). The adaptive value of humor and laughter. *Ethology and Sociobiology, 14,* 141–169.

Williams, C. E., & Stevens, K. N. (1972). Emotions and speech: Some acoustical correlates. *Journal of the Acoustical Society of America, 52,* 1238–1250.

Zajonc, R. B. (1980). Feeling and thinking: Preferences need no inferences. *American Psychologist, 35,* 151–175.

CHAPTER 13

Facial Expressions of Emotion

DAVID MATSUMOTO, DACHER KELTNER, MICHELLE N. SHIOTA,
MAUREEN O'SULLIVAN, and MARK FRANK

Within the field of emotion, the study of facial expressions has been notable both for empirical advances and for theoretical controversy. In this chapter, we draw upon an "evolutionist" approach to emotion, inspired by Charles Darwin, to draw together recent studies of facial expression. This literature indicates that facial expressions of emotion, as described by Darwin over 135 years ago, (1) include universal, reliable markers of discrete emotions when emotions are aroused and there is no reason to modify or manage the expression; (2) covary with distinct subjective experience; (3) are part of a coherent package of emotion responses that includes appraisals, physiological reactions, other nonverbal behaviors, and subsequent actions, as well as individual differences and mental and physical health; (4) are judged as discrete categories; and (5) as such, serve many interpersonal and social regulatory functions.

PERSPECTIVE AND ASSUMPTIONS

An evolutionist approach to facial expression has its roots in the work of Darwin (1872/1998) and of those who have refined and elaborated upon his evolutionist claims (Ekman, 1992b; Izard, 1971). Darwin claimed, in his principle of serviceable habits, that facial expressions are the residual actions of more complete behavioral responses, and occur in combination with other bodily responses—vocalizations, postures, gestures, skeletal muscle movements, and physiological responses. For example, we express anger by furrowing the brow and tightening the lips with teeth displayed, because these actions are part of an attack response; we express disgust with an open mouth, nose wrinkle, and tongue protrusion as part of a vomiting response. Facial expressions, then, are elements of a coordinated response involving multiple response systems.

As part of our evolutionary heritage, according to Darwin, all people, regardless of race or culture, should express emotions in the face and body in similar fashion. Darwin wrote *The Expression of the Emotions in Man and Animals* to refute the claims of Sir Charles Bell, the leading facial anatomist of his time and a teacher of Darwin's, about how God designed humans with unique facial muscles to express uniquely human emotions.[1] Relying on advances in photography and anatomy (Duchenne de Boulogne, 1862/1990), Darwin engaged in a detailed study of the muscle actions involved in emotion (see Table 13.1); he concluded that the muscle actions are universal, and their precursors can be seen in the expressive behaviors of nonhuman primates and other mammals.

Within the evolutionist framework that guides our analysis, facial expressions should covary with emotional experience, in large part because the signals that accompany involuntary experience give additional credibility to the display (Ekman, 1989; Ekman & O'Sullivan, 1991; although see Fridlund, 1994; Hauser, 1993; Krebs & Dawkins, 1984, for alternative perspectives). Those facial expressions that covary with emotion, it has been found, have certain properties, including brief duration, symmetry of muscle actions, and the presence of involuntary muscle actions (Ekman & Friesen, 1982; Ekman & Rosenberg, 2005). Facial expressions that accompany actual emotional experience are more reliable signals; they act as commitment devices to likely courses of action that are momentarily beyond the individual's volitional control (R. H. Frank, 1988; Gonzaga, Keltner, & Londahl, 2001).

The evolutionist perspective also suggests that facial expressions are more than simple readouts of internal states; they coordinate social interactions through their informative, evocative, and incentive functions (Keltner & Kring, 1998). They provide information to perceivers about the individual's emotional state (Ekman, 1993; Scherer, 1986), behavioral intentions (Fridlund, 1994), relational status vis-à-vis the target of the expression (Keltner, 1995; Tiedens, Ellsworth, & Mesquita, 2000), and objects and events in the social environment (Mineka & Cook, 1993). This view of facial expressions emerged from developmental studies of emotional exchanges between parents and children (Hertenstein & Campos, 2004; Klinnert, Campos, & Sorce, 1983; Klinnert, Emde, Butterfield, & Campos, 1986),

as well as from ethological studies of such social behaviors as flirting, reconciliation, aggression, and play. It is consistent with claims regarding the coevolution of signal and perceiver response to displays (Eibl-Ebesfeldt, 1989; Hauser, 1993). Thus an individual's emotional expression serves as a "social affordance" that evokes "prepared" responses in others (Esteves, Dimberg, & Öhman, 1994). Anger, for example, may have evolved to elicit fear-related responses and the inhibition of inappropriate action (Dimberg & Öhman, 1996); note that the Japanese often label another person's angry expression as "scary" (Matsumoto, 2006). Distress calls may have evolved to elicit sympathetic responses in observers (Eisenberg et al., 1989). Through these processes, emotional communication helps individuals in relationships—parents and children, mates, bosses and subordinates—respond to the demands and opportunities of their social environment. They are basic elements of social interaction, from flirtatious exchanges to greeting rituals. This perspective provides a compelling rationale for the prediction that people should be reliable judges of emotional displays, and sets the stage for the claim that deficits in expression are associated with psychological disorders.

The evolutionist perspective that we have described thus far leads to the following five claims, for which we review the most recent findings. Specially, an evolutionist approach to facial expression holds that discrete facial expressions of emotion (1) occur universally in emotionally arousing situations; (2) are linked with subjective experience; (3) are part of a coherent package of emotional responses; (4) are judged universally and discretely; and (5) have important social functions. In the discussion that follows, we bring together recent evidence that bears upon these claims.

THE CLAIMS OF THE EVOLUTIONIST PERSPECTIVE: AN EMPIRICAL REVIEW

Universality of Facial Emotional Expressions in Emotionally Arousing Situations

Claims concerning the universality of facial expressions of emotion are rooted in the notion that the facial anatomy is brought into service in expressions to solve similar problems across

TABLE 13.1. Descriptions of Facial Muscles and Other Nonverbal Behaviors Involved in the Emotions Darwin Considered Universal

Emotion	Darwin's description (nonfacial elements in parentheses)	Action units (AUs) associated with Darwin's description	AUs found to be associated with this emotion in research with humans (optional AUs in parentheses)	Homologous or analogous AUs found in chimpanzees
Anger	Nostrils raised, mouth compressed, furrowed brow, eyes wide open, head erect, (chest expanded, arms rigid by sides, stamping ground, body swaying backward/forward, trembling]	4; 5; 24; 38	4; 5 or 7; 22; 23; 24	4; 22; 23; 24
Contempt	Lip protrusion, nose wrinkle, partial closure of eyelids, turning away eyes, upper lip raised, (snort, body expiration, expiration)	9; 10; 22; 41; 61 or 62	Unilateral 12; unilateral 14	9; 10
Disgust	Lower lip turned down, upper lip raised, expiration, mouth open, spitting, blowing out, protruding lips, throat-clearing sound, lower lip and tongue protruding	10; 16; 22; 25 or 26	9 or 10; (25 or 26)	9; 10
Fear	Eyes open, mouth open, lips retracted, eyebrows raised, (crouching, paleness, perspiration, hair standing on end, muscles shivering, yawning, trembling)	1; 2; 5; 20	1; 2; 4; 5; 20; (25 or 26)	1; 2; 4
Happiness	Eyes sparkling, skin under eyes wrinkled, mouth drawn back at corners	6; 12	6; 12	6; 12
Joy	Zygomatic and orbicularis muscles contracted, upper lip raised, nasolabial fold formed, (muscles trembling, purposeless movements, laughter, clapping hands, jumping, dancing about, stamping, chuckling/giggling)	6; 7; 12	6; 12	6; 12
Sadness	Corners of mouth depressed, inner corner eyebrows raised, (low spirits)	1; 15	1; (4); 15; (17)	1; 4; 15; 17
Surprise	Eyebrows raised, mouth open, eyes open, lips protruding, (expiration, blowing/hissing, open hands high above head, palms toward person with straightened fingers, arms backwards)	1; 2; 5; 25 or 26	1; 2; 5; 25 or 26	1; 2

Note. The action unit (AU) numbers are those of Ekman and Friesen's (1978) Facial Action Coding System (FACS).

cultures related to social living, such as restoring justice, attending to others in need, signaling danger, expressing sexual or affiliative interest, and so on. By implication, the facial muscles themselves should be universal, and indeed they are. All humans around the world, regardless of race or culture, have the same facial anatomy (Gray & Goss, 1966). This universal facial musculature, furthermore, appears to be activated in emotion-specific ways across cultures.

Evidence from Adult Humans across Cultures

The strongest evidence for the universality of facial expressions of emotion comes from studies that directly measure facial behaviors when emotions are elicited. The first was Ekman's (1972) well-known study involving American and Japanese participants who viewed neutral and stressful films, and whose facial behaviors were recorded throughout the experiment (unbeknownst to them). Ekman coded the last 3 minutes of facial behavior during the neutral films, and the entire 3 minutes of the last stress film clip, using a modified version of the Facial Affect Scoring Technique (FAST), a precursor to the Facial Action Coding System (FACS; Ekman & Friesen, 1978). The FAST identified facial configurations of six emotions—anger, disgust, fear, happiness, sadness, and surprise— in different regions of the face. Two sets of analyses were performed on the facial codes: one involving separate facial areas, and one involving the whole face. The rank-order correlations on the facial behavior codes from the separate areas between the American and Japanese participants ranged from .72 for the eyes–lids area to .92 for the brows–forehead area. When the codes were combined into emotion-related configurations, the correlations ranged from .86 in the brows–forehead region to .96 in the lower face. Disgust, sadness, anger, and surprise were the most frequently displayed emotions, but fear and happiness were also evident. When facial codes were combined for whole-face emotions, according to the theoretical rationales of Darwin and of Tomkins (1962, 1963), the correlation between the Americans and the Japanese on the frequencies of whole-face emotions expressed spontaneously was .88.

Subsequent research has yielded further evidence supportive of the notion that theoretically relevant, universal facial expressions are elicited by specific emotionally evocative stimuli. There are at least 25 published studies in which the facial behaviors of individuals who participated in emotionally arousing conditions were coded reliably with the FACS and matched to the universal facial configurations of emotion (see Table 13.2). These studies demonstrate that the facial configurations of at least seven emotions, as postulated by Darwin and Tomkins, are produced when emotion is aroused and there is no reason to modify the expression because of social circumstances. (See also Eibl-Ebesfeldt, 1989, for an ethological perspective.)

The range of cultures in the 26 studies (25 in Table 13.2 and Ekman, 1972) is extensive. Matsumoto and Willingham's (2006) study, for instance, involved 84 athletes from 35 countries. Participants in other studies were Americans, Japanese, Germans, Canadians, and French. Collectively, these studies demonstrate that the facial expressions reported originally by Ekman actually do occur when emotion is aroused in people of different cultures. Table 13.1 contrasts the specific facial muscles originally proposed by Darwin (1872/1998) with the facial action units (AUs) that have been shown to be related to various emotions according to Ekman and Friesen's (1978) FACS.

Evidence from Nonhuman Primates

For years, ethologists (Chevalier-Skolnikoff, 1973; Geen, 1992; Hauser, 1993; Snowdon, 2003; Van Hoof, 1972) have noted the morphological similarities between human expressions of emotion and nonhuman primate expressions displayed in similar contexts. Van Hoof (1972) described the evolution of the smile and laugh along two different evolutionary tracks across early mammals, monkeys, apes, chimpanzees, and humans. Redican (1982) suggested that among nonhuman primates, facial displays described as grimaces and open-mouth grimaces are akin to the human emotions of fear and surprise; that the tense-mouth display is similar to anger; and that grimaces and a tense mouth combined form the often identified threat display. Redican also noted that nonhuman primates show a play face similar to the happy face of humans, and he suggested that the nonhuman pout serves a similar function to the human sad face. Ueno, Ueno, and Tomonaga (2004) demonstrated that both infant rhesus macaques

TABLE 13.2. Studies Examining Spontaneous Facial Expressions of Emotion

Citation	Participants	Eliciting stimuli or situation	Measurement system	Emotions corresponding to the facial muscle configurations in universal expressions
Bonanno & Keltner (1997, 2004); Keltner & Bonanno (1997)	German schizophrenic and psychosomatic patients, and healthy controls	Engaging in a political conversation with a partner they had never met before	EMFACS	Contempt, disgust, anger, sadness, fear, surprise, happiness
Bonanno et al. (2002)	Conjugally bereaved individuals	Interviews about their deceased spouses or ongoing important relationships	EMFACS	Anger, contempt, disgust, fear, sadness, Duchenne smiles
Camras et al. (1992)	Individuals with experience of childhood sexual abuse	Narrative interviews about the most distressing event or series of events in their lives	EMFACS	Anger, disgust, sadness, fear, Duchenne smiles
Chesney et al. (1990)	American and Japanese infants	Arm restraint, which produces distress	FACS	Anger, sadness, fear, and happiness
Ekman et al. (1980)	American salaried employees in managerial positions at an aerospace firm	Structured interview designed to assess Type A behavior	FACS	Disgust, fear, sadness, happiness, anger, contempt, surprise
Ekman et al. (1988)	American college students	Films designed to elicit positive and negative emotion	FACS	Happiness, unspecified negative emotions
Ekman et al. (1990)	Student nurses	Films designed to elicit strong negative emotions	FACS	Happiness
Ekman et al. (1997)	American college students	Two film clips designed to elicit positive emotions, and two designed to elicit negative emotions	FACS	Happiness
Ellgring (1986)	Depressed inpatients	Intake and discharge interviews	FACS and EMFACS	Happiness, contempt, anger, disgust, fear, sadness
Frank et al. (1993)	German depressed patients	Interviews	FACS	Happiness
Gosselin et al. (1995)	American University students	Films designed to elicit various emotions	FACS	Happiness
Harris & Alvarado (2005)	Actors from the Conservatory of Dramatic Arts in Québec	Interpreting 2 of 24 scenarios designed to elicit happiness, fear, anger, surprise, sadness, and disgust	FACS	Happiness, fear, anger, surprise, sadness, and disgust

(continued)

TABLE 13.2. (continued)

Citation	Participants	Eliciting stimuli or situation	Measurement system	Emotions corresponding to the facial muscle configurations in universal expressions
Heller & Haynal (1994)	American college students	Either being tickled, listening to an audiotape of jokes, or placing a hand in ice water	FACS	Duchenne smiles
Keltner et al. (1995)	French depressed patients	Interviews with the patients' psychiatrists	FACS and EMFACS	Contempt
Lerner et al. (2005)	American adolescents with behavior problems	Administration of the Wechsler Intelligence Scale for Children—Revised	EMFACS	Anger, fear, and sadness
Matsumoto & Willingham (2005)	American college students	Induction of three kinds of stress	EMFACS	Fear, anger, and disgust
Mauss et al. (2005)	Olympic medalists	Immediately after winning or losing a medal in competition, and on the podium	FACS	Six different types of smiles, contempt, disgust, fear, and sadness
Gross & Levenson (1993)	American college students	Films designed to elicit amusement and sadness	Emotion Expressive Behavior Coding (Messinger et al., 2001)	Amusement and sadness
Rosenberg & Ekman (1994)	Infants and their mothers	Play sessions between infants and mothers	FACS and Baby FACS	Duchenne smiles of happiness
Ruch (1995)	American university students	Videos selected for their ability to elicit primarily disgust and secondarily fear	FACS	Disgust, sadness, fear, happiness, contempt, and anger
Ruch (1993)	German university students	Slides of jokes and cartoons	FACS	Happiness
Soto et al. (2005)	German university students	Slides of jokes and cartoons	FACS	Happiness
Gross & Levenson (1993)	Chinese American and Mexican American college students	Aversive acoustic startle	Emotion Expressive Behavior Coding (Levenson, 2003b)	Anger, anxiety, disgust, confusion, contempt, interest, embarrassment, fear, happiness, sadness, surprise, crying, laughter

and infant chimpanzees showed different facial expressions to sweet and bitter tastes, but that the chimps' facial expressions were more similar to human facial expressions than to those of the macaques. However, even some of the smaller apes, such as siamangs (*Symphalangus syndactylus*), noted for their limited facial expression repertoire, have distinguishable facial expressions accompanying sexuality, agonistic behavior, grooming, and play (Liebal, Pika, & Tomasello, 2004). De Waal (2002) suggests that for some states a species less closely related to humans than chimpanzees, the bononos, may have more emotions in common with humans.

The most recent research has gone beyond demonstrating equivalence in morphological descriptions of expressions to identifying the exact facial musculature involved in the display behavior.[2] Indeed, the strongest support for the biological bases of facial expression would be a demonstration of homology in facial expressions between humans and related species, such as chimpanzees (*Pan troglodytes*). This would suggest that as humans evolved during the 120 million years of primate evolution, similar facial muscles developed, presumably to serve similar social functions. The newest work in this area, by Waller and colleagues (2006), reported that the forehead musculature of chimps is less well developed than that of humans. (They speculate that the greater hairiness of chimps makes eyebrow movements less visible, and hence less communicative.) But many other facial muscles and expressions have homologues and analogues comparable to those defined in the human FACS (Ekman & Friesen, 1978). For example, Waller et al. (2006) report that many of the muscles coded on the human face have the same location and functional effect in humans and chimpanzees (see Table 13.1). Based on this work, there is now a ChimpFACS that allows for identification of the specific AUs chimpanzees use in producing facial expressions (see Vick, Waller, Parr, Pasqualini, & Bard, 2007).[3]

Linkages between Facial Emotional Expressions and Subjective Experience

The evolutionist perspective suggests a linkage between each universal signal of emotion and a subjective experience, in particular when there is no reason to manage or modify the expression because of social circumstances. Eleven studies reported in Table 13.2 report correlations between emotion-specific facial behaviors and self-reports of the experience of the discrete emotion (these findings are summarized in Table 13.3). It is noteworthy that linkages between discrete facial expressions of emotion and self-reports of the same emotional states are stronger in within-subject designs that involve precise, second-to-second measurement of both expression and experience, such as Rosenberg and Ekman's (1994) study and that by Mauss, Levenson, McCarter, Wilhelm, and Gross (2005). In the latter, cross-lag correlations indicated very high within-individual correlations between facial behavior and experience intensity for both amusing and sadness-eliciting films (*r*'s = .73 and .74, respectively). When correlations were corrected for disattenuation, they were even higher (*r*'s = .89 and .97).

Moreover, important *nonfindings* not reflected in Table 13.3 need to be considered. In Bonanno and Keltner's (1997) study, for instance, anger, contempt, and sadness were positively correlated with reports of grief, but fear and disgust were not. In Ekman, Friesen, and Ancoli's (1980) study, expressions of disgust were positively correlated with disgust but negatively correlated with anger and sadness. In Harris and Alvarado's (2005) study, Duchenne smiles were correlated with happiness and amusement, but not with reports of feeling anxious, angry, or embarrassed.

Complementing the studies listed in Table 13.3 are several lines of research that provide convergent evidence. Matsumoto and Kupperbusch (2001) reported significant correlations between judged expressions and self-reported experience. Duchenne smiles have been correlated with the experience of positive emotion in young and old adults (Frank, Ekman, & Friesen, 1993; Hess, Banse, & Kappas, 1995; Keltner & Bonanno, 1997; Smith, 1995). Duchenne and non-Duchenne smiles distinguished nonharassed and harassed job applicants (Woodzicka & LaFrance, 2001), as well as honest and deceptive interviewees (Ekman, Friesen, & O'Sullivan, 1988). Frank and Ekman (1997) reported predicted differences in fear between honest and deceptive men. The facial signals related to embarrassment and amusement (e.g., gaze aversion and smile controls vs. the open-mouthed smile) were correlated with self-reports of these emotions (Keltner, 1995). Spontaneous laughter and

TABLE 13.3. Studies Reporting Significant Correlations between Spontaneous Facial Expressions of Emotion and Self-Reports of Specific Emotions

Citation[a]	Facial expressions measured	Self-reports obtained	Correlation
Bonanno & Keltner (1997)	Duchenne laughing	Grief (concurrent)	−.39*
	Anger		.36*
	Contempt		.31*
	Sadness		.34*
Keltner & Bonanno (1997)	Duchenne smiles	Distress	−.49**
		Fear	−.31*
		Enjoyment	.35*
	Duchenne laughing	Distress	−.36*
		Enjoyment	.34*
Bonanno & Keltner (2004)	Duchenne smiles	Distress	−.44*
	Duchenne laughing	Anger	−.51**
Ekman et al. (1980)	Smiling (frequency)	Happiness	.60**
	Smiling (duration)	Happiness	.35*
	Smiling (intensity)	Happiness	.34*
	Disgust (frequency)	Disgust	.37*
		Anger	−.35*
		Sadness	−.46**
	Disgust (duration)	Disgust	.55**
		Fear	.46*
		Pain	.41*
Ekman et al. (1990)	Duchenne smiles	Amusement	.70*
		Happiness	.59*
		Excitement	.39***
		Interest	.40***
		Anger	−.38***
		Sadness	−.44***
Harris & Alvarado (2005)	Duchenne smiles	Happiness	.19† (humor condition)
		Amusement	.28**
Mauss et al. (2005)	Duchenne smiles	Amusement	.73***
	Sadness	Sadness	.74***
Rosenberg & Ekman (1994)[b]	Disgust and fear	Disgust and fear	.71 (rat film)
			.90 (amputation film)
			.83 (amputation film)
Ruch (1993)	Duchenne smiles	Positive affectivity	.33* (experimental group)
			.52* (control group)
			.78* (rank order of cell means)
		Verbal enjoyment	.28*
Ruch (1995)	Duchenne smiles	Funniness	.55 (between-subjects design, aggregate data)
			.96 (within-subjects design, aggregate data)
			.61 (between-subjects design, raw data)
			.71 (within-subjects design, raw data)
			.63 (across all stimuli and designs)

[a]Gosselin et al. (1995) obtained self-reports but did not report correlations between the ratings and facial expressions.
[b]The statistics reported for this study are the probabilities of co-occurrence between the ratings of specific emotion categories and the corresponding facial expressions.
*$p < .05$; **$p < .01$; ***$p < .001$; †$p < .10$

smiling were found to have some distinct expe-riential correlates (Keltner & Bonanno, 1997). The intensity of laughter or smiling correlated with self-reports of the funniness of the humor-ous stimuli (McGhee, 1977; Ruch, 1995).

Facial Expressions as Part of a Coherent Package of Emotional Responses

Darwin (1872/1998) suggested, in his principle of serviceable habits, that facial expressions are the residual actions of more complete behav-ioral responses. By implication, facial expres-sions not only should be related to emotional experience; they should also be coordinated with other components, such as autonomic or neuroendocrine changes, that enable the organ-ism to respond adaptively. Researchers refer to this possibility in terms of "emotion pack-ages," "emotion response system coherence," or "response covariation" (Bonanno & Kelt-ner, 2004; Ekman, 1992a; Lazarus, 1991; Levenson, 1994). Distinct lines of evidence sug-gest that brief facial expressions of emotion covary in systematic fashion with appraisal processes, physiological responses, specific ac-tions (e.g., aggressive behavior or cooperation), broad individual differences in emotionality, and measures of physical and mental health.

Co-occurrence with Distinct Appraisals

If facial expressions are part of a coherent re-sponse profile, they should covary with emotion-specific appraisal processes. Evidence suggests that this is the case. For example, be-reaved adults' facial expressions of anger and sadness while discussing their deceased spouses co-occurred with distinct appraisal themes (jus-tice and loss) coded from participants' sponta-neous narratives that were contemporaneous with the facial expressions (Bonanno & Keltner, 1997). Another study found that pos-ing facial expressions of anger was related to the appraisal that others were responsible for social events, whereas posing facial sadness was associated with the appraisal that the same events were due to situational causes (Keltner, Ellsworth, & Edwards, 1993). Moreover, spontaneous facial expressions reliably differ-entiate whether Olympic athletes have won or lost a medal, and differences in their smiling behavior differentiate what kind of medal they won (Matsumoto & Willingham, 2006). As a final example, expressions of anger, contempt,

and disgust are reliably associated with ap-praisals related to moral violations of autonomy, community, and divinity, respec-tively (Rozin, Lowery, Imada, & Haidt, 1999). Taken together, these studies suggest that facial expressions of distinct emotions covary with specific appraisals.

Covariance with Distinct Physiological Responses

Facial expressions are also coordinated with physiology. When emotions are aroused and fa-cial expressions are used as markers of those emotions, discrete physiological signatures oc-cur in both the autonomic nervous system and the brain (Davidson, 2003; Ekman, Davidson, & Friesen, 1990; Ekman, Levenson, & Friesen, 1983; Levenson, Carstensen, Friesen, & Ekman, 1991; Levenson & Ekman, 2002; Levenson, Ekman, & Friesen, 1990; Levenson, Ekman, Heider, & Friesen, 1992; Mauss et al., 2005; Tsai & Levenson, 1997). Table 13.4, adapted from Levenson (2003b), summarizes the major findings in this area and highlights how emotions signaled in facial expression are associated with activity in other physiological systems. These patterns have been found in people from cultures as widely divergent as the United States and the Minangkabau of West Sumatra, Indonesia.

Alongside these findings, it is important to note that the coherence of facial expression and physiology has not always been consistent. Some studies (Brown & Schwartz, 1980; Cacioppo, Martzke, Petty, & Tassinary, 1988) demonstrated only low correlations between expression and physiological response, and some found no relationship (Buck, 1977; Mauss, Wilhelm, & Gross, 2004). These nega-tive findings are the likely results of several methodological factors: (1) the fact that the oc-currence of an emotion is sometimes defined by the attempt to manipulate it, instead of the in-dependent confirmation of its elicitation; (2) the type of emotion elicited; (3) the nature of the measures of emotional responding used; (4) the temporal resolution of the measurement (Mauss et al., 2005; Rosenberg & Ekman, 1994); (5) the fact that the laboratory may not be the optimal context in which to elicit adap-tive physiological responses; and (6) the differ-ence between between- and within-subjects de-signs. The Mauss et al. (2005) study described earlier highlights the importance of the last is-sue. They measured facial behaviors, emotional

TABLE 13.4. Changes in Appearance and Autonomic Nervous System (ANS) Activity Associated with the Discrete Emotional States Darwin Considered Universal

Emotion	AUs associated with the physiological changes reported	Type of change	Change	ANS mediation
Anger	1; 4; 5; 17; 23 or 24	Coloration	Reddening	Vasodilation, increased contractability
		Moisture and secretions	Foaming	Salivary glands
		Protrusions	Piloerection	Muscle fibers at base of hair follicles
			Blood vessels bulging	Vasodilation
		Eye appearance	Constriction	Pupils
			Bulging	Eyelid muscles
Disgust	9 or 10	Moisture and secretions	Salivating, drooling	Salivary glands
Fear	1; 2; 4; 5; 7; 20	Coloration	Blanching	Vasoconstriction
		Moisture and secretions	Sweating, clamminess	Sweat glands
		Protrusions	Piloerection	Muscle fibers at base of hair follicles
		Eye appearance	Dilation	Pupils
			Bulging	Eyelid muscles
Happiness	6; 12	Eye appearance	Twinkling	Lacrimal glands plus contraction of orbicularis oculi
Sadness	1 (or 1 + 4); 15	Moisture and secretions	Tearing, crying	Lacrimal glands
Embarrassment		Coloration	Blushing	Vasodilation

Note. Adapted with permission from Levenson (2003b). Changes from the original table include the reorganization of contents according to emotion, the addition of action units (AUs) associated with physiological changes, minor wording changes, and the removal of sexual arousal from the emotion category.

experience, and three types of physiological response (skin conductance, cardiovascular activation, and somatic activity) with second-by-second precision while participants watched films designed to elicit amusement and sadness. The results indicated clear, moderate-sized, within-individual correlations between facial behavior and the various physiological response components.

Most recently, Lerner, Gonzalez, Dahl, Haririr, and Taylor (2005) demonstrated that the discrete facial expressions of fear, anger, and disgust were reliably linked not only to cardiovascular responses, but to neuroendocrine activity as well. Participants were exposed to three different types of stressors during which they were videotaped, and their cardiovascular and hypothalamic–pituitary–adrenocortical (cortisol) responses were measured. Fear expressions were associated with elevated cardiovascular and cortisol levels; anger and disgust were linked with reduced responses. Matsumoto, Nezlek, and Koopmann (2007) reported moderate-sized correlations between self-reported expressive behavior and three types of physiological sensations (ergotropic, trophotropic, and felt temperature) in approximately 3,000 respondents from 27 countries. They also reported consistent correlations between verbal and nonverbal expressions, as well as between emotion intensity and physiological sensations, all of which suggest coherence in an underlying neurophysiological reality.

Covariance with Subsequent Behaviors

Another source of evidence supporting the links between expressions and emotional responses comes from studies that demonstrate covariance between facial expressions of emotion and subsequent behaviors. Facial expressions of emotion can signal behavioral intent. In the first study to demonstrate this effect, Ekman, Liebert, et al. (1972) examined the relationship between facial expressions of emotion produced by children as they watched television and their subsequent hurtful behaviors and aggressive play. Children were videotaped as they watched either a violent scene from a movie or competitive sports. Afterwards, they were placed in a situation where they could either help or hurt another child, and then engaged in a free-play period. Boys who smiled during the violent scenes engaged in more hurtful behavior and aggressive play afterwards; boys who showed sadness during the violent scenes engaged in more helpful behavior and less aggressive play when the video was finished.

Matsumoto, Haan, Gary, Theodorou, and Cooke-Carney (1986) videotaped the facial behaviors of preschool dyads as they either cooperated or competed in a Prisoner's Dilemma game, and used the Emotion Facial Action Coding System (EMFACS) to code facial behaviors. The children displayed varied emotional responses, and these were reliably linked to the actions of the game. Cooperative behaviors elicited decreased negative emotion, whereas children who were defected against expressed more non-Duchenne smiles and positive–negative blends. Most importantly, facial expressions that occurred after an action—cooperation or competition—predicted subsequent behavior. Children who expressed Duchenne smiles after their partners cooperated were more likely to cooperate also; those who expressed anything else after cooperation were more likely to defect. Defections that were followed by non-Duchenne smiling were more likely to lead to subsequent, repeated defections; when defections were followed by Duchenne smiling, however, the subsequent act was likely to be cooperative.

More recently, Keltner, Moffitt, and Stouthamer-Loeber (1995), in their study of adolescent boys, examined relations between facial expressions of emotion observed in a 2-minute interaction and teacher reports of social behavior. Facial displays of anger observed in an interactive IQ testing context correlated significantly with teacher ratings of delinquent and aggressive behavior at school; facial displays of fear correlated negatively with these behaviors, and positively with withdrawal-related behaviors.

Covariance with Broad Individual Differences

Further evidence consistent with the claim that facial expressions covary with multisystem responses comes from studies linking facial expressions to measures of individual differences in emotionality. For example, as noted earlier, Bonanno and Keltner (1997) used the FACS to code bereaved adults' facial expressions as they talked about their recently deceased spouses. Facial expressions of anger predicted increased grief severity 14 and 25 months after loss; laughing and smiling, however, predicted reduced grief over time. Importantly, facial expressions predicted long-term adjustment, independently of initial levels of grief and individual differences in the tendency to report high levels of distress. These findings suggest that brief measures of facial expressions (in this study, 6 minutes of behavior were coded) predict broad patterns of adaptation to important life events.

Harker and Keltner (2001) coded women's college yearbook photos with the FACS, and showed that Duchenne smiling was positively correlated with multiple measures of personality (i.e., affiliation, warmth, competence), personal well-being, and marital satisfaction at various times over the next 30 years. And Abe and Izard (1999) measured discrete facial expressions of emotion in 18-month-old infants during episodes of the Strange Situation procedure, and correlated these with maternal ratings of the five-factor model of personality when the children were 3.5 years old. Negative expressions were strongly correlated with Neuroticism and inversely related to Agreeableness and Conscientiousness; full-face positive expressions were positively correlated with Extraversion and Openness to Experience. These findings suggest that facial expressions of discrete emotions systematically covary with coherent patterns of thought, feeling, and action as captured in personality measures.

Covariance with Measures of Mental and Physical Health

If facial expressions are part of more coherent responses to the environment, they should likewise be related to measures of mental and physical health, which capture maladaptive patterns of thought, action, and feeling. Several studies indicate that fleeting facial expressions of emotion are telling clues about personal adjustment. Anger displays are related to the incidence of ischemia in patients with coronary artery disease (Rosenberg et al., 2001). The oblique eyebrows and pressed lips of sympathy correlate with reduced heart rate, whereas winces of pain are related to elevated heart rate (Eisenberg et al., 1989). Facial expressions differentiate among genuine pain, masked pain, and faked pain (Craig, Hyde, & Patrick, 1991; Prkachin, 1992), as well as between healthy individuals and psychiatric patients (Ellgring, 1986; Steimer-Krause, Krause, & Wagner, 1990), schizophrenic and psychosomatic patients (Steimer-Krause et al., 1990), schizophrenic and depressed patients (Berenbaum & Oltmanns, 1992; Ekman, Matsumoto, & Friesen, 1997; Ellgring, 1986), suicidal and nonsuicidal depressed patients (Heller & Haynal, 1994), and patients with major versus minor depression (Ekman et al., 1997). In Ekman et al.'s (1997) study, for instance, patients with major depression showed more sadness and disgust and fewer non-Duchenne smiles than those with minor depression. Manic patients showed more Duchenne and non-Duchenne smiles, and less anger, disgust, or sadness than either group with depression. Schizophrenic patients showed more fear and fewer displays of all other emotions. Moreover, expressions of contempt and unfelt happiness measured during intake interviews of the depressed patients predicted improvement at discharge. In another study, facial expressions of disgust (and glaring) differentiated between individuals with Type A and Type B personalities, and facial expressions of contempt, anger, and disgust were all correlated with various speech indices of hostility, anger, competitiveness, and despondency (Chesney et al., 1990). Moreover, Duchenne smiles differentiated whether depressed patients were improving as a result of treatment (Ekman et al., 1997), and patients with right-hemisphere damage were impaired in the production of facial expressions of emo-

tions, particularly positive emotion (Borod, Koff, Lorch, & Nicholas, 1986).

Pathologies also affect the ability to pose and recognize emotional expressions. Abused children, for instance, have difficulties both posing and recognizing facial expressions (Camras et al., 1988; Pollak, Cicchetti, Hornung, & Reed, 2000; Pollak & Sinha, 2002). Severely autistic children have broad and pervasive deficits in recognizing emotions (Hobson, 1986; Ozonoff, Pennington, & Rogers, 1990). Children with high-functioning autism or Asperger's syndrome have emotion-specific deficits: They are generally able to recognize happiness, sadness, fear, and anger (Capps, Yirmiya, & Sigman, 1992), but not facial signals of embarrassment or shame (Heerey, Keltner, & Capps, 2003). Individuals with high trait anxiety recognize fearful faces better than those without such anxiety (Surcinelli, Codispoti, Montebarocci, Rossi, & Baldaro, 2004), and individuals who are depressed are generally worse at recognizing all facial emotions (Persad & Polivy, 1993). Individuals with current substance dependence and a history of alcohol dependence are also generally worse at recognizing facial emotions (Foisy et al., 2005). And patients with myotonic dystrophy Type 1 have difficulty recognizing angry, disgusted, and fearful faces (Winblad, Hellstrom, Lindberg, & Hansen, 2006).

More than 135 years ago, Charles Darwin claimed that brief facial expressions are really tokens of more complex, multisystem responses to specific environmental demands or opportunities. The literature we have reviewed in this section elaborates upon this early evolutionist claim, indicating that facial expressions of distinct emotions covary systematically with distinct appraisals, physiological response, social behavior, stable individual differences, and markers of physical and mental health.

Recognition of Facial Emotional Expressions: Universality and Brain Involvement

Universal Recognition

Early studies supporting the universal recognition of facial expressions of emotion were judgment studies, in which observers of different cultures viewed facial stimuli and judged the emotions portrayed in them. The earliest studies by Ekman and Izard demonstrated the existence of six universal expressions—anger, disgust, fear, happiness, sadness, and surprise—in literate and preliterate cultures (Ekman, 1972, 1973; Ekman & Friesen, 1971; Ekman, Sorenson, & Friesen, 1969; Izard, 1971). Even when low-intensity expressions were used (Ekman et al., 1987; Matsumoto et al., 2002), there was strong agreement across cultures about the emotion in the expression.

Since the original studies by Ekman and Izard, 27 studies examining judgments of facial expressions have replicated the finding of universal recognition of facial expressions of emotion (Matsumoto, 2001). In addition, a meta-analysis of 168 datasets examining judgments of emotion in the face and other nonverbal stimuli indicated universal emotion recognition at well above chance levels (Elfenbein & Ambady, 2002b). Even after correction for chance guessing, this statistic was associated with a very large effect size, consistently supporting the findings that expressions are universally recognized.

More recent research continues to complement this conclusion. Horstmann (2003), for instance, asked approximately 2,000 online participants whether the universal facial expressions signaled feeling states, behavioral intentions, or action requests. The majority of the observers chose feeling states as the primary message of the expressions of disgust, fear, sadness, surprise, and happiness. (Participants did choose behavioral intentions or action requests as the message of angry expressions.) Lawrence et al. (2005) asked 484 children between 6 and 16 years of age to judge the universal faces. All of these children were able to judge the emotions accurately beyond chance levels, and the accuracy rates increased linearly across age for happiness, surprise, fear, and disgust; for sad and angry expressions, accuracy rates remained constant across age. And Parr (2003) has demonstrated that chimpanzees are able to discriminate five emotional expressions with similarities to human expressions (relaxed-lip face, pant-hoot, play face/relaxed open-mouth face, scream face, and bared-teeth face) and a neutral face. Moreover, chimpanzees are able to match different emotional faces with specific behaviors—a finding suggesting that they understand specific meanings associated with facial expressions, much

as humans do in matching faces with emotional stories (Matsumoto & Ekman, 2004; Rosenberg & Ekman, 1995). These findings suggest strongly that chimpanzees, like humans, respond to different faces as categories.

There have been various methodological critiques of the studies of face recognition (e.g., Russell, 1991a, 1994; Russell, Bachorowski, & Fernandez-Dols, 2003). This body of criticism has been addressed in a number of studies (e.g., Ekman et al., 1987; Matsumoto, 2005; Matsumoto & Ekman, 1989, 2004; Yrizarry, Matsumoto, & Wilson-Cohn, 1998; Frank & Stennett, 2001; Rosenberg & Ekman, 1995). These studies demonstrate that the original findings of universality in judgments of discrete emotion categories were not artifacts of the forced-choice judgment task and are, in fact, quite robust across different judgment tasks and cultures. The literature we review below indicates that the recognition of distinct facial expressions activates specific regions of the brain.

Brain Activation Produced by Perceiving Facial Expressions

Electroencephalographic and brain imaging studies demonstrate brain specificity in judgments of discrete emotions. The perception of fearful faces activates regions in the left amygdala (Breiter et al., 1996; Phillips et al., 1997; Whalen et al., 2004), even when the presentation of a fearful face is masked by the presentation of an immediately ensuing neutral expression (Whalen et al., 1998), or by other, consciously perceived expressions in the face or voice (de Gelder, Morris, & Dolan, 2005). This neural network is modulated by the right prefrontal cortex (Hariri, Mattay, Tessitore, Fera, & Weinberger, 2003) and by the peptide oxytocin (Kirsch et al., 2005). The perception of sad faces activates the left amygdala and right temporal lobe (Blair, Morris, Frith, Perrett, & Dolan, 1998). The perception of angry faces activates the right orbito-frontal cortex and cingulate cortex (Blair et al., 1998; Sprengelmeyer et al., 1996). The perception of disgusted faces activates the basal ganglia, anterior insula, and frontal lobes (Phillips et al., 1997; Sprengelmeyer et al., 1996). Duchenne smiles activate the left side of the lateral frontal, midfrontal, anterior temporal, and central anterior scalp regions (Davidson et al., 1990;

Ekman & Davidson, 1993). Some evidence suggests that the brain areas involved when emotion is elicited are the same areas involved in judging emotions in others (Calder, 2003; Calder, Keane, Manes, Antoun, & Young, 2000).

Disease and lesion studies indicate that the perception of different emotions is associated with different brain regions. Bilateral lesions to the amygdala impair the ability to recognize fearful faces and vocalizations, but not the ability to recognize facial expressions of sadness, disgust, or happiness (Adolphs, Tranel, Damasio, & Damasio, 1994, 1995; Adolphs et al., 1999; Broks et al., 1998; Calder, Young, & Perrett, 1996; Sprengelmeyer et al., 1996; Young, Hellawell, Van de Wal, & Johnson, 1996). Individuals suffering from Huntington's disease, which affects the basal ganglia, are unable to recognize disgusted expressions accurately but are accurate in judging facial expressions of other negative emotions (Sprengelmeyer et al., 1996). Even carriers of Huntington's disease are unable to recognize facial expressions of disgust (Gray, Young, Barker, Curtis, & Gibson, 1997).

The last 10 years, then, have seen the emergence of two robust literatures converging upon the conclusion that evolution has shaped the capacity, universal to humans, to reliably recognize distinct facial expressions of emotion. The first is the new wave of studies of emotion recognition, which have dealt with confounds and problems in interpretation of the influential Ekman and Izard studies, and found consistently that the recognition of facial emotion expressions is universal. A second literature has shown that different patterns of regional activation in the brain occur when individuals perceive distinct facial expressions, raising the possibility that we humans have evolved distinct emotion perception systems or circuits.

Important Social Functions of Facial Emotional Expressions

Central to an evolutionist analysis of emotion is the premise that the emotions evolved to help solve social problems (e.g., Ekman, 1992; Keltner, Haidt, & Shiota, in press; Tooby & Cosmides, 1992). Expressions are central to these processes in three ways (Keltner, 2003). First, they provide information about the expressor's emotions, intentions, relationship with the target, and relationship with the environment. Second, they evoke responses, particularly emotions, from others. Third, they provide incentives for desired social behavior. The research reviewed above supports the first contention. Research reviewed in this section supports the second two.

Facilitating Specific Behaviors in Perceivers

Because facial expressions of emotion are universal social signals, they contain meaning not only about the expressor's intent and subsequent behavior, but also about what the perceiver is likely to do. Marsh, Ambady, and Kleck (2005) showed observers fearful and angry faces, and asked them either to push or to pull a lever when they saw them. Anger facilitated avoidance-related behaviors, whereas fear facilitated approach-related behaviors. Winkielman, Berridge, and Wilbarger (2005) found that subliminal presentation of smiles produced increases in how much of a beverage people poured and consumed, and how much they were willing to pay for it; presentation of angry faces decreased these behaviors. Also, emotional displays evoke specific, complementary emotional responses from observers. For example, anger has been found to evoke fear (Dimberg & Öhman, 1996; Esteves et al., 1994), whereas distress evokes sympathy and aid (Eisenberg et al., 1989).

Signaling the Nature of Interpersonal Relationships

Some of the more important and provocative set of findings in the area of facial emotional expressions and interpersonal relationships come from Gottman and Levenson's (Gottman & Levenson, 1992; Gottman, Levenson, & Woodin, 2001) studies involving married couples. In their research, married couples visited their laboratory after the spouses had not seen each other for 24 hours, and then the spouses engaged in intimate conversations about daily events, issues of conflict, and so forth. Discrete expressions of contempt, especially by the men, and disgust, especially by the women, predicted later marital dissatisfaction and even divorce.

Regulating Social Interaction

Facial expressions of emotion, and other facial behaviors, are important regulators of social interaction. In the developmental literature, this concept has been investigated under the rubric of "social referencing" (Klinnert et al., 1983)—that is, the process whereby infants seek out emotional information from others to interpret ambiguous objects and events, and then use that information to act (see also Hertenstein & Campos, 2004).

The Importance of Judging Emotions Accurately

Because facial expressions are reliable markers of emotion, and because they serve important social functions, the ability to judge them accurately may be linked to important intra- and interpersonal processes. In exploring this thesis, Matsumoto and his colleagues addressed this problem in the creation of the Japanese and Caucasian Brief Affect Recognition Test (JACBART), which was based on Ekman and Friesen's (1969) observation of microexpressions (described earlier). In the JACBART, seven universal facial expressions are presented very briefly (for 0.20 second), embedded within a 1-second presentation of the same expressor's neutral face.[4] Matsumoto et al. (2000) demonstrated the internal and temporal reliability of the emotion recognition scores produced; sufficient item discrimination and range; convergent validity among emotions; and reliability across response alternatives. Construct validity was established by correlations between emotion recognition accuracy scores and the personality constructs Openness and Conscientiousness in multiple measures of personality. Moreover, emotion recognition accuracy scores were independent of visual acuity in judging general facial stimuli presented at high speeds. The findings on Openness have been replicated by others (Terracciano, Merritt, Zonderman, & Evans, 2003).

Emotion recognition ability has been theoretically linked to the concept of emotional intelligence (Mayer, Salovey, Caruso, & Sitarenios, 2001; Salovey & Mayer, 1990). In fact, in a study using behavioral measures to test the predictive validity of the JACBART, emotion recognition accuracy was correlated with Problem Solving, Goal Setting, and total Effectiveness as measured by an In-Basket task (Matsumoto, LeRoux, Bernhard, & Gray, 2004). And Yoo, Matsumoto, and LeRoux (2006) used the JACBART to demonstrate that emotion recognition abilities of international students measured at the beginning of the school year were correlated with various ad-

justment indices at the beginning of the year (anxiety, homesickness, culture shock), as well as at the end of the year (anxiety, contentment). Recognition ability was also correlated with students' end-of-year grade point averages and with ratings of their participation in the behavioral task obtained in the laboratory session.

The hypothesis that microexpressions are related to deception, outlined above, suggests that the ability to recognize emotions from microexpressions should be related to the ability to detect lies. In fact, using an early microexpression test (the Brief Affect Recognition Test), Ekman and Friesen (1974) did indeed find that the ability to recognize microexpressions was significantly correlated with lie detection accuracy. Ekman and O'Sullivan (1991) replicated this finding. Most recently, Ekman (2003) has developed the Micro Expression Training Tool (METT), which allows individuals to test themselves on their ability to identify correctly basic expressions of anger, fear, sadness, disgust, happiness, contempt, and surprise. Training with this technique significantly increases the accurate recognition of deceptive items in which microexpressions occur (Ekman & Frank, 2005), and these results have been replicated across cultures (Frank, 2007). Recent research has indicated that schizophrenic individuals trained with the METT improved to a level that was not significantly different from the performance of pretrained controls (Russell, Chu, & Phillips, 2006).

In concluding our empirical review, we suggest that the studies brought together here, for the first time, strongly support the five claims made from an evolutionist approach to facial expression. The data suggest that facial expressions of emotion, as originally described by Darwin, are universally aroused in specific situations (Claim 1); linked to subjective experience (Claim 2); part of a coherent, multisystem response package (Claim 3); judged across different cultures in similar fashion (Claim 4); and associated with social functions (Claim 5).

A RESEARCH AGENDA FOR THE FUTURE

Evolutionist approaches to facial expression, and the methods and findings inspired by this perspective, have been integral to the development of the field of emotion. This perspective has inspired coherent lines of empirical inquiry on the universality, coherence, recognition, and social functions of facial expression. All remain fruitful areas of exploration. We close this chapter by referring briefly to questions where the need for empirical research is great, and where opportunities for discovery are clear.

When Do Discrete Facial Expressions of Emotion Appear in Development?

There is continuing controversy about whether newborns signal discrete emotions in the face. The biologically based programs that lead to the regular occurrence of facial expressions may unfold later according to maturational or developmental milestones, especially milestones in cognitive abilities. Few longitudinal data in early infancy, however, shed light on the developmental timetable for discrete facial expressions, and future research is needed in this area.

What Other Emotions May Be Expressed in the Face?

Anger, disgust, fear, happiness, sadness, and surprise are the only emotions for which evidence has been found to date demonstrating their universal signal characteristics, unique physiological signatures, universal appraisal mechanisms, and presence in other primates. But they may not be the only emotions with such qualities. Unfortunately, evidence for others is suggestive but incomplete. For instance, preliminary data suggest that candidates include displays of contempt (Ekman & Friesen, 1986; Ekman & Heider, 1988); embarrassment (Keltner & Buswell, 1997) and pride (Tracy & Robins, 2004) and positive emotions such as awe, desire, and love (Gonzaga, Keltner, & Londahl, 2001; Gonzaga et al., 2006; Shiota, Campos, & Keltner, 2003). Future studies will need to address the possibility that other emotions are also displayed in the face, as well as variants of the same emotion.

In What Other Channels Can Emotions Be Expressed?

It is certain that emotions are expressed in channels other than the face and voice, the two most studied to date. Both the well-studied emotions, such as anger and disgust, and the less investigated emotions, such as embarrass-

ment and love, are certain to involve expressive behavior in other channels, such as gaze, head position, posture, touch, or proximity. Recent research suggests such possibilities. New research in this area includes studies on embarrassment (Keltner, 1995), shame (Halisch & Halisch, 1980; Lewis, Alessandri, & Sullivan, 1992; Stipek & Gralinski, 1991), pride (Tracy & Matsumoto, 2005; Tracy & Robins, 2004), romantic love (Gonzaga et al., 2001), and sympathy (Eisenberg et al., 1989).

These new findings suggest that more emotions than previously thought can be communicated in brief expressive behaviors. These findings raise important questions to pursue. To what extent do the different channels—facial expression, gaze, posture, touch—covary in coherent fashion? To what extent to these channels of emotion communication convey distinct emotion-relevant information (e.g., about felt experience or behavioral intention), and to what extent is the information they convey redundant?

What Factors Moderate Facial Expressions and Their Linkages with Other Emotion Responses?

Regulation of facial expressions in humans is a complex neuropsychological phenomenon that can occur outside of conscious awareness (Matsumoto & Lee, 1993). Expression regulation via display rules provides an opportunity to understand how the linkage between expression and experience can be systematically decoupled. The coherence between emotion and expression is moderated by context, and contexts that require the modification of expression may result in decoupling of the linkage between experience and display. Research on this topic, however, is still in its infancy.

What Factors Moderate the Production of Facial Prototypes of the Universal Emotions?

The full-face, high-intensity facial prototypes of the basic emotions do not always occur when emotion is aroused. Facial expression prototypes, we suggest, are more likely to be seen when strong emotions are aroused and the context allows for their expression, such as when married couples fight (Gottman & Levenson, 1992), or athletes win or lose a medal at the Olympic Games (Matsumoto &

Willingham, 2006). When the full-face prototypes are not expressed, partial facial expressions may occur. In addition to the influence of
context and emotion intensity, partial expressions occur in part because of the different neural wiring of the facial muscles (Matsumoto &
Lee, 1993). Lower-face muscles are represented
more fully in the motor cortex than those of the
upper face, allowing for more control of the
lower face. Moreover, the number of bilateral
versus contralateral fibers to the facial muscles
differs depending on region, with the lower
face being primarily contralateral and bilateral
fibers increasing in the upper face. And voluntary and involuntary expressions are under the
control of different neural tracts. These factors
strongly suggest that the lower-face components of facial expressions are more likely to be
moderated by various factors, including culture
and individual differences.

How Many Variants of Each Facial Emotional Expression Exist?

The original studies documenting universality
of facial expressions, as well as subsequent research, indicate that many of the emotions
have variants in expressions. With some exceptions (Matsumoto, 1989; Rozin, Lowery, &
Ebert, 1994), research has not examined the
nature of these variants. Different variants may
be associated with different intentions; for instance, anger may lead to a joke, walking away,
or physical aggression, and it is possible that
these different behavioral consequences are signaled by different variants of anger expressions. Similar differences may exist for the
other emotions as well, and future studies will
need to explore these possibilities.

The only emotion that appears to have a single facial muscle action is that of enjoyment,
which is signaled by the Duchenne smile. There
are, however, many kinds of enjoyment
(Ekman, 2003), and it is likely that these different kinds of enjoyment are signaled through
different expressive channels, such as postural
behavior and gaze activity. This research is just
getting underway.

CONCLUSION

An evolutionist approach to facial expression
has generated vibrant empirical literatures,
which allow for the following conclusions:

1. Some facial expressions are universal, reliable markers of discrete emotions when
emotions are aroused and there is no reason
to modify or manage the expressions.
2. Discrete facial expressions generally correspond to discrete underlying subjective experiences.
3. Discrete facial expressions are part of a coherent package of emotion responses that
includes appraisals, physiological reactions,
other nonverbal behaviors, and subsequent
actions; they are also reliable signs of individual differences and of mental and physical health.
4. Discrete facial expressions are judged reliably in different cultures.
5. Discrete facial expressions serve many interpersonal and social regulatory functions.

Numerous questions of theoretical significance
remain, and await a next wave of empirical
studies.

NOTES

1. To wit, Darwin penciled in the margin of Bell's book,
"He never looked at a monkey" (Darwin, 1872/
1998).
2. The importance of specifying the exact muscles underlying facial expressions can be understood by recognizing the difference in ethologists' verbal descriptions of fear, play, and threat faces of apes. A
nonfearful threat involves a tense mouth (AU 23)
with no teeth showing. When fear is involved, as is
common when subordinate animals are threatening
those superior to them in the social hierarchy, the lips
are stretched back (AU 20), thereby showing teeth.
This seeming smile is not a smile at all, but a fear grimace. By contrast, in the commonly reported "play
face" of apes, the corners of the lips go up (AU 12) as
they do in human smiles. The difference between AU
20 (a tense lateral stretch) and AU 12 (a relaxed upward pull) is crucial.
3. In analyzing the facial musculature of human infants,
Oster (2004) found that adjustments had to be made
to the human adult FACS to account for the greater
degree of subcutaneous fat in infants. Similarly, the
Waller et al. (2006) chimpanzee FACS has just been
completed, and several adjustments had to be made
to this as well. With this tool, future researchers will
be able to ascertain for sure which muscles are
innervated in which types of expressions in chimpanzees.
4. Many other tests have been developed over the years
to assess related concepts, such as the Profile of Nonverbal Sensitivity (Rosenthal, Hall, DeMatteo, Rogers, & Archer, 1979), the Social Skills Inventory

(Riggio, 1986), the Social Interpretations Test (Archer & Akert, 1977), and the Diagnostic Analysis of Nonverbal Accuracy Scale (Nowicki & Duke, 1994). These, however, do not focus on the recognition of discrete emotional states. Other tests are more emotion-focused, such as the Communication and Reception of Affect Test (Buck, 1976), the Test of Emotional Styles (Allen & Hamsher, 1974), the Understanding our Feelings Test (Elmore, 1985), the Feldstein Affect Judgment Test (Wolitzky, 1973), the Affect Communication Test (Friedman, Prince, Riggio, & DiMatteo, 1980), the Contextual and Affective Sensitivity Test (Trimboli & Walker, 1993), and the Perception of Affect Task (Lane, Sechrest, & Reidel, 1996). These, however, suffer from questionable validity of the expressions used to portray emotion, the inability to produce scores on discrete emotions, and the lack of balance in encoder characteristics.

REFERENCES

Abe, J. A. A., & Izard, C. E. (1999). A longitudinal study of emotion expression and personality relations in early development. *Journal of Personality and Social Psychology, 77*(3), 566–577.

Adolphs, R., Tranel, D., Damasio, H., & Damasio, A. R. (1994). Impaired recognition of emotion in facial expression following bilateral damage to the human amygdala. *Nature, 372,* 669–672.

Adolphs, R., Tranel, D., Damasio, H., & Damasio, A. R. (1995). Fear and the human amygdala. *Journal of Neuroscience, 15,* 5879–5891.

Adolphs, R., Tranel, D., Hamann, S., Young, A. W., Calder, A. J., Phelps, E. A., et al. (1999). Recognition of facial emotion in individuals with bilateral amygdala damage. *Neuropsychologia, 37,* 1111–1117.

Allen, J. R., & Hamsher, J. H. (1974). The development and validation of a test of emotional styles. *Journal of Consulting and Clinical Psychology, 42,* 663–668.

Archer, D., & Akert, R. (1977). Words and everything else: Verbal and nonverbal cues in social interaction. *Journal of Personality and Social Psychology, 35,* 443–449.

Berenbaum, H., & Oltmanns, T. (1992). Emotional experience and expression in schizophrenia and depression. *Journal of Abnormal Psychology, 101,* 37–44.

Blair, R. J. R., Morris, J. S., Frith, C. D., Perrett, D. I., & Dolan, R. J. (1998). Dissociable neural responses to facial expressions of sadness and anger. *Brain, 122*(5), 883–893.

Bonanno, G. A., & Keltner, D. (1997). Facial expressions of emotion and the course of conjugal bereavement. *Journal of Abnormal Psychology, 106,* 126–137.

Bonanno, G. A., & Keltner, D. (2004). The coherence of emotion systems: Comparing "on-line" measures of appraisal and facial expressions, and self-report. *Cognition and Emotion, 18*(3), 431–444.

Bonanno, G. A., Keltner, D., Noll, J., G., Putnam, F. W., Trickett, P. K., LeJeune, J., et al. (2002). When the face reveals what words do not: Facial expressions of emotion, smiling, and the willingness to disclose childhood sexual abuse. *Journal of Personality and Social Psychology, 83*(1), 94–110.

Borod, J. C., Koff, E., Lorch, M. P., & Nicholas, M. (1986). The expression and perception of facial emotion in brain-damaged patients. *Neuropsychologia, 24,* 169–180.

Breiter, H. C., Etcoff, N. L., Whalen, P. J., Kennedy, W. A., Rauch, S. L., Buckner, R. L., et al. (1996). Response and habituation of the human amygdala during visual processing of facial expression. *Neuron, 17,* 875–887.

Broks, P., Young, A. W., Maratos, E. J., Coffey, P. J., Calder, A. J., Isaac, C. I., et al. (1998). Face processing impairments after enchephalitis: Amygdala damage and recognition of fear. *Neuropsychologia, 36,* 59–70.

Brown, A., & Schwartz, G. E. (1980). Relationship between facial electromyography and subjective experience during affective imagery. *Biological Psychology, 11,* 49–62.

Buck, R. W. (1976). A test of nonverbal receiving ability: Preliminary studies. *Human Communication Research, 2,* 162–171.

Buck, R. W. (1977). Nonverbal communication of affect in preschool children: Relationships with personality and skin conductance. *Journal of Personality and Social Psychology, 35,* 225–236.

Cacioppo, J. T., Martzke, J. S., Petty, R. E., & Tassinary, L. G. (1988). Specific forms of facial emg response index emotions during an interview: From Darwin to the continuous flow hypothesis of affect-laden information processing. *Journal of Personality and Social Psychology, 54,* 592–604.

Calder, A. J. (2003). Disgust discussed. *Annals of Neurology, 53*(4), 427–428.

Calder, A. J., Keane, J., Manes, F., Antoun, N., & Young, A. W. (2000). Impaired recognition and experience of disgust following brain injury. *Nature Neuroscience, 3*(11), 1077–1078.

Calder, A. J., Young, A. W., & Perrett, D. I. (1996). Categorical perception of morphed facial expressions. *Visual Cognition, 3*(2), 81–117.

Camras, L. A., Oster, H., Campos, J., Miyake, K., & Bradshaw, D. (1992). Japanese and American infants' responses to arm restraint. *Developmental Psychology, 28,* 578–583.

Camras, L. A., Ribordy, S., Hill, J., Martino, S., Spaccarelli, S., & Stefani, R. (1988). Recognition and posing of emotional expressions by abused children and their mothers. *Developmental Psychology, 24*(6), 776–781.

Capps, L., Yirmiya, N., & Sigman, M. (1992). Understanding of simple and complex emotions in nonretarded children with autism. *Journal of Child Psychology and Psychiatry, 33,* 1169–1182.

Chesney, M. A., Ekman, P., Friesen, W. V., & Black, G. W. (1990). Type A behavior pattern: Facial behavior and speech components. *Psychosomatic Medicine, 52*(3), 307–319.

Chevalier-Skolnikoff, S. (1973). Facial expression of emotion in nonhuman primates. In P. Ekman (Ed.), *Darwin and facial expression* (pp. 11–89). New York: Academic Press.

Craig, K., Hyde, S., & Patrick, C. (1991). Genuine, suppressed, and fake facial behavior during exacerbation of chronic low back pain. *Pain, 46,* 161–171.

Darwin, C. (1998). *The expression of emotion in man and animals.* New York: Oxford University Press. (Original work published 1872)

Davidson, R. J. (2003). Parsing the subcomponents of emotion and disorders of emotion: Perspectives from affective neuroscience. In R. J. Davidson, K. R. Scherer, & H. H. Goldsmith (Eds.), *Handbook of affective sciences* (pp. 8–24). New York: Oxford University Press.

de Gelder, B., Morris, J. S., & Dolan, R. J. (2005). Unconscious fear influences emotional awareness of faces and voices. *Proceedings of the National Academy of Sciences USA, 102*(51), 18682–18687.

De Waal, F. B. M. (2002). Apes from Venus: Bonobos and human social evolution. In F. B. M. De Waal (Ed.), *Tree of origin: What primate behavior can tell us about human social evolution* (pp. 39–68). Cambridge, MA: Harvard University Press.

Dimberg, U., & Öhman, A. (1996). Behold the wrath: Psychophysiological responses to facial stimuli. *Motivation and Emotion, 20*(2), 149–182.

Duchenne de Boulogne, G. B. (1990). *The mechanism of human facial expression.* New York: Cambridge University Press. (Original work published 1862)

Eibl-Ebesfeldt, I. (1989). *Human ethology.* New York: Aldine de Gruyter Press.

Eisenberg, N., Fabes, R. A., Miller, P. A., Fultz, J., Shell, R., Mathy, R. M., et al. (1989). Relation of sympathy and distress to prosocial behavior: A multimethod study. *Journal of Personality and Social Psychology, 57,* 55–66.

Ekman, P. (1972). Universal and cultural differences in facial expression of emotion. In J. R. Cole (Ed.), *Nebraska symposium on motivation, 1971* (Vol. 19, pp. 207–283). Lincoln: University of Nebraska Press.

Ekman, P. (Ed.). (1973). *Darwin and facial expression.* New York: Academic Press.

Ekman, P. (1989). Why lies fail and what behaviors betray a lie. In J. C. Yuille (Ed.), *NATO Advanced Science Institutes Series. Series D: Behavioural and social sciences. Vol. 47. Credibility assessment* (pp. 71–81): Dordrecht, The Netherlands: Kluwer.

Ekman, P. (1992a). Are there basic emotions? *Psychological Review, 99*(3), 550–553.

Ekman, P. (1992b). Facial expressions of emotion: New findings, new questions. *Psychological Science, 3*(1), 34–38.

Ekman, P. (1993). Facial expression and emotion. *American Psychologist, 48*(4), 384–392.

Ekman, P. (2003). *Emotions revealed.* New York: Times Books.

Ekman, P., & Davidson, R. J. (1993). Voluntary smiling changes regional brain activity. *Psychological Science, 4*(5), 342–345.

Ekman, P., Davidson, R. J., & Friesen, W. V. (1990). The Duchenne smile: Emotional expression and brain physiology: II. *Journal of Personality and Social Psychology, 58*(2), 342–353.

Ekman, P., & Frank, M. G. (2005). *The ability to detect deception improves with microexpression recognition training.* Manuscript submitted for publication.

Ekman, P., & Friesen, W. (1969). The repertoire of nonverbal behavior: Categories, origins, usage, and coding. *Semiotica, 1,* 49–98.

Ekman, P., & Friesen, W. (1971). Constants across culture in the face and emotion. *Journal of Personality and Social Psychology, 17,* 124–129.

Ekman, P., Friesen, W., & Ancoli, S. (1980). Facial signs of emotional experience. *Journal of Personality and Social Psychology, 39,* 1125–1134.

Ekman, P., & Friesen, W. V. (1974). Nonverbal behavior and psychopathology. In R. J. Friedman & M. Katz (Eds.), *The psychology of depression: Contemporary theory and research* (pp. 3–31). Washington, DC: Winston.

Ekman, P., & Friesen, W. V. (1978). *Facial Action Coding System: Investigator's guide.* Palo Alto, CA: Consulting Psychologists Press.

Ekman, P., & Friesen, W. V. (1982). Felt, false, and miserable smiles. *Journal of Nonverbal Behavior, 6*(4), 238–258.

Ekman, P., & Friesen, W. V. (1986). A new pan-cultural facial expression of emotion. *Motivation and Emotion, 10*(2), 159–168.

Ekman, P., Friesen, W. V., & O'Sullivan, M. (1988). Smiles when lying. *Journal of Personality and Social Psychology, 54*(3), 414–420.

Ekman, P., Friesen, W. V., O'Sullivan, M., Chan, A., Diacoyanni-Tarlatzis, I., Heider, K., et al. (1987). Universals and cultural differences in the judgments of facial expressions of emotion. *Journal of Personality and Social Psychology, 53*(4), 712–717.

Ekman, P., & Heider, K. G. (1988). The universality of a contempt expression: A replication. *Motivation and Emotion, 12*(3), 303–308.

Ekman, P., Levenson, R. W., & Friesen, W. V. (1983). Autonomic nervous system activity distinguishes among emotions. *Science, 221*(4616), 1208–1210.

Ekman, P., Liebert, R. M., Friesen, W., Harrison, R., Zlatchin, C., Malmstrom, E. J., et al. (1972). Facial expressions of emotion while watching televised violence as predictors of subsequent aggression. In G. A. Comstock, E. A. Rubinstein, & J. P. Murray (Eds.), *Television and social behavior: A technical report to* the *Surgeon General's Scientific Advisory Committee on Television and Social Behavior. Vol. 1. Television's effects: Further explorations* (pp. 22–58). Washington, DC: U.S. Government Printing Office.

Ekman, P., Matsumoto, D., & Friesen, W. (1997). Facial expression in affective disorders. In P. Ekman & E. L. Rosenberg (Eds.), *What the face reveals: Basic and applied studies of spontaneous expression using the Facial Action Coding System (FACS)* (pp. 331–341). New York: Oxford University Press.

Ekman, P., & O'Sullivan, M. (1991). Who can catch a liar? *American Psychologist, 46*(9), 913–920.

Ekman, P., & Rosenberg, E. L. (Eds.). (2005). *What the face reveals: Basic and applied studies of spontaneous expression using the Facial Action Coding System (FACS)* (2nd ed.). New York: Oxford University Press.

Ekman, P., Sorenson, E. R., & Friesen, W. V. (1969). Pancultural elements in facial displays of emotion. *Science, 164*(3875), 86–88.

Elfenbein, H. A., & Ambady, N. (2002b). On the universality and cultural specificity of emotion recognition: A meta-analysis. *Psychological Bulletin, 128*(2), 205–235.

Ellgring, H. (1986). Nonverbal expression of psychological states in psychiatric patients. *European Archives of Psychiatry and Neurological Sciences, 236,* 31–34.

Elmore, B. C. (1985). Emotionally handicapped comprehension of nonverbal communication. *Journal of Holistic Medicine, 7,* 194–201.

Esteves, F., Dimberg, U., & Öhman, A. (1994). Automatically elicited fear: Conditioned skin conductance responses to masked facial expressions. *Cognition and Emotion, 8*(5), 393–413.

Foisy, M.-L., Philippot, P., Verbanck, P., Pelc, I., Van Der Straten, G., & Kornreich, C. (2005). Emotional facial expression decoding impairment in persons dependent on multiple substances: Impact of a history of alcohol dependence. *Journal of Studies on Alcohol, 66,* 673–681.

Frank, M. G. (2007). *Decoding deception and emotion by Americans and Australians.* Manuscript in preparation.

Frank, M. G., & Ekman, P. (1997). The ability to detect deceit generalizes across different types of high-stake lies. *Journal of Personality and Social Psychology, 72,* 1429–1439.

Frank, M. G., Ekman, P., & Friesen, W. V. (1993). Behavioral markers and recognizability of the smile of enjoyment. *Journal of Personality and Social Psychology, 64*(1), 83–93.

Frank, M. G., & Stennett, J. (2001). The forced-choice paradigm and the perception of facial expressions of emotion. *Journal of Personality and Social Psychology, 80*(1), 75–85.

Frank, R. H. (1988). *Passions without reason.* New York: Norton.

Fridlund, A. (1994). *Human facial expression: An evolutionary view.* San Diego: Academic Press.

Friedman, H. S., Prince, L. M., Riggio, R. E., & DiMatteo, M. R. (1980). Understanding and assessing nonverbal expressiveness: The Affective Communication Test. *Journal of Personality and Social Psychology, 39*(2), 333–351.

Geen, T. (1992). Facial expressions in socially isolated nonhuman primates: Open and closed programs for expressive behavior. *Journal of Research in Personality, 26,* 273–280.

Gonzaga, G. C., Keltner, D., & Londahl, E. A. (2001). Love and the commitment problem in romantic relationships and friendship. *Journal of Personality and Social Psychology, 81*(2), 247–262.

Gonzaga, G. C., Turner, R. A., Keltner, D., Campos, B., & Altemus, M. (2006). Romantic love and sexual desire in close relationships. *Emotion, 6*(2), 163–179.

Gosselin, P., Kirouac, G., & Dore, F. (1995). Components and recognition of facial expression in the communication of emotion by actors. *Journal of Personality and Social Psychology, 68,* 83–96.

Gottman, J. M., & Levenson, R. W. (1992). Marital processes predictive of later dissolution: Behavior, physiology, and health. *Journal of Personality and Social Psychology, 63*(2), 221–223.

Gottman, J. M., Levenson, R. W., & Woodin, E. (2001). Facial expressions during marital conflict. *Journal of Family Communication, 1,* 37–57.

Gray, H., & Goss, C. M. (1966). *Anatomy of the human body* (28th ed.). Philadelphia: Lea & Febiger.

Gray, J. M., Young, A. W., Barker, W. A., Curtis, A., & Gibson, D. (1997). Impaired recognition of disgust in huntington's disease gene carriers. *Brain, 120,* 2029–2038.

Gross, J. J., & Levenson, R. W. (1993). Emotional suppression: Physiology, self-report, and expressive behavior. *Journal of Personality and Social Psychology, 64*(6), 970–986.

Halisch, C., & Halisch, F. (1980). Cognitive assumptions of young children's self-evaluation reactions after success and failure. *Entwicklungspsychologie und Pädagogische Psychologie, 12*(3), 193–212.

Hariri, A. R., Mattay, V. S., Tessitore, A., Fera, F., & Weinberger, D. R. (2003). Neocortical modulation of the amygdala response to fearful stimuli. *Biological Psychiatry, 53,* 494–501.

Harker, L. A., & Keltner, D. (2001). Expressions of positive emotion in women's college yearbook pictures and their relationship to personality and life outcomes across adulthood. *Journal of Personality and Social Psychology, 80,* 112–124.

Harris, C. R., & Alvarado, N. (2005). Facial expressions, smile types, and self-report during humous, tickle, and pain. *Cognition and Emotion, 19*(5), 655–669.

Hauser, M. (1993). Right hemisphere dominance for the production of facial expression in monkeys. *Science, 261,* 475–477.

Heerey, E. A., Keltner, D., & Capps, L. M. (2003). Making sense of self-conscious emotion: Linking theory of mind and emotion in children with autism. *Emotion, 3*(4), 394–400.

Heller, M., & Haynal, V. (1994). Depression and suicide faces. *Cahiers Psychiatriques Genevois, 16,* 107–117.

Hertenstein, M. J., & Campos, J. J. (2004). The retention effects of an adult's emotional displays on infant behavior. *Child Development, 75*(2), 595–613.

Hess, U., Banse, R., & Kappas, A. (1995). The intensity of facial expression is determined by underlying affective states and social situations. *Journal of Personality and Social Psychology, 69,* 280–288.

Hobson, P. R. (1986). The autistic children's appraisal of expressions of emotion: A further study. *Journal of Child Psychology and Psychiatry, 27,* 671–680.

Horstmann, G. (2003). What do facial expressions convey?: Feeling states, behavioral intentions, or action requests? *Emotion, 3*(2), 150–166.

Izard, C. E. (1971). *The face of emotion.* New York: Appleton-Century-Crofts.

Keltner, D. (1995). The signs of appeasement: Evidence for the distinct displays of embarrassment, amusement, and shame. *Journal of Personality and Social Psychology, 68,* 441–454.

Keltner, D. (2003). Expression and the course of life: Studies of emotion, personality, and psychopathology from a social-functional perspective. *Annals of the New York Academy of Sciences, 1000,* 222–243.

Keltner, D., & Bonanno, G. A. (1997). A study of laughter and dissociation: The distinct correlates of laughter and smiling during bereavement. *Journal of Personality and Social Psychology, 73,* 687–702.

Keltner, D., & Buswell, B. N. (1997). Embarrassment: Its distinct form and appeasement functions. *Psychological Bulletin, 122*(3), 250–270.

Keltner, D., Ellsworth, P. C., & Edwards, K. (1993). Beyond simple pessimism: Effects of sadness and anger on social perception. *Journal of Personality and Social Psychology, 64,* 740–752.

Keltner, D., Haidt, J., & Shiota, M. N. (2006). Social functionalism and the evolution of emotions. In M. Schaller, J. A. Simpson, & D. T. Kenrick (Eds.), *Evolution and social psychology.* New York: Psychology Press.

Keltner, D., & Kring, A. M. (1998). Emotion, social function, and psychopathology. *Review of General Psychology, 2*(3), 320–342.

Keltner, D., Moffitt, T., & Stouthamer-Loeber, M. (1995). Facial expressions of emotion and psychopathology in adolescent boys. *Journal of Abnormal Psychology, 104,* 644–652.

Kirsch, P., Esslinger, C., Chen, Q., Mier, D., Lis, S., Siddhanti, S., et al. (2005). Oxytocin modulates neural circuitry for social cognition and fear in humans. *Journal of Neuroscience, 25*(49), 11489–11493.

Klinnert, M. D., Campos, J. J., & Sorce, J. F. (1983). Emotions as behavior regulators: Social referencing in infancy. In R. Plutchik & H. Kellerman (Eds.), *Emotion: Theory, research, and experience* (pp. 57–86). New York: Academic Press.

Klinnert, M. D., Emde, R. N., Butterfield, P., & Campos, J. (1986). Social referencing: The infant's use of emotional signals from a friendly adult with a mother present. *Developmental Psychology, 22*(4), 427–432.

Krebs, J. R., & Dawkins, R. (1984). Animal signals: Mind reading and manipulation. In J. R. Krebs & R. Dawkins (Eds.), *Behavioural ecology: An evolutionary approach* (pp. 380–402). Sunderland, MA: Sinauer Associates.

Lane, R. D., Sechrest, L., & Reidel, R. (1996). Impaired verbal and nonverbal emotion recognition in alexithymia. *Psychosomatic Medicine, 58,* 203–210.

Lawrence, K., Bernstein, D., Pearson, R., Mandy, W., Brand, S., Wade, A., et al. (2005). *Age, gender and puberty influence the development of facial emotion recognition.* Manuscript submitted for publication.

Lazarus, R. (1991). *Emotion and adaptation.* New York: Oxford University Press.

Lerner, J. S., Gonzalez, R. M., Dahl, R. E., Haririr, A. R., & Taylor, S. E. (2005). Facial expressions of emotion reveal neuroendocrine and cardiovascular stress responses. *Biological Psychiatry, 58,* 743–750.

Levenson, R. W. (1994). Human emotions: A functional view. In P. Ekman & R. J. Davidson (Eds.), *The nature of emotion: Fundamental questions* (pp. 17–42). New York: Oxford University Press.

Levenson, R. W. (2003b). Blood, sweat, and fears: The autonomic architecture of emotion. *Annals of the New York Academy of Sciences, 1000,* 348–366.

Levenson, R. W., Carstensen, L. L., Friesen, W. V., & Ekman, P. (1991). Emotion, physiology, and expression in old age. *Psychology and Aging, 6*(1), 28–35.

Levenson, R. W., & Ekman, P. (2002). Difficulty does not account for emotion-specific heart rate changes in the directed facial action task. *Psychophysiology, 39*(3), 397–405.

Levenson, R. W., Ekman, P., & Friesen, W. V. (1990). Voluntary facial action generates emotion-specific autonomic nervous system activity. *Psychophysiology, 27*(4), 363–384.

Levenson, R. W., Ekman, P., Heider, K., & Friesen, W. V. (1992). Emotion and autonomic nervous system activity in the Minangkabau of West Sumatra. *Journal of Personality and Social Psychology, 62*(6), 972–988.

Lewis, M., Alessandri, S. M., & Sullivan, M. W. (1992). Differences in shame and pride as a function of children's gender and task difficulty. *Child Development, 63*(3), 630–638.

Liebal, K., Pika, S., & Tomasello, M. (2004). Social communication in siamangs (*Symphalangus syndactylus*): Use of gestures and facial expressions. *Primates, 45*(1), 41–57.

Marsh, A. A., Ambady, N., & Kleck, R. E. (2005). The effects of fear and anger facial expressions on approach- and avoidance-related behaviors. *Emotion, 5*(1), 119–124.

Matsumoto, D. (1989). Face, culture, and judgments of anger and fear: Do the eyes have it? *Journal of Nonverbal Behavior, 13*(3), 171–188.

Matsumoto, D. (2001). Culture and emotion. In D. Matsumoto (Ed.), *The handbook of culture and psychology* (pp. 171–194). New York: Oxford University Press.

Matsumoto, D. (2005). Scalar ratings of contempt expressions. *Journal of Nonverbal Behavior, 29*(2), 91–104.

Matsumoto, D. (2006). Culture and cultural worldviews: Do verbal descriptions of culture reflect anything other than verbal descriptions of culture? *Culture and Psychology, 12*(1), 33–62.

Matsumoto, D., Consolacion, T., Yamada, H., Suzuki, R., Franklin, B., Paul, S., et al. (2002). American–Japanese cultural differences in judgments of emotional expressions of different intensities. *Cognition and Emotion, 16*(6), 721–747.

Matsumoto, D., & Ekman, P. (1989). American–Japanese cultural differences in intensity ratings of facial expressions of emotion. *Motivation and Emotion, 13*(2), 143–157.

Matsumoto, D., & Ekman, P. (2004). The relationship between expressions, labels, and descriptions of contempt. *Journal of Personality and Social Psychology, 87*(4), 529–540.

Matsumoto, D., Haan, N., Gary, Y., Theodorou, P., & Cooke-Carney, C. (1986). Preschoolers' moral actions and emotions in Prisoner's Dilemma. *Developmental Psychology, 22*(5), 663–670.

Matsumoto, D., & Kupperbusch, C. (2001). Idiocentric and allocentric differences in emotional expression and experience. *Asian Journal of Social Psychology, 4*, 113–131.

Matsumoto, D., & Lee, M. (1993). Consciousness, volition, and the neuropsychology of facial expressions of emotion. *Consciousness and Cognition: An International Journal, 2*(3), 237–254.

Matsumoto, D., LeRoux, J. A., Bernhard, R., & Gray, H. (2004). Personality and behavioral correlates of intercultural adjustment potential. *International Journal of Intercultural Relations, 28*(3–4), 281–309.

Matsumoto, D., LeRoux, J. A., Wilson-Cohn, C., Raroque, J., Kooken, K., Ekman, P., et al. (2000). A new test to measure emotion recognition ability: Matsumoto and Ekman's Japanese and Caucasian Brief Affect Recognition Test (JACBART). *Journal of Nonverbal Behavior, 24*(3), 179–209.

Matsumoto, D., Nezlek, J., & Koopmann, B. (2007). Evidence for universality in phenomenological emotion response system coherence. *Emotion, 7*(1), 57–67.

Matsumoto, D., & Willingham, B. (2006). The thrill of victory and the agony of defeat: Spontaneous expressions of medal winners at the 2004 Athens Olympic Games. *Journal of Personality and Social Psychology, 91*(3), 568–581.

Mauss, I. B., Levenson, R. W., McCarter, L., Wilhelm, F. L., & Gross, J. J. (2005). The tie that binds?: Coherence among emotion experience, behavior, and physiology. *Emotion, 5*(2), 175–190.

Mauss, I. B., Wilhelm, F. L., & Gross, J. J. (2004). Is there less to social anxiety than meets the eye?: Emotion experience, expression, and bodily responding. *Cognition and Emotion, 18*(5), 631–662.

Mayer, J. D., Salovey, P., Caruso, D. R., & Sitarenios, G. (2001). Emotional intelligence as a standard intelligence. *Emotion, 1*(3), 232–242.

McGhee, P. E. (1977). Children's humour: A review of current research trends. In A. J. Chapman & H. C. Foot (Eds.), *It's a funny thing, humour* (pp. 199–209). Oxford: Pergamon Press.

Messinger, D. S., Fogel, A., & Dickson, K. L. (2001). All smiles are positive, but some smiles are more positive than others. *Developmental Psychology, 37*(5), 642–653.

Mineka, S., & Cook, M. (1993). Mechanisms involved in the observational conditioning of fear. *Journal of Experimental Psychology: General, 122*(1), 23–38.

Nowicki, S. J., & Duke, M. P. (1994). Individual differences in the nonverbal communication of affect: The Diagnostic Analysis of Nonverbal Accuracy Scale. *Journal of Nonverbal Behavior, 18*, 9–35.

Oster, H. (2004). *Baby FACS: Facial Action Coding System for infants and young children.* Unpublished manuscript, New York University.

Ozonoff, S., Pennington, B. F., & Rogers, S. J. (1990). Are there emotion perception deficits in young autistic children? *Journal of Child Psychology and Psychiatry, 31*, 343–361.

Parr, L. (2003). The discrimination of faces and their emotional content by chimpanzees (*Pan troglodytes*). *Annals of the New York Academy of Sciences, 1000* 56–78.

Persad, S. M., & Polivy, J. (1993). Differences between depressed and non-depressed individuals in the recognition of and response to facial emotional cues. *Journal of Abnormal Psychology, 102*(3), 358–368.

Phillips, M. L., Young, A. W., Senior, C., Brammer, M., Andrew, C., Calder, A. J., et al. (1997). A specific neural substrate for perceiving facial expressions of disgust. *Nature, 389*, 495–498.

Pollak, S. D., Cichetti, D., Hornung, K., & Reed, A. (2000). Recognizing emotion in faces: Developmental effects of child abuse and neglect. *Developmental Psychology, 36*(5), 679–688.

Pollak, S. D., & Sinha, P. (2002). Effects of early experience on children's recognition of facial displays of emotion. *Developmental Psychology, 38*(5), 784–791.

Prkachin, K. (1992). The consistency and facial expressions of pain: A comparison across modalities. *Pain, 51*, 297–306.

Redican, W. K. (1982). An evolutionary perspective on human facial displays. In P. Ekman (Ed.), *Emotion in the human face* (pp. 212–280). New York: Cambridge University Press.

Riggio, R. E. (1986). Assessment of social skill. *Journal of Personality and Social Psychology, 51*, 649–660.

Rosenberg, E. L., & Ekman, P. (1994). Coherence between expressive and experiential systems in emotion. *Cognition and Emotion, 8*(3), 201–229.

Rosenberg, E. L., & Ekman, P. (1995). Conceptual and methodological issues in the judgment of facial expressions of emotion. *Motivation and Emotion, 19*(2), 111–138.

Rosenberg, E. L., Ekman, P., Jiang, W., Babyak, M., Coleman, R. E., Hanson, M., et al. (2001). Linkages between facial expressions of anger and transient myocardial ischemia in men with coronary heart disease. *Emotion, 1*(2), 107–115.

Rosenthal, R., Hall, J. A., DeMatteo, M. R., Rogers, P. L., & Archer, D. (1979). *Sensitivity to nonverbal communication: The PONS test.* Baltimore: Johns Hopkins University Press.

Rozin, P., Lowery, L., & Ebert, R. (1994). Varieties of disgust faces and the structure of disgust. *Journal of Personality and Social Psychology, 66*(5), 870–881.

Rozin, P., Lowery, L., Imada, S., & Haidt, J. (1999). The CAD triad hypothesis: A mapping between three moral emotions (contempt, anger, disgust) and three moral codes (community, autonomy, divinity). *Journal of Personality and Social Psychology, 75*(4), 574–585.

Ruch, W. (1993). Extraversion, alcohol, and enjoyment. *Personality and Individual Differences, 16*, 89–102.

Ruch, W. (1995). Will the real relationship between facial expression and affective experience stand up?: The case of exhilaration. *Cognition and Emotion, 9*, 33–58.

Russell, J. A. (1991a). Culture and the categorization of emotions. *Psychological Bulletin, 110*, 426–450.

Russell, J. A. (1994). Is there universal recognition of emotion from facial expression?: A review of cross-cultural studies. *Psychological Bulletin, 115*, 102–141.

Russell, J. A., Bachorowski, J.-A., & Fernandez-Dols, J. M. (2003). Facial and vocal expressions of emotion. *Annual Review of Psychology, 54*, 329–349.

Russell, T. A., Chu, E., & Phillips, M. L. (2006). A pilot study to investigate the effectiveness of emotion recognition mediation in schizophrenia using the microexpression training tool. *British Journal of Clinical Psychology, 45*, 579–583.

Salovey, P., & Mayer, J. D. (1990). Emotional intelligence. *Imagination, Cognition, and Personality, 9*(3), 185–211.

Scherer, K. R. (1986). Vocal affect expression: Review and a model for future research. *Psychological Bulletin, 99*, 143–165.

Shiota, M. N., Campos, B., & Keltner, D. (2003). The faces of positive emotion: Prototype displays of awe, amusement, and pride. In P. Ekman, J. Campos, R. J. Davidson, & F. B. M. De Waal (Eds.), *Emotions inside out: 130 years after Darwin's The Expression of Emotions in Man and Animals* (pp. 296–299). New York: The New York Academy of Sciences.

Smith, M. C. (1995). Facial expression in mild dementia of the Alzheimer type. *Behavioural Neurology, 8*, 149–156.

Snowdon, C. T. (2003). Expression of emotion in nonhuman animals. In R. J. Davidson, K. R. Scherer, & H. H. Goldsmith (Eds.), *Handbook of affective sciences* (pp. 457–480). New York: Oxford University Press.

Soltysik, S., & Jelen, P. (2005). In rats, sighs correlate with relief. *Physiology and Behavior, 85*(5), 598–602.

Soto, J. A., Levenson, R. W., & Ebling, R. (2005). Cultures of moderation and expression: Emotional experience, behavior, and physiology in Chinese Americans and Mexican Americans. *Emotion, 5*(2), 154–165.

Sprengelmeyer, R., Young, A. W., Calder, A. J., Karnat, A., Lange, H., Homberg, V., et al. (1996). Loss of disgust: Perceptions of faces and emotions in Huntington's disease. *Brain, 119*, 1647–1665.

Steimer-Krause, E., Krause, R., & Wagner, G. (1990). Interaction regulations used by schizophrenic and psychosomatic patients: Studies on facial behavior in dyadic interactions. *Psychiatry, 53*, 209–228.

Stipek, D. J., & Gralinski, J. H. (1991). Gender differences in children's achievement-related beliefs and emotional responses to success and failure in mathematics. *Journal of Educational Psychology, 83*(3), 361–371.

Surcinelli, P., Codispoti, M., Montebarocci, O., Rossi, N., & Baldaro, B. (2004). Facial emotion recognition in trait anxiety. *Anxiety Disorders, 20*, 110–117.

Terracciano, A., Merritt, M., Zonderman, A. B., & Evans, M. K. (2003). Personality traits and sex differences in emotion recognition among African Americans and Caucasians. *Annals of the New York Academy of Sciences, 1000*, 309–312.

Tiedens, L. Z., Ellsworth, P. C., & Mesquita, B. (2000). Stereotypies about sentiments and status: Emotional expectations for high- and low-status group members. *Personality and Social Psychology Bulletin, 26*(5), 560–574.

Tomkins, S. S. (1962). *Affect, imagery, and consciousness: Vol. 1. The positive affects.* New York: Springer.

Tomkins, S. S. (1963). *Affect, imagery, and consciousness: Vol. 2. The negative affects.* New York: Springer.

Tooby, J., & Cosmides, L. (1992). Psychological foundations of culture. In J. Barkow, L. Cosmides, & J. Tooby (Eds.), *The adapted mind* (pp. 19–136). New York: Oxford University Press.

Tracy, J. L., & Matsumoto, D. (2005). *Unique expressions of pride and shame: Evidence from the 2004 Athens Olympic games.* Manuscript submitted for publication.

Tracy, J. L., & Robins, R. W. (2004). Show your pride: Evidence for a discrete emotion expression. *Psychological Science, 15*(3), 104–197.

Trimboli, A., & Walker, M. (1993). The CAST test of nonverbal sensitivity. *Journal of Language and Social Psychology, 12*, 49–65.

Tsai, J. L., & Levenson, R. W. (1997). Cultural influences of emotional responding: Chinese American and European American dating couples during interpersonal conflict. *Journal of Cross-Cultural Psychology, 28,* 600–625.

Ueno, A., Ueno, Y., & Tomonaga, M. (2004). Facial responses to four basic tastes in newborn rhesus macaques (*Macaca mulatta*) and chimpanzees (*Pan troglodytes*). *Behavioural Brain Research, 154*(1), 261–271.

Van Hoof, J. A. R. A. M. (1972). A comparative approach to the phylogeny of laughing and smiling. In R. A. Hinde (Ed.), *Nonverbal communication* (pp. 209–241). Cambridge, UK: Cambridge University Press.

Vick, S.-J., Waller, B. M., Parr, L. A., Pasqualini, M. S., & Bard, K. A. (2007). A cross species comparison of facial morphology and movement in humans and chimpanzees using the Facial Action Coding System (FACS). *Journal of Nonverbal Behavior, 31,* 1–20.

Waller, B. M., Vick, S.-J., Parr, L., Bard, K. A., Pasqualini, M. S., Gothard, K. M., et al. (2006). Intramuscular electrical stimulation of facial muscles in humans and chimpanzees: Duchenne revisited and extended. *Emotion, 6*(3), 367–382.

Whalen, P. J., Kagan, J., Cook, R., Davis, F. C., Kim, H., Polis, S., et al. (2004). Human amygdala responsivity to masked fearful eye whites. *Science, 306,* 2061.

Whalen, P. J., Rauch, S. L., Etcoff, N. L., McInerney, S. C., Lee, M. B., & Jenike, M. A. (1998). Masked presentations of emotional facial expressions modulate amygdala activity without explicit knowledge. *Journal of Neuroscience, 18,* 411–418.

Winblad, S., Hellstrom, P., Lindberg, C., & Hansen, S. (2006). Facial emotion recognition in myotonic dystrophy type 1 correlates with CTG repeat expansion. *Journal of Neurology, Neurosurgery and Psychiatry, 77,* 219–223.

Winkielman, P., Berridge, K. C., & Wilbarger, J. L. (2005). Unconscious affective reactions to masked happy versus angry faces influence consumption behavior and judgments of value. *Personality and Social Psychology Bulletin, 31*(1), 121–135.

Wolitzky, D. (1973). Cognitive control and person perception. *Perceptual and Motor Skills, 36,* 619–623.

Woodzicka, J., & LaFrance, M. (2001). Real versus imagined gender harassment. *Journal of Social Issues, 57*(1), 15–30.

Yoo, S. H., Matsumoto, D., & LeRoux, J. A. (2005). *Emotion regulation, emotion recognition, and intercultural adjustment.* Manuscript submitted for publication.

Yoo, S. H., Matsumoto, D., & LeRoux, J. A. (2006). Emotion regulation, emotion recognition, and intercultural adjustment. *International Journal of Intercultural Relations, 30*(3), 345–363.

Young, A. W., Hellawell, D. J., Van de Wal, C., & Johnson, M. (1996). Facial expression processing after amygdalotomy. *Neuropsychologia, 34,* 31–39.

Yrizarry, N., Matsumoto, D., & Wilson-Cohn, C. (1998). American-Japanese differences in multiscalar intensity ratings of universal facial expressions of emotion. *Motivation and Emotion, 22*(4), 315–327.

CHAPTER 14

A "Nose" for Emotion
Emotional Information and Challenges in Odors and Semiochemicals

JEANNETTE M. HAVILAND-JONES
and PATRICIA J. WILSON

Suppose you could walk into an empty theater, sniff the air, and know that it had staged a horror production. Would the departed actors and audience leave behind "mood chemicals" in the air? Would audiences coming to a later show find the show more horrible because of lingering chemicals? **What does the nose sense?**

It is surprising that olfaction has waited so long to be considered an important sensory system for the field of emotion, since experts in olfaction largely regard the primary response to odorants as "emotional" (see Van Toller & Dodd, 1988, 1992). This odd incongruity can probably be attributed to the persistent belief that olfaction is a primitive and vestigial system (Schaal & Porter, 1991). As Cain (1978) noted 30 years ago, many significant scientists in the Western world have attended to odors and "semiochemicals" (message-bearing chemicals), but seldom for very long. The result is a distinguished historical literature largely unknown to modern psychologists, even though some of the great historical psychologists or prepsychologists—such as Galen, Boring, Ellis,

and Titchener—made contributions. The last 30 years have seen astonishing developments in the research on smell, but much of what is in the psychological realm remains devoted to what Cain (1978) has called "industrial endeavors"—perfumery, malodor control, and food products.

In this chapter, we focus on the emerging research on humans, semiochemicals, and moods or emotions. This means that we only use the vast literature on the influence of semiochemicals on insects' and other animals' behavior to inform our presentation, but do not review it. We begin with a brief review of the new developments in the physiology of olfaction, including the olfactory, trigeminal, and vomeronasal systems, because this opens up the diversity of research related to odors and semiochemicals. From there, we move to the growing body of work revealing the profound influence that pheromones and odors (both manufactured and body odors) have been found to have on human moods and cognitive processes. Next, we cover research showing the effects that flowers and floral odors have on human cognition and emotion, and we propose an evolutionary explanation for those effects. This part of the chapter is included because it contributes to our hypotheses about how semiochemicals function in human performance. We then strive to integrate the full range of sometimes quirky findings on humans, odors, and emotions into a system demonstrating how humans might make sense of the ubiquitous presence of semiochemicals in their daily lives.

NEW DISCOVERIES AND THE HUMAN GENOME CHALLENGE

In 2004 the Nobel Prize for medicine was awarded to Buck and Axel for their discovery of the genes (accounting for 3% of the human genome) that express for the receptors detecting odors in the nose (see Buck & Axel, 1991). Although 3% may seem small, the olfactory system is second in size only to the immune system. It can detect and discriminate many hundreds of different odors at remarkably low concentrations (less than one part per trillion for mercaptan, for example), due to the pattern of activation of some 1,000 odor receptors. It appears that olfaction may have greater status in human perceptual experience than previous researchers ever suspected. Given this new perspective on olfaction, we have an extraordinarily limited understanding of the psychology of olfaction compared with other sensory modalities. Knowing what we now do, it is time for psychology to expand its training and research programs in this area.

Odors can both attract and repel. The historical record reveals an ancient human awareness of odors and use of odorants to create healthy and attractive personal, physical, and social environments, and to mask the unpleasant and the foul. In ancient times, the best of Persian scientists worked with aromas both as physicians and as social managers. Lavender oil was used to cleanse a sick room, while fragrances used at a wedding had complex meanings for the expected future of the couple. Perfumers were prized enough in ancient Egypt to be favored with their own god, Nefertum. Pharaohs were buried surrounded by flowers and perfumes, the better to be accepted into the afterlife (Steele, 1992). Cleopatra adorned herself with fragrant oils to seduce Marc Antony

(Stoddart, 1990), and lovers created wreaths of scented flowers to adorn the beloved's hair (Classen, Howes, & Synnott, 1994). During the Middle Ages, it was believed that foul air carried the plague, so people fumigated their homes with all manner of scents to counteract it. Odor, then, was seen as both potentially dangerous and potentially beneficial. (The gold head of a physician's cane originally contained aromatics to cleanse and heal.) Fragrance as a personal adornment was thought to stimulate the mind as well as the emotions (Classen et al., 1994).

In the modern day, we know that environmental pollutants and malodors do pose health risks (Schiffman & Williams, 2005; Rosenkranz & Cunningham, 2003). Some of these risks are present in seemingly innocuous settings. For example, a recent study found that exposure to the solvents typically found in nail salons can lead to a decline in cognitive and neurosensory performance over time (LoSasso, Rapport, Axelrod, & Whitman, 2002). LoSasso and her colleagues note that these changes are consistent with those found in workers exposed to industrial levels of such solvents. Rotton (1983) found that exposure to uncontrollable unpleasant odors decreased performance on complex tasks, increased negative judgments on evaluative tasks, and decreased tolerance levels after performing such tasks. Furthermore, the state of Pennsylvania has invested heavily in finding solutions to the odors generated by mushroom and pig farming, because of the negative impact on most people exposed to these odors (Rouhi, 2002).

What we already know suggests the pervasive importance of olfactory processes for both emotion and cognition. Yet, although testing for vision and hearing is fairly routine (especially among children), and although the first olfactometer came into use in the late 1880s, olfactory tests are not normally used. This is a potentially important omission, as impaired sense of smell is associated in at least some cases with disease processes; it occurs early in the onset of both Alzheimer's and Parkinson's disease (Mesholam, Moberg, Mahr, & Doty, 1998). People who lose their olfactory sense commonly become profoundly depressed. Olfactory loss also appears to be associated with a decline in verbal memory (Swan & Carmelli, 2000) and may be predictive of general cognitive decline (Graves et al., 1999).

The possible associations between olfaction and emotional and cognitive processes hold implications for research environments, yet we are not careful about the quality of air or odor compounds in those research environments. The importance of air control in research environments has not been self-evident outside smell and taste laboratories. We know that malodors adversely affect human responses, but what of the many omnipresent odors that drift innocently through a research environment: coffee, microwaved lunches, a strong shampoo, perfumes or colognes? Other sorts of "air control" are less obvious but equally (perhaps even more) important—for example, anxiety of researchers and participants, or continued use of the same space for negative (or positive) emotion investigations.

THE BIOLOGY OF SEMIOCHEMICALS

Not only the genetics of olfaction, but even the physiology, has undergone a change. The Woodworth and Schlosberg text *Experimental Psychology* (1955) simply stated that "the receptors for smell are found in two small patches of yellowish olfactory epithelium" (p. 304). We now know that not one system, but three, respond to airborne chemical signals: (1) the olfactory system, (2) the trigeminal system, and (3) the vomeronasal system (VNS). In this section, we quickly highlight pertinent aspects of each system that help to inform emotion research. We focus on the odor discrimination feature of what is traditionally called the olfactory sensory system (e.g., is an odor bananas or gardenias?); for the trigeminal system, we focus on somatic arousal detection (e.g., is an odor irritating?); for the still-controversial VNS, we focus on "putative" pheromones.

The Olfactory System

The popular wisdom that odor and emotion share a privileged link is supported by evidence from neuroscience; they share common pathways within the limbic system. Succinctly, odor information is detected by the olfactory epithelium in the nasal cavity and relayed to the main olfactory bulb, which in turn projects directly to the ipsilateral primary olfactory cortex (Brand, 2006). The olfactory tract projects to, among other brain regions, the amygdala and the orbito-frontal cortex. Both of these have been implicated in emotion processing (Baas, Aleman, & Kahn, 2004; Britton et al., 2006; Rolls, 1996; Zald, 2003). It is particularly noteworthy that the projections are bidirectional (Zald & Pardo, 1997). Recent brain imaging studies of olfactory processes suggest that olfactory information is processed both hierarchically and in a parallel fashion, as are data from other sensory systems (Savic, 2005). However, Savic notes that immediate emotional response is commonly associated with odor perception. The amygdala, she notes, is activated at the most primary level of odor perception. As the odor-related task becomes more semantic (i.e., odor memory), additional brain structures become engaged. Later in this chapter, we present a functional approach to the olfactory system, which suggests that semantic and memory functions of odors or semiochemicals may also occur after emotional or mood changes have begun. In effect, odors may potentiate emotional responses even when there is no attentional focus on the odor or it is below the threshold for detection.

Olfaction, in contrast to the other sensory modalities, does not affect the thalamus initially, but instead innervates the central nervous system (CNS) (Stockhorst & Pietrowsky, 2004). It is further distinguished by its externally exposed neurons, which die and renew themselves on a regular basis (Carleton, Petreanu, Lansford, Alvarez-Buylla, & Lledo, 2003). The generative nature of the system has led several researchers, including us, to wonder whether "learning" to discriminate some airborne chemicals might involve building a structure to key onto previously undiscriminated molecules. This would account for reports that people who are anosmic to certain odors become sensitive over a period of several weeks or months of exposure. These unique features of the olfactory system imply fundamental neural and CNS differences from other sensory modalities.

Another interesting feature of the olfactory system is that organisms may respond physiologically and emotionally in the presence of semiochemicals even when they do not notice the presence of any odor. Apparently, conscious awareness, much less the identification of odors, is not a prerequisite for eliciting a physiological or behavioral emotional response (e.g., Bensafi et al., 2003). Once again this observation lends itself to the hypothesis that semio-chemicals may influence emotional preatten-tive processes and affect both mind and body.

People seem largely unaware that they them-selves produce chemosignals. This is not to say that people are not aware of body odors, but this awareness seems to be limited to special cases, such as bad odors on the negative side or the odor of clean infants on the positive side. People seem equally unaware that they are de-tecting and processing these chemical messages coming from others. Our review (below) shows that some mood signals as well as sexual ones are communicated largely without awareness.

The Trigeminal System

The trigeminal system serves somatosensory (e.g., temperature or pain) and motor (e.g., bit-ing and chewing) functions for the face and head (see Brand, 2006, for a review). The trigeminal nerve, the fifth cranial nerve, is com-posed of three branches—the ophthalmic, the maxillary, and the mandibular—each of which innervates different parts of the face. These nerves project eventually to the thalamus and then to the cortex. Only the mandibular nerve carries motor information. The first two branches exhibit complex interactions with the olfactory system as these branches of the trigeminal nerve extend into the nasal lining. Among its functions is to detect chemical irrita-tion. The typical reaction of recoiling from the smell of ammonia, for example, is due to acti-vation of the trigeminal system. The emotional reaction to such irritation is usually negative, but it can be uplifting or exciting, as when a sniff of strong peppermint is "fresh" and ap-pealing. It is noteworthy that the trigeminal nerve relays proprioceptive stimulation to the sensory cortex. This is part of the facial feed-back of emotional expression in the facial mus-culature. Emotional expression is part of this system as well.

The Vomeronasal System

A third system receptive to specific airborne semiochemicals—"pheromones"—is the VNS. Present in a wide variety of species, neurons from the vomeronasal organ (VNO) form the vomeronasal nerve, which synapses in the ac-cessory olfactory bulb (Halpern, 1987). Herein lies controversy. Although a VNO is observable in the human fetus and in many adult humans,

its existence may not be universal; when it is present, it may not be functional (see Meredith, 2001, for a review). A neural pathway has not been observed in humans. Since the purpose of the VNO in most animals seems to be detection of pheromones, this suggests that humans may not respond to pheromones, at least not with the VNO.

Pheromones are specific subsets of semio-chemicals that are emitted by members of a species and elicit behavior change in recipients of the same species (Karlson & Luscher, 1959). Although pheromones are most often consid-ered in terms of sexual attraction, they serve other functions as well. For example, the ant that has discovered a new food source leads its colony to that source via a pheromone trail. Research has demonstrated that humans are influenced by chemical stimuli from other humans—findings we will return to later. Are such semiochemicals pheromones? The present general suspicion is that pheromone reaction is very limited or nonexistent in humans; how-ever, there are many reasons to consider this question open to new experimentation and techniques. What about the lack of conclusion regarding a functional VNO? Animal research suggests that a VNO is not necessary for pheromone detection (Dorries, Adkins-Regan, & Halpern, 1997), diminishing the importance of the VNO question and placing detection back into the olfactory system. In any case, there has been only a modest research effort to examine the effect of "putative" human phero-mones on emotional reactions.

Our early understanding of olfaction has been replaced with a more nuanced apprecia-tion that expands the neural impact of olfac-tory responses, considers the impact of at least the trigeminal system in the olfactory experi-ence, and raises tantalizing questions when the VNS is considered as well. This begins to inter-sect with folk wisdom and naïve psychology beliefs that smell matters in mood and emo-tional behavior. The question to be resolved is in what ways and to what extent it matters.

EMOTIONAL AND COGNITIVE PROCESSES: MEMORY

In the novel *Swann's Way* (Proust, 1913/1957), the protagonist experiences a profound emo-tional experience while sipping tea and dunk-ing *madeleines* (French tea cakes):

... I raised to my lips a spoonful of the tea in which I had soaked a morsel of the cake. No sooner had the warm liquid, and the crumbs with it, touched my palate than a shudder ran through my whole body, and I stopped, intent upon the extraordinary changes that were taking place. An exquisite pleasure had invaded my senses, but individual, detached, with no suggestion of its origin. And at once the vicissitudes of life had become indifferent to me, its disasters innocuous, its brevity illusory—this new sensation having had on me the effect which love had of filling me with a precious essence; or rather this essence was not in me, it was myself. I had ceased now to feel mediocre, accidental, mortal. Whence would it have come to me, this all-powerful joy? (p. 56)

After much struggle, a memory reaches "the clear surface of [his] consciousness" (p. 57), and his reminiscence begins. The phenomenon that Proust describes resonates with many people (see Gilbert & Wysocki, 1987). (The experience of Proust's protagonist is primarily a flavor experience. Flavor is the result of the integration of taste and smell, with olfaction supplying about 70% of the sensory information.) Although this particular taste/odor produces an idiosyncratic intense "joy" response, the Proust tale has led to a general hypothesis that odors can stimulate the intense recall of events, particularly childhood events, better than other stimuli and with rich emotional content. The underlying argument is that odors have a privileged function in memory. Research offers support for this hypothesis, but it must be qualified.

Discussing her work investigating odor–memory links, Herz (2000) posits that odors trigger memories that are more emotional than memories triggered by other sensory modalities. In one study (Herz & Cupchik, 1995), odors described as either positive or negative, or their verbal odor labels, were paired with paintings described as either positive or negative. Participants wrote a description of the paintings after viewing them in the presence of either the actual odor or the verbal cue. Participants were tested 2 days later for recall of the description of the paintings. Odor was associated with greater emotional content in the recollections, but not greater accuracy.

In another test of the Proust phenomenon, Aggleton and Waskett (1999) recruited participants who had taken from one to three guided tours of the Jorvik Viking Centre in York, Great Britain. The underground Centre recreates 10th-century York, complete with distinctive smells of that period. The tours are scripted and the smells are consistent. In the study, participants were exposed to either Jorvik's distinctive smells, novel odors, or no odors while completing questionnaires that probed for things they might have remembered from their visits. Those exposed to the Jorvik smells recalled significantly more details about their previous visits to the Centre, compared to those in both the novel-odor and no-odor conditions. The Jorvik smells elicited more detailed recall of the memory of the visit. In this case, the odor association did improve accuracy.

The previously mentioned studies investigated recall as a result of the associations between odor and an autobiographical memory. Odors may evoke more than learned associations, however, and may frequently affect nonattentive or preattentive processes. In fact, one of the issues concerning odor-evoked memories is that the full range of odor effects may be masked by a tendency to focus only on learned, semantic processes. Semantic processes, as higher-order, explicit processes, may override other processes linking emotion and odors when explicit verbal responses are used as a measure (see Savic, 2005). Implicit processing may be equally or more effective for odors evoking both emotion and behavior, and may lead to responses that are not easily linked to previous experience (Degel & Koster, 1999; Hudson, Wilson, Freyberg, & Haviland-Jones, 2007).

As an example of odor exposure leading to subconscious behavioral change, Holland, Hendriks, and Aarts (2005) showed that exposure to undetected citrus cleaner led participants in a word recognition task to respond faster to words related to cleanliness. They also spontaneously cleaned up their own cookie crumbs in the next phase of the study. This is a fascinating example of unconscious searches for congruent information related to undetected odors. (Similar effects are described below in the section on pheromones.) This study does not address the question of learning—participants may have learned the link between the odor of cleaner and cleanliness—but it does speak to the question of whether an odor must be identified before it can affect behavior. In this case, the odor was not identified. This makes us suspect with amusement and alarm that our human moods and actions are continuously influenced by chemicals (both natural and artificial) that evoke a search for congruent information and behavior.

Phillips and Cupchik's (2004) work on odors facilitating memory for textual material also demonstrates that explicit semantic processing is not necessary to evoke congruent search and behavior. They found that lower-intensity odors may be more influential in heightening recollection, hinting that the explicit semantic associations may sometimes take precedence when attention is brought to them and then may block other aspects of odors. Phillips and Cupchik found that pleasant paragraphs read in the presence of a pleasant floral odor were more likely to be remembered for affiliative and social content. Accuracy of recall was enhanced if the participants perceived the odor to be of low intensity. The authors suggested that an odor that is too intense may distract from the inherent unity between odor and experience. One of the important results of this study is the link not just between valences (pleasant to pleasant), but also of the particular pleasant floral odor to social memory. This association raises the possibility that some odors may carry vestiges of communicative messages that are not necessarily learned. As some flowers emit odors that mimic the social odors of a mammalian species in order to attract them (von Helversen, Winkler, & Bestmann, 2000), it is possible that odors produced by a variety of plants and animals may have some element of intra- or interspecies information.

ODORS AS COMMUNICATION

We know that odors are meaningful to us; we just do not appreciate the breadth of their meanings. Chemical signals serve a wide variety of communicative functions, ranging from the mundane to the profound. Some of these we hold in common wisdom: Holiday smells may evoke festivity, while medicinal smells may specify illness and (we hope) healing. New mothers like infant body odors more than nonmothers do (Fleming et al., 1993). And infants sleep better if they have an object with their mothers' odor on it (Goodlin-Jones, Eiben, & Anders, 1997). These observations make sense to us. Who would not associate holiday smells with specific emotional responses? Or who would challenge the idea that an infant is comforted by its mother's smell? Such associations seem reasonable, even

though we would also not be surprised if the association were absent.

But there is evidence for other kinds of meaning in odors. For example, several studies have demonstrated that relatives can identify the clothing of other relatives: Mothers can identify the clothing of their neonates (Russell, Mendelson, & Peeke, 1983), and siblings can identify clothing of siblings (Porter, Balogh, Cernoch, & Franchi, 1986). At first glance, one might say that these could very well be learned associations. But grandparents seem to be able to find the hospital shirts of their newborn grandchildren before meeting the infants (Porter et al., 1986). These are "family" identifications. Strangers also can match the worn t-shirts of mothers and their children, but not the t-shirts of husbands and wives (Porter, Cernoch, & Balogh, 1985). These studies suggest that body odors provide kinship information, and thus communication functions, at a deep genetic level.

Related to this idea of genetic information is the research on the major histocompatibility complex (MHC). The MHC is a group of genes that code for the immune system, as well as for one's unique odor signature. In humans, this signature is expressed as human leukocyte antigen (HLA) type. Studies have demonstrated that in closed populations, people are more likely to prefer partners with an HLA type different from their own, thus incurring the genetic advantages of a more diverse gene pool for the immune systems of their offspring (Ober et al., 1997). Another study shows that women prefer the scent of t-shirts worn by men with an HLA type other than their own (Wedekind, Seebeck, Bettens, & Paepke, 1995). These areas are still in their infancy and remain controversial, but suggest more influences of human semiochemicals.

Pheromones

As mentioned earlier, pheromones are chemical compounds secreted into the environment by members of a species and detected by other members of the same species, in whom they trigger behavioral, physical, and/or neuroendocrine responses (Karlson & Luscher, 1959). The studies to date that present the strongest evidence for pheromonal influences in humans are menstrual synchrony studies (McClintock, 1971; Stern & McClintock, 1998) and studies of the effects of male axillary compounds on women's cycles and reported mood (Preti, Wysocki, Barnhart, Sondheimer, & Leyden, 2003). Women exposed to the axillary secretions of other women (Stern & McClintock, 1998) or even of men (Preti et al., 2003) will have changes in their menstrual cycle. Our basic biological regulatory cycles are influenced by exposure to the body chemicals of others, even when the persons themselves are absent.

In behavioral research, studies have focused most often on the 16 androstene steroids as pheromone candidates. Between the mid-1970s and the mid-1990s, androstenone and androstenol were targets of research because the quantities of these steroids present in adult males are roughly equivalent to those produced by boars, and these compounds reliably function as pheromones in pigs (Dorries, Adkins-Regan, & Halpern, 1995). The results of this body of work are contradictory. For example, although women who wore necklaces laced with androstenol while they slept reported more social encounters with men the next day (Cowley & Brooksbank, 1991), other women exposed to androstenol did not report an increased sexual response to erotic passages (Benton & Wastell, 1986). Women exposed to androstenone rated themselves as less sexy than women exposed to other compounds (Filsinger, Braun, Monte, & Linder, 1984)—not the result one would expect.

It has been suggested that androstenol and androstenone may serve territorial functions, rather than sexual attraction functions. Women waiting in a dentist's office preferred chairs sprayed with androstenone (Kirk-Smith & Booth, 1980), while men tended to avoid bathroom stalls sprayed with androstenol (Gustavson, Dawson, & Bonett, 1987). Again, these were instances in which exposure to an undetected airborne chemical influenced behavior.

There are also reports that emotions may be influenced by these putative pheromones. The focus of research since the mid-1990s has been on androstadienone (AND), another 16 androstene steroid. Work with AND was sparked by the still controversial finding that AND elicited reaction in the VNO of females, but not males (Grosser, Monti-Bloch, Jennings-White, & Berliner, 2000). The same research reported a decrease in negative affect associated with AND. The Grosser et al. study delivered AND directly to the nasal cavity via a vapor pulse. Using a different methodology, Jacob and McClintock (2000) suggested that AND "modulates" negative mood in women. These researchers disguised the AND with clove oil and exposed the women to the stimuli by wiping a solution beneath the nose. The women in the control condition reported increased negativity and decreased positive mood over several hours; the women in the AND condition remained stable over time. Although these studies suggest that AND may indeed have mood effects, any conclusion that AND is a human pheromone remains speculative. Nevertheless, while the question of whether people respond to classical pheromones is debated, the emotional responses of humans to some semiochemicals is less dubious.

Mood Odors

There is accumulating evidence that humans communicate *emotionally* with body odors. One of the earliest studies to reveal this was conducted by Chen and Haviland-Jones (1999). As a part of this study, the effect of human odors on mood reports and dream memories was investigated. To this end, underarm pads (absorbing axillary odors) were collected from nightshirts (provided and laundered with unscented products) worn for a number of days by male and female odor donors who were young children, young adults, or older adults. Participants who were exposed to these odors later were asked to report their moods and to write a dream memory. No reference to the odor pads was made; they were simply placed on the working desk in an open glass container (the jar held the pads of one set of donors—same age and gender). Despite the fact that the odors of the young men and older women were not discriminated and were both rated as most unpleasant and intense, they affected the moods and dream memories of the detectors very differently. Specifically, the odors from the young men elicited more negative moods on a rating scale and more aggressive dream content. The older women's odors elicited more positive moods and more affiliative dream content. This initial study raised two key questions. First, it appears to be a challenge to any generalization of the Proust association effect. The odors were not identified or discriminated as old versus young or as male versus female, and yet there were different mood effects. Second, both odors were intense and unpleasant, and yet one evoked fairly pleasant responses. This is also a challenge to the associative explanations.

Because the odors judged to be the same had different mood effects, Chen and Haviland-Jones (1999, 2000) hypothesized that mood was being communicated. The young men in the study who were donors were all college students and at a time in their lives that was inherently stressful and required a goal-oriented attitude. Even their participation in our study was motivated by a course requirement rather than personal interest. It seemed likely that these young men might experience higher levels of frustration and aggression than other groups while wearing our axillary pads. On the other hand, the older women, who were all very healthy and retired, were probably living their lives at a more peaceful pace, focused on personal fulfillment and possibly nurturing activities. As such, the moods and emotions they experienced while wearing the axillary pads could have been more positive than those of the young males.

This led to a more direct investigation of the possibility that mood can be communicated with chemosensory products in axillary perspiration. To produce the mood odors, donors (nonsmokers, not wearing deodorant) came into the lab, placed the axillary pads under their arms, and watched a short video that showed repeated brief clips from popular movies of actors showing an emotional reaction (e.g., fear, anger, or happiness). Detectors were later asked to match the axillary pads to a mood name (e.g., "fear," "happy," "control"). The detectors were able to identify the mood at levels significantly above chance. A subsequent study by another lab (Ackerl, Atzmueller, & Grammer, 2002) has at least partially replicated the Chen and Haviland-Jones (1999) findings.

Additional studies have expanded our understanding of the effects that body odors have on those exposed to them. For example, Chen, Katdare, and Lucas (2006) asked how cognitive processing might be influenced by the presence of mood odors. Participants were given a word association task in the presence of axillary pads from donors who watched a scary or neutral video. The word task paired neutral and/or threat words in a counterbalanced design. Although threat-related words were processed equally fast in all mood odor conditions, participants were more accurate in the fear condition. On the other hand, in ambiguous pairings (threat-neutral, for example), the fear odor slowed processing. According to Chen et al., exposure to the fear odor led the subjects to adopt a more efficient yet cautious cognitive strategy for the task. In a similar vein, DeGroat and Haviland-Jones (2005) found a difference in reaction time between the fear and happy odor conditions in a visual image reaction task. Here the images were mixed, pleasant and unpleasant. Again, the fear odor was associated with slower reaction times than the happy odor.

It seems counterintuitive that the fear odors sometimes would lead to slower responding. One explanation might be that sensing an odor without having a visual or auditory match leads to a slow, cautious search for a match rather than the rapid "fear–flight" response. In fact, it is possible that sensing a fear odor with no obvious source would lead to "freezing" rather than flight, because the direction of flight toward safety would not be known.

OF FLOWERS AND HUMANS

Turning to the influence of more pleasant odors on moods, we serendipitously had begun a research program in positive psychology that had broad environmental goals and implications. We (Haviland-Jones, Rosario, Wilson, & McGuire, 2005) investigated how flowers, some of which were fragrant, as compared with other objects in the environment, evoke positive emotional and social responses in humans. The 2005 article describes three different studies conducted over several years. The first study in the series riveted our attention, because 100% of the participants exposed to a mixed flower bouquet responded with the Duchenne (zygomatic/orbicularis orbis) smile.

In the first study (Haviland-Jones et al., 2005) two members of the research team (one to code, one to present) brought a flower bouquet, a fruit basket, or a pillar candle to each participant to thank him or her for participation. The stimulus was closed in a box to hide it from the coder (so the coding would be double-blind), as well as to prevent anticipatory responses from the participant. All the participants who received the floral stimulus responded with the Duchenne smile within 5 seconds of the door on the box opening to reveal the stimulus. The group receiving the flowers also had a pre- to poststimulus mood change; only the group receiving the flowers reported more positive emotion over a 3-day period.

In the second study (Haviland-Jones et al., 2005), participants received "doses" of floral bouquets. Those who received more than one over several weeks had the lowest reports of depression. Participants in this study, who were all over age 60, scored higher on an episodic memory task after receiving the bouquets. This may indicate some potential motivational effects on cognitive tasks as well as emotional responses.

In the third study, there were more positive social interactions when a single flower was given to a person in an elevator than when a pen was given (or nothing). Not only were participants in the elevator more likely to respond with a Duchenne smile, but they were more likely to move closer to the experimenter, initiate new conversations, and look directly at the experimenter when a flower was given. This was the case for men as well as women, even though most people in modern Western culture associate flowers with women and predominantly give flowers to women.

A closer examination of earlier research (Dimberg & Thell, 1988) also suggested that flower photographs presented subliminally may elicit a positive response. Dimberg and Thell exposed participants to fear stimuli (e.g., snakes) and a "neutral" stimulus (flowers) tachistoscopically. They found that exposure to flowers elicited electromyographic (EMG) activation of the zygomatic muscles (a smile), referring to this as a positive response. They did not, however, measure the EMG activation of the orbicularis orbis muscles, also required for the Duchenne or "true" smile, so they could not conclude that flowers elicited happiness. The Duchenne smile reliably indicates happiness and positive affect, even in the absence of a self-report of happiness (Dimberg, Thunberg, & Elmehed, 2000). Such a smile activates both the zygomatic muscles of the cheeks and the orbicularis orbis muscles of the eyes.

There are several explanations for the flowers and positive emotion effect, only one of which involves semiochemicals. There are some theories that flowers mark the places where fruit would be harvested, and thus are

an evolutionary food signal (Pinker, 1997) and naturally associated with positive feelings. But in that case, one would have expected the fruit gift itself to produce as much happiness as the flowers (if not more), and this was not the case. On its own, the flowers' association with potential food cannot explain our results. Alternatively, it may be that the symmetry of flowers—a cue for memory and recognizability, and an evolutionary signal for detecting food and other significant events (Enquist & Arak, 1994)—led to the smiles and happiness. This idea is also captured by Cupchik (2006), who presents arguments for the evolutionary significance of aesthetics. However, it would be difficult to argue that the floral bouquet had more symmetry than the fruit basket or the pillar candle. It is possible that the semiochemicals and the fragrance of the flowers alone might have produced smiles and happy moods. Or all of the proposed effects may be synergistic, lending flowers a quality of "superstimulus"— appropriate odors, colors, symmetry, and association with food rewards. The significance of the studies seems to be that a naturally occurring stimulus such as flowers, not necessarily rewarding in any biological sense (not food, shelter, etc.), can affect mood rather dramatically.

We do not dismiss the possibility that learned associations accounted for some of the effects. However, learned associations alone cannot explain why the effect of the flowers was so much greater than that of the fruit and candles. The reactions of participants who received flowers was astonishing; they invited the experimenters into their homes and sent thank-you cards, sometimes with photographs of the flowers. In the elevator study, several participants who received nothing or a pen were disappointed upon seeing other people emerging from the elevator with flowers and returned repeatedly in an attempt to receive a flower themselves; no one returned for the attractive pen, seemingly more useful in the library.

It is likely that odor plays a very significant role in the human preference for flowers. Not only do people choose flowers because they like the odor, but they also perfume themselves and their personal belongings with floral odors. In one set of studies, both men and women who wore floral and other colognes for a month reported better moods than a similar group of people who did not have this treatment (Schiffman, Sattely-Miller, Suggs, & Graham, 1995; Schiffman, Suggs, & Sattely-Miller, 1995). The pleasant odors of flora may alone account for the positive mood effects we have described above. Cupchik has reported that pleasant floral odors used when people were reading a passage from literature influenced the episodes remembered from that passage (Cupchik & Phillips, 2005; Phillips & Cupchik, 2004). Those exposed to such odors remembered the positive emotional material better, as well as some types of social information. This once again suggests a strong associative effect, because there is an association between the pleasantness of the odor and the positive nature of the episode.

In a report prepared for the Sense of Smell Institute, we (Haviland-Jones & Wilson, 2005) found that the odors of some flowers (gardenia and others), even when present at such a low level as to be undetected by the participants, prevented negative emotional responses to stressful video material and also sent people to "search" their own memories for more positive emotional associations. We have argued that because the mood-enhancing effects of these odors were found even when the participants could not detect the presence of any odor, a nonsemantic, possibly nonassociative process is necessary to explain the mood effects of floral odors.

We suggest that flowering plants have found a positive "mood niche" to exploit: Humans provide propagation and care for these special flowering plants, which in turn improve moods. Positive mood itself has survival benefits (see Lucas & Diener, Chapter 29; Fredrickson & Cohn, Chapter 48; and Panksepp, Chapter 4, this volume). There may be some places in the world or some plants or animals that evoke or provide more happiness for people than other places, plants, or animals. Some aspects of this process are likely to include semiochemicals and odors.

Interspecies communication through chemosensory signals is not uncommon in the insect phyla (Weller, Jacobson, & Conner, 2000) and is even noted in mammals (von Helversen et al., 2000). Some flowers give off an odor that brings large gatherings of bats to "party," as von Helversen et al. (2000) report. These flowers require multiple pollinators, and the swarms of bats comply in the requisite numbers. They come in response to a chemo-sensory, airborne signal that mimics bat odors used for gathering. When the flowers no longer require pollination, they cease to put out the chemosensory signal. So it is known that plants and mammals may have coevolved systems that require chemosensory information. Humans and flowers may also be involved in such a system, demonstrating another avenue for olfactory and semiochemical functions—no matter whether this effect is unknown to the recipient of the chemical, amusingly suspected, or actually demonstrated as in our (Haviland-Jones et al., 2005) research.

OUR HYPOTHESES ABOUT THE NOSE AND EMOTION

We humans are overwhelmed with semiochemicals at all times in our lives. Some like to say that we live in a "chemical soup"—not referring to factory wastes, but to the everyday chemical information that plants, storms, babies, books, foods, and so forth produce. For the most part, it seems that we do not need to attend to the specific information; it sums itself as congruent or incongruent with other cues and is generally part of the background rather than the foreground. Some of this "soup" apparently cues us about the moods in the air, but not in such a way that we are usually aware of it.

A number of studies have led us to a hypothesis we have called the "search" function of semiochemicals. The puzzle is that small, fairly consistent responses to semiochemicals or odorants are found in many behaviors, such as reaction times or semantic constructions. These behaviors are not noticed by the people producing them, and in fact may be denied. For example, even though some say they can smell fear, for the most part they do not claim to be made afraid by that. Almost no one claims to smell happiness, and the potentiating effects of a happy odor are summarily dismissed. Yet these odors may in fact have unnoticed, small, consistent effects. The general phenomenon that behavior may occur without actual understanding of its stimulus is known in several systems.

There is ample evidence that we can respond to stimuli that we do not recognize (e.g., Öhman & Mineka, 2001; Zajonc, 1980), and that we may attribute our responses—memories, associations—to the wrong stimulus (Tversky & Kahneman, 1992). Öhman (see Chapter 44, this volume) points out that there are likely to be different brain structures involved in preattentive, potentiating stimulus processing versus focused attentive processes. In the case of long-term anxiety versus fear of a particular stimulus, he argues that it is possible to influence or potentiate the search for anxiety-causing stimuli, independently of attention to an actual fearful stimulus. The potentiation seems quite likely to interfere with processing nonfearful stimuli. In the case of our mostly pleasant chemosensory stimuli, we suspect that even other emotions may be similarly "potentiated." Pleasant stimuli with social significance may well lend themselves to the search for congruent information and may inhibit the search for incongruent stimuli.

We propose that there must be an ongoing, not-quite-conscious match–mismatch system that is correlating bits of information across the sensory systems. It is actively searching for existing associations and making new associations. If the semiochemical stimulus indicates a romantic possibility, the behavior of the person exposed to a romantic semiochemical may become more congruent with a search for romance—a bit of leaning forward, a little touch of the hair, as in a tiny display. It is unlikely that anyone would be aware of this shift in behavior. If there is no receptive person, or no time and place for romance, the behaviors elicited by the semiochemicals are short-circuited. There is not enough concurrence to support a romantic interlude. On the other hand, if the search finds a response, a person, or an event, we conclude that the words of the potential partner, or the mood music, or some other visible or audible event precipitated romance, not the semiochemical and our own subtle "search" behavior. We seldom refer to the romance in semiochemicals, even though we say colloquially that "romance was in the air." As another example, a man who searches for something pleasing to concur with a pleasant odor may think of an upcoming vacation. If asked why he is happy, he refers to the vacation, not to what the nose has sensed. He credits the result of a search, not the impetus for the search.

Whether a search is initiated and aborted when no other sensory or ideational system confirms the search, or whether the search leads to a target that is then presumed to be the evoker, the information from the nose is not credited. In the theater, if an odor lingering after a horror movie showing was different from the odor lingering after the comedy theater patrons departed, the nose might well know, but the narrative mind behind the nose would take all the credit for knowing and attributing the extra "frisson" to other things.

NEW DIRECTIONS

Based on the available research it is reasonable to believe that we humans have some chemosensory signals that contain mood information, and that we are generally able to have our moods influenced by a variety of natural and constructed odorants. We are a considerable distance from knowing how influential such communication might be, whether it is learned differently for men and women and in different cultures, or whether there are universal elements. The genetic components of the chemical aspects are also still to be discovered. Could we vary behavioral tendencies or attitudes as well as mood by changing the chemosensory environment? To suggest that the environment, chemosensory or otherwise, is psychologically unimportant assumes that we are separate and apart from the environment. But we are not separate; we interact with the environment, and such interaction by definition is bidirectional. That we can come to understand the influences of such bidirectionality on mood, behaviors, or human performance in general enhances our well-being and is essential to understanding the nature of who we are.

ACKNOWLEDGMENT

We would like to thank Linnea R. Dickson for her expert commentary on and editing of this chapter.

REFERENCES

Ackerl, K., Atzmueller, M., & Grammer, K. (2002). The scent of fear. *Neuroendocrinological Letters, 23,* 79–84.

Aggleton, J. P., & Waskett, L. (1999). The ability of odours to serve as state-dependent cues for real-world memories: Can Viking smells aid the recall of Viking experiences? *British Journal of Psychology, 90,* 1–7.

Baas, D., Aleman, A., & Kahn, R. S. (2004). Lateralization of amygdala activation: A systematic review of functional neuroimaging studies. *Brain Research: Brain Research Reviews, 45*(2), 96–1003.

Bensafi, M., Brown, W. M., Tsutsui, T., Mainland, J. D., Johnson, B. N., Bremner, E. A., et al. (2003). Sex-steroid derived compounds induce sex-specific effects on autonomic nervous system function in humans. *Behavioral Neuroscience, 117*(6), 1125–1134.

Benton, D., & Wastell, V. (1986). Effects of androstenol on human sexual arousal. *Biological Psychology, 22,* 141–147.

Brand, G. (2006). Olfactory/trigeminal interactions in nasal chemoreception. *Neuroscience and Biobehavioral Reviews, 30,* 908–917.

Britton, J. C., Phan, K. L., Taylor, S. F., Welsh, R. C., Berridge, K. C., & Liberzon, I. (2006). Neural correlates of social and nonsocial emotions: An fMRI study. *NeuroImage, 31*(1), 397–409.

Buck, L., & Axel, R. (1991). A novel multigene family may encode odorant receptors: A molecular basis for odor recognition. *Cell, 65,* 175–187.

Cain, W. S. (1978). History of research on smell. In E. C. Carterette & M. P. Friedman (Eds.), *Handbook of perception* (Vol. 6, pp. 197–229). New York: Academic Press.

Carleton, A., Petreanu, L. T., Lansford, R., Alvarez-Buylla, A., & Lledo, P. (2003). Becoming a new neuron in the adult olfactory bulb. *Nature Neuroscience, 6*(5), 507–518.

Chen, D., & Haviland-Jones, J. (1999). Rapid mood change and human odors. *Physiology and Behavior, 68,* 241–250.

Chen, D., & Haviland-Jones, J. (2000). Human olfactory communication of emotion. *Perceptual and Motor Skills, 91,* 771–781.

Chen, D., Katdare, A., & Lucas, N. (2006) Chemosignals of fear enhance cognitive performance in humans. *Chemical Senses, 31,* 415–423.

Classen, C., Howes, D., & Synnott, A. (1994). *Aroma: The cultural history of smell.* London: Routledge.

Cowley, J. J., & Brooksbank, B. W. L. (1991). Human exposure to putative pheromones and changes in aspects of social behaviour. *Journal of Steroid Biochemistry and Molecular Biology, 39*(4), 647–659.

Cupchik, G. C. (2006). Emotion in aesthetics and the aesthetics of emotion. In P. Locher, C. Martindale, & L. Dorfman (Eds.), *New directions in aesthetics, creativity and the arts* (pp. 209–224). Amityville, NY: Baywood.

Cupchik, G. C., & Phillips, K. (2005). The scent of literature. *Cognition and Emotion, 19*(1), 101–119.

Degel, J., & Koster, E. P. (1999). Odors: Implicit memory and performance effects. *Chemical Senses, 24*(3), 317–325.

DeGroat, D. A., & Haviland-Jones, J. (2005, April). *Exposure to human emotion semiochemicals (mood odors) affects behavior.* Poster presented at the annual meeting of the Association for Chemoreception Sciences, Sarasota, FL.

Dimberg, U., & Thell, S. (1988). Facial electromyography, fear relevance and the experience of stimuli. *Journal of Psychophysiology, 2,* 213–219.

Dimberg, U., Thunberg, M., & Elmehed, K. (2000). Unconscious facial reactions to emotional facial expressions. *Psychological Science, 11*(1), 86–89.

Dorries, K. M., Adkins-Regan, E., & Halpern, B. P. (1995). Olfactory sensitivity to the pheromone, androstenone, is sexually dimorphic in the pig. *Physiology and Behavior, 57*(2), 255–259.

Dorries, K. M., Adkins-Regan, E., & Halpern, B. P. (1997). Sensitivity and behavioral responses to the pheromone androstenone are not mediated by the vomeronasal organ in domestic pigs. *Brain, Behavior and Evolution, 49,* 53–62.

Enquist, M., & Arak, A. (1994). Symmetry, beauty and evolution. *Nature, 372,* 169–172.

Filsinger, E. E., Braun, J. J., Monte, W. C., & Linder, D. E. (1984). Human (*Homo sapiens*) responses to pig (*Sus scrofa*) sex pheromone 5 alpha-androst-16-en-3-one. *Journal of Comparative Psychology, 98*(2), 219–222.

Fleming, A. S., Corter, C., Franks, P., Surbey, M., Schneider, B., & Steiner, M. (1993). Postpartum factors related to mother's attraction to newborn infant odors. *Developmental Psychobiology, 26*(2), 115–132.

Gilbert, A. N., & Wysocki, C. J. (1987) The smell survey. *National Geographic, 172,* 514–525.

Goodlin-Jones, B. L., Eiben, L. A., & Anders, T. F. (1997). Maternal well-being and sleep–wake behaviors in infants: An intervention using maternal odor. *Infant Mental Health Journal, 18*(4), 378–393.

Graves, A. B., Bowend, J. D., Rajaram, L., McCormich, W. C., McCurry, S. M., Schellenberg, G. D., et al. (1999). Impaired olfaction as a marker for cognitive decline: Interaction with apolipoprotein E ε4 status. *Neurology, 53*(7), 1480–1487.

Grosser, B., Monti-Bloch, L., Jennings-White, C., & Berliner, D. (2000). Behavioral and electrophysiological effects of androstadienone, a human pheromone. *Psychoneuroendocrinology, 25,* 289–299.

Gustavson, A. R., Dawson, M. E., & Bonett, D. G. (1987). Androstenone, a putative human pheromone, affects human (*Homo sapiens*) male choice performance. *Journal of Comparative Psychology, 101*(2), 210–212.

Halpern, M. (1987). The organization and function of the vomeronasal system. *Annual Review of Neuroscience, 10,* 325–362.

Haviland-Jones, J., Rosario, H. H., Wilson, P. J., & McGuire, T. (2005). An environmental approach to positive emotion: Flowers. *Evolutionary Psychology, 3,* 104–132.

Haviland-Jones, J., & Wilson, P. J. (2005). *Fragrance: Emotion, sensuality and relationships.* New York: Sense of Smell Institute.

Herz, R. S. (2000, July–August). Scents of time. *The Sciences,* pp. 34–39.

Herz, R. S., & Cupchik, G. C. (1995). The emotional distinctiveness of odor-evoked memories. *Chemical Senses, 20*(5), 517–528.

Holland, R. W., Hendriks, M., & Aarts, H. (2005). Smells like clean spirit: Nonconscious effects of scent on cognition and behavior. *Psychological Science, 16*(9), 689–693.

Hudson, J. A., Wilson, P. J., Freyberg, R., & Haviland-Jones, J. (2007). *Scents and sensibility: Effects of implicit odor exposure on autobiographical memory.* Manuscript submitted for publication.

Jacob, S., & McClintock, M. K. (2000). Psychological state and mood effects of steroidal chemosignals in women and men. *Hormones and Behavior, 37*(1), 57–78.

Karlson, P., & Luscher, M. (1959). Pheromones: A new term for a class of biologically active substances. *Nature, 183,* 55–56.

Kirk-Smith, M. D., & Booth, D. A. (1980). Effects of androstenone on choice of location in others' presence. In H. van der Starre (Ed.), *Olfaction and taste* (Vol. 7, pp. 397–400). London: IRL Press.

LoSasso, G. L., Rapport, L. J., Axelrod, B. N., & Whitman, R. D. (2002). Neurocognitive sequelae of exposure to organic solvents and (meth)acrylates among nail-studio technicians. *Neuropsychiatry, Neuropsychology, and Behavioral Neurology, 15*(1), 44–55.

McClintock, M. (1971). Menstrual synchrony and suppression. *Nature, 229,* 244–245.

Meredith, M. (2001). Human vomeronasal organ function: A critical review of best and worst cases. *Chemical Senses, 26,* 433–445.

Mesholam, R. I., Moberg, P. J., Mahr, R. N., & Doty, R. L. (1998). Olfaction in neurodegenerative disease: A meta-analysis of olfactory functioning in Alzheimer's and Parkinson's diseases. *Archive of Neurology, 55,* 84–90.

Ober, C., Weitkamp, L. R., Cox, N., Dytch, H., Kostyu, D., & Elias, S. (1997). HLA and mate choice in humans. *American Journal of Human Genetics, 61,* 497–504.

Öhman, A., & Mineka, S. (2001). Fears, phobias and preparedness: Toward an evolved module of fear and fear learning. *Psychological Review, 108,* 438–522.

Phillips, K., & Cupchik, G. C. (2004). Scented memories of literature. *Memory, 12*(3), 366–375.

Pinker, S. (1997). *How the mind works.* New York: Norton.

Porter, R. H., Balogh, R. D., Cernoch, J. M., & Franchi, C. (1986). Recognition of kin through characteristic body odors. *Chemical Senses, 11,* 389–395.

Porter, R. H., Cernoch, J. M., & Balogh, R. D. (1985). Odor signatures and kin recognition. *Physiology and Behavior, 34,* 445–448.

Preti, G., Wysocki, C. J., Barnhart, K. T., Sondheimer, S. J., & Leyden, J. J. (2003). Male axillary extracts contain pheromones that affect pulsatile secretion of luteinizing hormone and mood in women recipients. *Biology of Reproduction, 68*(6), 2107–2113.

Proust, M. (1957). *Swann's way* (C. K. S. Moncrieff, Trans.). New York: Penguin Books. (Original work published 1913)

Rolls, E. T. (1996). The orbitofrontal cortex. *Philosophical Transactions of the Royal Society of London: Series B. Biological Sciences, 351*(1346), 1433–1443.

Rosenkranz, H. C., & Cunningham, A. R. (2003). Environmental odors and health hazards. *The Science of the Total Environment, 313,* 15–24.

Rotton, J. (1983). Affective and cognitive consequences of malodorous pollution. *Basic and Applied Social Psychology, 4,* 171–191.

Rouhi, A. M. (2002). Exploring the chemical senses. *Chemical and Engineering News, 80*(1), 24–29.

Russell, M., Mendelson, T., & Peeke, H. (1983). Mother's identification of their infant's odors. *Ethology and Sociobiology, 4,* 29–31.

Savic, I. (2005). Brain imaging studies of the functional organization of human olfaction. *Chemical Senses, 30*(Suppl. 1), i222–i223.

Schaal, B., & Porter, R. H. (1991). "Microsmatic humans" revisited: The generation and perception of chemical signals. In P. J. B. Slater & J. S. Rosenblatt (Eds.). *Advances in the study of behavior* (Vol. 20, pp. 135–199). San Diego, CA: Academic Press.

Schiffman, S. S., Sattely-Miller, E. A., Suggs, M. S., & Graham, B. G. (1995). The effect of pleasant odors and hormone status on mood of women at mid-life. *Brain Research Bulletin, 36,* 19–29.

Schiffman, S. S., Suggs, M. S., & Sattely-Miller, E. A. (1995). Effects of pleasant odors on mood of males at mid-life: Comparison of African-American and European-American men. *Brain Research Bulletin, 36*(1), 31–37.

Schiffman, S. S., & Williams, C. M. (2005). Science of odor as a potential health issue. *Journal of Environmental Quality, 34*(1), 129–138.

Steele, J. J. (1992). The anthropology of smell and scent in ancient Egypt and modern South American shamanism. In S. Van Toller & G. H. Dodd (Eds.), *Fragrance: The psychology and biology of perfume* (pp. 287–303). London: Elsevier.

Stern, K., & McClintock, M. K. (1998). Regulation of ovulation by human pheromones. *Nature, 392,* 177–179.

Stockhorst, U., & Pietrowsky, R. (2004). Olfactory perception, communication, and the nose-to-brain pathway. *Physiology and Behavior, 83,* 3–11.

Stoddart, D. M. (1990). *The scented ape.* Cambridge, UK: Cambridge University Press.

Swan, G. E., & Carmelli, D. (2000). Impaired olfaction predicts cognitive decline in nondemented older adults. *Neuroepidemiology, 21*(2), 58–67.

Tversky, A., & Kahneman, D. (1992). Advances in prospect theory: Cumulative representation of uncertainty. *Journal of Risk and Uncertainty, 5,* 297–323.

Van Toller, S., & Dodd, G. H. (Eds.). (1988). *Perfumery: The psychology and biology of fragrance.* London: Chapman & Hall.

Van Toller, S., & Dodd, G. H. (Eds.). (1992). *Fragrance: The psychology and biology of perfume.* London: Elsevier.

von Helversen, O., Winkler, L., & Bestmann, S. J. (2000). Sulfur containing "perfumes" attract flower visiting bats. *Journal of Comparative Physiology A: Neuroethology, Sensory, Neural, and Behavioral Physiology, 186*(2), 143–153.

Wedekind, C., Seebeck, T., Bettens, F., & Paepke, A. J. (1995). MHC-dependent mate preferences in humans. *Proceedings of the Royal Society of London: Biological Sciences, 260,* 245–249.

Weller, S. J., Jacobson, N. L., & Conner, W. E. (2000). The evolution of chemical defenses and mating systems in tiger moths. *Biological Journal of the Linnaean Society, 68,* 557–558.

Woodworth, R. S., & Schlosberg, H. (1955). *Experimental psychology.* London: Methuen.

Zajonc, R. B. (1980). Feeling and thinking: Preferences need no inferences. *American Psychologist, 35,* 151–175.

Zald, D. H. (2003). The human amygdale and the emotional evaluation of sensory stimuli. *Brain Research Reviews, 41,* 88–123.

Zald, D. H., & Pardo, J. V. (1997). Emotion, olfaction, and the human amygdala: Amygdala activation during aversive olfactory stimulation. *Proceedings of the National Academy of Sciences of the USA, 94,* 4119–4124.

CHAPTER 15

The Neuroimaging of Emotion

TOR D. WAGER, LISA FELDMAN BARRETT,
ELIZA BLISS-MOREAU, KRISTEN A. LINDQUIST, SETH DUNCAN,
HEDY KOBER, JOSH JOSEPH, MATTHEW DAVIDSON,
and JENNIFER MIZE

Questions about the nature of emotion have existed since psychology emerged as a scientific discipline in the late 19th century (Darwin, 1872/1998; Dewey, 1895; Irons, 1897; James, 1884). For a century, scientists were unable to measure emotions at their source, and so they relied on measures of behavior, reported experience, and activity of the peripheral nervous system to address fundamental questions about what emotions are and how they function in the economy of the mind. Although much was learned that is of both scientific interest and practical value, questions about the nature of emotion remained fundamentally unresolved. The relatively recent introduction of neuroimaging techniques, particularly functional magnetic resonance imaging (fMRI) and positron emission tomography (PET), provide a new perspective on the emotion in the intact human brain, and have the potential to identify which brain areas are consistently and specifically associated with particular types of emotional states. Fifteen years' worth of neuroimaging research has investigated the neural underpinnings of emotions—including responses to ba-

sic affective stimuli such as pictures or odors; the experience and regulation of the discrete emotional events that we refer to as "disgust," "anger," and "desire"; and the perception of emotion in others. These findings have the potential to shed new light on what emotions are and how they work.

We begin this chapter by sketching a hypothesized "neural reference space" for emotion (Barrett, Mesquita, Ochsner, & Gross, 2007; Edelman & Tononi, 2001), which refers to the set of brain structures thought to instantiate emotions and related affective states. We then examine how findings from neuroimaging studies map onto this space, and what they contribute to the understanding of the brain bases of affect and emotion. We take a meta-analytic approach, integrating the results obtained in 163 individual studies to locate the regions most consistently activated across a range of emotion-related tasks. We refer to this set of regions as the "observed neural reference space." Next, we bring meta-analytic evidence to bear on three unresolved issues in the emotion literature. First, we ask whether the experience and perception of emotion produce different patterns of brain activation. Second, we ask whether the experiences of pleasant and unpleasant affect are instantiated by distinct circuitry in the human brain. Third, we address the methodological question of whether PET and fMRI are equally suitable for studying emotion in the human brain, particularly in brainstem and midbrain areas. In addressing these three questions, we also touch on other issues, such as the centrality of the amygdala in emotion, the representation and lateralization of affect in the brain, and the validity of fMRI as a means of studying emotional experience. Other recent meta-analyses have tackled the structure of emotion (Murphy, Nimmo-Smith, & Lawrence, 2003; Phan, Wager, Taylor, & Liberzon, 2002), so we do not address this question here.

THE HYPOTHESIZED NEURAL REFERENCE SPACE FOR EMOTION-RELATED PHENOMENA

Animal and lesion studies guide and constrain current thinking about the neural systems that give rise to emotion. Animal models can provide exquisite neurophysiological detail that constrains theories about mental processes, and neuropsychology provides unique evidence on the brain components necessary for intact emotional processes in humans. Although neuroimaging offers unique advantages, in that it offers a probe of brain function in the intact human, interpretation of neuroimaging studies relies heavily on these complementary methods. Below, we provide a few pointers to the massive body of evidence on the affective brain that informs our interpretations of the body of neuroimaging studies to date. We begin in the oldest parts of the brain and work our way up to the cortical centers that so markedly differentiate humans from other species.

Brainstem

Brainstem nuclei form the oldest centers related to affective processing and generate autonomic output to regulate the heart, vasculature, and other visceral organs. Nuclei within these regions have generally bidirectional connections with other emotion-related structures, such as the medial prefrontal cortex (mPFC), insula (INS), and amygdala (Amy) (Amaral, Price,

Pitkanen, & Carmichael, 1992; Barbas, Saha, Rempel-Clower, & Ghashghaei, 2004; McDonald, 1998; Ongur, An, & Price, 1998; Ongur & Price, 2000). (For a listing of all abbreviations used for brain regions in this chapter, see Table 15.1.) A particularly important structure is the midbrain periaqueductal gray (PAG), which is thought to coordinate coherent physiological and behavioral responses to threat (Bandler & Shipley, 1994; Holstege & Georgiadis, 2004; Van der Horst & Holstege, 1998). Stimulation of different longitudinal columns of PAG elicits distinct coordinated, organism-wide response "modes" that mirror the natural affective reactions elicited by threat. For example, stimulation of lateral columns elicits "defensive" behaviors, such as facing and backing away from a perceived attacker, hissing, and attack when approached (Gregg & Siegel, 2001); it also elicits autonomic responses that include tachycardia, increased blood pressure and blood flow to the face, pupillary dilation, and piloerection (Lovick, 1992), as well as analgesia. Together, these effects are consistent with a defensive–aggressive emotional response. As PAG receives direct projections from numerous cortical regions, including the anterior cingulate cortex (ACC), mPFC, anterior INS (aINS), and medial temporal lobe (MTL) (Shipley, Ennis, Rizvi, & Behbehani, 1991), the PAG might be thought of as an integrative emotional center, and it plays a central role in some conceptions of emotion (Panksepp, 1998).

In spite of their prevalence in animal models, brainstem nuclei are rarely discussed in neuroimaging studies, partly due to their small size and difficulty in localization. Many studies report activation in these subcortical areas, however, and we analyze the specificity and reliability of these activations in this chapter. We find consistent activations around the human PAG, particularly in studies of negative emotional experience. These results underscore homologies between humans and other animals.

Diencephalon

The hypothalamus (Hy) and thalamus constitute most of the diencephalon. Like the PAG, the Hy is a major player in animal models of emotion. It governs the pituitary and thereby the body's endocrine system; plays a major role in the regulation of motivated behavior and homeostatic processes (Sewards & Sewards,

TABLE 15.1. Abbreviations for Brain Regions, Organized by Anatomical Structure

Localization prefixes/suffixes		Paralimbic	
v	ventral	Ins or INS	insula
a	anterior	Ag	agrancular region of insula
d	dorsal	mPFC	medical prefrontal cortex
r	rostral	vmPFC	ventromedial prefrontal cortex
s	superior	OFC	orbito-frontal cortex
i	inferior	ACC	anterior cingulate cortex
fr	frontal	rdACC	rostral dorsal anterior cingulate
lat.	Lateral	pgACC	pregenual cingulate
m or med.	Medial	sgACC	subgenual cingulate
BA	Brodmann's area	TP	temporal pole
		pHCMP	parahippocampal cortex
Brainstem		MTL	medial temporal lobe
Midb	midbrain		
PAG	periaqueductal gray	**Other cortical regions**	
VTA	ventral tegmental area	*Lateral frontal*	
		IFG	inferior frontal gyrus
Diencephalon		frOP	frontal operculum
Hy	hypothalamus	IFS	inferior frontal sulcus
Thalamus		*Medial wall*	
Thal	thalamus	dmPFC	dorsomedial prefrontal cortex
MD	mediodorsal nucleus	PCC	posterior cingulate cortex
MGN	medial geniculate nucleus	pre-SMA	pre-supplementary motor area
CM	centromedian nucleus	*Temporal*	
STN	subthalamic nucleus	MTL	medial temporal lobe
		TC	temporal cortex
Subcortical telencephalon		STS	sup. temporal culcus
Amy	amygdala	STG	sup. temporal gyrus
HCMP	hippocampus	*Occipital*	
BF	basal forebrain (cholinergic)	OCC	occipital cortex
BNST	bed nucleus of the stria terminalis	V1	primary visual cortex
Str	striatum (Cau/Put)		
Put	putamen	**Cerebellum**	
Cau	caudate	CB	cerebellum
GP	globus pallidus		
NAC	nucleus accumbens		

2003; Valenstein, Cox, & Kakolewski, 1970); and interacts with the autonomic nervous system through large reciprocal connections with the PAG and other brainstem nuclei (Saper, Loewy, Swanson, & Cowan, 1976). The lateral Hy receives projections from diverse limbic structures and projects to the midbrain (midb), middle hypothalamic zone, and medial Hy. The middle zone regulates autonomic functions and bottom-up forms of attention via connections to brainstem nuclei, including the PAG, reticular formation, parabrachial nucleus, ventral tegmental area (VTA), raphe nuclei, and spinal autonomic centers. And finally, the medial zone regulates endocrine function, such as

the release of cortisol during stress. As we show here, activations in the human Hy and surrounding structures are reliable across studies and show a preference in frquency of activation for studies of positive emotional experience.

The thalamus is perhaps best known for its role in sensory processing, but it contains over 30 distinct nuclei whose cortico-thalamic loops cover virtually the entire cortical mantle. The mediodorsal nucleus (MD) and the intralaminar nuclei are most closely associated with affective processes. Human thalamic activations are reliable in studies of emotion, and some parts show preference for emotional experience.

Subcortical Telencephalon

Overlying the brainstem and diencephalon are a group of subcortical areas that are typically identified as core limbic structures. These include the amygdala, hippocampus, cholinergic basal forebrain (BF) nuclei, and basal ganglia. The amygdala is well known for its role in emotion, particularly fear, though it also plays a prominent role in appetitive processes (Braesicke et al., 2005; Waraczynski, 2006). The basolateral complex plays a critical role in fear conditioning—the learning of associations between specific environmental cues and aversive outcomes (Anglada Figueroa & Quirk, 2005; Davis, 1992; Goosens & Maren, 2001; LeDoux, 2000; Nader, Majidishad, Amorapanth, & LeDoux, 2001). The central nucleus, at the dorsal end of the amygdala, is important for the physiological and behavioral expression of conditioned fear responses (Davis, 1992; Feldman, Conforti, & Saphier, 1990; Kalin, Shelton, & Davidson, 2004). However, the role of these structures in emotional experience (e.g., the *feeling* of fear) is less certain, as fear-like responses to naturally threatening stimuli do not always require the amygdala (Davis & Lee, 1998; Walker & Davis, 1997; Wallace & Rosen, 2001). As we show below, imaging studies suggest that activations observed in the human amygdala are more likely to relate to visual cues that signal affective significance than to those signaling negative experience.

The amygdala, like many gross anatomical structures in the "affective brain," plays roles in both positive and negative affective processes. It is critical for the evaluation of sensory cues associated with reward (Cador, Robbins, & Everitt, 1989; Everitt, Cador, & Robbins, 1989; Everitt et al., 1999) and the short-term updating of the reward value of cues in context (Baxter & Murray, 2002; Schoenbaum, Chiba, & Gallagher, 1998; Schoenbaum, Setlow, Saddoris, & Gallagher, 2003). Recently Paton, Belova, Morrison, and Salzman (2006) showed that separate populations of amygdala neurons respond to stimuli that predict positive and negative future outcomes.

Taken together, all of this research suggests that the amygdala is important to the evaluation of sensory cues for relevance to the organism, and directs an organism to learn more about a stimulus so as to better determine its predictive value for well-being and survival

(Davis & Whalen, 2001; Kim, Somerville, Johnstone, Alexander, & Whalen, 2003; Whalen, 1998). This is consistent with the idea that amygdala activations in human neuroimaging studies are related to the salience or potential information value of visual stimuli (Amaral, 2003; Liberzon, Phan, Decker, & Taylor, 2003; Whalen et al., 2004).

Interspersed with cell groups in the extended amygdala are a variety of cell groups spread throughout the BF. Some, such as the bed nucleus of the stria terminalis (BNST), are likely to be important for fear and anxiety (Davis & Lee, 1998; Davis & Shi, 1999; Walker & Davis, 1997). Other nuclei serve as suppliers of acetylcholine to the cortex and play a key role in motivational modulation of attention (Sarter, Hasselmo, Bruno, & Givens, 2005) and sensory plasticity (Bear & Singer, 1986; Weinberger, 1995). These or other nuclei may be important for human reward and pleasure: Early stimulation studies in humans suggested that stimulation of the septal region in the BF can produce pleasurable responses (Heath, 1972; Heath, Cox, & Lustick, 1974), though these early observations may have actually been related to seeking or appetitive behavior related to stimulation of the visual striatum rather than to "pleasure" per se. We show below that the BF and septal regions are consistently activated in neuroimaging studies of emotion, and that different parts of this region are selective for positive and negative affect. Midline structures around the septal nuclei are activated preferentially by studies of positive emotional experience, whereas more lateral areas around the BNST and extended amygdala are activated preferentially by studies of negative emotional experience.

The hippocampus, posterior to the amygdala, figures prominently in Gray's (1978) affective/motivational theory of behavioral inhibition in anxiety. However, recent studies documenting the role of the hippocampus in long-term memory formation and consolidation (Squire & Zola-Morgan, 1991) have led researchers to suspect that its role in emotional behavior is memory-related. Consistent with this view, the hippocampus is particularly important for contextual fear conditioning in rodents (e.g., Maren, Aharonov, & Fanselow, 1997). In humans, hippocampal and medial temporal activations are reliable in emotion-related tasks, but appear to be more related to perception of affective stimuli than to emotional experience.

The basal ganglia are a set of subcortical structures that are critical for planning and initiating motivationally relevant behaviors. Although they were once thought to be primarily related to motor control, their functional role is likely to extend to the computation of affective value in a more general sense. The striatum—consisting of the caudate, putamen, and nucleus accumbens (NAC)—and the globus pallidus (GP, not shown) constitute the major part of the basal ganglia. The ventral parts of the striatum—including NAC, ventral striatum (ventral caudate and putamen)—and ventral pallidum play important roles in motivation, reward, and learning. Along with VTA and lateral Hy, they form a network of regions rich in dopamine and opioid receptors that might be considered the appetitive motivational "backbone" of the brain (Berridge, 2004). Whereas this system was originally thought to mediate primary hedonic or "reward" responses, there is now substantial evidence that dopamine signaling in this network—particularly in the mesolimbic pathway from VTA to NAC—is more closely related to the generation of motivated behavior than to "pleasure" per se (Berridge & Robinson, 1998; Salamone, Cousins, & Snyder, 1997). These areas are some of the most frequently activated structures in studies of human emotion, and different portions of these structures are preferentially activated by positive versus negative emotional experience.

Paralimbic Cortex

The paralimbic "belt" is a set of phylogenetically older cortex with large, direct projections to subcortical and brainstem nuclei. These include the orbitofrontal cortex (OFC), rostral mPFC, aINS, and anterior temporal cortex (TC). Damage to OFC is associated with inappropriate generation and regulation of affect, which may take the form of flattened affect, increased expression and reports of negative emotion, or inappropriate emotion for the social context, depending on the case (Beer, Heerey, Keltner, Scabini, & Knight, 2003; Berlin, Rolls, & Kischka, 2004; Hornak et al., 2003). Damage is also associated with reduced physiological output (e.g., heart rate and skin conductance; Anderson, Damasio, Tranel, & Damasio, 2000; Angrilli, Palomba, Cantagallo, Maietti, & Stegagno, 1999; Roberts et al., 2004).

The ventral areas of the medial wall have direct projections to the Hy and lower brainstem autonomic effectors (Saper, 1995). Subgenual cingulate (sgACC) and ventromedial prefrontal cortex (vmPFC) are related to visceromotor control in a number of animal studies (Vogt, Finch, & Olson, 1992), and subregions appear to play different and perhaps opposing roles in the generation and regulation or extinction of hypothalamic–pituitary–adrenal "stress" responses (Sullivan & Gratton, 2002) and conditioned fear responses (Milad & Quirk, 2002). Rostral dorsal anterior cingulate (rdACC) and pregenual anterior cingulate (pgACC) have also been associated with diverse affect-related functions, including maternal bonding, pain, and emotion; the rostral cingulate may be subdivided into more rostral affect-related regions and more posterior response-selection-related regions (Devinsky, Morrell, & Vogt, 1995; Vogt, Nimchinsky, Vogt, & Hof, 1995). In human neuroimaging of emotion, distinct subregions of dorsal and ventral mPFC, rdACC, pgACC, and OFC are activated. Dorsomedial PFC and multiple regions within OFC are selective for studies of emotional experience, but ACC is not. Medial OFC and vmPFC are selective for positive emotion.

aINS, shown in the top left portion of Plate 15.1 (see color insert), is connected with diverse subcortical "limbic" regions and projects to brainstem autonomic centers. It has been associated with interoception of affect-related body states, including perception of pain and itch (Craig, 2002), and with visceromotor control (Yasui, Breder, Saper, & Cechetto, 1991). The aINS can be divided based on cytoarchitecture and function into ventral and dorsal regions (Mesulam & Mufson, 1982). The evolutionarily older ventral portion, agranular insula (Ag), is a core paralimbic region containing primary cortical regions for sensory–affective processing (taste and smell) and is particularly associated in human imaging studies with emotion (Wager & Barrett, 2004). The dorsal region, by contrast, is activated in a more diverse set of cognitive tasks; it contains the operculo-insular junction, commonly activated in tasks requiring the context-sensitive deployment of attention (Thompson-Schill, D'Esposito, Aguirre, & Farah, 1997; Wager, Reading, & Jonides, 2004). (In many cognitive studies, the area of operculo-insular activation is referred to as the inferior frontal gyrus [IFG]). This distinction turns out to be important for our analyses, as the human studies we review show preference for positive emotional experience in the ventral aINS (near OFC and primary taste and smell cortices), and preference for negative emotional experience in the dorsal aINS regions (which are most often activated by pain and tasks that elicit negative emotions).

The medial and lateral anterior TC are densely interconnected with OFC, and early studies of human TC stimulation produced particularly strong and vivid emotional experiences (Sem-Jacobsen, 1968). These experiences often took the form of reliving a period of the past (e.g., a scene from childhood) as though actually there, complete with emotive behavior appropriate for the situation. We find reliable activation of anterior TC in studies of emotional experience, with different portions preferentially activated by positive and negative emotions.

Above, we have summarized some of the broad roles thought to be played by the various structures that make up the affective brain. Next, we present the methods and results of our meta-analysis in more detail. Though the results are largely consistent with hypotheses based on animal and lesion data, they provide maps of the human affective brain that in many cases indicate that different regions within the broad structures discussed above may play different and even opposing roles.

THE META-ANALYTIC APPROACH

In spite of the growing literature on the neural bases of emotion, we still know very little about the precise functions of key brain regions in the affective brain that instantiate the emotional lives of humans. A major difficulty in human work is variability: Studies of what scientists assume are the same phenomenon (e.g., the experience of fear) can produce widely varying results both across participants within a study and across studies. For the most part, this variability is treated as error, even though it may reflect real and important differences in brain anatomy (at the individual participant level) or task requirements and therefore psychological process (at the level of the study). Single neuroimaging studies typically average signals across individuals to identify brain areas that show consistent activity across a group

of participants. Similarly, with the use of meta-analytic techniques, we can average results across studies to identify brain areas that show consistent activity across a group of studies. Meta-analyses allow us not only to identify consistent brain–process correspondences (i.e., the extent to which a brain area consistently shows increased activity with a psychological process), but also to identify the specificity of such correspondences. Of course, many of the details and nuances of individual studies are lost in a meta-analytic approach, but its strength is that it allows us to view the affective brain painted in broad strokes, and provides us with a means to address whether ask the major psychological categories that scientists typically rely on—perception versus experience, positive versus negative affect, or varieties of negative emotion (e.g., sadness vs. anger vs. fear)—produce reliable and specific differences in brain activity.

The Sample of Studies

We included findings from a total of 163 neuroimaging studies (57 PET and 106 fMRI) on unmedicated, healthy adults published between 1990 and 2005. These are summarized in Table 15.2 and described in detail in Appendix 15.1.[1] All studies were coded for whether they targeted "affect" (defined as a pleasant or unpleasant state arising from presentation of survival-related or social stimuli) or "emotion" (defined as instances of categories typically labeled by the English words "anger," "sadness," "fear," "disgust," and "happiness"). We also coded other relevant study properties, such as whether a study involved perception or experience, whether positive or negative feelings were evoked (for studies of experience), and whether PET or fMRI methods were used.[2] Papers were coded first by a team of four trained raters. Each paper was coded by two different coders. We included only activations (omitting deactivations, because they were less consistently reported).

Multilevel Analytic Strategy: Peak Density Analysis

Meta-analyses of neuroimaging studies do not usually compute average effect sizes, as is done with behavioral data, but instead summarize the frequency with which studies report peak activation coordinates in a particular brain location (Fox, Parsons, & Lancaster, 1998; Laird et al., 2005; Wager, Phan, Liberzon, & Taylor, 2003; Wager, Reading, et al., 2004).[3] Each study reports one or more contrasts that map the difference in brain activity for two conditions (e.g., positive vs. neutral picture viewing). By convention, activated regions in each contrast are summarized as coordinates in a standardized, three-dimensional brain space divided in millimeters: x (left–right), y (back–front), and z (top–bottom) coordinates. In a meta-analysis, the brain is divided up into a set of three-dimensional cubic volumes (called "voxels"; each is $2 \times 2 \times 2$ mm), and maps are constructed of the density of reported activation coordinates within a local volume (within 10 mm) around each voxel.

Previous meta-analyses used activation coordinates as the unit of analysis. For example, if 12 studies with one contrast map each reported 18 peak coordinates within 10 mm of a voxel in frontal cortex, the density for that voxel would be $18/(10 \text{ mm}^3)$. That value would be compared to the distribution of values expected by chance in order to assess significance. Rather than treating individual peaks as the unit of analysis, our meta-analyses treat a contrast as a random effect with activation coordinates nested within contrast.[4] Thus the density measure of interest is the number of *contrasts* (not the number of individual activation peaks) that produced activation near a voxel. In the example above, there were 12 contrasts that reported activations near the frontal voxel of interest, which amounts to 12 nominally independent pieces of information, and our density count is $12/(10 \text{ mm}^3)$. Studies might report multiple nearby peaks for the same contrast because of low spatial smoothness in the data, reporting conventions, low thresholds, or even voxel sizes used. Our method is insensitive to these types of variations across studies. As a result, a single study can no longer disproportionately contribute to the result by reporting many nearby peaks in an area.

For the present dataset, we included 437 contrasts, each associated with a set of reported coordinates. (Table 15.2 summarizes the contrasts we analyzed.) Each set of coordinates was transformed into a map of "active" voxels that were within 10 mm of a reported peak for that contrast. We then computed a summary density map of the proportion of contrasts activating near each voxel by taking a weighted average of contrast activation maps.

The weight for each study was the square root of the sample size, multiplied by an adjustment weight for type of the analysis used for population inference.[5] The values in this peak density map have a transparent interpretation: "Density" refers to the number of contrasts or statistical parametric maps with a nearby (within 10 mm) peak, weighted by the quality of information provided by the study.

Statistical Inference and Thresholding

The density map is then compared to Monte Carlo simulations to identify voxels with activations that exceed the frequency expected by chance (i.e., a uniform distribution of activation coordinates across the brain's gray matter). For the present dataset, using a Monte Carlo simulation in which the observed number of activation coordinates from the 437 activation maps were placed at random locations throughout the brain—and repeating this process 5,000 or more times—allowed us to determine which locations in the brain showed a greater-than-chance number of nearby activation coordinates, providing a stringent family-wise error rate correction for search across the locations within the brain. Our approach was first to locate regions that were consistently activated across a significant number of these studies (the "observed neural reference space"), and then to analyze the likelihood of activating a region in relation to different categories of emotional phenomena.

The maps in Plates 15.1, 15.2, and 15.3 (see color insert) and Figure 15.1 show voxels for which the density of reported peaks exceeded that expected by chance, corrected for search across the many voxels of the brain (i.e., family-wise error rate correction). The yellow color in the plates shows regions in which the peak density is high enough that the null-hypothesis chance of finding *a single significant voxel* anywhere in the gray matter of the brain is $p < .05$. The other colors use an "extent-based" threshold, in which the number of contiguous voxels above a primary threshold (e.g., $p < .001$) are counted and compared with the number of contiguous voxels expected by chance (Friston, Worsley, Frackowiak, Mazziotta, & Evans, 1994). Colored regions show areas in which a *cluster of voxels this large* is unlikely to occur by chance anywhere in the brain. We have used the Monte Carlo simulation to establish extent thresholds at $p <$

TABLE 15.2. Summary of Contrasts Analyzed

Experience versus perception

	Experience	Perception	Mixed
PET	109	28	11
fMRI	131	129	29

Affective/emotional valence

	Negative	Positive	Mixed/nonspecific
PET	94	30	24
fMRI	187	65	37

Specific emotion

	Happiness	Anger	Disgust	Fear	Sadness	Mixed/other
PET	17	10	4	11	23	9
fMRI	19	16	40	57	22	34

Correction for multiple comparisons

	Unknown	Corrected	Small-volume corrected	Uncorrected
PET	7	21	0	121
fMRI	8	73	28	186

Population inference

	No (infer *on* sample only)	Yes (infer *on* population)
PET	124	24
fMRI	74	215

Note. A summary of the 437 contrast maps from 163 studies used in the meta-analysis. Numbers reflect the number of contrasts in each category. "Population inference" refers to the number of contrasts that treated subject as a random effect, allowing valid population inference ("yes" in the table), as compared with contrasts that performed a "fixed-effects" analysis and whose results cannot be generalized beyond the sample studied. Lower weights were given to "fixed-effects" and smaller-sample studies in the meta-analysis.

.001 (orange in the plates) and $p < .005$ (pink in the plates). We report the significance of voxels at the highest primary threshold for which the significance criteria are met.

Visualization and Localization

The three-dimensional illustrations of brain slices presented in this chapter were reconstructed from a canonical MRI image (colin27.img, the single-subject template in SPM2; *www.fil.ion.ucl.ac.uk/spm/software/spm2*). This brain was coregistered with the international standard Montreal Neurologic Institute (MNI) brain template (avg152T1.img), which is itself based on the average of 152 brains registered roughly to landmarks from the atlas of Talairach and Tourneaux (1988). To localize highly replicable regions, we overlaid significant voxels on the MNI average template and determined their locations by using the atlases

of Duvernoy (Duvernoy, 1995; Duvernoy & Bourgouin, 1999), Martin (1996), Haines (2000), and Ongur, Ferry, and Price (2003); this method provided more accurate results than automated labeling systems. We use the single-subject brain only for visualization in our illustrations, because its anatomical detail makes brain landmarks more identifiable to readers. We do not report Brodmann's areas (BAs) because their boundaries cannot be identified with sufficient accuracy on this template brain (unless they are in regions shown in Ongur et al., 2003, who provide labels registered to the MNI brain). Although variation across labs and software packages in nominally similar warping to "Talairach space" produces inconsistencies among reported coordinates (Brett, Johnsrude, & Owen, 2002), the MNI template brain is the most popular template for electronic registration, so using it minimizes localization errors in the meta-analysis results.

THE OBSERVED
NEURAL REFERENCE SPACE FOR
EMOTION-RELATED PHENOMENA

Plate 15.1 summarizes the regions that were consistently activated in our database of neuro-imaging studies. (Stereotactic coordinates for the most consistent activation foci are listed in Appendix 15.2.) The right lateral surface of the brain (upper left panel), the left medial surface (upper right panel), the cerebellum (CB) (purple shading, lower left panel), and the brain-stem and prominent subcortical regions (lower right panel) are shown in three-dimensional rendering.

There was remarkable consistency between the hypothetical and observed neural reference spaces for emotion-related phenomena. As expected, we observed consistent activity in or closely associated with "limbic" areas. A striking feature of the map is the inclusion of diencephalic and brainstem regions that have been identified in animal models of affective behavior, but are infrequently discussed in human neuroimaging studies. In the brainstem, PAG and VTA were consistently activated, whereas lower brainstem centers in the pons and medulla were not consistently activated (though some pontine activations were consistent in other analyses presented below). Consistently activated diencephalic regions included the subthalamic nucleus (STN), Hy, and much of the dorsal thalamus, though the maximal consistency in the thalamus was in the central medial zone, around the "limbic" MD and centromedian (CM) nuclei. In the telencephalon, large significant regions of activation were observed in and around the amygdala extending into the BF, NAC, hippocampus, and vStr and vGP. In the paralimbic belt, consistent findings included vmPFC (10 m/r), multiple lateral OFC sites (42/12l and m; 13l), the aINS, and the medial and lateral anterior TC (pHCMP and temporal pole [TP]). Cingulate activations were largely limited to the rostral half of the ACC, corresponding to the so-called "affective" zone (Bush, Luu, & Posner, 2000). Strikingly, however, activations in the medial wall were clustered into at least three distinct groups, corresponding to pgACC, rACC, and sgACC.

The area of superior dmPFC above the cingulate sulcus (BA 9 extending back to BA 32) was consistently activated and distinct from ACC activation. The functional contributions of dmPFC have yet to be precisely deter-

mined, but recent research and theorizing suggest that these brain areas contribute jointly to making mental state attributions (for reviews, see Adolphs, 2001; Blakemore, Winston, & Frith, 2004; Lane & McRae, 2004)—such as when a person makes judgments about the psychological states of another person, or monitors, introspects, or makes inferences about his or her own moment-to-moment feelings (see also Mitchell, Banaji, & Macrae, 2005; Ochsner et al., 2004).

We also observed consistent activations in regions not traditionally considered part of the neural reference space for emotion, including those in the lateral frontal cortex, TC, occipital cortex (OCC), and cerebellum. These findings suggest that additional psychological processes involved in emotion-related phenomena may be overlooked in existing neuroscience models.

Although individual studies have reported lateral frontal activations in locations that span the expanse of cortex (see, e.g., Figure 15.1A), the only consistent activations across all studies lie in the bilateral IFG, extending from the pars opercularis (Broca's area, BA 44) through pars triangularis (BA 45) and pars orbitalis on the inferior frontal convexity (BA 47/lateral 12). The activated region also extended into the frontal operculum and was contiguous with activation in OFC and aINS. Neuroimaging studies of response inhibition, response selection, task switching, and working memory have commonly activated the area around BA 44–45 and the underlying operculum (Badre, Poldrack, Pare-Blagoev, Insler, & Wagner, 2005; Gabrieli, Poldrack, & Desmond, 1998; Martin & Chao, 2001; Poldrack et al., 1999; Wager, Jonides, Smith, & Nichols, 2005; Wagner, Maril, Bjork, & Schacter, 2001). Meta-analyses have suggested that the frontal operculo-insular border contiguous with the dorsal aINS, rather than the lateral surface, is the area most consistently activated across studies (Wager, Reading, et al., 2004; Wager & Smith, 2003). A general role for BA 44–45 and the operculum might be context-based selection among competing stimulus–response mappings or sets (Thompson-Schill et al., 1997). In emotion-related phenomena, this region may be important for the information selection processes critical for conceptual processing associated with meaning analysis (such as that associated with appraisal). In support of this notion, emotion- and pain-related activity in IFG and the operculum is modified by both manipulations of the meaning context in which affective stimuli are presented (Benedetti, Mayberg, Wager, Stohler, & Zubieta, 2005; Kong et al., 2006; Wager, Rilling, et al., 2004) and voluntary regulation of emotional responses (Ochsner, Bunge, Gross, & Gabrieli, 2002).

Activation of superior temporal sulcus/superior temporal gyrus (STS/STG) and inferior temporal and occipital "association" cortices could be related to enhanced sensory integration, but their precise role in affective processing is unclear. Although the function of the posterior cingulate cortex (PCC) remains unclear (Maddock, 1999), it may play a role in memory-guided representation of context important for conceptual processing in emotion (Maddock, 1999; Mantani, Okamoto, Shirao, Okada, & Yamawaki, 2005; Minoshima et al., 1997). Primary visual cortex (V1) also showed consistent activation, suggesting that early visual processing is enhanced when compared to neutral control conditions.

The consistent cerebellar activation we observed might be related to increased demands on motor planning during affective and emotional states, but there is accumulating evidence for a more direct cerebellar role in emotion-related phenomena. Electrical stimulation of deep cerebellar nuclei in humans, particularly the fastigial nucleus, has been shown to induce activity in mesolimbic affect-related areas (Heath, Dempesy, Fontana, & Myers, 1978), and in some cases it has elicited states of profound rage (Heath et al., 1974). Conversely, cerebellar damage often produces what might be considered a disorder of emotion regulation, characterized by fluctuations between flattened affect and inappropriate social behaviors (e.g., "trying to kiss the experimenter"; Schmahmann & Sherman, 1998) reminiscent of the social and emotional deficits with OFC damage. The cerebellum is connected with specific prefrontal regions in topographically mapped reciprocal circuits (Middleton & Strick, 1994, 2000) and with "limbic" regions, including the Hy (Haines & Dietrichs, 1984), OFC (BA 12), dmPFC (BA 9 and BA 32), portions of IFG (BA 46), and inferior frontal convexity (BA 46/12) (Middleton & Strick, 2001). Cerebellar efferents to these areas pass largely through DM in the thalamus, which we also find is consistently activated in human emotion. One hypothesis is that the cerebellum might contribute to the processing of situational context

(Schmahmann & Sherman, 1998) as part of a complex pattern recognition system (Albus, 1971).

COMPARING EXPERIENCE AND PERCEPTION

Studies of human affect and emotion (and their associated contrast maps) can be categorized as investigations of "experience" (involving the generation of feelings in response to pictures, sounds, memories, imagery, or other stimuli) or "perception" (involving observation and judgment about the normative content in a stimulus, such as whether a picture of facial behavior is classified as an "expression" that depicts "fear," "anger," or "disgust"). The critical conceptual difference separating experience from perception is whether a contrast (comparing activity in an experimental vs. a control condition) captures activity related to the generation of subjective feelings. Of course, this distinction is often a matter of degree, because the passive viewing of some stimuli that are used in perception-based studies (such as photos from the International Affective Picture System) will evoke an affective response regardless of whether participants are asked to report it, and stimuli used in experience-based studies (such as memories of social situations or sounds) require the perception of emotional content. To perform this analysis, however, we distinguished contrasts where affective experiences were being generated from those where changes in the perceiver's affect was unlikely.

Studies of *experience* in our sample (see Appendix 15.1) typically involved the recall of personal experiences, the viewing of strongly evocative visual or auditory stimuli, or exposure to pleasant or unpleasant tastes or odors. Studies of *perception* involved judgments about visual stimuli such as facial expressions that were unlikely to produce a strong change in experience (though such stimuli can serve as primes that may influence subsequent behavior). Papers with ambiguous status were excluded from this analysis.

Meta-analysis density maps showing significant differences between experience and perception are shown in Plates 15.2A and 15.2B. Some significant regions are shown on the same axial brain slices for direct comparison in Plate 15.2C, with experience versus perception in red and perception versus experience in blue. The density maps identified brain locations where there was a relative difference in peak activity between the experience and perception studies. Because the null hypothesis assumed that points from each condition were uniformly distributed throughout the brain, this analysis shows brain locations where differences in the *relative distribution* of peaks is large.[6]

The results show a striking dissociation. Contrasts for the *experience* of affect or emotion showed relatively greater activation for the medial subcortex (including Hy, VTA, PAG, dorsal pons, and surrounding reticular formation), the diencephalon (including the BF/extended amygdala, Hy, and thalamus), areas of paralimbic cortex (OFC, aINS, vmPFC, and TP), MTL, dmPFC, ventral IFG, and the deep regions of the CB surrounding the deep cerebellar nuclei. These findings are consistent with other work suggesting prominent roles for OFC (Kringelbach, 2005), aINS (Craig, Chen, Bandy, & Reiman, 2000), and dmPFC (Barrett et al., 2007) in the experience of affect and emotion. Moreover, they are consistent with stimulation studies in humans. Numerous case reports by Sem-Jacobsen (1968) and others show effects on experience of both positive and negative emotions with stimulation of the dorsal and orbital medial wall, and vivid emotional memories with anterior and medial temporal stimulation. Experience-related increases in subcortical and brainstem areas attest to the reliability of subcortical activation in neuroimaging studies, although they are less frequently discussed than cortical activations. Interestingly, rdACC did not differentiate between experience and perception; it was activated by both types of studies.

Perception-related contrasts more consistently activated amygdala, pHCMP, pgACC, dorsal IFG, inferior TC and OCC, and lateral cerebellum. These findings are consistent with the idea that amygdala activations in human neuroimaging studies are related to the salience or potential information value of visual stimuli (Liberzon et al., 2003), rather than playing some necessary role in emotional experience (Anderson & Phelps, 2002). Finding inferior temporal and occipital specialization for perception does not come as a surprise, given the strong relationship between these areas and visuospatial processing. Dorsal IFG and lateral cerebellum specialization for perception may relate to pattern recognition and conceptual processing that is necessary for normal emotion perception. These regions are connected in topographically mapped loops (Middleton & Strick, 2001), suggesting that they may be part of the same functional circuit. Of course, such conclusions about the precise function of these circuits are speculative, and they remain to be tested in focused individual studies. What is striking, however, is that different regions of the IFG seem to be differentially involved in experience and perception: the ventral and opercular parts for experience, and the more dorsal part for perception.

COMPARING PLEASANT AND UNPLEASANT EXPERIENCES

Using only the 240 contrasts (in 95 studies) involving experience, we next examined whether pleasant and unpleasant experiences were implemented in separable distributed systems. A previous meta-analysis tackled the positive–negative distinction (Wager et al., 2003), but did not separate experience from perception, as we do here.

Reported activation peaks for unpleasant (blue) and pleasant (yellow) contrasts are shown in Plates 15.3A and 15.3B, and meta-analysis density maps showing relative differences are shown in Plates 15.3C and 15.3D, with pleasant versus unpleasant in yellow and unpleasant versus pleasant in blue. Overall, the results suggest dissociations based on valence that are in general agreement with hypothesized specializations based on animal and lesion studies. Pleasant experiences were associated with relatively greater activation in medial dopamine-rich areas (VTA, NAC, and portions of vStr), as well as in Hy, vmPFC, and right OFC. Unpleasant experiences were associated with more consistent activation in amygdala, aINS, PAG, left OFC, and more posterior portions of vStr and vGP. The results provide a promising indication that different gross anatomical areas may be differentially sensitive to pleasant and unpleasant stimuli, although they do not imply that activation in any of these regions is uniquely associated with either category. In fact, chi-square tests revealed no region with greater absolute proportions of pleasant activations, primarily because unpleasant experiences elicit more robust responses that engage many parts of the brain. The relative specialization we report here is important, however, because studies of animal models have found that neurons and nuclear groups that are specialized according to valence are often contained within the same gross anatomical structure—for example, intermixed positive and negative expected-value neurons within the amygdala (Paton et al., 2006), or rostrocaudal negative–positive gradients within the NAC (Reynolds & Berridge, 2002). This raises the question of whether neuroimaging truly provides the resolution to separate representations of positive and negative affect. Our results are in line with the idea that different brain regions have different relative concentrations of specialized neurons, and that large-scale structure (aggregated across millions of neurons) in the affect system can be detected via neuroimaging.

An additional point worth noting is that while we did not compare left and right hemispheres using direct statistical contrasts, we did observe a pattern of lateralization in the OFC and basal forebrain (and a lack of lateralization in superior lateral cortex) that was different from that predicted by previous theories. Studies based on electroencephalography (EEG; for a review, see, e.g., Davidson, 2000), and lesion studies linking left-hemisphere damage to depression (Borod, 1992), suggest that the left lateral prefrontal cortex supports pleasant moods and reactions to pleasant stimuli, whereas the right lateral prefrontal cortex supports unpleasant moods processes. It is possible that lateralized EEG activity is predictive of mood or affective style, but the pattern of specific brain activation underlying those cortical potentials is more complex. Alternatively, arousal differences across studies might mask lateralized differences (Canli, Desmond, Zhao, Glover, & Gabrieli, 1998), or lateralization might be more closely related to approach–avoidance motivation than to affective valence per se, as suggested by our previous meta-analyses and recent work (Pizzagalli, Sherwood, Henriques, & Davidson, 2005; Wager et al., 2003). These caveats notwithstanding, the neuroimaging correlates of observed lateralization of affect in EEG studies remain to be elucidated.

THE SEARCH FOR SUBCORTICAL CIRCUITS: COMPARING PET AND fMRI STUDIES

Most emotion-related research on rats and primates pinpoints midbrain and brainstem areas as important for emotional behavior, and thus far our meta-analyses suggest that these areas are particularly active during the experience of affect and emotion. Compared to PET imaging, fMRI is less well suited to the study of the basal telencephalon and brainstem, due to magnetic susceptibility artifacts.[7] The hypothesis, then, is that fMRI studies of emotion-related phenomena may underestimate midbrain and brainstem contributions to affect and emotion. Alternatively, however, these issues may be counterbalanced by fMRI's greater spatiotemporal precision and potential to collect larger amounts of data.

Using chi-square analysis, we compared density maps for contrasts from PET and fMRI studies to determine whether one imaging method was more likely to activate particular brain regions in absolute rather than relative terms. The analysis tested the proportion of contrasts using each method that activated within 10 mm of each voxel, and thus controlled for overall differences in the frequency of use of PET and fMRI. The map of regions with significant chi-square statistics, shown in Figure 15.1, reveals no significant differences between PET and fMRI in the brainstem, BF, vStr, or OFC. Thus the benefits of fMRI in spatial resolution may compensate in part for increased artifacts, and thus fMRI can be a useful tool for examining the subcortex. Superior cortical regions, as well as amygdala and some other subcortical regions, appeared to be more consistent in fMRI studies (white in Figure 15.1)—though we suspect that effects in amygdala in particular may be related to the widespread use of a priori amygdala regions of interest, rather than to inherently more reliable activation.

GENERAL DISCUSSION

The meta-analyses reported in this chapter build on previously published metaanalyses of emotion (Murphy et al., 2003; Phan et al., 2002; Wager et al., 2003) in important ways. First, whereas those analyses combined perception and experience of emotion and affect, we explicitly compared the two types of studies and found that they were distinguished by their relative concentration of peak activations: brainstem, hypothalamic, and paralimbic selectivity for experience, and amygdalar complex and posterior cortex selectivity for perception.

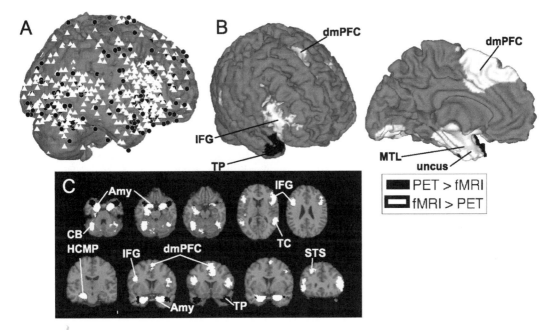

FIGURE 15.1. (A) Reported activation coordinates for contrasts using PET (black circles) and fMRI (white triangles) on the right lateral surface. (B) Meta-analysis results showing significant differences in absolute proportion of PET versus fMRI studies (black) and fMRI versus PET studies (white). The analysis used chi-square tests, controlling for the frequency of use of each method. (C) The comparisons in (C) shown on brain slices to reveal subcortical locations. Abbreviations are defined in the text and in Table 15.1.

Second, we compared studies of pleasant and unpleasant experiences; we found selectivity for pleasant experience in midline brainstem, hypothalamic, and ventromedial frontal regions, and selectivity for negative experience in distinct brainstem (PAG), insular, striatal, and orbital cortical regions. Third, we explicitly examined the suitability of fMRI as a method for investigating brainstem and basal telencephalon; we found that fMRI may be comparable to PET in its effectiveness as a tool for studying the brainstem and subcortex.

Of course, there is still much to be done. First, neuroimaging studies must continue to move away from referring to broad anatomical regions that in actuality perform different and often opposing functions. For example, the ACC encompasses about 15,000 $2 \times 2 \times 2$ voxels of brain tissue, but it is common for researchers to compare results from different studies at the gross structural level, trying to fit a single common interpretation to results that are in different areas with different anatomical projections and functional profiles. Using data across many studies to demarcate regions of

the brain precisely, as we have done here, is an essential step toward building a more systematic method. Once a set of regions is identified for study, it becomes possible to examine their dynamics (e.g., via connectivity analyses and structural models) in a much more meaningful way.

Second, in interpreting findings from our meta-analyses (or from any single neuroimaging study, for that matter), it is important to keep in mind that brain areas that span even a few millimeters are probably not consistently dedicated to any one process. Even individual neurons may participate in a number of functional circuits, and fMRI measures activity integrated over populations of neurons involved in different processes,[8] including different types of affect (Paton et al., 2006). The seminal work of Sem-Jacobsen (1968) in humans, and of Valenstein, Cox, and Kakolewski (1968) in rats, has shown strikingly that stimulation of brain sites very close together (no more than a few millimeters) can elicit vastly different emotional responses. In the words of Sem-Jacobsen (1976), "An electrode 0.5–1 cm from a positive point may give the opposite [emotional] response with about the same strength. There appears to be this dual arrangement in the ventromedial area of the frontal lobe, the central part of the temporal lobe, as well as other structures" (p. 516). In support of this notion, our summary of neuroimaging studies shows nearby regions with different functional specialization in the basal telencephalon, ventral basal ganglia, and inferior frontal cortex.

Furthermore, in early human electrical stimulation studies of emotion, although stimulation of the same site was often found to reproduce an emotional experience in the same session, elapsed time or variation of the behavioral contexts in which stimulation occurred markedly affected the emotional response. Documentation of this phenomenon in animals led Valenstein et al. (1970) to question the idea of fixed affective circuits. Thus, even with the relative precision of chronically implanted electrodes, the claim of Heraclitus that "you can never step into the same river twice" (Plato, 360 B.C.E.)may well apply to the emotional brain.

All these considerations lead us to believe that two kinds of paradigm shifts are essential for advancing the neuroimaging of emotion. One is that researchers need to move from studying brain areas in isolation to identifying interconnected, distributed circuits. Functional connectivity analysis may provide more precise information about brain processing related to various affective states and events, and confirm or constrain inferences about regional activations based on patterns of connectivity. In this respect, neuroimaging plays a unique and complementary role to lesion studies in animals, because neuroimaging alone allows the simultaneous measurement of the entire brain and dynamic patterns of functional connectivity across diverse systems. Another is that researchers should move beyond mapping brain responses to individual psychological phenomena to making inferences about psychological states based on brain activity. Neuroimaging provides unique and valuable information about the organization of the human brain; what is at stake here is the ability to learn about the organization of the mind from brain data. Making psychological inferences from brain activity is an extremely difficult task, and functional inferences in neuroimaging studies have often been made in an ad hoc fashion.

Valid psychological inference requires comparing activations across a number of psychological states; meta-analyses of the type we report here are one way to perform such comparisons. Formal inferences about psychological states from neuroimaging data can be made by using classifier systems, and this is a promising new direction.

Overall, the past 15 years have seen an explosion in the application of brain imaging methods to emotional phenomena. The emerging field of affective neuroscience has been engaged in a search for answers to two interdependent questions: the locations of brain regions that represent affective information, and the psychological distinctions that define the conditions for their activation. As information is accumulated, specific mappings can be made among studies of nondisabled humans, studies of humans with psychological and brain pathology, and animal models. Neuroimaging paves the way for synergy across these previously quite disparate fields by referring to the common "language" of the brain. When data are aggregated across neuroimaging studies, there is a remarkable and somewhat underappreciated consistency between animal and human stimulation work. As such data are accumulated, more elaborated and refined mappings between brain activity and affective processes will yield yet greater synergy across the neurosciences.

NOTES

1. In addition, there are certain methodological limitations to single neuroimaging studies that can be overcome with meta-analytic summaries. For example, current neuroimaging techniques are plagued by both low power and the presence of many false positives. Only 20% of the studies sampled corrected for multiple comparisons (i.e., tests of more than one brain region). Of these, many used inappropriate methods that did not provide adequate correction, yielding false-positive results.

2. Although emotions are the subset of affective responses that are elaborated with various sources of conceptual content (Barrett et al., 2007), we treated affect and emotion as separate categories in our analyses.

3. Effect size meta-analyses have been performed, but are problematic in general due to inconsistencies in data analysis across studies that can influence effect sizes. In addition, the peak density method avoids the need to estimate effect sizes in regions for which effects are not reported.

4. For simplicity, we assume that different contrasts reported by the same study are independent.

5. Larger studies have been weighted more heavily. The square root transformation provides a measure closer to effect size. Studies that used "random-effects" models appropriate for population inference were weighted 1.25 more heavily than those treating participants as a fixed effect. "Fixed-effects" models were commonly used in early neuroimaging studies, but are not appropriate for generalizing to a population. They generally produced much higher effect sizes (e.g., Z-scores) for the same data.

6. This analysis does not provide information about whether more studies of experience (or perception) activate an area in absolute terms. Information about the absolute frequencies of activation is provided by ^{2} (chi-square) analyses that test whether significantly more activation maps from experience studies versus perception studies activate an area. These analyses are available from Wager and Barrett, and were not included here because of space limitations; the results agree in large part with the areas shown here. Also, these maps do not provide direct inferences about the likelihood of experience (or perception), given activation in a particular area (Poldrack, 2006). Density-based maps of relative distributions are very useful, however, because they control for the overall frequency of activation across conditions, and therefore allow for more subtle differences to emerge. An example of this occurs in our analysis of pleasant versus unpleasant affective feelings.

7. Typical blood-oxygen-level-dependent (BOLD) fMRI measures functional activity by being sensitive to local field inhomogeneities (Ogawa et al., 1992). A difficulty is that transitions from air sinus space to tissue around the base of the brain create local field inhomogeneities, resulting in both signal loss and distortion, which limit both sensitivity and localization.

8. Counting neurons and synapses is difficult, but to provide a general idea of neural connectivity, some estimates are about 13.7×10^9 neocortical neurons (Braendgaard, Evans, Howard, & Gundersen, 1990) and 164×10^{12} synapses (Tang, Nyengaard, De Groot, & Gundersen, 2001), yielding an average of nearly 12,000 synapses per neuron. Many cortical areas have about 70,000–100,000 neurons per 1 mm^2 of tissue, an area substantially smaller than a voxel in human neuroimaging studies.

REFERENCES

Adolphs, R. (2001). The neurobiology of social cognition. *Current Opinion in Neurobiology, 11*(2), 231–239.

Albus, J. S. (1971). A theory of cerebellar function. *Mathematical Biosciences, 10*, 25–61.

Amaral, D. G. (2003). The amygdala, social behavior, and danger detection. *Annals of the New York Academy of Sciences, 1000*, 337–347.

Amaral, D. G., Price, J. L., Pitkanen, A., & Carmichael, S. T. (1992). Anatomical organization of the primate amygdaloid complex. In J. P. Aggleton (Ed.), *The amygdala: Neurobiological aspects of emotion, memory, and mental dysfunction* (pp. 1–66). New York: Wiley-Liss.

Anderson, A. K., & Phelps, E. A. (2002). Is the human amygdala critical for the subjective experience of emotion?: Evidence of intact dispositional affect in patients with amygdala lesions. *Journal of Cognitive Neuroscience, 14*(5), 709–720.

Anderson, S. W., Damasio, H., Tranel, D., & Damasio, A. R. (2000). Long-term sequelae of prefrontal cortex damage acquired in early childhood. *Developmental Neuropsychology, 18*(3), 281–296.

Anglada Figueroa, D., & Quirk, G. J. (2005). Lesions of the basal amygdala block expression of conditioned fear but not extinction. *Journal of Neuroscience, 25*(42), 9680–9685.

Angrilli, A., Palomba, D., Cantagallo, A., Maietti, A., & Stegagno, L. (1999). Emotional impairment after right orbitofrontal lesion in a patient without cognitive deficits. *NeuroReport, 10*(8), 1741–1746.

Badre, D., Poldrack, R. A., Pare-Blagoev, E. J., Insler, R. Z., & Wagner, A. D. (2005). Dissociable controlled retrievel and generalized selection mechanisms in ventrolateral prefrontal cortex. *Neuron, 47*, 907–918.

Bandler, R., & Shipley, M. T. (1994). Columnar organization in the midbrain periaqueductal gray: Modules for emotional expression? *Trends in Neurosciences, 17*(9), 379–389.

Barrett, L. F., Mesquita, B., Ochsner, K. N., & Gross, J. J. (2007). The experience of emotion. *Annual Review of Psychology, 58*, 7.1–7.31.

Baxter, M. G., & Murray, E. A. (2002). The amygdala and reward. *Nature Reviews Neuroscience, 3*(7), 563–573.

Bear, M. F., & Singer, W. (1986). Modulation of visual cortical plasticity by acetylcholine and noradrenaline. *Nature, 320*(6058), 172–176.

Beer, J. S., Heerey, E. A., Keltner, D., Scabini, D., & Knight, R. T. (2003). The regulatory function of self-conscious emotion: insights from patients with orbitofrontal damage. *Journal of Personality and Social Psychology, 85*(4), 594–604.

Benedetti, F., Mayberg, H. S., Wager, T. D., Stohler, C. S., & Zubieta, J. K. (2005). Neurobiological mechanisms of the placebo effect. *Journal of Neurosciences, 25*(45), 10390–10402.

Berlin, H. A., Rolls, E. T., & Kischka, U. (2004). Impulsivity, time perception, emotion and reinforcement sensitivity in patients with orbitofrontal cortex lesions. *Brain, 127*(Pt. 5), 1108–1126.

Berridge, K. C. (2004). Motivation concepts in behavioral neuroscience. *Physiology and Behavior, 81*(2), 179–209.

Berridge, K. C., & Robinson, T. E. (1998). What is the role of dopamine in reward: Hedonic impact, reward learning, or incentive salience? *Brain Research Reviews, 28*(3), 309–369.

Blakemore, S.-J., Winston, J., & Frith, U. (2004). Social cognitive neuroscience: Where are we heading? *Trends in Cognitive Sciences, 8,* 216–222.

Borod, J. C. (1992). Interhemispheric and intrahemispheric control of emotion: A focus on unilateral brain damage. *Journal of Consulting and Clinical Psychology, 60*(3), 339–348.

Braendgaard, H., Evans, S. M., Howard, C. V., & Gundersen, H. J. (1990). The total number of neurons in the human neocortex unbiasedly estimated using optical disectors. *Journal of Microscopy, 157*(Pt. 3), 285–304.

Braesicke, K., Parkinson, J. A., Reekie, Y., Man, M.-S., Hopewell, L., Pears, A., et al. (2005). Autonomic arousal in an appetitive context in primates: A behavioural and neural analysis. *European Journal of Neuroscience, 21*(6), 1733–1740.

Brett, M., Johnsrude, I. S., & Owen, A. M. (2002). The problem of functional localization in the human brain. *Nature Reviews Neuroscience, 3*(3), 243–249.

Bush, G., Luu, P., & Posner, M. I. (2000). Cognitive and emotional influences in anterior cingulate cortex. *Trends in Cognitive Sciences, 4*(6), 215–222.

Cador, M., Robbins, T. W., & Everitt, B. J. (1989). Involvement of the amygdala in stimulus–reward associations: Interaction with the ventral striatum. *Neuroscience, 30*(1), 77–86.

Canli, T., Desmond, J. E., Zhao, Z., Glover, G., & Gabrieli, J. D. (1998). Hemispheric asymmetry for emotional stimuli detected with fMRI. *NeuroReport, 9*(14), 3233–3239.

Craig, A. D. (2002). How do you feel? Interoception: The sense of the physiological condition of the body. *Nature Reviews Neuroscience, 3*(8), 655–666.

Craig, A. D., Chen, K., Bandy, D., & Reiman, E. M. (2000). Thermosensory activation of insular cortex. *Nature Neuroscience, 3,* 184–190.

Darwin, C. (1998). *The expression of the emotions in man and animals* (3rd ed.). New York: Oxford University Press. (Original work published 1872)

Davidson, R. J. (2000). Anterior electrophysiological asymmetries, emotion, and depression: Conceptual and methodological conundrums. *Psychophysiology, 35*(5), 607–614.

Davis, M. (1992). The role of the amygdala in fear and anxiety. *Annual Review of Neuroscience, 15*(1), 353–375.

Davis, M., & Lee, Y. L. (1998). Fear and anxiety: Possible roles of the amygdala and bed nucleus of the stria terminalis. *Cognition and Emotion, 12*(3), 277–305.

Davis, M., & Shi, C. (1999). The extended amygdala: Are the central nucleus of the amygdala and the bed nucleus of the stria terminalis differentially involved in fear versus anxiety? *Annals of the New York Academy of Sciences, 877,* 281–291.

Davis, M., & Whalen, P. J. (2001). The amygdala: Vigilance and emotion. *Molecular Psychiatry, 6*(1), 13–34.

Devinsky, O., Morrell, M. J., & Vogt, B. A. (1995). Contributions of anterior cingulate cortex to behaviour. *Brain, 118*(Pt. 1), 279–306.

Dewey, J. (1895). The theory of emotion: 2. The significance of emotions. *Psychological Review, 2,* 13–32.

Duvernoy, H. M. (1995). *The human brain stem and cerebellum: Surface, structure, vascularization, and three-dimensional sectional anatomy with MRI.* Vienna: Springer-Verlag.

Duvernoy, H. M., & Bourgouin, P. (1999). *The human brain: Surface, three-dimensional sectional anatomy with MRI, and blood supply.* Wien, Vienna: Springer-Verlag.

Edelman, G. M., & Tononi, G. (2001). *A universe of consciousness: How matter becomes imagination.* New York: Basic Books.

Everitt, B. J., Cador, M., & Robbins, T. W. (1989). Interactions between the amygdala and ventral striatum in stimulus–reward associations: studies using a second-order schedule of sexual reinforcement. *Neuroscience, 30*(1), 63–75.

Everitt, B. J., Parkinson, J. A., Olmstead, M. C., Arroyo, M., Robledo, P., & Robbins, T. W. (1999). Associative processes in addiction and reward. The role of amygdala–ventral striatal subsystems. *Annals of the New York Academy of Sciences, 877,* 412–438.

Feldman, S., Conforti, N., & Saphier, D. (1990). The preoptic area and bed nucleus of the stria terminalis are involved in the effects of the amygdala on adrenocortical secretion. *Neuroscience, 37*(3), 775–779.

Fox, P. T., Parsons, L. M., & Lancaster, J. L. (1998). Beyond the single study: function/location metanalysis in cognitive neuroimaging. *Current Opinion in Neurobiology, 8*(2), 178–187.

Friston, K. J., Worsley, K. J., Frackowiak, R. S. J., Mazziotta, J. C., & Evans, A. C. (1994). Assessing the significance of focal activations using their spatial extent. *Human Brain Mapping, 1,* 210–220.

Gabrieli, J. D., Poldrack, R. A., & Desmond, J. E. (1998). The role of left prefrontal cortex in language and memory. *Proceedings of the National Academy of Sciences of the USA, 95*(3), 906–913.

Goosens, K. A., & Maren, S. (2001). Contextual and auditory fear conditioning are mediated by the lateral, basal, and central amygdaloid nuclei in rats. *Learning and Memory, 8*(3), 148–155.

Gray, J. A. (1978). The neuropsychology of anxiety. *British Journal of Psychology, 69*(4), 417–434.

Gregg, T. R., & Siegel, A. (2001). Brain structures and neurotransmitters regulating aggression in cats: Implications for human aggression. *Progress in Neuropsychopharmacology and Biological Psychiatry, 25*(1), 91–140.

Haines, D. E. (2000). *Neuroanatomy: An atlas of structures, sections, and systems.* Philadelphia: Lippincott Williams & Wilkins.

Haines, D. E., & Dietrichs, E. (1984). An HRP study of hypothalamo-cerebellar and cerebellohypothalamic connections in squirrel monkey (*Saimiri sciureus*).

Journal of Comparative Neurology, 229(4), 559–575.

Heath, R. G. (1972). Pleasure and brain activity in man. Deep and surface electroencephalograms during orgasm. *Journal of Nervous and Mental Disease, 154*(1), 3–18.

Heath, R. G., Cox, A. W., & Lustick, L. S. (1974). Brain activity during emotional states. *American Journal of Psychiatry, 131*(8), 858–862.

Heath, R. G., Dempesy, C. W., Fontana, C. J., & Myers, W. A. (1978). Cerebellar stimulation: Effects on septal region, hippocampus, and amygdala of cats and rats. *Biological Psychiatry, 13*(5), 501–529.

Holstege, G., & Georgiadis, J. R. (2004). The emotional brain: Neural correlates of cat sexual behavior and human male ejaculation. *Progress in Brain Research, 143*, 39–45.

Hornak, J., Bramham, J., Rolls, E. T., Morris, R. G., O'Doherty, J., Bullock, P. R., et al. (2003). Changes in emotion after circumscribed surgical lesions of the orbitofrontal and cingulate cortices. *Brain, 126*(Pt. 7), 1691–1712.

Irons, D. (1897). The nature of emotion. *Philosophical Review, 6*(3), 242–256.

James, W. (1884). What is an emotion? *Mind, 9*(34), 188–205.

Kalin, N. H., Shelton, S. E., & Davidson, R. J. (2004). The role of the central nucleus of the amygdala in mediating fear and anxiety in the primate. *Journal of Neuroscience, 24*(24), 5506–5515.

Kim, H., Somerville, L. H., Johnstone, T., Alexander, A. L., & Whalen, P. J. (2003). Inverse amygdala and medial prefrontal cortex responses to surprised faces. *NeuroReport, 14*(18), 2317–2322.

Kong, J., Gollub, R. L., Rosman, I. S., Webb, J. M., Vangel, M. G., Kirsch, I., et al. (2006). Brain activity associated with expectancy-enhanced placebo analgesia as measured by functional magnetic resonance imaging. *Journal of Neuroscience, 26*(2), 381–388.

Kringelbach, M. L. (2005). The human orbitofrontal cortex: Linking reward to hedonic experience. *Nature Reviews Neuroscience, 6*(9), 691–702.

Laird, A. R., Fox, P. M., Price, C. J., Glahn, D. C., Uecker, A. M., Lancaster, J. L., et al. (2005). ALE meta-analysis: Controlling the false discovery rate and performing statistical contrasts. *Human Brain Mapping, 25*(1), 155–164.

Lane, R. D., & McRae, K. (2004). Neural substrates of conscious emotional experience: A cognitive-neuroscientific perspective. In M. Beauregard (Ed.), *Consciousness, emotional self-regulation and the brain* (pp. 87–122). Amsterdam: Benjamins.

LeDoux, J. E. (2000). Emotion circuits in the brain. *Annual Review of Neuroscience, 23*(1), 155–184.

Liberzon, I., Phan, K. L., Decker, L. R., & Taylor, S. F. (2003). Extended amygdala and emotional salience: A PET activation study of positive and negative affect. *Neuropsychopharmacology, 28*(4), 726–733.

Lovick, T. A. (1992). Inhibitory modulation of the cardiovascular defence response by the ventrolateral periaqueductal grey matter in rats. *Experimental Brain Research, 89*(1), 133–139.

Maddock, R. J. (1999). The retrosplenial cortex and emotion: New insights from functional neuroimaging of the human brain. *Trends in Neurosciences, 22*(7), 310–316.

Mantani, T., Okamoto, Y., Shirao, N., Okada, G., & Yamawaki, S. (2005). Reduced activation of posterior cingulate cortex during imagery in subjects with high degrees of alexithymia: A functional magnetic resonance imaging study. *Biological Psychiatry, 57*, 982–990.

Maren, S., Aharonov, G., & Fanselow, M. S. (1997). Neurotoxic lesions of the dorsal hippocampus and Pavlovian fear conditioning in rats. *Behavioral Brain Research, 88*(2), 261–274.

Martin, A., & Chao, L. L. (2001). Semantic memory and the brain: Structure and processes. *Current Opinion in Neurobiology, 11*, 194–201.

Martin, J. H. (1996). *Neuroanatomy: Text and atlas* (2nd ed.). Stamford, CT: Appleton & Lange.

McDonald, A. J. (1998). Cortical pathways to the mammalian amygdala. *Progress in Neurobiology, 55*(3), 257–332.

Mesulam, M. M., & Mufson, E. J. (1982). Insula of the Old World monkey: I. Architectonics in the insulo-orbito-temporal component of the paralimbic brain. *Jounral of Comparative Neurology, 212*(1), 1–22.

Middleton, F. A., & Strick, P. L. (1994). Anatomical evidence for cerebellar and basal ganglia involvement in higher cognitive function. *Science, 266*(5184), 458.

Middleton, F. A., & Strick, P. L. (2000). Basal ganglia and cerebellar loops: Motor and cognitive circuits. *Brain Research: Brain Research Reviews, 31*(2–3), 236–250.

Middleton, F. A., & Strick, P. L. (2001). Cerebellar projections to the prefrontal cortex of the primate. *Journal of Neuroscience, 21*(2), 700.

Milad, M. R., & Quirk, G. J. (2002). Neurons in medial prefrontal cortex signal memory for fear extinction. *Nature, 420*(6911), 70–74.

Minoshima, S., Giordani, B., Berent, S., Frey, K. A., Foster, N. L., & Kuhl, D. E. (1997). Metabolic reduction in the posterior cingulate cortex in very early Alzheimer's disease. *Annals of Neurology, 42*(1), 85–94.

Mitchell, J. P., Banaji, M. R., & Macrae, C. N. (2005). General and specific contributions of the medial prefrontal cortex to knowledge about mental states. *NeuroImage, 28*, 757–762.

Murphy, F. C., Nimmo-Smith, I., & Lawrence, A. D. (2003). Functional neuroanatomy of emotions: A meta-analysis. *Cognitive, Affective, and Behavioral Neuroscience, 3*(3), 207–233.

Nader, K., Majidishad, P., Amorapanth, P., & LeDoux, J. E. (2001). Damage to the lateral and central, but not other, amygdaloid nuclei prevents the acquisition of auditory fear conditioning. *Learning and Memory, 8*(3), 156–163.

Ochsner, K. N., Bunge, S. A., Gross, J. J., & Gabrieli, J. D. (2002). Rethinking feelings: An FMRI study of the cognitive regulation of emotion. *Journal of Cognitive Neuroscience, 14*(8), 1215–1229.

Ochsner, K. N., Knierim, K., Ludlow, D. H., Hanelin, J., Ramachandran, T., Glover, G., et al. (2004). Reflecting upon feelings: An fMRI study of neural systems supporting the attribution of emotion to self and other. *Journal of Cognitive Neuroscience, 16*(10), 1746–1772.

Ogawa, S., Tank, D. W., Menon, R., Ellermann, J. M., Kim, S., Merkle, H., et al. (1992). Intrinsic signal changes accompanying sensory stimulation: Functional brain mapping with magnetic resonance imaging. *Proceedings of the National Academy of Sciences of the USA, 89*(13), 5951–5955.

Ongur, D., An, X., & Price, J. L. (1998). Prefrontal cortical projections to the hypothalamus in macaque monkeys. *Jounrla of Comparative Neurology, 401*(4), 480–505.

Ongur, D., Ferry, A. T., & Price, J. L. (2003). Architectonic subdivision of the human orbital and medial prefrontal cortex. *Journal of Comparative Neurology, 460*(3), 425–449.

Ongur, D., & Price, J. L. (2000). The organization of networks within the orbital and medial prefrontal cortex of rats, monkeys and humans. *Cerebral Cortex, 10*(3), 206–219.

Panksepp, J. (1998). *Affective neuroscience: The foundations of human and animal emotions.* New York: Oxford University Press.

Paton, J. J., Belova, M. A., Morrison, S. E., & Salzman, C. D. (2006). The primate amygdala represents the positive and negative value of visual stimuli during learning. *Nature, 439*(7078), 865–870.

Phan, K. L., Wager, T., Taylor, S. F., & Liberzon, I. (2002). Functional neuroanatomy of emotion: A meta-analysis of emotion activation studies in PET and fMRI. *NeuroImage, 16*(2), 331–348.

Pizzagalli, D. A., Sherwood, R. J., Henriques, J. B., & Davidson, R. J. (2005). Frontal brain asymmetry and reward responsiveness: A source-localization study. *Psychological Science, 16*(10), 805–813.

Poldrack, R. A. (2006). Can cognitive processes be inferred from neuroimaging data? *Trends in Cognitive Sciences, 10*(2), 59–63.

Poldrack, R. A., Wagner, A. D., Prull, M. W., Desmond, J. E., Glover, G. H., & Gabrieli, J. D. (1999). Functional specialization for semantic and phonological processing in the left inferior prefrontal cortex. *NeuroImage, 10*(1), 15–35.

Reynolds, S. M., & Berridge, K. C. (2002). Positive and negative motivation in nucleus accumbens shell: Bivalent rostrocaudal gradients for GABA-elicited eating, taste "liking"/"disliking" reactions, place preference/avoidance, and fear. *Journal of Neuroscience, 22*(16), 7308–7320.

Roberts, N. A., Beer, J. S., Werner, K. H., Scabini, D., Levens, S. M., Knight, R. T., et al. (2004). The impact of orbital prefrontal cortex damage on emotional activation to unanticipated and anticipated acoustic startle stimuli. *Cognitive, Affective, and Behavioral Neuroscience, 4*(3), 307–316.

Salamone, J. D., Cousins, M. S., & Snyder, B. J. (1997). Behavioral functions of nucleus accumbens dopamine: Empirical and conceptual problems with the anhedonia hypothesis. *Neuroscience and Biobehavioral Reviews, 21*(3), 341–359.

Saper, C. B. (1995). Central autonomic system. In G. Paxinos (Ed.), *The rat nervous system* (2nd ed., pp. 107–135). San Diego: Academic Press.

Saper, C. B., Loewy, A. D., Swanson, L. W., & Cowan, W. M. (1976). Direct hypothalamoautonomic connections. *Brain Research, 117*(2), 305–312.

Sarter, M., Hasselmo, M. E., Bruno, J. P., & Givens, B. (2005). Unraveling the attentional functions of cortical cholinergic inputs: Interactions between signal-driven and cognitive modulation of signal detection. *Brain Research: Brain Research Reviews, 48*(1), 98–111.

Schmahmann, J. D., & Sherman, J. C. (1998). The cerebellar cognitive affective syndrome. *Brain, 121*(4), 561–579.

Schoenbaum, G., Chiba, A. A., & Gallagher, M. (1998). Orbitofrontal cortex and basolateral amygdala encode expected outcomes during learning. *Nature Neuroscience, 1*(2), 155–159.

Schoenbaum, G., Setlow, B., Saddoris, M. P., & Gallagher, M. (2003). Encoding predicted outcome and acquired value in orbitofrontal cortex during cue sampling depends upon input from basolateral amygdala. *Neuron, 39*(5), 855–867.

Sem-Jacobsen, C. W. (1968). *Depth-electrographic stimulation of the human brain and behavior: From fourteen years of studies and treatment of Parkinson's disease and mental disorders with implanted electrodes.* Springfield, IL: Thomas.

Sem-Jacobsen, C. W. (1976). Electrical stimulation and self-stimulation in man with chronic implanted electrodes. Interpretation and pitfalls of results. In A. Wauquier & E. T. Rolls (Eds.), *Brain-stimulation reward* (pp. 505–520). New York: Elsevier.

Sewards, T. V., & Sewards, M. A. (2003). Representations of motivational drives in mesial cortex, medial thalamus, hypothalamus and midbrain. *Brain Research Bulletin, 61*(1), 25–49.

Shipley, M. T., Ennis, M., Rizvi, T. A., & Behbehani, M. M. (1991). Topographical specificity of forebrain inputs to the midbrain periaqueductal gray: Evidence for discrete longitudinally organized input columns. In A. Depaulis & R. Bandler (Eds.), *The midbrain periaqueductal gray matter: Functional, anatomical, and neurochemical organization* (pp. 417–448). New York: Plenum Press.

Squire, L. R., & Zola-Morgan, S. (1991). The medial temporal lobe memory system. *Science, 253*(5026), 1380.

Sullivan, R. M., & Gratton, A. (2002). Prefrontal cortical regulation of hypothalamic–pituitary–adrenal function in the rat and implications for psychopathology: Side matters. *Psychoneuroendocrinology*, 27(1–2), 99–114.

Talairach, J., & Tournoux, P. (1988). *Co-planar stereotaxic atlas of the human brain: 3Dimensional proportional system. An approach to cerebral imaging*. Stuttgart: Thieme.

Tang, Y., Nyengaard, J. R., De Groot, D. M. G., & Gundersen, H. J. G. (2001). Total regional and global number of synapses in the human brain neocortex. *Synapse*, 41(3), 258–273.

Thompson-Schill, S. L., D'Esposito, M., Aguirre, G. K., & Farah, M. J. (1997). Role of left inferior prefrontal cortex in retrieval of semantic knowledge: A reevaluation. *Proceedings of the National Academy of Sciences of the USA*, 94(26), 14792–14797.

Valenstein, E. S., Cox, V. C., & Kakolewski, J. W. (1968). Modification of motivated behavior elicited by electrical stimulation of the hypothalamus. *Science*, 159(3819), 1119.

Valenstein, E. S., Cox, V. C., & Kakolewski, J. W. (1970). Reexamination of the role of the hypothalamus in motivation. *Psychological Review*, 77(1), 16–31.

Van der Horst, V. G., & Holstege, G. (1998). Sensory and motor components of reproductive behavior: Pathways and plasticity. *Behavioural Brain Research*, 92(2), 157–167.

Vogt, B. A., Finch, D. M., & Olson, C. R. (1992). Functional heterogeneity in cingulate cortex: The anterior executive and posterior evaluative regions. *Cerebral Cortex*, 2(6), 435.

Vogt, B. A., Nimchinsky, E. A., Vogt, L. J., & Hof, P. R. (1995). Human cingulate cortex: Surface features, flat maps, and cytoarchitecture. *Journal of Comparative Neurology*, 359(3), 490–506.

Wager, T. D., & Barrett, L. F. (2004). *From affect to control: Functional specialization of the insula in motivation and regulation*. Available online at *www.columbia.edu/cu/psychology.tor/*

Wager, T. D., Jonides, J., Smith, E. E., & Nichols, T. E. (2005). Towards a taxonomy of attention-shifting: Individual differences in fMRI during multiple shift types. *Cognitive, Affective, and Behavioral Neuroscience*, 5(2), 127–143.

Wager, T. D., Phan, K. L., Liberzon, I., & Taylor, S. F. (2003). Valence, gender, and lateralization of functional brain anatomy in emotion: A meta-analysis of findings from neuroimaging. *NeuroImage*, 19(3), 513–531.

Wager, T. D., Reading, S., & Jonides, J. (2004). Neuroimaging studies of shifting attention: A meta-analysis. *NeuroImage*, 22(4), 1679–1693.

Wager, T. D., Rilling, J. K., Smith, E. E., Sokolik, A., Casey, K. L., Davidson, R. J., et al. (2004). Placebo-induced changes in FMRI in the anticipation and experience of pain. *Science*, 303(5661), 1162–1167.

Wager, T. D., & Smith, E. E. (2003). Neuroimaging studies of working memory: A metaanalysis. *Cognitive, Affective, and Behavioral Neuroscience*, 3(4), 255–274.

Wagner, A. D., Maril, A., Bjork, R. A., & Schacter, D. L. (2001). prefrontal contributions to executive control: fMRI evidence for functional distinctions within lateral Prefrontal cortex. *NeuroImage*, 14(6), 1337–1347.

Walker, D. L., & Davis, M. (1997). Double dissociation between the involvement of the bed nucleus of the stria terminalis and the central nucleus of the amygdala in startle increases produced by conditioned versus unconditioned fear. *Journal of Neuroscience*, 17(23), 9375–9383.

Wallace, K. J., & Rosen, J. B. (2001). Neurotoxic lesions of the lateral nucleus of the amygdala decrease conditioned fear but not unconditioned fear of a predator odor: comparison with electrolytic lesions. *Journal of Neuroscience*, 21(10), 3619–3627.

Waraczynski, M. A. (2006). The central extended amygdala network as a proposed circuit underlying reward valuation. *Neuroscience and Biobehavioral Reviews*, 30, 472–496.

Weinberger, N. M. (1995). Dynamic regulation of receptive fields and maps in the adult sensory cortex. *Annual Review of Neuroscience*, 18(1), 129–158.

Whalen, P. J. (1998). Fear, vigilance, and ambiguity: Initial neuroimaging studies of the human amygdala. *Current Directions in Psychological Science*, 7(6), 177–188.

Whalen, P. J., Kagan, J., Cook, R. G., Davis, F. C., Kim, H., Polis, S., et al. (2004). Human amygdala responsivity to masked fearful eye whites. *Science*, 306(5704), 2061.

Yasui, Y., Breder, C. D., Saper, C. B., & Cechetto, D. F. (1991). Autonomic responses and efferent pathways from the insular cortex in the rat. *Journal of Comparative Neurology*, 303(3), 355–374.

APPENDIX 15.1. Studies Included in the Meta-Analysis

First author	Year	Imaging	Sex	N	Valence	Emotion						Induction method				
						Aff	Ang	Disg	Fear	Hap	Sad	Vis	Aud	T/Olf	Rec	Img
Studies of emotional experience																
Schafer	2005	fMRI	X	40	Neg			°	°			°				
Grimm	2005	fMRI	X	29	Neg	°						°				
Hutcherson	2005	fMRI	F	28	Neg	°						°				
Cato	2004	fMRI	X	26	Neg	°									°	
Eugene	2003	fMRI	F	20	Neg						°	°				
Lang	1998	fMRI	X	20	Neg				°			°				
Levesque	2003	fMRI	F	20	Neg	°						°				
Stark	2003	fMRI	X	19	Neg			°	°			°				
Aron	2005	fMRI	X	17	Pos	°										°
Simpson	2000	fMRI	X	17	Neg	°						°				
Anderson	2003	fMRI	X	16	Neg	°								°		
Dolcos	2004	fMRI	F	16	Neg	°						°				
Gottfried	2002	fMRI	X	15	Pos	°								°		
Stark	2005	fMRI	X	15	Neg	°						°				
Canli	1998	fMRI	F	14	Pos	°						°				
Goel	2001	fMRI	X	14	Pos	°							°			
Fulbright	1998	fMRI	X	13	Neg	°								°		
Goldin	2005	fMRI	F	13	Pos	°					°	°				
Heinzel	2005	fMRI	X	13	X	°						°				
Markowitch	2003	fMRI	X	13	Pos						°				°	
Moll	2005	fMRI	X	13	Neg			°	°							°
Northoff	2004	fMRI	X	13	X	°						°				
Shirao	2005	fMRI	F	13	Neg	°									°	
Elliott	2000	fMRI	X	12	Pos	°						°			°	
Fitzgerald	2004	fMRI	X	12	Neg			°							°	
Maratos	2001	fMRI	X	12	Pos				°	°		°				
Schienle	2006	fMRI	F	12	Neg			°	°			°				
Schienle	2002	fMRI	F	12	Neg			°				°				
DeAraujo	2003	fMRI	X	11	Pos	°								°		
Hariri	2003	fMRI	X	11	Neg							°				
Beauregard	2001	fMRI	M	10	Pos	°						°				
Canli	2000	fMRI	F	10	Neg	°						°				
Klein	2003	fMRI	F	10	Neg	°						°				
Lee	2004	fMRI	X	10	Pos						°	°				
Maddock	1997	fMRI	X	10	Neg	°							°			
Ruby	2004	fMRI	M	10	X		°								°	
Wrase	2003	fMRI	F	10	Neg			°	°			°				
Yamasaki	2002	fMRI	X	10	Neg	°						°				
Kringelbach	2003	fMRI	M	9	Pos	°								°		
O'Doherty (b)	2001	fMRI	X	9	Neg					°	°					
Small	2003	fMRI	X	9	Neg				°				°			
Whalen	1998	fMRI	M	8	Neg		°		°			°				
Wright	2004	fMRI	X	8	Neg							°				
Beauregard	1998	fMRI	X	7	Neg						°	°				
Moll	2002	fMRI	X	7	Neg			°				°				
O'Doherty (a)	2001	fMRI	?	7	Neg	°									°	
Phana	2004	fMRI	X	7	Neg			°	°			°				
Bystritsky	2001	fMRI	X	6	Neg				°						°	
Herpetz	2001	fMRI	F	6	Neg	°					°	°				
Nitschke	2004	fMRI	F	6	Pos	°	°					°				
Teasdale	1999	fMRI	X	6	Pos							°				
Francis	1999	fMRI	?	4	Pos	°								°		
Lorberbaum	1999	fMRI	F	4	Neg				°				°			
Damasio	2000	PET	X	25[a]	Pos		°		°	°	°				°	
George	1994	PET	X	21	Neg						°	°				
Kimbrell	1999	PET	X	16	Neg	°									°	
Paradiso	2003	PET	X	17	Neg	°		°		°		°				
Pietrini	2000	PET	X	15	Neg				°	°						°

(continued)

APPENDIX 15.1. *(continued)*

First author	Year	Imaging	Sex	N	Valence	Aff	Ang	Disg	Fear	Hap	Sad	Vis	Aud	T/Olf	Rec	Img
						| Emotion					|	| Induction method				|
Taylor	2000	PET	X	14	Neg	°						°				
Lane (a)	1997	PET	F	12	Pos	°						°				
Lane	1998	PET	F	12	X	°						°			°	
Partiot	1995	PET	°	12	Neg				°							°
Reiman	1997	PET	F	12	X				°			°			°	
Zaid	1997	PET	F	12	Neg	°							°			
Aalto	2002	PET	F	11	Neg					°	°	°				
Aalto	2005	Pet	F	11	Neg	°						°				
Gemar	1996	PET	M	11	Neg						°				°	
George	1995	PET	F	11	Neg						°				°	
Lane (c)	1997	PET	F	11	Pos	°						°			°	
Baker	1997	PET	M	10	Pos					°	°		°			
Beauregard	1997	PET	M	10	X	°						°				
Blood	2001	PET	X	10	Pos	°							°			
Blood	1999	PET	X	10	Pos	°							°			
Dolan	2000	PET	M	10	X	°						°				
George	1996	PET	M	10	Pos					°	°				°	
Lane (b)	1997	PET	M	10	X			°		°	°	°				
Liberzon	2000	PET	F	10	Neg	°						°				
Liberzon	2000	PET	F	10	Neg	°						°				
Liberzon	2003	PET	X	10	Neg				°			°				
Taylor	2003	PET	X	10	Neg	°						°				
Redoute	2000	PET	M	9	Pos	°						°				
Zald	1998	PET	F	9	Pos	°									°	
Doughtery	1999	PET	M	8	Neg		°									°
Liotti	2000	PET	F	8	Neg	°									°	
Mayberg	1999	PET	F	8	Neg										°	
Ottowitz	2004	PET	F	8	Neg						°					°
Paradiso	1997	PET	X	8	Pos	°						°				
Rauch	1999	PET	M	8	Pos	°									°	
Shin	2000	PET	M	8	Neg				°						°	
Taylor	1998	PET	F	8	Neg	°						°				
Kosslyn	1996	PET	M	7	Neg	°						°				
Pardo	1993	PET	X	7	Neg						°				°	
Fischer	1996	PET	X	6	Neg	°									°	
Isenberg	1999	PET	X	6	Neg		°	°	°	°		°				
Lane	1999	PET	M	6	X	°						°				

Studies of mixed or ambiguous perception/experience

First author	Year	Imaging	Sex	N	Valence	Aff	Ang	Disg	Fear	Hap	Sad	Vis	Aud	T/Olf	Rec	Img
Habel	2005	fMRI	M	26	Pos					°		°				
Kuchinke	2005	fMRI	X	20	Pos	°						°				
Crosson	1999	fMRI	X	17	X	°							°			
Wicker	2003	fMRI	M	14	Neg							°		°		
Hariri	2002	fMRI	X	12	Neg	°						°				
Zatorre	2000	fMRI	X	12	X								°			
Rolls	2003	fMRI	X	11	Neg	°							°			
Buchanan	2000	fMRI	M	10	X	°		°	°					°		
Tabert	2001	fMRI	F	9	Neg	°						°				
Paradiso	1999	PET	X	17	Pos							°		°		
Royet	2000	PET	M	12	X								°	°		
Royet	2001	PET	M	12	X	°								°		
Zatorre	2000	PET	X	12	X									°		
Frey	2000	PET	F	11	Neg	°							°			

Studies of emotional perception

First author	Year	Imaging	Sex	N	Valence	Aff	Ang	Disg	Fear	Hap	Sad	Vis	Aud	T/Olf	Rec	Img
Das	2005	fMRI	X	28	Neg			°				°				
Tessitore	2005	fMRI	X	27	X			°				°				

(continued)

269

First author	Year	Imaging	Sex	N	Valence	Emotion						Induction method				
						Aff	Ang	Disg	Fear	Hap	Sad	Vis	Aud	T/Olf	Rec	Img
Liddell	2005	fMRI	X	25	Neg				o		o	o				
Fischer	2004	fMRI	X	24	Neg		o					o				
Williams, L.	2004	fMRI	X	22	Neg				o			o				
Kesler-West	2001	fMRI	X	21	Neg					o	o	o				
Pessoa	2002	fMRI	X	21	Neg	o						o	o			
Fitzgerald	2005	fMRI	X	20	Pos		o	o	o	o	o	o				
Grobras	2005	fMRI	X	20	Neg		o					o				
Schroeder	2004	fMRI	X	20	Neg							o				
Hariri	2000	fMRI	X	16	X		o		o			o				
Somerville	2004	fMRI	X	16	Pos		o	o	o			o				
Fecteau	2005	fMRI	X	15	X								o			
Grandjean	2005	fMRI	X	15	Neg		o						o			
Reinders	2005	fMRI	X	15	Neg	o						o				
Gur	2002	fMRI	X	14	X			o	o	o		o				
Shin	2005	fMRI	M	13	Neg	o						o				
Williams, L.	2005	fMRI	X	13	Neg		o	o	o			o				
Williams, M.	2005	fMRI	X	13	X	o						o				
Dolan	2001	fMRI	X	12	Neg				o			o	o			
Iidaka	2001	fMRI	X	12	Neg							o				
Killgore	2004	fMRI	F	12	X		o			o		o				
Strange	2000	fMRI	X	12	Neg	o						o				
Vuilleumier	2001	fMRI	X	12	Neg						o	o				
Wang	2005	fMRI	X	12	Neg			o				o				
Adams	2003	fMRI	X	11	Neg							o				
Williams, L.	2001	fMRI	M	11	Neg				o			o				
Breiter	1996	fMRI	M	10	Pos				o	o		o				
Gorno-Tempini	2001	fMRI	X	10	Pos			o		o		o				
Hare	2005	fMRI	X	10	Pos									o		
Mccullough	2005	fMRI	X	10	X	o						o				
Sato	2004	fMRI	X	10	Neg			o	o			o				
Wildgruber	2005	fMRI	X	10	X								o			
Critchley	2000	fMRI	X	9	X							o				
Lange	2003	fMRI	?	9	Neg	o						o				
Nomura	2004	fMRI	X	9	Neg	o						o				
Dolan	1996	fMRI	M	8	Pos					o		o				
Narumoto	2000	fMRI	X	8	X	o						o				
Phillips	2004	fMRI	M	8	Neg			o	o			o				
Phillips (b)	1998	fMRI	X	8	Pos		o					o				
Whalen	2001	fMRI	X	8	Neg	o		o				o				
Phillips	1997	fMRI	X	7	Neg			o	o			o				
Phillips (a)	1998	fMRI	M	6	Neg				o			o	o			
Sprengelmeyer	1998	fMRI	X	6	Neg			o	o			o				
Blair	1999	PET	M	13	Neg		o				o	o				
George	1996	PET	X	13	X								o			
Kilts	2003	PET	X	13	Pos		o		o			o				
George	1993	PET	F	9	X							o				
Pourtois	2005	PET	M	8	Neg	o						o				
Sergent	1994	PET	M	8	X	o						o				
Nakamura	1999	PET	M	7	X	o						o				
Imaizumi	1997	PET	M	6	X	o							o			
Morris	1999	PET	M	6	X	o							o			
Morris	1996	PET	X	5	Pos	o			o	o		o				
Morris	1998	PET	X	5	X	o			o			o				
Totals		77	17	20	37	23	26	112	19	15	17	9				

Note. Emotions: Aff, affect (see text); Ang, anger; Disg, disgust; Fear, fear; Hap, happiness; Sad, sadness. Induction methods: Vis, visual; Aud, auditory; T/Olf, tactile/olfactory; Rec, recall; Img, mental imaging. X in Sex and Valence columns refers to "mixed" sex or valence.

[a]Damasio (2000) had differing numbers of subjects for each emotion, ranging from 16 for the lowest and 25 for the highest.

APPENDIX 15.2. Stereotactic Coordinates for Activation Foci

Name	Lat	X	Y	Z	Vol	%Act	Thr
Brainstem							
dPAG/SC	—	2	–30	–6	24	6	P
Diencephalon							
STN	R	12	–18	–6	280	14	P
Thal (DM, CM)	—	0	–16	4	1376	14	P
STN	R	16	–8	0	768	15	E
Hy	R	8	–10	–12	864	13	E
Hy	L	–10	0	–14	512	13	E
Subcortical telencephalon							
Amy/BF	R	20	–4	–20	5744	25	P
Amy/BF	L	–20	–6	–18	6800	30	P
HCMP/vGP	R	22	–12	–12	1944	21	P
vStr/BF	L	–30	2	–12	1832	26	P
vStr/vGP	R	26	0	–10	1704	24	P
vGP/vIns	L	–30	–8	–10	1984	24	P
vGP/Hy/STN	L	–10	–6	–6	1104	19	P
Amy (BL)	R	30	–2	–28	576	15	E
HCMP	L	–18	–14	–24	584	15	E
HCMP	L	–30	–12	–24	408	12	E
vStr/HCMP	R	32	–10	–8	624	14	E
vGP	R	14	6	–8	1208	17	E
vGP	L	–22	8	–12	432	13	E
Put	R	26	2	0	1936	15	E
Put	L	–28	0	0	1008	14	E
Para-HCMP	L	–28	–24	–18	200	5	E

Name	Lat	X	Y	Z	Vol	%Act	Thr
Paralimbic							
aIns	R	42	24	–8	1712	18	P
aIns	R	44	16	–2	2032	17	P
aIns/frOP	L	–40	24	–6	4248	25	P
vaIns (ag), TP	L	–28	6	–22	2344	25	P
mid-Ins	R	40	6	0	48	7	P
OFC (47/12m, 12l)	L	–28	34	–18	8	4	P
pgACC	—	2	40	2	168	8	P
dACC	—	0	24	32	64	8	P
rdACC	—	–4	34	8	8	4	P
TP (lat.)	R	50	8	–26	176	6	P
TP (med.)	R	38	12	–24	280	11	P
aIns	L	–34	12	–10	1160	19	E
aIns	L	–32	12	0	1224	15	E
vaIns (Ag)/TP	L	–40	10	–20	2040	18	E
vIns	R	40	4	–14	1040	17	E
mid-Ins	R	44	–4	0	1576	9	E
mid-Ins	L	–40	0	–2	1752	15	E
mid-Ins (dors.)	R	42	4	10	736	12	E
vmPGC (24, 10m/r)	—	2	32	–4	1672	11	E
dmPFC (BA 9)	—	–4	52	30	648	11	P
dmPFC (BA 9/32)	—	0	52	20	24	5	P
OFC (47/12m,l), vaIns	R	36	26	–16	2160	14	e
OFC (47/12L), IFG	L	–44	26	–16	1304	14	e
Uncus	R	12	–2	–26	480	12	E
Uncus	L	–12	0	–26	440	13	e
Other cortical regions							
IFG/frOP	R	48	22	12	1744	19	P
frOP	L	–46	16	0	552	12	P
IFS	L	–48	22	18	24	5	P
IFS	L	–46	10	24	48	6	P
PCC	—	2	–52	24	32	6	P
TC/OCC	R	52	–58	8	280	9	P
iTC	L	–36	–50	–20	8	5	P
iTC/sCBLM	R	40	–54	–22	2016	15	P
iTC/sCBLM	L	–38	–64	–18	936	10	P
STS (post.)	R	54	–46	10	720	10	P
OCC (lat.)	R	48	–70	–2	128	9	P
OCC (lat.)	L	–48	–70	10	48	5	P
iOCC	L	–32	–78	–18	16	6	P
IFG	L	–50	24	6	400	10	E
PCC	R	6	–60	18	176	6	E
pre-SMA	—	4	12	48	1208	8	E
pre-SMA	—	0	10	60	1280	8	E
TC/OCC	R	44	–60	–14	792	12	E
STG	L	–48	–8	–2	1096	10	E
V1 (BA 17)	L	–6	–88	0	1120	9	E

Note. Lat, lateralization; [X, Y, Z] are stereotactic coordinates; Vol, volume of region in mm^3; %Act, percentage of contrast maps activating within 10 mm; Thr, threshold type; P, primary height threshold; E, extent threshold.

CHAPTER 16

Interoception and Emotion
A Neuroanatomical Perspective

A. D. (BUD) CRAIG

When someone asks you, "How do you feel?," your answer includes your bodily feelings as well as your emotional feelings. Influential models of emotion view the embodiment of emotions as fundamental; that is, many observers believe that interoceptive awareness has a crucial role in emotional awareness (Barrett, Quigley, Bliss-Moreau, & Aronson, 2004; Damasio, 1994; James, 1890/2007; Philippot & Chalelle, 2002; Wiens, 2005). The neuroanatomical findings described in this chapter address the organization of pathways in the brain that engender feelings from the body, and they support the view that the neural substrates responsible for subjective awareness of your emotional state are based on the neural representation of your physiological state.

These data show that there is a phylogenetically novel homeostatic sensory afferent pathway in primates, especially in humanoid primates, that provides the basis for a sense of the physiological condition of the body ("the material me") in posterior insular cortex (Craig, 2002). A posterior-to-anterior progression of increasingly complex re-representations in the

human insula provides a foundation for the sequential integration of your homeostatic condition with your sensory environment, with your motivational condition, and with your social condition. Based on considerable evidence, I propose that this integration generates a unified penultimate metarepresentation of the global emotional moment at the junction of the anterior insula and the frontal operculum (Craig, 2004a, 2005). Convergent functional imaging findings reveal that the anterior insula and the anterior cingulate cortices are conjointly activated during all human emotions (e.g., Murphy, Nimmo-Smith, & Lawrence, 2003), which in my view indicates that the limbic sensory representation of subjective "feelings" (in the anterior insula) and the limbic motor representation of volitional agency (in the anterior cingulate) together form the fundamental neuroanatomical basis for all human emotions (Craig, 2002). This view is consistent with the definition of an emotion in humans as both a feeling and a motivation with concomitant autonomic sequelae (Rolls, 1999). In this view, emotions are not simply occasional events, but rather are ongoing and continuous, and emotional behaviors can occur without subjective feelings (as they do constantly in animals other than humanoid primates, or in unconscious human emotional acts).

Thus I concur with the idea that emotional behaviors evolved as energy-efficient means of producing goal-directed actions that fulfill homeostatic and social needs (Darwin, 1872/1965), and I believe that our capacity for awareness of our emotional behaviors (i.e., our subjective feelings) evolved because it enormously enhanced the efficiency and complexity of emotional communication. I propose in this chapter that a neuroanatomical substrate for subjective emotional awareness exists in fronto-insular cortex as a finite set of repeated penultimate metarepresentations of global emotional moments that extends across time, forming the basis not only for the continuity of subjective emotional awareness within a finite present, but also for the uniquely human faculty of music. In fact, there are numerous convergent observations that lead to this proposal. Finally, these considerations also provide a homeostatic model that can explain the asymmetrical roles of the left and right forebrain in human emotion (Craig, 2005). These ideas may seem heuristic, philosophical, and speculative, but they arise directly from experimental findings in cats, monkeys and humans, as I will explain. These insights afford an opportunity to reclassify functional psychiatric disorders on a neurobiological basis, and they identify interoceptive processing regions that can serve as treatment targets for emotional problems (e.g., Simmons, Strigo, Matthews, Paulus, & Stein, 2006).

As a functional neuroanatomist, I study the organization of the brain by using anatomical methods (e.g., tract tracing) and physiological methods (e.g., microelectrode recordings) in comparative animals. I also use psychophysical and functional imaging methods (e.g., functional magnetic resonance imaging, or fMRI) in humans to test the predictions from comparative animal studies and to extrapolate these findings into more highly evolved regions of the human brain. My research is based on the knowledge that the brain is not a mystical structure, but rather is reproducibly and evolutionarily well organized for the purpose of maintaining and advancing both the individual and the species. The brain is not color-

coded, its internal connections are not readily visible, its physiological operations are ephemeral, and it is organized in series of processing areas and nested hierarchies that form networks, so it is difficult to analyze. Studies of the effects of lesions and stimulation first identified the sensory regions (for vision, audition, and touch) and the motor regions (for skeletal movements and visceral activation) of the human cerebral cortex. Modern functional imaging studies, which produce color-coded maps of brain activation based on relative measurements of local cerebral blood flow during specific tasks, have validated these insights and are now being used in experimental psychology to reveal brain regions that are active during different cognitive and emotional tasks. However, such studies are constrained by inherent limitations in temporal, spatial, and statistical resolution, and most importantly by the fact that the underlying neural organization is generally not revealed by a top-down phenomenological approach (sometimes referred to as "blob-ology"; see Sternberg, 2000). By contrast, the findings described in this chapter begin with a bottom-up view of ascending pathways associated with the sensory representation of the physiological condition of the body.

The data indicate that these pathways represent the ongoing status of all tissues and organs of the body, including skin, muscle, and viscera. I use the term "interoception" specifically to denote this generalized homeostatic sensory capacity, redefining it from its original narrow usage to refer only to visceral sensation (Sherrington, 1948). The sensory afferents that represent the condition of the body subserve "homeostasis," which is the ongoing, hierarchically organized neurobiological process that maintains an optimal balance in the physiological condition of the body. Homeostasis in mammals comprises many integrated functions and includes autonomic, neuroendocrine, and behavioral mechanisms. Thermoregulation is a good example of a homeostatic function. The salient purpose of thermoregulation, as of homeostasis, is optimal energy management in support of life. All animals thermoregulate. The primordial means of thermoregulation in vertebrates is motivated behavior, similar to hunger and thirst. In humans, such affective motivations are accompanied by distinct homeostatic (interoceptive) "feelings"; these modalities include not only temperature, pain, itch, hunger, and thirst, but all feelings from the body, such as muscle ache, visceral urgency, and so-called "air hunger." Consistent with the view that an emotion in humans consists of a sensation and a motivation with direct autonomic sequelae (Rolls, 1999), I regard these feelings as "homeostatic emotions" that drive behavior. In my opinion, they are virtually equivalent to the "background emotions" of Damasio (1994), and they are incorporated in the concept of "core affect" (Russell & Barrett, 1999; Barrett et al., 2004). The neuroanatomy of the forebrain pathways described below provides compelling support for this concept.

Temperature sensation is an instructive example of a homeostatic emotion, because we normally think of it as an exteroceptive discriminative sensory capacity. However, the obligatory affect (pleasantness or unpleasantness) we feel with each temperature stimulus is the perceptual correlate of behavioral thermoregulatory motivation. This affect highlights the importance of temperature sensation for homeostasis, because its valence depends directly on your body's thermoregulatory needs (Cabanac, 1971; Mower, 1976). Thus the cool glass of water that feels wonderful if you are overheated feels gnawingly unpleasant if you are chilled. Conversely, if you are chilled, then a hot shower feels wonderful, even if it is stinging and prickly, but it would be called painful if you were too warm. Similarly, if you remain in a room that is too chilly (or too warm) for energy-efficient thermoneutrality (or if you place your hand on an object that is too cold or too hot), then you feel a growing discomfort (which as it increases may be called painful) until you respond in a behaviorally appropriate manner. In the same way, eating salt or sugar is pleasant (and thus motivated) if the body needs it, but it becomes unpleasant and distasteful after you've eaten enough. These affective feelings reflect behavioral motivations that are driven by the homeostatic needs of the body, and the human perception of this combination of a feeling and a motivation is a homeostatic emotion. Note that homeostatically motivated behaviors occur in all animals and require no awareness of accompanying feelings. In fact, the structural absence in subprimates of the forebrain homeostatic afferent pathways described below (specifically, the modality-selective interoceptive representation in the limbic sensory insular cortex, and the direct motivational pathway to the limbic behavioral motor cortex in the cingulate region) implies

that they cannot experience feelings from the body in the same way that humans do.

In what follows, I describe first the functional neuroanatomical evidence for an interoceptive (homeostatic afferent) pathway in primates, beginning with the development of spinal homeostatic afferent processing and the identified spinal neurons that represent each of the specific feelings from the body. I detail the projections of these neurons to spinal, brainstem, and thalamo-cortical levels in monkeys, and then I describe functional imaging studies in humans that validate these comparative findings. I emphasize a particular functional imaging experiment that demonstrates graded activation of the dorsal posterior insula by cooling stimuli, because this finding validates the identification of the ascending interoceptive pathway and because it provides compelling neuroanatomical evidence for the concept of homeostatic emotions. In addition, the data in this particular experiment reveal the neuroanatomical progression of activity to the anterior insula that underlies subjective awareness of feelings of temperature. Next, I summarize the convergent evidence for the role of anterior insula in all subjective emotional feelings, which substantiates the interoceptive basis for emotional awareness, and then I describe how repeated metarepresentations of global emotional moments can explain the observed role of this cortical region in awareness, time, and music. Finally, I summarize a neuroanatomical model for left–right emotional asymmetry based on the homeostatic afferent processing pathways.

THE FUNCTIONAL ANATOMY OF THE ASCENDING INTEROCEPTIVE PATHWAY IN PRIMATES

Specialized peripheral and central neural substrates that represent all homeostatic afferent activity generate the distinct feelings of pain, temperature, itch, muscle ache, sensual touch, and other bodily sensations by way of discrete sensory channels. This modality-selective sensory activity is conveyed first of all to hierarchically organized homeostatic integration and preautonomic response regions in the spinal cord and brainstem. An encephalized forebrain system that evolved virtually uniquely in primates surmounts the homeostatic response system; it provides a direct cortical sensory image of the physiological condition of the body in the limbic sensory insular cortex, and, in parallel, activates the limbic behavioral motor cortex in the medial frontal region (Figure 16.1; for complete descriptions, see Craig, 2002, 2003).

Small-Diameter Afferents

Small-diameter (A-delta and C) primary afferent fibers (which include nociceptors, thermoreceptors, osmoreceptors, and metaboreceptors) report the physiological status of the various tissues of the body. These fibers terminate monosynaptically on projection neurons in the most superficial layer of the spinal (and trigeminal) dorsal horn (which is called lamina I or the marginal zone). The way the spinal cord develops reveals the special role of these fibers in homeostasis. During development, these small-diameter afferents originate from a second wave of small neurons that emerge within the dorsal root ganglia subsequent to the large cells that generate the large-diameter fibers innervating mechanoreceptors and proprioceptors. The large-diameter fibers enter the spinal cord first and contact large dorsal horn neurons, and then the small-diameter fibers enter at the same time as the lamina I neurons appear. The lamina I neurons originate not from cells of the dorsal placode, but from progenitors of interneurons in the lateral horn (the sympathetic cell column), and they migrate to the top of the dorsal horn during a ventromedial rotation of the entire dorsal horn at precisely the right time during development to meet the incoming small-diameter afferents. This delicately coordinated ontogenetic sequence indicates that, together, the small-diameter afferents and the lamina I neurons constitute a cohesive system for homeostatic afferent activity that parallels the efferent sympathetic nervous system. In contrast, the large neurons that receive large-diameter fiber input come to lie at the base of the dorsal horn (because of the rotation) and serve as interneurons for skeletal motoneurons. The small-diameter afferent fibers in cranial parasympathetic nerves (e.g., vagus and glossopharyngeal) that innervate visceral organs terminate similarly in the nucleus of the solitary tract in the caudal medulla. These pathways represent, respectively, the afferent inputs for the sympathetic and the parasympathetic halves of the autonomic nervous system.

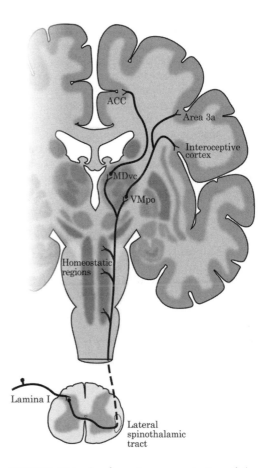

FIGURE 16.1. A schematic representation of the homeostatic (interoceptive) afferent pathway in primates that represents the physiological condition of the body. The main forebrain projections are to the dorsal posterior insula (interoceptive cortex) and to the medial frontal region (the anterior cingulate cortex, or ACC). The pathway that ascends from lamina I of the spinal cord via the lateral spinothalamic tract represents the sympathetic half of the homeostatic afferent system, and a parallel pathway via the nucleus of the solitary tract and the basal portion of the ventromedial nucleus in the thalamus represents its parasympathetic half (not depicted). From Craig (2003). Reprinted, with permission, from the *Annual Review of Neuroscience*, Volume 26. Copyright 2003 by Annual Reviews (*www.annualreviews. org*).

Lamina I Neurons

Consistent with this developmental view, the projections of lamina I neurons convey small-diameter homeostatic sensory afferent input directly to the homeostatic integration and control regions in the spinal cord and brainstem. Lamina I projections thus provide the substrate for the hierarchical, modality-selective somato-autonomic reflexes activated by spinal small-diameter afferents that are crucial for homeostatic function (Sato & Schmidt, 1973).

In the spinal cord, their major projection is to the autonomic cell column of the thoraco-lumbar spinal cord, where sympathetic preganglionic output neurons are located. In the brainstem, lamina I neurons project exclusively to recognized homeostatic integration sites, including the ventrolateral medulla, the catecholamine cell groups A1–A2 and A5–A7, the parabrachial nucleus (PB), and the periaqueductal gray (PAG). They converge at these sites with afferent activity associated with the parasympathetic system by way of the solitary nucleus. These sites are all heavily interconnected with the hypothalamus and amygdala. The crucial role of lamina I in homeostatic reflexes is highlighted by the fact that lamina I and the spinal autonomic cell columns are the only spinal sites that receive descending modulation directly from brainstem and hypothalamic preautonomic sources.

Lamina I neurons comprise several modality-selective classes that can be regarded as virtual "labeled lines" for distinct feelings from the body, such as first (sharp) pain, second (burning) pain, cool, warm, itch, sensual touch, muscle ache and cramp, and so on (although their activity must be integrated in the forebrain; see Craig, 2003). Each class consists of a morphologically distinct type of neuron that receives input from a specific subset of small-diameter afferents. Quantitative analyses using extracellular recordings from single lamina I neurons indicate that the response characteristics of these cells correspond very well with the psychophysical characteristics of these distinct sensations (Craig, Krout, & Andrew, 2001; Craig, 2004b). For example, the cooling-sensitive thermoreceptive-specific neurons that are uniquely found in lamina I respond linearly to innocuous cooling (Figure 16.2A) and saturate at noxious cold temperatures, as human cooling sensitivity does. Intracellular recording and staining showed that such cells are uniformly pyramid-shaped

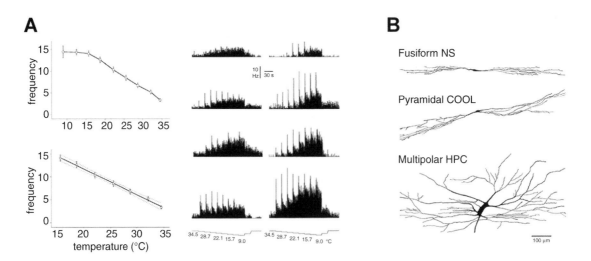

FIGURE 16.2. (A) Original data showing that thermoreceptive-specific lamina I spinothalamic neurons linearly encode skin temperature. The graphs on the left show the ensemble mean, and the graphs on the right show the responses of individual neurons to the characterizing staircase stimulus. From Craig, Krout, and Andrew (2001). Copyright 2001 by the American Physiological Society. Reprinted by permission. (B) Examples of lamina I neurons that were individually characterized and stained intracellularly, showing the correspondence of the three main physiological classes of cells with the three main morphological shapes. From Han, Zhang, and Craig (1998). Copyright 1998 by Nature Publishing Group. Reprinted by permission.

lamina I cells (Figure 16.2B). In contrast, the polymodal nociceptive lamina I cells are selectively sensitive to noxious heat, noxious pinch, and noxious cold, and are monosynaptically activated by C-fibers; their responses to repeated brief-contact heat and the thermal grill (an illusion of pain) correspond in all respects with the psychophysical characteristics of the human sensation of second ("burning") pain. Such cells are multipolar lamina I neurons (Figure 16.2B). The selectivity of lamina I spinothalamic tract neurons is convincingly demonstrated by the subpopulation of cells that have characteristics uniquely corresponding with the human sensation of itch (Andrew & Craig, 2001).

Whereas lamina I is usually thought of as a "pain and temperature" site, its role in homeostasis is clearly revealed by the neurons that respond selectively to small-diameter afferent input from muscle. Such afferents subserve ongoing homeostatic adjustments to muscular work, but when strongly activated they are also directly responsible for the feelings of muscle burn, pain, and cramping. The commingling of these muscle-selective neurons in lamina I with other cells selectively responsive to temperature or pain or itch emphasizes the fundamental perspective that lamina I neurons convey afferent activity representing all aspects of the physiological condition of all tissues of the body. It is also important to recognize that lamina I neurons do not simply provide emergency signals, but rather are engaged in homeostasis *on an ongoing basis*, just as cardiorespiratory activity is continuously affected by ongoing muscular activity and by ongoing temperature changes. Furthermore, many small-diameter afferents are sensitive to cytokines, opioids, steroids, hormones (e.g., somatostatin), and other local and circulating immune modulators, consistent with the role of sympathetic and parasympathetic autonomic efferents in the regulation of immune and neuroendocrine functions.

Lamina I Projections to the Primate Forebrain

High-resolution tract-tracing experiments have revealed that in primates, lamina I neurons project to the contralateral thalamus in the lateral spinothalamic tract, which ascends at the precise location within the spinal cord where cordotomy lesions in humans interrupt feelings from the body such as pain, temperature, itch, sensual touch, and so on (Figure 16.1; Craig, 2002, 2003). In subprimates, ascending lamina I activity is processed mainly in brainstem sites (e.g., A1, PB, and PAG), which then provide a highly integrated signal to emotional behavioral control regions in the forebrain. Encephalization in primates produced a somatotopographic, modality-selective lamina I spinothalamic projection to a specific thalamocortical relay nucleus (VMpo), which in turn projects to a discrete portion of dorsal posterior insular cortex (dpIns, or interoceptive cortex). A parallel pathway, also unique to primates, conveys afferent input from the vagal and glossopharyngeal nerves by way of the nucleus of the solitary tract to a rostrally adjacent thalamo-cortical relay nucleus (VMb), which in turn projects to a rostrally adjacent region of dorsal insular cortex. (The insula is a cortical "island" buried within the lateral sulcus that has intimate connections with amygdala, hypothalamus, and cingulate and orbito-frontal cortices.) Together, these pathways through VMpo and VMb provide a direct cortical image of all homeostatic afferent activity that mirrors the sympathetic and the parasympathetic halves of the efferent autonomic nervous system. The VMpo in the human thalamus is greatly enlarged relative to that of the macaque monkey.

The ascending projections of lamina I neurons in primates also provide a direct thalamo-cortical pathway that activates the anterior cingulate cortex (ACC) by way of a medial thalamic relay (MDvc). By contrast, in subprimates the medial thalamic sources of input to the ACC receive integrated homeostatic input from the brainstem (PB and PAG). (In cats and rats, there is instead a direct lamina I projection to a neighboring, developmentally related nucleus in medial thalamus [nucleus submedius], which projects to ventrolateral orbitofrontal cortex, associated with hedonic integration and descending antinociception, rather than to the ACC.) I concur with the suggestion made previously by several neuroanatomists (e.g., M. Mesulam, and G. Van Hoesen) that the insula can be regarded as limbic sensory cortex because of its association with homeostatic afferent activity and the amygdala, hypothalamus, and orbito-frontal cortex, and that the ACC can be regarded as limbic motor cortex because of its association with homeostatic efferent (autonomic) activity and its descending projections to the PAG in the brainstem. This fits well with the modern view of the overall organization of frontal cortex into limbic sensory and limbic motor networks (Ongur & Price, 2000).

FUNCTIONAL IMAGING OF INTEROCEPTION IN HUMANS

Activation of Dorsal Posterior Insula

Functional imaging, lesion, and stimulation studies in humans confirm the crucial role of the dorsal insula in graded pain, graded temperature, graded itch, dynamic or painful muscle sensation, sensual touch, hunger, thirst, gustation, cardiorespiratory activity, "air hunger," and so on (for references, see Craig, 2002, 2003). It serves as primary sensory cortex for each of these distinct interoceptive "feelings" from the body. Accumulating evidence indicates that it is activated in a graded manner during each of these sensations, that stimulation of this region (or VMpo/VMb) can produce these sensations, and that lesions including dpIns (or VMpo/VMb) can selectively disrupt these sensations. Notably, dpIns is delimited by labeling for the receptors of corticotropin-releasing factor, which many investigators regard as a definitive marker for homeostasis (Sanchez, Young, Plotsky, & Insel, 1999). The primordial role of the insular cortex is modulation of brainstem homeostatic integration sites, which are the main targets of its descending projections. Thus the interoceptive cortical image of the physiological condition of the body in humans emerged evolutionarily as an extension of the hierarchical homeostatic system. In other words, feelings from the body in humans reflect its homeostatic condition.

The experimental tract-tracing findings in monkeys indicate that the lamina I input to VMpo, and also the cortical projections of VMpo and VMb to dpIns, are topographically organized in the anterior-to-posterior direction (face to foot). The neuroanatomical findings in the monkey predict that all homeostatic afferent modalities will produce graded activation in dpIns that is arranged somatotopographically in the anterior-to-posterior direction. Recent fMRI evidence has demonstrated this somatotopic gradient for sensations of heat pain, innocuous cooling, and muscle pain in the dpIns of humans (Brooks, Zambreanu, Godinez, Craig, & Tracey, 2005; Hua, Strigo, Baxter, Johnson, & Craig, 2005; Henderson, Gandevia, & Macefield, 2007). Significantly,

this gradient is orthogonal to the lateral-to-medial (face-to-foot) organization of the main somatosensory thalamus and the S1 and S2 somatosensory cortices. This contrast substantiates the differentiation of dpIns; in particular, it highlights the distinction of dpIns from S2, to which pain-related activation in the operculo-insular region has often been incorrectly ascribed. This also means that the large-diameter afferent lemniscal pathway to the somatosensory thalamus (VPM/VPL) and the small-diameter afferent pathway to VMpo/VMb develop along different neurotrophic gradients, which substantiates the concept that the VMb and VMpo representation of homeostatic afferents (which control smooth muscle) is separate from the main somatosensory representation of mechanical and proprioceptive inputs (which control skeletal muscle). That is, there are two fundamentally different thalamocortical representations of somatic afferent activity in the human brain, and the primary interoceptive cortex in the posterior insula is a distinct entity.

Activation of Anterior Cingulate

Many functional imaging studies have documented the role of the human ACC in behavioral drive and volition (behavioral agency; which seems to be guided dynamically by error likelihood estimation, see Brown & Braver, 2005), and the ACC is activated by homeostatic afferent activity. The ACC is activated in nearly all functional imaging studies of pain, and it is similarly activated in studies of muscle and visceral sensation. Functional imaging studies of the thermal grill illusion of pain (Craig, Reiman, Evans, & Bushnell, 1996) and of hypnotically modulated pain unpleasantness (Rainville, Duncan, Price, Carrier, & Bushnell, 1997) associate ACC activity directly with the affective motivation of pain (unpleasantness), and they indicate that this pathway engenders the affect and motivation that render pain a homeostatic emotional drive. The conjoint activation of dpIns and ACC by the distinct homeostatic modalities seems to correspond well with the idea that the feelings from the body constitute homeostatic emotions that simultaneously generate both a sensation and a motivation. That is, temperature, pain, itch, and muscle ache are homeostatic emotions that drive behavior, just as hunger and thirst are, and the condition of our bodies directly affects our feelings and our motivations on an ongoing basis. The activation of the region of the ACC by innocuous thermal stimuli described in the next section is particularly instructive.

FUNCTIONAL IMAGING OF TEMPERATURE SENSATION: AN EXAMPLE OF A HOMEOSTATIC EMOTION

Activation of Posterior Insula and Anterior Cingulate

Temperature, like pain and itch, is a feeling from our bodies that we normally externalize. We readily detect the temperature of an object or of the environment. Temperature sensation has always been regarded as a discriminative exteroceptive cutaneous sensory capacity allied with the sense of touch. However, the thermoreceptors in our skin, muscles, and viscera actually report local tissue temperature, and thermoregulation is necessary for all animals to use energy most efficiently. The functional anatomy of temperature sensation in humans reflects the primordial importance of temperature sensibility for homeostasis. The location of the discriminative thermosensory cortex identified by the PET imaging data in Plate 16.1 (see color insert) fits precisely with the location of dpIns identified by the functional anatomical tracing studies in the monkey (Craig, Chen, Bandy, & Reiman, 2000; see also Maihöfner, Kaltenhäuser, Neundörfer, & Lang, 2004; Hua et al., 2005). Plate 16.1 shows three different analyses of brain activation observed with PET imaging during the application of six different cool temperatures on the palm of the hand. The first row, a simple contrast between the highest and lowest temperatures, served as a mask for subsequent analyses. The second row shows a regression analysis against thermode temperature, which reveals that activation of one site in the contralateral cortex was directly correlated with objective temperature (the red blob on the left side at level 24). This site can therefore be regarded as primary thermosensory cortex. Its location in dpIns explains clinical reports of stroke-induced lesions that produced thermanesthesia (Schmahmann & Leifer, 1992; Greenspan, Lee, & Lenz, 1999). Strikingly, this region is not part of the somatosensory cortices that represent touch sensation, which lie on the parietal surface (postcentral gyrus) and in the parietal operculum. Rather, the role of insular

cortex as limbic sensory cortex fits neatly with the view that temperature sensation is first and foremost of importance for homeostasis. In addition, more recent fMRI evidence reveals that dynamic cooling produces graded activation at a site in the medial frontal cortex (in the limbic behavioral motor cortex near the ACC) adjacent to the site that is activated during pain (Hua et al., 2005). Together, these findings support the view that temperature produces both a feeling and a behavioral motivation in humans—that is, a homeostatic emotion.

Activation of Anterior Insula Related to Subjective Feelings of Temperature

So how do we "feel" temperature? Our subjective sense of innocuous temperature is very linear, but it is not perfect. The deviation is sufficient to provide a robust statistical difference between cortical activation associated with subjective rather than objective temperature. The third row in Plate 16.1 shows a regression analysis of the same dataset against the participants' subjective ratings of coolness. A large area of activation in the anterior insula and orbito-frontal cortex on the right side is conspicuous in these data. Close comparison of the activation blobs at level 24 in rows 2 and 3 reveals that in the subjective regression analysis, a new activation site appears just anterior to the main site activated in dpIns in the objective temperature regression analysis. Thus these data indicate that there is an immediate re-representation of thermosensory activation in the middle insula on the homolateral side, just anterior to dpIns. This re-representation must be an abstracted or integrated re-representation in some sense, because its activity is significantly more closely related to subjective ratings than to objective temperatures. The data show a subsequent commissural transfer from the middle insula to a lateralized series of re-representations in the anterior insula and orbito-frontal cortex on the right side, which are much more strongly correlated with subjective feeling. This is a neurobiologically parsimonious pattern of activation, because progressive re-representations that combine feature extraction and cross-modality integration are present in the serial processing streams observed in the visual, auditory, and parietal somatosensory cortical regions, and are consistent with the evolutionary development of new processing regions in primate cortex (Krubitzer & Kaas, 2005). The lateralization is crucial evidence of hemispheric specialization; I return to this issue later in the chapter.

FUNCTIONAL IMAGING OF SUBJECTIVE FEELINGS IN HUMANS

Thus the PET imaging data on temperature sensation illuminate an anatomical model in which the subjective awareness of feelings from the body is generated directly from cortical re-representations of the interoceptive image of the body's homeostatic condition. The results of many other imaging studies of subjective feelings in humans correspond with this anatomical model. These convergent data suggest that the cortical interoceptive image of the body provides the basis for awareness of the "material me" or the sentient self.

The data show an anatomical progression of activity from dpIns, first to the middle insula on the homolateral side, and then, by way of a commissural lateralization, to the right anterior insula. The posterior-to-anterior progression of processing in the insular cortex is consistent with several neuroanatomical considerations, most particularly with the enormous phylogenetic expansion of anterior insula across humanoid primates (Allman, Watson, Tetrault, & Hakeem, 2005). (Notably, in monkeys, interoceptive cortex seems to project directly to orbito-frontal cortex and does not generate the successive re-representations in anterior insular cortex that seem to be unique to humanoid primates.) Other imaging findings support the convergence in the middle insula of activity associated with emotionally salient stimuli of all modalities, in part by way of interconnections with the amygdala. Figure 16.3 summarizes my view of the anatomical organization of progressive integration in insular cortex, which is based on numerous anatomical and imaging reports (e.g., Chikama, McFarland, Amaral, & Haber, 1997; Brooks,

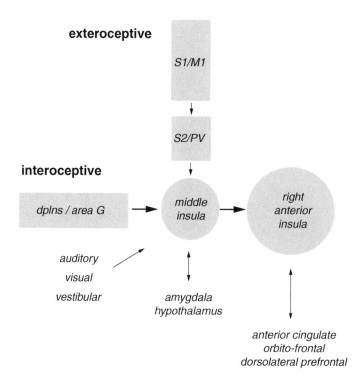

FIGURE 16.3. A conceptual diagram of the progressive integration in posterior, middle, and anterior insula of interoceptive state with the sensory, autonomic, motivational, and contextual conditions of the body and the brain to produce a finite set of global emotional representations. In this homeostatic model, the right anterior insula represents the energy-consuming (sympathetic) conditions, and the left anterior insula represents the energy-enriching (parasympathetic) conditions.

Nurmikko, Bimson, Singh, & Roberts, 2002; Adolphs, 2002; Schweinhardt et al., 2006; Henderson et al., 2007). This figure illustrates the concept that progressive re-representations of the physiological (interoceptive) condition of the body provide the basis for the integration of homeostatic afferent activity—first in the middle insula with emotionally salient inputs from all sensory modalities and from subcortical homeostatic control regions (hypothalamus and amygdala), and then in the anterior insula with emotionally salient activity in other limbic cortical regions (ACC, orbitofrontal cortex), as well as with the cortical region involved in contextual planning (dorsolateral prefrontal cortex). Thus this posterior-to-anterior progression of re-representations in the human insula provides a foundation for the sequential integration of the homeostatic condition of the body with the sensory environment, with internal autonomic state, with motivational conditions and finally with social conditions. This progression culminates in the most recently evolved regions of the anterior insula, situated at its junction with the frontal operculum and orbito-frontal cortex.

This anatomical view of homeostatic emotional integration is directly supported by evidence that activation of right anterior insula is correlated not only with subjective ratings of temperature, but also with subjective attention to pain (of either cutaneous, muscular, or visceral origin) (e.g., Brooks et al., 2002). The anatomical posterior-to-anterior progression can explain why activation associated with anticipation of pain and feelings of chronic pain localize in a more anterior portion of right anterior insula than activation during acute experimental pain (Schweinhardt et al., 2006). Furthermore, right anterior insula activation is correlated with subjective ratings of disgust or trustworthiness; with internally generated emotions like anger, sadness, happiness, lust, and fear; with imitation or empathic referral of these emotions; with empathic feelings of pain imputed to a loved one; and even with feelings of social exclusion (for references, see Craig, 2002). So the convergence of these findings supports the view that the cortical re-representations in right anterior insula of the interoceptive image of the body's physiological condition provides a basis for the subjective awareness of *all* emotional feelings. The culmination of this integration may involve different

modules that together produce a unified penultimate metarepresentation, which I refer to as a "global emotional moment." This convergent integration is supported by demonstrations of synergistic activation of anterior insula by interoceptive feelings and emotions (e.g., Phillips et al., 2003).

These neuroanatomical data substantiate the view that the cortical image of subjective feelings is built upon the homeostatic (interoceptive) hierarchy. The association of right anterior insula with subjective awareness of all emotions fits well with the idea that human emotions are based in part on feelings from the body, which is the essence of the James–Lange theory of emotion (James, 1890/2007). The metarepresentations of the state of the body in right anterior insula seem to differentiate inner from outer conditions (self from nonself) and to provide a subjective mental image of the material self as a feeling (sentient) entity that is utilized during all emotional states. In other words, it seems to provide the anatomical basis for emotional awareness. As discussed in greater detail in Craig (2002), this fits with the anatomical features of the so-called "somatic marker" hypothesis of consciousness (Damasio, 1994). The latter concept predicts that interoceptive state and emotional feelings are directly related, which is supported by recent evidence of distinct patterns of homeostatic activity during different emotions (Deichert, Flack, & Craig, 2005; Rainville, Bechara, Nagvi, & Damasio, 2006). The interoceptive re-representations in right anterior insula provide a substantive neural basis for these relationships, and also for the "as-if" loop that Damasio postulated would enable mental interoceptive predictions of the consequences of emotional behaviors based on prior experiences.

It is important to note explicitly that this integration in the anterior insula includes not only emotionally salient sensory inputs, but also the activity within the motivational regions of the brain itself (i.e., ACC, orbitofrontal cortex, ventral striatum). Notably, the integration of the behavioral agent with the "feeling self" can provide an anatomical basis for the representation in awareness of the illusory "I" postulated by Damasio. Interestingly, studies of placebo analgesia reveal coordinated activation of ACC and right anterior insula, suggesting that the integration in the latter of the activity in the former (the behavioral agent) not only produces a representation of motivation within subjective emotional awareness, but also enables motivation to modulate subjective feelings directly. This interpretation offers an explanation for the paradoxical finding in some studies that activity in right anterior insula *increases* with placebo analgesia, rather than being reduced (Petrovic, Kalso, Petersson, & Ingvar, 2002; Lieberman et al., 2004). This perspective also negates a main criticism of the James–Lange theory (i.e., that it did not allow for feelings of internally generated emotion), and by incorporating the likelihood that anterior insula stores representations of past interoceptive/emotional experiences, it enables ready explanations of the interactions between homeostatic functions and emotional states—for example, in anxiety, somatization and psychosomatic illness.

AN ANATOMICAL MODEL FOR SUBJECTIVE AWARENESS OF FEELINGS, AGENCY, AND TIME

Thus a refined and integrated image of the state of the body seems to provide the basis for awareness of the "feeling self." In this homeostatic model, the representation of the global emotional moment includes feelings about motivations, and it can be modified by expectations and motivations, based on interconnections between anterior insula and ACC (as well as subcortical structures, such as amygdala and ventral striatum, and the dorsolateral prefrontal cortex). In this view, the coactivation of the anterior insula and the ACC during all emotions not only corresponds with the view that an emotion is both a feeling and a motivation, but also provides the active behavioral agent that is missing from the "somatic marker" hypothesis. This interpretation is anatomically consistent with the dual lamina I spinothalamo-cortical projections (to insula and cingulate) and with the overall anatomical organization of primate frontal cortex into medial (limbic behavioral motor) and insular/orbital (limbic sensory) networks (Ongur & Price, 2000).

Anterior Insula and Awareness

The role of the right anterior insula in interoceptive awareness and subjective feelings is supported by the demonstration by Critchley, Weins, Rothshtein, Öhman, and Dolon (2004) that its activation is uniquely correlated with subjective perception of heartbeat timing, a classic test of interoceptive awareness (see discussion by Craig, 2004). This fits with psychological evidence associating interoceptive (heartbeat) awareness with self-reports of emotional experience (Barrett et al., 2004). Yet the analyses by Critchley et al. (2004) were based on subjective perceptions of cross-modal timing, and in fact, graded, selective activation of right anterior insula (and ACC) is produced during other cross-modal timing disparities—for instance, in the ventriloquism illusion (Bushara, Grafman, & Hallett, 2001). In addition, research has shown strong evidence of a direct relationship between right anterior insula activation and subjective awareness of timing: by using either long or short expected intervals, by using injections of clonidine to produce subjective temporal slowing, or by using graded attention to timing in a multicue task (summarized in Coull, 2004). Nevertheless, selective activation of anterior insula and ACC bilaterally was strongly *inversely* correlated with display time (and performance) in a backward-masking task that probed the temporal limits of visual observation during brief subsecond presentations (Deary et al., 2004); that is, activation increased with shorter presentation times. In my opinion, this very striking result, considered together with these other findings, indicates that the fundamental role of anterior insula may be described most simply as subjective awareness. This inference is supported by recent evidence indicating that the anterior insula and ACC are uniquely associated with lapses in attention (Weissman, Roberts, Visscher, & Woldorff, 2006), with "mind-wandering" (Mason et al., 2007), and with an intrinsic default network for "emotional salience" (Seeley et al., 2007). After highlighting a unique type of neuron in right anterior insula, I outline a structural proposal for this inference.

Von Economo Neurons

Allman et al. (2005) recently reported that a population of large spindle neurons, which they call "Von Economo neurons" (after an early neuroanatomist), is uniquely found in the anterior insula (or fronto-insular region) and ACC of humanoid primates. Most notably, they reported a trenchant phylogenetic correlation, in that spindle cells are most numerous in aged humans, but progressively less numerous in children, gorillas, bonobos, and chimpanzees, and nonexistent in macaque monkeys. This progression parallels the results of the mirror test for self-awareness (Macphail, 1998). Allman et al. hypothesize that the fronto-insular cortex may subserve "intuition," because it is activated in studies of uncertainty and anxiety, and they propose that the Von Economo spindle neurons provide the basis for large-scale integration and fast communication between the two sides of cortex. It seems likely to me that the numerous small clusters of Von Economo spindle neurons interconnect the most advanced portions of limbic sensory (anterior insula) and limbic motor (ACC) cortices, both ipsilaterally and contralaterally. The limbic cortices, in sharp contrast to the tightly interconnected and contiguous sensorimotor cortices, are situated physically far apart as a consequence of their pattern of evolutionary development. Analogous to the need for fast interconnections between somatosensory and motor cortices for playing the piano, the spindle neurons could enable fast, complex, and highly integrated emotional behaviors.

A Structural Model for Awareness and Music in the Anterior Insula

Thus an alternative hypothesis to the concept of "intuition" is the idea that the Von Economo spindle neurons, by interconnecting advanced limbic sensory and motor cortices, provide the anatomical basis for the generation of unified penultimate metarepresentations of global emotional moments, and indeed for a series of such metarepresentations across time. This hypothesis is based not only on the foregoing functional anatomical considerations, but also on growing evidence that the anterior insula is associated with music. Functional imaging studies indicate that listening to music or covertly imagining music strongly activates anterior insula (Ackermann & Riecker, 2004), and clinical studies indicate that restricted lesions of anterior insula can produce a condition known as "amusia," or disruption of the ability to appreciate the emotional content of music. Music is a uniquely human faculty that has the profound capacity to bind us together emotionally and to change both our emotions and our subjective perception of time. Music can be

described as the rhythmic temporal progression of emotionally laden moments—which suggests a very straightforward structural model for awareness, because a rhythmic progression of global emotional moments can easily be represented by a sequence of quantal anatomical units (Craig, 2004). (It is interesting to note here my observation that bonobos, who seem to me to be remarkably aware and who uniformly pass the mirror test, clearly use rhythm to communicate—synchronous rhythms for agreement and contrapuntal rhythms for disagreement and negotiation—whereas common chimpanzees do not; see also Macphail, 1998; De Waal, 2003; Williams, 1980.)

That is, if the progressive homeostatic emotional integration in the anterior insula does attain the concise representation of a global emotional moment (i.e., including all emotionally salient aspects of the homeostatic, sensory, autonomic, motivational, and social conditions, as described above), then development of the ability to represent each emotional moment *across time* would obviously be an enormous evolutionary advantage. A quantal series of such metarepresentations of feelings across time (from the past into the future) would directly enable the perception of autobiographical emotional continuity, the backward recognition of emotionally salient behavioral patterns, and the forward anticipation of emotional consequences (i.e., Damasio's "as-if" loop). Such an anatomical structure could engender awareness, because it would provide a cortical image of the self as a continuous sequence of sentient emotional moments (that could not "see" itself, just like "consciousness"). This anatomical structure could also directly underlie the rhythmic emotional progression of music. And, of course, repetition of the structural unit representing a global emotional moment (in this model, a cluster of Von Economo spindle neurons) to produce a sequence of such moments would be a natural and easily realizable neuroanatomical development evolutionarily. Evidence for the association of anterior insula with emotional value estimation in a temporal-difference model of interoceptive learning (Seymour et al., 2004) and with interoceptive prediction in anxiety (Paulus & Stein, 2006) provides support for this model.

Because the number of quantal representations of global emotional moments must be anatomically constrained and finite, its magnitude would correlate with the duration of the subjective emotional present (the "specious moment"). Thus one prediction of this model would be that moments of heightened awareness would be characterized by an altered perception of time. Intriguingly, the phrase "Time stood still" is often used to describe moments of heightened awareness. A finite absolute number of quantal global moments would mean that during such moments of heightened awareness, the absolute extent of the subjective perceptual present must be shortened: As finite resources were allocated to maximize representation of the present in real time, each global emotional moment would represent a shorter temporal duration, and the total extent of time represented across the total pool would be shorter. This seems intuitively obvious, and there are few quantitative psychometric data addressing this prediction (Tse, Intriligator, Rivest, & Cavanagh, 2004), but the only evidence of which I am aware associating the temporal focusing of awareness with neural activation is the aforementioned study by Deary et al. (2004).

Another prediction would be that the loss of such an anatomical structure would be associated not only with amusia, but also with a condition in which the self would not have emotional salience across time. In fact, whereas lesions of posterior insula can produce discrete loss of pain and temperature sensations, lesions of anterior insula can reportedly produce conditions regarded clinically as "anosognosia" (the lack of emotional awareness of oneself; Karnath, Baier, & Nagele, 2005) or "anergia" (complete listlessness; Manes, Paradiso, & Robinson, 1999) or "pain asymbolia" (Berthier, Starkstein, & Leiguarda, 1988), or "loss of the feeling of cigarette cravings" (Naqvi, Rudrauf, Damasio, & Bechara, 2007). Congenital disruption of the insula bilaterally is found in children with Smith–Magenis syndrome, which is characterized by mental retardation and lack of emotional coordination (Boddaert et al., 2004). Most striking is the direct association by recent clinical evidence of the selective degeneration of Von Economo neurons in the ACC and the anterior insula with the loss of emotional awareness that characterizes fronto-temporal dementia (Seeley et al., 2006). Of course, although I have focused my comments on the "feeling" side of the limbic cortical system, it is crucial to remember that if the Von Economo neurons interconnect anterior insula and ACC, consistent with the

conjoint activation of both sites during all emotions and during the experiment of Deary et al. (2004), then lesions of the ACC could produce closely related motivational dysfunctions. For example, the ACC has been associated with alexithymia in several studies (e.g., Kano et al., 2003). Further work in this direction is certainly needed.

HOMEOSTATIC AND EMOTIONAL ASYMMETRY IN THE FOREBRAIN

The homeostatic model of human emotional awareness presented in the preceding section is lateralized to the anterior insula and ACC on the right side. This fits with an established psychophysiological model, in which emotion is more strongly associated with the right forebrain. However, psychophysiological evidence has accumulated indicating that the left and right halves of the human forebrain are differentially associated with particular emotions and affective traits. That is, reviewers of literature relating affect and emotion to electroencephalographic activity, cortisol secretion, immune function, and functional imaging of brain activity have concluded that positive versus negative valence, approach versus withdrawal behavior, and/or affiliative versus personal relevance are associated with left- versus right-hemispheric forebrain activity, respectively, albeit with possible underlying circuits predominantly used for particular emotions (Heilman, 2000; Davidson, 2004; Allen & Kline, 2004; Wager, Phan, Liberzon, & Taylor, 2003; Murphy et al., 2003). I have recently proposed that forebrain emotional asymmetry in humans is anatomically based on an asymmetrical representation of homeostatic activity that originates from asymmetries in the peripheral autonomic nervous system (Craig, 2005).

Briefly, this proposal suggests that emotions are organized according to the fundamental principle of autonomic opponency for the management of physical and mental energy. In this homeostatic neuroanatomical model of emotional asymmetry, the left forebrain is associated predominantly with parasympathetic activity, and thus with nourishment, safety, positive affect, approach (appetitive) behavior, and group-oriented (affiliative) emotions; the right forebrain is associated predominantly with sympathetic activity, and thus with arousal, danger, negative affect, withdrawal (aversive) behavior, and individual-oriented (survival) emotions. In this model, management of physical and mental (meaning neural) energy is the salient organizational motif (as for homeostasis), such that energy enrichment is associated with the left forebrain and energy expenditure is associated with the right forebrain, consistent with the respective roles of the parasympathetic and sympathetic efferent systems. In this model, the evolution of matching homeostatic afferent and autonomic efferent asymmetries in the humanoid forebrain provided another substantial improvement in the efficiency of emotional control and communication, thereby facilitating increasingly complex social interaction (and leading ultimately to deictic signaling, language, and civilization). For example, it implies that the homeostatically parsimonious role of the left insula in (parasympathetic) emotional affiliation may be the basis for the crucial association of left anterior insula (which is now included in Broca's area) in verbal emotional communication and the predominant use of the contralateral (right) hand in deictic pointing among humanoid primates (De Waal, 2003).

Coordinated opponent interactions between the two hemispheres, mirroring the autonomic principle of coordinated opponency, can provide a fundamental management process. The analogy of driving a car is useful: Rather than placing your hands at opposite sides of the steering wheel, it is more efficient if you place your hands at the 2:00 and 10:00 positions, because then you can drive by exerting a steady downward pressure with one hand and simply varying the downward pressure with the other hand. This is exactly how the coordinated autonomic control of the heart functions; tonic sympathetic drive is modulated by rapid variations in parasympathetic drive. I propose that the forebrain coordinates emotional control in the same manner. Notably, the salient purpose of homeostasis is optimal energy management, and the efficient use of energy in the brain, which overall consumes about 25% of the body's entire energy budget, must be a potent evolutionary pressure. This model instantiates neurobiologically the psychological proposal that a hypothetical "calm and connection system" opposes the arousal–stress system (Uvnas-Moberg, Arn, & Magnusson, 2005). It can incorporate the bivalent concept of emotion, in which positive and negative affects are different psychological dimensions, and also

the core affect concept, in which energization is a key dimension (Barrett et al., 2004; Zautra, 2003; Philippot & Chalelle, 2002).

Thus the model provides a structural basis for suggesting that coordinated opponent interactions between left and right insula and cingulate are fundamentally important. Positive and negative affect interact in an opponent fashion; for example, it is well documented that social engagement (and oxytocin) can suppress arousal, stress, depression, and cortisol release, whereas, conversely, the latter factors can reduce mood, sociability, and immune function (Heinrichs, Baumgartner, Kirschbaum, & Ehlert, 2003; Zautra, 2003). This model proposes that the relative balance of activity within symmetrical modules in the left and right insula and cingulate may be of critical significance for neurophysiologically coordinated emotional complexity, or mental health.

For further elucidation of this proposal, see Craig (2005). Recent findings add to the evidence cited in that article by showing (1) that asthmatic (vagal bronchiopulmonary) afferent activity is associated with left insular activation (Rosenkrantz et al., 2005); (2) that emotionally pleasing music, if chosen individually by the subjects, activates the left anterior insula more strongly than the right (Koelsch et al., 2006); (3) that a patient with a selective lesion of the left anterior insula experienced a selective loss of musical enjoyment (Griffiths, Warren, Dean, & Howard, 2005); and (4) that covert singing at different tempos produces a strikingly clear asymmetry in anterior insula activation, consistent with the temporal effects of sympathetic and parasympathetic activity on heart rate (Ackermann & Riecker, 2004). Finally, these considerations provide a solid neurobiological foundation for explaining how increases in parasympathetic afferent activity can synergistically enhance positive emotion and reduce negative emotion, for example by slow meditative breathing (e.g., Brown & Gerbarg, 2005) or by electrical stimulation of the vagus nerve (Nemeroff et al., 2006).

ACKNOWLEDGMENTS

I thank Lisa Feldman Barrett for her editorial suggestions, Martin Paulus and Alex Zantra for comments on the final draft, and the National Institutes of Health and the Barrow Neurological Foundation for support.

REFERENCES

Ackermann, H., & Riecker, A. (2004). The contribution of the insula to motor aspects of speech production: A review and a hypothesis. *Brain and Language, 89,* 320–328.

Adolphs, R. (2002). Trust in the brain. *Nature Neuroscience, 5,* 192–193.

Allen, J. J., & Kline, J. P. (2004). Frontal EEG asymmetry, emotion, and psychopathology: The first, and the next 25 years. *Biological Psychology, 67,* 1–5.

Allman, J. M., Watson, K. K., Tetreault, N. A., & Hakeem, A. Y. (2005). Intuition and autism: A possible role for Von Economo neurons. *Trends in Cognitive Sciences, 9,* 367–373.

Andrew, D., & Craig, A. D. (2001). Spinothalamic lamina I neurons selectively sensitive to histamine: A central neural pathway for itch. *Nature Neuroscience, 4,* 72–77.

Barrett, L. F., Quigley, K. S., Bliss-Moreau, E., & Aronson, K. R. (2004). Interoceptive sensitivity and self-reports of emotional experience. *Journal of Personality and Social Psychology, 87,* 684–697.

Berthier, M., Starkstein, S., & Leiguarda, R. (1988). Asymbolia for pain: A sensory-limbic disconnection syndrome. *Annals of Neurology, 24,* 41–49.

Boddaert, N., De Leersnyder, H., Bourgeois, M., Munnich, A., Brunelle, F., & Zilbovicius, M. (2004). Anatomical and functional brain imaging evidence of lenticulo-insular anomalies in Smith–Magenis syndrome. *NeuroImage, 21,* 1021–1025.

Brooks, J. C., Nurmikko, T. J., Bimson, W. E., Singh, K. D., & Roberts, N. (2002). fMRI of thermal pain: Effects of stimulus laterality and attention. *NeuroImage, 15,* 293–301.

Brooks, J. C., Zambreanu, L., Godinez, A., Craig, A. D., & Tracey, I. (2005). Somatotopic organisation of the human insula to painful heat studied with high resolution functional imaging. *NeuroImage, 27,* 201–209.

Brown, J. W., & Braver, T. S. (2005). Learned predictions of error likelihood in the anterior cingulate cortex. *Science, 307,* 1118–1121.

Brown, R. P., & Gerbarg, P. L. (2005). Sudarshan Kriya yogic breathing in the treatment of stress, anxiety, and depression: Part I. Neurophysiologic model. *Journal of Alternative and Complementary Medicine, 11,* 189–201.

Bushara, K. O., Grafman, J., & Hallett, M. (2001). Neural correlates of auditory–visual stimulus onset asynchrony detection. *Journal of Neuroscience, 21,* 300–304.

Cabanac, M. (1971). Physiological role of pleasure. *Science, 173,* 1103–1107.

Chikama, M., McFarland, N. R., Amaral, D. G., & Haber, S. N. (1997). Insular cortical projections to functional regions of the striatum correlate with cortical cytoarchitectonic organization in the primate. *Journal of Neuroscience, 17,* 9686–9705.

Coull, J. T. (2004). fMRI studies of temporal attention: Allocating attention within, or towards, time. *Brain Research: Cognitive Brain Research, 21,* 216–226.

Craig, A. D. (2002). How do you feel? Interoception: The sense of the physiological condition of the body. *Nature Reviews Neuroscience, 3,* 655–666.

Craig, A. D. (2003). Pain mechanisms: Labeled lines versus convergence in central processing. *Annual Review of Neuroscience, 26,* 1–30.

Craig, A. D. (2004a). Human feelings: Why are some more aware than others? *Trends in Cognitive Sciences, 8,* 239–241.

Craig, A. D. (2004b). Lamina I, but not lamina V, spinothalamic neurons exhibit responses that correspond with burning pain. *Journal of Neurophysiology, 92,* 2604–2609.

Craig, A. D. (2005). Forebrain emotional asymmetry: A neuroanatomical basis? *Trends in Cognitive Sciences, 9,* 566–571.

Craig, A. D., Chen, K., Bandy, D., & Reiman, E. M. (2000). Thermosensory activation of insular cortex. *Nature Neuroscience, 3,* 184–190.

Craig, A. D., Krout, K., & Andrew, D. (2001). Quantitative response characteristics of thermoreceptive and nociceptive lamina I spinothalamic neurons in the cat. *Journal of Neurophysiology, 86,* 1459–1480.

Craig, A. D., Reiman, E. M., Evans, A., & Bushnell, M. C. (1996). Functional imaging of an illusion of pain. *Nature, 384,* 258–260.

Critchley, H. D., Weins, S., Rotshtein, P., Öhman, A., & Dolan, R. J. (2004). Neural systems supporting interoceptive awareness. *Nature Neuroscience, 7,* 189–195.

Damasio, A. R. (1994). *Descartes' error: Emotion, reason, and the human brain.* New York: Putnam.

Darwin, C. (1965). *The expression of the emotions in man and animals.* Chicago: University of Chicago Press. (Original work published 1872)

Davidson, R. J. (2004). Well-being and affective style: neural substrates and biobehavioural correlates. *Philosophical Transactions of the Royal Society of London: Series B. Biological Sciences, 359,* 1395–1411.

Deary, I. J., Simonotto, E., Meyer, M., Marshall, A., Marshall, I., Goddard, N., et al. (2004). The functional anatomy of inspection time: An event-related fMRI study. *NeuroImage, 22,* 1466–1479.

Deichert, N. T., Flack, W. F., Jr., & Craig, F. W., Jr. (2005). Patterns of cardiovascular responses during angry, sad, and happy emotional recall tasks. *Cognition and Emotion, 19,* 941–951.

De Waal, F. B. M. (2003). Darwin's legacy and the study of primate visual communication. *Annals of the New York Academy of Sciences, 1000,* 7–31.

Greenspan, J. D., Lee, R. R., & Lenz, F. A. (1999). Pain sensitivity alterations as a function of lesion location in the parasylvian cortex. *Pain, 81,* 273–282.

Griffiths, T. D., Warren, J. D., Dean, J. L., & Howard, D. (2004). "When the feeling's gone": A selective loss of musical emotion. *Journal of Neurology, Neurosurgery and Psychiatry, 75,* 344–345.

Han, Z.-S., Zhang, E.-T., & Craig, A. D. (1998). Nociceptive and thermoreceptive lamina I neurons are anatomically distinct. *Nature Neuroscience, 1,* 218–225.

Heilman, K. M. (2000). Emotional experience: A neurological model. In R. D. Lane & L. Nadel (Eds.), *Cognitive neuroscience of emotion* (pp. 328–344). New York: Oxford University Press.

Heinrichs, M., Baumgartner, T., Kirschbaum, C., & Ehlert, U. (2003). Social support and oxytocin interact to suppress cortisol and subjective responses to psychosocial stress. *Biological Psychiatry, 54,* 1389–1398.

Henderson, L. A., Gandevia, S. C., & Macefield, V. G. (2007). Somatotopic organization of the processing of muscle and cutaneous pain in the left and right insula cortex: A single-trial fMRI study. *Pain, 128,* 20–30.

Hua, L. H., Strigo, I. A., Baxter, L. C., Johnson, S. C., & Craig, A. D. (2005). Anteroposterior somatotopy of innocuous cooling activation focus in human dorsal posterior insular cortex. *American Journal of Physiology: Regulatory, Integrative, and Comparative Physiology, 289,* R319–R325.

James, W. (2007). *The principles of psychology.* Retrieved from *psychclassics.yorku.ca.James/Principles/index.htm* (Original work published 1890)

Kano, M., Fukudo, S., Gyoba, J., Kamachi, M., Tagawa, M., Mochizuki, H., et al. (2003). Specific brain processing of facial expressions in people with alexithymia: An H2 15O-PET study. *Brain, 126,* 1474–1484.

Karnath, H. O., Baier, B., & Nagele, T. (2005). Awareness of the functioning of one's own limbs mediated by the insular cortex? *Journal of Neuroscience, 25,* 7134–7138.

Koelsch, S., Fritz, T., DY, V. C., Muller, K., & Friederici, A. D. (2006). Investigating emotion with music: An fMRI study. *Human Brain Mapping, 27,* 239–250.

Krubitzer, L., & Kaas, J. (2005). The evolution of the neocortex in mammals: How is phenotypic diversity generated? *Current Opinion in Neurobiology, 15,* 444–453.

Lieberman, M. D., Jarcho, J. M., Berman S., Naliboff, B. D., Suyenobu, B. Y., Mandelkern, M., et al. (2004). The neural correlates of placebo effects: A disruption account. *NeuroImage, 22,* 447–455.

Macphail, E. M. (1998). *The evolution of consciousness.* Oxford: Oxford University Press.

Maihöfner, C., Kaltenhäuser, M., Neundörfer, B., & Lang, E. (2002). Temporo-spatial analysis of cortical activation by phasic innocuous and noxious cold stimuli: A magnetoencephalographic study. *Pain, 100,* 281–290.

Manes, F., Paradiso, S., & Robinson, R. G. (1999). Neuropsychiatric effects of insular stroke. *Journal of Nervous and Mental Disease, 187,* 707–712.

Mason, M. F., Norton, M. I., Van Horn, J. D., Wegner, D. M., Grafton, S. T., & Macrae, C. N. (2007). Wandering minds: The default network and stimulus-independent thought. *Science, 315,* 393–395.

Mower, G. (1976). Perceived intensity of peripheral thermal stimuli is independent of internal body temperature. *Journal of Comparative and Physiological Psychology, 90,* 1152–1155.

Murphy, F. C., Nimmo-Smith, I., & Lawrence, A. D. (2003). Functional neuroanatomy of emotions: A meta-analysis. *Cognitive, Affective, and Behavioral Neuroscience, 3,* 207–233.

Naqvi, N. H., Rudrauf, D., Damasio, H., & Bechara, A. (2007). Damage to the insula disrupts addiction to cigarette smoking. *Science, 315,* 531–534.

Nemeroff, C. B., Mayberg, H. S., Krahl, S. E., McNamara, J., Frazer, A., Henry, T. R., et al. (2006). VNS therapy in treatment-resistant depression: Clinical evidence and putative neurobiological mechanisms. *Neuropsychopharmacology, 31,* 1345–1355.

Olausson, H., Lamarre, Y., Backlund, H., Morin, C., Wallin, B. G., Starck, G., et al. (2002). Unmyelinated tactile afferents signal touch and project to insular cortex. *Nature Neuroscience, 5,* 900–904.

Ongur, D., & Price, J. L. (2000). The organization of networks within the orbital and medial prefrontal cortex of rats, monkeys and humans. *Cerebral Cortex, 10,* 206–219.

Paulus, M. P., & Stein, M. B. (2006). An insular view of anxiety. *Biological Psychiatry, 60,* 383–387.

Petrovic, P., Kalso, E., Petersson, K. M., & Ingvar, M. (2002). Placebo and opioid analgesia: Imaging a shared neuronal network. *Science, 295,* 1737–1740.

Philippot, P., & Chalelle, G. (2002). Respiratory feedback in the generation of emotion. *Cognition and Emotion, 16,* 605–627.

Phillips, M. L., Gregory, L. J., Cullen, S., Cohen, S., Ng, V., Andrew, C., et al. (2003). The effect of negative emotional context on neural and behavioural responses to oesophageal stimulation. *Brain, 126,* 669–684.

Rainville, P., Bechara, A., Naqvi, N., & Damasio, A. R. (2006). Basic emotions are associated with distinct patterns of cardiorespiratory activity. *International Journal of Psychophysiology, 61,* 5–18.

Rainville, P., Duncan, G. H., Price, D. D., Carrier, B., & Bushnell, M. C. (1997). Pain affect encoded in human anterior cingulate but not somatosensory cortex. *Science, 277,* 968–971.

Rolls, E. T. (1999). *The brain and emotion.* Oxford: Oxford University Press.

Rosenkranz, M. A., Busse, W. W., Johnstone, T., Swenson, C. A., Crisafi, G. M., Jackson, M. M., et al. (2005). Neural circuitry underlying the interaction between emotion and asthma symptom exacerbation. *Proceedings of the National Academy of Sciences USA, 102,* 13319–13324.

Russell, J. A., & Barrett, L. F. (1999). Core affect, prototypical emotional episodes, and other things called emotion: Dissecting the elephant. *Journal of Personality and Social Psychology, 76,* 805–819.

Sanchez, M. M., Young, L. J., Plotsky, P. M., & Insel, T.

R. (1999). Autoradiographic and *in situ* hybridization localization of corticotropin-releasing factor 1 and 2 receptors in nonhuman primate brain. *Journal of Comparative Neurology, 408*, 365–377.

Sato, A., & Schmidt, R. F. (1973). Somatosympathetic reflexes: Afferent fibers, central pathways, discharge characteristics. *Physiological Reviews, 53*, 916–947.

Schmahmann, J. D., & Leifer, D. (1992). Parietal pseudothalamic pain syndrome: Clinical features and anatomic correlates. *Archives of Neurology, 49*, 1032–1037.

Schweinhardt, P., Glynn, C., Brooks, J., McQuay, H., Jack, T., Chessell, I., et al. (2006). An fMRI study of cerebral processing of brush-evoked allodynia in neuropathic pain patients. *NeuroImage, 32*, 256–265.

Seeley, W. W., Carlin, D. A., Allman, J. M., Macedo, M. N., Bush, C., Miller, B. L., et al. (2006). Early frontotemporal dementia targets neurons unique to apes and humans. *Annals of Neurology, 60*, 660–667.

Seeley, W. W., Menon, V., Schatzberg, A. F., Keller, J., Glover, G. H., Kenna, H., et al. (2007). Dissociable intrinsic connectivity networks for salience processing and executive control. *Journal of Neuroscience, 27*, 2349–2356.

Seymour, B., O'Doherty, J. P., Dayan, P., Koltzenburg, M., Jones, A. K., Dolan, R. J., et al. (2004). Temporal difference models describe higher-order learning in humans. *Nature, 429*, 664–667.

Sherrington, C. S. (1948). *The integrative action of the nervous system.* Cambridge, UK: Cambridge University Press.

Simmons, A., Strigo, I., Matthews, S. C., Paulus, M. P., & Stein, M. B. (2006). Anticipation of aversive visual stimuli is associated with increased insula activation in anxiety-prone subjects. *Biological Psychiatry, 60*, 402–409.

Sternberg, R. J. (2000). Cognition: The holey grail of general intelligence [Comment]. *Science, 289*, 399–401.

Tse, P. U., Intriligator, J., Rivest, J., & Cavanagh, P. (2004). Attention and the subjective expansion of time. *Perception and Psychophysics, 66*, 1171–1189.

Uvnas-Moberg, K., Arn, I., & Magnusson, D. (2005). The psychobiology of emotion: The role of the oxytocinergic system. *International Journal of Behavioural Medicine, 12*, 59–65.

Wager, T. D., Phan, K. L., Liberzon, I., & Taylor, S. F. (2003). Valence, gender, and lateralization of functional brain anatomy in emotion: A meta-analysis of findings from neuroimaging. *NeuroImage, 19*, 513–531.

Weissman, D. H., Roberts, K. C., Visscher, K. M., & Woldorff, M. G. (2006). The neural bases of momentary lapses in attention. *Nature Neuroscience, 9*, 971–978.

Wiens, S. (2005). Interoception in emotional experience. *Current Opinion in Neurology, 18*, 442–447.

Williams, L. (1980). *The dancing chimpanzee: A study of the origins of primitive music.* London: Allison & Busby.

Zautra, A. J. (2003). *Emotions, stress, and health.* New York: Oxford University Press.

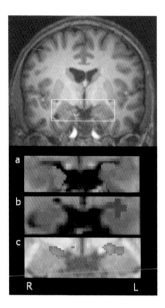

PLATE 10.1. Conditioned fear in the human brain. Above: Structural magnetic resonance image (MRI) of the human brain. The area containing the amygdala is within the box. (a) Fear conditioning. Functional MRI (fMRI) showing amygdala activation by a conditioned stimulus (CS) after pairing with an unconditioned stimulus (US). (b) Instructed fear. fMRI showing amygdala activation by a CS that was not directly paired with a US, but instead indirectly paired with the US via instructions to participants. (c) Observational fear learning. fMRI showing amygdala activation by a CS after the participants observed someone else undergoing fear conditioning where the CS was paired with a US.

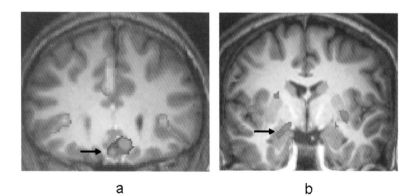

a   b

PLATE 10.2. Regions of activation during extinction of conditioned fear in humans. (a) Activation of the ventromedial prefrontal cortex (vmPFC) (arrow), indicating a decrease in blood-oxygenation-level-dependent (BOLD) signal to the CS+ (relative to a CS2) during acquisition. This vmPFC BOLD response increased as extinction training progressed, and the magnitude of this increase predicted the retention of extinction learning. (b) Amygdala activation (arrow) to the CS+ during acquisition versus early extinction, indicating that extinction training results in a reduction in BOLD signal to the CS+. This change in the amygdala response during extinction training predicted early extinction success. Adapted from Phelps, Delgado, Nearing, and LeDoux (2004). Copyright 2004 by Cell Press. Adapted by permission.

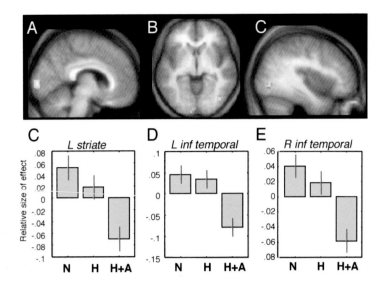

PLATE 10.3. Activation of visual cortex to fearful faces is diminished following amygdala damage. Statistical parametric maps of emotion three-group interaction (A–C) across the whole brain, showing the main effects for fearful versus neutral faces for patient groups in the (A) left striate cortex, (B) left and right inferior temporal lobe, and (C) right inferior temporal lobe. Parameter estimates for the relative size of effect in this analysis of variance (arbitrary units, mean centered) for peaks in (D) left striate cortex, (E) left inferior temporal lobe, and (F) right inferior temporal lobe, showing increased activation to fearful faces in both normal controls (N) and patients with damage confined to the hippocampus (H), but not patients with both hippocampal and amygdala damage (H + A). Adapted with permission from Vuilleumier, Richardson, Armony, Driver, and Dolan (2004) with permission from Macmillan Publishers Ltd. Copyright 2004.

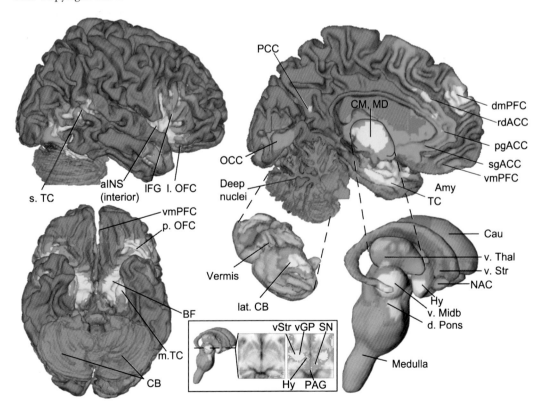

PLATE 15.1. Consistently activated regions in human neuroimaging studies of affect and emotion, shown as colored regions. Details are provided in the text. Abbreviations are defined in the text and in Table 15.1.

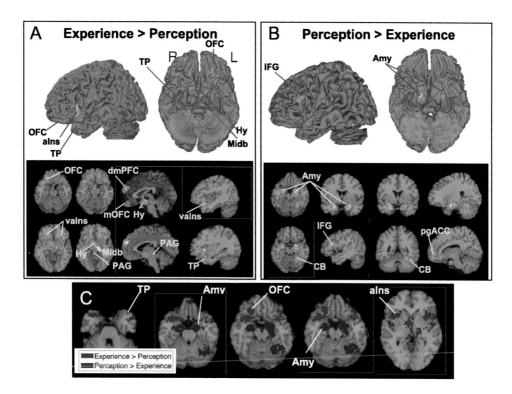

PLATE 15.2. Regions showing relatively more consistent activation for studies of experience versus perception (A) and perception versus experience (B). Some regions are shown on the same brain slices in C for direct comparison. Abbreviations are defined in the text and in Table 15.1.

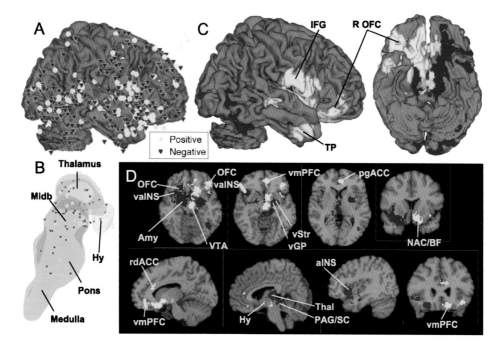

PLATE 15.3. (A) Reported activation coordinates for contrasts of pleasant experience ("positive," yellow circles) and unpleasant experience ("negative," blue triangles) on the right lateral surface. (B) Reported coordinates in the brainstem and diencephalon. (C) Significant regions showing relative differences in frequency of activation for positive versus negative (yellow) and negative versus positive (blue) comparisons. (D) The comparisons in C shown on brain slices to reveal subcortical locations. Abbreviations are defined in the text and in Table 15.1.

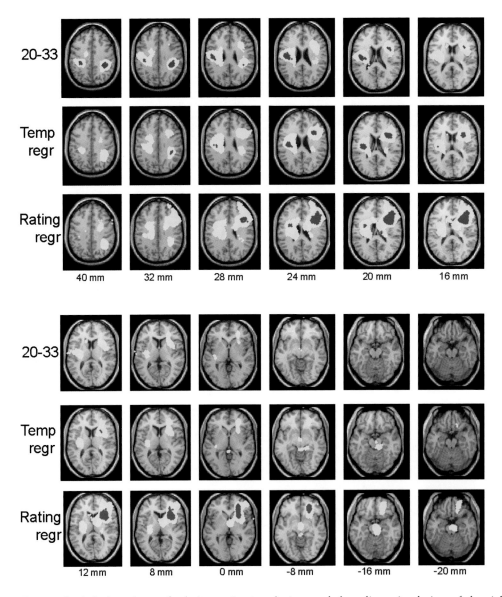

PLATE 16.1. Statistical analyses of relative activation during graded cooling stimulation of the right hand, showing the localization of primary discriminative thermosensory cortex in the contralateral (left) dorsal posterior insula (at levels 20 and 24) and the more extensive area associated with subjective feelings in the right anterior insula (levels 8 through 24) and orbito-frontal cortex (levels 0 and −8). The yellow and red blobs indicate two different statistical levels ($p < .005$ and $p < .0001$). From Craig, Chen, Bandy, and Reiman (2000). Copyright 2000 by Nature Publishing Group. Reprinted by permission.

PART III

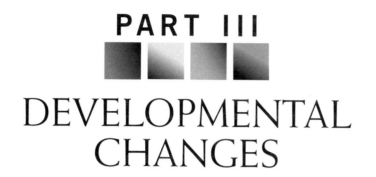

DEVELOPMENTAL CHANGES

CHAPTER 17

The Development of Facial Expressions
Current Perspectives on Infant Emotions

LINDA A. CAMRAS and SERAH S. FATANI

Although the relevance of facial expression to emotion is widely acknowledged, the nature of the relationship between them has been subject to considerable debate. Charles Darwin's *The Expression of the Emotions in Man and Animals* (Darwin, 1872/1998) is most often cited as the seminal work on emotional expression, providing a detailed account of expressive behavior across both animal species and human cultures. Darwin argued that expressive behavior in both animals and humans could be explained in terms of three principles: serviceable associated habits, antithetical actions, and nervous system excitation. According to the principle of serviceable associated habits, some expressive behaviors are derived from instrumental actions that can serve adaptive functions when carried out in their entirety. For example, one component of the anger expression (baring the teeth) originated in the action of biting. However, Darwin was notably ambiguous regarding the current adaptive value of emotional expressions and their relationship to

human motivation (see Fridlund, 1994, for discussion). Nonetheless, starting with Silvan Tomkins (1962), most recent and contemporary emotion theorists (e.g., Ekman, 1994, 2003; Izard & Ackerman, 2000; Izard, 1991) implicitly share the view that emotions are primary motivational forces in humans and that much of human behavior is organized in the service of emotion-related functions and goals.

In addition to advocating the central role of emotion in human motivation, Tomkins also revived scientific interest in emotional facial expression—a topic that had languished in the 20th century. As cogently reviewed and critiqued by Ekman (1982), several studies conducted from the 1920s through the 1950s had purported to find no systematic relationship between facial expression and emotion in either adults or infants. Nevertheless, Tomkins encouraged two young investigators, Paul Ekman and Carroll Izard, to pursue a series of studies on the recognition of emotional facial expressions in a variety of Western and non-

Western cultures. These investigations included Ekman, Sorenson, and Friesen's (1969) landmark study of emotion recognition by the Fore people, a preliterate New Guinea tribe. Since that time, considerable evidence (reviewed by Matsumoto, Keltner, Shiota, O'Sullivan, & Frank, Chapter 13, this volume) has been garnered in adult studies linking facial emotional expression to other components of emotion responding (in particular, self-reported feelings). Although there are vocal opponents to both the thesis of universality and the notion that facial expressions reflect one's emotions rather than more specifically serve as messages of social communication (Barrett, Lindquist, & Gendron, 2007; Fridlund, 1994; Russell, 1994), many contemporary psychologists still accept the premise that the prototypic emotional expressions described for adults are related to human emotions as motivational states.

EMOTIONAL EXPRESSION IN INFANCY

One plausible extension of the adult-based theories of facial expression is the proposal that a similar relationship between expression and emotion exists throughout the lifespan. Yet the implications of findings from the adult literature for the development of expressive behavior are not straightforward. More than one developmental pathway might lead to the outcomes reported for adults. In fact, as we describe below, a number of investigators hold that infant facial expressions do not correspond to adult-like discrete emotions and have proposed alternative developmental models.

In this chapter, we review a number of these theoretical models, focusing on three questions that are central to understanding the development of emotional expression during infancy and beyond: (1) How do facial expressions become organized during the course of development? (2) What is the relation between facial expressions and emotion-eliciting situations? (3) What is the relationship between facial expressions and other emotion-related behavioral responses (e.g., emotion "action tendencies")? These three questions are not unrelated. In particular, as described below, investigators often have sought to address the first one by examining evidence regarding the second and third questions across development.

DIFFERENTIAL EMOTIONS THEORY

Although several related versions of discrete-emotion theories have been proposed in the adult literature, only Izard's differential-emotions theory (DET; Ackerman, Abe, & Izard, 1998; Izard, 1991; Izard & Malatesta, 1987) includes an explicit developmental component. According to DET, each discrete emotion consists of three constituents—neural, expressive, and experiential—that operate as an integral hard-wired system. Following Tomkins (1962), Izard has argued that emotions (rather than drives) are the primary motivators of human behavior. Presumably an individual experiencing an emotion is motivated to pursue goals associated with its adaptive function. Thus emotions motivate the individual's selection and organization of behaviors around these adaptive goals. Selection and organization of such behaviors are also acknowledged to depend upon situational factors, the individual's personality, and other aspects of his or her developmental history.

As a core component of emotion, expressive behavior is generally not discretionary, but instead is an automatic readout of the emotion system. However, several important caveats to this principle are related to our three focal questions regarding expressive development. First, DET proponents acknowledge that some fleeting facial expressions observed in the first 2 months of life may not be expressions of emotion (Izard & Abe, 2004). According to DET, at this very early age the neural circuits involved in facial expressions at maturity are still lacking in infants, and infant expressions such as smiles during sleep or during transitional states (e.g., waking up from a nap) may reflect random central nervous system activity (Ackerman et al., 1998). Thus, in response to our first question concerning how facial expressions become organized, DET proponents propose that expressive reorganization occurs early in development as a result of neurological maturation.

The second exception to the automatic readout hypothesis suggests that expressive impulses sometimes may be too weak to produce observable expressive behavior. Presumably this might result in an absence of the predicted facial expression—but not in the production of a facial configuration corresponding to a different emotion. Lastly, according to DET, expression production may be regulated by older infants, children, and adults according to social and personal display rules that are acquired over the course of development. This is accomplished by overriding the automatic output of expressive behavior via a voluntary control system that exists separately from emotion. As a result, older infants, children, and adults may not always produce facial expressions corresponding to their true emotions. However, infants past the neonatal stage but younger than approximately 1 year are presumed not to exert such voluntary control over their facial behavior (Izard et al., 1995). Thus, in response to our second question concerning the relationship between expression and emotion-eliciting situations, DET proposes that observable facial expressions produced by infants during their first year of life may not always occur in emotion-eliciting situations, but those that do occur should invariably correspond to the elicited emotion. In contrast, older children and adults may voluntarily produce expressions corresponding to nonexperienced emotions.

Perhaps surprisingly, DET proponents have not specifically addressed our third focal question, concerning the relationship between infant facial expressions and emotion-related action patterns. Although DET acknowledges that emotional expression includes nonfacial behaviors (e.g., vocalizations), instrumental actions are not considered to be a core component of emotion. Thus relationships between facial expressions and action patterns in infancy have not been specified or subjected to investigation. Instead, as described below, the primary focus in DET-related research with infants has been on the patterning of emotional expression across development and the relationship between expressive behavior and emotion-eliciting incentive events.

To facilitate the study of infants' expressive development, Izard and his colleagues developed the MAX and AFFEX coding systems (Izard, 1995; Izard, Dougherty, & Hembree, 1983) for use in scoring infant expressive behavior and identifying facial configurations that are the expressions of discrete emotions or blends of such emotions. Using these systems, Izard and his colleagues have measured expressive behavior in response to a number of eliciting situations. In several of their studies (Abe & Izard, 1999; Izard & Abe, 2004; Izard, Hembree, & Huebner, 1987), they have reported that infants produce facial expressions representing appropriate emotion responses to

the incentive events. Izard et al. (1995) have also examined the relative frequency of full-face versus partial emotional expressions or blends in infants of different ages, as well as the stability of individual differences across infants in the production of various facial configurations. According to Izard's view, younger infants should produce more full-face expressions and fewer partial expressions or blends, because full-face expressions are presumed to be less controlled and regulated. Furthermore, morphological stability of the MAX-specified facial configurations across infancy has been reported (Izard et al., 1995) and is considered evidence for their sharing emotion meaning with the prototypic expressions described for adults. Lastly, Izard and colleagues have conducted a number of judgment studies in which they report that observers perceive the MAX-specified facial configurations to represent their presumed emotions (Huebner & Izard, 1988; Izard, 1971; Izard et al., 1995; Izard, Huebner, Risser, McGinnes, & Dougherty, 1980).

All of these forms of evidence are controversial. For example, Oster (2005) has pointed to important differences in the morphology of emotional expressions described for adults and those specified in the MAX and AFFEX coding systems. In addition, Oster's own judgment studies (Oster, Hegley, & Nagel, 1992) suggest that several MAX- and AFFEX-specified expressions are perceived as representing distress rather than discrete negative emotions. Other investigators (Matias & Cohn, 1993) have found that blends rather than full-face expressions are predominant during mothers' interactions with young infants. Lastly, observation of infant expressive behavior in response to a number of different eliciting situations has revealed patterns of expressive responses that do not appear to reflect the discrete negative emotions presumed to be experienced by the majority of infants. We return to these findings below.

DIFFERENTIATION THEORIES OF EMOTIONAL DEVELOPMENT

Prior to the advent of contemporary discrete-emotion theories, the most prominent view of infant emotional development portrayed ontogeny as a process of differentiation and integration. In 1932 Katherine Bridges published a highly influential monograph that dominated the literature on infant expressive development for several decades. In this monograph, she described infant emotions as originating in a state of diffuse excitement that differentiates first to generate delight and distress, and then to produce more distinct emotion states such as fear, anger, elation, and affection. More recently Alan Sroufe (1996) has produced a theory of emotional development that retains the notion of specific emotions deriving from less differentiated earlier reactions. According to Sroufe, the emergence of emotions can be described in terms of three developmental steps: pre-emotion reactions during the newborn period, precursor emotions during the first half year of life, and more mature emotions during the second half year. Although he describes these steps in detail only for joy, fear, and anger, Sroufe contends that the analysis can be extended to other emotions.

Differentiation theorists implicitly attribute the reorganization of emotional expression during early infancy to maturational processes. Thus their view of how expressions become organized (and reorganized) over the course of early development (i.e., the mechanisms of developmental change) is similar to that proposed by DET. However, in response to our second two questions, they describe very different patterns of relationships between facial expressions and emotion-eliciting situations, as well as between such expressions and emotion-related behavioral responses. Generally speaking, differentiation theorists have distinguished between positive and negative expressions and between positive and negative emotional states occurring early in development. However, beyond these broad-based valence distinctions, they do not propose a consistently tight correspondence between specific emotional expressions and the less differentiated emotional states that precede the development of mature discrete emotions. For example, Sroufe distinguishes between positive and negative facial expressions (i.e., smiles vs. distress expressions), but does not distinguish between distress expressions accompanying wariness (the precursor to fear) and frustration (the precursor of anger). Instead, wariness and frustration are distinguished in terms of both their eliciting circumstances and an infant's nonfacial responses (i.e., avoidance vs. diffuse attack). Thus facial expressions are systematically related to both

emotion-eliciting situations and emotion-related behaviors, but not in the manner proposed by DET (i.e., as involving a one-to-one correspondence between specific expressions and corresponding discrete emotions).

Because Sroufe has superseded Bridges as the most influential differentiation theorist, we present a more complete description of his model. According to Sroufe, neonatal pre-emotion reactions (i.e., smiling, distress) are automatic reflexive responses to quantitative, rather than qualitative, aspects of stimulation (e.g., temporal and intensity features of arousal). For example, smiling can be produced by gentle modulated arousal, while distress results from more intense arousal buildup. Because Sroufe believes that eliciting stimuli for these reactions can be identified that are somewhat analogous to the later elicitors of more mature emotions (e.g., physical restraint for anger), he considers these neonatal reactions to be prototypes for later-developing, more discrete emotions. Nonetheless, because Sroufe defines emotions as subjective reactions requiring some degree of cognitive evaluation, these early precognitive reactions are not themselves considered emotions.

Following the neonatal period, precursor emotions (e.g., pleasure, wariness, frustration) emerge. These are considered true emotions, because the infant has begun to develop the cognitive ability to process stimulus content; however, they are still regarded as precursors, because they involve only the simple cognitive process of relating present experiences to past experiences. Thus pleasure arises from stimulus recognition, wariness from recognition failure, and frustration from inability to execute a familiar (i.e., recognizable) behavioral routine. Of particular relevance to the topic of this chapter, Sroufe states that some precursor emotions are not distinguishable in terms of their facial or vocal expressive components. For example, wariness and frustration reactions are similarly manifested in crying and distress. After the first 6 months, basic emotions (e.g., joy, fear, and anger) begin to emerge. Sroufe views these as mature emotions, because they involve more complex cognitive evaluation processes. For example, fear is elicited by the perception of a threat, as opposed to a more general failure to recognize a stimulus. Fear and anger are differentially manifested in more specific behavioral responses (e.g., avoidance vs. diffuse attack).

Also of particular relevance for this chapter, Sroufe asserts that reliable differences in the facial expressions for these emotions emerge some time after the emergence of the emotions themselves. Thus Sroufe's theory is distinct from DET in its contention that there are not distinct facial expressions corresponding to distinct emotions at all ages. For example, according to Sroufe (1996), "few or no elements of the fear face are seen in the distress of wariness" (p. 65). Earlier and later forms of emotions and emotional expressions are related through their developmental history rather than through their morphology.

AN ONTOGENETIC VIEW OF EXPRESSIVE DEVELOPMENT

Focusing more specifically on expressive behavior rather than emotional development in general, Oster (2005) considers a broader range of facial expressions than either Sroufe or Izard does. Rather than confining her efforts to a search for the origins of adult emotional facial configurations, Oster seeks to investigate the infant's entire expressive repertoire. According to her ontogenetic view, an infant shows a variety of distinctive facial expressions that have important signal value within the context of the infant's world, going beyond or even irrespective of their relationship to discrete emotions. Because the adaptational demands of the environment differ for infants and adults, she argues that it is reasonable to believe that their emotional and expressive repertoires may differ accordingly.

Although Oster has not articulated a specific position on the question of how facial expressions get organized over the course of development (i.e., our first focal question), her view implicitly suggests that expressions are tied to emotion-related states from the beginning, but that emotion states themselves may change with development. In principle, this position is similar to Sroufe's, although Oster identifies a different set of emotion-related states preceding the development of discrete emotions (e.g., attempts by the infant to regulate negative affect). In response to our second focal question (regarding relations between situations and emotional expressions), Oster's discussion, like Sroufe's, implies that facial expressions are systematically related to situations that elicit these emotional states. Unlike Sroufe, Oster does not discuss relationships between expressions and nonfacial emotion-related actions on the part of the infant (our third focal question). Instead, she relies on analyses of the temporal patterning of facial expressions, their situational occurrence, and observers' interpretations of the expressions to make inferences about the emotion states underlying infants' expressive behavior.

As an example of her perspective in practice, Oster has studied the situational occurrence of "pouting," a mouth configuration that would be identified as a component of sadness according to the MAX and AFFEX coding systems. However, based on her observations, Oster proposes that "pouting" reflects an effort by the infant to regulate distress, and that the label of "sadness" fails to capture its more specific meaning and signal value. Examining infant expressions by means of her fine-grained Baby FACS (an infant-oriented version of Ekman, Friesen, & Hager's anatomically based Facial Action Coding System; Oster, 2006), Oster has also highlighted morphological differences between the discrete negative emotional expressions proposed for infants according to MAX and adult facial configurations corresponding to the same emotions (e.g., adult anger and fear prototypes). These morphological differences suggest that the meanings of adult and infant expressions may not be identical. In addition, Oster notes the broad situational occurrence of MAX-specified pain and anger faces that are often produced in the context of infant crying. Like several other investigators (e.g., Camras, 1991; Sroufe, 1996), she concludes that currently there is no convincing evidence that these MAX-specified expressions correspond to discrete adult-like emotions. Instead, they may reflect a more generalized distress reaction or a more specific level or type of distress that does not correspond to a discrete-emotion label (e.g., intense distress or modulated distress rather than "anger" or "sadness"). To determine the true meaning of infant emotional expressions, Oster advocates an empirical approach to expressive development that takes infancy itself as its point of origin, seeks to identify infants' repertoire of expressive behaviors, and attempts to determine their adaptive value for infants themselves as well as their ontogenetic relationship to expressive behavior in older individuals. According to Oster, whether or not this relationship involves a true differentiation process remains to be determined.

THE FUNCTIONALIST FRAMEWORK

The functionalist approach to emotion was proposed by Barrett and Campos (1987) to rectify discrete-emotion theories' tendency to focus narrowly on a set of core components situated within the person. According to the functionalist approach, an emotion is a relational process through which an individual attempts to establish, change, or maintain some significant aspect of his or her relationship to the external or internal environment. Emotions can acquire their significance via several processes. Perhaps the most important of these are social signaling (i.e., observation of others' expressive responses) and appraisal of the event's relevance to one's personal goals. The elicited emotion reflects the nature of that relationship and includes an open class of responses designed to attain (or maintain) a desired goal state. For example, an event appraised as involving a significant loss might evoke responses designed to recoup the loss or to acquire an acceptable substitute. Of importance, the specific responses themselves (e.g., crying, searching for the lost object, seeking comfort) are not predetermined by an innate emotion program, but are drawn from the individual's entire response repertoire in the service of achieving the person's particular goal for that emotion episode. That is, emotion responses are functional rather than fixed or preprogrammed. Nonetheless, the functionalist approach acknowledges that there may be intrinsic links between specific emotions (or emotion families) and particular responses (e.g., action tendencies, facial expressions, physiological patterning). However, these links are not invariant and are subservient to the context-dependent selection of responses designed to achieve the individual's emotion goals.

With respect to how infant expressions become organized (our first focal question), functionalists propose that this occurs in conjunction with infants' social development. Consistent with its overall conceptualization of the emotion process, functionalism views facial expressions primarily as social signals serving to communicate emotions to others, rather than as direct readouts of emotions themselves.

Thus regarding relationships between facial expressions and emotion situations (our second focal question), functionalists assert that facial expressions may or may not be generated, depending upon whether they would be serviceable in the particular emotion situation. Importantly, functionalists do not believe that the absence of facial signaling in an emotion episode necessarily reflects the suppression of "naturally" produced expressive behavior. Although expressive behavior indeed may sometimes be altered in accordance with social display rules, this reflects a change in the evaluation of the expression's functionality, rather than the suppression of an inherent automatic readout of the emotion. According to the functionalist perspective, socialization processes are important in establishing the conditions under which emotion signals (including facial expressions) are produced. Developmental changes in expression–emotion relationships reflect an individual's socialization experiences in conjunction with his or her evaluation of the effectiveness of expressive behavior.

In response to our third focal question, functionalists would propose an indirect rather than a direct relationship between facial expressions and other emotion-related behaviors. Because functionalists view all emotion-related behaviors as discretionary, co-occurrences of specific facial expressions and instrumental behaviors would not necessarily be expected. In fact, functionalists have argued that facial expressions and instrumental behaviors may be produced as alternative responses in emotion situations, depending upon the individual's assessment of their relative functionality. Thus, in response to our third focal question, functionalists would predict that relationships between facial expressions and other emotion-related behaviors might not be observed within an individual, but might be observed as substitute responses to the same emotion situation.

Functionalism represents an important advance in developmental theorizing about expressive behavior. Although it does not elaborate on the specific mechanisms of expression production (i.e., processes that determine whether expressions are generated, and if so, which ones), the functionalist approach has provided an important alternative to theories that focus on relatively rigid relationships among a set of core emotion components. It encourages investigators to view emotion as a more flexible system of responses oriented toward achieving an individual's goals.

A SOCIOCULTURAL INTERNALIZATION MODEL

More recently, Holodynski and Friedlmeier (2006) have presented an integrative model of expressive development spanning infancy and childhood. With respect to infancy, they propose, as differentiation theorists do, that infant facial expressions initially reflect precursor emotions (e.g., distress, pleasure, fearful tension) and are not selectively associated with discrete-emotion-specific causes or coordinated with emotion-specific behaviors. However, caregivers interpret these diffuse infant expressions within their contexts of occurrence and thus respond to infants with appropriate actions. At the same time, caregivers shape links between specific facial expressions and discrete emotions through their own behavior. That is, caregivers mirror infants' expressive behavior during their interactions with infants, but do so selectively and in exaggerated form. For example, when an infant cries in circumstances considered sadness-appropriate by the caregiver, then that caregiver may respond with an exaggerated sadness expression while offering comfort to the infant. That is, the caregiver displays both exaggerated (i.e., prototypic) facial expressions and emotion-appropriate motive-serving actions. Infants thus acquire these expression–emotion relationships, which are later reflected in their own expressive and emotional behavior. Holodynski and Friedlmeier's model therefore provides a clear proposal for each of the focal questions we address in this chapter. According to their model, socialization is the means through which diffuse expressions of positive affect or distress are organized into the specific facial configurations corresponding to discrete emotions that are selectively associated with emotion-related situations and behavior responses.

Holodynski and Friedlmeier's (2006) model incorporates a number of findings from the developmental literature regarding expressive mirroring during mother–infant interaction. At the same time, their proposals regarding the linking of discrete emotional expressions and emotion-specific functional actions requires further substantiation. In particular, given that

early social interactions may differ widely across cultures, further research involving non-Western mothers and infants is required to further substantiate their proposal regarding mechanisms of expressive development. Nevertheless, Holodynski and Friedlmeier present an intriguing model that has the potential to bridge the gap between infant and adult expressive behavior.

THE DYNAMICAL SYSTEMS PERSPECTIVE

Like the functionalist perspective, the dynamical systems approach to emotional development emphasizes flexibility in the organization of emotion responses and variability from individual to individual (Camras & Witherton, 2005; Haviland-Jones, Boulifard, & Magai, 2001; Magai & Haviland-Jones, 2002). Originating outside the social sciences, the dynamical systems framework has been proposed as a general model that can be used to account for the organization of complex systems of various sorts (see Kelso, 1995). Because it provides a unique and novel perspective on system organization and interrelationships among system components, the dynamical systems approach presents a provocative alternative to the theoretical models described above.

The dynamical systems perspective addresses the question of system organization (our first focal question) by asserting a broader principle of self-organization, rather than narrower principles of either maturational control or shaping via socialization (Fogel & Thelen, 1987; Fogel et al., 1992). With regard to relationships between facial expressions and both eliciting circumstances and emotion-related behavioral responses (i.e., our second and third focal questions), the principle of self-organization implies a flexible relationship among these systems components, as determined by the particulars of the situational context and the individual's developmental history. We expand upon these ideas below.

According to the dynamical systems perspective, emotions may be conceived of as "attractor states"—that is, frequently observed organizations of emotion system components (Fogel & Thelen, 1987). However, dynamical systems attractors may themselves involve considerable variability in their details. Thus in the case of emotion, the dynamical systems approach—like the functionalist approach—asserts that any specific episode may or may not include a particular emotion component (e.g., an emotional facial expression). Furthermore, at a lower level of analysis, emotion components themselves (e.g., facial expressions) may vary in their details. Such variability also may reflect the influence of lower-order contextual factors that influence the formation of an attractor. For example, Fogel, Nelson-Goens, Hsu, and Shapiro (2000) found that different types of mother–infant interactions are related to specific variants of infant smiling. Fogel, Messinger, and their colleagues (e.g., Messinger, Fogel, & Dickson, 1999, 2001) propose that such expressive variability engenders variability in emotional experience, because emotion itself emerges from the interaction of its constituent components.

Dynamical systems approaches are particularly concerned with processes leading to system change both across real time and across development (Fogel & Thelen, 1987; Thelen, 1989). According to this perspective, qualitative shifts in the organization of a system (termed "phase shifts") will occur when some key system component (termed the "control parameter") reaches a critical threshold. For example, Wolff (1987) observed that increasing the intensity of stimulus input sometimes itself produced a qualitative change in an infant's expressive behavior (e.g., from smiling to crying). Across development, a major reorganization of emotion responding may also occur when some developmental variable reaches its critical threshold. For example, a number of investigators (Camras, Oster, Campos, Miyake, & Bradshaw, 1992; Emde, Izard, Huebner, Sorce, & Klinnert, 1985; Fogel & Thelen, 1987; Sroufe, 1996) have noted heterochronicity in the development of infant emotional responses (e.g., the early appearance of smiles dissociated from other components of the presumed corresponding emotion). According to a dynamical systems perspective, such expressive components may become part of an organized emotional response when some (as yet unidentified) component of the system achieves threshold. Importantly, control parameters may differ across episodes occurring both within a narrow time frame and across development. For example, the intensification of either hunger or pain above a certain threshold may lead to infant distress. Across development, a major reorga-

nization of emotion responding may occur when motor development, language development, or some other developmental variable reaches a critical threshold (Campos, Kermoian, & Zumbahlen, 1992). Two unique features of dynamical systems models of change are these: (1) The system demonstrates increased instability as the control parameter reaches its critical threshold; and (2) as it approaches the point of transition, the system becomes more responsive to external perturbations. For example, as hunger increases, an infant may be more likely to cry in response to being accidentally poked by the caregiver.

Various scholars have applied dynamical systems principles somewhat differently to provide accounts of infant emotional development. For example, Fogel et al. (1992) view emotions as emerging de novo from the self-organized interactions of components, including some that are not emotion-specific (e.g., gaze, posture, instrumental actions). In contrast, Marc Lewis retains the notion that discrete emotions are preexisting hard-wired assemblies of expressive, physiological, and phenomenological components, but views these assemblies as components within larger self-organized dynamical systems (i.e., emotion–appraisal amalgams; Lewis & Douglas, 1998). With respect to emotional facial expressions, the former position implies that unique relationships between facial configurations and emotional experience should not be expected. The latter position implies that an invariant concordance between certain facial expressions and their corresponding affective experiences should exist.

Because advocates of both these positions can offer plausible (but different) sorts of evidence consistent with their view, we have sought to develop a third position that can accommodate the widest range of findings to date. This effort originated in Camras's (1992) observational study of her daughter's expressive behavior during the first 9 weeks of life. Initially adopting the perspective of discrete-emotion theories, Camras made a number of unexpected observations that could not easily be explained by DET's account of infant expressive behavior. Subsequent research (described below), as well as a review of the literature (Camras, Malatesta, & Izard, 1991), similarly revealed phenomena indicating that DET's initial account of infant expressive development required modification.

In particular, three anomalous phenomena were identified: (1) the systematic occurrence of codeable "emotional" expressions in situations unlikely to have elicited the corresponding discrete emotion (e.g., nonemotional neonatal smiling [Emde et al., 1985], "surprise" expressions produced by infants who were unlikely to be experiencing surprise [Camras, Lambrecht, & Michel, 1996]); (2) the nonoccurrence of emotional expressions corresponding to the emotion presumably experienced by infants (e.g., absence of fear expressions in infants judged to be afraid on the visual cliff [Hiatt, Campos, & Emde, 1979], absence of surprise expressions in infants judged to be surprised by an expectancy violation [Camras, 2000; Camras et al., 2002]); and (3) rapid shifts between MAX-designated facial expressions for anger, sadness, and physical distress/pain during bouts of intense crying occurring in response to almost any form of negative elicitor (including MAX-specified pain expressions in circumstances during which pain was unlikely to be experienced; Camras, 1992).

To explain these findings, Camras (2000) has proposed that infant emotions and infant facial expressions constitute overlapping but partly separate dynamical systems. More specifically, to explain the first anomaly described above, Camras and her colleagues (Camras et al., 1996; Michel, Camras, & Sullivan, 1992) drew upon dynamical systems research in the area of nonfacial motoric action, and in particular upon the concept of the "coordinative motor structure" (i.e., a grouping of muscle actions that are synergistically linked to each other; see also Fogel, 1985). Thus they proposed that infant facial expressions may sometimes be produced in non-emotion-related circumstances via self-organizing processes of recruitment among "lower-order" facial muscle movements. For example, Camras et al. (1996) showed that 5- and 7-month-old infants will raise their brows as they open their mouths to incorporate an object. That is, opening the mouth recruits a synergistically-related raised brow movement producing an expression of "surprise" in nonsurprising situations.

To explain the second set of anomalous findings, Camras (2000; Camras et al., 2002) proposed that facial expressions are nonobligatory components of emotion episodes and are produced only when their corresponding control parameters are present at the necessary threshold. In dynamical systems terms, discrete-

emotion attractors (i.e., larger ensembles of emotion components) can be variable and thus may or may not include a prototypic emotional expression in any one instance. This view is similar to the functionalists' notion that facial expressions are produced only when they serve a communicative function. However, dynamical systems proponents would recognize the potential for a broader set of control parameters (both social and nonsocial) to determine whether or not a facial expression is produced. For example, Michel et al. (1992) showed that infants raised their brows when looking upward to view an attractive object, but not when looking downward. In this case, head position and gaze direction served as "control parameters" determining whether or not the infant produced a facial expression codeable as "interest" in an interest-relevant situation.

To explain the third set of anomalous findings, Camras (1992) proposed that the facial configurations depicted by DET (see above) as reflecting discrete anger, sadness, or physical pain may represent negative affective states that do not correspond to traditional categories of discrete emotions. Like Oster (2005), she suggested that some of these expressions may reflect different intensities of a more general state of "distress"—in other words, negative emotion that is relatively undifferentiated with respect to distinguishable functional goals (e.g., removing an obstacle vs. escaping danger). Some forms of negative emotional expression also may reflect infants' efforts to modulate that distress (Oster, 2005) and/or the influence of non-emotion-related factors such as head position and gaze direction. For example, Camras et al. (2007) have suggested that differences in head position and/or gaze direction during negative emotion episodes may determine whether infants produces brow configurations associated with prototypic expressions of fear or sadness or anger.

Recent studies have continued to explore the relationship between negative facial expressions and negative emotion in infants. In a collaborative investigation of European American, Japanese, and Chinese infants, Camras et al. (2007) found that more 11-month-olds produced MAX-specified anger expressions than fear expressions in both anger/frustration-eliciting situations and fear-eliciting situations. Other mismatches between infant facial expressions and their situationally based predicted emotions have also been documented (Bennett, Bendersky, & Lewis, 2002, 2004). At the same time, some studies (Lewis, Alessandri, & Sullivan, 1990; Lewis & Ramsay, 2005; Sullivan & Lewis, 2003; Weinberg & Tronick, 1994) have found differential relationships between MAX-specified anger and sadness expressions and other components of infant responding. However, these important findings can be accommodated within both a discrete-emotion model and a model that links specific infant negative expressions to different levels of distress intensity and modulation. Because it can incorporate the wider range of findings reviewed above, we currently favor the latter interpretation.

Because at the present time there is no extant evidence suggesting that the "pain," "anger," and "sadness" configurations occur in infants when negative emotion is completely absent, we currently retain the notion of an invariant concordance between these expressions and some form of negative affect. This represents a compromise between the discrete-emotions perspective (with its emphasis on hard-wired relationships between specific expressions and specific negative emotions) and the purely dynamical systems view espoused by Fogel and his colleagues (a view that rejects the notion of invariant links controlled by preexisting emotion programs). However, we preserve the right to revise our present position in light of future research that may reveal examples of mismatches between negative emotion and negative infant facial expressions (e.g., analogous to crying from happiness in adults).

To summarize our view of expressive development, we concur with other dynamical systems thinkers in asserting that facial expressions and other components of discrete emotions develop heterochronically. That is, they are not initially associated with each other in young infants. We further propose that during the course of development, these facial configurations do eventually become linked to other components of their corresponding discrete emotions. For example, anger expressions become differentially linked to other components of anger rather than to more general distress.

Although the mechanisms involved in such a transformation are currently unknown, they may reasonably be proposed to involve infant–caregiver interactions such as those described by Holodynski and Friedlmeier (2006). Cast in dynamical systems terms, the control parameters producing a phase shift in expressive behavior would be embedded in such interactions. However, to justify employing dynamical systems concepts to describe this developmental change, researchers would need to demonstrate that such transformation involves the characteristics of a dynamical systems phase shift (e.g., increased instability and responsiveness to perturbations during the period of transformation).

Beyond these proposals, we also wish to suggest that a one-to-one invariant relationship between the prototypic facial expressions and other components of discrete emotions may never arise. In dynamical systems terms, discrete-emotion attractors (i.e., larger ensembles of emotion components) may be variable even in adulthood and thus may or may not include a prototypic emotional facial expression in any particular instance. In addition, as dynamical systems thinkers, we believe that prototypic "emotional" facial configurations may also serve as components of non-emotion-related "attractor states." Thus they may be systematically produced in non-emotion-related contexts (e.g., when women lift their brows and open their mouths to produce a "surprise" expression while putting on mascara).

FUTURE DIRECTIONS

Like the other theoretical perspectives reviewed above, the dynamical systems perspective has made a significant but limited contribution to our understanding of infant emotional and expressive development. Although it serves as a valuable heuristic to those seeking an alternative theory that can incorporate data not easily accommodated by other perspectives, currently proposed dynamical systems accounts are themselves incomplete. Thus, although we ourselves favor the dynamical systems perspective, we believe that it is premature to adjudicate definitively among the several theoretical approaches described above. Instead, we conclude by identifying some directions for future research that will enable scholars to develop their thinking further within each perspective and to evaluate the relative merits and limitations of each approach.

First, we believe that it is critically important for future researchers to more extensively document the factors associated with production of various emotional expressions across a wide variety of situations and across a broad developmental time period. This is an essential gap that must be filled in order to proceed to create an account of expressive development within any theoretical framework. To provide a specific example from the dynamical systems perspective, once we determine the age and circumstances under which prototypic fear expressions are produced, we can seek to identify developmental phase shifts and determine the relevant "control parameters" for this expression. Similarly, investigators utilizing other approaches can determine whether the eliciting factors for this expression are consistent with their own theoretical perspective.

Second, we wish to reemphasize our belief that a satisfactory account of emotional expression must also explain the variability described for the emotional expression prototypes themselves. For example, as highlighted by Oster (2005), several different facial configurations are included as "sad" expressions within the MAX and AFFEX coding systems, and these may have very different meanings. With respect to smiling, Fogel and his colleagues have conducted exemplary work in identifying contextual factors systematically associated with variants of this expression. Further studies should focus on explaining variability within the prototypic expressions described for other discrete emotions. One unique contribution of the dynamical systems approach to the development of emotional expression is to conceptualize both expressions and emotions as variable attractor states rather than fixed entities, and thus to motivate efforts to understand their variability.

In conclusion, we also feel it is important to emphasize that none of the developmental perspectives described above are necessarily inconsistent with findings in the adult literature of correspondences between emotional expressions and self-reported feeling states (Matsumoto et al., Chapter 13, this volume). However, we also call for studies that further explore the relationship between facial expression and emotion in older children and adults. By generating more extensive data on children's and adults' production of facial expressions in a wide range of circumstances, we can best ensure that our models accurately reflect the true relationship between expression and emotion throughout the lifespan.

REFERENCES

Abe, J. A., & Izard, C. E. (1999). A longitudinal study of emotion expression and personality relations in early development. *Journal of Personality and Social Psychology, 77*(3), 566–577.

Ackerman, B. P., Abe, J. A., & Izard, C. E. (1998). Differential emotions theory and emotional development: Mindful of modularity. In M. F. Mascolo & S. Griffin (Eds.), *What develops in emotional development?* (pp. 85–106). New York: Plenum Press.

Barrett, K. C., & Campos, J. J. (1987). Perspectives on emotional development: II. A functionalist approach to emotions. In J. Osofsky (Ed.), *Handbook of infant development* (2nd ed., pp. 555–578). New York: Wiley.

Barrett, L. F., Lindquist, K., & Gendron, M. (2007). Language as a context for emotion perception. *Trends in Cognitive Sciences, 11*, 327–332.

Bennett, D., Bendersky, M., & Lewis, M. (2002). Facial expressivity at 4 months: A context by expression analysis. *Infancy, 3*(1), 97–113.

Bennett, D., Bendersky, M., & Lewis, M. (2004). On specifying specificity: Facial expressions at 4 months. *Infancy, 6*(3), 425–429.

Bridges, K. M. B. (1932). Emotional development in early infancy. *Child Development, 3*, 324–341.

Campos, J., Kermoian, R., & Zumbahlen, M. (1992). Socioemotional transformations in the family system following infant crawling onset. In N. Eisenberg & R. Fabes (Eds.), *New directions for child development: Vol. 55. Emotion and its regulation in early development* (pp. 25–40). San Francisco: Jossey-Bass.

Camras, L. A. (1991). Conceptualizing early infant affect: View II and reply. In K. Strongman (Ed.), *International review of studies on emotion* (pp. 16–28, 33–36). New York: Wiley.

Camras, L. A. (1992). Expressive development and basic emotion. *Cognition and Emotion, 6*(3/4), 269–283.

Camras, L. A. (2000). Surprise!: Facial expressions can be coordinative motor structures. In M. Lewis & I. Granic (Eds.), *Emotion, development and self-organization* (pp. 100–124). New York: Cambridge University Press.

Camras, L. A., Lambrecht, L., & Michel, G. (1996). Infant "surprise" expressions as coordinative motor structures. *Journal of Nonverbal Behavior, 20*, 183–195.

Camras, L. A., Malatesta, C., & Izard, C. (1991). The development of facial expressions in infancy. In R. Feldman & B. Rime (Eds.), *Fundamentals of nonverbal behavior* (pp. 73–105). Cambridge, UK: Cambridge University Press.

Camras, L. A., Meng, Z., Ujiie, T., Dharamsi, S., Miyake, K., Oster, H., et al. (2002). Observing emotion in infants: Facial expression, body behavior and rater judgments of responses to an expectancy-violating event. *Emotion, 2*, 178–193.

Camras, L. A., Oster, H., Bakeman, R., Meng, Z., Ujiie,

T., & Campos, J. J. (2007). Do infants show distinct negative facial expressions for different negative emotions?: Emotional expression in European-American, Chinese, and Japanese infants. *Infancy*, *11*(2), 131–155.

Camras, L. A., Oster, H., Campos, J., Miyake, K., & Bradshaw, D. (1992). Japanese and American infants' responses to arm restraint. *Developmental Psychology*, *28*(4), 578–583.

Camras, L. A., & Witherington, D. C. (2005). Dynamical systems approaches to emotional development. *Developmental Review*, *25*, 328–350.

Darwin, C. (1998). *The expression of the emotions in man and animals*. New York: Oxford University Press. (Original work published 1872)

Ekman, P. (1982). *Emotion in the human face* (2nd ed.). Cambridge, UK: Cambridge University Press.

Ekman, P. (1994). All emotions are basic. In P. Ekman & R. Davidson (Eds.), *The nature of emotion: Fundamental questions* (pp. 15–19). New York: Oxford University Press.

Ekman, P. (2003). *Emotions revealed: Recognizing faces and feelings to improve communication and emotional life*. New York: Holt.

Ekman, P., Sorenson, E., & Friesen, W. (1969). Pan-cultural elements in facial display of emotion. *Science*, *164*, 86–88.

Emde, R. N., Izard, C., Huebner, R., Sorce, J. F., & Klinnert, M. (1985). Adult judgments of emotions: Replication studies within and across laboratories. *Infant Behavior and Development*, *8*, 79–88.

Fogel, A. (1985). Coordinative structures in the development of expressive behavior in early infancy. In G. Zivin (Ed.), *The development of expressive behavior* (pp. 249–267). New York: Academic Press.

Fogel, A., Nelson-Goens, G., Hsu, H., & Shapiro, A. (2000). Do different infants smiles reflect different positive emotions? *Social Development*, *9*(4), 497–520.

Fogel, A., Nwokah, E., Dedo, J., Messinger, D., Dickson, K., Matusov, E., et al. (1992). Social process theory of emotion: A dynamic systems approach. *Social Development*, *1*(2), 122–142.

Fogel, A., & Thelen, E. (1987). The development of early expressive and communicative action. *Developmental Psychology*, *23*, 747–761.

Fridlund, A. (1994). *Human facial expression*. San Diego, CA: Academic Press.

Haviland-Jones, J. M., Boulifard, D., & Magai, C. (2001). Old–new answers and new–old questions of personality and emotion: A matter of complexity. In H. A. Bosma & E. S. Kunnen (Eds.), *Identity and emotion: Development through self-organization* (pp. 151–171). Cambridge, UK: Cambridge University Press.

Hiatt, S., Campos, J., & Emde, R. (1979). Facial patterning and infant emotional expression: Happiness, surprise, and fear. *Child Development*, *50*, 1020–1035.

Holodynski, M., & Friedlmeier, W. (2006). *Development of emotions and their regulation: A socio-culturally based internalization model*. Boston: Kluwer Academic.

Huebner, R. R., & Izard, C. E. (1988). Mothers' responses to infants' facial expressions of sadness, anger, and physical distress. *Motivation and Emotion*, *12*, 185–196.

Izard, C. E. (1971). *The face of emotion*. New York: Appleton-Century-Crofts.

Izard, C. E. (1991). *The psychology of emotions*. New York: Plenum Press.

Izard, C. E. (1995). *The Maximally Discriminative Facial Movement Coding System*. Unpublished manuscript.

Izard, C. E., & Abe, J. A. (2004). Developmental changes in facial expression of emotions in the strange situation during the second year of life. *Emotion*, *4*(3), 251–265.

Izard, C. E., & Ackerman, B. P. (2000). Motivational, organizational, and regulatory functions of discrete emotions. In M. Lewis & J. M. Haviland-Jones (Eds.), *Handbook of emotions* (2nd ed., pp. 253–264). New York: Guilford Press.

Izard, C. E., Dougherty, L., & Hembree, E. (1983). *A system for identifying affect expressions by holistic judgments (AFFEX)*. Newark: Instructional Resources Center, University of Delaware.

Izard, C. E., Fantauzzo, C. A., Castle, J. M., Haynes, O. M., Rayias, M. F., & Putnam, P. H. (1995). The ontogeny and significance of infants' facial expressions in the first 9 months of life. *Developmental Psychology*, *31*(6), 997–1013.

Izard, C. E., Hembree, E. A., & Huebner, R. R. (1987). Infants' emotion expression to acute pain: Developmental changes and stability of individual differences. *Developmental Psychology*, *23*(1), 105–113.

Izard, C. E., Huebner, R. R., Risser, D., McGinnes, G. C., & Dougherty, L. M. (1980). The young infant's ability to produce discrete emotion expressions. *Developmental Psychology*, *16*, 132–140.

Izard, C. E., & Malatesta, C. (1987). Perspectives on emotional development I: Differential emotions theory of early emotional development. In J. Osofsky (Ed.), *Handbook of infant development* (2nd ed., pp. 494–554). New York: Wiley.

Kelso, J. (1995). *Dynamic patterns*. Cambridge, MA: MIT Press.

Lewis, M., Alessandri, S. M., & Sullivan, M. W. (1990). Violation of expectancy, loss of control, and anger in young infants. *Developmental Psychology*, *26*, 745–751.

Lewis, M., & Ramsay, D. (2005). Infant emotional and cortisol responses to goal blockage. *Child Development*, *76*, 518–530.

Lewis, M. D., & Douglas, L. (1998). A dynamic systems approach to cognition–emotion interactions in development. In M. F. Mascolo & S. Griffin (Eds.), *What develops in emotional development?* (pp. 159–188). New York: Plenum Press.

Magai, C., & Haviland-Jones, J. M. (2002). *The hidden genius of emotion.* Cambridge, UK: Cambridge University Press.

Matias, R., & Cohn, J. (1993). Are MAX-specified infant facial expressions during face-to-face interaction consistent with differential emotions theory? *Developmental Psychology, 29*(3), 524–531.

Messinger, D., Fogel, A., & Dickson, K. (1999). What's in a smile? *Developmental Psychology, 35*(3), 701–708.

Messinger, D., Fogel, A., & Dickson, K. (2001). All smiles are positive, but some smiles are more positive than others. *Developmental Psychology, 37*(5), 642–653.

Michel, G., Camras, L., & Sullivan, J. (1992). Infant interest expressions as coordinative motor structures. *Infant Behavior and Development, 15,* 347–358.

Oster, H. (2005). The repertoire of infant facial expressions: An ontogenetic perspective. In J. Nadel & D. Muir (Eds.), *Emotional development* (pp. 261–292). Oxford: Oxford University Press.

Oster, H. (2006). *Baby FACS: Facial Action Coding System for infants and young children.* Unpublished manuscript, New York University.

Oster, H., Hegley, D., & Nagel, L. (1992). Adult judgments and fine-grained analysis of infant facial expressions: Testing the validity of *a priori* coding formulas. *Developmental Psychology, 28,* 1115–1131.

Russell, J. A. (1994). Is there universal recognition of emotion from facial expression?: A review of the cross-cultural studies. *Psychological Bulletin, 115,* 102–141.

Sroufe, L. A. (1996). *Emotional development.* New York: Cambridge University Press.

Sullivan, M., & Lewis, M. (2003). Contextual determinants of anger and other negative expressions in young infants. *Developmental Psychology, 39,* 693–705.

Thelen, E. (1989). Self-organization in developmental processes: Can systems approaches work? In M. R. Gunnar & E. Thelen (Eds.), *Minnesota Symposium on Child Psychology: Vol. 22. Systems and development* (pp. 77–118). Hillsdale, NJ: Erlbaum.

Tomkins, S. (1962). *Affect, imagery, consciousness: Vol. 1: The positive affects.* New York: Springer.

Weinberg, K., & Tronick, E. (1994). Beyond the face: An empirical study of infant affective configurations of facial, vocal, gestural, and regulatory behaviors. *Child Development, 65,* 1503–1515.

Wolff, P. (1987). *The development of behavioral states and the expression of emotions in early infancy.* Chicago: University of Chicago Press.

CHAPTER 18

The Emergence of Human Emotions

MICHAEL LEWIS

Observation of newborn infants reveals a rather narrow range of emotional behavior. They cry and show distress when pained, lonely, or in need of food and attention. They look attentive and focused on objects and people in their world. They appear to listen to sounds, to look at objects, and to respond to tickle sensations. Moreover, they seem to show positive emotions, such as happiness and contentment. When fed, picked up, or changed, they show relaxed body posture, smile, and appear content. Although they show a wide range of postural and even facial expressions, the set of discrete emotions that they exhibit is rather limited. Yet, in a matter of months and indeed by the end of the third year of life, these same children display a wide range of emotions. In fact, by this age, almost the full range of adult emotions can be said to exist (Lewis, 1992b). In 3 years, the display and range of human emotions go from a few to the highly differentiated many, as well as from action patterns to feelings. In order to understand this rapid development, it is necessary for us to consider the set of issues that will enable a careful articula-

tion of their development. The first issue to be discussed, therefore, is the topic of the topology of emotional features. Embedded within this is a consideration of the development of these features. Finally, the developmental sequence over the first 3 years of life is considered.

THE TOPOLOGY OF EMOTION

In order to talk about developmental issues involved in the study of emotion, it is important that we first make clear what we mean by the term "emotion." "Emotion," like the term "cognition," refers to a class of elicitors, behaviors, states, and experiences. If we do not distinguish among these features of emotion, the study of them and their development becomes difficult. For example, Zajonc (1980)—and, more recently, Barrett (see Lindquist & Barrett, Chapter 34, this volume) and Niedenthal (see Chapter 36, this volume)—argued that emotions can occur without cognitions, while Lazarus (1982) argued that emotions require cognitions. As we shall see, Zajonc and Lazarus were describing different features of emotional life. Because of this, each could arrive at diametrically opposing positions without endangering his own argument. The reasons for this are quite simple: As we shall see, one was arguing for emotions as states, perhaps connected to action patterns and environmental triggers, whereas the other argued for emotions as experiences.

Emotional Elicitors

In order for an emotion to occur, some stimulus event—what I will call the "emotional elicitor"—must trigger a change in the state of the organism. The state of the organism can be a change in an idea, or it can be a change in the physiological state of the organism. The triggering event may either be an external or internal stimulus. External elicitors may be nonsocial (e.g., loud noise) or social (e.g., separation from a loved one). Internal elicitors may range from changes in specific physiological states to complex cognitive activities. Since it is obviously much harder to identify and manipulate an internal elicitor than an external one, it is not surprising that most research deals with external stimuli; that is, it attempts to determine precisely which features of the elicitor activate the emotion.

A major problem in defining an emotional elicitor is that not all stimuli can be characterized as emotional elicitors. For example, a blast of cold air may cause a drop in body temperature and elicit shivering, but one is reluctant to classify this occurrence as an emotional event. In general, we use our "common sense" to define an event as an emotional elicitor. Thus, for example, the approach of a stranger or experience on a visual cliff apparatus is usually the eliciting event for fear in the very young. The approach of a familiar parent is not used for fear, but is used as an elicitor to measure joy or happiness. Events that we use to elicit particular emotions grow out of our common experiences. Unfortunately, such experiences may not be correct. As we can see in studies on fear, not all children show fear at a stranger's approach (Lewis & Rosenblum, 1974).

The problem of the nature of elicitors becomes even more serious when we try to measure physiological reactions to emotional events. For example, in the presentation of a horror film and the measurement of physiolog-ical response to that horror film, one assumes that the elicitor is a fearful one. What physiologically appears is then taken as the response to fear. When subjects are questioned as to the nature of the elicitor and what emotions it produces, it is often the case that (1) they do not produce the emotion believed associated with the elicitor, or (2) they produce a diverse set of emotional reactions. Schwartz and Weinberger (1980), for example, asked subjects what emotions they had to a set of different events and found that they offered a variety of emotions for the same elicitor. Likewise, a colleague and I asked adults to mention the emotions produced by such elicitors as going to the wedding of their child or the death of a parent, and found that they gave a variety of emotions as their responses (Lewis & Michalson, 1983). Such research as this suggests that we have little information, excluding our common experience, in regard to the nature of emotional elicitors.

While from a scientific viewpoint little information about which emotions are elicited by which stimulus events is available, it appears to be the case that within a culture adult individuals seem to possess common knowledge in regard to how they should react emotionally to particular stimulus events. So, for example, at the death of a friend's parent, we know the emotion others either are likely to have or are expected to show. The script learning of appropriate emotions by stimulus conditions, whether these are "true" emotions or simply play-acting, informs us that knowledge about emotional elicitors and appropriate emotional responses is something that is acquired. In reviews of this subject (see Harris, 1989; Lewis, 1989), data on children's acquisition of such knowledge reveal that by the age of 10 years children have a good sense of the appropriate emotions for appropriate stimulus elicitors. The learning of these emotional scripts appears to take place quite early. For example, when children were asked to choose which emotional expression was likely to go with a set of stories that included receiving gifts at a birthday party, being lost from your mother in a grocery store, and falling and hurting yourself, children as young as 3–5 years were already capable of responding appropriately—that is, the way adults would respond to these same emotional scripts (Lewis, 1989). Learning what is appropriate vis-à-vis the culture is important for children, and they acquire such knowledge early.

Serious child maltreatment results in failures in this domain (Pollak, Cicchetti, Hornung, & Reed, 2000). The acquisition of such knowledge does not necessarily imply that the situations do not produce the emotions that are commonly believed to occur under such conditions. All that needs to be pointed out is the possibility that specific stimulus events are more likely to elicit some emotions rather than others. The emotion elicitors can be a function of what a child has learned in terms of how to behave, as well as a function of some automatic process whereby specific events elicit specific emotions.

Development of Elicitors

The problem of the development of elicitors raises an important issue: Namely, what is the relation between emotions (states, experiences, and expression) and elicitors? Darwin (1872/1965), arguing for the bioevolutionary approach, suggested that emotional behaviors or action patterns are adaptive responses to specific events (or elicitors). Thus one might suggest that anger is the result of a blocked goal, sadness the result of loss, and fear the result of uncertainty or loss of control. Izard's (1977) original differential-emotions theory held to this view, although there may not be as close to a one-to-one relation as he proposed. To test this view, my colleagues and I (Bennett, Bendersky, & Lewis, 2005; Lewis, Hitchcock, & Sullivan, 2004; Lewis & Ramsay, 2005; Lewis, Ramsay, & Sullivan, 2006; Sullivan & Lewis, 2003) examined 4-month-old infants' response to frustration. Darwin argued that anger is the action pattern that evolved to enable humans to overcome a barrier to a goal. After the infants in our study were taught to pull a string to get to see a picture, and after they had learned the response to the goal, the pull no longer resulted in the picture's coming on (frustration or goal blockage). Across many studies, we found that the action pattern most frequently associated with this elicitor was an anger-like face, increased pulling, increases in autonomic nervous system (ANS) response, and no increase in stress hormone. Children who showed not anger-like faces but sadness-like faces showed no increases in pulling nor in ANS response, but did show significant increases in stress hormone levels. Such findings support Darwin's idea that emotions—action patterns—evolved as adaptive responses to particular events (elicitors).

Although these studies of anger in response to a blocked goal appear clear in showing a perhaps innate connection between elicitor and action pattern, more work with other elicitors is needed. The difficulty is in the need to specify the elicitor carefully—a problem that is not readily addressed, and one that Gibson (1960) expressed concern about over 45 years ago in his paper on the nature of the stimulus. Unless we can specify the elicitor carefully, much difficulty in understanding emotional behavior and its development will continue.

It would appear, therefore, that there is a class of elicitors that has little developmental history. A blocked goal causes angry action patterns in organisms throughout their lives. The looming of a visual event causes startle and attention, and perhaps fear as well. The sight of food always serves as a positive elicitor, if one is hungry. It would therefore seem possible to imagine a class of events, biologically connected, that would produce a particular emotional state. Even for this class of more automatic-seeming elicitors, the developmental events of the organisms may be such as to inhibit or restrict the elicitors from operating in their natural way.

In the class of elicitors with a developmental course, the structure that supports the elicitor–response connection is likely to undergo change. Within this class are elicitors that are biologically connected to a response, as well as elicitors that are connected to a response through learned associations. For example, infants' fear of strangers may be biologically programmed; over time, stranger fear may decline because the biological structure supporting the elicitor–response connection has broken down or has been altered by experience. Learned associations between elicitors and responses may also be subject to developmental change because new structures are formed or old ones are extinguished; for instance, the formation of new structures can be predicated on cognitive changes. The data from numerous sources suggest that important cognitive factors play a role in mediating the effects of classes of events in the elicitation of fear (see, e.g., Campos & Stenberg, 1981; Feinman & Lewis, 1984). Several of these cognitive processes are considered here, and more could probably be added to the list. These capacities are regarded as critical and serve as examples of the role that cognitive development may play in mediating the development of fear elicitors. First, memory must play an important role in the elicitation of fear. Children must be able to recognize and associate past events that were noxious. The white coats of doctors may be associated with pain and thus acquire the capacity to elicit fear. In terms of cognitive expectancy, violation per se does not seem to be a fear elicitor. In fact, violation of expectancy may be arousing, and the particular emotion produced may depend on whether the organism can assimilate and control the event (Lewis & Goldberg, 1969). Some events that are uncontrollable are likely to elicit fear as well (see Gunnar, 1980).

Tracing the developmental course of elicitors is a difficult task to do. The development of other cognitive processes—categorization, classification, reasoning, and the like—is also likely to influence which elicitors produce what emotional responses; for example, failure in a task produces sadness in children prior to 24 months of age, while failure at a task after 24 months is likely to produce shame or guilt, as well as sadness. The same elicitor produces different emotions, depending upon children's cognitive capacity. Before children can evaluate their actions against some standard, the success at achieving a goal results in happiness. Once children are capable of this evaluation of self, the emotion as a consequence of the success is likely to be pride (Lewis, 1992b). Such findings as these alert us to several problems concerning emotional elicitors. These include (1) that specific elicitors may have an automatic biological adaptive connection to specific emotions, whereas others are connected through learned associations; (2) that individuals may differ in the extent to which the same elicitor produces different emotions; and (3) that the relation between emotional elicitors and emotional outcomes changes as a function of the meaning system of a particular individual.

Emotional States

Emotional states are inferred constructs. These states are defined as particular constellations of changes in somatic and/or neurophysiological activity. Emotional states can occur without organisms' being able to perceive these states. Individuals can be angry as a consequence of a particular elicitor and yet not perceive the angry state that they are in. An emotional state may involve changes in neurophysiological and hormonal responses, as well as changes in facial, bodily, and vocal behavior. As Darwin

(1872/1965) and more recently I (Lewis, 2005a; Lewis et al., 2006) have discussed, states are considered action patterns that include facial changes and physiological responses.

Two views exist concerning emotional states. According to the first, states are associated with specific receptors; indeed, they constitute the activation of these receptors (Izard, 1977; Tomkins, 1962, 1963). In the second, emotional states are not associated with specific receptors and stimuli and do not exist as specific changes; instead, they are general response tendencies associated with specific cognitions (Mandler, 1975, 1980; Ortony, Clore, & Collins, 1988; Schachter & Singer, 1962).

In the first view, specific emotional states or action patterns are postulated that have concomitant physiological components and that are expressed in specific facial and bodily behaviors. There is a one-to-one correspondence between an emotion, such as anger, fear, sadness, or happiness, and some internal specific state that matches this emotion. This view of specific emotional states has served, since Darwin's (1872/1965) initial formulation, as the basis of what we believe to be the correspondence between the specific emotions we experience and the functions of our bodies (see Niedenthal, Chapter 36, this volume). Except for bodily and facial expressions, no one-to-one correspondence has been found in adults between such inferred physiological changes and emotions. Investigators exploring brain function (Davidson & Fox, 1982; Nelson & Bosquet, 2000; Nelson & Bloom, 1997) and those looking at specific ANS changes (Ekman, 1989) argue for some correspondence between specific internal states and specific emotions. Even so, the evidence for specific states remains lacking.

The nonstate theories, cognitive in nature, argue less for a specific correspondence between an internal state and emotions; rather, cognitive activity is seen as the determiner of specific emotions. Either general arousal models, such as Schachter and Singer's (1962) model, or cognitive theory models have as their basic tenet a denial of the existence of specific states; rather, emotions occur as a consequence of thinking (Elster, 1999; Lazarus, 2001; Ortony et al., 1988).

Specific states, having specific stimuli that elicit them, have been suggested. The theory of innate releasing mechanisms (IRMs) suggests that animals will show a fear response, given a particular stimulus event. Thus one argument is that there is a direct correspondence between a specific elicitor and a specific state. Watson (1919) argued that there are specific elicitors in infants; fear is produced by a falling sensation or by loud noises. Likewise, attachment theorists argued that children show joy or attachment to the object that takes care of them (Bowlby, 1969). Anger as a consequence of a blocked goal has been shown in animals and infants.

On the other hand, it is quite clear that certain specific emotions can be produced only through cognitive processes. For example, certain elicitors invoke cognitive processes, which in turn may elicit or produce specific emotional states. In such cases, cognition is necessary for the elicitation of a specific state, but may not be the material of that state. Consider the emotion of shame. One must have certain cognitions for shame to occur. Shame occurs when persons evaluate their behavior against some standard and find that they have failed (Lewis, 1992b and Chapter 46, this volume). Such cognitions can lead to a specific emotional state, which is likely to have specific bodily activity. In these cases cognitions are the elicitors of the emotion, the state being brought into existence by thoughts; thus there are many possibilities:

1. An emotional state or action pattern can be elicited in some automatic fashion by certain stimulus events—for example, the case of fear when an animal sees a predator (IRM).

2. Emotional states can be elicited through cognitive evaluative processes. They may be automatic—that is, may be action patterns to certain thoughts. Darwin believed that the self-conscious emotions are elicited by thoughts about others' thinking about us. Plutchik (1980) and I (Lewis, 1992b) have argued for distinguishing between different emotional states by using the difference between the levels of cognitive activity involved in their elicitation. Fear of falling is elicited by little cognition, shame by much cognition.

3. Alternatively, there are no specific emotional states or action patterns, but only general arousal, which is interpreted vis-à-vis the events surrounding the arousal (Clore & Ortony, 1991; Schachter & Singer, 1962). In this model, there is an emotional state, but not specific action patterns associated with it.

What is clear is that even if there are specific emotional states, they may bear little correspondence to our emotional lives—either emotional expressions or our experience of emotions. So, for example, it may be quite possible to have a specific emotional state but to be unaware of it, ignore it, or even deny it. Likewise, we may have a specific emotional state but choose not to express it. Thus, for example, I may be angry at my dean for not giving me a raise, but I am not likely to express that anger when I see her. Emotional states, then, are inferred, and whether they are specific, general, or nonexistent awaits further research.

If we hold to the existence of emotional states, then for the most part they must be viewed as transient action patterns that are alterations in ongoing levels of neurophysiological and/or somatic activity. These transient, ongoing changes in our neurophysiological and somatic activity levels imply that there is a constant stream of change. It becomes difficult to imagine, therefore, being awake and not being in some emotional state or some level of arousal. However, since there need not be any correspondence between an emotional state and emotional experience and expression, there is no reason to assume that we are aware of the states that we are in. This does not mean that these states are not affecting our ongoing behavior—only that they are not apparent (Lewis, 1991).

Development of Emotional States

In a discussion of the developmental issues pertaining to emotional states, two issues need to be addressed. The first concerns the nature of the different states and how they are derived; the second pertains to the developmental course of states once they emerge. For example, if emotional states are viewed as specific, the question of how specific states develop needs to be addressed. Two general models are possible. According to one, specific emotional states are derived from developmental processes. Such processes may be purely maturational, or they may be interactive, involving the organism with its environment. The second model does not depict a role for development in the emergence of specific states; rather, discrete emotional states are assumed to be innate.

In the first model, the infant has two basic states or one bipolar state at birth: a negative or distress state and a positive or satiated state. Subsequent states emerge through the differentiation of this basic bipolar state. Differentiation theories focus on the modulation of both the bipolar state and general arousal state. Hedonic tone and arousal may be the dimensions necessary to generate specific emotional states. This idea was proposed by Bridges (1932) and is considered a differentiation hypothesis. This theory has been adopted by others, including Spitz (1965), and more recently Sroufe (1996).

The way in which the interface of arousal and hedonic tone develops into specific emotional states remains speculative. It has been argued that both mother–child interaction and maturation underlie the process of differentiation (Als, 1975; Brazelton, Koslowski, & Main, 1974; Sander, 1977). The regulation of the child's state may be the mechanism leading to differentiation. Although some theorists stress that emotional differentiation is determined more by biological than by interactive factors, the combination of the two forces seems most likely. While such a theory is appealing, the derivation of specific emotional states remains without empirical support.

A much simpler developmental model concerning differentiation can be considered from a purely biological perspective. Such a biological model can be imagined in which undifferentiated emotion becomes differentiated as a function of maturation. According to such a view (see Lewis & Michalson, 1983), the rate of differentiation and the unfolding of differentiated emotion states are programmed according to some physiological timetable. The differentiation from general to specific structures is a common process in morphology; there is no reason not to consider such a possibility in emotional development. The most likely explanation of emotional development is the differentiation of emotion states that occurs as a function of maturation, socialization, and cognitive development. Whatever processes underlie this differentiation, the model is developmental in nature.

An alternative model is that some discrete states are preprogrammed in some sense and need not be further differentiated (Izard, 1978). They exist at birth, even though they may not emerge until a later point in development. The view is unlike the differentiation model in that discrete emotional states do not develop from an original undifferentiated state, but are innate at birth in already differentiated form. In this discrete-systems model, specific emotion states emerge either in some predetermined order or as needed in the life of the infant. They may co-occur with the emergence of other structures, although they are independent of them. The emotional system essentially operates according to biological directives.

These different models address the conceptual difference between experience and structure found in the arguments of Hume and Kant. In one case, experience produces a structure (Hume, 1739/1888). In the other case, experience is assimilated into innate structures (Kant, 1781/1958). In the study of emotional development, the question is whether emotional states are preformed and depend only on the development of cognitions, or whether cognitions themselves produce the emotional states or structures. Such a distinction is rather fine, but has important theoretical implications. Such a distinction can be seen in the study of fear: Is each fear state the same as other fear states, regardless of the circumstances, or do fear states differ as a function of the elicitors? For example, is the fear state produced by a loud noise the same as the fear state produced by the association of a doctor's white coat with the pain of a needle? Are emotional states independent of or dependent on particular cognitions? If emotional states are independent, they need not be created by the cognitions.

The first issue in the development of states concerns the origin of discrete emotional states. The second issue focuses on the developmental changes in emotional states once they have emerged. For example, 8-month-old children may show behaviors reflecting fear at the appearance and approach of strangers, and 2-year-old children may exhibit fear behaviors when they have broken their parents' favorite lamp. Do similar fear states underlie the fear expressions in both cases? Although the elicitors of states and the children's cognitive capacities are different in these two cases, the underlying emotional states may be similar.

Major developmental changes may occur in (1) the events that produce emotional states, (2) the behavioral responses used to reference states, and (3) the cognitive structures of children. Whether the emotional state itself changes as a function of development is difficult to determine. However, there may well be important physiological and neural changes that differentiate young and old organisms. Given that important physiological changes occur over age, the physiological processes associated with emotional states may change over time. If this were the case, then the consistency of an emotion may be a function of our experience of it more than the underlying state. What is clear and what will be shown below is that the appearance of particular emotions may depend on new cognitions, as well as the fact that new cognitions may allow for the development of new emotions. The former case can be seen again in the example of fear. While 1-year-old infants may fear falling off a "visual cliff," they do not fear failing an exam or being caught cheating on their income tax. Such fears in an adult are due to elaborate social and cognitive development. An example of the latter—that is, cognitions producing new emotions—has to do with classes of emotions called "self-conscious evaluative emotions." These emotions, such as pride and shame, cannot occur until elaborate cognitive processes have occurred (see Stipek, Recchia, & McClintic, 1992). Although cognitions are related to new emotions, the materials of these emotional states or action patterns are not likely to be the materials of the emotional states. As such, it is hard to believe that experiences or even cognitions (thoughts) create the states. If that is the case, than states are a feature of human life having an evolutionary developmental history.

Emotional Expressions

Emotional expressions are those potentially observable surface changes in face, voice, body, and activity level. Emotional expressions are seen by some as the manifestations of internal emotional states (Ekman & Friesen, 1974; Levenson, Ekman, & Friesen, 1990). In fact, no single measure of emotional states or action patterns is more differentiating than emotional expressions. The problem with emotional expressions is that they are soon capable of being masked, dissembled, and in general controlled by an individual (Saarni, 1999). Moreover, emotional expressions are subject to wide cultural and socialization experiences. Thus the relationship between expressions and states remains somewhat vague (Lewis & Saarni, 1993). The measurement of emotional expression is reviewed in detail in other chapters, so I

spend little time on the definition of emotional expression except to make several points.

First, emotional expressions tend to be studied in terms of facial expression, and while body postures have been studied (see, e.g., Argyle, 1975), the study of children's emotional expressiveness in terms of body postures and activity has received little attention. Vocalizations are one of the least understood aspects of emotional expression, although they seem to be important conveyors of emotional states. Indeed, vocal expressions are extremely powerful and may have the ability to elicit similar emotional states in others. Vocalizations may be much more contagious than facial or bodily expressions. For example, movies are much funnier when seen with others who laugh out loud than when seen by oneself. Because of the contagious nature of vocalization, vocal expression may be the target of early socialization efforts. Crying is a case in point. Crying behavior is quickly brought under control as parents socialize their children not to cry when distressed or in need. Locomotion may be another mode of expressing emotions. For example, moving away from and moving toward an object are physical responses associated with different emotional states (Schneirla, 1959). Indeed, an infant's movement away from an unfamiliar toy or person, independent of facial expression, is often used to reference fear (Schaffer, Greenwood, & Parry, 1972). Interestingly, movement toward can be part of two different action patterns: It can reflect either joy or anger.

Although there are some data on emotional expressions in each of these four modalities (facial, postural, vocal, and locomotor), the relations among them have received almost no attention. It seems reasonable to assume that sobering, crying, and running away form a coherent response that reflects the emotional state of fear. The particular modality used to express an emotion may be a function of specific rules of socialization or of a response hierarchy in which one modality has precedence over another. Such a hierarchy may be determined either by a set of biological imperatives or by a set of socialization rules. The use of one or more channels to express a particular emotion may be determined by a complex set of interactions. One issue of particular interest is the effect on some expressions when one modality is inhibited. Inhibition in a particular modality can be experimentally produced, for example, by preventing a child from moving about. For instance, if children are prevented from running away from an approaching stranger because they are restrained in a high-chair, they may express their internal state more intensely through alternative means, such as changes in facial musculature. Another example of the use of differential modalities in expressing emotions occurs in the work on stress. We (Lewis, Ramsay, & Kawakami, 1993), for example, found that infants who do not express distress when pained by inoculation are more likely to show large adrenocortical responses. Suomi (1991) and Levine and Wiener (1989) have found that monkeys that do not show loud cries of distress upon being separated from their mothers are much more likely to show higher adrenocortical responses. Thus the relations among modalities of expression may play an important role in determining what emotional expressions are presented and the intensity of them.

Development of Emotional Expressions

The question concerning the development of emotional expressions takes many forms. First and foremost is the question of whether a particular emotional expression—the synchronization of a set of particular facial musculature movements—appears de novo or has a developmental course (see Camras & Fatani, Chapter 17, this volume). Izard (1977), for one, argued for their appearing as part of the adaptive evolutionary history of humans, while others (Camras, Lambrecht, & Michel, 1996; Oster, 2005) have shown changes in the facial neuromusculature synchronization. This controversy is all the more interesting, given that there are no theories suggesting how the synchronization takes place except for proposals of some environmental organizer. There are no data on how environments organize these muscle movements, although there is a suggestion that environments affect individual differences in facial expressions—that is, in the likelihood of an expression, given the same elicitor. For example, some infants show more joy than others at the approach of their mothers, and this difference may be a function of the infants' interaction with their environments. Even so, there is no evidence for environments' organizing the neuromusculature. Alternatively, the belief in a connection between elicitors and specific action patterns leads to the belief that the action pattern itself is a given, established by adaptive evolutionary processes.

Another issue related to the facial musculature question is the nature of the association among facial, vocal, and physiological behaviors that make up an action pattern. As described earlier, my colleagues and I have shown that an anger-like face, increased action toward a goal, lower stress response, and greater ANS organization appear to be such an action pattern evolved as an adaptive emotional response to the blockage of a goal. How does the organization of multiple modalities come about? The full developmental course of emotional expressions, then, is uncharted.

We are much more inclined to believe that particular emotional expressions reflect a specific underlying state in infants and young children when we see particular faces in particular contexts. Thus, for example, when children show wary or fearful faces at the approach of a stranger, we are more apt to credit those faces as meaning that the children are in a fear state than if the children show those same faces toward their mothers, who are sitting next to them. Faces, expressed in the context of particular situations, lend validating meaning to the connection between facial expression and internal state. Nevertheless, the question of whether a facial expression truly reflects an emotional state cannot be readily answered, except through phenomenological report.

Emotional Experiences

Emotional experiences are the interpretations and evaluations by individuals of their perceived situations, emotional states, and expressions. Emotional experiences require that individuals attend to their emotional states (i.e., changes in their neurophysiological behavior), as well as the situations in which the changes occur, the behaviors of others, and their own expressions. Attending to these stimuli is neither automatic nor necessarily conscious. An emotional experience may not occur because of competing stimuli to which the organism's attention is drawn. For example, consider the following scenario: The car a woman is driving suddenly has a blowout in the front tire; the car skids across the road, but the woman succeeds in bringing it under control and stopping the car on the shoulder. Her physiological state as well as her facial expression may indicate that while she is bringing the car under control, her predominant emotional state is fear. Because her attention is directed toward controlling the car, however, she is not aware of her internal state or of her expressions. She only experiences fear after she gets out of the car to examine the tire. Emotional experiences thus require people to attend to a select set of stimuli. Without attention, emotional experiences may not occur, even though an emotional state may exist. Many other examples are possible. From the clinical literature, a patient may be in a particular emotional state (e.g., depression), but may attend to select features of that state (e.g., fatigue), and so may only experience tiredness. Or a patient may not experience pain at the dentist when distraction is provided through the use of earphones and loud music.

An emotional experience may not necessarily be conscious, either. If one is willing to distinguish between explicit and implicit experiences, emotional experiences may occur at different levels of consciousness. Such an analysis forms the basis of much psychoanalytic thought. For example, individuals may be in an emotional state of anger. That is, with proper measurement techniques, one would find a pattern of internal physiological responses indicative of anger. Moreover, these persons may act toward those objects that or persons who have made them angry in a way that suggests they are intentionally behaving in response to an internal state of anger. Nonetheless, the persons may deny that they feel anger or are acting in an angry fashion. Within the therapeutic situation, such people might be shown that (1) they are angry, and (2) they are responding intentionally as a consequence of that anger. The therapeutic process may further reveal that unconscious processes are operating in a fashion parallel to conscious ones. Defense mechanisms, for example, function to separate levels of awareness. Although awareness may not be at a conscious level, unconscious awareness may still exert powerful effects. Slips of the tongue, accidents, and classes of unintentional conscious behavior may all be manifesting intentional unconscious awareness (Freud, 1901/1960). Thus people may experience their internal states and expressions and be aware of this experience, or they may experience them in an unconscious mode in which the conscious perception of the experience is unavailable.

Up until this point, we have assumed that there exists an internal state that is experienced. As some have argued, the experiencing of an emotion does not have to rely upon any internal state at all. In fact, no internal state

may exist. For those who do not believe in the construct of a unique set of variables marking a specific state (Clore & Ortony, 1991; Ortony et al., 1988), the experience of the state is nothing more than a cognitive construction, utilizing such perceptions as the nature of the experience, past history, the responses of others, and so on. Under such a view, emotional experiences are the unique and specific states themselves. From a cognitive-constructive perspective, such a view of emotions is quite reasonable. In fact, data on patients with spinal injuries suggest that emotional experiences can occur without specific physiological states. For example, patients with such injuries who are incapable of receiving neural messages from below the waist report sexually orgasmic experiences, even though no state information is available to them. They construct the experience from their past knowledge and not from any change in their neurophysiological state.

Emotional experiences occur through the interpretation and evaluation of states, expressions, situations, behaviors of others, and beliefs about what ought to be happening. Emotional experiences therefore depend on cognitive processes. Cognitive processes involving interpretation and evaluation are enormously complex and involve various perceptual, memory, and elaborating processes. Evaluation and interpretation not only involve cognitive processes that enable organisms to act on information, but are very much dependent on socialization to provide the content of the emotional experience. The particular socialization rules are little studied and not well understood (Lewis & Saarni, 1985; Saarni, 1999).

Not all theories of emotional experience need be tied to the context, nor do all suggest that there is an underlying emotional state. However, all emotional experience does involve an evaluative interpretive process, including the interpretation of internal states, context, behavior of others, and meaning given by the culture.

Development of Emotional Experiences

The development of emotional experiences is one of the least understood aspects of emotion. Emotional experiences require an organism to possess some fundamental cognitive abilities, including the ability to perceive and discriminate, recall, associate, and compare. Emotional experiences also require a particular cognitive ability—that is, the development of a concept of self. Emotional experiences take the linguistic form "I am frightened" or "I am happy." In all cases, the subject and object are the same: that is, oneself. Until an organism is capable of objective self-awareness (Duval & Wicklund, 1972), the ability to experience may be lacking. Emotional experience requires both general cognitive capacities—something I touch upon below—and the specific cognitive capacity of self-referential behavior, or what I have referred to as "consciousness" (Lewis, 1992b, 2003b).

General cognitive processes necessary for organisms to perceive and discriminate elicitors of particular behaviors (whether these be internal or external to them), as well as overt emotional expressions of themselves and of others, have a developmental course. For example, infants younger than 6 months are generally unable to discriminate between facial patterns and do so on the basis of discrete features (Caron, Caron, & Myers, 1982). Schaffer (1974) demonstrated that children cannot make simultaneous comparisons prior to 7 or 8 months of age. This would suggest that infants are not capable of experiencing emotions prior to this point. Moreover, some emotional experiences may require a higher level of cognitive processing than others, and some are likely to develop earlier than others. For example, fear probably emerges earlier than shame, since the former requires less cognitive and evaluative processing than the latter (Lewis, 1992b).

If emotional experience is the consequence of an evaluation of one's bodily changes, and also of the context and the behaviors of others, then two processes are necessary for most emotional experiences: (1) the knowledge that the bodily changes are uniquely different from other changes (i.e., they are internal rather than external), and (2) the evaluation of these changes. The internal–external distinction for emotional development is important, because it addresses the differences between experience and expression. If we believe that facial expression is equivalent to an emotional state or experience, then it is possible to infer an internal event by examining its external manifestation. If, however, we do not subscribe to the view of a one-to-one correspondence between expression and experience, then all we can say is that there is an external manifestation of some unperceived internal event. Emotional experi-

ences, by nature, are internal events. Moreover, the internal and external distinction can only be carried out by a self capable of making the distinction between the self and the other. Such evaluation may involve the process of self-awareness.

Self-awareness is an information-processing and decision-making event related to internal stimuli. It logically requires an organism to possess the notion of agency (Lewis, 2003a). The term "agency" refers to that aspect of action that makes reference to the cause of the action—not only who or what is causing the stimulus to change, but who is evaluating it. The stimulus change itself may have the effect of alerting the organism and forcing it to make some type of evaluation. Emotional experience requires that the organism be capable of attending to itself. Thus the statement "I am happy" implies two things: first, that I have an internal state called happiness, and second, that I perceive that internal state of myself. Until organisms are capable of this cognitive capacity, they should not be capable of emotional experiences (Lewis, 2003b, 2005b; Lewis & Brooks-Gunn, 1978, 1979). This does not mean that infants, prior to acquiring an objective self or consciousness of the self, do not have unique emotional states; they do. What seems reasonable to postulate is that an individual can be in a particular emotional state and yet not experience it. Just as we have seen in the example of the woman whose car slides off the road, an emotional state can exist without experience, so we can imagine an infant's having an emotional state without being able to experience it. This leads to the rather peculiar proposition that a child can be in a state of pain or can be in a state of fear, yet not experience that state, if by "experiencing it" we mean being able to make reference to the self as having that state. In a series of studies, my collaborators and I have demonstrated that the emergence of this self-conscious process does not occur prior to 15 months of age, and that it seems to emerge mostly as a function of maturation in the second half of the second year of life. It is only then that children can be both in a particular emotional state and can be said to experience that state. Moreover, the production of certain states requires self-awareness; therefore, certain emotions are unlikely to occur until this cognitive process emerges (Lewis, Sullivan, Stanger, & Weiss, 1989).

Once the basic cognitive processes that allow for objective self-awareness or consciousness occur, organisms are capable of experiencing emotions. As I have pointed out, they may be capable of experiencing existing emotional states as well as capable of experiencing emotions that have no internal state, either because internal emotional states do not exist or because the organisms are experiencing a different emotional state from that which exists. The rules that govern how we experience our emotional states or how we create emotional experiences themselves are complex and varied. Clearly, socialization rules are involved, on a cultural as well as on a familiar or individual level. For example, in cultures that do not tolerate interpersonal aggression—Japan, for example—the experiencing of anger is culturally inappropriate. It may be the case that Japanese children or adults may act in an angry way and may even have an emotional state of anger. However, because having such a state is inappropriate, they are not likely to have the emotional experience of anger. Exactly how the socialization process proceeds so as to influence, modify, alter, or accent emotional experiences is little understood. Clearly, the topic of the socialization of emotion involves the socialization of at least all four features of emotion discussed here. It affects the meaning of stimuli and what we allow events to do in terms of acting as elicitors of particular emotions. It affects the emotional-expressiveness dimension of emotion, and, finally, it affects the emotional experience.

From an interpersonal and intrapersonal point of view, the socialization rules that act on the experiencing of emotion are somewhat better articulated. Freud's theory of the unconscious and of defense mechanisms addresses this point. Defense mechanisms have as their chief function preventing individuals from experiencing emotions or, alternatively, from having emotions that they do not like to have. For example, denial and repression serve the function of preventing people from having particular emotional experiences that they deem unacceptable. They prevent it by not allowing them to become conscious or self-aware. Projection, on the other hand, allows for the experiencing of the emotion—not as the self's experiencing it, however, but as the self's experiencing it in another. As we can see in each defense mechanism, the major function is to provide means for altering emotional experience.

REINTEGRATING EMOTIONAL LIFE

In the preceding discussion, I focused upon specific features of emotional life in order to see how the developmental process can affect each of these components. Unfortunately, the focus on individual features does a disservice to the complexity of emotional life. Moreover, it does not allow us to look at developmental issues that may be related to the relationships between various components, such as the relation between emotional expression and state (Lewis & Michalson, 1983). Very early in life, emotional expressions and states may have little correspondence. At some point in development, there appears to be some coherence between emotional states and expressions—a young child smiling with joy at someone's joke. With socialization and further development, the disassembling of expression from internal state takes place. Children very quickly learn to detach expression from states, and thus to dissemble: Children as young as 2½ years of age are quite capable of successfully lying about committing a transgression, through verbal response as well as through facial response (Lewis, 1993). Thus there is a developmental course in the connection between expression and state. A similar analysis can be made for the coherence between internal state and experience. Earlier in the developmental process, children may have internal states that they do not experience. There may then be a period in which internal states and experiences form some coherence, only to change once again so that experiences of emotion can take place without internal states. These developmental sequences in the coherence between features of emotional life need more careful study.

A MODEL OF EMOTIONAL DEVELOPMENT

In what follows, I present a model of the emergence of different emotions over the first 3 years of life. I choose this period because it represents the major developmental leap of the majority of adult emotions in emotional development. This is not to say that past 3 years of age other emotions do not emerge, or that the emotions that have emerged are not elaborated more fully. I suspect that both are the case.

One problem with articulating a model of the emergence of emotional life has to do with the appropriate markers for the emotions. Are we making reference solely to emotional expressions, or are we talking about emotional states or experiences? The ability to do more than observe the emitted behaviors of the child is needed, but behavioral observation is often all that is possible. In order to get at emotional experiences, we need language in the form of "I am sad" or "I am ashamed." Since during this period the language of the child is quite limited, the study of emotional experience is difficult. Likewise, the study of emotional-state development is difficult because there has been little success to date in finding unique configurations of neurophysiological measures that mark unique emotions in adults, let alone children and infants.

What we are left observing are emotional expressions and behaviors in context. Observation of a behavior in context allows us, at least from the adult meaning system, to assume that the child's expression reflects an emotion. Observation of fear over the approach of a stranger, or joy when a mother appears, allows us to accept that an internal state of fear or joy exists. With these limitations in mind, the following discussion and mapping of emotional development can take place.

Following Bridges (1932), as well as others, we assume that at birth the child shows a bipolar emotional life. On the one hand, there is general distress marked by crying and irritability. On the other hand, there is pleasure marked by satiation, attention, and responsivity to the environment. Attention to/interest in the environment appears from the beginning of life, and we can place this in the positive pole; or, if we choose, we can separate this, thus suggesting a tripartite division with pleasure at one end, distress at the other, and interest as a separate dimension (Lewis & Michalson, 1983; see Figure 18.1).

By 3 months, joy emerges. Infants start to smile and appear to show excitement/happiness when confronted with familiar events, such as faces of people they know or even unfamiliar faces. Also by 3 months, sadness emerges, especially around the withdrawal of positive stimulus events. Three-month-old children show sadness when their mothers stop interacting with them. Disgust also appears in its primitive form—a spitting out and getting rid of unpleasant-tasting objects placed in the mouth. Thus by 3 months children are already showing interest, joy, sadness, and disgust, and

exhibiting these expressions in appropriate contexts.

Anger has been reported to emerge between 4 and 6 months (Stenberg, Campos, & Emde, 1983). Anger is manifested when children are frustrated—in particular, when their hands and arms are pinned down and they are prevented from moving. However, we (Lewis et al., 1990) have shown anger in 2-month-old infants when a learned instrumental act was removed. This study demonstrates the earliest known emergence of anger. Anger is a particularly interesting emotion, since, from Darwin (1872/1965) on, it has been associated with unique cognitive capacity. Anger is thought to be both a facial and motor/body response designed to overcome an obstacle. Notice that in this definition of anger the organism must have some knowledge regarding the instrumental activity toward a goal. For anger to be adaptive, it must be a response that attempts to overcome a barrier blocking a goal. In some sense, then, means–ends knowledge must be available, and the demonstration of anger at this early point in life reflects the child's early knowledge acquisition relative to this ability (Lewis, 1991).

Fearfulness seems to emerge still later. Again, fearfulness reflects further cognitive development. Schaffer (1974) has shown that in order for children to show fear, they must be capable of comparing the event that frightens them with some other event; for instance, in stranger fear, infants have to compare the face of a stranger to their internal representation or memory of faces. Fear occurs when the face is found to be discrepant or unfamiliar relative to all other faces that the child remembers. Children's ability to show fearfulness, therefore, does not seem to emerge until this comparison ability emerges. Children begin to show this behavior at about 7–8 months, although it has been reported by some to occur even earlier, especially in children who seem to be precocious. In the first 8–9 months of life, children's emotional behavior reflects the emergence of the six early emotions, called by some "primary emotions" or "basic emotions" (see, e.g., Izard, 1978; Tomkins, 1962).

Surprise also appears in the first 6 months of life. Children show surprise when there are violations of expected events; for example, when infants see a midget (a small adult) walking toward them, they are reported to show interest and surprise rather than fear or joy (Brooks & Lewis, 1976). Surprise can be seen either when

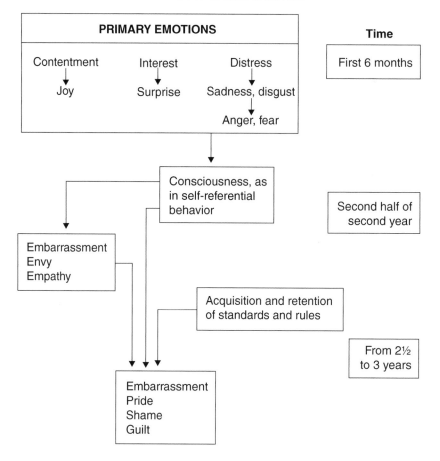

FIGURE 18.1. Development of emotions over the first 3 years of life.

there is violation of expectancy or as a response to discovery, as in an "Aha!" experience. We (Lewis, Sullivan, & Michalson, 1984) showed that when children were taught an instrumental arm-pulling response, they showed surprise at the point when they discovered that the arm pull could turn on a slide. Surprise can reflect either a violation or a confirmation of expectancy. Cognitive processes play an important role in the emergence of these early emotions, even though the cognitive processes are limited; this is not so for the next class of emotions.

Figure 18.1 indicates that a new cognitive capacity emerges somewhere in the second half of the second year of life. The emergence of consciousness or objective self-awareness (self-referential behavior) gives rise to a new class of emotions. These have been called "self-conscious emotions" and include embarrassment, empathy, and envy. Although little work exists in the development of these emotions,

several studies support the emergence of embarrassment at this point in development. We (Lewis et al., 1989) have shown that the emergence of embarrassment only takes place after consciousness or self-recognition occurs. Empathy, too, emerges in relation to self-recognition (Bischof-Köhler, 1991).

Two points are to be noticed about this class of emotions. First, the observation of these emotions requires measuring not only facial expressions, but also bodily and vocal behaviors. Whereas the earlier emotions can be observed readily in specific facial configurations, these new emotions require measurement of bodily behaviors. Embarrassment, for example, is best measured by nervous touching, smiling, gaze aversion, and return behaviors. The second important point related to the emergence of these emotions is that while they reflect self-consciousness, they do not require self-evaluation. The emergence of these self-conscious emotions is related uniquely to the cognitive milestone of paying attention to the self. This topic is taken up in more detail in another chapter (see Lewis, Chapter 46, this volume).

Figure 18.1 also shows a second cognitive milestone, which occurs sometime between 2 and 3 years of age. This ability is characterized by children's capacity to evaluate their behavior against a standard; the standard can be either external, as in the case of parental or teacher sanction or praise, or internal, as in the case of children's developing their own standards. This capacity to evaluate personal behavior in relation to a standard develops in the third year of life, and it gives rise to another set of emotions. We have called these "self-conscious evaluative emotions"; they include pride, shame, and guilt, among others. These emotions require that children have a sense of self and be capable of comparing their own behavior against standards. If children fail vis-à-vis the standard, they are likely to feel shame, guilt, or regret. If they succeed, they are likely to feel pride (Lewis, 1992a). It is important to note that pride and shame are quite different from happiness and sadness. For example, we can win a lottery and feel quite happy about winning the money; however, we would not feel pride, because we would not view the winning of the lottery as having anything to do with our behavior. The same is true for failure; we might feel sad if we were not able to do something, but if it was not our fault, then we would not feel shame or guilt. These complex social-evaluative emotions make their appearance at about 3 years of age (see Lewis, 1992b; Stipek et al., 1992).

Thus, by 3 years of age, the emotional life of a child has become highly differentiated. From the original tripartite set of emotions, the child comes within 3 years to possess an elaborate and complex emotional system. While the emotional life of the 3-year-old will continue to be elaborated and will expand, the basic structures necessary for this expansion have already been formed. New experiences, additional meaning, and more elaborate cognitive capacities will all serve to enhance and elaborate the child's emotional life. However, by 3 years of age, the child already shows those emotions that Darwin (1872/1965) characterized as unique to our species—the emotions of self-consciousness. With these, the major developmental activity has been achieved.

REFERENCES

Als, H. (1975). *The human newborn and his mother: An ethological study of their interaction.* Unpublished doctoral dissertation, University of Pennsylvania.

Argyle, M. (1975). *Bodily communication.* New York: International Universities Press.

Bennett, D. S., Bendersky, M., & Lewis, M. (2005). Does the organization of emotional expression change over time?: Facial expressivity from 4 to 12 months. *Infancy, 8*(2), 167–187.

Bischof-Köhler, D. (1991). The development of empathy in infants. In M. E. Lamb & H. Keller (Eds.), *Development: Perspectives from German-speaking countries* (pp. 245–273). Hillsdale, NJ: Erlbaum.

Bowlby, J. (1969). *Attachment and loss: Vol. 1. Attachment.* New York: Basic Books.

Brazelton, T. B., Koslowski, B., & Main, M. (1974). The origins of reciprocity: The early mother–infant interaction. In M. Lewis & L. A. Rosenblum (Eds.), *The effect of the infant on its caregiver* (pp. 49–76). New York: Wiley.

Bridges, K. M. B. (1932). Emotional development in early infancy. *Child Development, 3,* 324–334.

Brooks, J., & Lewis, M. (1976). Infants' responses to strangers: Midget, adult and child. *Child Development, 47,* 323–332.

Campos, J., & Stenberg, C. (1981). Perception, appraisal, and emotion: The onset of social referencing. In M. E. Lamb & L. R. Sherrod (Eds.), *Infant social cognition: Empirical and theoretical considerations* (pp. 273–314). Hillsdale, NJ: Erlbaum.

Camras, L. A., Lambrecht, L., & Michel, G. F. (1996). Infant "surprise" expressions as coordinative motor structures. *Journal of Nonverbal Behavior, 20*(3), 183–195.

Caron, R. F., Caron, A. J., & Myers, R. S. (1982). Abstraction of invariant face expressions in infancy. *Child Development, 53,* 1008–1015.

Clore, G. L., & Ortony, A. (1991). What more is there to emotion concepts than prototypes? *Journal of Personality and Social Psychology, 60,* 48–50.

Darwin, C. R. (1965). *The expression of the emotions in man and animals.* Chicago: University of Chicago Press. (Original work published 1872)

Davidson, R. J., & Fox, N. A. (1982). A symmetrical brain activity discriminate between positive versus negative affective stimuli in human infants. *Science, 218,* 1235–1237.

Duval, S., & Wicklund, R. A. (1972). *A theory of objective self-awareness.* New York: Academic Press.

Ekman, P. (1989). The argument and evidence about universals in facial expressions of emotion. In J. Wagner & A. Manstead (Eds.), *Handbook of social psychophysiology* (pp. 143–164). New York: Wiley.

Ekman, P., & Friesen, W. V. (1974). Detecting deception from the body or face. *Journal of Personality and Social Psychology, 29,* 288–298.

Elster, J. (1999). *Alchemies of the mind.* Cambridge, UK: Cambridge University Press.

Feinman, S., & Lewis, M. (1984). Is there social life beyond the dyad?: A social-psychological view of social connections in infancy. In M. Lewis (Ed.), *Beyond the dyad* (pp. 13–41). New York: Plenum Press.

Freud, S. (1960). *The psychopathology of everyday life* (A. Tyson, trans.). New York: Norton. (Original work published 1901)

Gibson, J. J. (1960). The concept of the stimulus in psychology. *American Psychologist, 15,* 694–703.

Gunnar, M. R. (1980). Control, warning signals and distress in infancy. *Developmental Psychology, 16,* 281–289.

Harris, P. (1989). *Children and emotion: The development of psychological understanding.* Oxford: Blackwell.

Hume, D. (1888). *A treatise of human nature* (L. A. Selby-Bigge, Ed.). Oxford: Clarendon Press. (Original work published 1739)

Izard, C. E. (1977). *Human emotion.* New York: Plenum Press.

Izard, C. E. (1978). Emotions and emotion–cognition relationships. In M. Lewis & L. A. Rosenblum (Eds.), *The genesis of behavior: Vol. 1. The development of affect* (pp. 389–413). New York: Plenum Press.

Kant, I. (1958). *Critique of pure reason* (N. Kemp Smith, Trans.). New York: Macmillan. (Original work published 1781)

Lazarus, R. S. (1982). Thoughts on the relations between emotion and cognition. *American Psychologist, 37,* 1019–1024.

Lazarus, R. S. (2001). Relational meaning and discrete emotions. In K. R. Scherer, A. Schorr, & T. Johnstone (Eds.), *Appraisal processes in emotion: Theory, methods, research* (pp. 37–67). New York: Oxford University Press.

Levenson, R. W., Ekman, P., & Friesen, W. V. (1990). Voluntary facial action generates emotion-specific autonomic nervous system activity. *Psychophysiology, 27,* 363–384.

Levine, S., & Wiener, S. G. (1989). Coping with uncertainty: A paradox. In D. S. Palermo (Ed.), *Coping with uncertainty: Behavioral and developmental perspectives* (pp. 1–16). Hillsdale, NJ: Erlbaum.

Lewis, M. (1989). Cultural differences in children's knowledge of emotional scripts. In P. Harris & C. Saarni (Eds.), *Children's understanding of emotion* (pp. 350–373). New York: Cambridge University Press.

Lewis, M. (1991). Ways of knowing: Objective self-awareness or consciousness. *Developmental Review, 11,* 231–243.

Lewis, M. (1992a). The self in self-conscious emotions. A commentary. In D. Stipek, S. Recchia, & S. McClintic (Eds.), *Self-evaluation in young children. Monographs of the Society for Research in Child Development, 57*(1, Serial No. 226), 85–95.

Lewis, M. (1992b). *Shame: The exposed self.* New York: Free Press.

Lewis, M. (1993). The development of deception. In M. Lewis & C. Saarni (Eds.), *Lying and deception in everyday life* (pp. 90–105). New York: Guilford Press.

Lewis, M. (2003a). The development of self-consciousness. In J. Roessler & N. Eilan (Eds.), *Agency and self-awareness: Issues in philosophy and psychology* (pp. 275–295). New York: Oxford University Press.

Lewis, M. (2003b). The emergence of consciousness and its role in human development. *Annals of the New York Academy of Sciences, 1001,* 1–29.

Lewis, M. (2005a, October 17). *Early individual differences in coping with stress: Emotional behavior, HPA and ANS reactivity.* Paper presented at the New York Academy of Sciences, Psychology Section, New York.

Lewis, M. (2005b). Origins of the self-conscious child. In W. R. Crozier & L. E. Alden (Eds.), *The essential handbook of social anxiety for clinicians* (pp. 81–98). Chichester, UK: Wiley.

Lewis, M., & Brooks-Gunn, J. (1978). Self-knowledge and emotional development. In M. Lewis & L. Rosenblum (Eds.), *The genesis of behavior: Vol. 1. The development of affect* (pp. 205–226). New York: Plenum Press.

Lewis, M., & Brooks-Gunn, J. (1979). *Social cognition and the acquisition of self.* New York: Plenum Press.

Lewis, M., & Goldberg, S. (1969). Perceptual–cognitive development in infancy: A generalized expectancy model as a function of the mother–infant interaction. *Merrill–Palmer Quarterly, 15,* 81–100.

Lewis, M., Hitchcock, D. F. A., & Sullivan, M. W. (2004). Physiological and emotional reactivity to learning and frustration. *Infancy, 6*(1), 121–143.

Lewis, M., & Michalson, L. (1983). *Children's emotions and moods: Developmental theory and measurement.* New York: Plenum Press.

Lewis, M., & Ramsay, D. S. (2005). Infant emotional and cortisol responses to goal blockage. *Child Development, 76*(2), 518–530.

Lewis, M., Ramsay, D. S., & Kawakami, K. (1993). Affectivity and cortisol response differences between Japanese and American infants. *Child Development, 64,* 1722–1731.

Lewis, M., Ramsay, D. S., & Sullivan, M. W. (2006). The relation of ANS and HPA activation to infant anger and sadness response to goal blockage. *Developmental Psychobiology, 48,* 397–405.

Lewis, M., & Rosenblum, L. (Eds.). (1974). *The origins of behavior: Vol. 2. The origins of fear.* New York: Wiley.

Lewis, M., & Saarni, C. (Eds.). (1985). *The socialization of emotion.* New York: Plenum Press.

Lewis, M., & Saarni, C. (Eds.). (1993). *Lying and deception in everyday life.* New York: Guilford Press.

Lewis, M., Sullivan, M. W., & Michalson, L. (1984). The cognitive–emotional fugue. In C. E. Izard, J. Kagan, & R. Zajonc (Eds.), *Emotions, cognition, and behavior* (pp. 264–288). New York: Cambridge University Press.

Lewis, M., Sullivan, M. W., Stanger, C., & Weiss, M. (1989). Self-development and self-conscious emotions. *Child Development, 60,* 146–156.

Mandler, G. (1975). *Mind and emotion.* New York: Wiley.

Mandler, G. (1980). The generation of emotion: A psychological theory. In R. Plutchik & H. Kellerman (Eds.), *Emotion: Theory, research, and experience* (Vol. 1, pp. 219–244). New York: Academic Press.

Nelson, C. A., & Bloom, F. E. (1997). Child development and neuroscience. *Child Development, 68,* 970–987.

Nelson, C. A., & Bosquet, H. (2000). Neurobiology of fetal and infant development: Implications for infant mental health. In C. H. Zeanah (Ed.), *Handbook of infant mental health* (2nd ed., pp. 37–59). New York: Guilford Press.

Ortony, A., Clore, G. L., & Collins, A. (1988). *The cognitive structure of emotions.* New York: Cambridge University Press.

Oster, H. (2005). The repertoire of infant facial expressions: An ontogenetic perspective. In J. Nadel & D. Muir (Eds.), *Emotional development: Recent research advances* (pp. 261–292). New York: Oxford University Press.

Plutchik, R. (1980). *Emotion: A psychoevolutionary synthesis.* New York: Harper & Row.

Pollak, S. D., Cicchetti, D., Hornung, K., & Reed, A. (2000). Recognizing emotion in faces: Developmental effects of child abuse and neglect. *Developmental Psychology, 36*(5), 679–688.

Saarni, C. (1999). *The development of emotional competence.* New York: Guilford Press.

Sander, L. W. (1977). Infant and caretaking environment: Investigation and conceptualization of adaptive behavior in a system of increasing complexity. In E. J. Anthony (Ed.), *The child psychiatrist as investigator* (pp. 170–183). New York: Plenum Press.

Schachter, S., & Singer, J. E. (1962). Cognitive, social, and physiological determinants of emotional state. *Psychological Review, 69,* 379–399.

Schaffer, H. R. (1974). Cognitive components of the infant's response to strangeness. In M. Lewis & L. A. Rosenblum (Eds.), *The origins of behavior: Vol.*

2. The origins of fear (pp. 11–24). New York: Wiley.

Schaffer, H. R., Greenwood, A., & Parry, M. H. (1972). The onset of wariness. *Child Development, 43,* 165–175.

Schneirla, T. C. (1959). An evolutionary and developmental theory of biphasic processes underlying approach and withdrawal. In M. R. Jones (Ed.), *Nebraska Symposium on Motivation* (Vol. 7, pp. 1–42). Lincoln: University of Nebraska Press.

Schwartz, G. E., & Weinberger, D. A. (1980). Patterns of emotional responses to affective situations: Relations among happiness, sadness, anger, fear, depression, and anxiety. *Motivation and Emotion, 4*(2), 175–191.

Spitz, R. A. (1965). *The first year of life.* New York: International Universities Press.

Sroufe, L. A. (1996). *Emotional development: The organization of emotional life in the early years.* New York: Cambridge University Press.

Stenberg, C. R., Campos, J. J., & Emde, R. N. (1983). The facial expression of anger in seven-month-old infants. *Child Development, 54,* 178–184.

Stipek, D., Recchia, S., & McClintic, S. (Eds.). (1992). Self-evaluation in young children. *Monographs of the Society for Research in Child Development, 57*(1, Serial No. 226).

Sullivan, M. W., & Lewis, M. (2003). Contextual determinants of anger and other negative expressions in young infants. *Developmental Psychology, 39*(4), 693–705.

Suomi, S. (1991). Primate separation models of affective disorders. In J. Madden (Ed.), *Neurobiology of learning, emotion and affect* (pp. 195–213). New York: Raven Press.

Tomkins, S. D. (1962). *Affect, imagery, consciousness: Vol. 1. The positive affects.* New York: Springer.

Tomkins, S. D. (1963). *Affect, imagery, consciousness: Vol. 2. The negative affects.* New York: Springer.

Watson, J. B. (1919). *Psychology from the standpoint of a behaviorist.* Philadelphia: Lippincott.

Zajonc, R. B. (1980). Feeling and thinking: Preferences need no inferences. *American Psychologist, 35,* 151–175.

CHAPTER 19

Children's Understanding of Emotion

PAUL L. HARRIS

AWARENESS OF EMOTION

In this chapter, I discuss children's developing awareness and understanding of emotions—both the emotions that they themselves feel and the emotions expressed by other people. I first describe children's changing ability to put feelings into words. Next, I consider how children's understanding of emotion changes with development. First, I emphasize that children cannot rely on a script-based conceptualization, but must attend to the relation between appraisal processes and ensuing emotion. More specifically, to understand how individuals may have different emotional reactions to the same situation, children need to understand the role of appraisal in the elicitation of emotion. Second, by way of a detailed illustration of this claim, I consider children's emerging understanding of a relatively complex but central emotion—namely, guilt. On the one hand, there are signs that children express guilt even in the preschool period. On the other hand, it is only in middle childhood that children systematically recognize when a person might be prone to guilty feel-

ings. I discuss possible reasons for this lag between the expression and the attribution of guilt, eventually highlighting the importance of understanding appraisal in the attribution of guilt. Finally, I turn to a discussion of individual differences in children's understanding of emotion. In that connection, I review the increasingly solid evidence that children who are given opportunities to engage in family conversation about emotion end up with a more accurate and comprehensive understanding.

TALKING ABOUT EMOTION

Psychological theories of emotion, whether focused on children or adults, have been influenced by Darwin's (1872/1998) emphasis on the continuities between human beings and nonhuman primates with respect to both the function and the communication of emotions. However, human beings, unlike other primates, can put their feelings into words. It could be argued that this capacity only serves to amplify a preexisting mode of nonverbal communication. However, it is more likely that it produces a psychological revolution. After all, it allows human beings to communicate what they feel not just about ongoing situations, but also about past, future, recurrent, or hypothetical situations. These conversations—which begin in early childhood—provide our species with a unique opportunity to share, understand, and reconstitute emotional experience.

To document young children's emerging ability to talk about emotion, we (Wellman, Harris, Banerjee, & Sinclair, 1995) studied a small group of children whose language production had been recorded on an intensive longitudinal basis from 2 to 5 years of age. We concentrated on all those utterances in which children referred either to an emotion or, for comparison purposes, to another subjective state that is not an emotion (namely, pain). The findings revealed that even 2-year-olds talk systematically about emotion. They refer to a small set of emotional states—both positive states (feeling happy or good; laughing; and feeling love or loving) and negative states (feeling angry or mad; feeling frightened, scared, or afraid; and feeling sad or crying). Although children talk most often about their own feelings, they also talk about the feelings of other people. Moreover, children's attributions of emotion are not triggered simply by the recognition of animate, expressive displays, because they readily attribute various emotions to dolls, stuffed animals, and made-up characters. In sum, almost as soon as they are able to talk, children begin to report on their own feelings and on those of other people, and they project such feelings onto nonhumans.

Despite this emerging communicative capacity, it could be argued that when children start to put their own feelings into words, they are not engaged in any self-conscious reporting of their experience. Thus Wittgenstein (1953) suggested that early emotion utterances should be seen not as reports of emotion, but as vocal expressions of emotion, on a par with exclamations such as "Ouch!" or "Ow!" A close examination of 2-year-olds' utterances shows that Wittgenstein's proposal does not capture the full complexity of young children's talk about emotion. If their references to emotion were simply supplements to, or substitutes for, the ordinary facial and behavioral indices of emotion, we would expect those utterances to be triggered more or less exclusively by ongoing or current emotions. However, about half of 2-year-olds' references to emotion are concerned with past, future, and recurrent feelings, and the distribution of references is similar among 3- and 4-year-olds.

This stable pattern shows that, from their earliest emergence, we can think of children's utterances about emotion as referential reports and not as lexical substitutes for scowls and smiles. Indeed, Wittgenstein's analysis is not even appropriate for children's pain utterances. Here too, children talk not only about current pains; they also refer to pains that they might experience in the future or have experienced in the past. More generally, analysis of children's references to emotion shows that these references can be mainly categorized as descriptive statements, even if they are sometimes used in an instrumental fashion—to obtain sympathy, or to influence the emotional state of another person (Dunn, Brown, & Beardsall, 1991; Wellman et al., 1995). Indeed, this bias toward commentary is evident even below 2 years of age. Dunn, Bretherton, and Munn (1987) found that children between 18 and 24 months used conversation about feelings primarily to comment on their own feelings or those of another person, even though their mothers—to whom most of these comments were directed—used such conversations in a more didactic or pragmatic fashion.

In a follow-up analysis of children's everyday conversations about emotion, Lagattuta and Wellman (2002) looked more closely at the way that children talk about negative as compared to positive emotions. As in the Wellman et al. (1995) study, they looked at the utterances produced by a small group of children whose language production had been studied on an intensive longitudinal basis from 2 to 5 years of age. Overall, children and their parents discussed positive and negative emotions at about the same rate. Nevertheless, when past emotions were discussed, there was a tendency to focus on negative rather than positive emotions. This bias toward the negative was true for children and adults alike. Talk about negative emotions also included about three times as many causal elaborations as talk about positive emotions did, and again this bias emerged among both children and adults. Moreover, when children and adults posed open-ended (as opposed to a closed-ended) questions about emotions, such questions were about three times more frequent for negative than for positive emotions. Overall, then, Lagattuta and

Wellman (2002) found that conversations about past emotional experiences are especially frequent, elaborate, and unconstrained in the case of negative emotions.

It seems plausible that conversations about past emotions may help children understand how an emotion can be reactivated long after the precipitating situation is over. This facilitation may occur in two ways. First, children may be drawn into conversation about past events and thereby experience a reactivation of the emotion that they felt earlier. To the extent that elaborate conversations about the past focus on negative events, children may be especially alert to the reactivation of negative emotion as compared to positive emotion. Second, when ruminating about a past event, children may display the emotion associated with that event and thereby puzzle their parents with a demeanor that is not consonant with present circumstances. Parental questioning may prompt children to think about their emotional state and its cause. Such questions ("What's the matter?", "What's bothering you?") are especially likely to occur when a child appears upset in otherwise positive circumstances. By contrast, a child who remains cheerful in the face of negative circumstances is less likely to provoke parental questioning. Thus if either of these speculations is correct, children may be especially aware of the way in which rumination about the past can evoke emotion in the case of negative as opposed to positive feelings.

Lagattuta and Wellman (2001) examined this issue with children ranging from 3 to 5 years of age. Children listened to stories in which the protagonist experienced an emotion that was either positive or negative and either did or did not match the current situation. Consider, for example, the following story about a negative emotion that did not match the current situation: "Suzie feels sad when the neighbor's black spotted dog scares away her rabbit. Many days later, the neighbor's dog slowly walks over, sits down, and wags his tail 'real friendly.' Suzie starts to feel sad. . . . Why does Suzie start to feel sad right now?" Children were scored for the frequency with which they produced so-called "cognitive cueing" explanations, involving references to a cue in the present situation that made the protagonist think about a past event—for example, "The dog makes her think about the lost rabbit." Lagattuta and Wellman (2001) found that children were especially likely to produce such cognitive cueing explanations for stories involving a negative mismatch, as exemplified by the story about Suzie's dog. For stories involving a positive emotion, such cognitive cueing explanations were less frequent, although among older children they became more frequent. By implication, conversations about negative emotions offer children an initial foothold toward the insight that one's current emotion is not tied to present circumstances, but is markedly influenced by thoughts and reminders of noncurrent situations.

Overall, the findings on children's conversations about emotion highlight the extent to which children's emotional experience and emotional reflection are not tied to the current moment. Language does, of course, allow children to put their ongoing feelings into words. In addition, however, it allows them to talk about future emotions and to revisit past emotions. It is probably by virtue of such conversations that children become aware of the fact that past emotion can be reactivated by reminders.

BEYOND SCRIPTS: DESIRES, BELIEFS, AND EMOTION

In the preceding section, I have talked in global terms about children's ability to report on and to understand emotion. In this section I consider in more detail the nature of this understanding and the way that it changes in the course of development. One simple and attractive proposal is that children develop an increasingly elaborate set of scripts for various emotions. Thus they identify and remember the type of situations that elicit particular emotions—fear, sadness, happiness, guilt, and so forth (Barden, Zelco, Duncan, & Masters, 1980; Harris, Olthof, Meerum Terwogt, & Hardman, 1987)—and they also identify and remember the typical actions and expressions that accompany a particular emotional state (Trabasso, Stein, & Johnson, 1981).

This notion of script-based knowledge has several advantages. It assimilates children's understanding of emotion to a wider body of research on children's recall and understanding of sequentially organized events (cf. Nelson & Gruendel, 1979). It highlights the fact that an understanding of emotion calls for a causal understanding of the connections among its sequential components. It is sufficiently flexible to be of service if we look outside the Western world to children's understanding of emotion in cultures where different emotional themes are prominent; for example, Lutz (1987) has used this approach in her analysis of the emotion concepts of children on the island of Ifaluk in the Western Pacific. Finally, the notion of an emotion script fits comfortably with a possibility raised in the preceding section—that children's understanding may be elaborated not just in the context of emotionally charged encounters, but in the context of family discussions in which past episodes are likely to be rehearsed and organized into a coherent narrative sequence.

However, closer scrutiny of the script concept reveals a conceptual difficulty. The same situation can elicit different emotions in different individuals, depending on the appraisal that a particular individual makes of the situation. This means that if a child attempts to store a list of scripts for emotion, it will be necessary to store different scripts for different people. An alternative, and more economical, solution is to define the eliciting situation in more abstract terms. For example, it is possible to define situations that provoke happiness as "situations that are judged by an actor to bring about the fulfillment of his or her goals." A move in this direction, however, tacitly acknowledges that emotions are very special kinds of scripts. They do not begin with the kind of objective event that we normally associate with scripts (e.g., the action of sitting down at a table might be seen as the first move in the dinner script). Rather, they begin with an event that is inherently psychological (namely, a person appraising a situation). A more fruitful approach to children's understanding of emotion, therefore, is to acknowledge that children may indeed construct scripts for given emotions—but that key elements of those scripts will include a diagnosis not of the objective situation that faces the actor, but rather an analysis of how the actor appraises that situation. To make the same point differently, it is not just psychologists who have to recognize the role of appraisal processes in emotion. Young children must do the same.

The limitations of the script-based approach can be highlighted in another way. Children with autism are often good at remembering recurrent sequences of events. Indeed, part of the clinical picture of autism is a disposition to become upset at an unexpected departure from a

routine sequence. Their script-sensitive memory appears to serve children with autism quite well with respect to emotion. Thus they readily judge that certain situations (getting nice things to eat, birthday parties) make people happy, whereas other situations (having to go to bed early, falling over) make people unhappy (Baron-Cohen, 1991; Tan & Harris, 1991). Using a different technique, Ozonoff, Pennington, and Rogers (1990) showed that autistic children could select the appropriate facial expressions to go with various emotionally charged pictures. For example, they chose a sad face for a picture of a child looking at a broken toy and an angry face for a picture of two children fighting. Despite this apparent familiarity with routine emotion scripts, children with autism perform poorly, compared with nonautistic controls, when a correct attribution of emotion requires them to go beyond the objective situation and to consider how a protagonist's beliefs influence his or her appraisal of that objective situation (Baron-Cohen, 1991; Harris, 1991). The clear implication is that nonautistic children do go beyond a script-based analysis and take into account the protagonist's appraisal of the situation.

If we accept this argument, we can ask in more detail how children make sense of the process of appraisal. First, 2- and 3-year-olds appreciate the role that desires or goals play in determining a protagonist's appraisal and ensuing emotion. For example, they understand that a toy elephant may feel happy to be given milk if she wants milk, whereas another animal may feel upset if he prefers juice instead (Harris, Johnson, Hutton, Andrews, & Cooke, 1989; Yuill, 1984). By 4 and 5 years of age, this simple desire-based concept of emotion is elaborated to include beliefs and expectations. Children realize that it is not the match between desire and actual outcome that triggers emotion, but the match between desire and expected outcome. Suppose, for example, that the elephant wants some milk and is about to get it, so that if the match between desire and actual outcome is the only factor taken into consideration, she should feel happy. Suppose further, however, that the elephant wrongly expects to get something other than milk. In that case, 4- and 5-year-olds realize that the elephant will feel upset rather than happy (Harris et al., 1989). They appreciate that her appraisal of the situation, and her ensuing emotion, are based on the mismatch between her desire and the expected outcome, even when the expectation is ill founded.

The shift from a desire to a belief–desire conception of mind and emotion is now well established. Emotion judgment tasks such as the one just described are useful sources of evidence, because whether children are asked to take only desires into account or beliefs and desires, they can still be asked to make the same simple binary judgment—namely, whether the animal is happy rather than sad. Another important source of evidence is children's spontaneous talk about psychological states. In the preceding section, I have described the way that children report on emotional states (Wellman et al., 1995). Using a similar database, Bartsch and Wellman (1995) have examined children's references to other mental states. Their analysis reveals that children talk systematically about desires and goals throughout most of the third year, chiefly using the term "want." Then, starting at about the third birthday, children also begin to make reference to beliefs, mainly using the terms "know" or "think." Eventually, by about the fifth birthday, talk about beliefs becomes as frequent as talk about desires.

This developmental pattern is probably universal. Tardif and Wellman (2000) report that children learning to speak Cantonese and Mandarin display a similar progression: Talk about goals and desires emerges early; talk about beliefs and expectations shows a later onset. These data help to rule out various possible interpretations of the lag between talk about desires and talk about knowledge and belief. For example, it might be argued that it arises because in English the predicate complement structure is simpler for the verb "want" than for the verbs "think" and "know." However, in Mandarin and Cantonese, the predicate complement structure is relatively simple across references to both desires and thoughts. Indeed, it is worth noting that in both Mandarin and Cantonese, some polysemous mental verbs can be used to indicate either desire or thought. Yet, despite the availability of the same lexical item for both meanings, the lag between references to desires and thoughts still emerges. In sum, whether we focus on children's emotion judgments by using experimental tasks involving a simple binary judgment, or on children's spontaneous references to mental processes in the course of their everyday conversation (be it in English, in Mandarin, or in Cantonese), the

evidence is robust that children focus initially on an agent's goals, but increasingly take into account his or her thoughts and beliefs.

It is worth noting that in the context of emotion judgments, the development of children's understanding of the role of thoughts and beliefs is quite protracted. Children ages 4–5 years are generally accurate in recognizing the impact of thoughts and beliefs on action (Wellman, Cross, & Watson, 2001). However, it is only at about 5–6 years of age that children recognize the impact of beliefs on emotion. Several studies support this conclusion. For example, Hadwin and Perner (1991) found that virtually all 5-year-olds could appreciate a story character's mistaken belief, but only at 6 years of age did a significant majority make correct attributions of surprise that were consistent with the story character's mistaken belief. Bradmetz and Schneider (1999) replicated the same lag between belief and emotion attributions across a series of five experiments. For example, when given a version of the story of Little Red Riding Hood, children frequently realized that Little Red Riding Hood mistakenly thinks it is her grandmother in the bed, but then went on to say that she was afraid—and invoked the wolf to explain her fear (e.g., "Because it is a wolf!" or "Because the wolf wants to eat her"). On the other hand, no child made a correct emotion attribution but failed the false-belief test. Finally, we (de Rosnay & Harris, 2002) compared children's performance on two versions of a nasty-surprise task (involving a protagonist's mistakenly expecting a positive outcome that turns out to be negative). Children frequently erred by incorrectly identifying the protagonist's emotion as negative, despite correctly identifying the protagonist's positive belief. In summary, whereas young preschoolers (ages 3–4 years) grasp that an individual will appraise a situation in terms of his or her desires—and will react with different emotions, depending on whether those desires are frustrated or fulfilled—children's appraisal of the impact of beliefs on emotion emerges more slowly. Only at about 5–6 years of age do they realize that the appraisal of frustration or fulfillment, rather than the objective situation, is what dictates emotional reactions.

Children's developing appreciation of appraisal processes can be further highlighted by taking a closer look at children's attributions of an important and complex social emotion—namely, guilt. In a pioneering study, Nunner-

Winkler and Sodian (1988) found a surprising age change. Children ages 4–5 years consistently claimed that a story protagonist who had committed a serious transgression (e.g., deliberately lied, pushed another child, or stolen something) would feel happy. The children justified this by noting that the outcome of the protagonist's transgression had produced positive results: He or she had successfully stolen something or had managed to displace another child on the swing. By about the age of 8 years, children were more likely to claim that the protagonist would feel bad and to refer to the story character's transgression in explaining that attribution.

One plausible explanation of this age change is that older children increasingly expect that a transgression will provoke a bad conscience; they have an understanding of what it means to feel guilty. Still, before focusing in more detail on that interpretation, I believe it is worth considering various alternatives. First, it is conceivable that younger children regard the transgressions as trivial. However, a long tradition of research on moral development shows that preschoolers actually think of lying, hitting, and stealing as serious transgressions (Smetana, 1981). Not surprisingly, therefore, Keller, Lourenço, Malti, and Saalbach (2003) could find no age change in children's castigation of such basic transgressions.

A second possibility is that older children expect the protagonist to feel bad because they are more alert to the risk of punishment. Indeed, because they are older and arguably expected to "know better," older children may expect more severe punishment for such transgressions than younger children. However, children's justifications lend little support to this explanation. They rarely refer to punishment or fear of punishment when explaining why the perpetrator feels bad.

A third possibility is that older children are more likely to interpret the question in terms of the emotion that the perpetrator *should* feel, whereas the younger children focus on what the perpetrator *does* feel. However, when Keller et al. (2003) asked children how they themselves would feel after such a transgression—a question format that should presumably have prompted the children to focus on socially desirable feelings—the familiar age change reemerged.

A fourth possibility is that older children have greater empathy: They may more readily acknowledge the suffering experienced by the victims of the transgressions, and they may attribute bad feelings to the person who has caused that distress. However, when Arsenio and Kramer (1992) explicitly asked children of various ages about the feelings of the victim, all age groups acknowledged his or her distress. A further problem for the empathy hypothesis is that a similar age change in children's emotion attributions emerges when they are asked about transgressions that do not involve any suffering by a victim. Lagattuta (2005) presented children from 4 to 7 years of age with stories involving a conflict between the protagonist's desire and various nonmoral rules concerning, for example, safety ("Don't run into the street") or nutrition ("Don't eat cookies before dinner"). Older children were more likely to acknowledge that the protagonist could feel bad after breaking the rule. Equally important, they were also more likely to acknowledge that the protagonist could feel good about resisting the temptation to break the rule. Clearly, in neither of these cases is it feasible to explain the age change in terms of increased empathy for a victim. In these episodes, there was no third party in the role of victim.

The most plausible explanation of the findings is that older children increasingly conceive of agents as engaging in a particular kind of appraisal process. Whereas younger children are inclined to think that wrongdoers focus mainly on their goals and feel happy or sad depending on whether those goals are fulfilled or not, older children increasingly acknowledge an additional appraisal process in which the wrongdoer appraises his or her actions in terms of whether or not they conform to various rules and obligations (Harris, 1989). In probing children's explanations for the emotion felt by the story characters, Lagattuta (2005) obtained firm support for this interpretation. Older children were more likely than younger children to focus on rules and obligations. They said, for example, "She feels a little bad because she shouldn't have done that," or " . . . because his mom said he had to stay out of the street.")

If the analysis above is correct, it implies that children come to attribute guilt only in middle childhood. Yet recent evidence suggests that even preschool children feel and express guilt. For example, Kochanska, Gross, Lin, and Nichols (2002) report that preschoolers show a fairly stable tendency toward displays of discomfort following a mishap; these displays correlate moderately with maternal ratings of a child's tendency to feel guilt; and children who display more discomfort are more likely to conform to adult-imposed rules. Taken together, these results suggest that even preschoolers do feel guilt. If that is the case, why do children only start to attribute guilt several years later? The most plausible explanation is that this lag is simply one more example of a very general developmental pattern. Children enter into a variety of mental states quite early in life: They entertain false beliefs, they experience surprise, and they feel badly about a misdemeanor. The ability to make sense of and attribute those mental states—whether to the self or to another person—is far from being an automatic accompaniment. It is only after constructing a theory or model of those mental states, including the appraisal processes that give rise to them, that children can make appropriate attributions of belief, surprise, or guilt.

INDIVIDUAL DIFFERENCES IN UNDERSTANDING EMOTION

So far, I have focused on important age changes in children's understanding of emotion. This emphasis reflects the research program that has dominated research for the past 20 years or more: Investigators have aimed to identify a succession of conceptual insights that children come to master in the course of development. However, more recently, attention has increasingly turned to individual differences in children's mastery of those insights. On the one hand, investigators have developed tools to measure variation in children's understanding of emotion; on the other hand, they have begun to analyze the reasons why some children are advanced in their understanding, whereas others are much slower.

We (Pons, Harris, & de Rosnay, 2004) have reported on a Test of Emotion Comprehension (TEC) composed of nine different components: (1) recognizing facial expressions of emotion; (2) understanding situational causes; (3) understanding the effect of external reminders on emotion; (4) understanding the link between desire and emotion; (5) understanding the link between belief and emotion; (6) understanding the potential discrepancy between felt and expressed emotion; (7) understanding guilt; (8) understanding the regulation of emotion; and

(9) understanding mixed or ambivalent emotions. We tested children between 3 and 11 years of age for their mastery of each component. The main findings were that children displayed a clear improvement with age on each component, and that the components themselves can be plausibly grouped into three developmental phases. The first period is characterized by the understanding of key public aspects of emotion—their mode of expression, their situational causes, and the effect of external reminders. The second period is characterized by mastery of the mentalistic nature of emotion—the role of desires and beliefs, and the distinction between felt and expressed emotion. The third period is characterized by an understanding of how the same individual can reflect on a situation from different points of view or in terms of different criteria and thereby evoke different feelings—either at the same time or successively. We (Pons et al., 2004) observed a hierarchical relationship among these three phases. By implication, understanding key external aspects of emotion is a prerequisite for understanding the more mentalistic aspects, which in turn is a prerequisite for understanding the impact of reflection and rumination on emotion.

In a follow-up study, we (Pons & Harris, 2005) looked at longitudinal change and stability in children's performance on the TEC. Children ages 7, 9, and 11 years at Time 1 were retested 13 months later at Time 2. More than half of the 7- and 9-year-olds showed gains at retest (although the majority of 11-year-olds performed about the same—probably reflecting the absence of challenging components for this older group). Individual differences were considerable at both Times 1 and 2 for all three age group. Thus children in the youngest group varied by as much as six components, and children in the two older groups varied by as much as four components. Moreover, when adjacent age groups were compared, the highest-scoring children in the younger group scored higher than the lowest-scoring children in the older group (by two to three components, depending on which two age groups were compared). Indeed, some of the 7-year-olds had an overall level of emotion understanding that was higher than some of the 11-year-olds'. These individual differences remained quite stable over the 13-month period. Thus, despite the gains over time made by many children in their understanding of emotion, their level of understanding at Time 1 was a good predictor of their understanding at Time 2.

Do these marked and stable individual differences in children's understanding of emotion have any implications for their behavior? In particular, we may ask whether children's understanding of emotion has an impact on their social relationships when they move outside the family and start to form relationships with peers. Several studies have explored this possibility. Denham, McKinley, Couchoud, and Holt (1990) tested preschoolers (mean age = 44 months) for their emotion knowledge: Children had to identify a puppet's emotion (of happiness, sadness, anger, or fear), both when it exhibited a prototypical reaction (e.g., fear during a nightmare) and when it showed an atypical reaction (e.g., sadness at going to preschool). In addition, a sociometric measure was used to assess children for their acceptance as playmates among their peers. Children with higher scores on the emotion test proved to be more popular among their peers, even when the contributions of age and gender were removed. Cassidy, Parke, Butkovsky, and Braungart (1992) obtained very similar results with first-grade children. Children's overall score in an interview about the causes, consequences, and associated expression of emotion was correlated with popularity. Finally, in a longitudinal study of 4- and 5-year-olds, Edwards, Manstead, and MacDonald (1984) found that children who were accurate at identifying facial expressions of emotion proved to be more popular 1–2 years later (even when their initial popularity was taken into account). The consistency among these three studies is striking.

Nevertheless, caution is needed in interpreting the findings (Manstead, 1994). First, we do not yet understand the causal link between the understanding of emotion and peer relationships. Acceptance by peers may increase children's opportunities for learning about emotion. Thus children's understanding of emotion may not promote their friendships; rather, causal arrow may move in the reverse direction. Alternatively, a third variable (such as intelligence or verbal ability) may underpin both emotion understanding and popularity.

Second, it would be premature to conclude that children with more advanced insight into emotion inevitably end up having healthy and positive relationships with their peers. Consider the thought-provoking study of bullying carried out by Sutton, Smith, and Swettenham (1999). Bullies are sometimes characterized as awkward children who resort to aggression because of their limited social skills. Yet it is also conceivable that bullying calls for an astute analysis of whom to victimize and how bystanders will react. With this in mind, Sutton et al. (1999) administered a set of stories designed to assess the understanding of emotions and cognitions among 7- to 10-year-olds. Children who were "ringleader" bullies scored higher than several other groups: "follower" bullies (i.e., those who helped or supported the ringleaders), victims, and defenders of the victims.

The implication of all these studies is that insight into other children's emotional and mental states is associated with social adroitness. Thus it is linked to popularity and acceptance, but also to leadership in the context of bullying. Although it is tempting to assume that a more advanced or precocious understanding of emotion invariably yields positive social outcomes, such an assumption is probably too optimistic.

To turn now to the origins of such individual differences, recent evidence increasingly points to a key role for family conversation. Consider a child with a parent who frequently discusses emotion—by drawing out the child's own feelings, by calling attention to the way that his or her actions may have emotional implications for other members of the family, or by elaborating on the feelings of story characters. Consider, on the other hand, a parent who is more constrained in talking about emotion, whether with respect to the child or to other people. These two different conversation partners might be expected to have a differential impact on the extent to which the child understands how an emotion comes about, or is prepared to talk about emotion, or both.

Certainly there is marked variation among families in the frequency with which emotions are discussed. Dunn, Brown, and Beardsall (1991) found that some children never made any mention of emotion during an hour-long home visit, whereas others made more than 25 such references; variation among the mothers was equally great. Accumulating evidence indicates that the frequency with which preschool children engage in family discussion about emotions and their causes is correlated with their later ability to identify how someone feels. The link has been found over a relatively short period straddling the third birthday—that is, from 33 to 40 months (Dunn, Brown, Slomkowski, Tesla & Youngblade, 1991)—as well as over a more extended period from 3 to 6 years (Dunn et al., 1991; Brown & Dunn, 1996).

Such correlational data are, of course, open to various interpretations. One possibility is that the correlation reflects some stable attribute of the child that manifests itself both in psychological talk and in sensitivity to emotion. For example, some children may be naturally empathic: They may seek out and elicit more conversations about emotion, and also display a keen ability to assess how other people feel, as measured by standard tests of emotion understanding. However, it is also plausible to suppose that the correlation reflects the didactic role that conversation can play for children. Frequent family discussion, particularly when parents are involved, may prompt children to talk about emotion and to increase their understanding and perspective taking. One piece of evidence that fits this second proposal has been reported by Garner, Jones, Gaddy, and Reddie (1997): They found that children's perspective taking is correlated with family discussion of emotion that focuses not simply on *what* a person feels, but rather on *why* someone feels a given emotion. We (de Rosnay, Pons, Harris, & Morrell, 2004) obtained a second piece of evidence consistent with the didactic role of family members: Mothers' use of mentalistic terms when describing their children (i.e., references to their children's psychological characteristics, rather than their physical characteristics or their behavior) were positively correlated with children's correct emotion attributions to story protagonists. Thus, even when a mother was not engaged in conversation with her child, characteristics of her discourse style nevertheless predicted the child's understanding of emotion.

Such an emphasis on the didactic role of parental conversation (especially maternal conversation) is consistent with a larger body of research that has investigated children's developing understanding of various mental states, including beliefs as well as emotions. Three important conclusions have emerged from these studies. First, when longitudinal data are collected, they confirm that the mothers' discourse is what predicts children's later understanding of mental states; there is no indication that children's understanding of mental states predicts later patterns of discourse by their mothers. Second, it is the mothers' focus on mental states that appears to be critical, rather than any generalized disposition to engage children in conversation. Third, this influence appears to have a sustained impact; it is evident among 3- and 6-year-olds alike (Harris, de Rosnay, & Pons, 2005; Ruffman, Slade, & Crowe, 2002).

In the coming years, we may expect to see more research on the questions of how children come to vary in their understanding of emotion, and what part family talk may play in promoting that variation. In that regard, we can anticipate an increasing confluence of findings from research on early attachment, on children's conversations about emotionally charged events (especially past negative events), and on individual differences in children's understanding of mental states (including emotion). For the most part, these topics have been studied independently of one another, but that is likely to change. Such a confluence is likely to yield practical as well as theoretical benefits. If we know more about how children's understanding of emotion can be facilitated in the context of the family, especially family conversation, we may be able to reproduce some of those beneficial effects through deliberate and systematic therapeutic intervention.

CONCLUSIONS

In this chapter, I have examined several interrelated aspects of children's understanding of emotion: their ability to report emotion in words and to understand the way that past emotions can be reactivated; their sensitivity to key components of the appraisal processes that modulate a person's emotional response to a given situation (namely, the person's desires, the person's beliefs, and the person's evaluation of his or her own standing in relation to various rules and obligations); and individual differences in emotion understanding, their links with peer relationships, and the key role of family conversation in promoting children's understanding of emotion.

At certain points, I have touched on a larger theme that deserves more attention in future research. Arguably, children's developing understanding of emotion is simply an epiphenomenon of the underlying process. This understanding may operate at a "meta" level, sealed off from the underlying emotional process that is its subject matter. To take a concrete example, it is possible to assert that a child functions at two separate levels: On one level, there is the child's experience and display of guilt; at a separate level, there is the child's capacity for reporting on, attributing, and ruminating about the experience of guilt. Increased sophistication at the "meta" level may have few or no effects on processing at the primary, lower level.

Such a clear-cut separation between levels of processing may simplify our analysis of development, but it probably distorts or ignores some important features of human emotion. It effectively predicts that a disruption or delay in the development of an understanding of emotion need have no repercussions for the basic emotional processes themselves. However, there are several reasons for thinking that such repercussions do exist. First, there is a therapeutic tradition suggesting that intense emotional experiences that are reworked in the context of communication and rumination have different sequelae from those that are not. Such reworking need not be in the context of discussion with a trained therapist; it can also occur in the context of a privately written narrative (Pennebaker, 1996). One plausible extrapolation of these findings is that the emotional lives of children who grow up in homes where there is open discussion of emotionally charged encounters will be different from those where such discussion does not occur. They are likely to be prompted to engage in the type of insightful thinking about the causes of their emotions that has been shown to be beneficial for adults' physical and mental health (Pennebaker, Barger, & Tiebout, 1989).

Second, this capacity for communication and rumination dramatically alters the contexts in which children can seek support and reassurance. Attachment theorists have emphasized the ways that a caretaker may or may not provide reassurance at moments of distress. Typically, they have focused on those moments when the precipitating factor is fairly easy for the caretaker to discern: The child is unnerved by a stranger, or distressed by the caregiver's recent absence, or fretful about the caregiver's imminent departure. However, the emotional horizon of an older child is much larger; he or she can be distressed or fearful about events that might happen in the future or happened in the more distant past. In such contexts, children who can articulate their anxieties and discuss their causes are clearly better placed to receive reassurance.

Finally, children's ability to understand and predict their own emotions likely effects their decision making about what course of action to take. In its turn, this chosen course of action will lead to—or prevent—certain emotional consequences. For example, the ability to anticipate guilt can serve as a brake or warning signal when a guilt-inducing transgression is contemplated (Lake, Lane, & Harris, 1995). This warning signal is sufficient to help children to inhibit the transgression, and to avoid any subsequent guilt. Stated in more general terms, children's insight into their emotional lives does not simply enable them to foresee the inevitable; it allows them to look into the future and to make choices about what their emotional life should be like. In that respect, children's understanding of emotion enables them to alter their experience of emotion.

REFERENCES

Arsenio, W. F., & Kramer, R. (1992). Victimizers and their victims: Children's conceptions of the mixed emotional consequences of moral transgressions. *Child Development*, 63, 915–927.

Barden, R. C., Zelko, F. A., Duncan, S. W., & Masters, J. C. (1980). Children's consensual knowledge about the experiential determinants of emotion. *Journal of Personality and Social Psychology*, 39, 968–976.

Baron-Cohen, S. (1991). Do people with autism understand what causes emotion? *Child Development*, 62, 385–395.

Bartsch, K., & Wellman, H. M. (1995). *Children talk about the mind*. New York: Oxford University Press.

Bradmetz, J., & Schneider, R. (1999). Is Little Red Riding Hood afraid of her grandmother?: Cognitive vs. emotional response to a false belief. *British Journal of Developmental Psychology*, 7, 501–514.

Brown, J. R., & Dunn, J. (1996). Continuities in emotion understanding from three to six years. *Child Development*, 67, 789–802.

Cassidy, J., Parke, R. D., Butkovsky, L., & Braungart, J. M. (1992). Family–peer connections: The roles of emotional expressiveness within the family and children's understanding of emotions. *Child Development*, 63, 603–618.

Darwin, C. (1998). *The expression of the emotions in man and animals* (3rd ed.). London: HarperCollins. (Original work published 1872)

Denham, S. A., McKinley, M., Couchoud, E. A., & Holt, R. (1990). Emotional and behavioral predictors of preschool peer ratings. *Child Development,* *61,* 1145–1152.

de Rosnay, M., & Harris, P. L. (2002). Individual differences in children's understanding of emotion: The roles of attachment and language. *Attachment and Human Development,* *4,* 39–54.

de Rosnay, M., Pons, F., Harris, P. L., & Morrell, J. M. B. (2004). A lag between understanding false belief and emotion attribution in young children: Relationships with linguistic ability and mothers' mental state language. *British Journal of Developmental Psychology,* *22,* 197–218.

Dunn, J., Bretherton, I., & Munn, P. (1987). Conversations about feeling states between mothers and their young children. *Developmental Psychology,* *23,* 132–139.

Dunn, J., Brown, J., & Beardsall, L. (1991). Family talk about feeling states and children's later understanding of others' emotions. *Developmental Psychology,* *27,* 448–455.

Dunn, J., Brown, J., Slomkowski, C., Tesla, C., & Youngblade, L. (1991). Young children's understanding of other people's feelings and beliefs: Individual differences and their antecedents. *Child Development,* *62,* 1352–1366.

Edwards, R., Manstead, A. S., & MacDonald, C. (1984). The relationship between children's sociometric status and ability to recognize facial expressions. *European Journal of Social Psychology,* *14,* 235–238.

Garner, P. W., Jones, D. C., Gaddy, G., & Rennie, K. M. (1997). Low-income mothers' conversations about emotions and their children's emotional competence. *Social Development,* *6,* 37–52.

Hadwin, J., & Perner, J. (1991). Pleased and surprised: Children's cognitive theory of emotion. *British Journal of Developmental Psychology,* *9,* 215–234.

Harris, P. L. (1989). *Children and emotion: The development of psychological understanding.* Oxford: Blackwell.

Harris, P. L. (1991). The work of the imagination. In A. Whiten (Ed.), *Natural theories of mind* (pp. 283–304). Oxford: Blackwell.

Harris, P. L., de Rosnay, M., & Pons, F. (2005). Language and children's understanding of mental states. *Current Directions in Psychological Science,* *14,* 69–73.

Harris, P. L., Johnson, C. N., Hutton, D., Andrews, G., & Cooke, T. (1989). Young children's theory of mind and emotion. *Cognition and Emotion,* *3,* 379–400.

Harris, P. L., Olthof, T., Meerum Terwogt, M., & Hardman, C. E. (1987). Children's knowledge of the situations that provoke emotion. *International Journal of Behavioral Development,* *10,* 319–343.

Keller, M., Lourenço, O., Malti, T., & Saalbach, H. (2003). The multifaceted phenomenon of 'happy victimizers': A cross-cultural comparison of moral emotions. *British Journal of Developmental Psychology,* *21,* 1–18.

Kochanska, G., Gross, J. N., Lin, M.-H., & Nichols, K. E. (2002). Guilt in young children: Development, determinants, and relations with a broader system of standards. *Child Development,* *73,* 461–482.

Lagattuta, K. H. (2005). When you shouldn't do what you want to do: Young children's understanding of desires, rules and emotions. *Child Development,* *76,* 713–733.

Lagattuta, K. H., & Wellman, H. M. (2001). Thinking about the past: Early knowledge about links between prior experience, thinking, and emotion. *Child Development,* *72,* 82–102.

Lagattuta, K. H., & Wellman, H. M. (2002). Differences in early parent–child conversations about negative versus positive emotions: Implications for the development of psychological understanding. *Developmental Psychology,* *38,* 564–580

Lake, N., Lane, S., & Harris, P. L. (1995). The expectation of guilt and resistance to temptation. *Early Development and Parenting,* *4,* 63–73.

Lutz, C. (1987). Goals, events, and understanding in Ifaluk emotion theory. In D. Holland & N. Quinn (Eds.), *Cultural models in language and thought* (pp. 290–312). Cambridge, UK: Cambridge University Press.

Manstead, A. S. R. (1994). Children's understanding of emotion. In J. J. Russell, J.-M. Fernández-Dols, A. S. R. Manstead, & J. C. Wellenkamp (Eds.), *Everyday conceptions of emotion* (pp. 315–331). Dordrecht, The Netherlands: Kluwer.

Nelson, K., & Gruendel, J. (1979). At morning it's lunchtime: A scriptal view of children's dialogues. *Discourse Processes,* *2,* 73–94.

Nunner-Winkler, G., & Sodian, B. (1988). Children's understanding of moral emotions. *Child Development,* *59,* 1323–1338.

Ozonoff, S., Pennington, B. F., & Rogers, S. J. (1990). Are there emotion perception deficits in young autistic children? *Journal of Child Psychology and Psychiatry,* *31,* 343–361.

Pennebaker, J. W. (1996). Cognitive, emotional, and language processes in disclosure. *Cognition and Emotion,* *10,* 601–626.

Pennebaker, J. W., Barger, S. D., & Tiebout, J. (1989). Disclosures of traumas and health among Holocaust survivors. *Psychosomatic Medicine,* *51,* 577–589.

Pons, F., & Harris, P. L. (2005). Longitudinal change and longitudinal stability of individual differences in children's emotion understanding. *Cognition and Emotion,* *19,* 1158–1174.

Pons, F., Harris, P. L., & de Rosnay, M. (2004). Emotion comprehension between 3 and 11 years: Developmental periods and hierarchical organization. *European Journal of Developmental Psychology,* *1,* 127–152.

Ruffman, T., Slade, L., & Crowe, E. (2002). The relation between children's and mother's mental state language and theory-of-mind understanding. *Child Development,* *74,* 734–751.

Smetana, J. G. (1981). Preschool children's conception of moral and social rules. *Child Development, 52,* 1333–1336.

Sutton, J., Smith, P. K., & Swettenham, J. (1999). Social cognition and bullying: Social inadequacy or skilled manipulation? *British Journal of Developmental Psychology, 17,* 435–450.

Tan, J., & Harris, P. L. (1991). Autistic children understand seeing and wanting. *Development and Psychopathology, 3,* 163–174.

Tardif, T., & Wellman, H. M. (2000). Acquisition of mental state language in Mandarin- and Cantonese-speaking children. *Developmental Psychology, 36,* 25–43.

Trabasso, T., Stein, N. L., & Johnson, L. R. (1981). Children's knowledge of events: A causal analysis of story structure. In G. Bower (Ed.), *Learning and motivation* (Vol. 15, pp. 237–282). New York: Academic Press.

Wellman, H. M., Cross, D., & Watson, J. (2001). Meta-analysis of theory-of-mind development: The truth about false belief. *Child Development, 72,* 655–684.

Wellman, H. M., Harris, P. L., Banerjee, M., & Sinclair, A. (1995). Early understanding of emotion: Evidence from natural language. *Cognition and Emotion, 9,* 117–149.

Wittgenstein, L. (1953). *Philosophical investigations.* Oxford: Blackwell.

Yuill, N. (1984). Young children's coordination of motive and outcome in judgments of satisfaction and morality. *British Journal of Developmental Psychology, 2,* 73–81.

CHAPTER 20

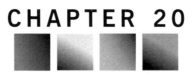

The Interface
of Emotional Development
with Social Context

CAROLYN SAARNI

When the second edition of this handbook was published in 2000, I wrote a chapter with a similar title, and at that time I thought I knew something about the reciprocal influence of context and emotion (i.e., contexts provide the "stage" as well as the "audience" for emotions, and emotions influence both the "audience" and the selection of "stages" to play themselves out upon). Although I did not use that particular dramaturgical metaphor in the earlier chapter, it sums up what I thought captured the reciprocity between context and emotion. Now my thoughts about the relationship between context and emotion, especially from a developmental perspective (i.e., how this relationship changes over time), have taken a definite turn: Action—and thus motivation—play a larger role in my construal of how emotions depend upon context and vice versa. I now assign a larger role to intentionality, to self-organizing principles, and to *systems* of interaction. In short, emotional development needs to be considered from within a "bioecological" framework; this conceptual platform regards living organisms as dynamic systems reciprocally embedded in a community. Clements and Shelford (1939), early plant and animal bioecologists, provided the theoretical underpinnings for the concept of bioecology, and their emphasis was very clearly on the synthesis of habitat and organism. Habitat for plant and animal communities is analogous to context for human communities (ranging from families to societies), and the adjustments and adaptation made by plants and animals in tandem with their habitats correspond to the developmental relationships between genotypes and likely or possible phenotypes in human development that are manifested in particular social contexts (Bronfenbrenner & Ceci, 1994).

In this chapter, I review some of the traditional and contemporary viewpoints on the relationship between context and emotional development. I include some particularly interesting studies that illustrate the bioecological framework for understanding emotional development in its social context. I also discuss several features of the cultural context that constitute important aspects of the bioecological framework.

WHY IS CONTEXT SIGNIFICANT FOR EMOTIONAL DEVELOPMENT?

Some studies explicitly invoke the role of context as an illustration of the plasticity of emotional development. For example, the classic longitudinal research by Murphy and Moriarty (1976) provided many rich descriptions of children who maintained a distinctive style of emotional regulation that at its core contained some degree of continuity; yet across varying contexts and developmental stages, the children's actual expression of their regulatory style was quite variable. I quote one such description below:

> Moreover, forms of expression of reaction changed while the essential reaction continued. Sheila protested loudly, vociferously, and decisively as an infant; at three she was equally decisive in her unequivocal "no!"; by age ten she could cooperate yet still convey her clear negative reaction by "making a face." In other words, feelings and attitude patterns could persist in very different forms. (Murphy & Moriarty, 1976, p. 197)

In this example (and many others like it provided by the authors), I see plasticity of emotional development as reflecting a style of emotional responding that has multiple manifestations, which vary with development and eliciting situation. Murphy and Moriarty also described a different sort of plasticity of emotional development *across* children, whereby the same stimulus elicited widely differing emotional-expressive behavior. Some children reacted to a stressful stimulus by becoming rigid, as though freezing; other children revealed more disorganized cognitive functioning, manifested in slow, fuzzy speech or increased stammering. In this case, emotional plasticity is reflected in the same elicitor's being responded to by different emotional coping styles. Relative to a bioecological approach toward emotional development, I found Murphy's and Moriarty's work also firmly anchored in an appreciation of the infant's "organicity"—that is, its temperamental dispositions for how to respond to variable contexts. They too saw how the subsequent development of any given infant depended on the daily interactions, both social and object-oriented, that the infant experienced. Opportunities to access social and inanimate environments were possible insofar as these contexts provided "affordances" for interaction (Gibson, 1982),

and affordant characteristics of an environment were often made feasible by sensitive caregivers who could determine when a baby was overstimulated or understimulated.

Still another kind of emotional plasticity is described in early work by Fraiberg (1971). She found that infants with very low vision were minimally facially expressive in interactions with their caregivers, but they were very active with their fingers; indeed, they relied on their fingers' sensory capacities to explore their worlds. Thus, for a more typical expressive part of the body (the face), these infants substituted other parts of their body that remained maneuverable by them—namely, their fingers. These visually impaired infants were experienced by their parents as somehow emotionally unresponsive, which was a judgment or "rating" of their facial expressiveness in contexts deemed by "raters" (their parents) as somehow atypical. This idea that a judgment of emotion is made in the eyes of the beholder has been at the center of much debate in the field of emotion, pitting universalists (e.g., Ekman, 1989) against cultural relativists (e.g., Russell, 1991). The former minimize the role of context as well as the plasticity of emotion; the latter emphasize the significance of context, including culture, in understanding emotion and the plasticity of emotion expression, appraisal, and meaning (Fernández-Dols, 1999; White, 2000; Wierzbicka, 1999).

A relevant study by Camras et al. (2002) examined directly the role of context and culture on raters' judgments of the emotion surprise in infants close to 1 year of age. The data were collected in Japan, in China, and in the United States with European American infants. The naive raters (in the United States) were to judge when the infants reacted with surprise when a toy they had seen on four previous trials after lifting off a cloth covering it was covertly replaced with a new toy. This expectancy-violating event was thought to elicit surprise, but the infants showed classic surprise expressions about as often in the four baseline sessions as they did in the "surprising-toy-switch" condition (about 30%). More often, the Japanese and European American infants showed a body stilling (a cessation of movement), accompanied by a sober facial expression. The Chinese infants did not show this bodily stilling or sobering of facial expression, because for these two behaviors to be observed, there must be more body activity and expressivity preceding the expectancy-violating event for stilling or sobering to be judged as occurring. The Chinese infants appeared more placid or "self-contained," or perhaps their behavioral cues for reacting to a discrepancy were too subtle to be observed by Western judges. Were the Japanese and European American babies actually surprised by the toy switch, or were they just focusing their attention on this discrepancy as they stopped wiggling and displayed a somber expression? They already possessed object permanence, but perhaps surprise is an emotion that develops later and may well depend on contextual features such as proximity to caregivers (because otherwise an "impossible event" could be experienced as a source of distress), temperamental proclivities toward reactivity, and the extent to which the individual has some control over the elicitor of the surprising event (e.g., the classic Jack-in-the-Box, which pops out of the lid when the crank handle is turned and after the music plays to a certain point). Maybe we need to watch 15- to 18-month-olds play with the Jack-in-the-Box and, with caregivers nearby, watch how the toddlers respond to Jack reliably popping out from under the open lid as *they themselves* crank the handle the requisite number of times. I predict that by the second or third pop-up, we might see more classic surprise faces, but then with subsequent repetition (again under the toddlers' control), there would be a transformation of the expressive response toward positive anticipation and eventually habituation. Surely there is a thesis somewhere in such a follow-up project; for a related study with much younger infants with a Jack-in-the-Box manipulated by *and coached by* their mothers to associate surprise with the popping up of Jack's head, see research undertaken by Reissland and Shepherd (2002).

To sum up, plasticity of emotional development relative to context can be seen in four ways: (1) in a particular style of emotion regulation manifesting itself in different forms in the same individual at different developmental periods, whereby the eliciting situations share some common relational theme for the individual; (2) in the same or very similar emotion-evoking context eliciting different expressive reactions, suggestive of the same hedonic tone but with varying manifestations across different individuals (e.g., a "freezing" reaction to a stressful stimulus vs. an agitated reaction); (3) in the "equipotentiality" of emotion-expressive channels (e.g., facial expressions vs. vocal

channel or kinesthetic channel); and (4) in judges' ratings of emotion in others that are informed by the context in which the others appear to be responding to relational goals. These four different ways of looking at plasticity in emotional development vis-à-vis shifting contexts are compatible with functionalist (Campos, Mumme, Kermoian, & Campos, 1994) and dynamic-systems (Camras, 1991, 1992) theoretical perspectives. Each of the four ways is linked to how the developing child responds to the environment in an intentional, goal-directed way, thus rendering that environment emotion-evocative, which feeds back into the child's repertoire of what he or she brings to the contextual interaction. This notion of a feedback system is not new; indeed, it is part of the self-organizing approach to emotional development (e.g., Fogel et al., 1992), and is also reflected in Larsen and Prizmic-Larsen's (2006) discussion of the necessity for multimethod measurement in emotion research. These authors all address emotion as a multiresponse system in which the various components of emotion interact with one another (e.g., facial expressions may amplify subjective experience of emotion). Larsen and Prizmic-Larsen (2006) also raise further measurement issues of whether emotion is being investigated categorically (e.g., discrete or basic emotions) or dimensionally (e.g., hedonic tone, degree of arousal), and whether emotion is viewed from a state or trait perspective. Context further complicates the measurement of emotion and undoubtedly contributes to the fluidity or loose coupling of the varied response systems subsumed under the construct "emotion."

CONTEXT AND ITS ATTRIBUTES

Many studies emphasize how emotional development is simultaneously embedded in both verbal and nonverbal interpersonal exchanges, and in contexts that children respond to in relationship to their goals (for reviews, see Denham, 1998; Saarni, Campos, Camras, & Witherington, 2006). We can look at emotional development as a series of accumulated changes that reflect past opportunities for learning emotion-laden meaningful connections, but that only become manifest or expressed in the context of the moment. Such a viewpoint has been adopted by theorists such as Lerner and Kauffman (1985), who have described contextualism relative to development as a view that emphasizes successive (as opposed to progressive or endpoint-oriented) probabilistic change in the transactions between individual and environment over time. This view allows for more plasticity in development than do more constrained developmental models, which focus primarily on structural change (e.g., a cognitive-developmental approach assumes that the endpoint is the acquisition of formal operations). Contextualism may also be thought of as pragmatic and instrumental, with philosophical roots in the work of William James (1907/1975) and especially John Dewey (1925, 1934). To understand the pragmatics of a given instance of behavior, we need to consider the interpenetration of subject and context; that is, the person acts on his or her world even as the world reciprocally acts on the person. This again echoes the relational–functionalist position in developmental theory, insofar as behavior is responsive to an affordant environment and behavior functions so as to engage instrumentally with that affordant environment (Campos et al., 1994).

Time and Context

Lewis (1997) has argued that a contextual view of development means that earlier events are unlikely to have much relation to later ones. This is especially so "if the earlier events that are studied are not related to the needs and plans of the individual as they exist now or in the future" (p. 68). This is a potent idea for emotional development, for it means that emotion-related behavior at Time 1 need not influence or be related to emotion-related behavior at Time 2, *unless* Time 1 and Time 2 are both occasions that are defined by the same needs and plans of the individual expressing the emotion-related behavior. But this raises a double-barreled question: How might needs and plans be continuous across time and thus recurrently elicit similar emotional responses, and exactly how much time are we talking about? One possible solution is to think in terms of how the future can be embedded in the present: Our emotional functioning is revealed in how we strive to reach our goals, or are faced with having to revise them, or may be blocked from attaining them. This process may yield consequences that prove to be relatively desirable or undesirable in the here-and-now, but we do not live only in the present. The very fact that we have goals and intentions means

that the future affects our present actions. Our wants and desires are the sources of our motives, and thus they orient us toward the future—providing us, so to speak, with some navigational strategies for making it through the contextual landscape presently facing us (see also the discussion by Josephs, 1998). Thus, although we may debate whether the only known endpoint toward which our development "progresses" is our own death, we are not devoid of a future in the shorter run. It is firmly entrenched in our goals, and from this standpoint, our present adaptive efforts are wedded to our future. How far into the future—10 seconds or 10 years—is not known, for the dynamic flux inherent in context (especially in those circumstances not under our control) can intervene and lay waste to the best of our long-range plans. This is not to imply that contextual shifts are somehow undesirable; indeed, they can also provide unexpected opportunities for change or even release from an otherwise dreary and emotionally numbing life situation.

To complicate our thinking about emotional development still further, Lewis (1997) has also argued that a given behavior can instrumentally serve as the means to multiple goals, just as a variety of different behaviors may be useful for reaching the same goal. An example common in Western societies that illustrates the first point is crying: Tears may be shed in response to a loss or in response to being deeply moved (as in awe-inspiring events). Similarly, a social smile may function as a metacommunicative comment about one's own minor social gaffe or as a signal to another that his or her social gaffe was noticed but excused. As a further illustration, different emotional-expressive behaviors may be recruited to reach the same general goal; for example, when children want to be accepted by their friends (the goal), they variously adopt "cool emotional fronts" (Gottman, Katz, & Hooven, 1997; Saarni & von Salisch, 1993) but can also smile engagingly and genuinely (von Salisch, 1996). Both strategies are useful for fostering relationships with peers.

Communication of Emotion and Context

A number of developmental theorists have asserted that emotion communication cannot be separated from its context (Barrett, 1993; Fabes, 2002; Saarni, 1989, 1990; Trevarthen, 1984, 1993). Certainly the meaning of a particular facial expression is qualified by the context in which it occurs, as was described by Camras (1991): Her young daughter's expression of disgust was revealed both when her face was washed and when she was merely pulled into an upright position. It is the onlooker or recipient of the communicative message who must infer what the sender is communicating about his or her emotional experience. Did little Justine Camras experience both face washing and being pulled upright as distressingly aversive, or were these events simply interrupting whatever she was doing at the time? Or was one aversive and the other effortful? It is the parents, upon witnessing their baby's emotional-expressive behavior in conjunction with some situation, who attribute distress, irritability, or effort to their infant. Thus emotion communication becomes more complicated, for now we must add to the context surrounding the sender's emotional-expressive message the context surrounding the recipient as he or she attributes meaningfulness to the message.

Illustrative of the kind of complexity that one encounters if one seriously wants to examine how context affects emotion communication is the investigation of family conflict undertaken by Noller, Feeney, Sheehan, and Peterson (2000) with two-parent households and their adolescent twins. Although neither conflict between the spouses nor a mother's reports of conflict with her twins correlated with styles of conflict *between* the twins, a father's report of negative emotional communication (demand–withdraw patterns that were experienced as hostile or invalidating) with his adolescent twins was associated with increased expression of negativity and hostility *between* the twins. Noller et al. argued that this style of emotion communication was largely transmitted in nonverbal emotionally expressive behaviors—unpleasant vocalics (e.g., a sarcastic tone of voice), negative facial expressions, and other nonsupportive behaviors (e.g., closed, rigid body posture). In short, participants in emotional communication are both "senders" and "receivers" of emotional-expressive messages, and these messages are imbued with the individuals' own emotional expectancies, projections, and associations. The emotional-expressive exchanges can themselves be elicitors of emotion in the participants that influence subsequent coping efforts (e.g., withdrawal after being the recipient of a sarcastic comment accompanied by a sneering fa-

cial expression), and obviously relationships acquire meaning and nuance as various styles of emotion communication are exchanged (see also Gottman et al., 1997; Katz & Woodin, 2002; Ratner & Stettner, 1991; Saarni & Weber, 1999; Steinberg & Laird, 1989).

Reciprocal Emotion Communication and Context

Cross-cultural research on emotion socialization suggests that "emotions can be seen as both the medium and the message of socialization. Their uniqueness, [as well as] their crucial importance for understanding development, lies in this dual and encompassing role" (Lutz, 1983, p. 60). Thus, even as we may observe emotional development *in* a child, those who interact with the child are communicating their own emotions *to* the child, often elicited by their evaluation of the child's emotional behavior (Fabes, Poulin, Eisenberg, & Madden-Derdich, 2002; McDowell, Kim, O'Neil, & Parke, 2002; Spinrad & Stifter, 2002). Parenthetically, infancy researchers have long noted this sort of complementary, reciprocal, and incremental "dovetailing" of infants' and mothers' responses to one another (e.g., Cappella, 1981; Wasserman & Lewis, 1982). In addition to parents and other family members who are engaged in this reciprocal emotion-socializing process with children, the larger world of peers, the mass media, and other adult figures (e.g., teachers) are also part of the emotionally communicative social context. Thus children acquire both emotion-laden beliefs and emotional-expressive behaviors that reflect these different influences. At the same time, their cultural beliefs about feelings and how they have learned to express their emotions converge toward (sub)cultural norms (Gallois, 1994; Kirouac & Hess, 1999; Wierzbicka, 1994). Children become culturally predictable—a view elaborated by McNaughton (1996) on parenting practices and cultural identity, and by Tomasello, Kruger, and Ratner (1993) on the significance of intersubjectivity in cultural learning and human development.

The Taxonomy of Context

In an early paper, Lewis (1978) noted how difficult was the task of creating a meaningful taxonomy of situations. One could do so by using physical properties, such as the location of a situation; the functional activities associated with situations, such as eating, playing, or working; or the social/relational aspect of situations, such as being with family members versus with peers. But these dimensions interact with one another as well: For instance, playing with peers may occur away from home more often for older children, but less often for younger children. The more complex interaction of situational features in older children's play means that there will be less adult supervision, whereas for younger children there is more supervision; what then are the implications for the nature of their emotional experience in these different play settings? This approach—taking salient features of a context and combining them to yield research questions—is less often pursued than the reverse, which is to compare older and younger children's play with peers and "discover" that the context affects what they do!

Examples of how investigators have examined emotional development relative to different definitions of context include emphasizing the verbal/sociolinguistic environment that the child is exposed to (e.g., Denham & Auerbach, 1995; Dunn, Brown, & Beardsall, 1991; Lewis & Freedle, 1973; Miller & Sperry, 1987), the peer group setting as a mutually influencing context for emotional experience and/or emotion understanding (e.g., Asher & Rose, 1997; Saarni, 1988; Underwood, Hurley, Johanson, & Mosley, 1999), and the influence of emotional-expressive signals on emotional functioning (e.g., Cassidy, Parke, Butkovsky, & Braungart, 1992; Halberstadt, 1991; Hubbard, 2001; Lewis & Michalson, 1985; Saarni, 1992).

Researchers often explicitly invoke context as a substantial part of their investigation into some emotional process, and in recent years a number of studies have been carried out in different social contexts (e.g., within the family, between peers), and others have described in detail the kinds of processes that characterize the emotion-laden transactional flow back and forth between child and context (for a review, see Saarni et al., 2006). Process-oriented research seems especially well suited to an examination of emotional development in context, but this sort of research approach is not common in investigations of emotional development (however, see Bainum, Lounsbury, & Pollio, 1984, for a naturalistic study of smiling and laughing in young children; Gentzler, Contreras-Grau, Kerns, & Weimer, 2005, for study of parent–child dyadic emotional com-

munication; and Saarni, 1992, for a study of school-age children's attempts to influence the emotional state of a depressed adult). In the next section, I review several relevant studies that seem particularly illustrative of how context has been incorporated into research on emotional development.

SOME EXEMPLARY STUDIES

I examine in this section several important categories of how investigators have integrated the critical role played by social context into their research on emotional development. The categories into which I have rather arbitrarily placed the sorts of context involved include (1) relationship processes and attributes (such as friendship) that overlap with relationship dimensions (such as degree of closeness or degree of conflict); (2) expressive behavior in the "sender" as context for the child recipient; (3) environmental contexts such as culture; and (4) dispositions in the child that interact with social contexts. Due to space constraints, I am not be able to address the rich literature on young children's acquisition of discourse strategies and narrative practices as they relate to a contextual view of emotional development (e.g., Fivush, 1991; Nelson, 1996; Oppenheim, Nir, Warren, & Emde, 1997). Nor can I review here the many fascinating investigations of how young children employ language to mediate their understanding of emotions in context (e.g., Bretherton, Fritz, Zahn-Waxler, & Ridgeway, 1986; Cervantes & Callanan, 1998; Denham & Auerbach, 1995; Dunn, Bretherton, & Munn, 1987).

Relationship Processes and Attributes as Mediating or Moderating Contexts

One of the major ways that relationships as contexts for emotional development have been studied in children has been to look at linkages between children's relationships (most often, those with their parents) and the sorts of emotional functioning the children subsequently learn or express. To illustrate, Cassidy (1994) has argued that attachment style is related to children's subsequent emotion regulation, and others suggest that parent–child relationships are linked to children's subsequent emotional competence (e.g., Denham, Mitchell-Copeland, Strandberg, Auerbach, & Blair, 1997), empathy (Strayer & Roberts, 2004), and vicarious emotional responses (Eisenberg, Fabes, Schaller, Carlo, & Miller, 1991). These relational linkages have been construed either as "moderators" (they enhance, amplify, decrease, or inhibit the expression of the relationship) or as "mediators" (they are more direct causal links in the relationship). A considerable literature exists on young children's attachment status (secure, insecure/resistant, insecure/avoidant) and their social-emotional competence (reviewed in Contreras & Kerns, 2000). However, it is not always clear how attachment exerts this influence on children's subsequent social competence; that is, is it mediated through some process of caregiving or through its influence on children's emotion regulation, or is it moderated by the child's temperamental proclivities? Thompson (2006) argues convincingly that attachment security predicts children's social competence (defined as enhanced understanding of others' feelings as well as sociometric status), and that this relationship is mediated by sensitive caregiving that emphasizes open discourse about emotions (Cassidy, Kirsh, Scolton, & Parke, 1996; Denham, Blair, Schmidt, & DeMulder, 2002; Raikes & Thompson, 2005). However, it should be pointed out that this relationship appears anchored in sensitive caregiving that is relatively stable and continuous in children's lives.

Further support for the important role that emotion communication plays in relationships for children and their subsequent emotional functioning comes from a recent study by Gentzler et al. (2005) and a related study (using the same sample of children and parents) by Contreras, Kerns, Weimer, Gentzler, and Tomich (2000). The sample consisted of 75 fifth graders and their parents, and in the Gentzler et al. (2005) study, the children and parents were videotaped dyadically while discussing a distressing episode. A couple of measures were given to the parents to report on their children's tendency to experience negative emotions and their children's likely use of various coping strategies. The children also completed a measure that indexed the degree to which they were comfortable in affectively sharing with their parents. The investigators globally scored the observational task, with the intent of establishing the degree to which the parent and child in each dyad could communicate emotions openly to one another. Their results indicated that parents' reports of their children's emotions and their openness with

their children in the observation task both correlated with their children's constructive coping: Those children who were the "best constructive copers" were those who were comfortable communicating their emotions to their parents, and their parents in turn were supportive and responsive in emotionally distressing contexts.

In the earlier Contreras et al. (2000) study, the investigators wanted to determine whether mother–child attachment would influence children's constructive coping strategies, and whether these in turn would influence the children's peer competence (judged by their teachers). The children's attachment security (assessed with a scale developed by Kerns, Klepac, & Cole, 1996) and attachment-related state of mind (assessed with a semistructured projective interview developed by Resnick, 1993) were indeed found to be related to their use of constructive coping strategies (reported by their mothers), which was found to partially mediate the children's peer competence. What occurred was that the children's degree of negative emotionality (here viewed as a temperamental disposition) moderated the association between constructive coping and peer competence. If children who were prone to negative emotionality could draw upon constructive coping strategies, they were as likely to be judged as having competent social behavior as children low in negative emotionality were. Their attachment relationship was related to their constructive coping repertoire, but not to their proneness to negative emotionality. Thus the attachment relationship buffered children who were disposed toward frequent experiences of negative emotion, such that they acquired constructive coping strategies that they could then access in their social relationships with peers.

From a very different perspective, the various strategies used by children and youths to regulate anger in the context of close friendship was examined by von Salisch (2005). She developed a self-report scale for use with children, and a slightly modified version for adolescents, that examined anger regulation strategies within friendships—specifically, the strategies of ignoring, confrontation, redirection of attention, self-blaming, explanation, reconciliation, and humor. Her scale differs from other scales assessing anger reactions because of its emphasis on relational context (friendship); also, it does not view anger reactions as a trait of the person, unlike measures such as the State–Trait Anger Expression Inventory (Forgays, Forgays, & Spielberger, 1997) or the Anger Response Inventory for children and adolescents, which is similarly decontextualized (Tangney et al., 1996).

Von Salisch followed 85 children longitudinally for 5 years, from late childhood to mid-adolescence, and found that the adolescents had changed their self-reported regulation strategies: They were significantly more likely to use explanation/reconciliation and humor, and less likely to use confrontation, ignoring, redirection of attention, and self-blaming. What this suggests about the developmental change in anger regulation is that when children and youths are invested in a relationship, they are more likely to use emotion regulation strategies that maintain the relationship. This is not to say that the more "childish" strategies of anger regulation that they reported using when they were younger disappear from their repertoire, but they do not think they work well for maintaining or enhancing a relationship that they care about. Thus relationship context cannot be separated from the emotion regulation strategies or coping strategies that an individual uses, even though the temperamental disposition for emotional reactivity may predispose the individual to more frequent emotionality. Perhaps when the relationship context is one of anonymity or of an "outsider group," then the more childish anger regulation strategies become more likely (e.g., as in road rage incidents).

Emotional-Expressive Behavior as Context

Here I describe three studies examining the influence of adult interactants' emotional-expressive behavior on children's emotional development, which in turn influenced the children's social behavior. The first study was undertaken by McDowell and Parke (2005) with 76 fourth-grade children and their parents. They used various global ratings of parents' interactive behaviors with their children when discussing a difficult and emotion-evocative topic, and developed from these ratings two general composite scores. The first was parental use of positive affect, consisting of positive emotional expressions, negative emotional expressions (reverse-coded), clarity of expression, intensity of expression, and awareness of a child's feelings. The second was degree of control, consisting of parental regulation of a

child's emotions and adopting a controlling/directive style with a child. The children also participated in a "disappointing-gift" experience (Saarni, 1984), yielding four ratings: positive expressive responses, negative expressive responses, degree of tension, and degree of social monitoring. Their social competence was also evaluated via both teacher ratings and peer sociometric ratings 1 year later.

The results indicated that parental positive affect in the parent–child interaction task strongly predicted their children's use of fewer negative expressive behaviors in the disappointing-gift situation; that is, the children were able to mask their disappointment at receiving an inappropriate toy, and thus to avoid violating the common etiquette rule of "Smile and be gracious when given a gift, even if you don't like it." The influence of the parental control variable was also significant, but varied by parental gender: Higher father control was associated with fewer child positive expressive behaviors, and higher mother control was associated with a greater degree of tension manifested by a child.

For the prediction of the children's social competence a year later, children's display rule use predicted both teacher and peer ratings: Children's positive expressive behaviors in the disappointing-gift situation were strongly associated with positive peer ratings, and their low use of negative expressive behaviors in the same situation was more strongly associated with their teachers' positive social competence ratings of them. Parental positive affect was also significantly associated with higher positive teacher ratings of social competence, whereas for the peer ratings only mothers' positive affect had some influence. The mediational analyses revealed that children's negative expressive behaviors mediated the effects that their parents' positive affect and control (especially for fathers) had on their social competence with peers. What this complex pattern of results suggests is that as children mature, their parents are less likely to be present when their children are engaged in peer interaction, and thus we would presume that they are less likely to *directly* influence their children's social competence with peers. However, the effects of parents' emotional-expressive style are still manifest in terms of how their children manage their own emotional-expressive style, and it is this style that in turn affects children's social skills and acceptance by their peers. Parents' influence on their children's socially competent behavior with their peers is thus indirect.

Another intriguing study on the effects of caregivers' emotional-expressive behavior on children's social behavior was undertaken by Karrass and Walden (2005). They exposed 4- and 5-year-old children to an experimenter who adopted either a warm, friendly, and responsive (nurturant) expressive style or a cold, unfriendly, and unresponsive (non-nurturant) style. The children's facial expressions were coded for 30 seconds during part of this interaction. Then a second experimenter came in and interacted with the child over a mock task, and the child's social initiatives toward the second experimenter were observed. Their results indicated that when children interacted with a nurturant adult, they then initiated significantly more overtures toward a second adult than did children exposed to a non-nurturant adult. The non-nurturant adult also elicited significantly less happy facial expressions. Lastly, the children's happiness (as indicated by facial expressions) with the first experimenter significantly predicted their social initiatives with the second experimenter, and, indeed, their expressed happiness partially mediated the relationship between nurturing caregiving style and number of social initiatives with the second adult. Interestingly, expressed sadness did not partially mediate the relationship between nurturing style and social initiation. From a contextual point of view, what was apparently happening for these children was that exposure to a short social interaction yielding a happy experience acted as a prime for subsequent sociability, whereas a distressing social interaction elicited a more cautious (perhaps tense or sad) response in subsequent social interaction with another, similar female adult.

Karrass and Walden's (2005) results have some parallels with data I obtained with elementary school children (Saarni, 1992) in an early observational study where the children were faced with having to cheer up a despondent "market researcher" who previously had been very friendly. Whereas Karrass and Walden had randomly assigned their children to either the nurturing or the non-nurturing style of interaction, I had children act as their own controls by having them interact twice with the same experimenter, who varied her expressive behavior from happy and friendly in the first meeting to sad and withdrawn in the

second. The social task to be accomplished seemed straightforward, but the management of one's own emotions and behavior presented complex challenges in this case. Being confronted with the social context of a depressed woman could make oneself sad, angered that one had glibly agreed to try to cheer her up, or challenged to try to make her happier. Eighty children across three age groups (7–8, 9–10, and 11–12 years) participated, and all sessions were held at their school. An assistant accompanied the children to and from their classrooms, and prior to the second ("sad") meeting asked the children to help cheer up her colleague, who was feeling quite "down." All agreed to do so.

The children were videotaped throughout their interaction with the market researcher while doing a task for her. This permitted the establishment of a base rate of emotional-expressive behaviors when the children were with the market researcher in her happy state. This base rate could then be compared to what they attempted to do when trying to cheer her up in her sad state. As a check on the manipulation, a mirror was placed behind the children in a slightly offset position, so that the video camera could also simultaneously capture the "market researcher's" expressive behavior toward the child.

Results indicated that the oldest children (11–12 years) were the most positive in their emotional-expressive behavior in both the happy and sad sessions, and that the middle age group (9–10 years) revealed a curiously flat emotional profile in response to the two emotional-state variations. Among the youngest children (7–8 years) were those who did appear to become "engulfed" by the sad researcher's demeanor and looked as though they would very nearly cry, crawl under the table, or try to leave. Interestingly, the preadolescents, while showing the most positive behavior toward the sad researcher, also revealed the most tension-filled expressive behaviors—for example, biting their lips, touching themselves, rubbing their fingers together, and so forth. From an impressionistic standpoint, these oldest children seemed more self-contained and less influenced by the sad researcher's emotional-expressive behavior, despite their tension-laden nonverbal behaviors. The content of their conversation with her was also more often "upbeat," and they talked more than the two younger groups, who tended to clam up when faced with the sad woman. Few gender differences were found in this study, but older girls did smile more at the sad market researcher as a strategy to try to cheer her up. In contrast, some of the older boys appeared annoyed at the prospect of having to help cheer someone up, despite having agreed to do so (e.g., they drummed their fingers on the table, bumped around in their seats).

This observational study raised many questions about the mutual interaction of two individuals' emotional-expressive cues, as well as the added effect on children when they are aware of being videotaped. The context manipulation—interacting with either a happy or a sad person—overlapped with other contextual features: This was a relatively unfamiliar individual, who was an adult (more powerful status relative to the child), and the larger setting was that the children were at their school. Dealing with a depressed adult well known to a child while the child and adult are at home is a very different context, and one that has been productively explored by Zahn-Waxler and her colleagues with younger children (Zahn-Waxler, Cole, & Barrett, 1991; Zahn-Waxler, Kochanska, Krupnick, & McKnew, 1990). But in both settings, the effect of having to interact with a depressed adult is noticeably more negative for younger children. Perhaps one of the emotional tasks that young adolescents in North American society begin to learn is how, when, and with whom to "disconnect" their emotions from those of another, so as to maintain their own emotional boundaries when it is adaptive for them to do so (e.g., adolescents are relatively less involved in parental conflict; Cummings, Ballard, & El-Sheikh, 1991).

Cultural Practices as Context

Miller and Goodnow (1995) have argued that the very "normativeness" of cultural practices means that they are embedded in expectations about appropriate behavior, and that such expected behavior is in turn embedded in values and assumed conventions that help to give the cultural group its identity. They have argued further that children's development cannot be separated from cultural context and its associated practices, for these constitute the route by which the children become members of a community, sharing its beliefs and values. At the same time, developing children have the poten-

tial to change or modulate cultural practices (perhaps especially in adolescence); in other words, cultural values, beliefs, and practices can and do change.

Richly illustrative of the importance of cultural values and practices on emotional development is a recent study by Cole, Tamang, and Shrestha (2006) with 3- to 5-year-old children from two subcultures within Nepal: the Tamang, who practice Tibetan Buddhism, and the Brahman, who are high-caste Hindus and have higher status in Nepal than the Tamang. I concur with Cole and her colleagues when they state that "cultural values, which organize a community's beliefs and practices for maintaining standards of conduct, penetrate caregiver behavior. In the process of childrearing [which itself reflects many diverse cultural practices] children's emotions are socialized" (p. 1239). Cole et al. found that the Tamang households were characterized by high adult nurturance and child trust toward adults, whereas the Brahman households were more likely to promote autonomy and differentiation between adults and children. When the researchers examined their exhaustive observations of emotion episodes within the households, Tamang adults were more likely to respond to children's shame with teaching and nurturing, and to their anger with rebuking and teasing. Consistent with some of Cole and colleagues' earlier work with this population, Tamang children's scripts for anger tended to dismiss or minimize anger (Cole, Brushi, & Tamang, 2002), and anger was viewed as undesirable and not socially competent by village elders. The Brahman adults were more likely to respond to their children' anger with positive attention, as in a "teachable moment," and to children's shame with ignoring. Not surprisingly, Tamang children expressed shame more frequently than anger, and Brahman children expressed anger more often than shame. Cole et al. (2006) have explained these subcultural differences as reflecting important values differences and status differences between the two communities. The Tamang value self-effacement and compassionate tolerance, and anger is viewed as destructive to social harmony. For the privileged Brahmans, properly regulated anger may help to establish dominance and competence; the adults attribute greater value to academic competence in their children, and regulated anger may play a part in establishing or claiming one's societal and educational success. Cole et al. have also noted that Brahmans' expression of anger to lower-status people would not be reacted to negatively, since they are the ones in power and thus in control. These political–societal differences and religious value differences play themselves out in culturally imbued caregiving practices, such that within only a few years the children of the Tamang and the Brahmans reflect these values in their own scripted emotional responses.

Child Disposition in Interaction with Context

Children's temperament and biological disposition toward "emotionality" or behavioral inhibition have been extensively investigated, and the reader is referred to two recent reviews for a far more complete discussion than will be provided here (Kagan & Fox, 2006; Rothbart & Bates, 2006). Recently Ellis, Boyce, and their colleagues have proposed that children can also differ in genetically linked reactivity to stressful contexts (Ellis, Essex, & Boyce, 2005; Ellis, Jackson, & Boyce, 2006); they suggest that "biological sensitivity to context confers fitness benefits not only in highly stressful environments (by augmenting vigilance to threats and dangers) but also in highly protective environments (by increasing permeability to social resources and support)" (Ellis et al., 2006, p. 205). Their data on preschool children and their families revealed a curvilinear relationship with reactivity: Disproportionately more children were highly reactive either in highly supportive families or in highly stressed and adverse family environments. In "average" family environments, children were relatively low in reactivity. Ellis et al.'s theoretical position is that in environments that offer many possibilities ("multiniche"), as found in family rearing situations, many phenotypic expressions of stress reactivity will be favored, and that at the extremes (highly supportive vs. highly adverse), gene-linked regulatory effects will be switched on (as in reaching a threshold).

Bugental and Beaulieu (2004) adopted this context sensitivity position to explain their results in following medically at-risk children (born prematurely or with poor Apgar scores). They found that as toddlers these children's health prospered if their mothers had learned to provide sensitive and supportive care (and to avoid depression) by having participated in a home visitation program. In a control group, mothers did not receive such support, and as a result their toddlers fared far worse in health outcomes. Bugental and Beaulieu interpreted their results as showing support for context sensitivity could be "switched on" by exposure to early stress. The toddlers' reactivity was moderated by supportive and sensitive parenting, such that very positive outcomes for the children were obtained as they thrived in this sort of protective family environment—in contrast to biologically vulnerable children reared in adverse family environments (see also Bugental, 2003). In a similar vein, early research by Riksen-Walraven (1978) had working-class mothers trained to provide particularly responsive and contingent caregiving to their infants, with the result that their infants demonstrated more exploratory behavior and learned more quickly on a contingency task than a similar sample of infants whose low-income mothers were not trained and whose caregiving was not optimal. The point to be made here is that these very immediate and contingent social-interactive responses provided an affordant environment for the infants to respond to, and thus to fulfill their potential. A low-affordance, reduced-contingency/nonstimulating social environment is simply not designed to maximize children's potential.

Two other studies deserve mention here in terms of how children's emotional dispositions interact with social contexts. The first study, by Arsenio, Cooperman, and Lover (2000), observed 4- to 5-year-olds' emotional dispositions in free-play situations at their preschool and categorized them into anger, happiness, sadness, and so forth. They also observed children's emotional displays during aggressive episodes (gleeful vs. angry); obtained a measure of children's understanding of emotion; and had their teachers rate them on social competence, as well as having their peers rate them sociometrically. Their results showed that the relationship among peer acceptance, emotion understanding, and emotional disposition was mediated by the children's aggression, and also that children's displays of happiness during aggression directly affected (negatively) their peer acceptance. These latter children appeared to enjoy being "mean" and may have been displaying instrumental, hostile aggression tendencies rather than the more ordinary reactive or provoked aggression. Not surprisingly, they were not well liked. However, this happiness displayed during aggressive interactions was it-self not related to the children's disposition toward happiness as displayed during the baseline observational period. Instead, what predicted aggression were the children's baseline disposition toward anger, displays of happiness during the aggressive episode, and deficient emotion understanding. This combination in preschool children of angry emotional propensities, gleeful victimization or hostile power assertion, and deficient emotion knowledge appeared to push the children toward increasingly negative social outcomes, with the result that their social context for emotional development becomes channeled into one of peer rejection (Dodge et al., 2003; Katz, 2000).

The second study was an examination of emotion-regulating strategy use relative to different emotion-evocative situations. Zimmermann and Stansbury (2003) exposed 53 young preschoolers to three different sorts of challenging or stress-inducing situations: two anxiety-inducing situations (approaching a male stranger, interrupting a busy female experimenter who did not want to be interrupted) and a frustration-inducing situation (delay of gratification with mother present). Their results indicated that both context and temperamental reactivity (jointly measured by parent report and a lab-based observation) influenced what sort of emotion-regulating strategy was used. Self-comforting emotion regulation was most often elicited in the approaching-male-stranger situation, and distraction and instrumental regulatory strategies were more often used in the busy-experimenter and delay-of-gratification situations, which were also viewed as less distressing to the young children. (More specifically, the busy experimenter was female, she was not trying to engage the child, and a box of toys was nearby; in the frustration task, the mother was in the room, and the child had been asked to wait before eating some candy.) Temperament influenced this general pattern, such that shyer children more often used the instrumental tactic of withdrawal. Bolder children more often used distraction tactics. Attentional focusing was also related to use of a self-comforting strategy (e.g., sucking one's thumb), and it appeared as though these children had less flexible deployment of attention; that is, they focused on the stress-inducing situation instead of accessing available options in the situation for distraction purposes (e.g., exploring the box of toys). The degree of challenge or stress in the situation tended to make the effect of temperament more salient, which makes sense insofar as low-challenge situations (e.g., the delay-of-gratification situation with mother present) are not likely to elicit dispositional biases for emotion regulation.

What is potentially of interest here is that temperament- or disposition-related emotional style may contribute to children's avoiding some situations and choosing other situations that are conducive to their experiencing less negative emotional arousal or distress. This tendency for emotional disposition and context to begin showing coherence is borne out in Fabes and his colleagues' research on preschoolers' negative emotionality and their increasing experience of social isolation over a 3-month period observation of their social interaction—or lack thereof (Fabes, Hanish, Martin, & Eisenberg, 2002). It was not clear in this research whether these children who were prone to negative affect were choosing to engage more in solitary activities, or whether they were increasingly being rejected by their peers and thus left alone, but the outcome was the same: A disposition to display strong and negative emotion was associated with aloneness. Indeed, Asher and colleagues' work has long indicated that rejected children do feel lonely (e.g., Asher, Parkhurst, Hymel, & Williams, 1990). Lastly, a longitudinal study of adolescents (Murphy, Shepard, Eisenberg, & Fabes, 2004) indicated considerable continuity among reduced social functioning, a bias toward negative emotionality, and reduced regulatory skills (according to parent and teacher reports), again implying an increasing coherence over time of disposition and social contexts in which reduced social skills are displayed.

CONCLUSION

The bioecological platform that I endorse for understanding the interface (indeed, the interpenetration) of emotional development and context rests upon the ideas put forward by Bronfenbrenner and Ceci (1994), who proposed that proximal processes mediate the links between genotype and phenotype. These proximal processes are the kinds of social-contextual variables that have been addressed in this chapter—namely, caregiver behaviors, communication within relationships, interaction with peers and siblings, and so forth.

These immediate and also *motivating* interactive processes create dynamic environments that become affordant for infants and children to respond to; these responses in turn change those dynamic environments, and the ensuing chain of affordances stimulates the interactants' responses to one another further over time (see also Larsen & Almeida, 1999). These affordant social contexts are often contingent on the dovetailing of interpersonal communicative behaviors, and thus the emotional displays of interactants play a very salient role in the proximal processes mediating between our genotypes and what we in fact reveal as our behavioral phenotypes. The research described previously by Ellis et al. (2005, 2006) on context sensitivity is relevant here as well: Emotional reactivity was elevated both in highly favorable environments and in adverse environments, but the former produced highly adaptive outcomes and the latter poor outcomes (see also Bugental & Beaulieu, 2004). It is my hope that researchers studying emotion development will remember that emotions do not occur only in regions of the brain. The developing brain, affected as it is by its genetic heritage, still needs an environment in which to grow and reveal its complexity and plasticity in dynamic interpersonal exchanges with others in an interpersonal context.

REFERENCES

Arsenio, W., Cooperman, S., & Lover, A. (2000). Affective predictors of preschoolers' aggression and peer acceptance: Direct and indirect effects. *Developmental Psychology, 36*, 438–448.

Asher, S., Parkhurst, J., Hymel, S., & Williams, G. (1990). Peer rejection and loneliness in childhood. In S. Asher & J. Coie (Eds.), *Peer rejection in childhood* (pp. 253–273). New York: Cambridge University Press.

Asher, S., & Rose, A. (1997). Promoting children's social-emotional adjustment with peers. In P. Salovey & D. Sluyter (Eds.), *Emotional development and emotional intelligence* (pp. 196–224). New York: Basic Books.

Bainum, C. K., Lounsbury, K., & Pollio, H. (1984). The development of laughter and smiling in nursery school children. *Child Development, 55*, 1946–1957.

Barrett, K. (1993). The development of nonverbal communication of emotion: A functionalist perspective. *Journal of Nonverbal Behavior, 17*, 145–169.

Bretherton, I., Fritz, J., Zahn-Waxler, C., & Ridgeway, D. (1986). Learning to talk about emotions: A functionalist perspective. *Child Development, 57*, 529–548.

Bronfenbrenner, U., & Ceci, S. J. (1994). Nature–nurture reconceptualized in developmental perspective: A bioecological model. *Psychological Review, 101*, 568–586.

Bugental, D. B. (2003). *Thriving in the face of childhood adversity.* New York: Psychology Press.

Bugental, D. B., & Beaulieu, D. (2004). Maltreatment risk among disabled children: A bio-social-cognitive approach. In R. Kail (Ed.), *Advances in child development and behavior* (Vol. 31, pp. 129–164). San Diego: Academic Press.

Campos, J., Mumme, D., Kermoian, R., & Campos, R. (1994). A functionalist perspective on the nature of emotion. In N. Fox (Ed.), The development of emotion regulation. *Monographs of the Society for Research in Child Development, 59(2–3, Serial No. 240), 284–303.*

Camras, L. (1991). Conceptualizing early infant affect: Emotions as fact, fiction or artifact? In K. T. Strongman (Ed.), *International review of studies on emotion* (Vol. 1, pp. 16–28). New York: Wiley.

Camras, L. (1992). Expressive development and basic emotions. *Cognition and Emotion, 6*, 269–283.

Camras, L., Meng, Z., Ujiie, T., Dharamsi, S., Miyake, K., Oster, H., et al. (2002). Observing emotion in infants: Facial expression, body behavior, and rater judgments of responses to an expectancy-violating event. *Emotion, 2*, 179–193.

Cappella, J. (1981). Mutual influence in expressive behavior: Adult–adult and infant–adult dyadic interaction. *Psychological Bulletin, 89*, 101–132.

Cassidy, J. (1994). Emotion regulation: Influences of attachment relationships. In N. Fox (Ed.), The development of emotion regulation. *Monographs of the Society for Research in Child Development, 59(2–3, Serial No. 240), 228–249.*

Cassidy, J., Kirsh, S., Scolton, K., & Parke, R. D. (1996). Attachment and representations of peer relationships. *Developmental Psychology, 32*, 892–904.

Cassidy, J., Parke, R., Butkovsky, L., & Braungart, J. (1992). Family–peer connections: The roles of emotional expressiveness within the family and children's understanding of emotions. *Child Development, 63*, 603–618.

Cervantes, C., & Callanan, M. (1998). Labels and explanations in mother–child emotion talk: Age and gender differentiation. *Developmental Psychology, 34*, 88–98.

Clements, F. E., & Shelford, V. E. (1939). *Bio-ecology.* New York: Wiley.

Cole, P. M., Brushi, C., & Tamang, B. (2002). Cultural differences in children's emotional reactions to difficult situations. *Child Development, 73*, 983–996.

Cole, P. M., Tamang, B., & Shrestha, S. (2006). Cultural variations in the socialization of young children's anger and shame. *Child Development, 77*, 1237–1251.

Contreras, J., & Kerns, K. (2000). Emotion regulation processes: Explaining links between parent–child attachment and peer relationships. In K. Kerns, J. Contreras, & A. Neal-Barnett (Eds.), *Family and peers: Linking two social worlds* (pp. 1–25). Westport, CT: Praeger.

Contreras, J., Kerns, K., Weimer, B., Gentzler, A., & Tomich, P. (2000). Emotion regulation as a mediator of associations between mother–child attachment and peer relationships in middle childhood. *Journal of Family Psychology, 14,* 111–124.

Cummings, E. M., Ballard, M., & El-Sheikh, M. (1991). Responses of children and adolescents to interadult anger as a function of gender, age, and mode of expression. *Merrill–Palmer Quarterly, 37,* 543–560.

Denham, S. (1998). *Emotional development in young children.* New York: Guilford Press.

Denham, S., & Auerbach, S. (1995). Mother–child dialogue about emotions. *Genetic, Social, and General Psychology Monographs, 121,* 311–338.

Denham, S., Blair, K., Schmidt, M., & DeMulder, E. (2002). Compromised emotional competence: Seeds of violence sown early? *American Journal of Orthopsychiatry, 72,* 70–82.

Denham, S., Mitchell-Copeland, J., Strandberg, K., Auerbach, S., & Blair, K. (1997). Parental contributions to preschoolers' emotion competence: Direct and indirect effects. *Motivation and Emotion, 21,* 65–86.

Dewey, J. (1925). *Experience and nature.* La Salle, IL: Open Court Press.

Dewey, J. (1934). *Art as experience.* New York: Berkeley.

Dodge, K. A., Lansford, J., Burks, V., Bates, J. E., Pettit, G., Fontaine, R., et al. (2003). Peer rejection and social information-processing factors in the development of aggressive behavior problems in children. *Child Development, 74,* 374–393.

Dunn, J., Bretherton, I., & Munn, P. (1987). Conversations about feeling states between mothers and their young children. *Developmental Psychology, 23,* 132–139.

Dunn, J., Brown, J., & Beardsall, L. (1991). Family talk about feeling states and children's later understanding of others' emotions. *Developmental Psychology, 27,* 448–455.

Eisenberg, N., Fabes, R., Schaller, M., Carlo, G., & Miller, P. A. (1991). The relations of parental characteristics and practices to children's vicarious emotional responding. *Child Development, 62,* 1393–1408.

Ekman, P. (1989). The argument and evidence about universals in facial expressions of emotion. In H. Wagner & A. Manstead (Eds.), *Handbook of social psychophysiology* (pp. 143–163). New York: Wiley.

Ellis, B. J., Essex, M. J., & Boyce, W. T. (2005). Biological sensitivity to context: II. Empirical explorations of an evolutionary-developmental theory. *Development and Psychopathology, 17,* 303–328.

Ellis, B. J., Jackson, J. J., & Boyce, W. T. (2006). The stress response systems: Universality and adaptive individual differences. *Developmental Review, 26,* 175–212.

Fabes, R. (Ed.). (2002). *Emotions and the family.* New York: Haworth Press.

Fabes, R., Hanish, L., Martin, C. L., & Eisenberg, N. (2002). Young children's negative emotionality and social isolation: A latent growth curve analysis. *Merrill–Palmer Quarterly, 48*(3), 284–307.

Fabes, R., Poulin, R., Eisenberg, N., & Madden-Derdich, D. (2002). The Coping with Children's Negative Emotions Scale (CCNES): Psychometric properties and relations with children's emotional competence. In R. Fabes (Ed.), *Emotions and the family* (pp. 285–310). New York: Haworth Press.

Fernández-Dols, J. M. (1999). Facial expression and emotion: A situationist view. In P. Philippot, R. S. Feldman, & E. J. Coats (Eds.), *The social context of nonverbal behavior* (pp. 242–261). Cambridge, UK: Cambridge University Press.

Fivush, R. (1991). The social construction of personal narratives. *Merrill–Palmer Quarterly, 37,* 59–82.

Fogel, A., Nwokah, E., Young-Dedo, J., Messinger, D., Dickson, K. L., Matusov, E., et al. (1992). Social process theory of emotion: A dynamic systems approach. *Social Development, 1,* 122–150.

Forgays, D., Forgays, D. K., & Spielberger, C. (1997). Factor structure of the State–Trait Anger Expression Inventory. *Journal of Personality Assessment, 69,* 497–507.

Fraiberg, S. (1971). *Insights from the blind.* New York: Basic Books.

Gallois, C. (1994). Group membership, social rules, and power: A social psychological perspective on emotional communication. *Journal of Pragmatics, 22,* 301–324.

Gentzler, A., Contreras-Grau, J., Kerns, K., & Weimer, B. (2005). Parent–child emotional communication and children's coping in middle childhood. *Social Development, 14,* 591–612.

Gibson, E. J. (1982). The concept of affordance in development: The renascence of functionalism. In A. W. Collins (Ed.), *Minnesota Symposium on Child Psychology: Vol. 13. Theoretical perspectives on development* (pp. 55–81). Hillsdale, NJ: Erlbaum.

Gottman, J., Katz, L. F., & Hooven, C. (1997). *Metaemotion.* Hillsdale, NJ: Erlbaum.

Halberstadt, A. G. (1991). Toward an ecology of expressiveness: Family socialization in particular and a model in general. In R. S. Feldman & B. Rime (Eds.), *Fundamentals of nonverbal behavior* (pp. 106–160). New York: Cambridge University Press.

Hubbard, J. (2001). Emotion expression processes in children's peer interaction: The role of peer rejection, aggression, and gender. *Child Development, 72,* 1426–1438.

James, W. (1975). *Pragmatism.* Cambridge, MA: Harvard University Press. (Original work published 1907)

Josephs, I. (1998). Constructing one's self in the city of the silent: Dialogue, symbols, and the role of "as-if" in self-development. *Human Development, 41,* 180–195.

Kagan, J., & Fox, N. A. (2006). Biology, culture, and

temperamental biases. In W. Damon & R. Lerner (Series Eds.) & N. Eisenberg (Vol. Ed.), *Handbook of child psychology: Vol. 3. Social, emotional, and personality development* (6th ed., pp. 167–225). New York: Wiley.

Karrass, J., & Walden, T. (2005). Effects of nurturing and non-nurturing caregiving on child social initiative: An experimental investigation of emotion as a mediator of social behavior. *Social Development, 14,* 685–700.

Katz, L. F. (2000). Living in a hostile world: Toward an integrated model of family, peer, and physiological processes in aggressive preschoolers. In K. Kerns, J. Contreras, & A. Neal-Barnett (Eds.), *Family and peers: Linking two social worlds* (pp. 115–136). Westport, CT: Praeger.

Katz, L. F., & Woodin, E. M. (2002). Hostility, hostile detachment, and conflict engagement in marriages: Effects on child and family functioning. *Child Development, 73,* 636–652.

Kerns, K., Klepac, L., & Cole, A. (1996). Peer relationships and preadolescents' perceptions of security in the child–mother relationship. *Developmental Psychology, 32,* 457–466.

Kirouac, G., & Hess, U. (1999). Group membership and the decoding of nonverbal behavior. In P. Philippot, R. S. Feldman, & E. J. Coats (Eds.), *The social context of nonverbal behavior* (pp. 182–210). Cambridge, UK: Cambridge University Press.

Larsen, R. W., & Almeida, D. (1999). Emotional transmission in the daily lives of families: A new paradigm for studying family process. *Journal of Marriage and the Family, 61,* 5–20.

Larsen, R. W., & Prizmic-Larsen, Z. (2006). Measuring emotions: Implications of a multimethod perspective. In M. Eid & E. Diener (Eds.), *Handbook of multimethod measurement in psychology* (pp. 337–351). Washington, DC: American Psychological Association.

Lerner, R. M., & Kauffman, M. (1985). The concept of development in contextualism. *Developmental Review, 5,* 309–333.

Lewis, M. (1978). Situational analysis and the study of behavioral development. In L. Pervin & M. Lewis (Eds.), *Perspectives in interactional psychology* (pp. 49–66). New York: Plenum Press.

Lewis, M. (1997). *Altering fate: Why the past does not predict the future.* New York: Guilford Press.

Lewis, M., & Freedle, R. (1973). Mother–infant dyad: The cradle of meaning. In P. Pliner, L. Krames, & T. Alloway (Eds.), *Communication and affect: Language and thought* (pp. 127–155). New York: Academic Press.

Lewis, M., & Michalson, L. (1985). Faces as signs and symbols. In G. Zivin (Ed.), *The development of expressive behavior: Biology–environment interactions* (pp. 153–182). New York: Academic Press.

McDowell, D. J., Kim, M., O'Neil, R., & Parke, R. D. (2002). Children's emotional regulation and social competence in middle childhood: The role of mater-

nal and paternal interactive style. In R. Fabes (Ed.), *Emotions and the family* (pp. 345–364). New York: Haworth Press.

McDowell, D. J., & Parke, R. D. (2005). Parental control and affect as predictors of children's display rule use and social competence with peers. *Social Development, 14,* 440–457.

McNaughton, S. (1996). Ways of parenting and cultural identity. *Culture and Psychology, 2,* 173–202.

Miller, P., & Sperry, L. L. (1987). The socialization of anger and aggression. *Merrill–Palmer Quarterly, 33,* 1–31.

Miller, P. J., & Goodnow, J. (1995). Cultural practices: Toward an integration of culture and development. *New Directions for Child Development, 67,* 5–16.

Murphy, B., Shepard, S., Eisenberg, N., & Fabes, R. (2004). Concurrent and across time prediction of young adolescents' social functioning: The role of emotionality and regulation. *Social Development, 13,* 56–86.

Murphy, L., & Moriarty, A. (1976). *Vulnerability, coping, and growth.* New Haven, CT: Yale University Press.

Nelson, K. (1996). *Language in cognitive development: Emergence of the mediated mind.* New York: Cambridge University Press.

Noller, P., Feeney, J. A., Sheehan, G., & Peterson, C. (2000). Marital conflict patterns: Links with family conflict and family members' perceptions of one another. *Personal Relationships, 7,* 79–94.

Oppenheim, D., Nir, A., Warren, S., & Emde, R. (1997). Emotion regulation in mother–child narrative co-construction: Associations with children's narratives and adaptation. *Developmental Psychology, 33,* 284–294.

Raikes, H. A., & Thompson, R. A. (2005). Links between risk and attachment security: Models of influence. *Applied Developmental Psychology, 26,* 440–455.

Ratner, H., & Stettner, L. (1991). Thinking and feeling: Putting Humpty Dumpty together again. *Merrill–Palmer Quarterly, 37,* 1–26.

Reissland, N., & Shepherd, J. (2002). Gaze direction and maternal pitch in surprise-eliciting situations. *Infant Behavior and Development, 24,* 408–417.

Resnick, G. (1993). *Manual for the administration, coding and interpretation of the Separation Anxiety Test for 11–14 Year Olds.* Rockville, MD: Westat.

Riksen-Walraven, J. M. (1978). Effects of caregiver behavior on habituation rate and self-efficacy in infants. *International Journal of Behavioral Development, 1,* 105–130.

Rothbart, M. K., & Bates, J. E. (2006). Temperament. In W. Damon & R. Lerner (Series Eds.) & N. Eisenberg (Vol. Ed.), *Handbook of child psychology: Vol. 3. Social, emotional, and personality development* (6th ed., pp. 99–166). New York: Wiley.

Russell, J. A. (1991). Culture and the categorization of emotion. *Psychological Bulletin, 110,* 426–450.

Saarni, C. (1984). An observational study of children's

attempts to monitor their expressive behavior. *Child Development, 55,* 1504–1513.

Saarni, C. (1988). Children's understanding of the interpersonal consequences of dissemblance of nonverbal emotional-expressive behavior. *Journal of Nonverbal Behavior, 12*(4, Pt. 2), 275–294.

Saarni, C. (1989). Children's understanding of strategic control of emotional expression in social transactions. In C. Saarni & P. Harris (Eds.), *Children's understanding of emotion* (pp. 181–208). New York: Cambridge University Press.

Saarni, C. (1990). Emotional competence: How emotions and relationships become integrated. In R. A. Thompson (Ed.), *Nebraska Symposium on Motivation: Vol. 36. Socioemotional development (pp. 115–182). Lincoln: University of Nebraska Press.*

Saarni, C. (1992). Children's emotional-expressive behaviors as regulators of others' happy and sad states. *New Directions for Child Development, 55,* 91–106.

Saarni, C., Campos, J., Camras, L., & Witherington, D. (2006). Emotional development: Action, communication, and understanding. In W. Damon & R. Lerner (Series Eds.) & N. Eisenberg (Vol. Ed.), *Handbook of child psychology: Vol. 3. Social, emotional, and personality development* (6th ed., pp. 226–299). New York: Wiley.

Saarni, C., & von Salisch, M. (1993). The socialization of emotional dissemblance. In M. Lewis & C. Saarni (Eds.), *Lying and deception in everyday life* (pp. 106–125). New York: Guilford Press.

Saarni, C., & Weber, H. (1999). Emotional displays and dissemblance in childhood: Implications for self-presentation. In P. Philippot, R. S. Feldman, & E. Coats (Eds.), *The social context of nonverbal behavior* (pp. 71–105). Cambridge, UK: Cambridge University Press.

Spinrad, T., & Stifter, C. (2002). Maternal sensitivity and infant emotional reactivity: Concurrent and longitudinal relations. In R. Fabes (Ed.), *Emotions and the family* (pp. 243–264). New York: Haworth Press.

Steinberg, S., & Laird, J. (1989). Parent attributions of emotion to their children and the cues children use in perceiving their own emotions. *Motivation and Emotion, 13,* 179–191.

Strayer, J., & Roberts, W. L. (2004). Children's anger, emotional expressiveness, and empathy: Relations with parents' empathy, emotional expressiveness, and parenting practices. *Social Development, 13,* 229–254.

Tangney, J. P., Hill-Barlow, D., Wagner, P., Marschall, D., Borenstein, J. K., Sanftner, J., et al. (1996). Assessing individual differences in constructive versus destructive responses to anger across the lifespan. *Journal of Personality and Social Psychology, 70,* 780–796.

Thompson, R. (2006). The development of the person: Social understanding, relationships, conscience, self. In W. Damon & R. Lerner (Series Eds.) & N. Eisenberg (Vol. Ed.), *Handbook of child psychology:*

Vol. 3. Social, emotional, and personality development (6th ed., pp. 24–98). New York: Wiley.

Tomasello, M., Kruger, A. C., & Ratner, H. H. (1993). Cultural learning. *Behavioral and Brain Sciences, 16,* 495–552.

Trevarthen, C. (1984). Emotions in infancy: Regulators of contact and relationships with persons. In K. Scherer & P. Ekman (Eds.), *Approaches to emotion* (pp. 129–157). Hillsdale, NJ: Erlbaum.

Trevarthen, C. (1993). The function of emotions in early infant communication and development. In J. Nadel & L. Cumaioni (Eds.), *New perspectives in early communicative development* (pp. 48–81). London: Routledge.

Underwood, M., Hurley, J., Johanson, C., & Mosley, J. (1999). An experimental, observational investigation of children's responses to peer provocation: Developmental and gender differences in middle childhood. *Child Development, 70,* 1428–1446.

von Salisch, M. (1996). Relationships between children: Symmetry and asymmetry among peers, friends, and siblings. In A. E. Auhagen & M. von Salisch (Eds.), *The diversity of human relationships* (pp. 59–77). New York: Cambridge University Press.

von Salisch, M. (2005). Anger regulation among friends: Assessment and development childhood to adolescence. *Journal of Social and Personal Relationships, 22,* 837–855.

Wasserman, G., & Lewis, M. (1982). The effects of situations and situation transitions on maternal and infant behavior. *Journal of Genetic Psychology, 140,* 19–31.

White, G. M. (2000). Representing emotional meaning: Category, metaphor, schema, discourse. In M. Lewis & J. M. Haviland-Jones (Eds.), *Handbook of emotions* (2nd ed., pp. 30–44). New York: Guilford Press.

Wierzbicka, A. (1994). Emotion, language, and cultural scripts. In S. Kitayama & H. Markus (Eds.), *Emotion and culture* (pp. 133–196). Washington, DC: American Psychological Association.

Wierzbicka, A. (1999). *Emotions across languages and cultures.* Cambridge, UK: Cambridge University Press.

Zahn-Waxler, C., Cole, P. M., & Barrett, K. C. (1991). Guilt and empathy: Sex differences and implications for the development of depression. In J. Garber & K. Dodge (Eds.), *The development of emotion regulation and dysregulation* (pp. 243–272). New York: Cambridge University Press.

Zahn-Waxler, C., Kochanska, G., Krupnick, J., & McKnew, D. (1990). Patterns of guilt in children of depressed and well mothers. *Developmental Psychology, 26,* 51–59.

Zimmermann, L. K., & Stansbury, K. (2003). The influence of temperamental reactivity and situational context on the emotion-regulatory abilities of 3-year-old children. *Journal of Genetic Psychology, 164,* 389–409.

CHAPTER 21

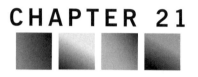

Young Children's Understanding of Others' Emotions

SHERRI C. WIDEN and JAMES A. RUSSELL

As adults, we not only have emotions but we try to understand emotions—in a variety of ways. We have concepts for mood and temperament and for specific categories of emotions (happiness, sadness, anger, hope, envy, etc.). We judge emotions along broad dimensions of valence (feeling good vs. feeling bad) and arousal (feeling low vs. high in energy). For each emotion, we know a script, including its eliciting event, conscious feeling, facial expression, vocalization, action, physiological manifestation, and so on, aligned in a causal and temporal order. We understand that one's emotional reaction to an event depends on how that event is appraised, and that the reaction can be regulated or faked. We use these various concepts to understand and predict emotional reactions and to guide our behavior accordingly.

Adult understanding of others' emotion is preceded by a long developmental path. Our chapter discusses that path from infancy through the preschool years, with a focus on issues of taxonomy. Do children begin with an innate, or at least prepared, set of mental categories for basic emotions? Or do these categories themselves develop out of an earlier, more primitive understanding? More generally, which aspects of this understanding develop earlier and thus are easier to acquire? And what then propels change down this path?

Our perspective in this chapter is unusual, in that we believe that understanding emotion in terms of adult-like discrete categories is a relatively late development—an endpoint of a process of differentiation rather than a starting point. We focus on 2-year-olds, who, we claim, see the emotional world largely in terms of broad dimensions of valence and arousal. We begin, however, by examining relevant research on infants and toddlers, and we provide an interpretation different from that usually offered. We end with a brief survey of development in children 3 years and older, including the formation of discrete emotion categories.

OUR CONCEPTUAL APPROACH

As adults, we place emotions in a hierarchy, a simplified version of which is shown in Figure 21.1. The broadest categories are at a superordinate level. These broad categories are subdivided into more specific ones (at a basic

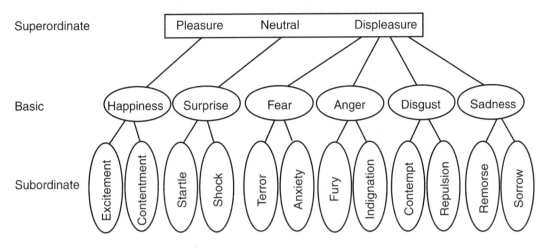

FIGURE 21.1. A hierarchical model of emotion.

level), which are further subdivided into even more specific ones (at a subordinate level). The question is where in this hierarchy children begin. Can they begin anywhere? Or do they begin in the middle (basic level) and only later acquire higher and lower levels? Or do they begin at the top and then differentiate (subdivide) the superordinate categories into ever more specific categories?

The most commonly assumed possibility is a discrete-category account. In this view, children initially understand emotions by means of discrete basic-level categories that can legitimately be labeled "angry," "scared," "sad," and the like. Children later come to understand that those emotions can be grouped together according to valence and arousal, thereby forming the superordinate level. They also subdivide the basic level to form a subordinate level (e.g., fear is subdivided into anxiety, panic, etc.). This basic-level account is consistent with the general idea that young children often start acquiring labels at the basic level of any conceptual hierarchy (e.g., Markman, 1989). For discrete-category accounts of emotion understanding, see Denham (1998), Izard (1994), Pons, Harris, and de Rosnay (2004), Saarni (1999), and Walker-Andrews (1997).

Another possibility, a differentiation account, is consistent with the general notion that cognitive development proceeds through differentiation (e.g., Werner, 1948) and is the basic assumption of our approach. Our specific differentiation account (Widen & Russell, 2003) is supplemented by a circumplex structural model (Bullock & Russell, 1984), according to

which the superordinate level of Figure 21.1 is actually more complex: It consists of the two broad dimensions of valence and arousal. The result can be thought of as four broad categories (Figure 21.2), although without sharp boundaries between them: On the pleasant side are pleasure + high arousal (which we might call "excitement" broadly construed) and pleasure + low arousal ("serenity"). On the unpleasant side are displeasure + high arousal ("distress") and displeasure + low arousal ("depression").

We believe that this simple scheme is a child's starting point and captures a 2-year-old's mental taxonomy for emotions. Children then differentiate within these broad categories, eventually arriving at discrete concepts such as anger and fear. Thus the mental categories of

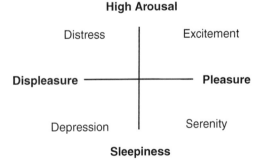

FIGURE 21.2. The circumplex model of emotion. Adapted from Bullock and Russell (1984). Copyright 1984 by the International Society for the Study of Behavioral Development. Adapted by permission of Sage Publications, Ltd.

anger, fear, jealousy, and so on are not pre-formed, but must be constructed though a process we describe as building a script.

Our topic in this chapter is the nature of children's *understanding* of emotion, rather than the nature of emotion per se or children's production of emotion. Still, we need to refer to emotions, and so, throughout this chapter, we write of emotions as if they could be unequivocally divided into discrete categories. We write of facial expressions as if a certain one conveyed exactly one discrete emotion. And we refer to happiness, surprise, fear, anger, disgust, and sadness as basic-level emotions. We write in this way not because we accept these assumptions, but for convenience, and to show that our developmental account of understanding is largely independent of assumptions about the emotions themselves.

INFANTS AND TODDLERS

Many researchers have claimed to find categorical understanding of emotion in infants and toddlers. In this section, we offer a different, more cautious interpretation of these studies. We rely on distinctions among "detection" (a sensory system is affected by information), "discrimination" (the ability to tell the difference between two stimuli), and "recognition" (the ability to attribute emotional meaning to a stimulus detected and discriminated); see Walker-Andrews (1997). It is recognition that corresponds to understanding.

Young Infants (<10 Months)

A common method used with the youngest infants is habituation: Infants are shown repeated trials of one kind of facial expression (e.g., happiness) until they habituate (i.e., until the time they spend looking at each face drops below a criterion). Then a different kind of facial expression (e.g., anger) is shown. Infants, including neonates, look longer at the new expression, indicating that they detect the change. Although it is tempting to suppose that the infants *recognize* happiness and anger from those expressions, the more justified interpretation is that they discriminate between features or patterns of features (e.g., see Caron, Caron, & Meyers, 1985). Perhaps infants begin by discriminating facial expressions on the basis of single features, such

as curvature of the mouth, openness of eyes, or shape of brows, and later discriminate on the basis of combinations of such features. The infants may thus have formed a category of "smile"—but without any corresponding recognition of its meaning or any understanding of happiness or feeling good.

Infants have also been said to *behaviorally* match the emotional display that is presented to them in a way that reveals their recognition of that display. Thus infants (as young as 10 weeks) smile more and show more interest when viewing a positive emotional display and hearing pleasant vocalizations; infants are more agitated and distressed when witnessing an adult frowning or crying (e.g., D'Entremont & Muir, 1999; Kahana-Kalman & Walker-Andrews, 2001). Most such studies have been restricted to a positive–negative coding of infants' responses, and thus, if the infants recognized the adult display, it might well have been in terms of valence. To our knowledge, only one such study coded infants' responses in terms of specific discrete emotions (Haviland & Lelwica, 1987). This study used Izard's (1979) Maximally Discriminative Facial Movement Coding System (MAX), and thus their results are based on the assumption that certain configurations of facial movements can be used to infer one specific, discrete emotion (for a challenge to this assumption, see Camras, 1992). Haviland and Lelwica found that 5-month-olds showed increased happiness and interest when their mothers displayed happiness; that they showed increased anger but decreased interest when their mothers displayed anger; but that they did not show sadness when their mothers displayed sadness. Indeed, the babies rarely showed sadness at all. Thus, although the results of this study give some support to a discrete category interpretation, the support is weak. Furthermore, infants' reactions may not require any *understanding* of the emotion displayed. That is, even if it could be shown that infants react with anger to adult anger displays, the adult displays may simply *elicit* emotional reactions from the infants—reactions not mediated or accompanied by understanding. In addition, in these studies, infants' reactions may also have included a component of imitation.

In *intermodal* matching, infants are simultaneously shown two videos of facial expressions (e.g., happiness and sadness), accompanied by a single voice that matches the emotion of one of the faces (e.g., Kahana-Kalman & Walker-Andrews, 2001; Soken & Pick, 1999). The measure of interest is whether infants look longer at the face that matches the emotion of the sound track than at the nonmatching face. Two conclusions emerge from this research: First, the youngest infants (from 3.5 to 5 months of age) do not show intermodal matching; instead, they show a preference for a smiling face or for the face on the right, regardless of vocalization. Second, infants about 5–7 months of age can match the voice to the target facial expression when given two emotions of opposite valence—evidence consistent with our dimensional view (e.g., Kahana-Kalman & Walker-Andrews, 2001; Walker-Andrews, 1986).

The key question is how infants respond to emotions of the same valence. To our knowledge, only one study provides such data. Soken and Pick (1999) investigated 7-month-olds' intermodal matching of all possible pairs of happiness, interest (a second positive emotion), anger, and sadness. Overall, there was a matching effect plus a preference for specific faces over others: The order of preference was interest, happiness, anger, and (least preferred) sadness. (In our account, this order translates to positive over negative and high- over low-arousal faces.) For our purposes, the interesting results came from the same-valence trials (happiness vs. interest, sadness vs. anger): Again, infants tended to match (i.e., they looked longer at the face whose emotion matched that of the voice). This finding can be interpreted as recognizing discrete emotion categories, but it could also be interpreted as matching by arousal (the second dimension in our circumplex). An even less generous interpretation is that, within valence, infants matched the level of animation in the face to the level of animation in the vocalization, without any reference to dimensions or categories of emotion.

To summarize, in our interpretation, adult emotional displays influence young infants (< 10 months) (Witherington, Campos, & Hertenstein, 2001). They respond behaviorally and emotionally to emotional actions of others. Vocal stimuli can capture their attention. Vocal, tactile, and visual displays alter their affective state (Owren, Rendall, & Bachorowski, 2003) and regulate their behavior (Campos, Thein, & Owen, 2003). Infants also evidence an early-emerging *perceptual* ability to detect

and to discriminate between classes of displays. If they recognize any emotional meaning in others' displays, that meaning is in terms of valence. But neither the infants' perceptions nor their emotional responses need be mediated by any understanding of the emotional meaning of the display. We question whether before about 10 months infants are in any way *recognizing* an emotional message conveyed by a facial or vocal communiqué.

Older Infants and Toddlers (10–24 Months)

By about 10 months, infants build on their perceptual abilities to begin to find emotional meaning in faces and voices. Infants use this information to guide their own behavior and to predict the behavior of another. At this age, infants begin triadic interactions: An infant and caregiver can jointly focus on a third stimulus. Infants use these interactions to aid them in learning which events are rewarding and which are punishing, which to approach and which to avoid. Infants begin to understand the referential nature of a caregiver's signals (Moses, Baldwin, Rosicky, & Tidball, 2001). Older infants and toddlers (10–24 months) adjust their behavior according to adults' emotional displays and thus allow a more convincing demonstration that they find emotional meaning in the events they witness. This adjustment can be seen in the social referencing paradigm.

In the typical social referencing study, an infant is presented with an ambiguous stimulus (e.g., a novel toy, a visual cliff). The infant tends to look to the caregiver for clarification. The caregiver, in turn, has been instructed to display a particular emotion (e.g., happiness or fear). The measure of interest is whether the infant then approaches or avoids the ambiguous stimulus, based on the caregiver's display (e.g., Feinman & Lewis, 1983; Klinnert, Emde, Butterfield, & Campos, 1986). By 10–12 months of age, infants can indeed use another's emotional display to guide their own behavior in this situation (e.g., Sorce, Emde, Campos, & Klinnert, 1985). As age increases, toddlers engage in social referencing more reliably and more quickly (e.g., Walden & Kim, 2005).

In most studies, the caregiver displays either a positive or negative (usually fear or disgust) signal. Thus the reliable finding that infants use this information is consistent with the idea that infants of this age interpret faces in terms of valence. For present purposes, the key question again is the infants' response to displays of the same valence. To our knowledge, only three social referencing studies have compared infants' responses to displays of more than one negative emotion (Bradshaw, 1986, as cited in Campos et al., 2003; Sorce et al., 1985; Svejda & Campos, 1982, as cited in Campos et al., 2003). Again, in these three studies, infants did respond differently to positive and negative displays. Indeed, from their review of how a caregiver's vocally expressed emotions regulated an infant's reaction to an ambiguous toy, Campos et al. (2003) concluded that "behavior regulation was a function only of the hedonic tone of the signal" (p. 117). None of the three studies found a clear behavioral difference in infants' responses to displays of the same valence, but the study by Sorce et al. (1985) comes closest. Sorce et al. included three negative emotions (fear, anger, sadness) and two positive ones (happiness, interest). The ambiguous stimulus was a visual cliff. The percentages of infants who crossed the visual cliff were 0% after a fear expression, 11% after an anger expression, 33% after a sadness expression, 74% after a happiness expression, and 73% after an interest expression. The large difference between negative and positive displays is again consistent with our dimensional perspective. The much smaller differences within the negative conditions provide limited support for a discrete-categories interpretation. Our alternative explanation for these within-valence differences is that sadness is a lower-arousal emotion than either anger or fear. Thus the sadness displays might have simply produced less of a response in infants. Recall that infants fail to respond to sadness faces in intermodal matching studies.

On one interpretation, social referencing studies suggest that toddlers find some meaning in adult displays. Because it is limited to a behavioral approach–avoidance measure, social referencing research cannot provide unequivocal evidence on just what the child understands. An alternative interpretation is that the adult facial display elicits a particular state in the infants (e.g., comfort or upset), which in turn influences their willingness to cross the visual cliff. If so, no understanding of emotion would be necessary in the social referencing situation.

The social referencing paradigm has been expanded to show that infants grasp the link between adult emotional displays and the object of that display (e.g., Moses et al., 2001; Mumme & Fernald, 2003). In these studies, infants witnessed an adult emotional display directed toward one of two objects but not the other. Both 12- and 18-month-olds were more likely to play with an object toward which the adult showed happiness and less likely to play with an object toward which the adult showed a negative emotion. None of these studies compared infants' reactions to different negative emotions. Thus these studies are again consistent with a valence interpretation and leave open the question of discrete emotion categories.

With another twist, the social referencing paradigm was used to examine children's understanding of the connection between an emotional display and the displayer's intentions or desires. In these referential understanding studies, infants (9–18 months of age) looked longer when a person's emotional display (e.g., sadness, happiness) did not predict their behavior (Barna & Legerstee, 2005; Phillips, Wellman, & Spelke, 2002). By 18 months, toddlers understood that someone could want more of a food that the children found undesirable (raw broccoli), based on emotional displays of pleasure and disgust (Repacholi & Gopnik, 1997). Thus in the second year of life, an infant is forging connections between others' emotional displays and their desires. But each of these studies again compared only happiness and one negative emotion—providing, in our interpretation, further support for the valence interpretation, but remaining silent on infants' and toddlers' understanding of discrete, basic-level emotions.

To summarize, it is plausible to suppose that older infants and toddlers (10–24 months) find meaning in emotional displays, but the question is the precise nature of that meaning. Of course, alternative interpretations are possible, and the studies reviewed here may not be capable of revealing an infant's full understanding of emotion. Still, it is interesting that in a literature with a fair number of studies conducted by researchers coming from a categorical perspective, there are no reports of infant behavior for which the only explanation would be couched in terms of their understanding discrete categories of emotions. The same data are consistent with a dimensional account.

TWO-YEAR-OLDS

Characterizing the emotion knowledge of 2-year-olds is key to capturing the developmental sequence of emotion understanding. Two-year-olds are beginning to talk, and we begin there.

Children typically begin using emotion labels at 18–20 months of age, but their use of these labels is infrequent (e.g., Bretherton, Fritz, Zahn-Waxler, & Ridgeway, 1986; Dunn, Bretherton, & Munn, 1987). Moreover, according to parental report, most children before their second birthday have only one emotion-related word in their vocabulary: "good" (Ridgeway, Waters, & Kuczaj, 1985). Between 24 and 36 months, children add "happy," "sad," "angry," and "scared" (Ridgeway et al., 1985). This, more generally, is a time when children describe others as the subjects of subjective experiences, such as feeling "sleepy," "tired," "hot," and "cold" (Huttenlocher & Smiley, 1990). Children also possess a lexical class of "feeling": When asked, "How does this person *feel*?" and shown facial expressions of emotions, 2-year-olds provided a feeling word on 70.2% of 336 trials; more telling, 92.8% of 153 "errors" (those trials on which they provided a non-target verbal response, other than "I don't know") were feeling words, including "tired," "bored," and other nonemotion words (Widen & Russell, 2007).

Longitudinal data on five children between their second and fifth birthdays provided by the Child Language Data Exchange System (CHILDES) allowed Wellman, Harris, Banerjee, and Sinclair (1995) to trace the development of emotion vocabularies in spontaneous speech and to infer some of the assumptions the children were making when they used emotion terms. Two-year-olds used not just "feel good" ("okay," "better") and "happy," but also "love" for positive feelings. They used "fear," "anger," and "sadness" for negative feelings. They understood that emotions are distinct from the causes eliciting them and from the behaviors and expressions resulting from them. These children did not simply use their emotion words to label their own reactions, but attributed emotions to other people, as well as to dolls and imaginary friends. They spoke of past and future emotions, not just present ones. The ways they spoke of emotions presupposed that emotions have "intentional objects" (things the emotions are about) and distin-

guished the objects of the emotions from their causes. In short, the CHILDES data showed that 2-year-olds evidenced a mentalistic conception of emotion.

What of their implicit emotion taxonomy? On the basis of evidence from spontaneous speech, Dunn et al. (1987) concluded that 2-year-olds could "distinguish and discuss" (p. 139) a variety of emotions. This conclusion is warranted to some degree, but the difficulty with studies of spontaneous speech is that we rarely know precisely what children mean by the emotion labels they use. When a child uses, say, "angry," the child has not been shown to mean the discrete emotion category of anger. We need experimental tasks that test this assumption.

Unfortunately, 2-year-olds are rarely included in experimental studies, and even when they are included, they produce so many "errors" that their results have been thought difficult to interpret. Traditionally, their responses are scored "correct" or "incorrect." When their "correct" responses are greater than expected by chance, this result too has been assimilated into the prevailing presumption that they understand the emotional world in terms of discrete emotions, albeit with many errors. When this assumption is examined in 2-year-olds, however, a very different conclusion emerges. When these children do not respond "correctly," they are not always silent. A closer look at 2-year-olds' responses, especially their "incorrect" ones, supports three complementary conclusions.

First, children add emotion words to their vocabulary in a systematic fashion. In a study in which children were asked to label the emotion conveyed by prototypical facial expressions of each of six basic-level emotions, children varied in the number of emotion labels they used (Widen & Russell, 2003). Some used none. Of those who used one label (regardless of age), that label was most likely to be "happy." Of those who used two, some used "happy" and "angry"; the others used "happy" and "sad." Children then added the other, either "angry" or "sad," as the third, but, on average, 10 months elapsed before the third label was added. The same pattern of results was found when children were told stories of prototypical emotional events and asked to label the emotion of the protagonist (Nelson, Widen, & Russell, 2006).

Second, when these children use the labels "sad" and "angry," they do not mean what adults mean. For example, in the free-labeling task just described, children use their few labels for all or most of the emotional stimuli presented, not just for the ones adults would label as happiness, sadness, or anger. The same conclusion is illustrated by a categorization task (Russell & Widen, 2002a). The category was presented as a box into which only people who felt a target emotion could go. The children were then shown, one at a time, photographs of various persons, each with a prototypical facial expression of an emotion, and asked whether each person should go into the box or be left out. The verbal demands were low, and children understood the task. But they did not show a discrete adult-like category of anger. Rather, for a 2-year-old, "angry" was much broader; they were as likely to include sad, fearful, and disgusted faces as angry ones (Figure 21.3). Similarly, shown an array of prototypical facial expressions and asked to find all the angry persons, 2-year-olds rarely selected positive faces, but did select the full range of negative ones, with about equal probability (Bullock & Russell, 1984; Denham & Couchoud, 1990).

The third conclusion from these studies is that 2-year-olds understand emotional stimuli mainly in terms of the broad dimensions of pleasure (valence) and arousal. In the studies described above, the breadth of the children's categories must be understood in terms of va-

lence. In Figure 21.3, for example, the "anger" category is extended to include all and only faces of negative valence. Other studies lead to the same conclusion. In a forced-choice study, each face was paired with each of eight other faces on different trials (Bullock & Russell, 1985). Two-year-olds' performance was above chance levels for "happy," "excited," "surprised," "scared, "mad," "disgusted," "sad," and "calm" (but not for "sleepy"). At first glance, this result seems to support a basic-level-categories approach: 2-year-olds could select the facial expression that matched the label for eight of nine emotion categories with above-chance accuracy. However, analyses of all their responses (both "correct" and "incorrect") suggests that the broad dimensions of valence and arousal may provide the better interpretation. Two-year-olds' performance was higher when the similarity of the pair of faces according to the circumplex model decreased. Similarity in the circumplex, in turn, can be interpreted in terms of similarity along the dimensions of valence and arousal. When the 2-year-olds were labeling facial expressions, their "incorrect" responses were more likely to be labels of the same valence than ones of the opposite valence in both free-labeling studies and forced-choice studies (Denham & Couchoud, 1990; Widen & Russell, 2003, Study 2; Nelson et al., 2006; Bullock & Russell, 1985).

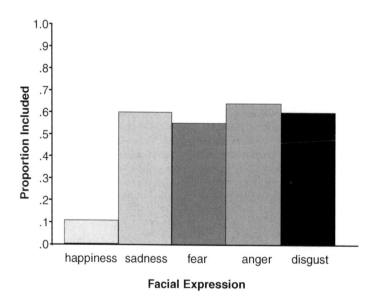

FIGURE 21.3. Faces that 2-year-olds included in the angry box.

The studies reviewed so far have relied on children's production or comprehension of emotion *words*. The fourth conclusion is that this evidence captures their underlying conceptual structure and not simply something of their word use. Recall the categorization task. An interesting feature of that study was that the anger box had been defined in two ways (Russell & Widen, 2002a): For half of the children the experimenter used the word "angry," and for the other half the experimenter used two photographs of prototypical anger facial expressions ("feel like this" [pointing]). Both ways of defining the angry box produced similar results—2-year-olds included the majority of all negative expressions in this box—even though, in the latter condition, the problem could have been solved for a discrete anger category simply by perceptual matching.

Bullock and Russell (1984; Russell & Bullock, 1986b) used yet another method that did not rely on emotion words: multidimensional scaling of judged similarity between facial expressions. Although the stimuli were facial expressions thought to convey basic discrete emotions, multidimensional scaling showed that 2-year-olds judge similarity on the basis of two broad dimensions—valence and arousal.

Two-year-olds are also learning about the causes and consequences of emotions. Wellman and Woolley (1990), in their research on understanding of desires, convincingly demonstrated that 2-year-olds can associate happiness with desired outcomes and sadness with undesired outcomes. In a study of slightly older children (as young as 3 years), Stein and Levine (1989) found that children could select a positive face for a positive outcome (e.g., receiving a toy) and a negative face for a negative outcome (e.g., losing a puppy); these same children did not, however, distinguish within negative outcomes. That is, they were as likely to select a sad as an angry face for outcomes that adults judged to elicit sadness, and the same for outcomes adults judged to elicit anger. Similarly, Trabasso, Stein, and Johnson (1981) found that 3- and 4-year-olds labeled events that frustrated their goals as both "sad" and "angry," and only older children distinguished the two. Other studies (e.g., Borke, 1971; Denham & Couchoud, 1990) have obtained similar results, again with children older than 2. We believe that 2-year-olds would show similar results, but the two studies we know of that actually tested 2-year-olds yielded mixed results (Denham & Couchoud, 1990; Widen & Russell, 2006)—presumably because tasks that are manageable for 3-year-olds might not be so for 2-year-olds.

Summary of the Research

Two-year-olds are surprisingly sophisticated in their mentalistic conception of emotion as a state separate from its causes and behavioral consequences. On the other hand, they are surprisingly limited taxonomically to the broad dimensions of valence and arousal. Children later move toward more specific discrete categories of emotion, but slowly and with difficulty (for more on this, see below). We found little evidence that children younger than 3 years understand anger, fear, and other discrete categories of emotion as such. When they use the words "scared," "angry," and so on, they seem to have in mind not discrete emotions but very broad categories of emotion, perhaps initially simply happy and unhappy ones. The evidence on 2-year-olds reinforces our cautious interpretation of evidence on those younger than 2 years.

This perspective is also consistent with the finding from the theory-of-mind perspective that 2-year-olds, lacking a full notion of belief, are limited to desire and perception (Wellman & Woolley, 1990). They attribute desires to others, and understand that fulfillment of desire leads to positive emotion, whereas unfulfilled desire leads to negative emotion. Furthermore, 2-year-olds understand desires as mental states, attributing different desires to different individuals. They therefore judge that "Bill who wants a bunny and finds one will be happy whereas Mary who wants a kitty and finds a bunny—the exact same bunny that Bill found—will be sad" (Wellman, 1995, p. 302). Two-year-olds also understand that others can perceive or fail to perceive an event (the bunny), but these children fail to understand that others can have different beliefs. To the extent that specific discrete emotions presuppose certain beliefs (Ortony, Clore, & Collins, 1987), the theory-of-mind research thus reinforces our doubts about how much 2-year-olds can understand about specific discrete emotions. That is, 2-year-olds routinely fail false-belief tasks, suggesting that they would fail to appreciate that a dog they know to be harmless could elicit fear in someone who believes it dangerous.

PRESCHOOLERS

In this section, we consider children 3 to 5 years of age, and build on the premise that 2-year-olds understand others' emotions in terms of the broad dimensions of pleasure and arousal—an understanding that complements their perception-and-desire theory of the minds of others. During their fourth year, children begin to evidence fuller understanding of beliefs (Wellman, 1995); this advance complements and perhaps underlies their fuller understanding of emotion concepts they already have in elementary form and their division of emotion into ever finer discrete categories. We present five hypotheses, which together constitute what we call the "differentiation model" of emotion understanding (Widen & Russell, 2003).

First Hypothesis

Valence and arousal dimensions continue to be important. When preschoolers make "errors," or when they judge similarity among emotions, they continue to show the influence of pleasure and arousal (Bullock & Russell, 1984, 1985; Widen & Russell, 2003). In all, seven studies to date have analyzed preschoolers' "incorrect" emotion responses on labeling faces (Bullock & Russell, 1984, 1985; Denham & Couchoud, 1990; Widen & Russell, 2002; 2003, Study 2, Study 3; 2004). At every age, valence continued to dominate children's "errors." Similar results occurred in two studies that specified the target emotion with stories rather than faces (Denham & Couchoud, 1990; Widen & Russell, 2004). Before children know other features of shame, gratitude, pride, and jealousy, they know their valence (Russell & Paris, 1994). Valence can be seen in even older children and adults (Bullock & Russell, 1984; Coren & Russell, 1992; Russell & Bullock, 1986a, 1986b; Russell & Fehr, 1994) and in a variety of cultures with a variety of languages (e.g., Russell, Lewicka, & Niit, 1989). Evidence for valence is ubiquitous.

Second Hypothesis

Children use different emotion labels with different frequencies. In spontaneous speech, children use some emotion labels more frequently than others. But the children may simply be experiencing or witnessing some emotions more frequently than others. However, in a study in which an equal number of emotions (represented as facial expressions) were presented (Widen & Russell, 2003, Study 3), the same differential frequency was found. Labels were used in the following rank order, starting with the most frequent: "happy," "sad," "angry," "scared," "surprised," and "disgusted." Differential frequency of label use for faces had been reported before (e.g., Gosselin & Simard, 1999; Izard, 1994), and the pattern was interpreted in one of two ways: (1) Some facial expressions (i.e., happiness, sadness, anger) are easier to recognize than others, or (2) some children lack some words in their vocabulary. We showed that the same order of use occurred for both "correct" and "incorrect" uses; differential use of labels was therefore not a result of the faces per se, but rather of children's interpretation of those faces. Furthermore, all children in the study had been shown in a prior task to have all six labels in their vocabulary. We thus interpret differential use of emotion labels as reflecting differences in accessibility of the emotion concepts, which in turn are correlated with the order in which the categories are acquired, as detailed in the next hypothesis.

Third Hypothesis

Emotion categories enter a child's taxonomy in a systematic order. As we have mentioned earlier, when children (2–5 years of age) were sorted, irrespective of age, by the number of different emotion category labels they used for facial expressions (or, in a separate study, emotion stories), labels were found to emerge in a systematic order (Figure 21.4) (Nelson et al., 2006; Widen & Russell, 2003). Earlier, we have described the steps up to three labels—"happy," "angry," and "sad." The next step allows two paths: Some children added "surprised," and some "scared." For five labels, the two paths merged. In the last step, "disgusted" was added. Age increased with the number of labels used, from a mean age of 30 months for those children producing no labels to 62 months for those producing five labels. Over 81% of the children (vs. the 23% expected by chance) fit the pattern of Figure 21.4. We have since replicated this result three times, and each time the proportion of children who fit the predicted pattern has been high: 78% (Widen & Russell, 2007), 86% (Widen & Russell, in press), and 91% (Nelson et al., 2006). Furthermore, children's position in the scheme of Figure 21.4 predicts their categorization of emotional stimuli in separate tasks (Widen & Russell, 2007, in press), even when age is controlled for.

In many studies, children have been asked to associate emotions with emotion labels. The ubiquitous conclusion, starting with Gates (1923), is that the proportion of correct associations increases with age. A second conclusion has been that the proportion correct varies with emotion. This latter finding provides an indirect test of our scheme in Figure 21.4. Earlier-emerging categories should be more practiced and accessible; if so, then we can expect that children will be more often correct with the earlier-emerging categories. In a review of 19 studies (Widen, 2005), preschoolers' performance was highest on happiness, sadness, and anger, followed by fear, disgust, and surprise, although the order within these two sets varied with task. This overall pattern held for three response formats, whether emotions were represented by facial expressions or stories, and whether emotion labels were the independent or dependent variable. Thus our developmental sequence shown in Figure 21.4 is probably not limited to the experimental context in which it was discovered (free labeling of faces and stories).

Of course, there are far more emotions than the six shown in Figure 21.4. The evidence suggests that additional emotion concepts enter the developmental picture after Labeling Level 5. For example, given stories about emotions, preschoolers were able to label our first five emotions (happiness, sadness, anger, fear, and surprise) earlier than shame, contempt, or love (e.g., Wintre & Vallance, 1994; cf. Brody & Harrison, 1987). Similarly, they are able to describe the causes for our first five emotions earlier than those for shame, gratitude, pride, or jealousy (Harris, Olthof, Meerum Terwogt, & Hardman, 1987; Russell & Paris, 1994).

Fourth Hypothesis

Categories begin broad, but then narrow. As is evident from Figure 21.4, emotion categories begin broad. During one period in the life of many 2-year-olds, the category labeled "angry" includes all negative emotions. With time, and as new categories emerge, this broad "anger" category gradually narrows. Children continue to use "angry" for the anger face, but are less likely to use it for sadness and fear faces on the labeling task (Widen & Russell, 2003) and on the box (categorization) task (Russell & Widen, 2002a). Narrowing has also been found when children were presented with an

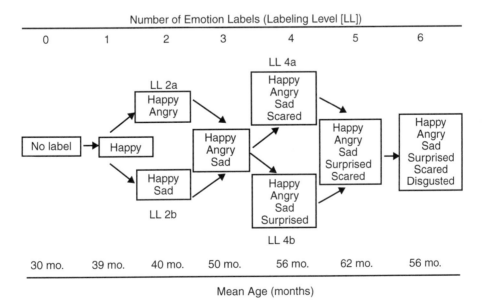

FIGURE 21.4. Systematic emergence of emotion labels. LL, Labeling Level. Adapted from Widen and Russell (2003). Copyright 2003 by the American Psychological Association. Adapted by permission.

array of facial expressions and asked to find all who displayed a particular emotion (Bullock & Russell, 1984, 1985; Bormann-Kischkel, Hildebrand-Pascher, & Stegbauer, 1990).

In our interpretation, narrowing begins when preschoolers begin to use the arousal dimension to distinguish between negative emotions. This process can be seen, for example, when preschoolers begin to exclude nontarget facial expressions from the anger box (Russell & Widen, 2002a). Thus, for the anger box, the order in which faces are excluded is predictable on the basis of arousal: Children first exclude sad faces, which are the most dissimilar to anger faces on arousal. They next exclude fearful faces and finally disgusted faces, although most 5-year-olds still include the disgusted face (narrowing is gradual and incomplete even at the end of the preschool years).

Later-emerging emotion categories also narrow with age. We had thought, based on children's free-labeling responses, that fear, surprise, and disgust began narrower (Widen & Russell, 2003), but a later categorization study showed that they begin just as broad as do happiness, anger, and sadness (Widen & Russell, 2007). Pride, jealousy, and so on similarly begin as broad concepts defined by nothing except valence, but then narrow as they take on more adult meaning (Russell & Paris, 1994). In these cases, narrowing is unlikely to be based on arousal but on other factors, as detailed next.

Fifth Hypothesis

Children form a script for each emotion category. As adults, we know that each emotion is a sequence of subevents. In fear, prototypically, a danger occurs; the person orients to it, freezes or flees, and feels unhappy; physiological arousal increases; face and voice change. The concept of fear is thus a script in which subevents unfold in a temporal and causal order. The script for sadness may include a loss, resulting in feeling bad, pouting or crying, whining, withdrawal, tears, and slow or suppressed movement. Children must acquire these scripts and their labels. In the studies described so far, it is not clear just how much of each script a child knows. For example, associating the word "scared" with a type of facial expression need not imply that the child knows other subevents of the fear script. Our fourth hypothesis suggests that scripts begin with few

components (which explains their initial breadth), but then acquire new components (and hence narrow).

How is a script built? Which parts enter the script earlier and which later? Answers to such questions can hint at the process of building a script. For example, some theorists have assumed that facial expressions are the bases for constructing scripts (e.g., Harris, 1989; Izard, 1994). If so, then a reasonable hypothesis would be that witnessing different facial expressions would compel the child to differentiate a currently broad script. According to this hypothesis, a child at Figure 21.4's Labeling Level 2a (who labels all negative emotions as "angry") would soon notice that some negative facial expressions involve downcast eyes, downturned mouth, and tears (or perhaps, more generally, facial signs of low arousal), whereas other faces involve knitted brows, staring eyes, bared teeth, and clenched jaw (or, more generally, facial signs of high arousal). As a consequence, the child would then divide the initially broad category into two separate categories and then become receptive to different labels ("sad," "angry") for this second category of negative emotions (although at this level both of these categories remain broader than the adult version).

Studies of children's scripts for emotions must present a child with one part of a script (mode of presentation) and ask the child for another part (mode of response). This face-early hypothesis can then be tested by including facial expressions in one mode or the other. For example, Camras and Allison (1985) told children (preschoolers to second graders) very brief stories about a girl (e.g., "Her mother has died"). Children were asked to identify the girl's emotion, using one of two response modes: an array of labels ("happy," "angry," "sad") or an array of corresponding faces (smiling, frowning, or crying). Much to everyone's surprise, children did better overall given the label response format than given the face response format. Ten studies have now compared facial expressions to at least one other mode: (1) emotion labels (Camras & Allison, 1985; Russell, 1990; Russell & Widen, 2002a, 2002b); (2) emotion stories describing the causes and/or consequences (Markham & Adams, 1992; Nelson et al., 2006; Widen & Russell, 2002, 2006); or (3) tone of voice (Stifter & Fox, 1987). All but one study (Stifter & Fox, 1987) found a difference between modes, but none found that facial expressions were the stronger cues to emotion. This face inferiority effect was particularly strong for fear. The inferiority of faces was robust whether mode was the independent or dependent variable, and whether children were asked to categorize, choose from an array, label, or describe the cause or consequence of the emotion.

Instead of faces as *the* bases of emotion scripts, there is emerging evidence that no one cue type is the strongest at all ages or for all emotions. We (Widen & Russell, 2004) asked children (3 or 4 years old) to describe the causes of six different emotions, specified by facial expressions, labels, or brief stories describing behavioral consequences. Again, faces were not the strongest cues for any emotion or for either age group. Behavioral consequences were the strongest cues for 3-year-olds, especially for anger. Emotion labels were the strongest cues for 4-year-olds, especially for fear and disgust. It remains possible that facial expressions are stronger cues for even younger children and for the earliest-emerging broad emotion categories (e.g., feeling good, feeling bad), however a child may label them.

Further evidence that faces are relatively weak cues to emotion is that, even given prototypical facial expressions of emotion, children take into account the apparent sex of the person whose emotion they are categorizing. We (Widen & Russell, 2002) asked children to label someone's emotion on the basis of either a prototypical facial expression or a brief stereotypical story. The "boy's" and the "girl's" faces and expressions were actually identical, but the faces were made to appear "male" and "female" by adding gender-appropriate hairstyles. The boy's and girl's stories for each emotion were also identical except for names and pronouns. Even given these clear cues to emotion, the perceived sex of the protagonist influenced children's emotion attributions. (This evidence also implies that scripts contain gender stereotypes and are thus not equivalent to scientific accounts of each emotion.)

Insufficient evidence is available to provide a clear account of how the scripts are acquired. Perhaps the scripts for happiness and sadness begin by linking facial expressions (smiling vs. crying) to feeling good versus bad, which then soon become linked to their causes (meeting vs. not meeting desires). For anger, the script may begin instead by linking hostile behavior to feeling bad. For fear and disgust, the script may begin with a child's hearing the labels "scared" and "disgusted," which prompts him or her to search for causes that differentiate these emotions from sadness and anger. In each case, once the first link is formed, the child can then add more components. Because different cues initiate the process for different emotions, different cues are more powerful in eliciting the concepts for different emotions. Because concepts for different emotions are acquired at different ages, different cues are more powerful at different ages.

Harris (2000) rightly objected to the notion of scripts as we have so far characterized them on the standard grounds offered for appraisal theories of emotion: The emotion that occurs depends not so much on the reality of the precipitating event as on how the precipitating event is appraised. An approaching dog elicits joy in the person who appraises the dog as playful, but elicits fear in the person who appraises it as dangerous. Understanding how emotions depend on appraisals is one of the tasks for the child developing an understanding of emotion. Although they are not physical events, appraisals can be considered as subevents of the emotion process and hence as elements in the script.

Appreciating the role of appraisals presupposes an understanding that different people can have different appraisals. A person's appraisal of an event is a belief about that event. Several sources of evidence hint at the dependence of emotion understanding on belief understanding. Of course, the two are correlated, but the dependency may go in one direction. First, belief understanding does not seem to depend on emotion understanding, as shown by evidence from children with developmental disorders (e.g., conduct disorder, autism) who can understand belief but not emotion (e.g., Blair, 2002). Second, there is clear evidence that children understand false beliefs before they can make the corresponding belief-based emotion attributions (e.g., Harris, Johnson, Hutton, Andrews, & Cooke, 1989; de Rosnay, Pons, Harris, & Morrell, 2004). For example, Bradmetz and Schneider (1999) demonstrated that children understood that when she first arrived, Little Red Riding Hood believed that the wolf was her grandmother. Nonetheless, these same children said that Little Red Riding Hood felt *afraid* rather than happy to see her grandmother. Thus they had mastered the false-belief task, but could not then attribute happiness to

Little Red Riding Hood at seeing her grandmother when they knew that it was in fact the wolf. Third, Rieffe, Meerum Terwogt, and Cowan (2005) asked children as young as 4 years to explain various emotional episodes. For happiness, anger, and sadness, children spontaneously referred to desires but not beliefs. In contrast, in explaining fear, they referred to beliefs. This evidence suggests that the three earliest concepts remain tied for a time to the desire psychology of their origin. In addition, many later, so-called "social" or "self-conscious" emotions are largely defined by beliefs about the eliciting situation. Regret, for instance, has no uniquely identifying facial, vocal, physiological, or behavioral action pattern associated with it, but centrally involves feeling bad based on the belief that a prior decision or event did not turn out well.

Of course, children's understanding of emotion continues to develop beyond what we have described so far. Pons et al. (2004) identified nine different components of children's understanding of emotion. In addition to the components we have already discussed here, children come to understand (1) how reminders of an event can reactivate an emotion, (2) how emotions can be controlled, (3) that there can be a discrepancy between outer appearance of emotion and inner experience, (4) that mixed emotions can exist, and (5) that emotions depend on the morality of the precipitating event.

CONCLUSION

One particularly interesting perspective on conceptual development in general is called "theory theory" (e.g., Gopnik & Wellman, 1994). From this perspective, a child's understanding of emotion is a theory; changes in understanding are changes in the theory. A child's initial theories are powerful, are often biologically given, and aid learning, but they are relatively simple and cannot explain all the evidence the child encounters. As children encounter unexplained events and even counterevidence, auxiliary hypotheses may be added to the original theory, without seriously altering it. But eventually, as in science, the old theory proves to be inadequate and a new theory is developed.

For emotion understanding, we propose that children's earliest theory includes the concepts of valence and arousal. As shown in Figure

21.2, these two dimensions can also be thought of as four broad categories: pleasure/high arousal, pleasure/low arousal, displeasure/high arousal, and displeasure/low arousal. Although simple, this theory allows a child to place the emotions of others in these broad categories and thus to anticipate the affective quality of their subsequent behavior, to acquire knowledge of the positive and negative quality of current events (such as a visual cliff), and to gain knowledge of the others' desires. Evidence indicates that this dimensional theory dominates the child's thinking about emotion for the second and most of the third years of life.

Emotion researchers have long debated whether emotions are understood in terms of dimensions or categories. When that debate is rephrased as a developmental question, the two sides of the debate can be reconciled. How does a child's initial broad dimensional understanding turn into the adult division of emotion into more discrete categories? Or, phrased in terms of the four broad categories, how are the broad categories differentiated into more specific ones? How are new categories acquired? And what propels these changes?

To answer the question of change, the theory theory points to the evidence facing the child. The four-category system does not allow sufficiently precise accounts of this evidence, and so the theory must be changed. The kind of evidence faced is what is eventually incorporated into emotion scripts: different kinds of emotion-eliciting situations, different overt behavior, different expressive behavior, and different labels used by the language community. This new theory still has valence and arousal as its bases, but can better accommodate the new evidence.

Another force on the child's developing theory of emotion is the development of other perceptual and cognitive abilities. Infants must acquire perceptual categories of facial actions before being able to attach emotional significance to those categories. Older children must develop a theory of mind. The concept of desire is needed for a child to understand why the same event can bring positive feelings to one but negative feelings to another. The concept of belief is needed to understand that different people can appraise the same situation differently and thus emotionally respond differently. Gopnik and Wellman (1994) contrasted the theory theory with two other broad perspectives on conceptual development, both of which could incorporate emotion understanding. According to the notion of innate modules, the prototype of which is a Chomskian account of language, more of emotion understanding would be universal and innate. If the categories for the basic emotions and their links to specific expressions are so viewed, then this perspective is similar to the usually encountered standard account of emotion understanding. In contrast, according to the simulation account (Harris, 1992), emotion understanding begins not with witnessing the emotions of others, but with experiencing them oneself. Presumably, the discrete categories of emotion experience are biologically given. In trying to anticipate the emotions of others, one does not rely on a conceptual theory or an innate module, but can simulate the experience in oneself. The contrast between the theory theory and the simulation theory points to the importance of studying personal experiences of emotion and their role in understanding others.

ACKNOWLEDGMENTS

We thank Lisa Feldman Barrett, Paul L. Harris, Mathew J. Hertenstein, Nicole L. Nelson, and Carolyn Saarni for their help and comments.

REFERENCES

Barna, J., & Legerstee, M. (2005). Nine- and twelve-month-old infants relate emotions to people's actions. *Cognition and Emotion, 19,* 53–67.

Blair, R. J. R. (2002). Theory of mind, autism, and emotional intelligence. In L. F. Barrett & P. Salovey (Eds.), *The wisdom in feeling: Psychological processes in emotional intelligence* (pp. 406–434). New York: Guilford Press.

Borke, H. (1971). Interpersonal perception of young children: Egocentrism or empathy? *Developmental Psychology, 5,* 263–269.

Bormann-Kischkel, C., Hildebrand-Pascher, S., & Stegbauer, G. (1990). The development of emotional concepts: A replication with a German sample. *International Journal of Behavioral Development, 13,* 355–372.

Bradmetz, J., & Schneider, R. (1999). Is Little Red Riding Hood afraid of her grandmother?: Cognitive vs. emotional response to a false belief. *British Journal of Developmental Psychology, 17,* 501–514.

Bretherton, I., Fritz, J., Zahn-Waxler, C., & Ridgeway, D. (1986). Learning to talk about emotions: A functionalist perspective. *Child Development, 57,* 529–548.

Brody, L. R., & Harrison, R. H. (1987). Developmental changes in children's abilities to match and label emotionally laden situations. *Motivation and Emotion, 11,* 347–365.

Bullock, M., & Russell, J. A. (1984). Preschool children's interpretation of facial expressions of emotion. *International Journal of Behavioral Development, 7,* 193–214.

Bullock, M., & Russell, J. A. (1985). Further evidence on preschoolers' interpretations of facial expressions of emotion. *International Journal of Behavioral Development, 8,* 15–38.

Campos, J. J., Thein, S., & Owen, D. (2003). A Darwinian legacy to understanding human infancy: Emotional expressions as behavior regulators. *Annals of the New York Academy of Sciences, 1000,* 110–134.

Camras, L. A. (1992). A dynamic systems perspective on expressive development. In K. Strongman (Ed.), *International review of studies on emotion* (pp. 16–28). New York: Wiley.

Camras, L. A., & Allison, K. (1985). Children's understanding of emotional facial expressions and verbal labels. *Journal of Nonverbal Behavior, 9,* 84–94.

Caron, R. F., Caron, A. J., & Myers, R. S. (1985). Do infants see emotional expressions in static faces? *Child Development, 56,* 1552–1560.

Coren, S., & Russell, J. A. (1992). The relative dominance of different facial expressions of emotion under conditions of perceptual ambiguity. *Cognition and Emotion, 6,* 539–556.

Denham, S. A. (1998). *Emotional development in young children.* New York: Guilford Press.

Denham, S. A., & Couchoud, E. A. (1990). Young preschoolers' ability to identify emotions in equivocal situations. *Child Study Journal, 20,* 153–169.

D'Entremont, B., & Muir, D. (1999). Infant responses to adult happy and sad vocal and facial expressions during face-to-face interactions. *Infant Behavior and Development, 22,* 527–539.

de Rosnay, M., Pons, F., Harris, P. L., & Morrell, J. M. B. (2004). A lag between understanding false belief and emotion attribution in young children: Relationships with linguistic ability and mothers' mental-state language. *British Journal of Developmental Psychology, 22,* 197–218.

Dunn, J., Bretherton, I., & Munn, P. (1987). Conversations about feeling states between mothers and their young children. *Developmental Psychology, 23,* 132–139.

Feinman, S., & Lewis, M. (1983). Social referencing at ten months: A second-order effect on infants' responses to strangers. *Child Development, 54,* 878–887.

Gates, G. S. (1923). An experimental study of the growth of social perception. *Journal of Educational Psychology, 14,* 449–461.

Gopnik, A., & Wellman, H. M. (1994). The theory theory. In L. A. Hirschfeld & S. A. Gelman (Eds.), *Mapping the mind: Domain specificity in cognition and culture* (pp. 257–293). New York: Cambridge University Press.

Gosselin, P., & Simard, J. (1999). Children's knowledge of facial expressions of emotions: Distinguishing fear and surprise. *Journal of Genetic Psychology, 160,* 181–193.

Harris, P. L. (1989). *Children and emotion: The development of psychological understanding.* Oxford: Blackwell.

Harris, P. L. (1992). From simulation to folk psychology: The case for development. *Mind and Language, 7,* 120–144.

Harris, P. L. (2000). *The work of the imagination: Understanding children's worlds.* Malden, MA: Blackwell.

Harris, P. L., Johnson, C. N., Hutton, D., Andrews, G., & Cooke, T. (1989). Young children's theory of mind and emotion. *Cognition and Emotion, 3,* 379–400.

Harris, P. L., Olthof, T., Meerum Terwogt, M., & Hardman, C. E. (1987). Children's knowledge of the situations that provoke emotion. *International Journal of Behavioral Development, 10,* 319–343.

Haviland, J. M., & Lelwica, M. (1987). The induced affect response: 10-week-old infants' responses to three emotion expressions. *Developmental Psychology, 23,* 97–104.

Huttenlocher, J., & Smiley, P. (1990). Emerging notions of persons. In N. L. Stein, B. Leventhal, & T. Trabasso (Eds.), *Psychological and biological approaches to emotion* (pp. 283–295). Hillsdale, NJ: Erlbaum.

Izard, C. E. (1979). *The Maximally Discriminative Facial Movement Coding System* (MAX). Newark: University of Delaware, Instructional Resources Center.

Izard, C. E. (1994). Innate and universal facial expressions: Evidence from developmental and cross-cultural research. *Psychological Bulletin, 2,* 288–299.

Kahana-Kalman, R., & Walker-Andrews, A. S. (2001). The role of person familiarity in young infants' perception of emotional expressions. *Child Development, 72,* 352–369.

Klinnert, M. D., Emde, R. N., Butterfield, P., & Campos, J. J. (1986). Social referencing: The infant's use of emotional signals from a friendly adult with mother present. *Developmental Psychology, 22,* 427–432.

Markham, R., & Adams, K. (1992). The effect of type of task on children's identification of facial expressions. *Journal of Nonverbal Behavior, 16,* 21–39.

Markman, E. M. (1989). *Categorization and naming in children: Problems of induction.* Cambridge, MA: MIT Press.

Moses, L. J., Baldwin, D. A., Rosicky, J. G., & Tidball, G. (2001). Evidence for referential understanding in the emotions domain at twelve and eighteen months. *Child Development, 72,* 718–735.

Mumme, D. L., & Fernald, A. (2003). The infant as onlooker: Learning from emotional reactions observed in a television scenario. *Child Development, 74,* 221–237.

Nelson, N. L., Widen, S. C., & Russell, J. A. (2006). *Children's understanding of emotions' causes and consequences: Labeling facial expression and stories.* Poster presented at the 18th Annual Convention of the American Psychological Society, New York.

Ortony, A., Clore, G. L., & Collins, A. (1987). *The cognitive structure of emotions.* New York: Cambridge University Press.

Owren, M. J., Rendall, D., & Bachorowski, J.-A. (2003). Nonlinguistic vocal communication. In D. Maestripieri (Ed.), *Primate psychology* (pp. 359–394). Cambridge, MA: Harvard University Press.

Phillips, A. T., Wellman, H. M., & Spelke, E. S. (2002). Infants' ability to connect gaze and emotional expression to intentional action. *Cognition, 85,* 53–78.

Pons, F., Harris, P. L., & de Rosnay, M. (2004). Emotion comprehension between 3 and 11 years: Developmental periods and hierarchical organization. *European Journal of Developmental Psychology, 1,* 127–152.

Repacholi, B. M., & Gopnik, A. (1997). Early reasoning about desires: Evidence from 14- and 18-month-olds. *Developmental Psychology, 33,* 12–21.

Ridgeway, D., Waters, E., & Kuczaj, S. A., II. (1985). Acquisition of emotion-descriptive language: Receptive and productive vocabulary norms for ages 18 months to 6 years. *Developmental Psychology, 21,* 901–908.

Rieffe, C., Meerum Terwogt, M., & Cowan, R. (2005). Children's understanding of mental states as causes of emotions. *Infant and Child Development, 14,* 259–272.

Russell, J. A. (1990). The preschooler's understanding of the causes and consequences of emotion. *Child Development, 61,* 1872–1881.

Russell, J. A., & Bullock, M. (1986a). Fuzzy concepts and the perception of emotion in facial expressions. *Social Cognition, 4,* 309–341.

Russell, J. A., & Bullock, M. (1986b). On the dimensions preschoolers use to interpret facial expressions of emotion. *Developmental Psychology, 22,* 97–102.

Russell, J. A., & Fehr, B. (1994). Fuzzy concepts in a fuzzy hierarchy: Varieties of anger. *Journal of Personality and Social Psychology, 67,* 186–205.

Russell, J. A., Lewicka, M., & Niit, T. (1989). A cross-cultural study of a circumplex model of affect. *Journal of Personality and Social Psychology, 57,* 848–856.

Russell, J. A., & Paris, F. A. (1994). Do children acquire concepts for complex emotions abruptly? *International Journal of Behavioral Development, 17,* 349–365.

Russell, J. A., & Widen, S. C. (2002a). A label superiority effect in children's categorization of facial expressions. *Social Development, 11,* 30–52.

Russell, J. A., & Widen, S. C. (2002b). Words versus faces in evoking children's knowledge of the causes of emotions. *International Journal of Behavioral Development, 26,* 97–103.

Saarni, C. (1999). *The development of emotional competence.* New York: Guilford Press.

Soken, N. H., & Pick, A. D. (1999). Infants' perception of dynamic affective expressions: Do infants distinguish specific expressions? *Child Development, 70,* 1275–1282.

Sorce, J. F., Emde, R. N., Campos, J. J., & Klinnert, M. D. (1985). Maternal emotional signaling: Its effect on the visual cliff behavior of 1-year-olds. *Developmental Psychology, 21,* 195–200.

Stein, N. L., & Levine, L. J. (1989). The causal organisation of emotional knowledge: A developmental study. *Cognition and Emotion, 3,* 343–378.

Stifter, C. A., & Fox, N. A. (1987). Preschool children's ability to identify and label emotions. *Journal of Nonverbal Behavior, 11,* 43–54.

Trabasso, T., Stein, N. L., & Johnson, L. R. (1981). Children's knowledge of events: A causal analysis of story structure. In G. H. Bower (Ed.), *The psychology of learning and motivation* (Vol. 15, pp. 237–282). New York: Academic Press.

Walden, T. A., & Kim, G. (2005). Infants' social looking toward mothers and strangers. *International Journal of Behavioral Development, 29,* 356–360.

Walker-Andrews, A. S. (1986). Intermodal perception of expressive behaviors: Relation of eye and voice? *Developmental Psychology, 22,* 373–377.

Walker-Andrews, A. S. (1997). Infants' perception of expressive behaviors: Differentiation of multimodal information. *Psychological Bulletin, 121,* 437–456.

Wellman, H. M. (1995). Young children's conception of mind and emotion: Evidence from English speakers. In J. A. Russell, J. M. Fernández-Dols, A. S. R. Manstead, & J. C. Wellenkamp (Eds.), *NATO ASI Series D: Behavioural and social sciences. Vol. 81. Everyday conceptions of emotion: An introduction to the psychology, anthropology and linguistics of emotion* (pp. 289–313). New York: Kluwer Academic.

Wellman, H. M., Harris, P. L., Banerjee, M., & Sinclair, A. (1995). Early understanding of emotion: Evidence from natural language. *Cognition and Emotion, 9,* 117–149.

Wellman, H. M., & Woolley, J. D. (1990). From simple desires to ordinary beliefs: The early development of everyday psychology. *Cognition, 35,* 245–275.

Werner, H. (1948). *Comparative psychology of mental development.* Oxford: Follett.

Widen, S. C. (2005). Preschoolers' use of emotion labels and understanding of emotion categories. *Dissertation Abstracts International, 65,* 6692.

Widen, S. C., & Russell, J. A. (2002). Gender and preschoolers' perception of emotion. *Merrill–Palmer Quarterly, 48,* 248–262.

Widen, S. C., & Russell, J. A. (2003). A closer look at preschoolers' freely produced labels for facial expressions. *Developmental Psychology, 39,* 114–128.

Widen, S. C., & Russell, J. A. (2004). The relative power of an emotion's facial expression, label, and behavioral consequences to evoke preschoolers' knowledge of its cause. *Cognitive Development, 19,* 111–125.

Widen, S. C., & Russell, J. A. (2006). *Free labeling of emotions by 2- and 3-year-olds: A face superiority effect.* Manuscript in preparation.

Widen, S. C., & Russell, J. A. (2007). Children's and adults' understanding of the "disgust face." *Cognition and Emotion.*

Widen, S. C., & Russell, J. A. (in press). *Evidence on the nature of children's understanding of emotion: The case of anger and disgust.* Manuscript submitted for publication.

Wintre, M. G., & Vallance, D. D. (1994). A developmental sequence in the comprehension of emotions: Intensity, multiple emotions, and valence. *Developmental Psychology, 30,* 509–514.

Witherington, D. C., Campos, J. J., & Hertenstein, M. J. (2001). Principles of emotion and its development in infancy. In G. Bremner & A. Fogel (Eds.), *Handbooks of developmental psychology: Blackwell handbook of infant development* (pp. 427–464). Malden, MA: Blackwell.

CHAPTER 22

Intermodal Emotional Processes in Infancy

ARLENE S. WALKER-ANDREWS

Very early in life, human infants interact with their caregivers in what is called "proto-conversation" (Rochat, Quierdo, & Striano, 1999; Trevarthen, 1979). In these social interactions, an infant and adult gaze, touch, smile, and vocalize toward one another in turn-taking sequences (Stern, Jaffe, Beebe, & Bennett, 1975). Some authors have likened this coregulated activity to a dance with a sense of shared rhythm and movement (e.g., Schore, 1994; Stern, 1985). Contingency is important to these interactions (Bigelow & Rochat, 2006), but perhaps more critical is that the members of the dyad are sharing affect.[1] Adult and infant do not merely mimic one another, nor do they respond randomly. Often they express the same affect but in different modalities; for example, the adult smiles, and the infant chortles in response. The interaction is multimodal. These temporally coordinated interactions between infants and adult caregivers have been described extensively (Trevarthen, 1993; Tronick, 1989). Furthermore, some studies have identified patterns indicating that the movements and vocalizations of infants are contingent with the temporal characteristics of the adults' actions (Jaffe, Beebe, Feldstein, Crown, & Jasnow, 2001; Stern, Hofer, Haft, & Dore, 1985). This process of mutual attunement "reflects the role of emotion in communication. It can be used to share feelings with another, to empathize, to mock, to respond contingently, to change the other's arousal level or emotion, to change the other's goal, to teach, or to play" (Fogel, 2000, p. 132). To summarize, infants are exposed to rich, multimodal affective displays in the first few months of life, and they respond reciprocally to that information. The experimental results to be summarized in this chapter support the premise that very young infants recognize the meaning of affective expressions, provided that the infants observe multimodal expressions in familiar contexts.

In an experimental study of affect as manifested in such social interactions, Haviland and Lelwica (1987) found that by 2½ months, infants are tiny experts in affective turn taking and sharing. Haviland and Lelwica videotaped mother–infant interactions in which mothers acted out three facial and vocal expressions, as assigned, for 20 seconds each. Infants responded differently to happy, angry, and sad facial–vocal expressions, sometimes matching or imitating. For example, to a maternal portrayal of sadness, an infant was likely to look down, show a sober face, and produce more mouthing. These responses were coordinated temporally with the mothers' affective displays, as indicated by event analyses. These authors concluded:

> First, by 10 weeks of age, infants respond differently to three maternal affect expressions when the presentation is simultaneously facial and vocal—joy, anger, and sadness. Second, these infants can match or mirror joy and anger expressions. Third, the infants' matching responses to the maternal affects are only part of complex but predictable behavioral patterns that seem to indicate meaningful affect states and possibly self-regulation in the infants. (Haviland & Lelwica, 1987, p. 102)

More recently, in another study of infants' responsiveness to live affective expressions, we (Montague & Walker-Andrews, 2001) conducted a study in which 4-month-olds were presented with affective expressions embedded in the familiar game of peek-a-boo. Peek-a-boo provides a rich natural context characterized by substantial multimodal information and spatiotemporal structuring, and in which the excitement builds on the expectation of the disappearance–reappearance of a face and the accompanying vocalizations. We asked a female experimenter unfamiliar to an infant to act out the typical happy–surprised facial–vocal expression used in the game as she hid her face and then reappeared with a vocalized "peek-a-boo." On designated reappearance trials, however, she portrayed an expression that would be unanticipated in the standard game (a sad, angry, or fearful expression). Infants reacted differently to the alteration of the typical peek-a-boo interaction. Infants in the angry and fearful conditions increased their looking time to these expressions, while those infants who viewed either typical happy–surprised or sad expressions on the designated trials decreased their looking time over the sequence. In addition, infants assigned to the angry condition increased their looking time on all trials subsequent to the first angry expression, as if the appearance of anger increased their overall level of arousal. Analysis of the infants' facial expressiveness demonstrated that infants in the

sad condition were more labile; they looked away more and they responded with more facial movements, as well as more expressions identifiable as interest (Izard, 1995). In summary, 2½-month-old infants who were presented with multimodal expressions by a familiar person (Haviland & Lelwica, 1987) and 4-month-olds presented with multimodal expressions by a stranger in a familiar setting (Montague & Walker-Andrews, 2001) discriminated the expressions. In addition, they responded differentially to those expressions in both contexts. These results show that young infants can discriminate and respond appropriately even during posed interactions, as long as affective information is multimodal and is presented in familiar contexts.

INFANTS' PERCEPTION OF EMOTION

That infants are successful participants in protoconversations suggests that the perception of affect occurs early in life and involves all of the senses. Despite this possibility, the study of infants' perception of affect in controlled experiments in the laboratory started with a focus on whether infants simply could tell the difference between posed facial expressions. As with much early infant research, the assumption was that one must simplify the stimuli for infants so as not to overwhelm their senses. Infants demonstrated an ability to discriminate such stimuli. For example, LaBarbera, Izard, Vietze, and Parisi (1976) presented infants with black-and-white slides of three facial expressions one at a time. They found that 4- and 6-month-olds looked longer at the joy expression than at anger and neutral expressions, but that there was no difference in looking time to the anger and neutral expressions. Similarly, Young-Browne, Rosenfeld, and Horowitz (1977) obtained some evidence of discrimination of facial expressions by 3 months. They reported that infants increased looking time to a slide of a surprised face after viewing a happy face and to a happy face after viewing a surprised face. Infants also increased their looking time when a surprised face followed a sad face, but not vice versa. No increments in looking time were found when happy and sad were contrasted in either order. Nevertheless, both studies showed that infants could discriminate photographed, static facial expressions.

Nelson, Morse, and Leavitt (1979) posed a more critical question: Can infants move beyond discrimination and actually recognize affective expressions? They argued that if infants could detect common information for affect across several photographed facial expression exemplars and generalize that information to a new exemplar, evidence of recognition of affect would be obtained. Seven-month-old infants viewed photographed facial expressions, but to introduce variability, several different persons posed for each photograph used during the familiarization interval. Infants increased their looking time to fearful expressions after viewing a set of happy expressions, although they did not look longer to a change in expression if these sets were presented in the reverse order. Nelson and Dolgin (1985) and others (e.g., Serrano, Iglesias, & Loeches, 1992) reported similar patterns with even younger infants (3 months), and concluded that young infants are sophisticated perceivers of facial affect. Reexamination of these results, however, suggested that infants might have been responding to feature differences between facial expressions rather than to affect. To test this alternative interpretation, Caron, Caron, and Myers (1985) varied the "toothiness" of various exemplars of angry and happy facial expressions. They found that infants grouped the expressions by the visibility of molars rather than the emotion displayed. In general, the early research on infants' recognition of affect indicated that infants relied primarily on feature information, unless affect was made much more salient (cf. Ludemann & Nelson, 1988). These findings appear to contradict data from mother–infant interaction studies suggesting that infants are quite accomplished at affect perception.

MULTIMODAL, DYNAMIC PRESENTATIONS

A major difference between the two types of studies summarized above—laboratory examinations of the visual perception of photographed facial expressions, and naturalistic observations of mother–infant interactions—can be found in the emotion exemplars presented. Infants appear more sophisticated when dynamic, live stimulus displays are used in supportive contexts. Although the cited laboratory studies provided stimulus control, they eradicated important information for affect. In the

natural world, a young infant usually observes unified expressive behaviors. That is, the infant typically views a person's face and gestures, hears that person's voice, and is touched by that person during an interaction. Rarely is an infant presented with only a voice or only a face and gestures when another person claims his or her attention. Infants do hear voices emanating from adjacent rooms on occasion, but these vocalizations are usually directed at someone else. Indeed, it is quite possible that a very young infant requires all of the information available multimodally for accurate discrimination and comprehension of expressions to develop. As Charlesworth and Kreutzer (1973) suggested, infants may need the "total expressive behavior (facial, vocal, verbal, and postural) of those around them before they can discriminate such behavior from other behaviors (e.g., instrumental behaviors such as chewing, drinking, reaching) and recognize their meaning" (p. 125). Facial expressions, which carry information about intentions, are a subset of facial actions that also include eye movements and instrumental behaviors such as eating, speaking, and sneezing. The infant must abstract the affectively relevant information from such facial actions.

The specific information available in a face or a voice and gestures is not precisely equivalent, but rather invariant, across behaviors. For example, the location in space of the voice and face are identical, and location is specified by both visual and auditory information. Furthermore, acoustic characteristics of the voice (e.g., volume, variability in pitch, rhythm, tempo) may be related to aspects of facial movements and gestures (e.g., extent, fluidity, tempo). The meaning of a behavior that is expressed orally is also expressed in behaviors that can be seen. With respect to affect, to perceive the unity of an expressive behavior, an infant must detect information that is invariant over more than one modality. The infant must perceive one event, specified multimodally, if that event is to have meaning. Evidence from studies conducted over the past 30 years suggests that the development of affect perception moves from detection of intermodal correspondences during multimodal interactions to the ability to recognize affect in almost any expression, including the information from gestures, brief vocal signals, or information preserved in a static drawing. For example, an adult observer can detect anger at a distance, as when witnessing someone slamming a fist on a surface. The gesture alone conveys the meaning to an adult.

Evidence for the early emergence of intermodal perception and sensitivity to amodal information for a property such as texture (which can be seen or felt) or affect (which can be seen or heard or felt) has grown dramatically over the past few decades. "There is compelling neural, electrophysiological, and behavior evidence of strong intermodal linkages in newborns and young of a variety of avian and mammalian species, including humans" (Lickliter & Bahrick, 2000, p. 644). Young infants are sensitive to correspondences between auditory, visual, and tactual stimulation (Gibson & Walker, 1984; Lewkowicz, 1992, 1996; Meltzoff & Borton, 1979; Pickens, 1994; Walker-Andrews & Lennon, 1985); they also show the effects of intersensory facilitation, in which stimulation in one modality enhances responsiveness to stimulation in other modalities (Bahrick, Flom, & Lickliter, 2002; Lewkowicz & Turkewitz, 1981; Lickliter & Stoumbos, 1991), across a range of situations.

Why multimodal presentations are more effective (especially during early development) remains an open question, however. Drawing from the theories of E. J. Gibson (1969) and J. J. Gibson (1979), I have proposed that detection of invariant relations underlies perceptual development and learning, including in the perception of emotion (Walker-Andrews, 1994). That is, the world itself is multimodal, with redundant information specifying objects and events. In the world of affect, shared meaning is carried by face, voice, gestures, posture, and touch. In some instances the correspondences are physical (such as synchrony between visible lip movements and onset of sounds), and in others they are more abstract. Infants appear to experience a world of perceptual unity based on the detection of amodal information and/ or intermodal correspondences that specify properties of objects and events and their "affordances":

> The infant does not begin by first discriminating the qualities of objects and then learning the combinations of qualities that specify them. Phenomenal objects are not built up of qualities; it is the other way around. The affordance of an object is what the infant begins by noticing. The meaning is observed before the substance and surface, the color and form, are seen as such. An affordance is an invariant combination of variables, and one might guess that it is easiest to perceive such an in-

variant unit than it is to perceive all the variables separately. (J. J. Gibson, 1979, pp. 134–135)

With experience, infants become sensitive to new invariant relationships and come to detect additional properties of objects and events, including social-emotional interactions. Learning itself results from changes in perceptual selection, leading to progressive differentiation of the environment. In essence, an infant perceives the meaning of an event prior to the separate physical properties of that event. The intermodal correspondences marking the visual and auditory information for a single affective expression allow or compel the infant to attend to that expression and explore it fully, even in the presence of other, competing events. When an infant observes someone laughing and speaking in an animated fashion, the shared properties are highlighted, while other information (such as the person's hair color or height) becomes background (Bahrick, Walker, & Neisser, 1981).

In summary, during multimodal stimulation, processing and learning of amodal properties is facilitated. Therefore, affective information, which is presented across modalities, should be easiest to detect when it is highlighted in multimodal presentations. Differentiation of the rhythm, animation, timing, and intensity of an affective expression is supported when the infant observes a speaking, gesturing, and frowning or smiling person during an interactive bout. Parten and Marler (1999) introduced a classification scheme for categorizing and comparing how the combination of unimodal signals detected in a multimodal communicative interaction is perceived across a wide range of species at all ages. They suggest that redundancy in meaning across the components of a multimodal signal may have one of several effects. The perceiver may respond to the redundant multimodal signals as if to any single component. Alternatively, the response may be enhanced. When the signals are nonredundant, there may be specific interactions: Each component may act independently, one may dominate or modulate another, or an entirely new response may emerge. An analogous example within vision only would be the presence of a smile in conjuction with fully crinkled eyes, compared to the smile unaccompanied by eye contractions.

Neurophysiological evidence suggests that the brain is set up for multimodal processing of the types of relationships Parten and Marler describe. For example, there are sites of multisensory convergence at the cortical level in cats (Wallace, Meredith, & Stein, 1992), monkeys (Mistlin & Perrett, 1990), and humans (Calvert, 2001), and many brain areas respond to multisensory inputs. For human infants, the perception of facial and vocal affective information may lead to greater responsiveness than the observation of either facial expressions or vocal expressions separately—a multiplicative or enhanced effect such as that found during neural processing of simultaneous visual and auditory stimuli in the superior colliculus of cats (Stein, Wallace, & Meredith, 1995). Finally, recent results suggest that humans and others experience an emotion upon viewing another's emotional response (Wicker et al., 2003).

INFANTS' PERCEPTION OF FACIAL–VOCAL EXPRESSIONS

Studies of infants' perception of affective expressions have borne out the proposal that infants are more sensitive to affective information when it is presented multimodally. For example, Caron, Caron, and MacLean (1988) showed infants videotapes of six women who acted out sad, happy, or angry facial–vocal expressions continuously until the infants lost interest in the specific expression (i.e., habituated). At that point, Caron et al. showed the infants a new set of videotaped expressions. The infants responded differently to this change, depending on their age and which expression they observed initially. Infants as young as 4 months of age could tell dynamic happy and sad expressions apart, and could distinguish angry and happy expressions by 7 months, as long as these expressions were presented in specific orders. That is, 4-month-olds discriminated happy and sad expressions when happy ones were presented first, and at 5 months when either order was used. Similarly, 7-month-olds discriminated angry and happy facial–vocal expressions when happy ones occurred first, but not without the presence of a voice. In each case, the presence of both face and voice was critical, as was the dynamic quality of the expressions. Infants failed to discriminate happy and angry facial expressions depicted in photographs at 9 months in an earlier study (Caron et al., 1985). More recently, my colleagues and I (Walker-Andrews,

Mayhew, Coffield, & Krogh-Jespersen, 2004) found that infants as young as 3½ months could recognize happy and sad expressions presented by their own parents. Infants were habituated to the face and voice of each parent acting out "happy" or "sad" in alternation. At testing, infants responded to a change in emotion, person, or emotion and person in either order. A second group of infants viewed the same videotaped expressions, but failed to show recognition of expressions presented by (to them) unfamiliar males and females. They dishabituated (i.e., regained visual interest) only to a change in both expression and person.

To determine how important it is that face and voice be presented together, we (Walker-Andrews & Lennon, 1991) studied the process by which 5-month-olds might come to discriminate happy and sad vocal expressions. We showed 5-month-olds a happy or angry vocal expression accompanied by an affectively matching, but static, facial expression; a facial expression depicting a different emotion; or a checkerboard until the infants' attention waned. Infants in this study increased their looking time to any change in vocal expression, except when a checkerboard had accompanied the vocal expression during the habituation phase. We speculated that the results reflected how infants might discover the different affordances of emotional expressions in their natural environment. This discovery would be made in the context of a communicative interaction where an infant is able to look at an adult's face while listening to the adult's voice. In this view, the face acts as a setting for attending to the affective quality of the voice.

Flom and Bahrick (2007) recently focused on the developmental course of infants' detection of affective information in bimodal (auditory–visual) and unimodal (auditory- or visual-only) displays. They presented infants of 3, 4, 5, and 7 months with dynamic color video films of an adult female portraying happy, angry, or sad affective expressions for habituation. Across experiments, infants were habituated to bimodal or unimodal presentations. At testing, they were presented a change in the habituated emotion expression. Flom and Bahrick found that infants discriminated affect by 4 months if bimodal displays were presented. For unimodal displays, affect discrimination did not appear until 5 months for auditory-only displays, and at 7 months for visual-only displays. Temporal synchrony was also necessary for the youngest infants' discrimination; 3-month-olds did not respond to a change in affect when the face and voice were temporally disaligned, although 4-month-olds were successful in this task.

Infants also show intermodal matching of affect expressions. In a series of studies, I (Walker, 1982; Walker-Andrews, 1986, 1988) showed infants ranging in age from 2 to 7 months pairs of facial expressions accompanied by a single vocal expression that affectively matched one of the facial expressions. For example, one infant saw a happy and an angry facial expression side by side while listening to an angry vocal expression for 2 minutes, followed by a second presentation in which the happy vocal expression was played. In such cases, 2-month-olds looked almost exclusively at the happy expression, regardless of which vocal expression was placed. Four-month-olds increased looking time to the happy facial expression when it was sound-matched, and 5- and 7-month-olds increased fixation to any of the facial expressions that were sound-matched. I (Walker, 1982) also conducted two experiments that focused on the role of temporal synchrony in intermodal matching of affective expressions. In one experiment, happy and angry facial expressions were presented upside down with a temporally synchronized vocal expression that affectively matched one of the faces. Infants failed to show a looking preference in this situation, although synchrony was present. In another experiment, temporal synchrony was disrupted, by delaying the voice by 2 seconds. In this case, infants failed to show visual preferences on the first trial, but on the second trial, the preference for the sound-matched facial expression emerged and increased steadily over the trial. In a final study (Walker-Andrews, 1986), 5- and 7-month-olds observed facial expressions in which the lower part of the face was blocked off, so that synchrony between lip movements and vocalizations was not visible. Older infants looked preferentially to the sound-matched facial expression, although 5-month-olds failed to do so.

These results, in combination with those of Flom and Bahrick (2007) and Caron et al. (1988), suggest that during the first year infants are developing the ability to detect common affect across bimodal, dynamic presentations of an emotional expression. Infants appear to detect affective information first in bimodal (face and voice) expressions, and they

seem to recognize happy expressions earliest. It is as if the redundancy between the sight and sound guides infants' perceptual selectivity and permits them to attend to the affective intent (see Bahrick et al., 1981; Bahrick, Lickliter, & Flom, 2004). The presence of temporal synchrony between face and voice contributes to perception in younger infants, but is neither imperative nor sufficient for matching to occur. For example, Soken and Pick (1992) demonstrated that 7-month-olds can match happy and angry facial expressions to their vocal counterparts based solely on motion information. They presented infants with point-light visual displays, created by placing luminescent dots on a blackened face, thereby eliminating feature information while preserving the motion information for affect. These displays were accompanied by affectively matching vocal expressions. Soken and Pick found that infants detected correspondences between facial and vocal expressions based on affective meaning, even when each component was produced by a different person.

As indicated earlier, when infants observe expressions presented by familiar persons such as their mothers, they show greater sensitivity. We (Kahana-Kalman & Walker-Andrews, 2001) found that infants could match happy and sad facial and vocal expressions that were presented by their own mothers. When 3-month-olds observed maternal affective expressions, they increased their looking time to the sound-specified film. Even when the face and voice were presented out of synchrony, 3-month-olds showed the matching effect. Infants failed to show intermodal matching when the expressions were portrayed by an unfamiliar woman, even when the vocal and facial displays were synchronized temporally. Infants' affective responsiveness also differed across emotions and according to the familiarity of the actress. When happiness was presented facially and vocally, infants were more expressive: They showed greater variability of affective expression and increased the number of expressions they showed. Judges rated infants as experiencing more positive affect and as more interested and engaged, especially when infants were viewing their mothers. Affect coding demonstrated that infants who viewed their mothers spent more time smiling at the happy sound-specified films than did infants viewing an unfamiliar woman. There were no differences in smiling duration when sadness was the sound-specified emotion. Infants produced more full and bright smiles when happiness was sound-specified, particularly for maternal happy expressions. Finally, the mean length of distress was protracted for infants who observed unfamiliar women, compared to those who observed their mothers. It is possible that the familiar context (mother) supports infants' perceptual skills, acting as a scaffold from which to explore other facets of the world. That infants respond affectively to their mothers' expressions underscores the conclusion that they detect affective meaning in those expressions.

We (Montague & Walker-Andrews, 2002) investigated infants' intermodal matching, using happy and angry as well as happy and sad expressions posed by both mothers and fathers. The participating 3-month-olds demonstrated intermodal matching for their mothers' expressions, but they did not make intermodal matches for expressions presented by unfamiliar males and females. For fathers, the pattern was more complex. Overall, the infants did not show intermodal matching for paternal expressions, but infants whose fathers engaged in 40% or more of routine caregiving activities showed the same intermodal matching for mothers and fathers. An ongoing longitudinal study (Montague, Kahana-Kalman, Goldman, Long, & Walker-Andrews, 2005) with infants at 3, 4, 5, and 7 months is aimed at documenting the developmental trajectory of such intermodal matching and expressiveness. At 4 months, infants smile more to maternal happy expressions (facial–vocal expressions with the voice presented out of synchrony) and show more lability to maternal sad expressions. No differences have been found in infants' responses to unfamiliar adults' expressions at this age.

Even older infants are more sensitive to the meanings expressed in multimodal portrayals. Vocal expressions alone, and vocal expressions combined with facial expressions, are more influential in regulating infants' behavior in social-referencing studies (Barrett, Campos, & Emde, 1996; Mumme, Fernald, & Herrera, 1996). Vaish and Striano (2004) examined the role of facial versus vocal information on infants' responses in a potentially threatening situation. Mothers acted out positive facial-only, vocal-only, or facial–vocal expressions toward their 12-month-olds on a visual cliff apparatus. Infants crossed the cliff more quickly in the facial–vocal and vocal-only conditions, and

looked more often to their mothers in the facial–vocal condition.

INFANTS' RESPONSES TO TACTUAL INFORMATION

Most studies that use multimodal expressions of emotion have used auditory–visual presentations. However, a few investigators have examined the effects of tactual information. For example, it has been established that contact (tactual stimulation) acts to soothe infants during still-face experiments, in which an infant becomes distressed when a caregiver becomes unresponsive facially and vocally (Gusella, Muir, & Tronick, 1988; Stack & Muir, 1990, 1992). Infants show more smiling, vocalizing, and gazing when touch is used in a still-face episode than when no touch is provided. Stack (2001) reported that mothers can modify their infants' behavior (e.g., elicit smiles) when the mothers are asked to do so by stroking or otherwise touching the infants. Recently, Moreno, Posada, and Goldyn (2006) explicitly examined the role of touch in the interactions of 3½-month-olds and their mothers. Mothers were asked to play with their infants in a face-to-face interaction for 3 minutes, once with touch and once without touch. Moreno et al. found, as in most studies investigating the perception of affect, that context is extremely important to affect recognition and regulation. Symmetry between mother and infant was influenced differentially, depending on the type of touch (playful vs. affectionate) and an infant's assigned condition. The authors concluded that dyads "make constant 'online' adjustments to their contribution of the interaction based on their own internal state as well as feedback they receive" (p. 16).

In summary, experimental studies suggest that infants can recognize emotional expressions early in development when affective information is presented multimodally. A number of factors influence the facility with which infants respond to that affective information, including the child's stage of development, the specific emotion, the familiarity of the person enacting an affective expression, and the context in which the expression is encountered. Pinning down the various factors and explicating mechanisms by which they act on infants' perception of affective information continue to be of interest to researchers.

CHILDREN'S PERCEPTION OF EMOTION

Although the focus of this chapter is on the development of affect understanding during infancy, it is worth noting that the understanding of emotional expressions also seems influenced by modality in young children. Children readily perceive, recognize, and label emotions across a wide range of conditions, and they show development in these abilities throughout childhood (Denham, 1998). Children are more capable of recognizing happy than sad expressions, and better at labeling both of these than angry and fearful expressions (Denham, Zoller, & Couchoud, 1994). Shackman and Pollak (2005), who examined learning factors that might influence the perception of multimodal affective expressions among school-age children conclude that contextual cues such as familiarity enhance children's ability to extract meaningful information from affective displays, as is the case with infants, and that the "importance of auditory versus visual percepts is influenced by the meaning attached to particular emotions contained in each expression and by the familiarity of the individual expressing emotion" (p. 1124).

SINGLE-MODALITY PRESENTATIONS

As alluded to in the review above, infants also come to recognize affective information in single-modality displays. The literature on the perception of facial expressions suggests that infants come to detect affective information in the face sometime in the second half of the first year, and in voices sometime before that. As described previously, Flom and Bahrick (2007) examined this development within a single study, finding that infants appear to recognize emotion in bimodal presentations first, followed by unimodal vocal expressions, and finally unimodal facial expressions. This is the sequence that Buhler (1930) and I (Walker-Andrews, 1997) have proposed, but there have been other proposals as well. Lewkowicz (1988a, 1988b) advanced a theory of early auditory dominance in infants' perception of social and nonsocial events, which was extended to the perception of affective expressions by Caron (1988). More recent results, however (e.g., Lewkowicz, 2000; Lewkowicz & Edmondson, 1993), have indicated that for

speech and affective information, the sequence originally proposed by Buhler (1930) is more likely to be the case. Although infants detect unimodal information that potentially specifies the meaning of an affective expression, there is no evidence that very young infants perceive this unimodal information as informative about affect. That is, although a neonate can discriminate the fundamental frequencies of two tones or the pitch of two different voices, or distinguish the upturned curve of a smile from the bared teeth of a snarl, the infant does not seem to perceive these differences as affective. Rather, the infant seems to rely on the redundant information in multimodal displays. Others (e.g., Klinnert, Campos, Sorce, Emde, & Svejda, 1983; Nelson, 1987) have alluded to this developmental pattern as well. As such, the developmental pattern may be no different from all sorts of perceptual learning in which information may be detected first in intermodal displays (Bahrick & Lickliter, 2002; Walker-Andrews, 1994).

EXPERIENCE OF EMOTION

The first part of this chapter has focused on the perception of emotions portrayed by others, as well as the responsiveness of infants and young children to that affective information. However, the ease with which human infants learn about emotion may stem from their own multimodal experience of emotion as well. At a minimum, the experience of anger at one's desires being thwarted can result in a plethora of physical and sensory signals: One's own angry cry is heard, the turmoil in the stomach is felt, the narrowing of one's eyes and hard stare are also perceived, and the consequences of one's actions are seen. Faced with an angry person, similar effects may occur. One hears the other's angry voice, sees the angry face, and feels one's own shrinking or firmly held stance. During protoconversations, the infant observes the typical happy facial expression, exaggerated pitch, and volubility of the happy voice, and may be tickled or playfully poked by a caregiver. The infant responds with a happy smile, energetic movements of his or her limbs, and laughter.

Stern (1985) has gone beyond this mere description of how one might experience an emotion multimodally, to the suggestion that the experience of emotion, because it is multimodal, provides a sense of self. He first talks of the multimodal experience of all kinds: "For instance, the actual experience of looking for the first time at something that, on the basis of how it felt to the touch, should look a certain way, and having it, indeed, look that way is something like a déjà vu experience" (p. 52). Moreover, what Stern calls "vitality affects" (feelings such as those experienced with the coming and going of emotions and thoughts) are experienced by the infant from within, as well as in the behavior of other persons. Recent evidence from Fogel and his colleagues demonstrates that infants have a rich emotional life, as demonstrated by the complexity of their smiles and other expressive behaviors in specific interactive contexts. In one study, Fogel et al. (2000) found that infants showed different types of smiles, depending on the context. That is, infants as young as 6 months emitted smiles—simple, Duchenne, play, and duplay—that varied with the game being played (peek-a-boo or tickle), portion of the game, trial, and direction of an infant's gaze. The authors concluded that when smiling, infants were experiencing "qualitatively different kinds of enjoyment during these two games" (p. 497)—enjoyment of readiness to engage in play, of relief, of participation and agency, of escape, and of buildup. The results indicate that the "same facial action, smiling, can reflect different positive emotions depending upon cooccurring facial actions and the dynamics of the social process, and that the positive emotional experience of infants as young as six months is more complex than previously reported" (p. 497). Of particular importance are (1) the demonstration that smiles are systematically related to context and have specific meanings during social communication, and (2) the suggestion that the smiles themselves are associated with feelings such as the enjoyment of relief or enjoyment of participation. The physical action of the tickle game is accompanied by the smiles of relief following the climax. The smile indexes a particular emotion. Again, as proposed by Stern (1985), infants have a sense of themselves as participants in an interaction. Infants' responses during interactions are coordinated, multimodal actions involving vocalizations, gaze, facial expressions, body movements, and gestures, which relay information to the other as well as to the infants themselves (Malatesta, 1981; Weinberg & Tronick, 1994) about internal states, and that regulate the behavior of both partners. Affective arousal may mediate

associations among infants' vocalizations, facial expressions, gaze, postural changes, and other responses (Fogel et al., 1997).

Smith (2005) speaks of the powerful computational system that is at work: "Developing in a social world does not just mean that development is guided by a mature partner. It also provides an additional level of higher-order multimodal correlations critical to concepts of self, other, intention, and what is commonly known in the literature as theory of mind" (p. 292). The interaction of baby and other provides multimodal, time-locked correlations that provide information about the appearance, actions, and internal states of the self and others. Perhaps one of the most remarkable demonstrations of the integration of information from the self and from others comes from the study of neonatal imitation. Meltzoff and Moore (1977) demonstrated that newborns can imitate simple movements of the face, head, and hand modeled by an adult. Meltzoff and Moore labeled this a "supramodal" process, because infants could imitate a seen protrusion of the tongue by an adult with their own (felt) tongue protrusion. Infants also mimic the phonetic and prosodic structure in their mothers' speech (Bloom, 1988; Kuhl & Meltzoff, 1996; Papousek & Papousek, 1989). Meltzoff and his colleagues suggest that information about facial acts is somehow fed into a supramodal representation that allows for imitation of what is modeled by another, even though one's own performance cannot be seen. Finally, recent findings regarding "mirror neurons" (e.g., Wicker et al., 2003) indicate that humans may respond with emotion to the observed emotional expressions of others. Whatever the mechanism, it is clear that intermodal processes play a critical role in imitation.

CONCLUSION

In conclusion, intermodal processes are critical to the development of emotion, including the perception of others' affective expressions and the growth of one's own emotional system. Infants are quick to detect amodal relations and intermodal correspondences in the fully multimodal packages presented during social interactions. The infant is gifted further with the experience of his or her own affective behavior, which includes facial, vocal, visceral, and kinesthetic responses. Just as an infant approaching the age of 1 is more influenced by vocal and facial expressions together than by either alone (Vaish & Striano, 2004), so is a young infant reliant on multimodal information for disambiguating or recognizing others' affective expressions. The term "resonance" as used by J. J. Gibson (1979) is apt for describing the perception–action coupling that is manifested in the perception and expression of affect. The emphasis on intermodal processes captures the fact that emotion is inherently multimodal. Infant and maternal facial expressions, gestures, and vocalizations are tightly coupled in a social interaction (Gogate, Walker-Andrews, & Bahrick, 2001). Moreover, a mother does not simply react to an infant's behavior; she also builds on it. Caregivers "create a conversation-like exchange by weaving their own behavior around the child's natural activity patterns. But babies' behaviors are both entrained by the mother's pattern and educated by the multimodal correspondences those interactions create" (Smith, 2005, p. 294). During the process, infants and caregivers react to, imitate, and scaffold their responses on one another, in ways that enrich the interaction and allow the infants to learn about emotion.

NOTE

1. In this example, the term "affect" is being used to describe more general states that include emotion and mood, and "affective information" the sensory stimuli specifying affect; "emotion" is being reserved for discrete experiences such as joy, anger, and fear.

REFERENCES

Bahrick, L. E., Flom, R., & Lickliter, R. (2002). Intersensory redundancy facilitates discrimination of tempo in 3-month-olds. *Developmental Psychology, 41*, 352–363.

Bahrick, L. E., & Lickliter, R. (2002). Intersensory redundancy guides early perceptual and cognitive development. *Advances in Child Development and Behavior, 30*, 153–187.

Bahrick, L. E., Lickliter, R., & Flom, R. (2004). Intersensory redundancy guides the development of selective attention, perception, and cognition in infancy. *Current Directions in Psychological Science, 13*(3), 99–102.

Bahrick, L. E., Walker, A. S., & Neisser, U. (1981). Selective looking by infants. *Cognitive Psychology, 13*, 377–390.

Barrett, K. C., Campos, J. J., & Emde, R. N. (1996). Infants' use of conflicting emotion signals. *Cognition and Emotion, 10*, 113–135.

Bigelow, A. E., & Rochat, P. (2006). Two-month-old infants' sensitivity to social contingency in mother–infant and stranger–infant interaction. *Infancy, 9*, 313–325.

Bloom, K. (1988). Quality of adult vocalizations affects the quality of infant vocalizations. *Journal of Child Language, 14*, 211–227.

Buhler, C. (1930). *The first year of life.* New York: John Day.

Calvert, G. A. (2001). Crossmodal processing in the human brain: Insights from functional neuroimaging studies. *Cerebral Cortex, 11*, 1110–1123.

Caron, A. J. (1988). *The role of face and voice in infant discrimination of naturalistic emotional expressions.* Paper presented at the International Conference on Infant Studies, Washington, DC.

Caron, A. J., Caron, R. F., & MacLean, D. J. (1988). Infant discrimination of naturalistic emotional expressions: The role of face and voice. *Child Development, 59*, 604–616.

Caron, R. F., Caron, A. J., & Myers, R. S. (1985). Do infants see emotional expressions in static faces? *Child Development, 56*, 1552–1560.

Charlesworth, W. R., & Kreutzer, M. A. (1973). Facial expressions of infants and children. In P. Ekman (Ed.), *Darwin and facial expression* (pp. 91–167). New York: Academic Press.

Denham, S. A. (1998). *Emotion development in young children.* New York: Guilford Press.

Denham, S. A., Zoller, D., & Couchoud, E. A. (1994). Socialization of preschooler's emotion understanding. *Developmental Psychology, 30*, 928–936.

Flom, R., & Bahrick, L. E. (2007). The development of infant discrimination of affect in multimodal and unimodal stimulation: The role of intersensory redundancy. *Developmental Psychology, 43*, 238–252.

Fogel, A., Dickson, K. L., Hsu, H., Messinger, D. S., Nelson-Goens, G. C., & Nwokah, E. E. (1997). Communication of smiling and laughter in mother–infant play: Research on emotion from a dynamic systems perspective. In K. Barrett (Ed.), *New directions for child development: No. 77. The communication of emotions: Current research from diverse perspectives* (pp. 5–24). San Francisco: Jossey-Bass.

Gibson, E. J. (1969). *Principles of perceptual learning and development.* Englewood Cliffs, NJ: Prentice Hall.

Gibson, E. J., & Walker, A. S. (1984). Development of knowledge of visual–tactual affordances of substance. *Child Development, 55*, 453–460.

Gibson, J. J. (1979). *The ecological approach to visual perception.* Hillsdale, NJ: Erlbaum.

Gogate, L. J., Walker-Andrews, A. S., & Bahrick, L. E. (2001). The intersensory origins of word comprehension: An ecological–dynamic systems view. *Developmental Science, 4*(1), 1–18.

Gusella, J. L., Muir, D. W., & Tronick, E. Z. (1988). The effect of manipulating maternal behavior during an interaction on 3- and 6-month-olds' affect and attention. *Child Development, 59*, 1111–1124.

Haviland, J. M., & Lelwica, M. (1987). The induced affect response: 10-week-old infants' responses to three emotion expressions. *Developmental Psychology, 23,* 97–104.

Izard, C. E. (1995). *The Maximally Discriminative Facial Movement Coding System (MAX)* (rev. ed.). Newark: University of Delaware, Information Technologies and University Media Services.

Jaffe, J., Beebe, B., Feldstein, S., Crown, C., & Jasnow, M. D. (2001). Rhythms of dialogue in infancy. *Monographs of the Society for Research in Child Development,* 66(2, Serial No. 265).

Kahana-Kalman, R., & Walker-Andrews, A. S. (2001). The role of person familiarity in young infants' perception of emotional expressions. *Child Development, 72,* 352–369.

Klinnert, M., Campos, J. J., Sorce, J., Emde, R. N., & Svejda, M. (1983). Emotions as behavior regulators: Social referencing in infancy. In R. Plutchik & H. Kellerman (Eds.), *The emotions: Vol. 2. Emotions in early development* (pp. 57–86). New York: Academic Press.

Kuhl, P. K., & Meltzoff, A. N. (1996). Infant vocalizations in response to speech: Vocal imitation and developmental change. *Journal of the Acoustical Society of America, 100,* 2425–2438.

LaBarbera, J. D., Izard, C. E., Vietze, P., & Parisi, S. A. (1976). Four- and six-month-old infants visual responses to joy, anger, and neutral expressions. *Child Development, 47,* 535–538.

Lewkowicz, D. J. (1988a). Sensory dominance in infants: 1. Six-month-old infants' response to auditory–visual compounds. *Developmental Psychology, 24,* 155–171.

Lewkowicz, D. J. (1988b). Sensory dominance in infants: 2. Ten-month-old infants' response to auditory–visual compounds. *Developmental Psychology, 24,* 172–182.

Lewkowicz, D. J. (1992). Infants' response to temporally based intersensory equivalence: The effect of synchronous sounds on visual preferences for moving stimuli. *Infant Behavior and Development, 15,* 297–324.

Lewkowicz, D. J. (1996). Infants' response to the audible and visible properties of the human face: I. Role of lexical/syntactic content, temporal synchrony, gender, and manner of speech. *Developmental Psychology, 32,* 347–366.

Lewkowicz, D. J. (2000). Infants' perception of the audible, visible, and bimodal attributes of multimodal syllables. *Child Development, 71,* 1241–1257.

Lewkowicz, D. J., & Edmondson, D. (1993). *Infants' responsiveness to the multimodal properties of the human face.* Paper presented at the biennial meeting of the Society for Research in Child Development, New Orleans.

Lewkowicz, D. J., & Turkewitz, G. (1981). Intersensory interaction in newborns: Modification of visual preferences following exposure to sound. *Child Development, 52,* 827–832.

Lickliter, R., & Bahrick, L. E. (2000). Perceptual development and the origins of multisensory responsive-

ness. In G. A. Calvert, C. Spence, & B. E. Stein (Eds.), *The handbook of multisensory processes* (pp. 643–654). Cambridge, MA: MIT Press.

Lickliter, R., & Stoumbos, J. (1991). Enhanced prenatal auditory experience facilitates species-specific visual responsiveness in bobwhite quail chicks (*Colinus virginianus*). *Journal of Comparative Psychology, 105,* 89–94.

Ludemann, P., & Nelson, C. (1988). Categorical representation of facial expressions by 7-month-old infants. *Developmental Psychology, 24,* 492–501.

Malatesta, C. A. (1981). Infant emotion and the vocal affect lexicon. *Motivation and Emotion, 5,* 1–23.

Meltzoff, A. N., & Borton, R. W. (1979). Intermodal matching by human neonates. *Nature, 282,* 403–404.

Meltzoff, A. N., & Moore, M. K. (1977). Imitation of facial and manual gestures by human neonates. *Science, 198,* 75–78.

Mistlin, A. J., & Perrett, D. I. (1990). Visual and somatosensory processing in the macaque temporal cortex: The role of 'expectation.' *Experimental Brain Research, 83,* 437–450.

Montague, D. P. F., Kahana-Kalman, R., Goldman, S., Long, L., & Walker-Andrews, A. S. (2005). *Infants' recognition of emotion expressions and the role of parental involvement and emotionality.* Poster presented at the biennial meeting of the Society for Research in Child Development, Atlanta, GA.

Montague, D. P. F., & Walker-Andrews, A. S. (2001). Peekaboo: A new look at infants' perception of emotion expression. *Developmental Psychology, 37,* 826–838.

Montague, D. P. F., & Walker-Andrews, A. S. (2002). Mothers, fathers, and infants: The role of familiarity and parental involvement in infants' perception of emotion expressions. *Child Development, 73,* 1339–1352.

Moreno, A. J., Posada, G. E., & Goldyn, D. T. (2006). Presence and quality of touch influence coregulation in mother–infant dyads. *Infancy, 9,* 1–20.

Mumme, D. L., Fernald, A., & Herrera, C. (1996). Infants' responses to facial and vocal emotional signals in a social referencing paradigm. *Child Development, 67,* 3219–3237.

Nelson, C. A. (1987). The recognition of facial expressions in the first two years of life: Mechanisms of development. *Child Development, 58,* 889–909.

Nelson, C. A., & Dolgin, K. (1985). The generalized discrimination of facial expressions by seven-month-old infants. *Child Development, 56,* 58–61.

Nelson, C. A., Morse, P. A., & Leavitt, L. A. (1979). Recognition of facial expressions by seven-month-old infants. *Child Development, 50,* 1239–1242.

Papousek, M., & Papousek, H. (1989). Forms and functions of vocal matching in interactions between mothers and their precanonical infants. *First Language, 9,* 137–158.

Parten, S., & Marler, P. (1999). Communication goes multimodal. *Science, 2823,* 1272–1273.

Pickens, J. (1994). Perception of auditory–visual distance relations by 5-month-old infants. *Developmental Psychology, 30,* 537–544.

Rochat, P., Quierdo, J. G., & Striano, T. (1999). Emerging sensitivity of the timing and structure of protoconversation in early infancy. *Developmental Psychology, 35,* 950–957.

Schore, A. (1994). *Affect regulation and the origins of the self: The neurobiology of emotional development.* Hillsdale, NJ: Erlbaum.

Serrano, J. M., Iglesias, J., & Loeches, A. (1992). Visual discrimination and recognition of facial expressions of anger, fear and surprise in four- to six-month-old infants. *Developmental Psychobiology, 25,* 411–425.

Shackman, J. E., & Pollak, S. D. (2005). Experiential influences on multimodal perception of emotion. *Child Development, 76,* 1116–1126.

Smith, L. B. (2005). Cognition as a dynamic system: Principles from embodiment. *Developmental Review, 25,* 278–298.

Soken, N. H., & Pick, A. D. (1992). Intermodal perception of happy and angry expressive behaviors by seven-month-old infants. *Child Development, 63,* 787–793.

Stack, D. M. (2001). The salience of touch and physical contact during infancy: Unraveling some of the mysteries of the somesthetic sense. In G. Bremner & A. Fogel (Eds.), *Handbooks of developmental psychology: Blackwell handbook of infant development* (pp. 351–378). Malden, MA: Blackwell.

Stack, D. M., & Muir, D. W. (1990). Tactile stimulation as a component of social interchange: New interpretations for the still-face effect. *British Journal of Developmental Psychology, 8,* 131–145.

Stack, D. M., & Muir, D. W. (1992). Adult tactile stimulation during face-to-face interactions modulates five-month-olds' affect and attention. *Child Development, 63,* 1509–1525.

Stein, B. E., Wallace, M. T., & Meredith, M. A. (1995). Neural mechanisms mediating attention and orientation to multisensory cues. In M. Gazzaniga (Ed.), *The cognitive neurosciences* (pp. 683–702). Cambridge, MA: MIT Press.

Stern, D. N. (1985). *The interpersonal world of the infant.* New York: Basic Books.

Stern, D. N., Hofer, L., Haft, W., & Dore, J. (1985). Affect attunement: The sharing by means of intermodal fluency. In T. M. Field & N. A. Fox (Eds.), *Social perception in infants* (pp. 249–286). Norwood, NJ: Ablex.

Stern, D. N., Jaffe, J., Beebe, B., & Bennett, S. L. (1975). Vocalizing in unison and alternation: Two modes of communication within the mother–infant dyad. *Annals of the New York Academy of Sciences, 263,* 89–100.

Trevarthen, C. (1979). Communication and cooperation in early infancy: A description of primary intersubjectivity. In M. Bullowa (Ed.), *Before speech:*

The beginning of interpersonal communication. Cambridge, UK: Cambridge University Press.

Trevarthen, C. (1993). The self born in intersubjectivity: The psychology of an infant communicating. In U. Neisser (Ed.) *Ecological and interpersonal knowledge of self* (pp. 121–173). New York: Cambridge University Press.

Tronick, E. Z. (1989). Emotions and emotional communication in infants. *American Psychologist, 44*(2), 112–119.

Vaish, A., & Striano, T. (2004). Is visual reference necessary? *Developmental Science, 7,* 261–269.

Walker, A. S. (1982). Intermodal perception of expressive behaviors by human infants. *Journal of Experimental Child Psychology, 33,* 514–535.

Walker-Andrews, A. S. (1986). Intermodal perception of expressive behaviors: Relation of eye and voice? *Developmental Psychology, 22,* 373–377.

Walker-Andrews, A. S. (1988). Infants' perception of the affordances of expressive behaviors. In C. K. Rovee-Collier (Ed.), *Advances in infancy research* (Vol. 5, pp. 173–221). Norwood, NJ: Ablex.

Walker-Andrews, A. S. (1994). Taxonomy for intermodal relations. In D. J. Lewkowicz & R. Lickliter (Eds.), *The development of intersensory perception* (pp. 39–56). Hillsdale, NJ: Erlbaum.

Walker-Andrews, A. S. (1997). Infants' perception of expressive behaviors: Differentiation of multimodal information. *Psychological Bulletin, 121,* 437–456.

Walker-Andrews, A. S., & Grolnick, W. (1983). Discrimination of vocal expression by young infants. *Infant Behavior and Development, 6,* 491–498.

Walker-Andrews, A. S., & Lennon, E. M. (1985). Auditory–visual perception of changing distance by human infants. *Child Development, 56,* 544–548.

Walker-Andrews, A. S., & Lennon, E. (1991). Infants' discrimination of vocal expressions: Contributions of auditory and visual information. *Infant Behavior and Development, 14,* 131–142.

Walker-Andrews, A. S., Mayhew, E., Coffield, C., & Krogh-Jespersen, S. (2004). *Familiarity allows contempt: Infants' understanding of the emotion of familiar people.* Poster presented at the meeting of the International Society for Infant Studies, Chicago.

Wallace, M. T., Meredith, M. A., & Stein, B. E. (1992). Integration of multiple sensory modalities in cat cortex. *Experimental Brain Research, 91,* 484–488.

Weinberg, M. K., & Tronick, E. Z. (1994). Beyond the face: An empirical study of infant affective configuration of facial, vocal, gestural, and regulatory behaviors. *Child Development, 65,* 1503–1515.

Wicker, B., Keysers, C., Plailly, J., Royet, J.-P., Gallese, V., & Rizzoulatti, G. (2003). Both of us disgusted in my insula: The common neural basis of seeing and feeling disgust. *Neuron, 40,* 655–664.

Young-Browne, G., Rosenfeld, H. M., & Horowitz, F. D. (1977). Infant discrimination of facial expressions. *Child Development, 48,* 555–562.

CHAPTER 23

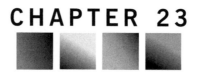

Long-Lived Emotions
A Life Course Perspective
on Emotional Development

CAROL MAGAI

INTERVIEWER: Do you believe there is such a thing as a limited life span
for humans?

MICHAEL R. ROSE, Professor of Evolutionary Biology: No. Life span is
totally tunable. In my lab, we tune it up and down all the time.
—DREIFUS (2006, reporting on life extension in fruit flies)

If we could physically retard the process of aging in humans, which appears increasingly likely, would the landscape of our emotional lives change? In this chapter, I argue that retarding physical aging would indeed alter the emotion system, though perhaps in some unanticipated ways. In order to assess my prediction, we need to start with what is already known about emotion and the aging process. Accordingly, I review the literature on theories of emotion and aging, as well as what is known about change and continuity in emotion across the adult lifespan based on the empirical literature.

ADULT DEVELOPMENTAL MODELS OF AFFECT AND AGING

Over the past several decades, three bodies of theory concerning emotion and aging have risen to prominence: (1) differential-emotions theory (DET) and related functionalist accounts, (2) optimization and selectivity theories, and (3) cognitive–affective developmental theory. DET is given prominence in this review because, of the three theories, it is the only one that actually has its empirical roots in infancy and early development, articulates with adult development and development in later life, and thus encompasses the lifespan. Because of space limitations, however, I attend mainly to its applicability to adulthood.

Differential-Emotions Theory

Although a number of theories regarding human emotions were propounded during the 1960s and 1970s, Carroll Izard's DET (Izard, 1971, 1977, 1991) was unique in that it had a distinctly developmental emphasis. My colleagues and I have made other contributions in this vein, especially in the area of adult development and aging (Magai & Haviland-Jones, 2002; Magai & Nusbaum, 1996; Malatesta-Magai, Jonas, Shepard, & Culver, 1992). DET, a variant of discrete-emotions theory, derives its name from the theory's emphasis on the qualitatively different nature of the primary or basic emotions: joy, interest, surprise, anger, contempt, disgust, fear, sadness, shame, and guilt, each with a distinctively different motivational, expressive, and phenomenological aspect. Although the preponderance of research and theory emanating from Izard's laboratory has dealt with infancy and early childhood, more recent formulations by Izard and colleagues—and related discrete-emotions accounts—have explicitly addressed the issue of adult development and aging (Consedine & Magai, 2006; Izard & Ackerman, 1998; Izard, Ackerman, Schoff, & Fine, 1999; Magai & Haviland-Jones, 2002; Magai & McFadden, 1995; Malatesta, 1982, 1990; Malatesta, Izard, Culver, & Nicolich, 1987; Malatesta & Wilson, 1988; Malatesta-Magai et al., 1992).

One aspect of the emotion system that is considered stable over developmental time involves the feeling states that accompany the primary or fundamental emotions. Each primary emotion is associated with a distinct qualitative feeling state, and each is paired with a particular motivational vector. These pairings are held to be hard-wired in the nervous system and to remain stable from infancy to old age. The constancy of emotional phenomenology across developmental epochs is attributed to the fact that feeling–motivation linkages are evolutionarily grounded and adaptive in nature. For example, the feeling of fear is fundamentally about the experience of threat and invokes the motivation to defend the self—at any stage of development. Similarly, the feeling of sadness involves sensations of loss, whether one is a child, a middle-aged adult, or an elderly person; these sensations of loss are accompanied by psychomotor slowing and, unless they are suppressed, facial expressions indicative of loss (horseshoe mouth and oblique brows). Expressive behavior—especially facial expressions of emotion—are also seen as hard-wired; that is, the basic neurological substrate of emotion gives rise to patterned facial expressions that are recognized universally (Izard, 1971), as in the sadness expression just described. According to the theory, facial expressive behavior acts as both a

signal to the self (motivating acquisitive, affiliative, or self-protective behavior) and as a signal to the social environment (communicating needs, desires, fears, and intentions). The critical motivational and communicative aspects of facial expressive behavior, as evolutionarily grounded, are basic to survival and adaptation (Darwin, 1872); what DET makes explicit is that these expressions are critical to adaptation and survival not only in infancy, but throughout the lifespan (Izard & Malatesta, 1987).

Going beyond these fixed elements of the emotion system, the theory specifies domains in which developmental changes are to be expected. Also, these changes are held to be inherent not at the local level of the hard-wired emotions themselves, but in their linkages with the cognitive and behavioral subsystems, which lead to elaboration and complexity. For example, individuals acquire an increasingly sophisticated ability to anticipate the emotional responses of others over time, which accrues from accumulated interpersonal experience and the increasingly dense and elaborated connections that are forged among the emotional, cognitive, and behavioral subsystems of personality. Thus, in theory, we may anticipate that greater age will be accompanied by an increasingly sophisticated and nuanced ability to recognize, appreciate, and relate to the emotions of others. As well, such experience-based and experience-enriched interconnections should enable the internal perception of a more richly textured emotional phenomenology—or greater emotional complexity—over developmental time.

Another aspect of the emotion system that undergoes change over developmental time occurs in the area of facial expressive behavior. Although the neuromuscular patterning of the basic emotions is hard-wired, expressive behavior becomes modulated in accord with familial and cultural norms and with advancing skill at understanding interpersonal process; while this appears to occur most strikingly in infancy and childhood, it is a lifespan process, according to research on younger, middle-aged, and older adults (Malatesta & Izard, 1984). In turn, these developmental acquisitions create feedback and feedforward loops that have an impact on interpersonal relations, potentially facilitating the development, maintenance, and protection of social relations and social support systems. These changes in the formal aspects of expressive behavior include the ability to minimize or amplify expressive behavior and the capacity to reflect mixed, nuanced, or more complex emotions.

Differential emotions theory also touches upon how emotions relate to the acquisition of personality traits, following on the work of Silvan Tomkins (1962, 1963, 1991, 1992) and his discussion of "ideo-affective structures." Izard's "affective–cognitive structures" (Izard, 1971, 1977), like Tomkins's ideo-affective structures, are construed as relatively stable aspects of personality in which early and repetitive emotional experiences result in structural changes that become consolidated in personality. These "structures," or internal models, give rise to enduring expectations that color the individual's affective world and bias information processing and behavior in predictable ways. It is this aspect of DET that has received particular elaboration in our work (e.g., Magai & Haviland-Jones, 2002; Magai & Nusbaum, 1996; Malatesta, 1982, 1990), where references to "structures" are exchanged for the more plastic concepts of "affective traits" or "biases." This work has detailed a set of patterned affect-specific perceptual biases and affect-specific productive biases or emotion-based personality traits (Malatesta, 1990; Magai & McFadden, 1995; Malatesta & Wilson, 1988), which are manifested in the behaviors, cognitions, and interpersonal processes of ordinary individuals in everyday life. Another derivation from DET leads us to expect that different emotion-based aspects of personality should lead to qualitatively different kinds of social relations (Magai, Hunziker, Mesias, & Culver, 2000; Izard, 1991). Because emotions are fundamentally social in nature, and because different emotions communicate qualitatively different kinds of social messages, they serve as important informational signals to social partners. If particular emotion biases are trait-like in nature and are emitted repetitively, they are likely to establish different patterns of social relations.

Our more recent work (e.g., Magai & Haviland-Jones, 2002; Magai & Nusbaum, 1996) has incorporated elements of dynamic-systems theory, such as attractors and repellors, phase shifts, and nonlinear effects, to model not only personality stability but also personality change. In brief, the theory suggests that when intense, unanticipated, or surprising emotional experiences of a positive or negative nature are encountered and are cognitively elaborated in the context of an interpersonally supportive environment, internal models of affect and interpersonal process can be substantively reworked and result in personality change.

In summary, DET postulates that feeling states and patterned expressive behavior are innate aspects of the emotion system; however, the latter retains some degree of plasticity, which results in cultural variants of expressive behavior, as well as idiosyncratic familial and individual variants. Because of the intrinsic interconnectivity of the nervous system and the linkages among the emotional, cognitive, and behavioral subsystems of personality (Izard, 1971, 1977), emotional experiences at the individual level over developmental time give rise to the capacity for increasingly complex emotional phenomenology and increasing sophistication in noticing, recognizing, and responding to the emotions of others. The capacity for change as a function of accumulative experience suggests that, all other things being equal, as people age they should show an enhanced capacity to experience and express more complex emotions, demonstrate greater emotion-regulatory capacities, experience and reflect greater empathy to the emotional distress of others, and sustain and enrich interpersonal relations with age. However, the theory also notes that the magnitude of these developmentally enabled capacities is, to a certain extent, constrained at the individual level by the formation of emotional biases in the personality. These biases, in turn, condition the extent to which, and manner in which, these capacities will be manifested. Finally, the biases themselves are also subject to modification over time, again depending on emotional events at the level of individual lives.

Optimization and Selectivity Theories of Emotion

Another set of theoretical formulations about affect and aging, which I refer to as "optimization and selectivity theories," has centered on emotional regulatory capacities of individuals across the adult years and their social environments. The works of Powell Lawton and Laura Carstensen are most noteworthy in this respect. Both authors propose that emotions are central psychological processes, and that adults become increasingly skilled emotion regulators over the lifespan, particularly in the later years.

Lawton (e.g., Lawton, 2001; Lawton, Kleban, & Dean, 1993; Lawton, Kleban, Rajagopal, & Dean, 1992; Lawton, Moss, Winter, & Hoffman, 2002; Lawton, Ruckdeschel, Winter, & Kleban, 1999) has proposed that there are three dimensions of affective experience that undergo change during adulthood, especially in later life: (1) responsiveness or reactivity to emotional stimuli, (2) dynamic features of affects (the frequency, rise time, duration, and intensity of emotions), and (3) self-regulatory processes. However, it is the third aspect of affective experience that has seen his greatest theoretical elaboration. According to Lawton, as adults age they acquire greater mastery over their emotions, and this occurs in the context of adaptations to changes in social contexts and life events. In this view, older adults are not only more skilled at emotion regulation; they deploy their regulatory skills deliberatively and proactively toward the general goal of "affective optimization." That is, they seek to create and maintain the kinds of social environments in which there is a balance between emotionally stimulating and insulating features, and in which they can avoid the occasion of conflict and negative affect. Although Lawton has viewed this as the normative developmental trajectory, he has also made allowances for individual differences. Indeed, Lawton et al. (1999) hypothesized that older people may vary in their mix of openness to the experience of emotion and in the degree to which they control emotional expression, and that these idiosyncratic patterns can conceivably affect what they actually experience.

Carstensen's socioemotional selectivity theory (Carstensen, 1988, 1992, 1993, 1995; Carstensen, Fung, & Charles, 2003), which takes its inspiration from a proposed model of successful aging (Baltes & Baltes, 1990)—selective optimization with compensation—is a lifespan theory of motivation focused primarily on how adults create conditions in which they may optimize their social and emotional lives. Starting with the well-established observation that the social networks of adults tend to narrow in the later part of the lifespan, Carstensen has proposed that social network attrition is an electively driven process that is related to changes in the nature of goals in later life. That is, according to Carstensen, there are three primary human motives: (1) emotion regulation, (2) development and maintenance of the individual's self-concept, and (3) information seeking. The priority of these motives changes in middle and later life, in the context of an age-related diminution in physiological and psychological resources. As such, information seeking recedes in importance, and emotional goals take on primacy; thus changes in emotions are consequences of motivational changes. Emotional goals include maintaining optimal emotion regulation directed at a positively valenced emotional life, and achieving emotional satisfaction in the context of close and emotionally gratifying interpersonal relationships.

These shifts in prioritization from knowledge acquisition to maintenance of social relations have three sources. One relates to the maturing individual's lifetime accrual of experience and knowledge, such that fewer and fewer people can provide information that is new and personally meaningful. A second source is the reality of physical aging, which results in energy depletion, heightened physiological arousability, and increased physical debilitation. A third source is the growing realization that the individual's remaining lifetime is finite. Although a sense of imminent mortality can be activated in adults of any age, it is held to be particularly salient in older adults and accentuates the need to prioritize emotional goals. Thus the theory provides a theoretical rationale for the narrowing of social networks in later life, as an alternative to disengagement theory (Cumming & Henry, 1961). Instead of a turning away from social engagement, as disengagement theory would have it, Carstensen's theory proposes that older adults selectively reduce their social networks at the service of investing in and deepening those that are most emotionally gratifying. That is, social contacts become limited to relationships that offer the opportunity to maximize positive outcomes—social support, companionship, and assistance—and to avoid or reduce resource-depleting negative affect and conflict (Carstensen, 1992; Carstensen, Graff, Levenson, & Gottman, 1996; Carstensen, Gottman, & Levenson, 1995). Controlling the quality of social engagements constitutes an adaptive strategy to regulate emotion, which is important to the maintenance of well-being in later life.

In summary, the theoretical formulations of Lawton and Carstensen have focused principally on emotion-regulatory characteristics, processes, and functions in the context of social relations over the adult years, especially in later life. Both view aging as involving shifts in goal priorities and the concurrent acquisition of more accomplished and efficient emotion regulatory skills. Together, these changes both motivate and assist aging individuals to reduce peripheral social interactions and avoid the experience of negative affect. Lawton's formulations acknowledge the existence of interpersonal differences in the qualities of affect regulation that distinguish individual personality profiles, and he proposes that this should have an impact on what different individuals actually experience. In contrast, Carstensen's theory assumes that adaptive mechanisms such as socioemotional selectivity operate in similar ways across different personality characteristics (Lang, Staudinger, & Carstensen, 1998; Mariske, Lang, Baltes, & Baltes, 1995). The theory assumes that all older individuals value close relations and are motivated to selectively cultivate those relationships that are the most emotionally gratifying. Both theories offer clear predictions regarding emotional experience and social behaviors in older adults. Older versus younger adults (or those confronted with the imminence of their own mortality) should orient more toward emotional stimuli, should place a priority on social versus informational goals, and should engage in activities that are likely to reduce negative affect and increase positive affect.

Cognitive–Affective Developmental Theory

Gisela Labouvie-Vief offers a theory of emotion and aging that situates emotional development within the context of evolving cognitive and ego processes (Labouvie-Vief, 2003; Labouvie-Vief, Chiodo, Goguen, Diehl, & Orwoll, 1995; Labouvie-Vief, DeVoe, & Bulka, 1989; Labouvie-Vief & Diehl, 2000; Labouvie-Vief, Hakin-Larson, DeVoe, & Schoeberlein, 1989; Labouvie-Vief & Medler, 2002). Based on neo-Piagetian and postformal cognitive models, her theory suggests that emotional experiences are qualitatively restructured as the maturing individual acquires more complex forms of cognition with which to evaluate the world and develops a more differentiated and integrated self-concept. The increasing cognitive sophistication that comes with

maturation provides ever more complex scaffolding for more differentiated experiences of emotion and for the development of more sophisticated emotion-regulatory capacities.

Although there are no fixed stages in Labouvie-Vief's theory, she proposes a trajectory of adult emotional development aligned with levels of cognitive and personality development. In infancy and early childhood, emotion regulation is said to operate at a presystemic cognitive level, being governed by the actions of external social agents. With the advent of formal operations during adolescence and early adulthood, an "intrasystemic" period emerges, allowing the individual to regulate emotions in the context of abstract ideals and cultural standards; here emotional process is characterized by internal regulation that remains highly dependent on social conventions which define standards of comportment with respect to emotional speech and behavior. As such, the cognitive–affective system remains bounded by conventional language, symbols, and norms; behavior is conformity-driven rather than oriented toward change and transformation. Labouvie-Vief asserts that for individuals to achieve true emotional maturity, they must advance beyond conventional governance of behavior to one in which the individuals integrate self-reflective internal subjectivity into the cognitive–emotional system.

From early adulthood through middle age, there is an emerging intersystemic level of integration, in which there is a gradual shift from the conventional to the contextualistic orientation. That is, rules and standards for behavior are no longer viewed as absolute, but rather as relativistic and moderated by context. Subjectivity, autonomy, and self-exploration increase as cognitions and behaviors become more individualized and less driven by convention. Such advances in cognitive and ego complexity are held to produce important reorganizations of the self that ultimately have an impact on emotional development. This description of a hierarchical integration represents what Labouvie-Vief calls the "de-repression of emotion," which comes to be more prominent during middle adulthood. In this normative-developmental aspect of the model, greater cognitive and emotional complexity during the middle years gives rise to enhanced flexibility of self-regulation and the capacity for more modulated emotion expression.

In more recent formulations, Labouvie-Vief's work on affective organization and change in cognitive–affective development differentiates between two aspects of affect regulation related to the self, having different aims and possibly different trajectories. One aspect seeks to maximize positive affect and minimize or attenuate negative affect; here the goal is to maintain a positively valenced self-concept that entails regulating behaviors and values so as to conform to social norms and to avoid interpersonal conflict. The other aspect of emotional development, affective complexity, involves intrapsychic differentiation, greater mixing of positive and negative affect, greater tolerance of ambiguity, and more flexible affect regulation. Its aim is to maintain an open and undistorted view of reality. The greater awareness of differentiated inner states and de-repression of affect during the middle years, in which opposing feelings may conflict with one another, is not without cost, as this situation makes for a certain degree of tension. Some individuals may not be capable of tolerating or resolving the tension, which may provoke a retreat into more defensive modes of coping. Other individuals may find that the internal tension intensifies their efforts at reconciliation and integration, producing advances in ego level and gains in emotional maturity. Moreover, as a developmental trajectory, the enhanced growth in cognitive–affective complexity may or may not continue to accrue beyond middle age, when fluid intelligence (i.e., abstract cognitive abilities) starts to decline, since emotional maturity in this theoretical context is defined as integrally interknit with cognitive capacities. Hence this kind of emotional complexity may peak in the middle years.

In summary, Labouvie-Vief's theory entertains the thesis that there may be both general, developmental trends reflecting improvement with age—although experience, ego level, and other cognitive phenomena, rather than age per se, are the agents of change—as well as individual differences in the extent to which an individual has a preference for positivity or complexity. The theory maintains that the course of emotional development over the adult years involves qualitative changes in the subjective aspects of emotional life that entail more complexly textured emotional experience and greater capacity for affect regulation. The latter changes accrue from more general developmental changes in cognitive capacities and ego development.

In concluding this section on theoretical contributions to the field of emotions and aging, we can see that there are a number of testable theoretical formulations about change and continuity in different components of the emotion system over the adult years. In broad strokes, the theories converge on aspects of phenomenology, expressive behavior, sensitivity to behavioral emotional cues, emotion regulation, and the role of emotions in personality consolidation and change. This then becomes the organizing framework for a review of the empirical literature.

EMPIRICAL WORK ON EMOTIONAL DEVELOPMENT OVER THE LIFE COURSE

Continuity and Change in Subjective Emotional Experience

Researchers have typically assessed age-related differences in the phenomenological experience of emotion through self-reports, using rating scales of emotional frequency or intensity. Another, less often used methodology is rating emotional experience by examining narratives about emotional experiences. At times the focus is on dimensional aspects of emotion; at other times the focus is at the discrete-emotion level. In the service of being comprehensive, in the present chapter I distinguish between age differences in terms of broad hedonic tone (positive vs. negative affect) and at the level of discrete or differential emotions. I also consider the case of blended or mixed emotions, to assess whether theoretical formulations about emotional complexity at the individual level can be supported.

Positive and Negative Affect

There is now a considerable literature on changes in positive and negative affect over the adult lifespan, though most of it is cross-sectional in nature. In brief, reviews of this literature (Consedine & Magai, 2006; Magai, 2001) indicate that positive affect increases over the adult years, and that negative affect decreases or remains level. Although the literature is more limited, longitudinal studies suggest a somewhat different picture. There are six such studies that have tracked changes over time, ranging from 4 to 22 years.

The Berlin Aging Study, which drew its participants from a stratified probability sample of older adults (Baltes & Mayer, 1999), yielded both cross-sectional and longitudinal data on age-related differences in levels of positive and negative affect as measured by the Positive and Negative Affect Schedules. Although cross-sectional data from this study indicated that positive affect scores declined across several groups of older adults, including individuals ages 70–75 and 90–100 years, and that these declines were substantial (Smith, Fleeson, Geiselmann, Settersten, & Kunzmann, 1999), longitudinal analyses over a 4-year period were interpreted as suggesting that positive and negative affect remain relatively stable (Kunzmann, Little, & Smith, 2000). Studies that have tracked changes over longer periods of time, however, tend to find a tapering off of positive and negative affect. The Los Angeles Longitudinal Study of Generations (Charles, Reynolds, & Gatz, 2001), which surveyed groups of individuals from young adulthood to the mid-80s, found that positive affect remained stable for young, middle-aged, and older adults, but decreased slightly among the oldest individuals (mid-60s to mid-80s) while negative affect declined in all groups, including the oldest sample. The Boston Department of Veterans Affairs-based Normative Aging Study (Mroczek & Spiro, 2005) assessed life satisfaction—a measure of global positive affect—over a 22-year period of time; the participants ranged in age from 40 to 85. The authors found that life satisfaction peaked at age 65 and then declined. The Baltimore Longitudinal Study of Aging (Davey, Halverson, Zonderman, & Costa, 2004; Terracciano, McCrae, Brant, & Costa, 2005) collected data on neuroticism and extraversion—which load on negative and positive affect, respectively—from 1958 to the most recent wave of investigation; the authors found declines in both measures (at least until age 80) in this highly educated cohort of adults.

In summary, although the data are not always consistent, cross-sectional data indicate that there are increases in positive affect and decreases in negative affect over the adult years, though some of these effects may be due to samples with a restricted age range or to the existence of cohort effects (Charles et al., 2001; Costa, McCrae, & Zonderman, 1987). The lon-

gitudinal data, especially data focused on the later years, suggests that there are declines in positive and negative affect toward the end of the lifespan, although there are exceptions to this general trend. Declines in the frequency or level of affect in the later years may be due to the depletion of physiological resources or to the narrowing of social networks in later life that occurs as a normative aspect of aging (Carstensen, 1992; Carstensen, Isaacowitz, & Charles, 1999); reduced social networks conceivably limit the occasion for the elicitation of emotion.

Changes in Discrete Emotions

In some ways it is harder to evaluate changes in emotion at the discrete level, because the methods of assessment are more varied, spanning retrospective ratings (e.g., Mroczek, 2001), experimental manipulations (e.g., Tsai, Carstensen, & Levenson, 2000), and online ratings (e.g., Carstensen, Mayr, Pasupathi, & Nesselroade, 2000). In general, when the research is cross-sectional and the measures are self-reports of emotions, the most reliable finding is a reduction in the frequency or level of anger with increasing age (Birditt & Fingerman, 2003; Gross et al., 1997; Lawton et al., 1993; Schieman, 1999; Stoner & Spencer, 1987). Other cross-sectional data suggest reductions in shame/shyness (Consedine & Magai, 2003; Lawton et al., 1993), and possibly in sadness and fear, but not in disgust (Gross et al., 1997). The literature on longitudinal studies of discrete emotions is far more limited. In fact, at this writing, there are only three relevant studies. One assessed changes in anxiety, sadness, interest, anger-in, anger-out, and total anger over an 8-year period of time in a sample of individuals whose mean ages were 56 years when first interviewed and 63 years at the second interview (Magai, 1999). Only anger-out showed a significant decline over the 8-year period, with no signs of change in the other emotions. Another study, the Baltimore Longitudinal Study of Aging Terracciano et al., 2005), tracked changes in the facets constituting the five dimensions of the NEO Personality Inventory over time. Self-consciousness, a facet of neuroticism, which is related to the discrete-emotion construct of shame, showed a linear decline with age, as did hostility; however, this effect appeared to taper off at the upper reaches of the age range (80–90 years), with the possible exception of anxiety.

This picture of decreases in a number of discrete negative emotions as based on retrospective self-reports is not sustained when one examines studies in which emotions are elicited under emotion induction conditions. Instead, this research indicates either no age differences in emotional experience or an enhanced effect among older adults once emotion is aroused. For example, one study found that older and younger adults reported equivalent levels of anger, sadness, fear, and interest in response to a relived-emotions task in which autobiographical memories involving anger, sadness, fear, and interest were elicited (Malatesta-Magai et al., 1992); in another study using the relived-emotions task for memories involving fear, sadness, anger, and happiness, there were no age-related differences for fear, sadness, and happiness ratings, though there was a reduction of anger ratings (Labouvie-Vief, Lumley, Jain, & Heinze, 2003). Several studies have used film stimuli to elicit emotions under laboratory conditions. One study found that older versus younger adults reported greater sadness in response to age-relevant sadness themes such as the loss of loved ones (Kunzmann & Grühn, 2005), whereas another found that younger and older adults had equivalent levels of subjective responses to sad and amusing films (Tsai et al., 2000). Finally, another study found that older adults had higher ratings on contempt than younger adults in response to film clips of injustice (Charles, 2005). Other studies have examined age differences in response to political or historical events. For example, older adults reported feeling just as sad, angry, and hopeful as middle-aged and younger adults in response to a political event (Levine & Bluck, 1997). Thus it appears that when discrete emotions are aroused, older adults experience the same or greater intensities or levels of such emotions as younger and middle-aged adults.

Emotional Experience as Sampled in Emotional Narratives

Another approach to assessing people's phenomenological experience of emotion is to evaluate the quality of narrative productions. Here an individual is not constrained by a fixed-format choice of items to rate, but generates spontaneous material that reflects directly on the nature of his or her inner affective world. I first summarize the findings with respect to positive and negative affect, and then turn to those studies that have examined discrete emotions.

In one of the most extensive analyses of narrative material, researchers culled through over 3,000 narrative transcripts of individuals ranging in age from 8 to 85 years for their use of affect words; this was complemented by a similar analysis of the collected works of 10 eminent authors across their professional lives (Pennebaker & Stone, 2003). The analysis of the self-disclosure material indicated that the use of positive affect increased with age, with the magnitude of the increase from ages 55–69 to age 70+ being quite pronounced; the use of negative affect words declined with age. In the analysis of the output of eminent authors such as Jane Austen, the researchers found a pattern similar to the findings based on the self-disclosure material. In another study (Schredl & Doll, 1998), the dream content of people ranging in age from adolescence to the 80s was content-analyzed; this research yielded data consistent with those from the foregoing study, in that age was once again negatively correlated with negative affect. Of particular interest is a study that compared the self-report ratings of emotion with those derived from narratives in a sample of 87 younger and older adults (mean ages of 20 and 62 years, respectively). In this study of reactions to the verdict of the O. J. Simpson trial as it was disclosed on TV, participants were interviewed and tape-recorded for later content analysis, and also rated the intensity and frequency of their anger, sadness, happiness, and surprise (Alea, Bluck, & Semegon, 2004). The researchers found that both scalar and narrative measures indicated a greater emotional response among the older adults and more frequent and more intense experience of sadness in the older adults; a similar trend occurred for anger, but it did not reach significance. Finally, my colleagues and I tabulated the number of instances of 10 discrete-emotion words in the narratives of young, middle-aged, and older adults in a relived-emotions task (Magai, Consedine, Krivoshekova, McPherson, & Kudadjie-Gyamfi, 2006). We found that 9 of the 10 emotion words were used at equivalent frequencies; the only exception was that younger adults used more expressions of contempt than the other two age groups.

In summary, the bulk of evidence from narrative analyses points to no real declines in the capacity for emotion across the adult years; if anything, older adults sometimes express more acute emotional experience than younger adults. Thus, if retrospective ratings of the frequency or level of emotion indicate greater placidity in older adults (lower positive and negative affect), this could be a function of fading memory due to the passage of time. In contrast, if the eliciting circumstances are immediate, are autobiographical, or involve personally meaningful life events, the emotional capacities of older adults appear to be preserved.

Emotional Complexity

In a recently developing line of research, investigators have sought to assess whether or not there are age-related changes in the complexity of people's emotional experiences. Research in this vein is variously referred to as research on "affective complexity" (Labouvie-Vief, Chiodo, et al. (1995) and Labouvie-Vief, Diehl, et al. (1995), "emotional heterogeneity" (Charles, 2005), and "emotional differentiation" (Carstensen et al., 2000; Ong & Bergeman, 2004). Labouvie-Vief views the ability to tolerate and sustain ambivalent or mixed emotions as a hallmark of cognitive–affective complexity (Labouvie-Vief, Chiodo, et al., 1995; Labouvie-Vief, DeVoe, et al., 1989; Labouvie-Vief, Diehl, Chiodo, & Coyle, 1995), and others have suggested that the capacity for more complex or variegated emotional experience may be functionally related to greater resiliency (Ong & Bergeman, 2004), increased life satisfaction (Carstensen et al., 2000, 2003), or the development of greater dialectical, conflict-engaging thinking over time (Magai & Haviland-Jones, 2002).

The relation between complexity and age is not altogether clear at this point, which in part may be related to the fact that emotional complexity has been measured in several different ways. In Labouvie-Vief's work, complexity scores are derived from the unique patterning of cognitive and affective processes as evinced in coded narratives. In her empirical work, complexity tends to increase over the adult years and peaks in middle adulthood, with some decline thereafter. The apparent decline in later life may be in part a function of the way in which the construct is measured. Because this index of affective complexity has a strong cognitive component, and because fluid intelligence declines in later life (as noted earlier), it is perhaps not surprising that this measure of affective complexity follows the trajectory of cognitive decline.

In other research on emotional complexity, there appear to be linear increases with age, although the relevant longitudinal work has yet to be done. In these studies, "complexity" is defined as involving an increased *range* of emotions, or as consisting of *blends or overlaps* among negative emotions or between positive and negative affects (Carstensen et al., 2000; Charles, 2005; Ong & Bergeman, 2004). Two studies have assessed this kind of complexity in the context of experience-sampling research (Carstensen et al., 2000; Ong & Bergeman, 2004). In both studies, the indices of blended or overlapping emotions were based on the average intraindividual correlation between positive and negative affect. Both found a linear increase in complexity/poignancy with age; that is, older respondents tended to relate more mixed and bittersweet emotions and more poignant experiences within the same sampled moment than younger respondents did. A related construct—"emotion heterogeneity," defined as an overlap between a dominant negative emotion (i.e., the most intense emotion) and other negative emotions—was found to characterize the experiences of older adults to a greater extent than those of younger adults (Charles, 2005; Magai et al., 2006). This kind of emotional complexity is apparently not limited to the subjective aspect of emotion, but is also found when experience is sampled from narrative reports (Magai et al., 2006), and also may be seen in expressive behavior (as detailed below).

Continuity and Change in Emotional Behavior

Although emotional behaviors encompass facial, vocal, bodily, and gestural expressions, the bulk of the literature on age-related differences in emotional behavior during the adult years involves research on facial expressions. Researchers have typically assessed age differences either in response to film stimuli, during the course of a relived-emotions task (autobiographical memories), or during *in vivo* interpersonal interactions. One research team studied the expressions of older and younger European and Chinese American adults in response to a film-based emotion induction (Tsai et al., 2000). The data indicated equivalent levels of expressed happiness, laughing, smiling, and crying in the two age groups. In addition, four studies have used autobiographical memories to elicit emotion. In one of the earlier studies, spontaneous facial activity was monitored during a relived-emotions task (Levenson, Carstensen, Friesen, & Ekman, 1991); no differences between younger and older adults were found. Another group of researchers (Moreno, Borod, Welkowitz, & Alpert, 1990) examined age differences in facial symmetry of expressive behavior in young, middle-aged, and older women during the induction of four emotions, surprise, joy, sadness, and disgust; though they found no age differences in laterality, they found that older faces were rated as showing more intense disgust. In a third study (Malatesta-Magai et al., 1992), younger adults (< 50 years old) and older adults (> 50 years old) were asked to recount four kinds of autobiographical emotional events involving interest, sadness, fear, and anger; older adults were found to express greater interest, sadness, fear, and anger, respectively, than younger adults. A more recent study in which young, middle-aged and older adults related sad and angry events (Magai et al., 2006) found similar durations of anger, sadness, disgust, fear, and interest in all three age groups. However, there were two departures from this general trend: a greater duration of shame, contempt, and joy expressions in the younger sample, and a greater duration of knit brow in the oldest adults. The shame–contempt–joy triad was interpreted as indexing a cynical/self-conscious, perhaps mocking, facial presentation—a pattern that is common in adolescents and young adults (Kahlbaugh & Haviland, 1994; Malatesta-Magai & Dorval, 1992). The greater duration of knit brow was interpreted as indexing greater concentration, thought, or conscientiousness on the part of older adults, or alternatively as indicating that the task was more demanding of the older adults' more limited cognitive resources.

Finally, in terms of *in vivo* interactions, a study of married couples showed that older couples relative to middle-aged couples displayed less anger and disgust during discussion of a marital problem (Carstensen et al., 1995), though there were no differences in joy, contempt, and sadness, and older adults displayed more expressions of affection. Another study, this time involving the coding of spontaneous facial expressions of emotion in patients with mid- to late-stage dementia during a family visit (Magai, Cohen, Gomberg, Malatesta, & Culver, 1996), found that negative emotions were preserved across levels of cognitive decline; only joy expressions were lower in frequency among the most deteriorated patients. In that study, facial expressions of emotions were also found to be functionally related to emotional contexts; that is, sadness expressions, which were rare during the beginning and middle stages of the visit, increased as family members prepared to leave. In general, then, the data from the above-described kinds of studies, although not always consistent at the level of discrete emotions—which may be attributable to differential eliciting conditions or to the number and types of expressions coded—suggest that there are no real decrements in the level of facial emotional expressivity across the adult years or in the capacity to express emotion in emotional contexts. Indeed, in some cases, older adults show more intense or more frequent emotional expressions than younger adults.

A smaller body of literature, however, points to a somewhat different aspect of facial expressions that may change with age. An early study (Malatesta & Izard, 1984), which involved filming young, middle-aged, and older women as they described emotional events in their lives, undertook a *component* versus a *global* analysis of facial expressions. This study found that although there were fewer component muscle movements in the facial expressions of the middle-aged and older women, their expressions were more complicated, with more instances of different emotions combined within the same coding unit. As well, in a second study, naïve judges found it more difficult to accurately judge the type of emotional events these women were talking about from their facial expressions (Malatesta, Fiore, & Messina, 1987).

Continuity and Change in Sensitivity to Emotion Signals

The literature on sensitivity to emotional information has ranged from studies of "emotional salience"—that is, the degree to which people orient to emotional content—to the perception of facial, vocal, and bodily expressions of emotion. Here I describe only studies of emotional salience and studies of sensitivity to facial expressions of emotion; studies of vocal and bodily expressions have tended to use nonstandard stimuli.

A limited body of research has indicated that emotional content may be more salient for older versus younger adults. In an incidental-memory paradigm, adults ranging from 20 to 83 years were asked to recall as much content as they could (Carstensen & Charles, 1994); the study found a linear increase with age in the proportion of emotional to neutral phrases that were recalled, which was interpreted as indicating that emotional content is more salient to older adults. A more recent study (May, Rahhat, Berry, & Leighton, 2005) assessed younger and older adults' ability to remember three types of contextual information about an event—perceptual, conceptual nonemotional, and emotional. Results indicated that younger adults were better than older adults at remembering perceptual and conceptual source information, but that the age difference in source memory was eliminated when the informational content was emotional, suggesting that emotional information differentially engages older adults. Other research that has examined younger and older adults' processing of emotionally positive versus negative material indicates that older adults tend to show a positivity bias. That is, they tend to orient to and remember positively valenced material more than negatively valenced material, while such a positivity effect does not seem to apply in younger adults (see Mather & Carstensen, 2005, for a review). Moreover, some have suggested that the older adults' tendency to orient to emotional material may help compensate for some of the losses in cognitive function that accrue with age, such as declines in working memory, attention, and sensory functioning (Blanchard-Fields, 2005; Carstensen & Mikels, 2005). However, there is also evidence that when the cognitive processing demands are too strong, and/or emotion is too arousing, it exerts a penalty on the executive functions of older adults. In a study of attentional processes involving emotion-laden words, known as the "emotional Stroop task" (Wurm, Labouvie-Vief, Aycock, Rebucal, & Koch, 2004), older adults showed poorer performance than younger adults. One form of the task required participants to make lexical decisions to emotion words spoken in several tones of voice; in the other form of the task, participants had to name the font color of emotionally arousing words displayed on a computer screen. Latencies were longer for test words spoken in an incongruent tone of voice and for test words high on arousal, but only in the case of older adults.

Studies have also examined adults' capacity to read the emotional content of faces accurately. Two studies have found that older adults are just as accurate as younger adults at recognizing a range of discrete emotions, but that they are poorer at recognizing sadness (MacPherson, Phillips, & Della Sala, 2002; Moreno, Borod, Welkowitz, & Alpert, 1993). Moreover, two studies of emotion recognition among patients in the early stages of Alzheimer's disease showed that these patients performed at a level comparable to that of older adult controls (Lavenu, Pasquier, Lebert, Petit, & Van der Linden, 1999). In contrast, another team of investigators (McDowell, Harrison, & Demaree, 1994) found that older adults were less accurate than younger adults in the identification of sad, angry, fearful, and neutral expressions, and one study of patients with dementia found that these patients recognized facial emotion at a lower rate than nondemented older adults and younger adults (Allen & Brosgole, 1993).

In summary, emotion appears to be particularly salient to older adults, and this appears to help offset declines in cognitive function. As well, although there is some inconsistency in the literature, there do not appear to be great age differences in the ability to recognize facial expressions of emotion, with the possible exception of sadness.

Continuity and Change in Emotion Regulation

A body of literature has been accumulating on the emotion regulation capacities of older adults. The term "emotion regulation" encompasses a range of behavioral responses, including deliberate suppression of ongoing experience and/or expression, as well as anticipatory regulation and the active avoidance of emotionally provocative situations. Self-report studies suggest that older adults control their emotions more than younger adults do (Gross et al., 1997; Labouvie-Vief, DeVoe, et al., 1989; Lawton et al., 1992), that they may be better at anticipating and avoiding interpersonal conflict (Birditt & Fingerman, 2005; Birditt, Fingerman, & Almeida, 2005; Birditt, Fingerman, & Almeida, 2005; Carstensen et al., 1995), and that they may be better at delaying emotion expression (Diehl, Coyle, & Labouvie-Vief, 1996). Self-report studies are, however, vulnerable to presentational biases. The few experimental studies in which participants have been required to control behavioral expressions of emotion have primarily been conducted with younger adults in response to film clips (Gross, 1998; Gross & Levenson, 1993, 1997). Only two studies have directly tested the thesis that the capacity to regulate emotion improves with age. In one study (Kunzmann, Kupperbusch, & Levenson, 2005), younger and older adults viewed three films designed to elicit disgust; no age differences were found in the ability to suppress or amplify emotional expression, nor in subjective emotional experience. In the second study (Magai et al., 2006), young, middle-aged, and older adults were asked to relate personal stories involving anger and sadness, but were told not to let their feelings show behaviorally. The impact of the experimental manipulation was only evident in the older adults; the inhibition instructions had no effect on young and middle-aged adults. Taken together, these studies suggest then that the ability to regulate emotion voluntarily does not decline with age and perhaps may even improve.

Continuity and Change in Emotion Traits

There is now fairly consistent evidence that broad dimensions of positive and negative affect are stable over both short and longer periods of time. Studies tracking change over a period of weeks in the frequency or intensity of emotion states have found test–retest reliabilities in the .70s and .80s (Diener & Larsen, 1984; Epstein, 1979). Longer-term studies have returned similar results. For example, a longitudinal study of subjective well-being in a national sample (Costa et al., 1987) showed substantial stability in positive and negative affect over a period of 7–12 years, and measures of extraversion and neuroticism (which tap positive and negative affect, respectively, as noted earlier) have also been found to be stable over a 10-year period (Costa & McCrae, 1980). In terms of discrete emotions, one study (Berenbaum, Fujita, & Pfennig, 1995) found stability coefficients in the .70s and .80s for sadness, anger, and fear over a period of weeks. A study of postpartum women (Izard, Libero, Putnam, & Haynes, 1993) assessed the stability of 12 emotions over 3 years; the stabil-

ities ranged from a low of .33 for fear to a high of .71 for contempt, with an average of .56. Another study (Magai, 1999) obtained 8-year stability coefficients for anxiety, depression, interest, anger-in, anger-out, and total anger, ranging from .47 to .75. Finally, the Baltimore Longitudinal Study of Aging, which assessed depressive symptoms at five occasions over an 8-year period of time, found that depressive symptoms were trait-like in nature (Davey et al., 2004).

Balancing this picture of general stability are a few studies that have examined interindividual differences in intraindividual stability and change. Such studies have indicated that changes do occur at the level of the individual over the adult years in such broad categories as positive–negative affect and neuroticism–extraversion (Charles et al., 2001; Kunzmann et al., 2000). Such changes have been attributed to changes in health, as well as to emotional events that involve the initiation or termination of intimate relationships or other intense affiliative experiences (Magai, 1999; Magai & Haviland-Jones, 2002), although additional longitudinal research is necessary to flesh out this very preliminary work.

SUMMARY OF SUPPORT FOR THEORETICAL MODELS

Three leading bodies of theory, although they have different emphases, collectively suggest (1) that the capacity for emotion regulation should improve over time, with a corresponding improvement in the balance of positive to negative affect; (2) that persons should orient more to the emotional aspects of life and human relations as they age; (3) that basic emotional processes, such as the ability to recognize emotion and the capacity to experience emotional arousal in response to emotional stimuli, should remain relatively intact; (4) that emotion experience and expression should become more complex, nuanced, and elaborated; and (5) that individual-level changes should consist of emergent stability in patterns of both emotion experience and expression, while still preserving the capacity for change.

The empirical literature, in the main, suggests broad support for these theoretical propositions, though more longitudinal and cross-sequential studies are necessary to confirm the patterns disclosed through cross-sectional work and the limited longitudinal studies that currently exist. With respect to changes in hedonic tone and discrete emotions, the most consistent findings indicate that there are increases in the level or frequency of positive emotion and declines in negative emotion broadly across the adult years, and especially a decrease in anger; these effects appear related to gains in the ability to regulate emotion over the adult years. However, among the oldest-old, there appear to be declines in both positive and negative emotions, which may be linked to the shrinkage of social networks or to the depletion of physiological resources in late life. In terms of the salience of emotion, age appears to bring with it an increasing appreciation for the affective aspects of life and social relations. The literature also seems to suggest greater emotional complexity with age, and these effects are found at the phenomenological and expressive levels; however, depending on how complexity is defined and measured, this greater affective complexity may continue across the life course or may taper off after middle age. Finally, it appears that emotional biases in experience and expression become consolidated in personality over developmental time, though change can occur at the level of individual lives under certain theoretically specified conditions.

CONCLUDING THOUGHTS: EMOTION, FRUIT FLIES, AND LIVES IN PROGRESS

The epigraph to this chapter alludes to the fact that recent advances in longevity-enhancing research have proven effective in retarding the aging process in fruit flies, not to mention in mammals (e.g., Rikke & Johnson, 2004; Weindruch, 1996), and hold promise for increasing the human lifespan in the not-too-distant future. In the event of an extended lifespan, would the landscape of our emotional lives change? In all likelihood, the answer is yes, on several counts. First, if time left to live is of the essence, as the formulations of socioemotional selectivity theory suggest, we might anticipate that the postponement of imminent mortality would raise the age of divestment in informational goals (pursuit of novelty, sensation seeking) in favor of socioemotional goals. In turn, the prolonged pursuit of novelty and sensation seeking might take a toll on pair-

bonded relationships and also lead to further changes in career paths, if trends over the last 50 years are any guide. But for the most part, the form of the emotional change would also "depend" on whether life extension would occur in the context of stretching out the years of physical decline—an extended-senescence model—or whether, like Oscar Wilde's character Dorian Gray, people would retain the health and physical vitality of their youth. In the past, life extension accruing from decreased mortality during infancy and life-saving medical advances prolonged the length of the adult years overall, but ultimately also led to lengthening the time spent in physical decline. Michael Rose's (Dreifus, 2006) research on fruit flies, in which he extended the age over which reproduction can occur through selective breeding over multiple generations, has shown that life can be significantly extended without incurring the ravages of senescence. Research may ultimately reveal the genetic mechanisms that underlie this Dorian Gray effect, and thus the prospect of a materially enhanced human lifespan is not inconceivable. In any case, it is clear that the extended-senescence effect would result in a different pattern of affective aging than the Dorian Gray effect would. The latter effect would preserve and extend all the benefits derived from the accumulated experience and emotional wisdom into grand old ages without the penalty of physical decline, whereas the former would not. In the senescence model, an extended proportion of the lifespan would be spent in disability, depletion of physiological resources, and narrowing of social networks, which would result in declines in levels of emotion and perhaps reductions in emotional complexity. Finally, one possibly unexpected effect of the Dorian Gray model—under conditions of an extended sexual and reproductive life, and the attendant vicissitudes of serial partnerships and blended families—would be greater bouts of human drama. But then, as some would say, what's wrong with that?

ACKNOWLEDGMENTS

Work on this chapter was supported by grants from the National Institute of General Medical Science and the National Institute on Aging (Nos. SO6 GM54650, 1KO7 AG00921, and RO1 AG021017).

REFERENCES

Alea, N., Bluck, S., & Semegon, A. B. (2004). Young and older adults' expression of emotional experience: Do autobiographical narratives tell a different story? *Journal of Adult Development, 11,* 235–250.

Allen, R., & Brosgole, L. (1993). Facial and auditory affect recognition in senile geriatrics, the normal elderly and young adults. *International Journal of Neuroscience, 68,* 33–42.

Baltes, P. B., & Baltes, M. M. (1990). Psychological perspectives on successful aging: The model of selective optimization with compensation. In P. B. Baltes & M. M. Baltes (Eds.), *Successful aging: Perspectives from the behavioral sciences* (pp. 1–34). New York: Cambridge University Press.

Baltes, P. B., & Mayer, K. U. (Eds.). (1999). *The Berlin Aging Study: Aging from 70 to 100.* New York: Cambridge University Press.

Berenbaum, H., Fujita, F., & Pfennig, J. (1995). Consistency, specificity, and correlates of negative emotions. *Journal of Personality and Social Psychology, 68,* 342–352.

Birditt, K., & Fingerman, K. L. (2003). Age and gender differences in adults' descriptions of emotional reactions to interpersonal problems. *Journal of Gerontology: Series B. Psychological Sciences, 58B,* 237–245.

Birditt, K., & Fingerman, K. L. (2005). Do we get better at picking our battles?: Age group differences in descriptions of behavioral reactions to interpersonal tensions. *Journals of Gerontology: Series B. Psychological Sciences and Social Sciences, 60B,* P121–P128.

Birditt, K., Fingerman, K. L., & Almeida, D. M. (2005). Age differences in exposure and reactions to interpersonal tensions: A daily diary study. *Psychology and Aging, 20,* 330–340.

Blanchard-Fields, F. (2005). Introduction to the special section on emotion–cognition interactions and the aging mind. *Psychology and Aging, 20,* 539–541.

Carstensen, L. L. (1988). A life-span approach to social motivation. In J. Heckhausen & C. S. Dweck (Eds.), *Motivation and self-regulation across the life span* (Vol. 9, pp. 341–364). New York: Cambridge University Press.

Carstensen, L. L. (1992). Social and emotional patterns in adulthood: Support for socioemotional selectivity theory. *Psychology and Aging, 7,* 331–338.

Carstensen, L. L. (1993). Motivation for social contact across the lifespan: A theory of socioemotional selectivity. In J. E. Jacobs (Ed.), *Nebraska Symposium on Motivation: Vol. 40. Developmental perspectives on motivation* (pp. 209–254). Lincoln: University of Nebraska Press.

Carstensen, L. L. (1995). Evidence for a life-span theory of socioemotional selectivity. *Current Directions in Psychological Science, 4,* 151–156.

Carstensen, L. L., & Charles, S. T. (1994). The salience of emotion across the adult life span. *Psychology and Aging, 9,* 259–264.

Carstensen, L. L., Fung, H. H., & Charles, S. T. (2003). Socioemotional selectivity theory and the regulation of emotion in the second half of life. *Motivation and Emotion, 27,* 103–123.

Carstensen, L. L., Gottman, J. M., & Levenson, R. W. (1995). Emotional behavior in long-term marriage. *Psychology and Aging, 10,* 140–149.

Carstensen, L. L., Isaacowitz, D. M., & Charles, S. T. (1999). Taking time seriously: A theory of socioemotional selectivity. *American Psychologist, 54,* 165–181.

Carstensen, L. L., Mayr, U., Pasupathi, M., & Nesselroade, J. R. (2000). Emotional experience in everyday life across the adult life span. *Journal of Personality and Social Psychology, 79,* 644–655.

Carstensen, L. L., & Mikels, J. A. (2005). At the intersection of emotion and cognition. Aging and the positivity effect. *Current Directions in Psychological Science, 14,* 117–121.

Carstensen, L. O., Graff, J., Levenson, R. W., & Gottman, J. M. (1996). Affect in intimate relationships: The developmental course of marriage. In C. Magai & S. McFadden (Eds.), *Handbook of emotion, adult development, and aging* (pp. 227–247). San Diego: Academic Press.

Charles, S. T. (2005). Viewing injustice: Greater emotion heterogeneity with age. *Psychology and Aging, 20,* 159–164.

Charles, S. T., Reynolds, C. A., & Gatz, M. (2001). Age-related differences and change in positive and negative affect over 23 years. *Journal of Personality and Social Psychology, 80,* 136–151.

Consedine, N. S., & Magai, C. (2003). Attachment and emotion experience in later life: The view from emotions theory. *Attachment and Human Development, 5,* 165–187.

Consedine, N. S., & Magai, C. (2006). Emotion development in adulthood: A developmental functionalist review and critique. In C. Hoare (Ed.), *The Oxford handbook of adult development and learning* (pp. 123–148). New York: Oxford University Press.

Costa, P. T., Jr., & McCrae, R. R. (1980). Influence of extraversion and neuroticism on subjective well-being: Happy and unhappy people. *Journal of Personality and Social Psychology, 38,* 668–678.

Costa, P. T., Jr., McCrae, R. R., & Zonderman, A. B. (1987). Environmental and dispositional influences on well-being: Longitudinal follow-up of an American national sample. *British Journal of Psychology, 78,* 299–306.

Cumming, E., & Henry, W. (1961). *Growing old.* New York: Basic Books.

Darwin, C. E. (1872). *The expression of the emotions in man and animals.* London: Murray.

Davey, A., Halverson, C. F., Jr., Zonderman, A. B., & Costa, P. T., Jr. (2004). Change in depressive symptoms in the Baltimore Longitudinal Study of Aging. *Journals of Gerontology: Series B. Psychological Sciences and Social Sciences, 59B,* P270–P277.

Diehl, M., Coyle, N., & Labouvie-Vief, G. (1996). Age and sex differences in strategies of coping and defense across the life span. *Psychology and Aging, 11,* 127–139.

Diener, E., & Larsen, R. J. (1984). Temporal stability and cross-situational consistency of affective, behavioral, and cognitive responses. *Journal of Personality and Social Psychology, 47,* 871–883.

Dreifus, C. (2006, December 6). Live longer with evolution?: Evidence may lie in fruit flies. *The New York Times,* p. 2.

Epstein, S. (1979). The stability of behavior: I. On predicting most of the people much of the time. *Journal of Personality and Social Psychology, 37,* 1097–1126.

Gross, J. J. (1998). Antecedent- and response-focused emotion regulation: Divergent consequences for experience, expression, and physiology. *Journal of Personality and Social Psychology, 74,* 224–237.

Gross, J. J., Carstensen, L. L., Pasupathi, M., Tsai, J., Goetestam-Skorpen, C. G., & Hsu, A. Y. C. (1997). Emotion and aging: Experience, expression, and control. *Psychology and Aging, 12,* 590–599.

Gross, J. J., & Levenson, R. W. (1993). Emotional suppression: Physiology, self-report, and expressive behavior. *Journal of Personality and Social Psychology, 64,* 970–986.

Gross, J. J., & Levenson, R. W. (1997). Hiding feelings: The acute effects of inhibiting negative and positive emotion. *Journal of Abnormal Psychology, 106,* 95–103.

Izard, C. E. (1971). *The face of emotion.* New York: Appleton-Century Crofts.

Izard, C. E. (1977). *Human emotions.* New York: Plenum Press.

Izard, C. E. (1991). *The psychology of emotions.* New York: Plenum Press.

Izard, C. E., & Ackerman, B. P. (1998). Emotions and self-concept across the life-span. *Annual Review of Gerontology and Geriatrics, 17,* 1–26.

Izard, C. E., Ackerman, B. P., Schoff, K. M., & Fine, S. E. (1999). Self-organization of discrete emotions, emotion patterns, and emotion–cognition relations. In M. D. Lewis & I. Granic (Eds.), *Emotion, development, and self-organization: Dynamic systems approaches to emotional development* (pp. 12–36). New York: Cambridge University Press.

Izard, C. E., Libero, D. Z., Putnam, P., & Haynes, O. M. (1993). Stability of emotion experiences and their relations to traits of personality. *Journal of Personality and Social Psychology, 64,* 847–860.

Izard, C. E., & Malatesta, C. (1987). Emotional development in infancy. In J. Osofsky (Ed.), *Handbook of infant development* (pp. 494–554). New York: Wiley.

Kahlbaugh, P. E., & Haviland, J. M. (1994). Nonverbal communication between parents and adolescents: A study of approach and avoidance behaviors. *Journal of Nonverbal Behavior, 18,* 91–113.

Kunzmann, U., & Grühn, D. (2005). Age differences in emotional reactivity: The sample case of sadness. *Psychology and Aging, 20,* 47–59.

Kunzmann, U., Kupperbusch, C., & Levenson, R. W. (2005). Behavioral inhibition and amplification during emotional arousal: A comparison of two age groups. *Psychology and Aging, 20,* 144–158.

Kunzmann, U., Little, T. D., & Smith, J. (2000). Is age-related stability of subjective well-being a paradox?: Cross-sectional and longitudinal evidence from the Berlin Aging Study. *Psychology and Aging, 15,* 511–526.

Labouvie-Vief, G. (2003). Dynamic integration: Affect, cognition, and the self in adulthood. *Current Directions in Psychological Science, 12,* 201–206.

Labouvie-Vief, G., Chiodo, L. M., Goguen, L. A., Diehl, M., & Orwoll, L. (1995). Representations of self across the life span. *Psychology and Aging, 10,* 404–415.

Labouvie-Vief, G., DeVoe, M., & Bulka, D. (1989). Speaking about feelings: Conceptions of emotion across the lifespan. *Psychology and Aging, 4,* 425–437.

Labouvie-Vief, G., & Diehl, M. (2000). Cognitive complexity and cognitive–affective integration: Related or separate domains of adult development? *Psychology and Aging, 15,* 490–504.

Labouvie-Vief, G., Diehl, M., Chiodo, L. M., & Coyle, N. (1995). Representations of self and parents across the life span. *Journal of Adult Development, 2,* 207–222.

Labouvie-Vief, G., Hakin-Larson, J., DeVoe, M., & Schoeberlein, S. (1989). Emotions and self-regulation: A lifespan view. *Human Development, 32,* 279–299.

Labouvie-Vief, G., Lumley, M. A., Jain, E., & Heinze, H. (2003). Age and gender differences in cardiac reactivity and subjective emotion responses to emotional autobiographical memories. *Emotion, 3,* 115–126.

Labouvie-Vief, G., & Medler, M. (2002). Affect optimization and affect complexity: Modes and styles of regulation in adulthood. *Psychology and Aging, 17,* 571–588.

Lang, F. R., Staudinger, U. M., & Carstensen, L. L. (1998). Perspectives on socioemotional selectivity in late life: How personality and social context do (and do not) make a difference. *Journal of Gerontology: Series B. Psychological Sciences, 53B,* P21–P30.

Lavenu, I., Pasquier, F., Lebert, F., Petit, H., & Van der Linden, M. (1999). Perception of emotion in frontotemporal dementia and in Alzheimer's disease. *Alzheimer's Disease and Associated Disorders, 13,* 96–101.

Lawton, M. P. (2001). Emotion later in life. *Current Directions in Psychological Science, 10,* 120–123.

Lawton, M. P., Kleban, M. H., & Dean, J. (1993). Affect and age: Cross-sectional comparisons of structure and prevalence. *Psychology and Aging, 8,* 165–175.

Lawton, M. P., Kleban, M. H., Rajagopal, D., & Dean, J. (1992). The dimensions of affective experience in three age groups. *Psychology and Aging, 7,* 171–184.

Lawton, M. P., Moss, M. S., Winter, L., & Hoffman, C. (2002). Motivation in later life: Personal projects and well-being. *Psychology and Aging, 17,* 539–547.

Lawton, M. P., Ruckdeschel, K., Winter, L., & Kleban, M. H. (1999). Affect-experiential personality types in middle and late adulthood. *Journal of Mental Health and Aging, 5,* 223–239.

Levenson, R. W., Carstensen, L. L., Friesen, W. V., & Ekman, P. (1991). Emotion, physiology, and expression in old age. *Psychology and Aging, 6,* 28–35.

Levine, L. J., & Bluck, S. (1997). Experienced and remembered emotional intensity in older adults. *Psychology and Aging, 12,* 514–523.

MacPherson, S. E., Phillips, L. H., & Della Sala, S. (2002). Age, executive function, and social decision making: A dorsolateral prefrontal theory of cognitive aging. *Psychology and Aging, 17,* 598–609.

Magai, C. (1999). Personality change in adulthood: Loci of change and the role of interpersonal process. *International Journal of Aging and Human Development, 49,* 339–352.

Magai, C. (2001). Emotions over the lifespan. In J. E. Birren & K. W. Schaie (Eds.), *Handbook of the psychology of aging* (5th ed., pp. 310–344). San Diego, CA: Academic Press.

Magai, C., Cohen, C., Gomberg, D., Malatesta, C., & Culver, C. (1996). Emotional expression during mid- to late-stage dementia. *International Psychogeriatrics, 8,* 383–395.

Magai, C., Consedine, N. S., Krivoshekova, Y. S., McPherson, R., & Kudadjie-Gyamfi, E. (2006). Emotion experience and expression across the adult lifespan: Insights from a multimodal assessment study. *Psychology and Aging, 21,* 303–317.

Magai, C., & Haviland-Jones, J. (2002). *The hidden genius of emotion: Lifespan transformations of personality.* New York: Cambridge University Press.

Magai, C., Hunziker, J., Mesias, W., & Culver, L. C. (2000). Adult attachment styles and emotional biases. *International Journal of Behavioral Development, 24,* 301–309.

Magai, C., & McFadden, S. H. (1995). *The role of emotions in social and personality development: History, theory, and research.* New York: Plenum Press.

Magai, C., & Nusbaum, B. (1996). Personality change in adulthood: Dynamic systems, emotions and the transformed self. In S. H. McFadden (Ed.), *Handbook of emotion, adult development, and aging* (pp. 403–420). San Diego: Academic Press.

Malatesta, C. (1982). The expression and regulation of emotion: A lifespan perspective. In T. Field & A. Fogel (Eds.), *Emotion and early interaction* (pp. 1–24). Hillsdale, NJ: Erlbaum.

Malatesta, C. (1990). The role of emotion in the development and organization of personality. In R.

Thompson (Ed.), *Nebraska Symposium on Motivation: Vol. 36. Socioemotional development* (pp. 1–56). Lincoln: University of Nebraska Press.

Malatesta, C., Fiore, M. J., & Messina, J. (1987). Affect, personality, and facial expressive characteristics of older individuals. *Psychology and Aging, 1,* 64–69.

Malatesta, C., & Izard, C. E. (1984). Facial expression of emotion in young, middle-aged, and older adults. In C. Malatesta & C. E. Izard (Eds.), *Emotion and adult development* (pp. 253–274). Beverly Hills, CA: Sage.

Malatesta, C., Izard, C. E., Culver, L. C., & Nicolich, M. (1987). Emotion communication skills in young, middle-aged, and older women. *Psychology and Aging, 2,* 193–203.

Malatesta, C., & Wilson, A. (1988). Emotion–cognition interactions in personality development: A discrete emotions, functionalist analysis. *British Journal of Social Psychology, 27,* 92–112.

Malatesta-Magai, C., & Dorval, B. (1992). Language, affect, and social order. In M. R. Gunnar & M. Maratsos (Eds.), *Modularity and constraints in language and cognition* (pp. 139–177). Hillsdale, NJ: Erlbaum.

Malatesta-Magai, C., Jonas, R., Shepard, B., & Culver, C. (1992). Type A personality and emotional expressivity in younger and older adults. *Psychology and Aging, 7,* 551–561.

Mariske, M., Lang, F. R., Baltes, P. B., & Baltes, M. M. (1995). Selective optimization with compensation: Life-span perspectives on successful human development. In L. Backman (Ed.), *Psychological compensation: Managing losses and promoting gains* (pp. 25–49). Hillsdale, NJ: Erlbaum.

Mather, M., & Carstensen, L. L. (2005). Aging and motivated cognition: The positivity effect in attention and memory. *Trends in Cognitive Sciences, 9,* 496–502.

May, C. P., Rahhat, T., Berry, E. M., & Leighton, E. A. (2005). Aging, source memory, and emotion. *Psychology and Aging, 20,* 571–578.

McDowell, C. L., Harrison, D. W., & Demaree, H. A. (1994). Is right hemisphere decline in the perception of emotion a function of aging? *International Journal of Neuroscience, 70,* 1–11.

Moreno, C., Borod, J. C., Welkowitz, J., & Alpert, M. (1990). Lateralization for the expression and perception of facial emotion as a function of age. *Neuropsychologia, 28,* 199–209.

Moreno, C., Borod, J. C., Welkowitz, J., & Alpert, M. (1993). The perception of facial emotion across the adult life span. *Developmental Neuropsychology, 9,* 305–314.

Mrozek, D. K. (2001). Age and emotion in adulthood. *Current Directions in Psychological Science, 10*(3), 87–90.

Mroczek, D. K., & Spiro, A. (2005). Change in life satisfaction during adulthood: Findings from the Veterans Affairs Normative Aging Study. *Journal of Personality and Social Psychology, 88,* 189–202.

Ong, A. D., & Bergeman, C. S. (2004). The complexity of emotions in later life. *Journals of Gerontology: Series B. Psychological Sciences and Social Sciences, 59B,* P117–P122.

Pennebaker, J. W., & Stone, L. D. (2003). Words of wisdom: Language use over the lifespan. *Journal of Personality and Social Psychology, 85,* 291–301.

Rikke, B. A., & Johnson, T. E. (2004). Lower body temperature as a potential mechanism of life extension in homeotherms. *Experimental Gerontology, 39,* 927–930.

Schieman, S. (1999). Age and anger. *Journal of Health and Social Behavior, 40,* 273–289.

Schredl, M., & Doll, E. (1998). Emotions in diary dreams. *Consciousness and Cognition, 7,* 634–646.

Smith, J., Fleeson, W., Geiselmann, B., Settersten, R. A., & Kunzmann, U. (1999). Sources of well-being in very old age. In P. B. Baltes & K. U. Mayer (Eds.), *The Berlin Aging Study: Aging from 70 to 100* (pp. 450–471). New York: Cambridge University Press.

Stoner, S. B., & Spencer, W. B. (1987). Age and gender differences with the Anger Expression Scale. *Educational and Psychological Measurement, 47,* 487–492.

Terracciano, A., McCrae, R. R., Brant, L. J., & Costa, P. T., Jr. (2005). Hierarchical linear modeling analyses of the NEO-PI-R scales in the Baltimore Longitudinal Aging Study. *Psychology and Aging, 20,* 493–506.

Tomkins, S. S. (1962). *Affect, imagery, consciousness: Vol. 1. The positive affects.* New York: Springer.

Tomkins, S. S. (1963). *Affect, imagery, consciousness: Vol. 2. The negative affects.* New York: Springer.

Tomkins, S. S. (1991). *Affect, imagery, consciousness: Vol. 3. The negative affects: Fear and anger.* New York: Springer.

Tomkins, S. S. (1992). *Affect, imagery, consciousness: Vol. 4. Cognition: Duplication and transformation of information.* New York: Springer.

Tsai, J., Carstensen, L. L., & Levenson, R. W. (2000). Automatic, subjective, and expressive responses to emotional films in older and younger Chinese Americans and European Americans. *Psychology and Aging, 15,* 684–693.

Weindruch, R. (1996). Caloric restriction and aging. *Scientific American, 274,* 46–52.

Wurm, L. H., Labouvie-Vief, G., Aycock, J., Rebucal, K. A., & Koch, H. E. (2004). Performance in auditory and visual emotional Stroop tasks: A comparison of older and younger adults. *Psychology and Aging, 19,* 523–535.

PART IV

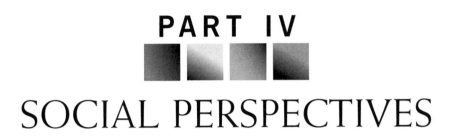

SOCIAL PERSPECTIVES

CHAPTER 24

Gender and Emotion in Context

LESLIE R. BRODY and JUDITH A. HALL

Gender differences in emotional functioning are widely documented, but are often inconsistent across personality, social, cultural, and situational variables, as well as types of emotional processes, quality of emotions, and task characteristics. This is not surprising, considering the adaptive communicative and motivational functions that emotions serve. Since males and females are often socialized to have different motives and goals—depending on their ages, cultural backgrounds, and socialization histories—gender differences should occur in emotional processes, but should also fail to generalize broadly, instead varying as a function of these same factors. Social/interpersonal goals that may differ for males and females include culturally prescribed gender roles (e.g., the role of child caretaker vs. economic provider); social motives, such as needs for intimacy versus control; and adapting to the power and status imbalances between the two sexes, in which men typically have higher power and status than do women (see Brody, 1999). Intrapersonal processes may also differ for males and females, including the ways in

which emotions and conflict are regulated and the types of self-schemas (e.g., independence vs. interdependence) that are maintained (Cross & Madson, 1997). Both interpersonal and intrapersonal processes may be influenced by a complex interaction or feedback loop between gender differences in underlying biological processes (such as temperament) and social and cultural responses to those differences (especially on the part of caretakers), which are in turn influenced by cultural values surrounding gender, gender roles, and differential emphases on collectivism versus individualism.

Recent research has focused on the complexities of when and how gender differences vary, with the theoretical frame being that gender differences in emotional functioning are both mediated and moderated by sociocultural, cognitive, biological, and behavioral variables. In turn, the variables that are found either to moderate or to mediate gender differences in emotional functioning give clues as to their etiology. In our chapter, we highlight contextual variations in gender differences in several different emotional processes, focusing on normal adult populations. We also present an updated theoretical model for the etiology of gender differences.

STEREOTYPES AND DISPLAY RULES

The stereotype that females are more emotional than men is pervasive across several different cultures (Timmers, Fischer, & Manstead, 2003). Among North American samples, women are believed to be more emotionally intense (Robinson & Johnson, 1997), as well as more emotionally expressive (e.g., smiling, laughing, crying) and more skilled in the use of nonverbal cues related to emotion (Briton & Hall, 1995). However, stereotypes are also emotion-specific: Happiness, embarrassment, surprise, sadness, fear, shame, and guilt are believed to occur more in women, and anger, contempt, and pride more in men (e.g., Hess et al., 2000; Plant, Hyde, Keltner, & Devine, 2000). Although the distinction between expression and experience is not always made, when it is, the results consistently show stereotypes to be stronger for expression than for experience (Plant et al., 2000).

How well are the stereotypes supported by self-reports and behavioral data? In general, rather well. Stereotypes about gender differences in expression tend to correspond with self-reports of expression (see below); stereotypes about gender differences in nonverbal behavior correspond well with measured gender differences (Briton & Hall, 1995); and the belief that gender differences in expression are stronger than gender differences in experience is corroborated when researchers measure both simultaneously. For example, Kring and Gordon (1998) documented gender differences in facial expressions, but not in self-reports of experience, in response to evocative films.

To find that stereotypes are somewhat confirmed in self-reports or in actual behavior should be relatively unsurprising, because our most automatically encoded and retrievable memories are based on frequently occurring behaviors, which may form the basis for many stereotypes (Hasher & Zacks, 1984). On the other hand, as pointed out by Brody (1997), gender and emotion stereotypes are imprecise, are overly general, and ignore the importance of the modality in which an emotion is expressed, as well as the situational and cultural context within which emotional expression occurs. Because stereotypes ignore both the social context and individual differences, they often lead to the erroneous assumption that gender differences are exclusively biological in origin.

Despite these cautions, stereotypes warrant a closer analysis, because they powerfully shape the reality of gender differences in at least two ways. First, in any given interaction, gender stereotypes can generate expectancies about our same- and opposite-sex partners that influence and elicit particular behaviors and emotional expressions, becoming self-fulfilling prophecies (Hall & Briton, 1993). Second, stereotypes have a strong implicit prescriptive aspect, taking the form of "display rules," which are cultural norms regulating how, when, and where emotions can be expressed by males and females in any particular culture. For example, across 48 countries, adults reported that happiness was more desirable for girls and that fearlessness and anger suppression were more desirable for boys (Diener & Lucas, 2004). Violating stereotypic display rules can lead to negative social consequences, such as social rejection and discrimination.

SELF-REPORT MEASURES

Self-report measures, though serving as the basis of much of the available evidence about emotion and expression, are problematic for three reasons. First, gender stereotypes may color participants' self-concepts and therefore their self-descriptions (Robinson & Clore, 2002). Some research supports this idea. The extent to which students endorsed gender stereotypes related to the extent to which they themselves reported experiencing different emotions from those of the opposite sex (Grossman & Wood, 1993). Second, stereotypical responding may be exacerbated by social desirability motives, which in turn may be influenced by display rules. And third, the important conceptual distinction between emotional experience and emotional expression is frequently blurred. The items to which participants are asked to respond may not make the distinction; the commonly used term "emotional," for example, implies both experience and expression. Or participants may have difficulty making this distinction even if they are asked to do so. With these cautions in mind, we review studies that have used self-report measures.

Self-Reports of General Emotional Experience and Expression

Many studies find that women rate themselves as more emotionally expressive than men report themselves to be (e.g., Simon & Nath, 2004). Gross and John (1998) factor-analyzed six frequently used self-report measures of emotional expression and identified five factors: positive expressivity, negative expressivity, the intensity of emotional expression, expressive confidence (such as enjoying acting), and masking or emotional regulation (such as suppressing anger). Women rated themselves significantly higher on the first three of these factors. Greater intensity is found for women both in their descriptions of specific emotional experiences (Hess et al., 2000; Tobin, Graziano, Vanman, & Tassinary, 2000) and on global self-report measures such as the Affect Intensity Measure (AIM; Diener, Sandvik, & Larsen, 1985). Intensity must be distinguished from frequency, however. In the 1996 General Social Survey, involving more than 1,300 respondents, there was no overall gender difference in reports of overall frequency of emotional experience (Simon & Nath, 2004). Estimates of overall frequency may mask differences for specific emotions, however, as we demonstrate in the next section.

Finally, there is emotional contagion: Women report a higher likelihood of "catching" the emotions of others than men report (Doherty, 1997). This self-reported difference is corroborated, for certain emotions, when facial muscle activity is recorded through electromyography (Dimberg & Lundquist, 1990). Emotional contagion combined with facial feedback processes (Strack, Martin, & Stepper, 1988) could contribute to women's greater reported intensity of experience.

Self-Reports of Specific Emotions

The specific positive emotions reported more intensely or more frequently by women include joy, love, affection, warmth, and feelings of well-being (see Brody, 1993; Fischer & Manstead, 2000). Higher female reporting of positive emotions emerges most clearly in situations involving intimate interpersonal relationships. When interpersonal situations are not the focus—for example, when participants are asked about total frequency in the past week—women report significantly less positive affect than men report (Simon & Nath, 2004). Females also generally report more empathy and sympathy than do males; these emotions are hard to classify as either positive or negative (see Lennon & Eisenberg, 1987). However, gender differences in empathy become smaller from ages 22 to 92 (Schieman & Van Gundy, 2000), reflecting either developmental or generational effects. Many negative emotions—including disgust; sadness; feelings of vulnerability, such as fear, anxiety, and hurt; and feelings of dysphoric self-consciousness, such as shame and embarrassment—are generally reported more by women than by men (see, e.g., Brody, 1999; Hess et al., 2000; Simon & Nath, 2004; Fischer, Rodriguez Mosquera, van Vianen, & Manstead, 2004), although gender differences in shame are inconsistent (Simon & Nath, 2004) and can vary depending on the gender-role-related relevance of the target situation (Ferguson, Eyre, & Ashbasker, 2000). Sadness, depression, and dysphoria are also reported to be more intense and of longer duration by women than by men (Scherer, Wallbott, & Summerfield, 1986).

Although men may express more anger through vocal, facial, and behavioral modalities than women, the data on gender differences in anger from research using self-report questionnaires are inconsistent. When asked general questions about how many days per week they get angry, men and women report no differences (Simon & Nath, 2004). However, when asked about the intensity of their anger, sometimes women report getting more intensely angry than men (e.g., Simon & Nath, 2004) and sometimes they show no gender differences, as was shown across 37 different countries (Fischer et al., 2004). Reports of anger are sometimes, but not always, heightened in women and girls when a situational context is specified, especially one involving interpersonal relationships (e.g., Buntaine & Costenbader, 1997; Chaplin, Cole, & Zahn-Waxler, 2005; Kring, 2000). Compared to men, women also report more enduring experiences of anger (Simon & Nath, 2004), are more likely to report hurt or disappointment in response to anger-inducing situations (Brody, 1993), and are more likely to report feeling ashamed after expressing anger (Kring, 2000), but are also more likely to view their anger as appropriate (Simon & Nath, 2004).

Emotions that males sometimes report expressing or are reported by others to express more frequently or intensely than females do are contempt, loneliness, pride, confidence, guilt, and excitement (Brody, 1993, 1999; Simon & Nath, 2004). However, gender differences in contempt, guilt, and loneliness have been inconsistent across studies, depending on situational circumstances, the characteristics of the particular samples assessed, and methodological variables (including differences between scenario-based methods and trait measures of these emotions) (Benetti-McQuoid & Bursik, 2005; Ferguson et al., 2000).

What Do Self-Reports Measure?

Women's reports of higher affective intensity on global self-report measures such as the AIM may not accurately reflect sex differences in emotion at the time feelings are initially expressed or evoked. When daily logs are used to report momentary emotions, either no gender differences have been found (Barrett, Robin, Pietromonaco, & Eyssell, 1998), or men have reported positive events in their lives to be more intense than women have reported theirs to be (Seidlitz & Diener, 1998). Moreover, subsequent global self-reports of emotion do not significantly relate to the intensity of emotional reactions reported at the time events occurred (Seidlitz & Diener, 1998). Robinson, Johnson, and Shields (1998) found that men and women retrospectively remembered their emotions as more gender-stereotypic than they actually were. In a theoretical review, Robinson and Clore (2002) argue that global and retrospective self-reports of emotion partially reflect memories for the contextual details of events. Women may have more sophisticated emotion concepts that can serve as retrieval cues, or they may encode emotional experiences in more detail than men do (Seidlitz & Diener, 1998). This may subsequently contribute to their reports of more intense emotions relative to men on global measures, even in the absence of gender differences in emotional intensity at the time feelings are actually expressed. These hypotheses are consistent with data that girls and women in the United States and Australia are faster in accessing, and are able to recall more, childhood memories of emotional experiences than their male counterparts (Davis, 1999), and also with data from Poland that women use more positive and negative emotion

words when recalling vivid memories than men do (Niedzwienska, 2003). It is also possible that there are gender differences in the mental imagery surrounding emotional events, and enhanced mental imagery has been found to be related to heightened affective responding (Miller et al., 1987).

Robinson and Clore (2002) also argue that as the delay lengthens between the occurrence of an emotional event and later recall, detailed memories fade, and self-reports of emotion increasingly rely on belief- and identity-consistent generalizations. Thus gender-stereotypic beliefs and identity may contribute to gender differences in global self-report measures. Alternative explanations for the discrepancy between global and specific measures are also possible, including the idea that in the time elapsed since an event, women may cumulatively experience more emotion than men—perhaps, for example, ruminating over the event, which retriggers emotional experiences. And, as pointed out earlier, global self-report measures often blur the distinction between emotional experience and emotional expressiveness.

However, the gender differences that appear on global self-report measures—with females reporting a wide range of both more frequent and more intense emotions than men—are unlikely to be solely determined by stereotypes, self-presentation biases, memory encoding, or other cognitive differences between males and females. Gender differences also appear on other measures of expressiveness, including observed interactions, the verbalization of emotion, facial expressiveness, and nonverbal measures.

VERBALIZATION OF EMOTION

Consistent with self-report data, women have been found to refer to both positive and negative emotions more often in conversations and in writing samples. For example, in writing a response story to a scenario in which they dealt with an obstructive travel agent, females made more emotional references than did males (Girdler, Turner, Sherwood, & Light, 1990; see also Brody, 1999). Female physicians have been found to engage patients in more talk about emotions than male physicians do (Roter, Hall, & Aoki, 2002).

In both self-descriptions and observations of marital interactions, wives are more willing to tell their husbands when they are feeling tense; they are more apt to disclose their feelings; and they are more apt to try to explain their feelings than are husbands (Burke, Weir, & Harrison, 1976). Observations of marriages corroborate that women express more emotions in words—especially more negative emotions, including more distress and anger—than men do. Men have been found to withdraw from criticism and marital conflict by "stonewalling," which involves inhibiting facial action and minimizing listening and eye contact, more than their wives do (Levenson, Carstensen, & Gottman, 1994). A recent study of dating couples indicates that gender differences in interactions are moderated by levels of stress/discomfort with the discussion: In high-stress situations, gender differences are maximized, with men expressing less emotion, more restricted affect, and more withdrawal (Vogel, Wester, Heesacker, & Madon, 2003).

FACIAL EXPRESSIONS AND OTHER NONVERBAL BEHAVIORS

Women are more accurate facial expressers of most emotions, both when posing deliberately and when being observed unobtrusively (Hall, 1984). A measure integrating facial, vocal, and postural expressions shows that girls express more sadness and anxiety than boys at ages 4 and 6, and over this 2-year period, boys decrease their expression of these emotions (Chaplin et al., 2005). Quantitative reviews have also concluded that women are more generally expressive with their faces and hands, and that they smile, laugh, and nod more than men do (Hall, 1984; LaFrance, Hecht, & Levy Paluck, 2003). It is important to note, however, that these behaviors do not have to reflect emotional states (Chovil, 1991–1992; Krauss, Chen, & Chawla, 1996). Smiling is notably ambiguous as to its "real" emotional meaning, with some authors suggesting the possibility that smiling in women reflects false positivity (women's smiles were less congruent with the content of verbal statements than was the case for men; Bugental, Love, & Gianetto, 1971). However, women's facial expressions were less discrepant from their words than were men's in the research of Halberstadt, Hayes, and Pike

(1988), and women and men displayed Duchenne (enjoyment) and non-Duchenne (social) smiles in approximately equal proportions in Hecht and LaFrance's (1998) study, meaning that women did not show an excessive proportion of emotionally artificial smiles.

Men may convey anger more clearly in their facial expressions than women do. For example, when participants were videotaped as they discussed angry, sad, and happy emotional memories, a panel of judges was subsequently able to identify men's facial displays of anger (independent of verbal content) more accurately than women's (Coats & Feldman, 1996). Men are also more facially reactive in response to angry stimuli than are women, as measured by facial electromyographic activity (Dimberg & Lundquist, 1990).

NONVERBAL DECODING SKILL

Across many studies, females score higher than males in identifying the meanings of nonverbal cues of face, body, and voice (Hall, 1978, 1984; McClure, 2000). Interestingly, most of the studies have tested sensitivity to expressions of affect, which is a female-stereotypic knowledge domain. When the knowledge domain is male-stereotypic (such as judging status or dominance), the differences appear to be much smaller or nonexistent (Schmid Mast & Hall, 2004). Evidence is also accumulating that performance on nonverbal decoding tasks is susceptible to motivational influences, which may have implications for the size of the obtained gender differences (Klein & Hodges, 2001).

EMOTIONAL COMPETENCE

Components of Emotional Competence

Theories of emotional intelligence define several emotion-related traits and skills to be important for adaptive functioning (Matthews, Zeidner, & Roberts, 2002), including perceiving emotions accurately, using emotion to facilitate thought, and understanding and managing emotion. Women score higher on all of these components on the Mayer, Salovey, and Caruso Emotional Intelligence Test (Day & Carroll, 2004; Mayer, Caruso, & Salovey, 2000). Consistent with this result is the large literature showing female advantage in perceiving nonverbally communicated emotions (see above).

Several other constructs can be seen as falling generally under the heading of emotional competence. Gohm and Clore (2000) found that women reported a greater tendency to pay attention to their emotions. When participants were clustered according to their pattern of scores on attention, clarity, and intensity, women predominated among those who were high on all three and those who were high on intensity but low on clarity (called "overwhelmed"), while men predominated among those who were low on all three and those who were low on intensity and high on clarity (called "cerebral").

Women and girls display more complex emotion knowledge than men and boys do when asked to describe emotional reactions of self and others in hypothetical scenarios (Ciarrochi, Hynes, & Crittenden, 2005). Ciarrochi et al. (2005) showed that a motivational manipulation brought men's performance up to the level of women's, but only after men spent a significantly longer amount of time on the task. As mentioned above with regard to nonverbal decoding accuracy, motivational factors may play an important role in emotion-related tasks.

Emotion Regulation

Emotion regulation or management consists of behavioral, cognitive, attentional, physiological, or emotional strategies to eliminate, maintain, or change emotional experience and/or expression (Ochsner & Gross, 2005), with closely related constructs being coping strategies and defense mechanisms. These constructs include the ideas that people attempt to control emotional processes in accordance with cultural pressures (display rules, stereotypes, and power/status imbalances), and/or in accordance with personality-related factors (self-construals, motives, conflicts and goals, with a primary goal being the avoidance of painful affect; Cramer, 2002; Matsumoto, Takeuchi, Andayani, Kouznetsova, & Krupp, 1998). Because cultural pressures and personality-related factors differ by gender, it should not be surprising to find gender differences in emotion regulation strategies. Men report or are observed to use more problem-solving, behavioral, suppression, and externalizing emotion regulation strategies than women do, including

blaming others, taking active steps, and engaging in distracting or avoidance activities such as exercise (Brody, Muderrisoglu, & Nakash-Eisikovits, 2002; Cramer, 2002; Gross & John, 2003). Women report or are observed to use more social support strategies; internalizing strategies, such as blaming themselves; and emotion-focused strategies, such as ruminating, consisting of passively focusing attention on negative affect rather than taking active steps (Cramer, 2002; Nolen-Hoeksema & Jackson, 2001; Thayer, Newman, & McClain, 1994). The gender difference in rumination has been found to be mediated by trauma and chronic strain histories (Nolen-Hoeksema, Larson, & Grayson, 1999), as well as by several attributions, including the uncontrollability of negative emotions and feelings of responsibility for social relationships (Nolen-Hoeksema & Jackson, 2001).

Gender differences in emotion regulation strategies need to be qualified by type of emotion and situation. For example, women report that they exert more control over anger, contempt, and disgust than do men, and men report that they exert more control over fear and surprise than do women across four different cultures (Matsumoto et al., 1998). Moreover, women choose rumination strategies when in neutral or depressed moods, but choose distraction when in angry moods (Rusting & Nolen-Hoeksema, 1998).

Personality factors, including motives, may also moderate gender differences in emotion regulation. Females report regulating anger and sadness to protect others' feelings, whereas males attempt to maintain control and to avoid nonsupportive interpersonal reactions (Timmers, Fischer, & Manstead, 1998; Zeman & Shipman, 1998). Agreeableness, one of the Big Five personality factors consisting of such characteristics as helpfulness and sympathy, is a stronger predictor of self-reported efforts to control emotions for women than for men (Tobin et al., 2000).

Although both avoidance and emotion-focused coping strategies tend to be nonadaptive for both sexes (Thayer et al., 1994), evidence indicates that some regulation and defense strategies may be differentially adaptive for each gender, varying in complex ways as a function of type of situation, how gender-stereotypic the defense is, and the quality of the emotion being regulated (Brody et al., 2002).

SITUATIONAL AND RELATIONSHIP SPECIFICITY

In What Situation Is Emotion Being Expressed?

Gender differences in each modality of emotional expression shift depending on the particular situation. For example, when participants recorded their emotions in response to random beeps by pagers for a 1-week period, women reported more positive affect states (e.g., happy and friendly, as opposed to unhappy and angry) while at work than they did while at home. The opposite was true of men: They reported more positive affect states while at home (Larson, Richards, & Perry-Jenkins, 1994). That women might experience more negative states in marriage than men do is consistent with Stets's (1997) observational study of married couples in videotaped discussions. Women's verbal and nonverbal behavior was much more negative than that of their husbands.

Studies also indicate that the meaning of a situation for the two sexes affects patterns of emotional expressiveness. For example, women reported relatively more hurt and sadness when partners rejected them, in accordance with interdependent self-construals, while men reported relatively more hurt and sadness when partners demanded more intimacy, in accordance with independent self-construals (Brody et al., 2002).

To Whom Is Emotion Being Expressed?

Some critical aspects of context affecting emotional expressiveness are the characteristics of the participants in the interaction and the nature of their relationship, including their level of familiarity and intimacy, their power and status with respect to each other, and their genders. For example, both men and women express more emotions and more intense emotions to people they know intimately and feel closer to (Barrett et al., 1998). Barrett et al. (1998) speculate that women's tendencies to rate their interpersonal interactions as more intimate than men's may partially mediate gender differences in emotional intensity. Women from a wide variety of cultures also express emotions to a greater number of people than men, who tend to limit themselves to expressing emotions only to intimate partners (Rimé, Mesquita, Philippot, & Boca, 1991). Women also report

controlling their emotions less with family members than males do (Matsumoto et al., 1998).

Both sexes are also more comfortable disclosing feelings (with the possible exception of anger) to women than to men (Timmers et al., 1998). In a meta-analysis of sex differences in self-disclosure (which includes but is not limited to the disclosure of feelings), women self-disclosed more to female partners, but not more to male partners, than males did (Dindia & Allen, 1992). Anger may be the only feeling that is verbally disclosed or directed more toward men than toward women, especially in situations in which no provocation is involved (Bettencourt & Miller, 1996).

CULTURAL SPECIFICITY

Across 37 countries, women report more intense emotions that last longer and are expressed more overtly than do men (Fischer & Manstead, 2000). In other cross-cultural studies, females express more nonverbal emotional reactions—including facial reactions, vocal reactions, body movements, laughing, and smiling—when expressing joy, sadness, fear, and anger than males do (Scherer et al., 1986). Moreover, in a six-nation study using U.S. and Japanese college students as posers of facial expressions, the emotions portrayed by females were more accurately judged by every cultural group, even though the photographs were intended to be standardized exemplars (Biehl et al., 1997). However, interactions among gender of judge, gender of poser, and culture have also been found to exist for at least some emotions (Matsumoto, 1992).

Gender differences in emotional expression across cultures are likely to vary as a function of cultural values, especially individualistic versus collectivistic values (giving priority to personal goals vs. loyalty to collective/group goals). Collectivism needs to be distinguished from relational values, which prioritize maintaining intimate relationships and which are more characteristic of women than men across cultures (Kashima et al., 1995). In Fischer and Manstead's (2000) data, the extent of gender differences in the intensity and duration of joy, shame, disgust, and guilt, and in the nonverbal behaviors associated with those emotions, were greater in individualistic than in collectivistic countries. Similarly, gender differences in the reported intensity of emotion in response to scenarios depicting joy, fear, and anger were not significant in a sample of American blacks, who are hypothesized to have more collectivistic values than other American ethnic groups (Vrana & Rollock, 2002). Fischer and Manstead (2000) theorize that males in individualistic cultures are especially likely to minimize emotional expressions, because expressing emotions might threaten the control that is critical to their status.

PHYSIOLOGICAL AROUSAL

Research suggests that gender differences in physiological arousal, including changes in heart rate, blood pressure, skin conductance, and levels of catecholamines (epinephrine and norepinephrine), are specific to particular physiological measures and emotions, as well as to particular tasks and circumstances (see Brody, 1999). In the same situations, some measures of arousal (such as neuroendocrine functioning or blood pressure) show men to be more aroused than women, while others (such as cardiovascular reactivity) show inconsistent or contradictory gender difference patterns (Polefrone & Manuck, 1987; Neumann & Waldstein, 2001). Type of emotion, age, and ethnicity may moderate gender differences. For example, men show higher levels of skin conductance to fearful films than women, but not to films evoking other emotions (Kring & Gordon, 1998). Although 15- to 50-year-old women show higher cardiac reactivity than same-age men when recalling angry or scary memories, no gender differences are evident when recalling sad or happy memories. In men and women over 50, no gender differences in cardiac reactivity are found across emotions (Labouvie-Vief, Lumley, Jain, & Heinze, 2003). The moderating effects of ethnicity are evident in a study showing that American black men exhibit greater cardiovascular reactivity to imagined emotional situations than other groups do (Vrana & Rollick, 2002).

Internalizers, Externalizers, Generalizers, and Low Responders

Gender differences in the patterns of correspondence between physiological arousal and other modes of emotional expression (e.g., self-reports) are consistent with gender differences

in emotion regulation, and in fact often provide clues as to emotion control strategies. Earlier work on gender differences in patterns of relationships (Buck, 1977; Manstead, 1991) suggested that men were more often "internalizers" (showing physiological arousal with no overt emotional expressions), whereas women were more often "externalizers" (showing overt emotional expressions with no corresponding physiological arousal). More recent studies confirm these patterns, but also indicate that women are relatively more likely than men to be "generalizers" (Brody, 1999)—that is, to show concordance in their expression of emotion, even at young ages (Quas, Hong, Alkon, & Boyce, 2000), and especially at high levels of physiological reactivity (Avero & Calvo, 1999). In contrast, men are more likely than women to be "low responders" (Kring & Gordon, 1998), showing no or low levels of expression across modalities. Discordance among males may be related to maintaining control or suppressing the behaviors and self-reports that correspond to arousal (Avero & Calvo, 1999), whereas concordance among females may be related to heightened emotional awareness of self and others and to female-stereotypic gender roles that encourage emotional expression.

Exceptions to these patterns have been noted in the literature on marital interaction, in which husbands' arousal has sometimes been found to be more likely to correspond to negative affect than wives' (Levenson et al., 1994, but see Kiecolt-Glaser et al., 1996). Moreover, men's cardiovascular reactivity is more often related to their expression and suppression of anger than is women's (Burns & Katkin, 1993).

NEURAL SUBSTRATES OF EMOTIONAL FUNCTIONING

With the advent of new technology, particularly functional magnetic resonance imaging (fMRI) and positron emission tomography (PET), researchers are studying potential gender differences in the brain regions involved in emotional expression, perception, and experience, especially in limbic system activation and brain lateralization (Schienle, Schafer, Stark, Watler, & Vaitl, 2005). Although recent fMRI and PET data are intriguing, they are also plagued with small sample sizes, the lack of a coherent theoretical model incorporating the idea that biological development is both influenced by and influences the social context, and inconsistencies in interpretation. Researchers often fail to consider that gender differences in the activation of a specific brain region in response to emotional stimuli can result from a multitude of processes, including differences in attention, the quality of emotional experience, the imagery associated with the experience, or the expression of emotion in different modalities (Wager & Ochsner, 2005). Activation itself has been confusingly interpreted to indicate that an area of the brain is both strong or weak for a particular function (Brody, 1999). We hope that these limitations will be addressed as the field progresses.

ETIOLOGY OF GENDER DIFFERENCES

Gender-role-related differences in motives, goals, and social status are consistent with many of the data we have reviewed about gender differences in emotional processes. For example, the emotions that women display more than men (e.g., warmth, happiness, shame, fear, and nervousness), their relatively stronger abilities in emotional decoding, and their higher facial and nonverbal expressiveness may be related to motives for affiliation and intimacy; to a self-schema based on interdependence; to perceived vulnerability in the face of lower power; and to their traditional gender roles (including child caretaking and social bonding, which necessitate reading others' emotion signals). Greater male pride, loneliness, and contempt are consistent with the male roles of differentiating from and competing with others; with maintaining a relatively high-status position; and with a self-schema based on individualism or independence. Moreover, the differing types of emotion regulation strategies used by women and men, and their differing rationales for using them (avoiding interpersonal conflict vs. maintaining control), are also consistent with gender-role-related motives and undoubtedly contribute to some of the gender differences in patterns of expressiveness, including concordance/externalizing and discordance/internalizing. That gender differences in various aspects of emotional functioning become minimized as adults age is also consistent with the idea that emotions are adaptive for gender roles, which become less rigid in later life (Gutmann, 1987).

However, social and gender-role-related variables cannot always account for gender differences in emotion. For example, evidence indicates that status differences do not account well for gender differences in nonverbal behavior (Hall, Coats, & Smith LeBeau, 2005). In our view, multiple interrelated factors contribute to the etiology of gender differences that span cultural, biological, societal, interpersonal, and intrapersonal levels of analysis. Furthermore, these multiple causes coexist with multiple moderating factors. We propose two etiological models that encompass proximal and distal factors; interpersonal and intrapersonal feedback processes; and the complex intertwining of situational, sociocultural, biological, personality, and cognitive factors both over time and in specific situations.

A Developmental Perspective

The first model includes distal factors, such as gender differences in temperament, family socialization history, gender-segregated play patterns, and cultural values, all of which contribute to the nature of gender differences. An integration of these factors involves a feedback loop in which differing temperamental characteristics of male and female infants elicit differential responses from caretakers and peers, who are also conforming to cultural pressures and display rules for gender socialization. Differing temperamental characteristics include higher activity and arousal levels in males and faster maturation rates for effortful control processes in females (see Brody, 1999; Else-Quest, Hyde, Goldsmith, & Van Hulle, 2006). Although in the past this model also included higher levels of sociability/empathy in females as a gender difference possibly rooted in temperament (Brody, 1999; Brody & Hall, 2000), a recent meta-analysis (Else-Quest et al., 2006) suggests that there are gender differences in infant arousal (favoring boys) and in infant effortful control processes, including inhibitory control and attention focusing (favoring girls), but not in infant sociability. Infant gender differences in self-control may partly contribute to the higher levels of agreeableness and sociability characterizing females later in development (Goodwin & Gotlib, 2004) because higher levels of self-control (along with early language development) would make it more likely that girls would attend to socioemotional relationships and rules. In turn, agreeableness is a significant predictor of other emotional processes that are heightened in women, including emotional intensity and efforts to regulate emotions (Tobin et al., 2000).

The socialization of emotion is especially influenced by characteristics of the family system, including the parents' own temperaments, their gender role attitudes and behaviors, the quality of their marital relationships, their cultural and socioeconomic backgrounds, and the gender constellation of the children in their families (Brody, 1999). The quality of parent–child narrative discourse and interaction has been found to vary as a function of the gender composition of the parent–child dyad and the type of emotion displayed or discussed. For example, fathers attend more to their preschool daughters' emotions of sadness and anxiety than to their sons', and to their sons' expressions of anger than to their daughters'; parental attention also predicts the later expression of sadness and anxiety 2 years later (Chaplin et al., 2005). This and other research suggests that boys learn to be less expressive of, and more controlling of, emotions communicating vulnerability as they develop. Mothers use more emotion labels in conversations with preschool daughters than with sons, and mothers' use of emotion labels significantly predicts individual differences in children's use of emotion labels (Cervantes & Callanan, 1998). And, consistent with feminist object relations analyses of development, when fathers are more involved in child care, sons and daughters express less gender-role-stereotypic emotions (Brody, 1997). Finally, gender-segregated peer groups and differentiated patterns of play both elicit and reinforce gender-role-specific emotional styles (Rose & Rudolph, 2006).

Putting Distal and Proximal Causes Together: The Example of Smiling

The second model integrates distal factors (such as gender differences in social roles and cultural values, social knowledge, and developmental history) with proximal factors (including characteristics of the situation, especially quality of affect and others' expectations and treatment by others) to account for gender differences in expressiveness, using smiling as an illustration (Hall, Carter, & Horgan, 2000). A key feature is a set of feedback processes that intensify women's positive affect during social interaction and thereby increase their smiling.

Smiling itself enhances positive affect through both physiological mechanisms and attributional processes (Strack et al., 1988).

If we take women's greater smiling as a starting point, regardless of its immediate cause, facial feedback would produce more positive affect in women than in men. Positive psychological feedback can also follow from smiling due to gender-related motives and traits. For example, if women smile partly to fulfill their internalized conception of "femininity," this would reinforce their feelings of femininity and generate positive affect, which would produce more smiling. Other gender-related motives are interpersonal trust, liking for others, and capacity for intimacy. Some of these motives intrinsically imply more positive affect and smiling (such as liking others). But, in addition, the knowledge that one has acted on these motives (showing that one is trusting, that one likes others, etc.) produces positive affect, because one is acting in concordance with a gender-relevant value (Wood, Christensen, Hebl, & Rothgerber, 1997). In turn, others respond favorably, contributing to the cycle. Women may also use smiling in the service of social skills to put others at ease, facilitate interaction, and defuse conflict. Again there would be positive feedback, because it is reinforcing to feel socially competent and to know that one has promoted comfort and communication, which in turn promotes more smiling. And others' favorable reactions produce positive affect and more smiling. Finally, smiling itself is highly reciprocal: The more one is smiled at, the more one will smile back (Hinsz & Tomhave, 1991). Reciprocity, combined with emotional contagion, should increase the intensity of women's positive affect and smiling.

Thus women experience numerous positive feedback cycles involving their own behavior, their cognitions, their physiological processes, and others' behaviors. These sum to create enhanced positive affect in their immediate social interactions compared to men's, which ultimately influences how much they smile relative to men.

Hankin and Abramson's (2001) model for women's heightened depression is also based on feedback cycles involving frequent exposure to negative events, heightened negative affect, and cognitive vulnerability factors. The similarity between the two models highlights the need for research on how the quality of immediate social interactions relates to or predicts long-term emotional styles, as well as how non-verbal expressions (such as smiling) relate to generalized affective states (such as depression).

CONCLUDING THOUGHTS

As in our chapters in the first two editions of this volume (Brody & Hall, 1993, 2000), we have continued to find consistent gender differences in several different emotional processes across several types of data. For example, gender stereotypes have frequently been borne out by data on actual patterns of behavior. We have also emphasized that gender differences in any particular modality of emotional expression are culturally and situationally specific. We have argued that the differential expression of emotions for the two sexes is adaptive for the successful fulfillment of gender roles, and we have alluded to a developmental etiological model that integrates a multiplicity of variables, including temperament and socialization factors. Finally, using smiling as an example, we have shown that proximal affective experiences, including motivational, personality, and cognitive determinants and feedback cycles, are likely to be important determinants of differential affective experiences.

The numerous variables involved in understanding both how and when gender differences occur, as well as their origins, make the research process in this area particularly complex. The most productive research strategy in this area is one that investigates how the correlates and patterns of emotional functioning differ for each gender, incorporating a diverse set of biological, personality, social, cognitive, and cultural variables as both mediators and moderators.

REFERENCES

Avero, P., & Calvo, M. G. (1999). Emotional reactivity to social-evaluative stress: Gender differences in response systems concordance. *Personality and Individual Differences, 27,* 155–170.

Barrett, L. F., Robin, L., Pietromonaco, P. R., & Eyssell, K. M. (1998). Are women the more emotional sex?: Evidence from emotional experiences in social context. *Cognition and Emotion, 12,* 555–578.

Benetti-McQuoid, J., & Bursik, K. (2005). Individual differences in experiences of and responses to guilt and shame: Examining the lenses of gender and gender role. *Sex Roles, 53,* 133–142.

Bettencourt, B. A., & Miller, N. (1996). Gender differences in aggression as a function of provocation: A meta-analysis. *Psychological Bulletin, 119,* 422–447.

Biehl, M., Matsumoto, D., Ekman, P., Hearn, V., Heider, K., Kudoh, T., et al. (1997). Matsumoto and Ekman's Japanese and Caucasian Facial Expressions of Emotion (JACFEE): Reliability data and cross-national differences. *Journal of Nonverbal Behavior, 21,* 3–21.

Briton, N. J., & Hall, J. A. (1995). Beliefs about female and male nonverbal communication. *Sex Roles, 32,* 79–90.

Brody, L. R. (1993). On understanding gender differences in the expression of emotion: Gender roles, socialization and language. In S. Ablon, D. Brown, E. Khantzian, & J. Mack (Eds.), *Human feelings: Explorations in affect development and meaning* (pp. 89–121). Hillsdale, NJ: Analytic Press.

Brody, L. R. (1997). Beyond stereotypes: Gender and emotion. *Journal of Social Issues, 53,* 369–393.

Brody, L. R. (1999). *Gender, emotion and the family.* Cambridge, MA: Harvard University Press.

Brody, L. R., & Hall, J. A. (1993). Gender and emotion. In M. Lewis & J. M. Haviland (Eds.), *Handbook of emotions* (pp. 447–460). New York: Guilford Press.

Brody, L. R., & Hall, J. A. (2000). Gender, emotion, and expression. In M. Lewis & J. M. Haviland-Jones (Eds.), *Handbook of emotions* (2nd ed., pp. 338–349). New York: Guilford Press.

Brody, L. R., Muderrisoglu, S., & Nakash-Eisikovits, O. (2002). Emotions, defenses, and gender. In R. F. Bornstein & J. M. Masling (Eds.), *The psychodynamics of gender and gender role* (pp. 203–249). Washington, DC: American Psychological Association.

Buck, R. (1977). Nonverbal communication accuracy in preschool children: Relationships with personality and skin conductance. *Journal of Personality and Social Psychology, 33,* 225–236.

Bugental, D. E., Love, L. R., & Gianetto, R. M. (1971). Perfidious feminine faces. *Journal of Personality and Social Psychology, 17,* 314–318.

Buntaine, R. L., & Costenbader, V. K. (1997). Self-reported differences in the experience and expression of anger between girls and boys. *Sex Roles, 36,* 625–637.

Burke, R. J., Weir, T., & Harrison, D. (1976). Disclosure of problems and tensions experienced by marital partners. *Psychological Reports, 38,* 531–542.

Burns, J. W., & Katkin, E. S. (1993). Psychological, situational, and gender predictors of cardiovascular reactivity to stress: A multivariate approach. *Journal of Behavioral Medicine, 16,* 445–465.

Cervantes, C. A., & Callanan, M. A. (1998). Labels and explanations in mother–child emotion talk: Age and gender differentiation. *Developmental Psychology, 34,* 88–98.

Chaplin, T. M., Cole, P. M., & Zahn-Waxler, C. (2005). Parental socialization of emotion expression: Gender differences and relations to child adjustment. *Emotion, 5,* 80–88.

Chovil, N. (1991–1992). Discourse-oriented facial displays in conversation. *Research on Language and Social Interaction, 25*, 163–194.

Ciarrochi, J., Hynes, K., & Crittenden, N. (2005). Can men do better if they try harder?: Sex and motivational effects on emotional awareness. *Cognition and Emotion, 19*, 133–141.

Coats, E. J., & Feldman, R. S. (1996). Gender differences in nonverbal correlates of social status. *Personality and Social Psychology Bulletin, 22*, 1014–1022.

Cramer, P. (2002). The study of defense mechanisms: Gender implications. In R. F. Bornstein & J. M. Masling (Eds.), *The psychodynamics of gender and gender role* (pp. 81–128). Washington, DC: American Psychological Association.

Cross, S. E., & Madson, L. (1997). Models of the self: Self-construals and gender. *Psychological Bulletin, 122*, 5–37.

Davis, P. J. (1999). Gender differences in autobiographical memory for childhood emotional experiences. *Journal of Personality and Social Psychology, 76*, 498–510.

Day, A. L., & Carroll, S. A. (2004). Using an ability-based measure of emotional intelligence to predict individual performance, group performance, and group citizenship behaviors. *Personality and Individual Differences, 36*, 1443–1458.

Diener, E., Sandvik, E., & Larsen, R. J. (1985). Age and sex effects for emotional intensity. *Developmental Psychology, 21*, 542–546.

Diener, M. L., & Lucas, R. E. (2004). Adults' desires for children's emotions across 48 countries. *Journal of Cross-Cultural Psychology, 35*, 525–547.

Dimberg, U., & Lundquist, L. (1990). Gender differences in facial reactions to facial expressions. *Biological Psychology, 30*, 151–159.

Dindia, K., & Allen, M. (1992). Sex differences in self-disclosure: A meta-analysis. *Psychological Bulletin, 112*, 106–124.

Doherty, R. W. (1997). The Emotional Contagion Scale: A measure of individual differences. *Journal of Nonverbal Behavior, 21*, 131–154.

Else-Quest, N. M., Hyde, J. S., Goldsmith, H. H., & Van Hulle, C. A. (2006). Gender differences in temperament: A meta-analysis. *Psychological Bulletin, 132*, 33–72.

Ferguson, T. J., Eyre, H. L., & Ashbasker, M. (2000). Unwanted identities: A key variable in shame–anger links and gender differences in shame. *Sex Roles, 42*, 133–157.

Fischer, A. H., & Manstead, A. S. R. (2000). The relation between gender and emotion in different cultures. In A. H. Fischer (Ed.), *Gender and emotion: Social psychological perspectives* (pp. 71–98). New York: Cambridge University Press.

Fischer, A. H., Rodriguez Mosquera, P. M., van Vianen, A. E. M., & Manstead, A. S. R. (2004). Gender and culture differences in emotion. *Emotion, 4*, 87–94.

Girdler, S. S., Turner, J. R., Sherwood, A., & Light, K. C. (1990). Gender differences in blood pressure control during a variety of behavioral stressors. *Psychosomatic Medicine, 52*, 571–591.

Gohm, C. L., & Clore, G. L. (2000). Individual differences in emotional experience: Mapping available scales to processes. *Personality and Social Psychology Bulletin, 26*, 679–697.

Goodwin, R. D., & Gotlib, I. H. (2004). Gender differences in depression: The role of personality factors. *Psychiatry Research, 126*, 135–142.

Gross, J. J., & John, O. P. (1998). Mapping the domain of expressivity: Multimethod evidence for a hierarchical model. *Journal of Personality and Social Psychology, 74*, 170–191.

Gross, J. J., & John, O. P. (2003). Individual differences in two emotion regulation processes: Implications for affect, relationships, and well-being. *Journal of Personality and Social Psychology, 85*, 348–362.

Grossman, M., & Wood, W. (1993). Sex differences in intensity of emotional experience: A social role interpretation. *Journal of Personality and Social Psychology, 65*, 1010–1022.

Gutmann, D. (1987). *Reclaimed powers: The new psychology of men and women in later life.* New York: Basic Books.

Halberstadt, A. G., Hayes, C. W., & Pike, K. M. (1988). Gender and gender role differences in smiling and communication consistency. *Sex Roles, 19*, 589–604.

Hall, J. A. (1978). Gender effects in decoding nonverbal cues. *Psychological Bulletin, 85*, 845–857.

Hall, J. A. (1984). *Nonverbal sex differences: Communication accuracy and expressive style.* Baltimore: Johns Hopkins University Press.

Hall, J. A., & Briton, N. J. (1993). Gender, nonverbal behavior, and expectations. In P. D. Blanck (Ed.), *Interpersonal expectations: Theory, research, and applications* (pp. 276–295). Cambridge, UK: Cambridge University Press.

Hall, J. A., Carter, J. D., & Horgan, T. G. (2000). Gender differences in the nonverbal communication of emotion. In A. H. Fischer (Ed.), *Gender and emotion: Social psychological perspectives* (pp. 97–117). New York: Cambridge University Press.

Hall, J. A., Coats, E. J., & Smith LeBeau, L. (2005). Nonverbal behavior and the vertical dimension of social relations: A meta-analysis. *Psychological Bulletin, 131*, 898–924.

Hankin, B. L., & Abramson, L. Y. (2001). Development of gender differences in depression: An elaborated cognitive vulnerability–transactional stress theory. *Psychological Bulletin, 127*, 773–796.

Hasher, L., & Zacks, R. T. (1984). Automatic processing of fundamental information: The case of frequency of occurrence. *American Psychologist, 39*, 1372–1388.

Hecht, M. A., & LaFrance, M. (1998). License or obligation to smile: The effect of power and sex on amount and type of smiling. *Personality and Social Psychology Bulletin, 24*, 1332–1342.

Hess, U., Senecal, S., Kirouac, G., Herrera, P., Philippot, P., & Kleck, R. E. (2000). Emotional expressivity in men and women: Stereotypes and self-perceptions. *Cognition and Emotion, 14*, 609–642.

Hinsz, V. B., & Tomhave, J. A. (1991). Smile and (half) the world smiles with you, frown and you frown alone. *Personality and Social Psychology Bulletin, 17*, 586–592.

Kashima, Y., Yamaguchi, S., Kim, U., Choi, S., Gelfand, M. J., & Yuki, M. (1995). Culture, gender and self: A perspective from individualism–collectivism research. *Journal of Personality and Social Psychology, 69*, 925–937.

Kiecolt-Glaser, J. K., Newton, T., Cacioppo, J. T., MacCallum, R. C., Glaser, R., & Malarkey, W. B. (1996). Marital conflict and endocrine function: Are men really more physiologically affected than women? *Journal of Consulting and Clinical Psychology 64*, 324–332.

Klein, K. J. K., & Hodges, S. D. (2001). Gender differences, motivation, and empathic accuracy: When it pays to understand. *Personality and Social Psychology Bulletin 27*, 720–730.

Krauss, R. M., Chen, Y., & Chawla, P. (1996). Nonverbal behavior and nonverbal communication: What do conversational hand gestures tell us? In M. P. Zanna (Ed.), *Advances in experimental social psychology* (Vol. 28, pp. 389–450). San Diego, CA: Academic Press.

Kring, A. M. (2000). Gender and anger. In A. H. Fischer (Ed.), *Gender and emotion: Social psychological perspectives* (pp. 211–231). New York: Cambridge University Press.

Kring, A. M., & Gordon, A. H. (1998). Sex differences in emotion: Expression, experience, and physiology. *Journal of Personality and Social Psychology 74*, 686–703.

Labouvie-Vief, G., Lumley, M. A., Jain, E., & Heinze, H. (2003). Age and gender differences in cardiac reactivity and subjective emotion responses to emotional autobiographical memories. *Emotion 3*, 115–126.

LaFrance, M., Hecht, M. A., & Levy Paluck, E. (2003). The contingent smile: A meta-analysis of sex differences in smiling. *Psychological Bulletin, 129*, 305–334.

Larson, R. W., Richards, M. H., & Perry-Jenkins, M. (1994). Divergent worlds: The daily emotional experience of mothers and fathers in the domestic and public spheres. *Journal of Personality and Social Psychology, 67*, 1034–1046.

Lennon, R., & Eisenberg, N. (1987). Gender and age differences in empathy and sympathy. In N. Eisenberg & J. Strayer (Eds.), *Empathy and its development* (pp. 195–217). Cambridge, UK: Cambridge University Press.

Levenson, R. W., Carstensen, L. L., & Gottman, J. M. (1994). The influence of age and gender on affect, physiology, and their interrelations: A study of long-term marriages. *Journal of Personality and Social Psychology, 67*, 56–68.

Manstead, A. S. R. (1991). Expressiveness as an individual difference. In R. S. Feldman & B. S. Rimé (Eds.), *Fundamentals of nonverbal behavior* (pp. 285–328). Cambridge, UK: Cambridge University Press.

Matsumoto, D. (1992). American–Japanese cultural differences in the recognition of universal facial expressions. *Journal of Cross-Cultural Psychology, 23*, 72–84.

Matsumoto, D., Takeuchi, S., Andayani, S., Kouznetsova, N., & Krupp, D. (1998). The contribution of individualism vs. collectivism to cross-national differences in display rules. *Asian Journal of Social Psychology, 1*, 147–165.

Matthews, G., Zeidner, M., & Roberts, R. D. (2002). *Emotional intelligence: Science and myth*. Cambridge, MA: MIT Press.

Mayer, J. D., Caruso, D. R., & Salovey, P. (2000). Emotional intelligence meets traditional standards for an intelligence. *Intelligence, 27*, 267–298.

McClure, E. B. (2000). A meta-analytic review of sex differences in facial expression processing and their development in infants, children, and adolescents. *Psychological Bulletin, 126*, 424–453.

Miller, G. A., Levin, D. N., Kozak, M. J., Cook, E. W., McLean, A., & Lang, P. J. (1987). Individual differences in imagery and the psychophysiology of emotion. *Cognition and Emotion, 1*, 367–390.

Neumann, S. A., & Waldstein, S. R. (2001). Similar patterns of cardiovascular response during emotional activation as a function of affective valence and arousal and gender. *Journal of Psychosomatic Research, 50*, 245–253.

Niedzwienska, A. (2003). Gender differences in vivid memories. *Sex Roles, 49*, 321–331.

Nolen-Hoeksema, S., & Jackson, B. (2001). Mediators of the gender difference in rumination. *Psychology of Women Quarterly, 25*, 37–47.

Nolen-Hoeksema, S., Larson, J., & Grayson, C. (1999). Explaining the gender difference in depressive symptoms. *Journal of Personality and Social Psychology, 77*, 1061–1072.

Ochsner, K. N., & Gross, J. J. (2005). The cognitive control of emotion. *Trends in Cognitive Sciences, 9*, 242–249.

Plant, E. A., Hyde, J. S., Keltner, D., & Devine, P. G. (2000). The gender stereotyping of emotions. *Psychology of Women Quarterly, 24*, 81–92.

Polefrone, J. M., & Manuck, S. B. (1987). Gender differences in cardiovascular and neuroendocrine response to stressors. In R. Barnett, L. Biener, & G. Baruch (Eds.), *Gender and stress* (pp. 13–38). New York: Free Press.

Quas, J., Hong, M., Alkon, A., & Boyce, W. T. (2000). Dissociations between psychobiologic reactivity and emotional expression in children. *Developmental Psychobiology, 37*, 153–175.

Rimé, B., Mesquita, B., Philippot, P., & Boca, S. (1991). Beyond the emotional event: Six studies on the social sharing of emotion. *Cognition and Emotion, 5*, 435–465.

Robinson, M. D., & Clore, G. L. (2002). Belief and feeling: Evidence for an accessibility model of emotional self-report. *Psychological Bulletin, 128,* 934–960.

Robinson, M. D., & Johnson, J. T. (1997). Is it emotion or is it stress?: Gender stereotypes and the perception of subjective experience. *Sex Roles, 36,* 235–258.

Robinson, M. D., Johnson, J. T., & Shields, S. A. (1998). The gender heuristic and the database: Factors affecting the perception of gender-related differences in the experience and display of emotions. *Basic and Applied Social Psychology, 20,* 206–219.

Rose, A. J., & Rudolph, K. D. (2006). A review of sex differences in peer relationship processes: Potential trade-offs for the emotional and behavioral development of girls and boys. *Psychological Bulletin, 132,* 98–131.

Roter, D. L., Hall, J. A., & Aoki, Y. (2002). Physician gender effects in medical communication: A meta-analytic review. *Journal of the American Medical Association, 288,* 756–764.

Rusting, C. L., & Nolen-Hoeksema, S. (1998). Regulating responses to anger: Effects of rumination and distraction on angry mood. *Journal of Personality and Social Psychology, 74,* 790–803.

Scherer, K. R., Wallbott, H. G., & Summerfield, A. B. (1986). *Experiencing emotion: A cross-cultural study.* New York: Cambridge University Press.

Schieman, S., & Van Gundy, K. (2000). The personal and social links between age and self-reported empathy. *Social Psychology Quarterly, 63,* 152–174.

Schienle, A., Schafer, A., Stark, R., Walter, B., & Vaitl, D. (2005). Gender differences in the processing of disgust and fear-inducing pictures: An fMRI study. *NeuroReport, 16,* 277–280.

Schmid Mast, M., & Hall, J. A. (2004). Who is the boss and who is not?: Accuracy of judging status. *Journal of Nonverbal Behavior, 28,* 145–165.

Seidlitz, L., & Diener, E. (1998). Sex differences in the recall of affective experiences. *Journal of Personality and Social Psychology, 74,* 262–271.

Simon, R. W., & Nath, L. E. (2004). Gender and emotion in the United States: Do men and women differ in self-reports of feelings and expressive behavior? *American Journal of Sociology, 109,* 1137–1176.

Stets, J. E. (1997). Status and identity in marital interaction. *Social Psychology Quarterly, 60,* 185–217.

Strack, F., Martin, L. L., & Stepper, S. (1988). Inhibiting and facilitating conditions of the human smile: A nonobtrusive test of the facial feedback hypothesis. *Journal of Personality and Social Psychology, 54,* 768–777.

Thayer, R. E., Newman, J. R., & McClain, T. M. (1994). Self-regulation of mood: Strategies for changing a bad mood, raising energy, and reducing tension. *Journal of Personality and Social Psychology, 67,* 910–925.

Timmers, M., Fischer, A. H., & Manstead, A. S. R. (1998). Gender differences in motives for regulating closeness. *Personality and Social Psychology Bulletin, 24,* 974–985.

Timmers, M., Fischer, A. H., & Manstead, A. S. R. (2003). Ability versus vulnerability: Beliefs about men's and women's emotional behavior. *Cognition and Emotion, 17,* 41–63.

Tobin, R. M., Graziano, W. G., Vanman, E. J., & Tassinary, L. G. (2000). Personality, emotional experience, and efforts to control emotions. *Journal of Personality and Social Psychology, 79,* 656–669.

Vogel, D. L., Wester, S. R., Heesacker, M., & Madon, S. (2003). Confirming gender stereotypes: A social role perspective. *Sex Roles, 48,* 519–528.

Vrana, S. R., & Rollock, D. (2002). The role of ethnicity, gender, emotional content, and contextual differences in physiological, expressive, and self-reported emotional responses to imagery. *Cognition and Emotion, 16,* 165–192.

Wager, T. D., & Ochsner, K. N. (2005). Sex differences in the emotional brain. *NeuroReport, 16,* 85–87.

Wood, W., Christensen, P. N., Hebl, M. R., & Rothgerber, H. (1997). Conformity to sex-typed norms, affect, and the self-concept. *Journal of Personality and Social Psychology, 73,* 523–535.

Zeman, J., & Shipman, K. (1998). Influence of social context on children's affect regulation: A functionalist perspective. *Journal of Nonverbal Behavior, 22,* 141–165.

CHAPTER 25

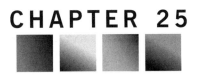

The Cultural Psychology of the Emotions
Ancient and Renewed

RICHARD A. SHWEDER, JONATHAN HAIDT, RANDALL HORTON,
and CRAIG JOSEPH

> *Great, deep, wide and unbounded, the ocean is nevertheless drunk by*
> *underwater fires; in the same way, Sorrow is drunk by Anger.*
> —Translation of an unidentified Sanskrit stanza from India
> in the early Middle Ages (GNOLI, 1956, p. 35)

This chapter elaborates, revises, and partially recapitulates an evolving description of the cultural psychology of the emotions, versions of which appeared in the first two editions of this handbook. We define and illustrate a cultural/ symbolic/meaning-centered approach to the study of the emotions, using some sources that are quite ancient (e.g., the 3rd-century A.D. Sanskrit text, the "Rasādhyāya" of the *Nāṭyaśāstra*) and others that are quite new. The chapter updates a componential approach to the cultural study of emotions, with special attention to comparative analyses of two emotion categories: those often translated and labeled in English as "anger" and "shame." The chapter also examines the moral context of emotional functioning in different cultural and religious traditions (e.g., Hinduism, Buddhism, and Islam), while suggesting that the character

and meaning of particular emotions are systematically related to the ethics (e.g., the ethics of autonomy, community, or divinity) prevalent in a cultural community (Haidt, 2001, 2003; Haidt, Koller, & Dias, 1993; Haidt & Joseph, 2004; Jensen, 1995, 1998, 2005; Shweder, 1990b, 1994a, 2002; Shweder & Haidt, 1993; Shweder, Much, Mahapatra, & Park, 1997).

The major goals of "cultural psychology" are to spell out the implicit meanings that give shape to psychological processes, to examine the distribution of those meanings across ethnic groups and temporal–spatial regions of the world, and to identify the manner of their social acquisition. Related goals are to reassess the principle of psychic unity or uniformity, and to develop a credible theory of psychological diversity or pluralism. The emphasis in cultural psychology is upon the way the human

409

mind can be transformed and made functional in a number of different ways, which are not equally distributed across ethnic and cultural communities around the world (see Markus & Kitayama, 1991; Markus, Kitayama, & Heiman, 1998; Shweder, 1991, 1996; Shweder & LeVine, 1984; Shweder et al., 1998).

One hallmark of cultural psychology is a conception of "culture" that is symbolic and behavioral at the same time. Culture, so conceived, can be defined as the range of ideas about what is true, good, beautiful, and efficient that are made manifest in the speech, laws, customary practices, and other purposive actions of the members of any norm-sensitive and self-policing group (Goodnow, Miller, & Kessel, 1995; Shweder et al., 1998; Shweder, 1999a, 1999b). In research on cultural psychology, "culture" thus consists of meanings, conceptions, and interpretive schemes that are activated, constructed, or brought "online" through participation in normative social institutions and routine practices (including linguistic practices) (see, e.g., D'Andrade, 1984; Geertz, 1973; LeVine, 1984; Miller, Potts, Fung, Hoogstra, & Mintz, 1990; Shweder, 1991, 1999a, 1999b). According to this view, a culture is the subset of humanly possible or available meanings that, by virtue of enculturation (informal or formal, implicit or explicit, unintended or intended), has become valued and active in giving shape to the psychological processes of the individuals in a particular norm-sensitive group.

A second hallmark of cultural psychology is the idea that interpretation, conceptualization, and other "acts of meaning" can take place rapidly, automatically, and un-self-consciously. Indeed, it is assumed that "acts of meaning" (e.g., the judgment that the human body may become polluted or desanctified because it is a temple for the soul; or that illness is a means of empowerment because it unburdens a person of accumulated spiritual debts; or that shyness, shame, modesty, and embarrassment are good and strong emotions because they are displays of civility signaling that people are playing their part in upholding and controlling the social order) can take place so rapidly, automatically, and un-self-consciously that from the point of view of an individual person they are indistinguishable from "raw" experience or "naked" consciousness itself (see, e.g., Geertz, 1984, on "experience-near" concepts, and Kirsh, 1991, on "thought in action"; see also

Fish, 1980; Nisbett & Wilson, 1977). According to this view, many rapid, automatic, and un-self-conscious psychological processes are best understood not as "pure," "basic," "fundamental," or "intrinsic" processes, but rather as content-laden processes, which are contingent on the implicit meanings, conceptual schemes, and ideas that give them life (Haidt, 2001; Markus et al., 1998; Mesquita, 2003; Nisbett & Cohen, 1995; Shweder, 1990a; Stigler, 1984; Stigler, Chalip, & Miller, 1986; Stigler, Nusbaum, & Chalip, 1988).

As an initial illustration of these points, we begin our discussion in the 3rd century A.D. in India with a brief examination of a Sanskrit text (the "Rasādhyāya" of the *Nāṭyaśāstra*) that was written relatively early in the historical record of systematic human self-consciousness about the emotions. It is through an analysis of this venerable text—an ancient example of a cultural psychology—that we address contemporary concerns. The "Rasādhyāya" is a useful intellectual pole star on which to concentrate a discussion of the cultural psychology of the emotions, for three reasons: (1) The text, although ancient, compares favorably with any contemporary treatise on the symbolic character of emotional experience; (2) the text, although famous among Sanskritists and scholars of South Asian civilization, is hardly known at all by emotion researchers in anthropology and psychology; and (3) the text provides the opportunity for an object lesson about the universally appealing yet, in some sense, culture-specific character of all accounts about what is "basic" to the emotional nature of human beings.

THE CULTURALLY CONSTRUCTED "BASIC EMOTIONS" OF THE "RASĀDHYĀYA"

Between the 3rd and 11th centuries A.D., Hindu philosophers of poetics and drama, interested in human emotions as objects of aesthetic pleasure, posited the existence of eight or nine basic emotions (*sthāyi-bhāva*) and developed a relatively detailed account of the symbolic structures that give them shape and meaning. There is no standard English translation of the Sanskrit terms for the postulated basic emotions. Indeed, there is no agreement about whether they should be translated as "emotions," "mental states," or "feelings," or about whether they should be translated as "basic," "dominant," "permanent," "universal," "natural," or "principal" emotions (or mental states or feelings). The eight basic (or dominant) emotions (or mental states or feelings) are variously translated as follows: (1) sexual passion, love, or delight (*rati*); (2) amusement, laughter, humor, or mirth (*hāsa*); (3) sorrow (*śoka*); (4) anger (*krodha*); (5) fear or terror (*bhaya*); (6) perseverance, energy, dynamic energy, or heroism (*utsāha*); (7) disgust or disillusion (*jugupsā*); and (8) amusement, wonder, astonishment, or amazement (*vismaya*). Some early medieval commentators mention an additional basic (or dominant) emotion (or mental state or feeling), (9) serenity or calm (*sama*). To simplify our exegesis, we refer to the eight (or nine) as "basic emotions," and we label them "sexual passion," "amusement," "sorrow," "anger," "fear," "perseverance," "disgust," "wonder," and "serenity."

The canonical Sanskrit text on the "emotions," attributed to Bharata, is the sixth chapter, the "Rasādhyāya," of the *Nāṭyaśāstra*, which is a book about drama. In Sanskrit drama, the primary aim of the aesthetic experience was psychological; indeed, it was the symbolic representation of emotional states per se that set the stage for aesthetic and revelatory experience (see Dimock et al., 1974). The famous sixth chapter of the *Nāṭyaśāstra* is about the narrative structure (the causes, consequences, and concomitants) of eight basic emotional states and the most effective means (via facial expression, voice, posture, setting, character, action, and physiological response) of their representation in the theatre. The *Nāṭyaśāstra* was probably written some time between the 3rd and 5th centuries A.D. The most famous of several commentaries on the text is by the 10th- and 11th-century Kashmiri Brahman philosopher Abhivanagupta (partial translations and contemporary commentaries can be found in Masson & Patwardhan, 1970, and Gnoli, 1956; see also Dimock et al., 1974, and Keith, 1924).

THE WONDER OF THE SANSKRIT EMOTIONS: A CULTURAL ACCOUNT

Contemporary non-Hindu researchers in the United States and Europe are likely to find the account of the "basic emotions" in the "Rasādhyāya" both familiar and strange. Indeed, one of the hazards of doing research on the emotions is the temptation to presumptively universalize a content-laden and culture-specific mental process and theorize that it is a basic or intrinsic mental process. Here we find it instructive (and a useful corrective to unbounded generalizations) to compare two such posited theories about "basic emotions" across historical time and cultural space. If we compare the Sanskrit list of nine (eight plus one) basic emotions (sexual passion, amusement, sorrow, anger, fear, perseverance, disgust, wonder, and sometimes serenity) with Paul Ekman's well-known contemporary list of nine (six plus three) basic emotions (anger, fear, sadness, happiness, surprise, and disgust, plus interest, shame, and contempt), which Ekman (1980, 1984) has derived from the analysis of everyday facial expressions, the two lists do not seem to us to be closely coordinated, although they are not totally disjoint either.

In his volume *Performance Theory*, Richard Schechner (1988) presents a series of photographs of facial expressions that he claims are iconic representations of the nine basic emotions of the *Nāṭyaśāstra*. This, of course, is a risky thing to do. The *Nāṭyaśāstra* never abstracts out facial expressions as the key markers of the basic emotions, but rather treats them as one element in an array of constituents; and there is every reason to believe that in Hindu drama facial expressions unfold dynamically in a sequence of movements, which are not easily frozen into a single frame (Hejmadi, Davidson, & Rozin, 2000). Nevertheless, Schechner posits direct analogies between six of his facial expressions for the Sanskrit basic emotions and the six facial expressions from Ekman's primary scheme—equating, for example, Ekman's representation of the face of surprise with the Sanskrit face of wonder, and Ekman's representation of the face of happiness with the Sanskrit face of sexual passion. Schechner thinks he sees a universal pattern reflected in the two schemes: He states, "Humankind has countless gods, but I would be very surprised if there were not some agreement concerning the basic emotions" (1988, p. 266). But how much agreement?

In our view, several of Schechner's equations are dubious. For example, in Ekman's face of surprise, the mouth is wide open; it is not similar to the mouth of the Sanskrit emotion of wonder, which is closed and faintly suggestive of a smile. (The mouth is closed in all of the facial expressions of the medieval Hindu emotions, which, we speculate, may be related to a cultural evaluation concerning the vulgarity of an open mouth.) And in Ekman's photo of the face of happiness, the eyes are directly frontal; they are not similar to the eyes of the Sanskrit emotion of sexual passion, where the gaze is conspicuously averted to one side, perhaps suggestive of coyness, secrecy, or conspiracy. More importantly, because Schechner's equation of American "happiness" with Sanskrit "sexual passion" seems peculiar from the start, it should also be noted that Ekman's photo of the face of happiness bears no resemblance whatsoever to the face of amusement, which is the Sanskrit emotion one might have intuitively expected to be connected to the Western conception of "happiness."

We doubt that most Americans could spontaneously generate accurate descriptions for the majority of the nine facial icons of the Sanskrit "basic emotions" displayed in Schechner's book. (Curiously, one of the faces that American graduate students seem to identify without much difficulty is the Sanskrit face of serenity, which as far as we know is not a "basic emotion" on any Western list. In informal experiments conducted in classes at the University of Chicago, they also converge in their responses to faces of fear, disgust, and sorrow, but not to the other five.) Indeed, we believe one can plausibly argue that happiness, surprise, and most of the other basic emotions on Ekman's list do not have close analogues among the basic emotions of the "Rasādhyāya," and any sense of easy familiarity with the Sanskrit list is more apparent than real.

As we read the "Rasādhyāya" and commentaries, three of the nine basic emotions (anger, fear, and sorrow) are genuinely familiar, in the sense of possessing an equivalent shape and meaning for medieval Hindus and contemporary Americans. Of course, to acknowledge those three points of dense similarity is not to suggest that those three emotional meanings must be cross-cultural universals. Wierzbicka (1992) has brought to a halt facile claims about translation equivalence by showing that "sadness" as understood in European and American conceptions of the emotions is not an empirical universal and is neither lexicalized, important, nor salient in most of the languages of the world. She claims that from the point of view of the study of the linguistic semantics of emotion terms around the world, there may be

no basic or universal emotions, although she allows that feelings that are more or less "shame-like" are quite widespread.

Nevertheless, anger, fear, and sorrow are easy to recognize in the "Rasādhyāya." Sorrow, for example, is said to arise from misfortune, calamity, and destruction, and from "separation from those who are dear, [their] downfall, loss of wealth, death and imprisonment." "It should be acted out by tears, laments, drying up of the mouth, change of color, languor in the limbs, sighs, loss of memory, etc." (Masson & Patwardhan, 1970, p. 52). Sorrow is said to be accompanied by other mental states, including world-weariness, physical weariness, lifelessness, tears, confusion, dejection and worry. Anger and fear are also easy to recognize in the text (see Masson & Patwardhan, 1970, pp. 52–53).

For three of the nine basic emotions described in the "Rasādhyāya," it is easy to recognize the underlying script, to readily see the self in the other, and to arrive at a cross-cultural and transhistorical agreement about what is basic in emotional functioning (at least for them and us). Yet as one moves beyond sorrow, anger, and fear to disgust, amusement, wonder, perseverance, sexual passion, and serenity, the way in which consciousness is partitioned or hierarchically structured into basic and nonbasic states in the "Rasādhyāya" seems less and less familiar, despite any initial appearances to the contrary. This decline in familiarity is similar to the "gradient of recognition" that Haidt and Keltner (1999) found when studying facial expressions in India and the United States: Some expressions are very well recognized across cultures, some are less well recognized, and there is no neatly bounded set of "universal" facial expressions.

Thus it becomes clear upon examination of the relevant Sanskrit texts and commentaries that medieval Hindu "disgust" overlaps with but also differs from modern American "disgust." Medieval Hindu disgust is partitioned into two subtypes. The first includes aspects of horror and disillusionment, as well as world-weariness associated with the quest for detachment, transcendence, and salvation; the second includes horror at the sight of blood. Medieval Hindu disgust is, as the anthropologist McKim Marriott has suggested to us, more like a domain of the loathsome, and it gathers together within its territory a broad range of human responses to the ugly, the nasty, and the odious.

It also becomes clear upon close examination that nuances make a difference, and that medieval Hindu "wonder" is not contemporary American "surprise," but rather a state of mind closer to admiration than to startle or shock. For Hindu wonder has less to do with a sudden violation of expectations and more to do with one's reactions to the opportunity to witness divine, heavenly, or exalted feats, events, or beings (including, e.g., the amazing feats of a juggler). It is even possible to do such witnessing with the mouth closed, as long as the eyes are wide open!

Upon closer examination, it becomes apparent as well that medieval Hindu "amusement" (which includes contemptuous, indignant, or derisive laughter at the faults and inferior status of others) is not contemporary American "happiness," which has celebratory implications. Indeed, happiness, shame, indignation, arrogance, and some contempt-like emotions are explicitly mentioned in the "Rasādhyāya" for inclusion among 33 nonbasic ("accompanying") mental states. Thus it seems reasonable to assert that the basic emotion designated by medieval Hindu philosophers as "amusement" is not adequately translated as "happiness" or as "contempt." (It should be noted that while the text provides little basis for determining equivalence of meaning for the terms used to translate the 33 nonbasic mental states, there is good reason to doubt that "shame" or "happiness" have the same implications and associations, or play the same psychological role, in India as they do in the contemporary United States. See Menon & Shweder, 1994, and Shweder, 1996, 2003, on the positive qualities of "shame" in India, where it is a virtue associated with civility, modesty and an ability to rein in one's destructive powers in support of the social order rather than with the diminishment of the ego; see also Parish, 1991, and below.)

Similarly, it becomes clear upon examination of the text that medieval Hindu "perseverance" is not contemporary American "interest," but is rather deeply connected to heroic determination and a willfulness to engage in acts requiring endurance and self-sacrifice. In the context of the early medieval Hindu scriptures, when the Hindu goddess Durga (or Kali) endures trials and tribulations yet persists in a seemingly hopeless battle against uncountable demons in an effort to save the world, her efforts are said to display the heroic *rasa* of perseverance. Mere interest has very little to do with it. She

would probably rather be doing something else (see below).

In summary, the two lists of nine basic human emotions closely and truly overlap at only three points. All the other apparent points of similarity (amusement as happiness, their disgust as our disgust, wonder as surprise, perseverance as interest) turn out to be merely apparent; and for several of the emotions (sexual passion, serenity, shame, contempt), there is not even an illusion of transcultural equivalence. In the end, most of the items cannot be easily mapped across the two lists without a good deal being lost in translation.

There are other ways in which the "Rasādhyāya" presents us with a somewhat unfamiliar portrait of the way consciousness is organized. According to the text and commentaries, the four primary basic emotions are sexual passion, anger, perseverance, and disgust. The four secondary basic emotions are amusement, sorrow, wonder, and fear. The ninth basic emotion, serenity, is sometimes viewed as a primary basic emotion and either substituted for disgust or associated with disgust (through a causal sequence that begins with horror and revulsion over attachments in the world, and ends with the serenity of ego alienation, detachment, and salvation).

In commenting on this scheme, it is worth noting that Sigmund Freud might find much of value in a conception of human personality that treats sexual passion and anger (and perseverance and disgust) as the deepest aspects of human experience. One wonders whether Freud would have interpreted perseverance and disgust as analogues to the life and death instincts. More notable, however, is the fact that the primary basic emotions are thus named because they are the "emotions" associated in classical and folk Hindu thought with the four worthy ends or goals of life. One of those goals of life—pleasure (*kāma*)—is linked to sexual passion. A second goal—control, autonomy, and power (*artha*)—is linked to anger. A third goal—social duty and moral virtue (*dharma*)—is linked to perseverance. The forth and perhaps highest goal—purity, sanctity, salvation, or the attainment of divinity (*moksha*)—is linked to disgust and/or serenity. In other words, presupposed by this famous formulation about the organization of human emotions is a special and local theory of morality and human motivation and a specific way of life. Thus it is hardly surprising that this particular medieval South Asian conception of the hierarchical structuring of consciousness into basics versus nonbasics and primary basics versus secondary basics should seem somewhat strange or alien to emotion researchers in North America, and vice versa. In other words, in the "Rasādhyāya" one finds a relatively elaborate account of the symbolic structures that give shape and meaning to a selected subset of mental experiences, which, because they have been privileged for local symbolic elaboration, have become transformed into mental experiences that people regard as "basic" in their particular culturally constituted world.

COMPARING AMERICAN "ANGER" AND TIBETAN *LUNG LANG*

The strategy adopted in the "Rasādhyāya" is to define a basic emotion by the implicit symbolic structure that gives shape and meaning to that emotion, and then to define that symbolic structure by resolving it into its determinants, consequences, and accompanying side effects. This strategy is directly parallel to various contemporary approaches to the cultural psychology of the emotions.

One aspect of this symbolic (or "cognitive," "interpretive," or "meaning-centered") approach is the view that kinds of emotions are not kinds of things like plants or animals. Instead, they are embodied interpretive schemes of a particular script-like or narrative form that give shape and meaning to the human experience of those conditions of the world that have a bearing on self-esteem (see Shweder, 1994b). The components that are proposed as slots in these emotion schemes may vary slightly from scholar to scholar, although most of the components or slots in use today can be found in the "Rasādhyāya."

Mesquita and Frijda (1992; see also Ellsworth, 1991; Frijda, 1986; Lazarus, 1991; Lewis, 1989; Lewis, Sullivan, & Michalson, 1984; Lutz, 1985; Russell, 1991; Stein & Levine, 1987), for example, parse each emotion script into a series of components including "antecedent events," "event coding" (type of condition of the world), "appraisal" (judged implications for self-esteem and well-being), "physiological reaction patterns," "action readiness," "emotional behavior," and "regulation." Shweder (1994b) suggests a parsing of emotion scripts into components such as "self-involving conditions of the world" (e.g., loss and gain, protection and threat), "somatic feelings" (e.g., muscle tension, pain, dizziness, nausea, fatigue, breathlessness), "affective feelings" (e.g., agitation, emptiness, expansiveness), "expressive modes" (e.g., face, posture, voice), and "plans for self-management" (e.g., to flee, to retaliate, to celebrate, to invest). (See also Shweder, 1991, where a slot is provided in the emotion narrative for variations in "social regulation" or the normative appropriateness of certain emotions being experienced or expressed.)

The primary assumption of the symbolic approach is that the "emotion" (e.g., sadness, fear, or love) is not something independent of or separable from the conditions that justify it, from the somatic and affective events that are ways of being touched by it, from the actions it demands, or the like. The "emotion" is the whole story: a kind of somatic event (fatigue, chest pain, goose flesh) and/or affective event (panic, emptiness, expansiveness) experienced as a perception of some antecedent conditions (death of a friend, acceptance of a book manuscript for publication, a proposition to go out to dinner) and their implications for the self (e.g., as loss, gain, threat, possibility), and experienced as well as a social judgment (e.g., of vice or virtue, sickness or health) and as a kind of plan for action to preserve one's self-esteem (attack, withdraw, confess, hide, explore). The "emotion" is the entire script. It is the unfolding experience of all the components, or, perhaps more accurately, the cohesive experience of the whole package deal.

A second aspect of the symbolic approach is the view that any "emotion" is decomposable into its components, and that these components are what must be compared when we ask whether two emotion experiences are the same or different across cultures. Based on earlier work by Shweder (1994b) and recent work by Horton (2006) attempting to integrate perspectives on emotion from across the fields of cognitive psychology and psychological anthropology, we find it useful to posit eight relevant components, which we describe below. We then illustrate the utility of this approach by using it to compare the emotion of "anger" (as it is experienced and understood by a sample of urban American adults) with the Tibetan emotion *lung lang* (as it is experienced and understood by Tibetan refugees [laity and religious virtuosos] settled in India). The eight components are as follows:

- *Component 1: Somatic experience.* Are people alike or different in introspectively and objectively observable physical changes (e.g., muscle tension, headaches, blood pressure shifts, activation of specific neural pathways) when they experience the emotion?
- *Component 2: Affective phenomenology.* Are people alike or different in their affective experiences (e.g., feelings of emptiness, calm, pleasantness, derealization, soul loss) when they experience the emotion?
- *Component 3: Environmental determinants.* Are people alike or different in the antecedent conditions associated with the emotion (e.g., winning the lottery, a remark from a subordinate, birth of a child, physical contact with a member of an outcaste group)?
- *Component 4: Appraisals of significance.* Are people alike or different in the appraisals of the antecedent conditions that elicit the emotion, and in ongoing construals that may inflect, extend, transform, or truncate the experience (e.g., others' actions were intentional, unwanted, goal-enhancing, expected, disrespectful, or status-degrading; the outcome can or cannot be changed)?
- *Component 5: Normative social appraisals.* Are people alike or different in the extent to which showing, displaying, or merely experiencing the emotion has been socially designated as a vice or virtue or as a sign of sickness or health?
- *Component 6: Self-management.* Are people alike or different in the impulses to action and plans for self-management that get activated in association with the emotion (e.g., to celebrate, to attack, to disengage and avoid the other person, to engage in problem solving)?
- *Component 7: Communication and symbolization.* Are people alike or different in the iconic and symbolic vehicles used for giving expression to the emotion (e.g., facial expressions, voice, posture, and action)?
- *Component 8: Social management.* Are people alike or different in the ways they respond to and manage the communication and symbolization of the emotion *by others* (e.g., empathically mirroring the emotion, cowering, withdrawing, discussing an individual's behavior with others, collectively shunning the individual)?

Depending on the interests and methodological commitments of investigators, any of these eight domains can be elaborated further. In extending the seventh component domain (communication and symbolization), for instance, one could ask: Are the cultures alike or different in the symbolic resources they accord their members for naming, evoking, and manipulating discrete facets of the emotional experience for the achievement of important social and individual goals (e.g., through meditations on compassion, death metal concerts, workshops on assertiveness training or anger management, mass political demonstrations, initiation rites, or vulnerability to dissociative states in which the emotion is prominent)?

We recognize that this componential model includes facets of emotion-related experience that many psychological researchers might resist including in a conceptual or analytic definition of emotion. From the perspective of the hybrid symbolic/interpretive/meaning-centered view of emotion that we are advancing, emotional experience is not analytically dissoluble from either the conditions that justify it or the social meaning systems that sustain it. This model offers a context-rich, maximally inclusive characterization of emotional experience—one in which elements of sociocultural and linguistic context provide the necessary background against which one can perceive local variations and transformations of the figural center of emotive processes.

The model can provide a useful framework for comparing emotional experiences not just across cultures, but within cultures as well. Horton (2006) has recently used the model to compare "anger" across three groups of individuals: a sample of American adults living in a mixed urban ethnic community, a sample of lay Tibetan refugees living in long-term settlements in India, and a sample of Tibetan Buddhist monks and nuns living in the same Indian communities.

The Tibetan emotion term *lung lang* (Wylie, 1959, gives it as *rlung langs*) is used by all classes of Tibetans living in the exile settlements of South Asia. It has a denotative breadth similar to that of the English "anger," and almost all modern bilingual dictionaries render it in English as simply "to get angry." The Tibetan expression, however, is actually a conceptual composite derived from two lexemes. The term *rlung*, which denotes the wind humor in the Tibetan ethnomedical system, is joined with the intransitive verb *langs pa*, which means "to rise." The combined expression *lung lang* thus invokes an underlying psychophysiological model of the emotion as a rising movement of the wind that animates consciousness, upward from the chest. This underlying model articulates with cultural understandings of the sources of vulnerability to chronic anger, the expected long-term effects, and the phenomenology of the experience of the emotion.

In the following discussion, we compare anger and *lung lang*, using the eight components listed above to reveal a complex pattern of similarities and differences. We begin with the domain of normative social appraisals. We do so because we believe that examining the moral and ethical construals of anger in American culture versus *lung lang* in Tibetan culture provides a crucial background for understanding observations in the other component domains.

Component 5: Normative Social Appraisals

Tibetan and American respondents were asked, "In general, if you think about anger/*lung lang*, do you think of it as a good or a bad thing?" They were then asked, "For what reasons is it good or bad?" Citing views grounded in Mahayana Buddhist ethical and metaphysical thought, Tibetan respondents, both lay and clerical, unequivocally viewed *lung lang* as morally bad. They assimilated it to the sentiment *she dangs* (anger/hatred), one of the "three moral poisons" (*dug gsum*) that are commonly accepted by Buddhists to be the root sources of all suffering for sentient beings. Americans, by contrast, viewed anger as a morally ambivalent, neutral, or natural process. Although Americans recognized the potential harmful effects of anger for others, they were less likely than Tibetans to insist on its harmful effect for the person who experiences it. Indeed, Americans emphasized several positive aspects of anger: It gives one an energy that can be used in a positive way; it can lead to problems' being addressed that might otherwise persist; it can be beneficial to society. Tibetans, by contrast, viewed *lung lang* as a fundamentally destructive sentiment, equally harmful to self and others. They viewed it as arising from an intrinsically flawed motivational state (a desire to harm another sentient being) and generative of ultimately bad results. Reflecting upon metaphysical understandings of *karma*, they insisted upon the symmetry of *lung lang*'s ill effects for all parties involved.

In response to the question "If a person gets angry a lot, over and over again, what kinds of things might happen to that person?", Tibetans and Americans were alike in predicting adverse social and health effects. In fact, the most common metaphorical expressions for the anticipated adverse social effects of chronic anger/*lung lang* in the two cultures were identical. Tibetans and Americans agreed that people will "become more distant" (Tibetan: *thags ring po chags*) from the chronically angry individual. For Tibetans, these predicted social effects tended to involve community-level judgments and processes.

Although norms and expectancies were relatively easy to compare across cultural groups, comparing the two emotions across many of the remaining component domains required a somewhat different procedure. The researcher asked American and Tibetan respondents to discuss in detail a recent situation in which they had felt anger/*lung lang*. The interviewer probed for background information on the circumstances in which an incident occurred, who was involved, and particular judgments and appraisals that might have guided respondents as they felt the emotion. The interview assessed their subjective physical and affective feelings in the situation, as well as their fantasies, actions and impulses, the reactions of bystanders and other individuals in the situation, and the eventual resolution of the situation. Coded and scored, these data provided the basis for systematic tests of differences across sample groups.

Component 1: Somatic Experience

Tibetan *lung lang* and American anger displayed considerable overlap in the domain of somatic experience. Feelings of tension, shaking/nervousness, and heat were reported as common somatic feelings experienced with anger/*lung lang* in all three groups. Americans, however, produced a broader, more detailed range of descriptions of physical feelings associated with anger.

In terms of the long-term anticipated somatic effects of anger/*lung lang*, individuals from both cultures predicted bad health effects for chronically angry individuals. Some predicted effects were common across all three groups (e.g., heart disease, blood pressure problems) while some differed. Many Tibetans predicted that such individuals would suffer from *srog lungs na tsha* (literally, a life-wind illness), a serious condition defined in Tibetan ethnomedical tradition. Several Tibetan respondents also asserted that the chronically angry individuals would be likely to die prematurely. Given the list of illnesses that Americans associate with chronic anger, it likewise would have been logically consistent for Americans to connect chronic anger directly with premature morbidity. Yet no American respondents made this connection.

Component 2: Affective Phenomenology

In contrast with other groups, several individuals from the Tibetan clerical sample described the experience of anger in dissociative terms (e.g., "It felt as though I were drunk or crazy at the time"). When asked, "When that situation had just ended, how did you feel?", Americans were far more likely than were Tibetans to report feelings of lingering anger. Tibetans (particularly the Buddhist clergy) were more likely than Americans to report feeling a host of other dysphoric emotional states at the end of the anger incidents. These included emotions similar to the sentiments lexicalized in English as "regret," "shame," and "unhappiness."

Lingering differences in the encoding and retrieval of memories of experiences of anger/*lung lang* were suggested by the fact that when respondents were asked, "If you think about that situation now, do you still feel a little angry?", Americans were much more likely than Tibetans were to say that they still felt angry when recalling the original situations. Americans did so whether the original feelings of anger were intense or mild. For Tibetans, the likelihood of feeling *lung lang* upon recalling the situation appeared driven by the strength of the feelings of *lung lang* in the original situation. Only in situations where original feeling of *lung lang* had been strong were Tibetan respondents likely to feel anger on recall.

Component 3: Environmental Determinants

The failure to meet obligations and disrespectful treatment by others were among the most common provocations to anger/*lung lang* in both cultures. For Tibetans, the experience of public criticisms and teasing (*kyag kyag*) that

had gotten out of hand played a disproportionate role as provocations. For Americans, a waste of the respondents' time served as a more common provocation. Tibetans reported particular difficulties with outgroup incidents of anger, reflecting tensions between the themselves and members of the local ethnically Indian communities where they how live. Socially, *lung lang* incidents displayed an asymmetric, hierarchical character not apparent in American anger incidents. Lay Tibetan respondents reported no incidents of feeling the emotion toward Buddhist monks or nuns, yet Tibetan monks and nuns readily reported such feelings toward lay individuals.

Component 4: Appraisals of Significance

Respondents from both cultures showed a reluctance to attribute a deliberate intent to harm the other party in the incidents they described. Across all groups, however, respondents rated their feelings of anger/*lung lang* as stronger when they said they had made such an attribution. Cultural differences in at least one variety of secondary appraisals were evident as well. Tibetans, both lay and clergy, were much less likely than Americans to judge the other person's provocative actions as typical or usual for that person. American respondents, by contrast, tended—chronically and spontaneously in open narratives—to connect the other person's provocative behavior in the current situation with the person's past behavior, and to assert that a dispositional pattern existed for the individual to act in that way. This attribution bias is consistent with prior cross-cultural research on the fundamental attribution error (cf. Shweder & Bourne, 1984; Miller, 1984). Collectively, this line of emerging research suggests that Americans make character-based, enduring dispositional attributions far more frequently than members of certain other cultural groups do.

Component 6: Self-Management

Tibetans were much more likely than Americans to believe that anger/*lung lang* can be prevented and even permanently transcended. Furthermore, many were able to point to individuals whom they believed had achieved such a state. Americans, by contrast, doubted whether anger-free living was either possible or desirable. When the hypothetical question "What kind of person would it be who never becomes angry?" was posed, Americans offered responses like these: "People who don't show it and then one day they explode," or "Maybe someone who was severely abused as a child." Some rejected the question outright, saying, for example, "We shouldn't be talking about this like it's a good thing." American respondents thus actively pathologized the hypoexpression of anger; in contrast, the notion that the absence of feelings of anger could be pathological was rejected quite thoroughly by the Tibetans.

Although Americans and Tibetans endorsed different ideal strategies for managing the emotion, in practice they appeared similar in many of the action tendencies and behaviors they reported engaging when the emotional experience had been triggered. Actions ranged from taking time out, practicing patience (a set of specific Tibetan Buddhist techniques), and seeking mediation, to issuing open criticisms or threats and (in some cases) exchanging blows with the other party. Tibetans reported a significantly shorter duration for feeling anger/*lung lang* than Americans in the incidents they described. Tibetan clergy reported significantly less intensity of anger/*lung lang* feelings than Americans or lay Tibetans.

Component 7: Communication and Symbolization

The two cultures accord their members radically different resources for naming, evoking, and manipulating discrete facets of the experience of anger/*lung lang*. If one considers the diverse American social practices in which anger plays a central role (e.g., in spectacle entertainments like *The Jerry Springer Show*, death metal concerts, or professional wrestling; in therapeutic contexts like psychotherapy groups for children of alcoholics or anger management classes; or in diagnostic categories like intermittent explosive disorder), the ambivalent quality of the American view of anger is apparent. These widely differing American cultural practices offer individuals varied opportunities to engage in expressing, channeling, harnessing, directing, and controlling anger.

Tibetans, by contrast, possess a conceptually rich and elaborate tradition of Buddhist ideas and ethical practices—such as the mind-training (*blo sbyong*) tradition—and a set of

cultural institutions and rituals dedicated to the goal of eliminating or transforming *lung lang*. Heavy metal and gangster rap have not caught on with Tibetan settlement youths, among whom performers like the Backstreet Boys and Bryan Adams represent the transgressive edge of global youth culture impingements. Conceptual resources and social practices in Tibetan exile society reflect an unequivocal moral condemnation of anger/*lung lang* and related sentiments. Particularly through the institutional structures and practices of Buddhist monasticism, resources in Tibetan exile society are dedicated to transforming, calming, preventing, and extinguishing *lung lang*, rather than channeling, cultivating, harnessing, expressing and directing it effectively.

Component 8: Social Management

Consistent with the normative ethical rejection of anger in Tibetan culture, during incidents in which anger/*lung lang* was openly expressed and witnesses were present, Tibetan bystanders were more likely to show disapproval of open displays of anger than were American bystanders.

These comparisons have been extended with ethnographic and ethnolinguistic data (see Horton, 2006). We believe that they illustrate the value of adopting a componential, symbolic/interpretive model of emotions when one is seeking to compare emotional experiences across cultural groups.

BITE YOUR TONGUE: THE CASE OF HINDU *LAJJA*

When emotions are analyzed in terms of their constituent components, the issue of translation equivalence for mental states becomes a matter of pattern matching. One tries to determine whether the variables in each of those component slots are linked in similar ways across cultures. One benefit of this approach is that it makes it possible to elucidate the way the abstract conceptual or definitional core of any particular emotion takes on a culture-specific character in different historical traditions and is associated with a somewhat different set of mental states across cultural groups. Consider, for example, the contemporary Hindu conception of *lajja* (or *lajya*), which has been explicated for two communities in South Asia: the Newars of Bhaktapur in Nepal (Parish, 1991), and the Oriyas of Bhubaneswar in Orissa, India (Menon & Shweder, 1994, 1998; Shweder, 2004). *Lajja* is often translated by bilingual informants and dictionaries as though it were equivalent in meaning to the English word "shame"; it is also sometimes translated as though it meant the same thing as the American English words "embarrassment," "shyness," "modesty," or "coyness." Yet, as should become obvious from the following bit of cultural exegesis, the translation of the meaning of mental states across languages and cultures is a far more subtle and hazardous process than many suppose.

For starters, somewhat unlike the meaning of "shame" current in contemporary Anglo-American circles, *lajja* is something one deliberately shows or puts on display the way we might show our "gratitude," "loyalty," or "respect." It is a state of consciousness that has been elevated in South Asia as a supreme virtue, especially for women, and it is routinely exhibited in everyday life—for example, every time a woman covers her face or ducks out of a room to avoid direct affiliation with those members of her family she is supposed to avoid. Parish (1991, p. 324) describes it as an emotion and a moral state. It is by means of their *lajja* that those who are civilized uphold the social order by showing perseverance in the pursuit of their own social role obligations; by displaying respect for the hierarchical arrangement of social privileges and responsibilities; by acting shy, modest, or deferential and not encroaching on the prerogatives of others; or by covering one's face, remaining silent, or lowering one's eyes in the presence of superiors. Like gratitude, loyalty, or respect, *lajja* (which is a way of showing one's civility and commitment to the maintenance of social harmony through displays of respectful restraint) is judged in South Asia to be a very good thing.

While *lajja* may be experienced by both men and women, it is an emotion and a virtue associated with a certain feminine ideal. It is talked about as a lovely ornament worn by women. *Lajja* is the linguistic stem for the name of a local creeper plant (a "touch-me-not"), which is so demure that upon the slightest contact it closes its petals and withdraws into itself. To say of a woman that she is full of *lajja* is a very positive recommendation. Here is one reason why.

Perhaps the most important collective representation of *lajja* in various regions of eastern India is the Tantric icon portraying the mother goddess Kali, brandishing weapons and a decapitated head in her 10 arms, eyes bulging and tongue out, with her foot stepping on the chest of her husband, the god Siva, who is lying on the ground beneath her. Based on interviews with 92 informants in Orissa, India, Menon and Shweder (1994, 1998, 2003) have examined the meaning of this icon and its significance for our understanding of *lajja*.

The gist of the story, as it is narrated by local experts, is that once upon a time the male gods gave a boon to a minor demon, Mahisasura, to the effect that he could only be killed at the hands of a naked female. They thereby turned Mahisasura into a major demon capable terrorizing all the male gods. In order to destroy the demon, the male gods pooled all their energy and powers to create the goddess Durga and arm her with their own weapons. On their behalf, they sent Durga into battle against Mahisasura, but they neglected to tell her about the boon. She fought bravely, but could not kill the demon; he was too strong and clever. In desperation, Durga appealed for guidance from an auspicious goddess, who let her in on the secret. As one informant narrated the story:

> So Durga did as she was advised to [she stripped], and within seconds after Mahisasura saw her [naked], his strength waned and he died under her sword. After killing him a terrible rage entered Durga's mind, and she asked herself, "What kinds of gods are these that give to demons such boons, and apart from that what kind of gods are these that they do not have the honesty to tell me the truth before sending me into battle?"

Durga felt humiliated by her nakedness and by the deceit. She decided that such a world with such gods did not deserve to survive; she took on the form of Kali and went on a mad rampage, devouring every living creature that came in her way. The gods then called on Siva, Kali's husband, to do something to save the world from destruction at the hands of the mother goddess. Siva lay in her path as she came tramping along, enraged. Absorbed in her wild dance of destruction, Kali accidentally stepped on Siva and placed her foot on her husband's chest, an unspeakable act of disrespect. When she looked down and saw what she had done she came back to her senses—in particular to her sense of *lajja*, which she expressed by biting her tongue between her teeth. She reined in her anger and became calm and still. To this day in Orissa, India, "Bite your tongue" is an idiomatic expression for *lajja*, and the biting of the tongue is the facial expression used by women as an iconic apology when they realize or are confronted with the fact that they have failed to uphold social norms.

One moral of the story is that men are incapable of running the world by themselves, even though they are socially dominant. They rely on women to make the world go 'round. Yet in a patriarchal society, men humiliate women by the way they exploit female power, strength, and perseverance. This leads to anger or rage in women, which is highly destructive of everything of value and must be brought under control for the sake of the social order. *Lajja* is a salient ideal in South Asia, because it preserves social harmony by helping women to swallow their rage.

If we decompose *lajja* into its component domains, it becomes apparent just how hazardous it can be to assume that one can render the emotional meanings of others with terms from our received English lexicon for mental states. One is reminded here of Geertz's discussion (1984, p. 130) of the difficulties of translating the Balinese term *lek*. Balinese *lek* seems much like Hindu *lajja*. Geertz notes that *lek* has been variably translated and mistranslated, and that "shame" is the most common attempt. He tries to render it as "stage fright." Hindu *lajja* does not map well onto words like "shame," "embarrassment," "shyness," "modesty," or even "stage fright." An analysis of the constituents of *lajja* helps us see why.

The normative social appraisal of *lajja*, for example, is quite positive. To be full of *lajja* is to possess the virtue of behaving in a civilized manner and in such a way that the social order and its norms are upheld. It is not a neurosis, and it does not connote a reduction in the strength of the ego. Indeed, *lajja* promotes self-esteem. To experience *lajja* is to experience that sense of graceful submission and virtuous, courteous, well-mannered self-control that led Kali to rein in her rage. One might try to render its meaning as "respectful restraint."

The environmental determinants of *lajja* as a sense of one's own virtue and civility are as varied as the set of actions that are dutiful and responsible, given one's station in life in a world

in which all people are highly self-conscious about their social designation (see Geertz, 1984, for a brilliant attempt to capture the dramatic qualities of such a world). They include events that we would find familiar (not being seen naked by the wrong person in the wrong context), as well as many events that might seem alien or strange (never talking directly to one's husband's elder brother or to one's father-in-law; never being in the same room with both one's husband and another male to whom he must defer).

In terms of self-management strategies, South Asian *lajja* may appear at first glance to be similar to American shame or embarrassment. It activates a habit or routine that sometimes results in hiding, covering up, and withdrawing from the scene. Yet what is really being activated by *lajja* is a general habit of respect for social hierarchy and a consciousness of one's social and public responsibilities, which in the context of South Asian norms may call for avoidance, silence, withdrawal, or other deferential, protective, or nonaggressive gestures and actions.

Finally, consider the semantic structure of the American English word "shame" and the Indian Oriya word *lajja* in the minds of particular informants. When middle-class Anglo-American college students are presented with the triad of terms "shame–happiness–anger" and asked, "Which is most different from the other two?", they are most likely to respond that either "happiness" or "shame" is most different from the other two, perhaps on the hedonic grounds that "shame" and "anger" go together (in contrast to "happiness") because they are both unpleasant feelings, or that "happiness" and "anger" go together (in contrast to "shame") because they are both ego-expanding emotions. Neither response is typical of responses in the South Asian community where Menon and Shweder (1994) have worked, where *lajja* (shame?) and *suka* (happiness?) are thought to go together in the triad test, and *raga* (anger?), perceived Tibetan-like as destructive of society, is viewed as the odd emotion out. Here something seems to be amiss in the translation process. Something may well have been amiss in most past attempts to equate emotions across languages and across local cultural worlds (see Lutz, 1985, 1988; Lutz and White, 1986; Rosaldo, 1984; Wierzbicka, 1990, 1992, 1997).

THE SOCIAL AND MORAL CONTEXT OF EMOTIONAL EXPERIENCE

The cases of *lung lang* and *lajja* illustrate the dependence of emotional experience on its social and moral context. To understand *lajja*, for example, one must understand the moral goods that Oriyas strive to achieve. This strategy of viewing emotions against the background of their associated moral goods can be extended to other emotions by using a framework that has proved useful in cultural psychological work. Shweder et al. (1997; see also Shweder, 1990b; Haidt, 2001; Haidt & Joseph, 2004; Haidt et al., 1993; Jensen, 1995, 1998, 2005) suggest that moral goods do not vary randomly from culture to culture, but rather tend to cluster into three sets of related goods or three ethics, known as the ethics of "autonomy," the ethics of "community," and the ethics of "divinity." Cultures rely upon the three ethics to varying degrees. The relative weights of the three ethics within a culture appear to affect the experience and expression of emotion, as well as the way emotions are conceptualized by both local folk and local experts.

In cultures that emphasize an ethic of autonomy, the central object of value is the individual conceptualized as a preference structure. Within that type of cultural world, the most salient moral goods are those that promote the autonomy, freedom, and well-being of the individual, with the result that nothing can be condemned that does not demonstrably harm others, restrict their freedom, or impinge on their rights. Haidt et al. (1993), for example, found that American college students (a population steeped in the ethics of autonomy) responded to stories about violations of food and sexual taboos (e.g., eating one's already dead pet dog) with disgust. Nevertheless, these students felt compelled by the logic of their ethical stance to separate their feelings of disgust from their moral judgments. As a result, they held firmly to the view that their personal emotional reactions did not imply that the actions were wrong. They spoke exclusively in the language of the ethics of autonomy, pointing out that nobody was hurt, and that the people involved had a right to do as they pleased in a private setting. Disgust plays an ambiguous role in such an autonomy-based cultural world (see Rozin, Haidt, & McCauley, Chapter 47, this volume). In such a world, the moral domain is limited to issues of harm, rights, and justice

(Turiel, 1983), and the emotions that are experienced as moral emotions (e.g., anger, sympathy, and guilt) are those that respond to a rather narrow class of ethical goods (e.g., justice, freedom, and the avoidance of harm). In such a world, the focus of ordinary folk and social scientists alike is upon individuals' striving to maximize their personal utility (e.g., Lazarus, 1991; Plutchik, 1980; Stein, Hernandez, & Trabasso, Chapter 35, this volume). Happiness, sadness, pride, and shame are viewed as responses to individual gains and losses, successes and failures. Other moral goods (such as loyalty, duty, and respect for status) that might be linked to the emotions are either lost or undertheorized.

Nevertheless, in many parts of the world the moral domain has been constructed in such a way that it is broader than, or at least different from, an ethic of autonomy. In cultures that emphasize an ethic of community, ontological priority is given to collective entities (the family, guild, clan, community, corporation, or nation), and the central moral goods are those that protect these entities against challenges from without and decay from within (e.g., goods such as loyalty, duty, honor, respectfulness, chastity, modesty, and self-control). In such a world, individual choices (what to wear, whom to marry, how to address others) take on a moral significance (Shweder, Mahapatra, & Miller, 1987), and the successful pursuit of individual goals may even be a cause for embarrassment or shame. Haidt et al. (1993), for example, found that outside of college samples, people of lower socioeconomic status generally thought it was morally wrong to eat one's already dead pet dog or to clean one's toilet with the national flag. Even when these actions were judged to be harmless, they were still seen as objectively disgusting or disrespectful and hence as morally wrong. In a cultural world based on an ethics of community, emotions may exist that are not fully felt by those whose morality is based on an ethics of autonomy. *Lajja* is a clear example, since it is not the type of emotion that will be experienced in a world that sees hierarchy and the exclusive prerogatives of others as unjust or as a form of oppression, rather than as a powerful and legitimate object of admiration and/or respect (Menon & Shweder, 1998).

Similarly, emotions related to honor and heroism may require a strong attachment and dedication to a collectivity or group, for whom the hero lays down his or her life. The *Nāṭyaśāstra*'s otherwise puzzling inclusion of perseverance or heroism as a basic emotion, equal to anger and fear, seems more intelligible against the backdrop of the ethics of community. A James Bond-type hero may display perseverance as he battles to save the "free world," yet we do not think he inspires the same emotional experience in an American audience that an Indian audience savors when a Hindi film hero battles to avenge the death of his father. Many older classic American films raised themes of family honor, but such themes have become less common in recent decades, as the ethics of autonomy has pushed back the ethics of community. Unlike Hindi films, modern American films rarely embed the hero in the thick traditions and obligations of family history. It is a rare movie indeed when we meet the hero's parents.

The third ethic, the ethic of divinity, may have a similar differential activation and enabling effect on emotional life. In the ethic of divinity, people (and sometimes animals) are seen as containing a bit of God (or a god) within them, and the central moral goods are those that protect and dignify the person's inherent divinity. The body is experienced as a temple, so matters that seem to be personal choices within the ethics of autonomy (e.g., food and sexual choices, personal hygiene) become moral and spiritual issues associated with such goods as sanctity, purity, and pollution. Given such an ethic, cleanliness is indeed next to godliness.

Within the terms of a cultural world focused on an ethic of divinity, even love and hate may lose their simple positive versus negative hedonic valences. A modern spiritual guide for Hindus (Yatiswarananda, 1979, p. 187) says that hatred and attachment are both fetters that "degrade the human being, preventing him from rising to his true stature. Both must be renounced." Hindu scriptures contain many stories about people who come to feel disgust at their own greedy and carnal attachments. This disgust helps them to renounce their attachments, and the renunciation floods them with a positive feeling. Of course, the very idea of an emotion connected with renunciation seems paradoxical, since spiritual progress in many Eastern religions is measured by the degree to which one moves beyond the experience of emotions. Only once this paradox is grasped does the mysterious ninth emotion of the *Nāṭyaśāstra*—serenity—begin to make sense, along with its otherwise puzzling textual association with disgust. Serenity or calmness is an important part of Hindu emotional life and emotional discourse precisely because of the centrality of an ethics of divinity in everyday Hindu life. Not surprisingly, it is on no Western lists of basic emotions.

THE MORAL CONTEXT OF EMOTIONAL EXPERIENCE IN ISLAMIC THOUGHT

Emotions can be moralized in various ways. One can formulate *rules* for the experiencing or expression of an emotion; one can make them the subject of *obligations*; one can frame their ethical significance in terms of their *consequences*; and so on. But perhaps the most powerful and pervasive way of moralizing emotions is by linking them with *virtues*—morally good traits or states of character.

The classic Western statement of the relationship between emotions and virtues is Aristotle's formulation:

> . . . fear and confidence and appetite and anger and pity and in general pleasure and pain may be felt both too much and too little, and in both cases not well; but to feel them at the right times, with reference to the right objects, towards the right people, with the right motive, and in the right way, is what is both intermediate and best, and this is characteristic of virtue. (*Nichomachean Ethics*, 1106b)

For Aristotle, emotions are not morally significant per se, but rather with respect to their alignment with ethical imperatives indexed by such phrases as "the right times," "the right objects," and so on. Virtue consists in large part of being "properly affected," which is a product of moral training and habituation.[1]

The great moral and religious traditions have been especially concerned with the moral significance of emotions. Here we briefly examine Islam's long-standing "hypercognition" (Levy, 1984) of the virtues and highly elaborated concern with the development of character, which is still very much alive and kept in the mainstream of everyday Islamic discourse through the foundational texts of the religion (the Qur'an and the *hadith*, or sayings of the Prophet), as well as through the many contemporary popular works of devotional literature that deal with ethics.[2]

An understanding of Islamic morality might usefully begin with the concept of *akhlaq*. For the vast majority of Muslims, morality or ethics *is* simply *akhlaq*, and *akhlaq* is almost universally the translation offered by Muslims for both "morality" and "ethics." This is significant for a study of virtue concepts in Islam because of the etymology of *akhlaq* and its related words. *Akhlaq* comes from the Arabic root *kh-l-q*, which means "to create, shape, make, form, or mold." *Akhlaq* is the plural form of *khuluq*, which denotes "an innate peculiarity, natural disposition, character, or nature." The Arabic translation of "ethics" in the sense of a philosophical discipline is *'ilm al-akhlaq*, or "science of *akhlaq*." Thus, while there are several Arabic words that translate "morality," the predominant one reflects an identification of morality and ethics with human nature as authored or divinely created with a specific *telos*, function, end, or purpose in mind that is definitive of the full realization of one's nature.

Since the time of Muhammad, Muslims have seen Islam as being, in some significant measure, a means for the transformation of emotional life from one of ignorance and backwardness to one appropriate to a divinely created nature. This theme has been elaborated throughout Islamic history by some of its greatest philosophers, some of whom even adopted Aristotelian ways of thinking about emotion and virtue. For example, the great Muslim philosopher al-Ghazali offered a typology of the virtues organized around three cardinal virtues: wisdom, courage, and temperance (Sherif, 1975). Table 25.1 shows al-Ghazali's typology. The translations of some of al-Ghazali's terms may seem somewhat stilted, being literal translations without the nuance that comes with context. But one thing that is immediately striking is how many of the virtues listed here are directly concerned with emotional states and their management (we have put them in **bold** type). This is especially the case with the category connected with "temperance," which is perhaps not surprising, since temperance in general connotes moderation.

al-Ghazali was also a Sufi—a Muslim mystic—and thus was especially concerned with the fusion of the mind and the soul, and with the practices through which perfect Gnostic communion with God could be achieved. Naturally, one of the aspects of the self that must be worked on in pursuit of this goal is

TABLE 25.1. al-Ghazali's Classification of Virtues

Cardinal virtue	Related virtues
Wisdom	Discretion
	Excellence of discernment
	Penetration of thought
	Correctness of opinion
Courage	Magnificence
	Intrepidity
	Greatness of soul
	Endurance
	Gentleness
	Fortitude
	Suppression of anger
	Correct evaluation of self
	Amiability
	Nobility
	Manliness
Temperance	**Modesty**
	Shame
	Remission
	Patience
	Liberality
	Good calculation
	Contentment
	Abstinence
	Cheerfulness
	Joy
	Tenderness of character
	Self-discipline
	Good appearance
	Tranquility
	Honest dealing
	Righteous indignation
	Wit

Note. Virtues directly related to emotional states and their management are given in **bold**.

emotional experience, and elsewhere in his work al-Ghazali elaborates on the need for "disciplining the heart," "breaking desires," and "cultivating the emotions."

There are some surprising, or at least counterintuitive, aspects of al-Ghazali's system. For example, it is probably not obvious (at least to contemporary Western readers) why "gentleness" would be classified under "courage," or why "righteous indignation" would be listed as a form of "temperance." For contemporary American English speakers, "courage" seems to be about the management of fear in the service of (reasonable) action, and indignation hardly seems to be a temperate emotion—though perhaps "righteous" is meant to indicate the right and just kind of moderation required. But this initial opacity is itself an illustration of the entanglement of moral concepts with emotion concepts. Part of the explanation of the classification of gentleness (as courage) and righteous indignation (as temperance) is Islam's conception of itself as a divinely given means for reforming what the early followers of Muhammed perceived to be the immoral, undisciplined ways of the pre-Islamic Bedouin. It becomes easier to promote the virtue of gentleness if it can be persuasively classified as a form of courage.

al-Ghazali's table of the virtues is only one instance of a widespread preoccupation with virtue ethics among Muslim philosophers. Miskawayh, for example, in his treatise *Tahdhib wal-Akhlaq*, offered a somewhat different classification, while other authors contributed in-depth analyses of specific virtues, such as patience (*sabr*) and gratitude (*shukr*) (Miskawayh, 1968). One might well wonder whether these medieval theories have any relevance for the moral thinking and emotion concepts of contemporary Muslims. Joseph (2001) studied the semantic organization of the virtue concepts of contemporary Arab Muslims living in the Bridgeview suburbs of Chicago. Using free-listing and similarity-sorting tasks and hierarchical cluster analysis, he found an intuitively available typology of the virtues in which, again, the emotions play a prominent role. The study discovered seven clusters of virtue concepts, which are listed below with their constituents. Concepts that seem clearly related to emotion are underlined.

Intellectual: wisdom and reason

Patience: optimism and patience

Self-control: strength, self-control, modesty, cleanliness, courage

Forbearance: humility, respect, gentleness, tolerance, forbearance, forgivingness

Attitudes toward others: good neighbor, love of others, good relations with kin, compassion

Altruistic: generosity, helping others, doing good works, sacrifice, gratitude

"Religious" virtues: sincerity, fidelity, truthfulness, trustworthiness, justice, *taqwa*[3]

As with al-Ghazali's philosophical classification of the virtues, the latent or implicit typology revealed here reinforces the observation that many emotion concepts, and the com-

ponents of them described above, are deeply teleological: They reveal the goals or ends toward which human beings are meant to strive by virtue of their supposed divinely authored nature, and at the same time identify defects and excesses that must be corrected if their *teloi* are to be achieved. As our discussion of emotion concepts like *lajja* and *lung lang* has suggested, components such as environmental determinants, appraisals of significance, self-management, social management, and communication are significantly constituted by normative ideals and concrete strategies for aligning emotional experience with ethical constraints.

Virtues, of course, are not themselves emotions. Rather, they constitute one powerful normative language for articulating and thinking about the ethical and moral dimensions of emotional experience.

CONCLUSION: THE CULTURAL PSYCHOLOGY OF THE EMOTIONS RENEWED

As we enter a new era of collaborative research among anthropologists, psychologists, linguists, philosophers, and biologists concerned with similarities and differences in emotional functioning on a worldwide scale, a major goal for the cultural psychology of the emotions will be to decompose the emotions (and the languages of the emotions) into multiple components for the sake of comparative understanding. We hope that by means of this decomposition of the emotions' symbolic structure (and the recognition of the connection between local moral worlds and the social construction of emotional experience), it will be possible to render the meaning of other people's mental states without assimilating them in misleading ways to an a priori set of lexical items available in the language of the researchers. In connection with this chapter, we hope the reader will have become somewhat more alert to all that is potentially lost or misleadingly accrued in the process of translation—as, for example, when Hindu *lajja* is rendered as American "shame," or Tibetan *lung lang* as American "anger."

It is one of the great marvels of life that across languages, cultures, and history, it is possible, with sufficient knowledge, effort, and insight, to truly understand the meanings of other people's emotions and mental states. Yet one must also marvel at one of the great ironies of life—namely, that the process of understanding the consciousness of others can deceptively appear to be far easier than it really is, thereby making it even more difficult to achieve a genuine understanding of "difference." Thus, in the end, this chapter is really a plea for a decomposition of emotional states into their multiple components of cultural meaning (from normative social appraisals to somatic and affective experience and more) and the application of those components of meaning in comparative research. Unless we take that step, we will continue to be prone to the bias that the emotional life of human beings is "basically" the same around the world. The truth may well be that when it comes to "basic emotions," we (medieval Hindus and contemporary secular Anglo-Americans, Tibetan Buddhists living in India and Arab Muslims living in Chicago, aboriginal Pintupis and indigenous Russians, migratory Inuit and settled Balinese) are not only basically alike in many ways, but are also basically different from each other in many significant ways as well.

NOTES

1. For general discussions of Aristotle's views of emotions and virtues, see, for example, Kosman (1980) and Roberts (1989).
2. For some classical and modern treatments of the Islamic concept of akhlaq and of the role of the virtues in morality, see, for example, Busool (1998), Lemu (1997), and Sherif (1975).
3. *Taqwa* is a difficult-to-translate term that roughly means "God-consciousness" and serves for many as the ultimate virtue—the one to which all the others are means.

REFERENCES

Aristotle. (1961). *Nichomachean Ethics* (W. D. Ross, Trans.). Oxford: Oxford University Press.

Busool, A. N. (1998). *Prophet Muhammad's high manners: Theory and practice.* Chicago: Qur'an Society.

D'Andrade, R. G. (1984). Cultural meaning systems. In R. A. Shweder & R. A. LeVine (Eds.), *Culture theory: Essays on mind, self, and emotion* (pp. 88–119). Cambridge, UK: Cambridge University Press.

Dimock, E. C., Gerow, E., Naim, C. M., Ramanujan, A. K., Roadarmel, G., & van Buitenen, J. A. B. (1974). *Literatures of India: An introduction.* Chicago: University of Chicago Press.

Ekman, P. (1980). Biological and cultural contributions to body and facial movement in the expression of emotions. In A. Rorty (Ed.), *Explaining emotions* (pp. 73–101). Berkeley: University of California Press.

Ekman, P. (1984). Expression and the nature of emotion. In K. Scherer & P. Ekman (Eds.), *Approaches to emotion* (pp. 319–343). Hillsdale, NJ: Erlbaum.

Ellsworth, P. (1991). Some implications of cognitive appraisal theories of emotion. In K. Strongman (Ed.), *International review of studies on emotion* (Vol. 1, pp. 143–161). Chichester, UK: Wiley.

Fish, S. (1980). *Is there a textbook in this class?: On the authority of interpretive communities.* Cambridge, MA: Harvard University Press.

Fridja, N. (1986). *The emotions.* Cambridge, UK: Cambridge University Press.

Geertz, C. (1973). *The interpretation of culture.* New York: Basic Books.

Geertz, C. (1984). From the nature point of view. In R. A. Shweder & R. A. Levine (Eds.), *Culture theory: Essays on mind, self, and emotion* (pp. 123–136). Cambridge, UK: Cambridge University Press.

Gnoli, R. (1956). *The aesthetic experience according to Abhinavagupta.* Rome: Istituto Italiano per Il Medio ed Estremo Oriente.

Goodnow, J., Miller, P., & Kessel, F. (Eds.). (1995). *New directions for child development: Vol. 67. Cultural practices as contexts for development.* San Francisco: Jossey-Bass.

Haidt, J. (2001). The emotional dog and its rational tail: A social intuitionist approach to moral judgment. *Psychological Review, 108,* 814–834.

Haidt, J. (2003). The moral emotions. In R. J. Davidson, K. R. Scherer, & H. H. Goldsmith (Eds.), *Handbook of affective sciences* (pp. 852–870). Oxford: Oxford University Press.

Haidt, J., & Joseph, C. (2004, Fall). Intuitive ethics: How innately prepared intuitions generate culturally variable virtues. *Daedalus,* pp. 55–66.

Haidt, J., & Keltner, D. (1999). Culture and facial expression: Open-ended methods find more faces and a gradient of recognition. *Cognition and Emotion, 13,* 225–266.

Haidt, J., Koller, S., & Dias, M. (1993). Affect, culture, and morality, or is it wrong to eat your dog? *Journal of Personality and Social Psychology, 65,* 613–628.

Hejmadi, A., Davidson, R. J., & Rozin, P. (2000). Exploring Hindu Indian emotion expressions: Evidence for accurate recognition by Americans and Indians. *Psychological Science, 11,* 183–187.

Horton, R. (2006). *Refining theory and practice in the cultural psychology of emotion: Tibetan "anger" and the roots of the modern Tibetan commitment to nonviolence.* Unpublished doctoral dissertation, University of Chicago.

Jensen, L. A. (1995). Habits of the heart revisited: Autonomy, community, divinity in adults' moral language. *Qualitative Sociology, 18,* 71–86.

Jensen, L. A. (1998). Different habits, different hearts: The moral languages of the culture war. *American Sociologist, 29,* 83–101.

Jensen, L. A. (2005). *Through two lenses: A cultural-developmental approach to moral psychology.* (Available from Lene Jensen, Department of Psychology, Clark University, Worcester, MA)

Joseph, C. (2001). *The virtues as a cultural domain: A study of Arabic speaking Muslims.* Unpublished doctoral dissertation, University of Chicago.

Keith, A. B. (1924). *The Sanskrit drama.* London: Oxford University Press.

Kirsh, D. (1991). Today the earwig, tomorrow man? *Artificial Intelligence, 47,* 161–184.

Kosman, L. A. (1980). Being properly affected: Virtues and feelings in Aristotle's ethics. In A. Rorty (Ed.), *Essays on Aristotle's ethics* (pp. 103–116). Berkeley: University of California Press.

Lazarus, R. S. (1991). Progress on a cognitive–motivational–relational theory of emotion. *American Psychologist, 46,* 819–834.

Lemu, B. A. (1997). *Islamic tahdhib and akhlaq: Theory and practice.* Chicago: IQRA' International Educational Foundation.

LeVine, R. A. (1984). Properties of culture: An ethnographic view. In R. A. Shweder & R. A. LeVine (Eds.), *Culture theory: Essays on mind, self, and emotion* (pp. 67–87). Cambridge, UK: Cambridge University Press.

Levy, R. I. (1984). Emotion, knowing, and culture. In R. A. Shweder & R. A. LeVine (Eds.), *Culture theory: Essays on mind, self, and emotion* (pp. 214–237). Cambridge, UK: Cambridge University Press.

Lewis, M. (1989). Cultural differences in children's knowledge of emotional scripts. In P. Harris & C. Saarni (Eds.), *Children's understanding of emotion* (pp. 350–374). New York: Cambridge University Press.

Lewis, M., Sullivan, M., & Michalson, L. (1982). The cognitive–emotional fugue. In C. E. Izard, J. Kagen, & R. Zajonc (Eds.), *Emotions, cognition, and behavior* (pp. 264–288). New York: Cambridge University Press.

Lutz, C. (1985). Depression and the translation of emotional worlds. In A. Kleinman & B. Good (Eds.), *Culture and depression: Studies in the anthropology and cross-cultural psychiatry of affect and disorder* (pp. 63–100). Berkeley: University of California Press.

Lutz, C. (1988). *Unnatural emotions: Everyday sentiments on a Micronesian atoll and their challenge to Western theory.* Chicago: University of Chicago Press.

Lutz, C., & White, G. (1986). The anthropology of emotions. *Annual Review of Anthropology, 15,* 405–436.

Markus, H. R., & Kitayama, S. (1991). Culture and the self: Implications for cognition, emotion and motivation. *Psychological Review, 98,* 224–253.

Markus, H. R., Kitayama, S., & Heiman, R. (1998). Culture and "basic" psychological principles. In E. T. Higgins & A. W. Kruglanski (Eds.), *Social psychology: Handbook of basic principles* (pp. 857–913). New York: Guilford Press.

Masson, J. L., & Patwardhan, M. V. (1970). *Aesthetic rapture: The Rasādhyāya of the Nāṭyaśāstra.* Poona, India: Deccan College.

Menon, U., & Shweder, R. A. (1994). Kali's tongue: Cultural psychology and the power of "shame" in Orissa, India." In S. Kitayama & H. Markus (Eds.), *Emotions and culture* (pp. 241–284). Washington, DC: American Psychological Association.

Menon, U., & Shweder, R. A. (1998). The return of the "white man's burden": The encounter between the moral discourse of anthropology and the domestic life of Hindu women. In R. A. Shweder (Ed.), *Welcome to middle age! (and other cultural fictions)* (pp. 139–188). Chicago: University of Chicago Press.

Menon, U., & Shweder, R. A. (2003). Dominating Kali: Hindu family values and Tantric power. In R. F. McDermott & J. J. Kripal (Eds.), *Encountering Kali: In the margins, at the center, in the west* (pp. 80–99). Berkeley: University of California Press.

Mesquita, B. (2003). Emotions as dynamic cultural phenomena. In R. J. Davidson, K. R. Scherer, & H. H. Goldsmith (Eds.), *Handbook of affective sciences* (pp. 871–890). Oxford: Oxford University Press.

Mesquita, B., & Frijda, N. (1992). Cultural variations in emotions: A review. *Psychological Bulletin, 112,* 179–204.

Miller, J. G. (1984). Culture and the development of everyday social explanation. *Journal of Social and Personality Psychology, 46,* 961–978.

Miller, P., Potts, R., Fung, H., Hoogstra, L., & Mintz, J. (1990). Narrative practices and the social construction of self in childhood. *American Ethnologist, 17,* 292–311.

Miskawayh, A. M. (1968). *The refinement of character* (C. Zurayk, Trans.). Beirut: The American University of Beirut.

Nisbett, R. E., & Cohen, D. (1995). *The culture of honor: The psychology of violence in the South.* Boulder, CO: Westview Press.

Nisbett, R. E., & Wilson, T. D. (1977). Telling more than we can know: Verbal reports on mental processes. *Psychological Review, 84*(3), 231–259.

Parish, S. (1991). The sacred mind: Newar cultural representations of mental life and the production of moral consciousness. *Ethos, 19*(3), 313–351.

Plutchik, R. (1980). *Emotion: A psychoevolutionary synthesis.* New York: Harper & Row.

Roberts, R. C. (1989). Aristotle on virtues and emotions. *Philosophical Studies, 56*(3), 293—306.

Rosaldo, M. Z. (1984). Toward an anthropology of self and feeling. In R. A. Shweder & R. A. LeVine (Eds.), *Culture theory: Essays on mind, self, and emotion* (pp. 137–157). Cambridge: Cambridge University Press.

Russell, J. A. (1991). Culture and the categorization of emotions. *Psychological Bulletin, 110*(3), 426–450.

Schechner, R. (1988). *Performance theory*. London: Routledge.

Sherif, M. A. (1975). *Ghazali's theory of virtue*. Albany: State University of New York Press.

Shweder, R. A. (1990a). Cultural psychology: What is it? In J. Stigler, R. A. Shweder, & G. Herdt (Eds.), *Cultural psychology: Essays on comparative human development* (pp. 1–43). New York: Cambridge University Press.

Shweder, R. A. (1990b). In defense of moral realism. *Child Development*, 61, 2060–2068.

Shweder, R. A. (1991). *Thinking through cultures: Expeditions in cultural psychology*. Cambridge, MA: Harvard University Press.

Shweder, R. A. (1994a). Are moral intuitions self-evident truths? *Criminal Justice Ethics*, 13(2), 24–31.

Shweder, R. A. (1994b). You're not sick, you're just in love": Emotion as an interpretive system. In P. Ekman & R. Davidson (Eds.), *The nature of emotions: Fundamental questions* (pp. 32–44). New York: Oxford University Press.

Shweder, R. A. (1996). True ethnography: The lore, the lure and the law. In R. Jessor, A. Colby, & R. A. Shweder (Eds.), *Ethnography and human development: Context and meaning in social inquiry* (pp. 15–52). Chicago: University of Chicago Press.

Shweder, R. A. (1999a). Cultural psychology. In R. A. Wilson & F. Keil (Eds.), *MIT encyclopedia of cognitive sciences* (pp. 211–213). Cambridge, MA: MIT Press.

Shweder, R. A. (1999b). Why cultural psychology? *Ethos*, 27, 62–73.

Shweder, R. A. (2002). The nature of morality: The category of bad acts. *Lahey Clinic Medical Ethics Newsletter*, 9, 6–7.

Shweder, R. A. (2003). Toward a deep cultural psychology of shame. *Social Research*, 70, 1109–1130.

Shweder, R. A. (2004). Deconstructing the emotions for the sake of comparative research. In A. S. R. Manstead, N. Frijda, & A. Fischer (Eds.), *Feelings and emotions: The Amsterdam Symposium* (pp. 81–97). New York: Cambridge University Press.

Shweder, R. A., & Bourne, E. (1984). Does the concept of the person vary cross-culturally? In R. A. Shweder & R. A. LeVine (Eds.), *Culture theory: Essays on mind, self, and emotion* (pp. 158–199). Cambridge, UK: Cambridge University Press.

Shweder, R. A., Goodnow, J., Hatano, G., LeVine, R. A., Markus, H. R., & Miller, P. (1998). The cultural psychology of development: One mind, many mentalities. In W. Damon (Series Ed.) & R. Lerner (Vol.

Ed.), *Handbook of child psychology: Vol. 1. Theoretical models of human development* (5th ed., pp. 865–937). New York: Wiley.

Shweder, R. A., & Haidt, J. (1993). The future of moral psychology: Truth, intuition and the pluralist way. *Psychological Science*, 4, 360–365.

Shweder, R. A., & LeVine, R. A. (Eds.). (1984). *Culture theory: Essays on mind, self and emotion*. Cambridge, UK: Cambridge University Press.

Shweder, R. A., Mahapatra, M., & Miller, J. G. (1987). Culture and moral development. In J. Kagan & S. Lamb (Eds.), *The emergence of morality in young children* (pp. 1–83). Chicago: University of Chicago Press.

Shweder, R. A., Much, N. C., Mahapatra, M., & Park, L. (1997). The "big three" of morality (autonomy, community, divinity) and the "big three" explanations of suffering. In A. M. Brandt & P. Rozin (Eds.), *Morality and health* (pp. 119–169). New York: Routledge.

Stein, N., & Levine, L. J. (1987). Thinking about feelings: The development and organization of emotional knowledge. In R. E. Snow & M. J. Farr (Eds.), *Aptitude, learning and instruction*. Hillsdale, NJ: Erlbaum.

Stigler, J. (1984). Mental abacus: The effect of abacus training on Chinese children's mental calculation. *Cognitive Psychology*, 16, 145–176.

Stigler, J., Chalip, L., & Miller, K. (1986). Culture and mathematics learning. *Review of Research in Education*, 15, 253–306.

Stigler, J., Nusbaum, H., & Chalip, L. (1988). Developmental changes in speed of processing: Central limiting mechanisms on shell transfer. *Child Development*, 59, 1144–1153.

Turiel, E. (1983). *The development of social knowledge: Morality and convention*. Cambridge, UK: Cambridge University Press.

Wierzbicka, A. (Ed.). (1990). The semantics of the emotions [Special issue]. *Australian Journal of Linguistics*, 10(2).

Wierzbicka, A. (1992). Talk about emotions: Semantics, culture and cognition. *Cognition and Emotion*, 6(3–4), 285–319.

Wierzbicka, A. (1997). *Understanding cultures through their key words: English, Russian, Polish, German and Japanese*. New York: Oxford University Press.

Wylie, T. (1959). A standard system of Tibetan transcription. *Harvard Journal of Asiatic Studies*, 22, 261–267.

Yatiswarananda, S. (1979). *Meditation and spiritual life*. Bangalore, India: Sri Ramakrishna Ashrama.

CHAPTER 26

Intergroup Emotions

ELIOT R. SMITH and DIANE M. MACKIE

Current emotion research and theory generally assume that emotions are adaptive and functional, with a strong focus on their functionality at the biological or individual level. This focus has often involved the use of nonsocial "prototype" emotion situations (such as encountering a bear while walking in the woods) as conceptual touchstones. However, social aspects of emotions are increasingly being investigated, following from the recognition that (in humans) emotions involve socially constructed meanings and most often occur in a social context. In this chapter, we describe one specific class of social emotions, which we have called "intergroup emotions"—emotions that arise when people identify with a social group and respond emotionally to events or objects that impinge on the group. After introducing the concept of intergroup emotions, we describe its relationship to theoretical models of emotions in general. We review evidence (from our own work and that of others) regarding the key properties of intergroup emotions, and conclude by summarizing the implications of this conceptualization, both for emotion theory in general and for intergroup relations. As we will

show, this model shares the assumption that emotions are generally functional, but at the level of social groups and not solely at the level of the individual.

WHAT ARE INTERGROUP EMOTIONS?

Group Identification and Depersonalization

The fundamental insight underlying the concept of intergroup emotions derives from a major line of social-psychological theory and research inspired by social identity theory (Tajfel, 1978) and self-categorization theory (Turner, Hogg, Oakes, Reicher, & Wetherell, 1987). This is the idea that important group memberships (those with which people psychologically identify) become a part of a person's identity, along with the person's unique, personal, individuating attributes. The "group" in this conceptualization can be a relatively small number of people who interact face to face (such as a committee or a sports team), or a larger social category of people who do not interact face to face (such as a national, ethnic, gender, or religious identity). Either type of group can serve as a vehicle for social identification and can constitute an important and meaningful aspect of people's identity.

Under circumstances that make a particular group membership or social identity salient, people do not think of themselves as unique individuals, but rather as relatively interchangeable members of the group (a process known as "depersonalization"). This occurs primarily in what is termed an "intergroup situation," one in which social comparisons, competition, or conflict between groups are salient—hence the name of our theoretical model, "intergroup emotions theory" (IET). The consequences of depersonalization are many (for a review, see Oakes, Haslam, & Turner, 1994). People conform to the norms of the activated group in their beliefs, attitudes, and behaviors. They become motivationally aligned with the group, so they see actions that advance the group's interests as desirable and beneficial. They perceive other members of the same group (the "ingroup") as similar to themselves and as likable, and tend to treat them with justice and fairness, while withholding these benefits from members of outgroups.

Tajfel's (1978) original formulation of social identity theory included the idea that when group identification turns a group into an important social identity for an individual, the group takes on emotional significance. However, compared to the cognitive, motivational, and behavioral consequences of group identification, emotional consequences received almost no theoretical or empirical attention until recently in the large literature inspired by social identity theory. This seems odd in view of the obvious fact that intergroup conflicts (whether labor–management disputes, ethnic or religious conflicts, clashes between street gangs and police, or international wars) are regularly characterized by extreme levels of emotion. Both direct participants and bystanders who identify with one of the groups involved but are not directly affected tend to experience strong negative feelings, including anger, fear, resentment, contempt, and so on.

Group Identification as a Basis for Intergroup Emotions

The core concepts underlying IET, introduced by Smith (1993), flow from this theoretical background. The fundamental idea is that

when someone in an intergroup situation is responding in terms of a social identity, objects or events that affect the ingroup will elicit emotional responses, because the group becomes in a real sense an aspect of the person's psychological self (Smith & Henry, 1996). Simply put, under these conditions depersonalization causes the person to react to the world as a group member rather than a unique individual, and thus objects and events have emotional consequences based on the way they relate to the group, not the individual. These group-based emotions can be understood and analyzed in the same way as any others—by using theories of emotions in general, such as appraisal theories. At the heart of IET, therefore, is the distinction between intergroup emotions and the more commonly studied individual-level emotions.

Let us clarify two important points. First, in our conceptualization, intergroup emotions are experienced by individuals (when they identify as members of a group), not by some kind of group mind. Whether intergroup emotions are actually shared across many members of a group is an empirical question, and we present relevant evidence later. Second, we assume that intergroup emotions are generally similar to individual-level emotions in the ways they are experienced, the effects they have on cognitive, perceptual, and motor processes, and so forth. They differ in the ways they are elicited (i.e., by group-relevant rather than personally relevant events) and in their functions (i.e., in regulating group-related or collective behavior rather than purely individual behavior).

As background for IET, the broad idea that intergroup relations and especially intergroup conflict might trigger emotional responses has been investigated since the middle 1980s, with seminal work by Dijker (1987), Gaertner and Dovidio (1986), and Stephan and Stephan (1985). Their research examined the usually negative emotions that people can experience when encountering individual members of outgroups, triggered by cultural differences (e.g., the outgroup member may violate ingroup norms) or by an anxiety-toned desire to make the interaction go smoothly and not to give offense. Research has amply demonstrated that these emotional reactions can occur and can motivate avoidance of outgroup members—demonstrating that avoidance need not necessarily be attributed to sheer antipathy for the outgroup.

From the standpoint of IET, an important question is whether these negative emotions experienced during intergroup contact are individual-level or intergroup emotions. They may often remain at the individual level, if the emotions are generated by perceptions of an outgroup member's *individual* annoying or offensive characteristics, or by one's perceived *personal* lack of knowledge about the outgroup and uncertainty about how to interact appropriately. Still, the definition of a situation as interpersonal or intergroup depends on the way the perceiver thinks about it. So a white person's concern about personally appearing prejudiced in a cross-group interaction would be an individual emotion, but if he or she feels like a representative of the entire white group and is concerned about confirming the stereotype that whites are generally racist, this would be a group-level emotion. A woman's anger at being made to look stupid by a man's cutting comment might be individual, but if she feels that she was made to look stupid *because* she was a woman, the emotion might be group-based. Whether the emotion is individual or intergroup, if repeated encounters with members of a particular group consistently give rise to feelings of annoyance, anxiety, and the like, the emotion may become associated with the mental representation of the group in general (just as for some individuals feelings of anxiety may become associated with dentists in general). As a result, the perceiver might start to experience anxiety, irritation, and so forth, on any thought about or encounter with that particular outgroup.

Intergroup Emotions and the Regulation of Behavior

Just as any emotion motivates people to take specific sorts of action (Frijda, Kuipers, & ter Schure, 1989), intergroup emotions should do the same. Generally, intergroup emotions should lead to actions specifically related to the intergroup situation. Examples include desires to confront or attack an outgroup, to avoid an outgroup, to affiliate with ingroup members, or to support or oppose government policies that have an impact on entire social groups. In this way, intergroup emotions involve appraisals, feelings, and action tendencies that are all at the group level: The individual who identifies with an ingroup may feel that *they* are

threatening *us*; *we* feel angry at *them*; *we* support policies designed to keep *them* from immigrating to our country, cut off their government benefits, and so on. The distinction between individual and intergroup emotions is parallel to that between individual and fraternal (i.e., group-based) relative deprivation (Runciman, 1966). The former is the perception that one is not doing as well as other individuals, and the latter is the perception that one's group is not doing as well as other groups; fraternal deprivation has more potent effects on political and social attitudes.

Two Foci of Intergroup Emotions

The fundamental idea that group identification can lead to group-level emotional responses has both a narrower and a broader version. First, emotions such as anger, fear, disgust, or envy targeted *specifically at an outgroup* may relate to perceptions, prejudiced attitudes, or discriminatory behaviors directed at the outgroup. This line of thinking leads to the important hypothesis that all negatively evaluated outgroups are not treated the same way. For example, outgroups that are targets of anger may be actively attacked or confronted, while outgroups that are targets of disgust may be avoided (see Mackie & Smith, 2002, for relevant evidence). Outgroup-directed emotions need not always be negative, for in some circumstances people feel sympathy or pity toward an outgroup, leading to desires to offer help.

Second, people may experience more general emotional feelings when they are thinking of themselves in terms of a particular social identity. These may include not only emotions directed at outgroups, but also positive or negative ingroup-directed emotions (such as group-based pride or collective guilt) and general affective feelings (such as happiness, anxiety, or irritation) that are based on group membership. Thus each group may have a typical "profile" of emotional tendencies, such that when thinking of themselves in terms of that group membership, people often feel proud, irritated, anxious, and so on, in a pattern that systematically differs from what they would report when thinking of themselves as individuals (Smith, Seger, & Mackie, 2007).

The same distinction between specifically targeted emotions and general feeling states also characterizes individual-level emotions, of course. Individuals at times experience emotions targeted at specific other individuals or objects (e.g., anger at a threatening rival, sympathy for a person in distress), and also possess relatively stable profiles of emotional feelings (e.g., general tendencies to feel angry, anxious, or happy) that relate to their personality characteristics (Watson & Clark, 1992).

RELATION OF IET TO EMOTION THEORY IN GENERAL

Appraisal Theories of Emotion

Our original outline of IET (Smith, 1993) and subsequent work (Mackie, Devos, & Smith, 2000; Mackie, Silver, & Smith, 2004; Smith, 1999) adopted the assumptions of appraisal theories of emotions, because they seemed to us to fit well with our general theoretical structure. Our sole modification to appraisal theory was the assumption that in an intergroup situation, events, objects, and groups are appraised in terms of their implications for the ingroup (not just the individual self). Intergroup emotions are generated by this appraisal process, just as individual-level emotions are generated by appraisals of objects or events that impinge on the individual self (Scherer, 1984; Roseman, 1984). For example, a person who identifies with a group and sees the ingroup as threatened by a powerful outgroup's actions may experience intergroup anxiety or fear. One consequence may be a desire or impulse to avoid or escape from the outgroup. As we have discussed earlier, intergroup emotions may be directed at the ingroup as well. For example, in an intergroup situation that makes social comparisons between groups salient, people may feel collective pride if they believe that their group has succeeded in an important task. Or feelings of collective guilt may result if people appraise their group as having violated important moral principles (Doosje, Branscombe, Spears, & Manstead, 1998).

Although many appraisal theories (e.g., Roseman, 1984) suggest that appraisals cause emotional states, the causal direction is not one-way. Tiedens and Linton (2001) have demonstrated that emotional states influence people's judgments on appraisal-related dimensions; for example, because anxiety is related to the appraisal of uncertainty, people in an anxious state judge events as highly uncertain. Although research has not yet tested this idea, there is every reason to think that this process should operate in the same way with regard to intergroup emotions as it does with individual-level emotions.

Finally, appraisal theories suggest that emotions lead to specific behavioral action tendencies (Frijda, 1986). Intergroup anger may lead to a desire to attack or confront the outgroup, disgust to a desire to avoid, or guilt to a desire to make reparations for the ingroup's actions. By adopting the assumptions of appraisal theories in this way, IET makes predictions about linkages of appraisals of the intergroup situation, specific emotional experiences that people report when they are thinking of themselves as group members, and motives or tendencies to engage in collective (group-level) actions (these predictions have been tested; see, e.g., Mackie et al., 2000).

Core Affect Model of Emotion

However, IET does not necessarily rest solely on appraisal theories. Its fundamental insight is the idea that group identification makes the ingroup part of the psychological self and hence makes group-relevant events or objects able to trigger emotions (just as self-relevant events or objects always do). The process of "triggering" could be described by using the concepts of appraisal theories, as in our earlier presentations of the IET model, or can be described in alternative ways. As an illustration, we consider the "core affect" model (Russell & Barrett, 1999; Russell, 2003; Barrett, 2006). In this model, states of core affect, which are described in a two-dimensional space whose axes are pleasantness and arousal, are fundamental components of all experienced emotions (as well as moods). Core affect can change for many reasons: in response to external stimuli such as pleasant or unpleasant environmental states or positive or negative events, or in response to internal physiological processes such as diurnal rhythms. Core affect is assumed to be subjectively perceptible (as the sense of feeling good, bad, energized, tired, etc.).

An experienced episode of emotion begins with a change of core affect that is consciously noted and attributed to some cause. This attribution makes the difference between just feeling negatively aroused and feeling negatively aroused *because* of a specific event. Attributing affective states to external objects or events is often unproblematic, because of the frequent close co-occurrence in time of external events and the affective reactions that they cause. And these attributions are adaptive, for they allow the perceiver to direct attention and behavior appropriately with regard to the object that is responsible for the feeling. However, the true causes of affective states are not always obvious, so people may make misattributions. A feeling of negative arousal that is actually due to irrelevant reasons (such as unpleasantly hot temperatures) may be misattributed to another person's annoying behavior, leading to the experience of anger, and potentially to aggression (Berkowitz, 1998).

How is an emotional experience labeled as an instance of a specific emotion such as anger, fear, sadness, or guilt? The core affect model holds that various factors—including the core affect and its perceived cause, as well as the situational context, one's overt behaviors, and bodily experiences (such as physiological changes)—become input to a perceptual categorization process in which the experience is categorized as a discrete emotion. Russell (2003) holds that the episode is categorized on the basis of the resemblance between these factors and the person's mental representation of a given emotion's prototype. Barrett's (2006) model differs in postulating not a fixed prototype representation, but a situated reconstruction—an emotion representation that is created online and flexibly tuned to the constraints and goals of the situation. In either case, these mental representations (prototype or situated reconstruction) can and will vary between people because of individual experiences and cultural differences. As a result of the categorization, a person could say that he or she feels *afraid* of the specific object. This labeling process produces the conscious awareness of having an emotional episode.

The core affect model incorporates many substantive predictions of appraisal theories, by postulating that appraisals (the person's interpretations of various aspects of the situation) relate to the process of categorization and self-perception of a specific emotion, rather than seeing appraisals as initiating the emotional state with all its concomitants (subjective feelings, autonomic changes, instrumental actions, etc.). See Russell (2003) for further discussion of relations between the core affect model and appraisal theories.

IET is broadly consistent with the core affect model as well as with appraisal theories. How might the process differ if a group (rather than an individual) identity is at stake? First, let us assume that an event occurs with implications for a person's important group membership, such as a reminder of a nation's colonial past for a person who identifies strongly with the national group. The event may lead to changes in core affect—in this example, negative arousal. Next, the person may search for a cause of that change, perhaps making a misattribution or perhaps correctly attributing it to the event in question. The individual will then draw on his or her affective feelings and attributions, as well as other aspects of the situation, to label the emotion as an instance of guilt—in this case, collective guilt. Desires to take collective actions, such as to make reparations or to offer aid to the victims of the ingroup's actions, may ultimately result. The overall process is not greatly different from that postulated by the core affect model in general; the key differences are that the self-relevance that triggers affective changes in the first place is relevance to a collective (rather than an individual) self, and that the interpretive and categorization processes that follow identify the emotion as an intergroup rather than individual-level emotion. In our example, the perceiver will be readily able to categorize the experience as one of collective guilt, because he or she will have no reason to feel *individually* guilty about ingroup actions that occurred perhaps hundreds of years ago.

Another example illustrates how the process of making an attribution can switch a perceiver between an individual or intergroup emotion. Someone who learns that he or she was not chosen for a much-wanted promotion (and hence feels strong negative arousal) may decide that the reason was his or her boss's ignorance and failure to recognize talent—and may thus experience anger or disappointment at the individual level. Alternatively, the same event may be attributed to minority groups' pressing for affirmative action through the promotion of underqualified minority candidates—in which case the individual's anger may be at the intergroup level (directed at the minority outgroup in general). The action tendencies will be quite different in this case than in the case of individual anger.

One test of whether an emotion is individual or intergroup is to ask this question: Would the emotional response be similar if the same event happened to some *other* ingroup member? For an intergroup emotion, the answer is probably yes; someone might be angered by perceiving that another ingroup member was "victimized" by an unfair affirmative action program, even if the perceiver was personally unaffected. In fact, U.S. Senator Jesse Helms ran a TV ad in his 1990 campaign, showing a pair of white hands crumpling a letter (presumably a rejection letter) while a voice-over stated, "You needed that job, but they had to give it to a minority" (the ad can be viewed at *www.pbs.org/ 30secondcandidate/timeline/years/1990.html*). Evidently the intention was to anger many white viewers at the thought that other members of their ingroup were being treated unfairly.

As this discussion indicates, each of the three main elements of the core affect model can be influenced by a person's group identifications. Core affect changes can arise from events that have an impact on the ingroup and not just the person as an individual (a common example is the way we feel great when our team wins). Attributions concerning the cause of a change in core affect may implicate social groups—for example, when we decide that an outgroup member is treating us unfairly because he or she is prejudiced against our group, not just for idiosyncratic personal reasons. And categorization processes may tell us that we are feeling an emotion as an individual (e.g., individual guilt for some personal action) or as a group member (e.g., collective guilt for an ingroup's historical acts).

EVIDENCE REGARDING INTERGROUP EMOTIONS

In this section, we review evidence regarding the properties of intergroup emotions, especially those that distinguish them from individual emotions. We describe recent studies that offer evidence on four fundamental questions: (1) Are intergroup emotions distinct from the same person's individual emotions? (2) Are they related to group identification? (3) Are they shared among members of the same group? (4) Do they functionally regulate intragroup and intergroup attitudes and behaviors? Our discussion also emphasizes studies that

demonstrate roles for intergroup emotions in several specific phenomena relevant to prejudice and intergroup relations.

Differences from Individual-Level Emotions

One important distinction between intergroup and individual emotions is demonstrated by findings that people can experience emotions on behalf of a group or fellow group members even when the perceivers are not personally affected (e.g., Mackie et al., 2004; Yzerbyt, Dumont, Wigboldus, & Gordijn, 2003). For example, people report feeling unhappy and angry when they learn of an event that harms other members of a situationally salient ingroup, even though the event has no conceivable implications for the perceivers as individuals (Yzerbyt et al., 2003).

In a more direct examination of relations between group and individual-level emotions, we (Smith et al., 2007) had students report the extent to which they generally felt 12 specific emotions, as individuals and as members of several different ingroups (university, national, and political party groups). As might be expected, reports of emotions at the individual and group level were correlated at about the .3 level (e.g., people who reported feeling more angry as individuals also tended to report feeling more angry as group members). Despite this correlation, analyses showed that profiles of group emotions and individual emotions were meaningfully distinct—qualitatively different, not merely differing in the overall level or intensity of individual versus group emotions.

Relationship to Group Identification

For all groups, we (Smith et al., 2007) found a strong relation between positive group emotions and ingroup identification. This makes sense both because group identification is a condition that enables the experience of intergroup emotions, and because positive intergroup emotions such as pride and satisfaction are likely to reward and encourage strong identification with a particular group. The relation of anger at the outgroup to group identification was also positive, consistent with some other research (Kessler & Hollbach, 2005). In contrast, negative group emotions other than outgroup anger (such as guilt, anxiety, and irritation) were more weakly and generally negatively related to identification. The data patterns suggest that the negative correlation is largely due to a type of motivated cognition: Strong group identification leads people to reinterpret and reappraise group-related events to avoid negative feelings (Doosje et al., 1998). An additional process that may contribute to the negative correlation is that negative emotions may motivate a decrease in identification with the particular group.

Social Sharing within an Ingroup

Our results (Smith et al., 2007) also demonstrate that people's group-level emotions are socially shared, and shared more strongly by people who identify more with the group. That is, each social group (Americans, Democrats, university students, etc.) has a specific profile of group-level emotions (e.g., high happiness, low anger, moderate guilt). When reporting their emotions for that particular group, members tend to converge toward the group profile, and those who identify more strongly with the group converge to a greater extent.

Three distinct processes may contribute to this convergence. First, the convergence may be due to "emotional contagion" (Neumann & Strack, 2000), meaning that people tend to take on the emotions displayed by fellow ingroup members with whom they interact. However, the contagion mechanism may be more relevant to face-to-face interacting groups than to the social category groups used in this study. Still, members of larger groups may be affected by emotional contagion when leaders or prototypical members are portrayed in the media and other group members model their emotions. Second, people could be regarded as conforming to ingroup norms with regard to their group-level emotions. It has long been known that when people strongly identify with a group, and their membership is made salient in a specific situation, they tend to conform to group norms or move closer to the group prototype in their behaviors and their attitudes (Hogg & Turner, 1987; Simon & Hamilton, 1994). Although existing research has not considered emotions as a domain in which people move toward a group prototype, the same process should operate with emotions. Finally, a third possibility is that group emotion convergence occurs because thinking about a group membership makes the same key group-relevant events and appraisals salient to different perceivers, so that emotional responses to such events are generally shared among group members. For example, when many individual Americans think of themselves as Americans, the same limited number of events and situations may be salient, such as attacks by militant anti-Americans. So these individuals may all report feeling angry as Americans because they are all responding to more or less the same salient events in more or less the same way. In general, all three of these processes (emotional contagion, conformity to emotion profiles that function as group norms, and shared reactions to salient group-relevant objects or events) may be important causes of group emotion convergence.

Regulation of Intergroup and Intragroup Attitudes/Behaviors

We (Smith et al., 2007) found that group emotions predicted both ingroup-directed and outgroup-directed action tendencies, above and beyond the relatively weak predictive power of individual-level emotions. These studies investigated a wide range of specific action tendencies involving ingroup support and solidarity, outgroup confrontation, and outgroup avoidance. The results suggested that anger at the outgroup (and, to a lesser extent, anger at the ingroup) was the most powerful predictor across all categories of action tendencies. The fact that anger at the outgroup predicts the desire to engage in confrontational behavior would be expected from standard theories relating emotion to action tendencies (Frijda et al., 1989; Mackie et al., 2000). The relation of anger at the outgroup to tendencies to support and affiliate with the ingroup is also consistent with previous research (Kessler & Hollbach, 2005) showing that this group emotion tends to increase ingroup identification. It is less clear why outgroup anger leads to tendencies to avoid the outgroup. We (Smith et al., 2007) suggested that this effect could also be regarded as part of a behavioral regulation strategy: Someone who thinks that being around outgroup members might cause anger may choose to avoid such situations, to minimize those negative feelings and perhaps the danger of acting inappropriately.

The regulation of intergroup behavior by intergroup emotions has also been demonstrated in other research (Maitner, Mackie, & Smith, 2007). Three studies investigated the role of intergroup satisfaction in intergroup conflict. After reading about real acts of aggression committed by an ingroup, participants reported how those actions made them feel and how much they would support similar aggression in the future. In all three studies, experiencing intergroup satisfaction increased support for similar aggression, whereas experiencing intergroup guilt decreased support for similar aggression. Study 2 showed that ingroup identification increased appraisals of the aggression as justified, which increased satisfaction and decreased guilt, and thus increased support for future aggression. Study 3 provided an experimental test of the model: When justification appraisals were manipulated, emotion and support for further aggression changed accordingly. These findings demonstrate conditions under which intergroup satisfaction can influence people's support for their group's aggression, and therefore can facilitate and sustain intergroup conflict.

Yet another aspect of behavioral regulation by intergroup emotions is that if intergroup emotions are functional, successfully implementing an emotion-linked behavioral tendency should allow the emotional feelings to dissipate, whereas impeding the behavioral tendency should intensify the emotion. We (Maitner, Mackie, & Smith, 2006) investigated the emotional consequences of satisfying or thwarting behavioral intentions related to intergroup emotions. Study 1 showed that if an attack on the ingroup produced anger, retaliation increased satisfaction, but if an attack produced fear, retaliation increased fear and guilt. Study 2 showed that outgroup-directed anger instigated via group insult dissipated when the ingroup successfully responded, but was exacerbated by an unsuccessful response. Responding in an emotionally appropriate way was satisfying, but ingroup failure to respond elicited anger directed at the ingroup. Study 3 showed that intergroup guilt following aggression was diminished when the ingroup made reparations, but was exacerbated when the ingroup aggressed again. These findings demonstrate that satisfying behavioral intentions associated with intergroup emotions fulfills a regulatory function.

Besides these examples from our own research, many other studies show that intergroup emotions are related to desires to take actions relevant to group memberships. For example, feelings of fear versus anger as Ameri-

cans experienced in response to the attacks of September 11, 2001, predicted respondents' support for restrictions on civil liberties measured several months later (Skitka, Bauman, & Mullen, 2004). A number of other researchers have demonstrated potent effects of group-level guilt and ingroup-directed anger on action tendencies related to apologizing and making reparations for past group-based offenses (Branscombe & Doosje, 2004; Leach & Iyer, 2006).

Relations of Intergroup Emotions to Prejudice

The theme that intergroup emotions regulate and direct people's attitudes and behaviors toward an outgroup has specific implications for understanding prejudice—a topic that has been the focus of much of our research. We (Miller, Smith, & Mackie, 2004) examined the role of intergroup emotions directed at a specific outgroup (African Americans) in predicting European Americans' prejudice against that group. The studies replicated large bodies of research that show effects of past intergroup contact on reducing prejudice, and of "social dominance orientation" (SDO), a personality-like individual difference reflecting desires to maintain hierarchies of group inequality, on increasing prejudice. The studies also demonstrated that intergroup emotions (self-reports of different emotions experienced by European Americans when encountering or thinking about African Americans) played a major role in mediating both of those effects. Specifically, the effect of past intergroup contact was mediated by positive intergroup emotions, and there was more tentative evidence suggesting mediation by negative emotions. In other words, intergroup contact increases positive emotions and decreases negative emotions, and both of these effects tend to reduce prejudice against the outgroup. The effect of SDO was mediated by both positive and negative intergroup emotions. People high in SDO tended to perceive certain outgroups as threatening, leading to negative emotions such as fear, anger, or resentment, which in turn increased prejudiced attitudes. Those high in SDO also appeared to experience fewer positive emotions such as sympathy or pride with regard to outgroups. Thus intergroup emotions play a key role in mediating the known powerful effects of both intergroup contact and SDO on prejudice.

The Miller et al. (2004) studies also examined stereotypes of the outgroup as an alternative potential mediator, permitting a comparison of their role with that of intergroup emotions. Stereotypes had no significant role in mediating the effects of past intergroup contact, and mediated part of the effect of SDO in one of the two studies. These results fit with the existing empirical and conceptual evidence for the priority of affective (emotional) over cognitive (stereotype beliefs) mediators of effects on prejudice. Pettigrew (1998), for example, noted that effects of intergroup contact on affective dependent variables are generally stronger than effects on measures of stereotypes, underlining the importance of understanding group-level emotions as part of the entire picture of prejudice and intergroup relations.

SUMMARY AND IMPLICATIONS

The perspective described in this chapter rests on the simple yet powerful idea that a social identity based on group identification—not just a biological/individual self—can have emotional implications. Many concrete research hypotheses can be generated by combining this fundamental idea with assumptions based on emotion theory in general, yielding the insight that appraisals of social situations, experienced emotions, and emotion-driven desires for action can all occur at the level of the social group as well as the individual.

Implications for the Study of Intergroup Relations

This set of ideas has several implications for our understanding of prejudice and intergroup relations. First, let us consider the relations of group-based emotions directed at a particular outgroup and the more traditional concept of stereotypes of the outgroup. IET holds that stereotypes are far from irrelevant, for they may feed into appraisals. For example, an outgroup may be seen as hard-working and achievement-oriented, which could lead to its being appraised as a potent threat to the ingroup's economic status in society. Note that, as this example implies, there is no necessary direct relationship between the valence of stereotypes and the valence of people's emotional responses to groups. Positive traits ascribed to the outgroup can lead to negative responses, because emotional responses rest on relational appraisals (what does the outgroup mean for us?) rather than on the valence of the outgroup's characteristics in isolation.

A related point is that, as mentioned previously, IET predicts that people may have qualitatively different types of prejudices against different groups, which may typically lead to different types of actions. We may wish, for example, to discriminate angry/resentful prejudice from anxious/fearful prejudice from disgust-based prejudice. The appraisals that relate to these, the individual-difference characteristics that may moderate them, and the action tendencies that will result may all look strikingly different from one another (see Neuberg & Cottrell, 2002). In this way, IET takes us beyond the simpler idea that prejudice is simply a negative attitude or antipathy toward a group, and toward a more specific, differentiated understanding of prejudice and its causes and effects (Mackie & Smith, 2002).

Finally, thinking about emotions as an important component of people's reactions to outgroups also leads to new conceptions regarding time. In traditional views, stereotypes and prejudiced attitudes toward an outgroup are typically regarded as highly stable (in fact, their resistance to change has been a core issue motivating much research). In contrast, emotions are labile, varying over seconds and minutes. This raises new research questions, such as whether someone's thoughts, evaluations, and behaviors toward an outgroup may differ specifically when the individual is in an emotional state from when he or she is not. At least one study suggests that the answer to this question may be yes (DeSteno, Dasgupta, Bartlett, & Cajdric, 2004).

Implications for Emotion Theory and Research

Just as IET encourages a rethinking of some issues related to prejudice and intergroup behavior, it also has implications for theory and research regarding emotion more generally. Perhaps the most fundamental implication is the idea that emotions pertain to an *identity* and not to a biological individual. An individual typically has multiple identities (including a personal self, many group memberships that may become salient in different circumstances, and possibly several important relational identities as well; Sedikides & Brewer, 2001). Each of these identities is an aspect of the self, so it remains true that, as emotion researchers assume, emotions always implicate the self. In addition, there will generally be a degree of continuity between emotions experienced in different identities (illustrated by the .3 correlations between group-level and individual-level emotions; Smith et al., 2007), perhaps partly due to biologically based differences in emotional reactivity. Still, each identity may have a distinctive emotion profile, both short-term and chronically. This idea has many as-yet-unexplored implications—for example, in regard to emotional vulnerability.

The idea that emotions are rooted in identities also has implications for emotion regulation: Because people can shift rapidly between identities (e.g., between one group membership and another, or between a group-level and an individual-level identity), such shifts can be part of an emotion regulation process (Smith & Mackie, 2006). People may be expected to adopt identities associated with positive group emotions or disidentify from groups associated with negative group emotions, and there is evidence consistent with this idea (Kessler & Hollbach, 2005). Research might productively examine more deta ils of this identity-based emotion regulation strategy, and compare its effectiveness against other strategies on which the literature has focused (Gross, 1998).

IET encourages theorists and researchers to look into social influences (especially influences of the intergroup context) on all aspects of emotional responding. Whereas a number of theorists (e.g., Smith & Lazarus, 1991; Mesquita, 2003) have argued that emotions are inherently relational or interpersonal in nature, our argument is slightly different—that emotions arise from group memberships or collective (not only relational) aspects of the self (Sedikides & Brewer, 2001). Group memberships may influence all aspects of emotional responding: changes in core affect, the causal attributions people make for such changes, the way they categorize their emotional experiences, and the types of actions that they may seek to perform when in emotional states. Investigations of these issues may clarify the ways emotions are functional at the level of groups and not solely individuals. Indeed, such group-level functionality is to be expected, for group

living is evolutionarily ancient in humans as well as related primate species, and it would be surprising indeed if emotions did not play a role in shaping our feelings about and reactions to other ingroup members as well as outgroup members (Cottrell & Neuberg, 2005; Caporael, 1997).

We close with one obvious point. For emotion researchers, intergroup relations offers a powerful venue in which to investigate emotions and their effects. This is a domain of social life in which emotions are often intense, compelling—and highly consequential (with effects including persecutions, pogroms, and genocides). It is also a domain in which, as we argue, emotions are often driven by people's self-identification with important social groups, rather than by their individual selves. Increases in our understanding of emotions themselves, as well as understanding of the social phenomena to which they contribute, may result from an increased focus on social group memberships as bases for emotions.

ACKNOWLEDGMENTS

Preparation of this chapter was supported by Grant No. R01 MH-63762 from the National Institute of Mental Health. We are grateful to Lisa Feldman Barrett, Angie Maitner, and Charlie Seger for helpful comments and assistance.

REFERENCES

Barrett, L. F. (2006). Solving the emotion paradox: Categorization and the experience of emotion. *Personality and Social Psychology Review, 10*(1), 20–46.

Berkowitz, L. (1998). Affective aggression: The role of stress, pain, and negative affect. In R. G. Geen & E. Donnerstein (Eds.), *Human aggression: Theories, research, and implications for social policy* (pp. 49–72). San Diego: Academic Press.

Branscombe, N. R., & Doosje, B. (Eds.). (2004). *Collective guilt: International perspectives*. Cambridge, UK: Cambridge University Press.

Caporael, L. R. (1997). The evolution of truly social cognition: The core configurations model. *Personality and Social Psychology Review, 1*, 276–298.

Cottrell, C. A., & Neuberg, S. L. (2005). Different emotional reactions to different groups: A sociofunctional threat-based approach to "prejudice." *Journal of Personality and Social Psychology, 88*, 770–789.

DeSteno, D., Dasgupta, N., Bartlett, M. Y., & Cajdric, A. (2004). Prejudice from thin air: The effect of emotion on automatic intergroup attitudes. *Psychological Science, 15,* 319–324.

Dijker, A. J. (1987). Emotional reactions to ethnic minorities. *European Journal of Social Psychology, 17,* 305–325.

Doosje, B., Branscombe, N. R., Spears, R., & Manstead, A. S. R. (1998). Guilty by association: When one's group has a negative history. *Journal of Personality and Social Psychology, 75,* 872–886.

Frijda, N. H. (1986). *The emotions.* Cambridge, UK: Cambridge University Press.

Frijda, N. H., Kuipers, P., & ter Schure, E. (1989). Relations among emotion, appraisal, and emotional action readiness. *Journal of Personality and Social Psychology, 57,* 212–228.

Gaertner, S. L., & Dovidio, J. F. (1986). The aversive form of racism. In J. F. Dovidio & S. L. Gaertner (Eds.), *Prejudice, discrimination, and racism* (pp. 61–90). Orlando, FL: Academic Press.

Gross, J. J. (1998). Antecedent- and response-focused emotion regulation: Divergent consequences for experience, expression, and physiology. *Journal of Personality and Social Psychology, 74,* 224–237.

Hogg, M. A., & Turner, J. C. (1987). Intergroup behavior, self-stereotyping and the salience of social categories. *British Journal of Social Psychology, 26,* 325–340.

Kessler, T., & Hollbach, S. (2005). Group-based emotions as determinants of ingroup identification. *Journal of Experimental Social Psychology, 41,* 677–685.

Leach, C. W., & Iyer, A. (2006). Anger and guilt about in-group advantage explain the willingness for political action. *Personality and Social Psychology Bulletin, 32,* 1232–1245.

Mackie, D. M., Devos, T., & Smith, E. R. (2000). Intergroup emotions: Explaining offensive action tendencies in an intergroup context. *Journal of Personality and Social Psychology, 79,* 602–616.

Mackie, D. M., Silver, L. A., & Smith, E. R. (2004). Intergroup emotions: Emotion as an intergroup phenomenon. In L. Z. Tiedens & C. W. Leach (Eds.), *The social life of emotions* (pp. 227–245). Cambridge, UK: Cambridge University Press.

Mackie, D. M., & Smith, E. R. (Eds.). (2002). *From prejudice to intergroup emotions: Differentiated reactions to social groups.* New York: Psychology Press.

Maitner, A. T., Mackie, D. M., & Smith, E. R. (2006). Evidence for the regulatory function of intergroup emotion: Emotional consequences of implemented or impeded intergroup action tendencies. *Journal of Experimental Social Psychology, 42,* 720–726.

Maitner, A. T., Mackie, D. M., & Smith, E. R. (2007). Antecedents and consequences of satisfaction and guilt following ingroup aggression. *Group Processes and Intergroup Relations, 10,* 223–237.

Mesquita, B. (2003). Emotions as dynamic cultural phenomena. In R. J. Davidson, K. R. Scherer, & H. H. Goldsmith (Eds.), *Handbook of affective sciences* (pp. 871–890). New York: Oxford University Press.

Miller, D. A., Smith, E. R., & Mackie, D. M. (2004). Effects of intergroup contact and political predispositions on prejudice: Role of intergroup emotions. *Group Processes and Intergroup Relations, 7,* 221–237.

Neuberg, S. L., & Cottrell, C. A. (2002). Intergroup emotions: A biocultural approach. In D. M. Mackie & E. R. Smith (Eds.), *From prejudice to intergroup emotions: Differentiated reactions to social groups* (pp. 265–283). New York: Psychology Press.

Neumann, R., & Strack, F. (2000). "Mood contagion": The automatic transfer of mood between persons. *Journal of Personality and Social Psychology, 79,* 211–223.

Oakes, P., Haslam, S. A., & Turner, J. C. (1994). *Stereotyping and social reality.* Oxford: Blackwell.

Pettigrew, T. F. (1998). Intergroup contact theory. *Annual Review of Psychology, 49,* 65–85.

Roseman, I. J. (1984). Cognitive determinants of emotion: A structural theory. *Review of Personality and Social Psychology, 5,* 11–36.

Runciman, W. G. (1966). *Relative deprivation and social justice.* Berkeley: University of California Press.

Russell, J. A. (2003). Core affect and the psychological construction of emotion. *Psychological Review, 110,* 145–172.

Russell, J. A., & Barrett, L. F. (1999). Core affect, prototypical emotional episodes, and other things called emotion: Dissecting the elephant. *Journal of Personality and Social Psychology, 76,* 805–819.

Scherer, K. R. (1984). Emotion as a multicomponent process: A model and some cross-cultural data. *Review of Personality and Social Psychology, 5,* 37–63.

Sedikides, C., & Brewer, M. B. (Eds.). (2001). *Individual self, relational self, collective self.* Philadelphia: Psychology Press.

Simon, B., & Hamilton, D. L. (1994). Self-stereotyping and social context: The effects of relative in-group size and in-group status. *Journal of Personality and Social Psychology, 66,* 699–711.

Skitka, L. J., Bauman, C. W., & Mullen, E. (2004). Political tolerance and coming to psychological closure following the September 11, 2001 terrorist attacks: An integrative approach. *Personality and Social Psychology Bulletin, 30,* 743–756.

Smith, C. A., & Lazarus, R. S. (1991). Appraisal components, core relational themes, and the emotions. *Cognition and Emotion, 7,* 233–269.

Smith, E. R. (1993). Social identity and social emotions: Toward new conceptualizations of prejudice. In D. M. Mackie & D. L. Hamilton (Eds.), *Affect, cognition, and stereotyping: Interactive processes in group perception* (pp. 297–315). San Diego: Academic Press.

Smith, E. R. (1999). Affective and cognitive implications of a group becoming part of the self: New models of prejudice and of the self-concept. In D. Abrams & M. A. Hogg (Eds.), *Social identity and social cognition* (pp. 183–196). Oxford: Blackwell.

Smith, E. R., & Henry, S. (1996). An in-group becomes

part of the self: Response time evidence. *Personality and Social Psychology Bulletin, 22,* 635–642.

Smith, E. R., & Mackie, D. M. (2006). It's about time: Intergroup emotions as time-dependent phenomena. In R. Brown & D. Capozza (Eds.), *Social identities: Motivational, emotional, cultural influences* (pp. 173–187). New York: Psychology Press.

Smith, E. R., Seger, C., & Mackie, D. M. (2007). Can emotions be truly group-level? Evidence regarding four conceptual criteria. *Journal of Personality and Social Psychology, 93,* 431–446.

Stephan, W. G., & Stephan, C. W. (1985). Intergroup anxiety. *Journal of Social Issues, 41,* 157–175.

Tajfel, H. (1978). *Differentiation between social groups: Studies in the social psychology of intergroup relations.* London: Academic Press.

Tiedens, L. Z., & Linton, S. (2001). Judgment under emotional certainty and uncertainty: The effects of specific emotions on information processing. *Journal of Personality and Social Psychology, 81,* 973–988.

Turner, J. C., Hogg, M. A., Oakes, P. J., Reicher, S. D., & Wetherell, M. S. (1987). *Rediscovering the social group: A self-categorization theory.* Oxford: Blackwell.

Watson, D., & Clark, L. A. (1992). On traits and temperament: General and specific factors of emotional experience and their relation to the five-factor model. *Journal of Personality, 60,* 441–476.

Yzerbyt, V. Y., Dumont, M., Wigboldus, D., & Gordijn, E. (2003). I feel for us: The impact of categorization and identification on emotions and action tendencies. *British Journal of Social Psychology, 42,* 533–549.

CHAPTER 27

Empathy and Prosocial Behavior

MARTIN L. HOFFMAN

The interest in empathy is an offshoot of research on helping others in distress that took off with the brutal murder of a young woman in Queens, New York in the mid-1960s, in full view of 30 people watching from their apartments. The early research on why bystanders don't help focused on the context and found that the presence of others can interfere with one's helping by activating assumptions of "diffusion of responsibility" ("I'm sure someone called the police") or "pluralistic ignorance" ("No one is doing anything, so it can't be an emergency").

Subsequent research has focused on prosocial motivation, mainly affective empathy. This chapter is concerned with empathy's arousal, development, and contribution to helping. It highlights the role of cognition in arousing empathy, developing it, and shaping it into related emotions (sympathy, empathic anger and feeling of injustice, guilt). It briefly summarizes gender differences and the role of socialization, and points up empathy's limitations. Finally, new directions for research are suggested.

EMPATHY DEFINED

"Empathy" can be defined as an emotional state triggered by another's emotional state or situation, in which one feels what the other feels or would normally be expected to feel in his situation. Since empathic moral issues involve people in distress (pain, danger, poverty), our primary concern is empathic distress. Finally, mature empathy is metacognitive: One is aware of empathizing—that is, one feels distressed but knows this is a response to another's misfortune, not one's own. One also has a sense of how one as well as others might feel in the victim's situation, and awareness that a victim's outward behavior and facial expression may not reflect how he or she feels.

EMPATHY AS A MORAL MOTIVE

One might expect some people to feel pleasure at another's misfortune, and some do under certain conditions, such as anger, dislike, and competition (Hareli & Weiner, 2002). The overwhelming evidence, however, is that most people feel empathically distressed and motivated to help (Hoffman, 1978, 2000; Eisenberg & Miller, 1987): The greater and the more intense their empathic distress is, and the more intense the victim's actual distress is, the quicker they are to help. Moreover, their empathic distress decreases more quickly and they feel better when they help than when they don't. Empathic distress, in short, has all the attributes of a prosocial moral motive.

There are also evolutionary grounds for empathy's being necessary for human survival and therefore part of human nature (Hoffman, 1981). Experiments have suggested empathy's presence in primates (Brothers, 1989), and there is recent evidence that primates and humans share "mirror neurons," which may be the neural substrate for mimicry (Iacoboni & Lenzi, 2002; Iacoboni et al., 2005). Finally, brain scan experiments and clinical studies show empathy's neural basis (Gallese, 2003); identical-twin research supports a hereditary component for empathy (Zahn-Waxler, Robinson, Emde, & Plomin, 1992); and evidence has been found for an empathy precursor at birth (Martin & Clark, 1982; Simner, 1971; Sagi & Hoffman, 1976). It seems reasonable to conclude that human nature is not just egoistic, as long assumed in Western psychology, but includes an empathic moral dimension—a built-in "empathic morality."

MODES OF EMPATHIC AROUSAL

Five empathy-arousing modes have been identified (Hoffman, 1978, 2000). The first three—mimicry, conditioning, and direct association—are automatic and preverbal.

Mimicry

Mimicry was intuitively understood by Adam Smith (1759/1976, p. 4): "The mob, when they are gazing at a dancer on the slack rope, naturally writhe and twist and balance their own bodies as they see him do." It was defined over 100 years later by Lipps (1906) as an innate, involuntary, isomorphic response to another's expression of emotion that occurs in two steps operating in close sequence: One automatically changes one's facial expression, voice, and posture in synchrony with slightest changes in the model's facial, vocal, postural expressions of

feeling; the resulting muscle movements trigger afferent feedback to the brain, producing feelings in observers that match the model's. The discovery of mirror neurons (noted above) suggests a simpler neural substrate: The same neural pattern is involved in feeling an emotion and observing someone else feeling it; therefore, observing another's emotional expression is all it takes to feel it. This may also explain infants' imitating their mothers' facial and hand gestures and the synchronicity of changes in facial expressions between infants and mothers, each responding to affect exhibited by the other (Jaffe, Beebe, Feldstein, Crown, & Jasnow, 2001; Stern, Hofer, Haft, & Dore, 1985).

Conditioning

One can acquire empathic distress as a conditioned response when one's actual distress is paired with another's expression of distress. This is inevitable in mother–infant interactions, as when a mother's distress stiffens her body and is transferred to the infant in the course of physical handling. The mother's facial and verbal expressions of distress then become conditioned stimuli that can subsequently evoke distress in the child even in the absence of physical contact. They can also be generalized, so that facial and verbal signs of distress from *anyone* can arouse distress in the infant.

Direct Association

Direct association does not require prior pairing with another's distress—just having distress feelings that can subsequently be evoked in similar situations by another's expression of distress. For example, having the experience of being separated from one's parents may help one empathize with a friend in the midst of a separation experience.

Empathy aroused by these three modes is passive, involuntary, and based on surface cues; it requires little cognitive processing or awareness that the source of one's distress is someone else's pain. Still, these modes are important, because they enable a primitive form of empathy in young infants. And since they continue beyond infancy, they give empathy an involuntary dimension through life. They are limited, however, because the victim must be present, and they only allow empathy with very simple emotions. These limitations are overcome by language and cognitive development, which support the two remaining modes of empathy arousal.

Verbally Mediated Association

In verbally mediated association, the victim's distress is communicated through language. When it is communicated *only* through language (a letter from the victim or someone else's description of the victim's plight), semantic processing is necessary to mediate the connection between the victim's feeling and the observer's empathic response. This semantic processing may put distance between observer and victim; however, this distancing is reduced when the decoded message enables the observer to construct visual or auditory images of the victim (sad face, blood, cries, moans) and respond empathically to these images through the preverbal modes. When the victim is present, the distancing effect is mitigated by preverbal arousal modes activated directly by the facial and other expressions of distress that accompany the victim's verbal communication. Or one's empathy may first be aroused by the relatively quick-acting preverbal modes and then fine-tuned by semantic processing.

Perspective Taking

The mode of perspective taking is not new. David Hume (1751/1957) thought that because people are constituted similarly and have similar life experiences, imagining oneself in another's place converts the other's situation into mental images that evoke the same feeling in oneself. Adam Smith (1759/1976, p. 261) went further: "By the imagination we place ourselves in the other's situation, we conceive ourselves enduring all the same torments, we enter, as it were, into his body, and become in some measure the same person with him, and thence form some idea of his sensations, and even feel something which, though weaker in degree, is not altogether unlike them." The modern research, begun in the 1950s, reveals three types of perspective taking. The first is self-focused: Imagining that the stimuli impinging on the victim are impinging on oneself evokes an empathic response, which can be enhanced by association with similar events in one's own past. The second is other-focused; it consists of attending to the victim's feelings, current life

condition, and behavior in similar situations. This may be more cognitive than affective empathy, except when the victim is present and affect is recruited from preverbal modes activated by the victim's face, voice, and posture. Research by Batson, Early, and Salvarani (1997) suggests that self-focused perspective-taking arouses more intense empathic distress (including its physiological manifestations), perhaps because self-focused perspective taking is more likely to evoke associations with painful events in one's own past. The third type of perspective taking focuses on both self and other; it consists of co-occurring, parallel processes that benefit from the emotional intensity of self-focused and the sustained attention to the victim of other-focused perspective taking. All three types of perspective taking are under voluntary control and may be drawn out over time, although they can also be triggered immediately on witnessing another's distress or by preverbal modes that draw attention to the victim's distress.

To summarize, empathic distress is a multidetermined and hence reliable prosocial motive (Hoffman, 2000). The arousal modes can operate alone or in any combination. The preverbal modes allow empathic arousal in infants, but continue operating in childhood and add an important involuntary dimension to empathy in adults. The cognitive modes enlarge empathy's scope to include subtle types of distress (e.g., disappointment) and allow empathy with victims who are absent. Multiple modes thus enable one to respond empathically to whatever distress cues are available: Facial, vocal, and postural cues are picked up through mimicry; situational cues through conditioning and association; distress expressed orally, in writing, or by someone else can arouse empathy through the cognitive modes. Multiple modes not only enable but often compel one to respond empathically—instantly, automatically, with or without conscious awareness. Even the cognitive modes, often drawn out and voluntarily controlled, can kick in immediately if one attends closely to the victim.

EMPATHIC OVERAROUSAL

Though empathic distress increases with the intensity of victims' distress it can become so aversive—a condition I have termed "empathic overarousal" (EOA)—that bystanders shift attention to their own distress, leave the victim, or think of other things to turn off the image of the victim (Hoffman, 1978). Strayer (1993) showed 5- to 13-year-olds film clips of distressed children (one child was unjustly punished; another was forcibly separated from family; a disabled child was climbing stairs). Subjects' empathic distress and attention to victims increased with the intensity of victims' distress until the subjects' empathic distress reached the level of victims' distress, after which subjects' focus shifted to themselves. Bandura and Rosenthal (1966) gave adults watching someone being given electric shocks a drug that intensified their empathic distress, which the subjects reduced by engaging in distracting thoughts and attending to lab details.

People are more vulnerable to EOA when they feel unable to reduce victims' distress or to confine empathic distress within a tolerable level of arousal. In one study, nursing trainees new to hospital wards were so empathically overaroused by terminally ill patients that they tried to avoid them; they changed when they found they could improve patients' quality of life (Williams, 1989). Children who exert emotional control and are taught coping strategies for handling anxiety by their parents are less vulnerable to EOA, can keep empathic distress within a tolerable range, and focus more on the victim's than on their own distress (Eisenberg, Fabes, Schaller, Carlo, & Miller, 1991; Fabes, Eisenberg, Karbon, Troyer, & Switzer, 1994; Valiente et al., 2004).

VICARIOUS TRAUMATIZATION OF CLINICIANS

I originally advanced the concept of EOA to explain bystanders' turning away from victims. But this does not hold for certain highly committed people ("witnesses"; see below) or people whose role requires staying and helping (clinicians, nurses, rescue workers). There is a growing literature on trauma clinicians' "compassion fatigue" and "vicarious trauma" (Figley, 1995; Pearlman & Saakvitne, 1995), which I have suggested may be due to EOA (Hoffman, 2000, 2002). I asked 125 clinicians how they felt and coped in their last therapy session with a trauma patient.[1] They reported a lot of EOA, with cognitive disruptions and horrible images, nightmares, and physical symp-

toms, which were often hard to shake off afterward ("I felt the sadness resurge and envelop me . . . almost impossible to concentrate and attend properly," "My neck felt strained, tired, stomach ached, dizzy"). Proximal causes of this EOA were patients' facial, vocal, and postural expressions of pain ("Her tears, description of childhood events, crying, and saying, 'Why don't they understand how what they do affects me?' "); vivid trauma narratives that evoked painful images, especially when associated with clinicians' own past traumas ("I still see the picture I saw as she spoke of the man who hurt her. He looks so malevolent. I imagined her small body size with a grown adult, her grimace of pain"); and some patients' calm demeanor that masked intense suffering ("Oh, my God, he's speaking as though he were describing the weather [drunken father threatened patient and mother with gun]. He's fully dissociated from the feelings, been wounded so badly"). The last example shows that a clinician's empathic distress can be more intense than the patient's actual distress that evoked it.

The coping strategies clinicians reported using to keep EOA under control included various information-processing techniques: gaining distance by imagining that a patient's trauma narrative was just a movie; splitting one's focus so that one was partly an "objective observer"; taking time out by pushing trauma images aside, thinking about other things, and then regrouping; and reminding oneself of past successes. These clinicians also used breathing and other relaxation techniques; consulted with colleagues and supervisors; talked things over with their therapists, spouses, and/or friends ("If I can't get the terrible images out of my mind, I seek coworkers for debriefing"); joined or started self-help groups; did volunteer community service; or started a strenuous exercise routine. One clinician (a witness?—see below) took to political action on behalf of people with her patient's problem ("I pictured that terrified child who had been physically and sexually abused, neglected, being threatened with removal from her foster/adoptive family. I had thoughts of lashing out at the system, and as a result of many such cases, I did work to change it").

Clinicians' EOA may best be viewed as part of an interactive process between intense empathic distress and attempts to control it to maintain their professional focus. That most clinicians stay with patients despite the sometimes intense pain of EOA suggests that trauma therapy is a prosocial moral encounter and should perhaps be added to the five types of such encounters previously identified (Hoffman, 2000). It also suggests that the answer to the question "Does empathy lead to anything more than superficial helping?" (Neuberg et al., 1997), is yes.

EMPATHY DEVELOPMENT

Mature empathy, as noted earlier, has a metacognitive dimension. This requires having a cognitive sense of oneself and others as separate beings with independent inner states (feelings, thoughts, perceptions) that are only partly reflected in outward behavior, and with separate identities and life conditions. Before 4 or 5 years of age, one can empathize, but with little or no metacognitive awareness. This suggested to me that empathy develops along with the development of cognitive self–other concepts, in six stages (Hoffman, 1978, 2000).

Global Empathic Distress: Newborn Reactive Cry

The well-known cry in response to the sound of another's cry by alert, content newborns is not simply imitation of the cry sound or a painful reaction to a noxious stimulus. It is vigorous, intense, and identical to spontaneous cries of infants in actual distress (Sagi & Hoffman, 1976; Simner, 1971). Martin and Clark (1982) found the same thing and also that infants cry less in response to the sound of their own cry (tape-recorded as in the previous cry research) or to a chimpanzee's (which adults find more aversive than human infant cries). This may mean that the cry is an innate, isomorphic response to a conspecific's cry, which presumably survived natural selection. The underlying mechanism could be mimicry, which would suggest that mirror neurons are in place at birth; or it could be conditioning, which newborns are also capable of (Blass, Ganchrow, & Steiner, 1984).

Whatever the cause, newborns respond to another's distress by feeling distressed. This suggests that the newborn cry may be the first instance of empathy without awareness. We might expect it to be undermined by around 6 months, due to the dawning awareness of others as physically separate from oneself. Indeed,

Hay, Nash, and Pedersen (1981) found that 6-month-olds looked at a crying child without immediately crying; in response to prolonged cries, they looked sad and puckered up their lips before starting to cry.

Egocentric Empathic Distress

By 11–12 months, infants do the same as Hay et al.'s (1981) 6-month-olds, but they also whimper and silently watch the victim (Radke-Yarrow & Zahn-Waxler, 1984). Some act, but their actions seem designed to reduce their own distress. A 1-year-old daughter of a student of mine saw a friend fall and cry, stared at the friend, began to cry, then put her thumb in her mouth and buried her head in her mother's lap—as she did when she hurt herself. A parsimonious explanation would be that like most infants her age, she still hadn't fully "graduated" from global empathic distress and remained unclear about the difference between something happening to another and to herself. Distress cues from others still elicited global empathic distress—a fusion of unpleasant feelings and stimuli from the dimly perceived other, her own body, and the situation. She felt upset and sought to comfort herself. I call this type of reaction "egocentric empathic distress," because it is both egocentric (there is a motive to reduce one's own distress) and empathic (it is contingent on another's distress). The contingency is what justifies calling it a precursor of empathic morality.

Quasi-Egocentric Empathic Distress

About 2 months later, still early in the second year, children's empathic crying, whimpering, and staring become less frequent. They begin making helpful advances toward a victim (tentative physical contact such as a pat or touch), which soon give way to more differentiated positive interventions: kissing, hugging, getting someone else to help, physically assisting, advising, reassuring. A 14-month-old boy responded to a crying friend with a sad look, and then gently took the friend's hand and brought him to his own mother, although the friend's mother was present (Hoffman, 1978). A 15-month-old girl "watches a visiting baby who is crying: she watched him carefully, followed him around, kept handing him toys and other items she's fond of (her bottle, a string of beads)" (Radke-Yarrow & Zahn-Waxler,

1984). These actions showed that the children now realized that others were physical entities independent of themselves, though they did not yet grasp that others have their own independent inner states. The actions were clearly designed to help another in distress and thus showed empathic distress operating as a prosocial motive.

Beginning wiht sympathetic distress, what happens when children realize that it is another who in distressed? They may feel relieved and turn away, but the mental image of the victim may still feed their empathic distress. In any case, the evidence is that children generally continue to feel distressed and offer help. The combination of feeling distressed, knowing this feeling is due to another's actual distress, and trying to help suggested to me (Hoffman, 1975a) that empathic distress is changing from a feeling more or less like the victim's feeling to a more reciprocal *feeling of concern for* the victim. This fits how most people report they feel when seeing someone in distress: They feel distressed themselves, but also feel "sympathetic distress" and a desire to help the victim. In any case, from then on through life, empathic distress may include a sympathetic component; people want to help because they feel sorry for the victim, not just to relieve their own empathic distress. *The sympathetic component of empathic distress may be the child's first truly prosocial motive.*

Qualitative-change hypotheses like this are difficult to test. At first there was just anecdotal evidence (Hoffman, 1975a), but three independent investigations have since provided more convincing support: Self–other differentiation (measured indirectly by mirror self–other recognition) predates sympathetic distress and helping (Bischof-Köhler, 1991; Johnson, 1992; Zahn-Waxler, Radke-Yarrow, & King, 1979). Explaining the underlying process is even more difficult (see Hoffman, 1976, 2007, for my attempt to do this). In any case, from now on in this chapter, the term "empathic distress" stands for empathic/sympathetic distress.

Veridical Empathy

Major advances in the self–other concept occur near the end of the second year and continue into the third. Children recognize themselves in a mirror (Lewis & Brooks-Gunn, 1979), revealing a sense of the body as a physical entity

that exists outside one's subjective self and can be seen by others. Children are also becoming aware that others have inner states (thoughts, feelings, desires) independent of their own. This allows more accurate empathy and effective helping behavior. Sarah, age 2 years 3 months, was riding in a car when her cousin became upset at losing his teddy bear. Someone said that it was in the trunk and could be retrieved when they get home. About 10–15 minutes later, when the car approached the house, Sarah said, "Now you can get your bear" (Blum, 1987).

The transition from quasi-egocentric to veridical empathic distress is illustrated by a slightly younger child, 2-year-old David, who brought his own teddy bear to comfort a crying friend. When it didn't work, he paused, ran to the next room, and returned with the friend's teddy bear; the friend hugged it and stopped crying. I suggest that David was cognitively advanced enough to wonder why his teddy didn't stop his friend's crying, to realize that he would want his own teddy and so might his friend, and to remember seeing his friend playing happily with his own teddy in the next room. His behavior may show how cognitively ready children learn from "quasi-egocentric" mistakes and corrective feedback (in David's case, the friend's continued crying) that another's needs may at times differ from theirs, and thus advance to veridical empathy.

Children can now empathize with awareness, take others' perspectives, and help more appropriately. Veridical empathy has the basic features of mature empathy, but becomes more complex with age. The growing understanding of causes, consequences, and correlates of emotions allows one to empathize not only with simple but with subtle distress feelings: Preschoolers can empathize with missing one's parents, older children with mixed feelings or disappointment in one's performance. Adolescents can empathize with another's need for independence, and even with fear of losing face by accepting help. Moreover, from 14 to 20 years of age they learn about many complex, highly specific distresses, such as failing tests important for one's future, parents' divorcing, or having less sexual experience than one's peers (Pasupathi, Staudinger, & Baltes, 2001). Apart from content, children in time realize that their inner self has a reflective part—an "I" that thinks, feels, plans, and remembers—and that other people do too. Their empathy is affected by knowing that people can display emotions not felt and feel emotions not displayed.[2]

Empathic Distress beyond the Situation

At some point, due to the emerging conception of self and others as continuous persons with separate histories and identities, children become aware that others feel joy, anger, sadness, fear, and low esteem not only in a particular situation, but also in their lives. Consequently, they not only respond empathically to another's immediate distress, but also to what they imagine is the other's chronically sad or unpleasant life.

When can they do this? The research on gender and ethnic identity suggests that children's sense of self as coherent, continuous, and stable is hazy until about 6–9 years (Ruble & Martin, 1998). We might expect them to know that others have identities soon afterward. This fits Gnepp and Gould's (1985) research: They described a child's prior experience (bitten by a gerbil or rewarded for an excellent dive), then asked subjects to predict the child's emotional reaction in a related subsequent event (e.g., the previously bitten child's turn to feed the class gerbil). Half the second graders and most of the fifth graders correctly used the prior information (e.g., realized that the previously bitten child would be afraid to feed the gerbil). This suggests that the ages of 7–10 years may be when knowledge of others' lives starts affecting a child's empathic responses. The child can then empathize with people who are chronically ill, emotionally deprived, or hopelessly poor—regardless of the others' immediate state. If they seem sad, knowing that their lives are sad may intensify the child's empathic distress. If they seem happy, the contradiction may stop the child short; rather than feeling empathic joy, he or she may realize that a sad life is a more compelling index of well-being and respond with empathic sadness, or with a mixture of joy and sadness (Szporn, 2001). Mature empathy is thus a response to a network of cues from others' behavior, emotional expression, immediate situation, and life condition.

Empathy for Distressed Groups

It is likely that when children are able to form social concepts and classify people, they can comprehend the plight not only of an individual but also of an entire group or class of people (e.g., victims/survivors of chronic illness, poverty, the Holocaust and other instances of ethnic cleansing, hurricanes and other natural disasters, war, and terrorism). At empathy's highest level, then, one can empathize not only with an individual's but also with a group's distressing life condition ("empathy narrative"). These may go together, as when empathy is generalized from a victim to a group—for example, from the famous picture of a burned baby in a fireman's arms to all of the Oklahoma City bombing victims (media-enhanced empathic distress for a group). Indeed, it may be difficult to empathize with a mass without first empathizing with individual victims; then, realizing that others are in the same boat, one can generalize one's empathy to the group.

As with a single victim, one can empathize with a group's life condition that contradicts its behavior. A student of mine wrote in a term paper:

> When I read accounts of slaves in America who were extremely religious and joyful in religious ceremonies, I feel sort of happy that they were doing something that gave them a sense of joy, even ecstasy, but I am reminded that they were oppressed and this is a false sense of joy or hope in the midst of a distressing, unfair life. I feel happy that they're happy despite being enslaved, but I feel bad for them too because this religious hope or joy is really a false sense of security. It was a bitter irony that they took joy from the promised salvation of this religion, given them by the slave owners whom they wanted to be liberated from.

Empathy for distressed groups has influenced U.S. politics and law (Hoffman, 2006). Harriet Beecher Stowe, whose 1852 novel *Uncle Tom's Cabin* humanized and described the living conditions of slaves in the South, was motivated to write it by intense empathic distress (especially for slave mothers forcibly separated from their children) and by empathic anger at the Fugitive Slave Law, as shown in this summary of an incident from the novel. An affluent, politically uninvolved housewife's deeply felt empathy for slaves she personally knows who "have been abused and oppressed all their lives" motivates her to oppose a new law against giving food, clothes, or shelter to escaping slaves. She argues with her husband, a government official who supports the law, noting that the Bible says people should "feed the hungry, clothe the naked, and comfort the desolate . . . folks don't run away when they are happy, but out of suffering." She becomes intensely opposed to the "shameful, wicked, abominable" law and vows to break it at the earliest opportunity (Stowe, 1852/1938, pp. 99–100).

The book served its purpose: "While no one should underestimate the great services of [William Lloyd] Garrison [and other abolitionists] in their effort to free the slaves it is truth to say that all their efforts were but a drop in the bucket compared with the stir and power that were in Uncle Tom's Cabin. . . . Never in human history has a work devoted to a great cause had such an instantaneous effect" (Ward, 1896). This is surely an exaggeration, but historians do agree that Stowe's book, motivated by empathic distress for slaves, did play a significant role in preparing the country psychologically for emancipation.

Another example is the work of Yale Kamisar, a law professor known by his colleagues as a scholar and enemy of injustice, who combined empathy with a logical, rational approach to constitutional law. His intense empathy for people accused of crimes and bullied into confessing by police interrogation procedures led to articles that gave rise to the 1966 *Miranda v. Arizona* decision, which linked these procedures to the Fifth Amendment's clause against self-incrimination and gave the accused the right to remain silent and have a lawyer present during interrogation. He continued supporting *Miranda* after it was attacked by judges and Congressmen for interfering with criminal investigations (Kamisar, 2000).

HOW EMPATHY IS SHAPED BY CAUSAL ATTRIBUTION

Adults spontaneously attribute causality to events (Weiner, 1985). So do 3-year-olds, who attribute and ask questions about causality, especially regarding people's actions, intentions, and feelings (Hickling & Wellman, 2001). We may therefore assume that most people attribute causality when witnessing someone in distress. If they blame the victim, empathic distress is reduced. Otherwise, depending on the attribution, empathic distress may be transformed in whole or in part into (1) sympathetic distress when the cause is unknown (as in the

developmental transition I have described earlier) or beyond the victim's control (e.g., illness, accident, loss; Weiner, Graham, Stern, & Lawson, 1982); (2) empathy-based guilt when one is the cause, when one's efforts to help have not prevented or alleviated the victim's distress (Batson & Weeks, 1996), or guilt over inaction when one has not tried to help, which would allow victims to suffer and which may have motivated some 1960s civil rights activists (Keniston, 1968) and Germans who saved Jews from Nazis (Oliner & Oliner, 1988); (3) empathic anger when someone else is the cause, even if the victim is distressed and not angry; or (4) empathy over injustice, when there is a discrepancy between a victim's fate and what he or she deserves. The last two of these are central to morality, law, and society, but have been little researched. They deserve further discussion, which now follows.

Empathy over Injustice and Empathic Anger

Humans seem to have a natural preference for fairness, reciprocity, and equity (Peterson & Cary, 2002). From this preference stem the beliefs that people should get what they deserve on the basis of performance, effort, good deeds, and character; that people's legal rights as citizens should be respected; and that punishment should be commensurate with a crime. When one sees others being treated unfairly or unjustly—getting less than they deserve, being deprived of their rights, or being punished too severely—the preference for fairness is violated, and this may transform empathic distress into a feeling of injustice, including motivation to right the wrong.

If a perpetrator is involved, one may feel empathic anger toward the perpetrator, whether this is an individual, a group, the law, or the state. John Stuart Mill (1861/1952, p. 469) connected empathic anger, empathy over injustice, and laws as follows: " . . . the natural feeling of retaliation . . . rendered by intellect and sympathy applicable to . . . those hurts that wound us through wounding others . . . serves as the guardian of justice." This suggests that empathy over injustice and empathic anger may be crucial links between individuals and laws by providing the voices needed to uphold justice, object to people and laws that abuse others, and be ready to punish or change them.[3]

An example of empathy over injustice is Supreme Court Justice Harlan's lone dissent in *Plessy v. Ferguson*, which made "separate but equal" education the law in 1896. His dissent expressed anger at racial discrimination and white dissembling about racial motivations. It was also suffused with empathic concern for suffering black Americans, and clearly linked this to injustice and the law: "We boast of the freedom enjoyed by our people. But it is difficult to reconcile that boast with a law which, practically, puts the brand of servitude and degradation upon a large class of our fellow citizens . . . our equals before the law" (Kluger, 1977, p. 82).

SOCIALIZATION

The role of parent has three facets: discipline, model, and nurture. The research, done mostly in the 1960s through 1990s and reviewed elsewhere (Hoffman, 2000), is here summarized. The discipline method most likely to foster empathy, helping, and guilt over harming others is a type of reasoning called "induction," often used by educated middle-class parents when children harm or are about to harm someone. Inductions direct a child's attention to the other's distress, and may thus engage and strengthen the empathy-arousing modes described above. By highlighting the child's role in causing the other's distress, inductions also contribute to empathy-based guilt. Power-assertive discipline (physical force, threats, commands) is associated with low empathy, helping, and guilt, although it may be needed at times to get children to attend to and process an induction's message.

Parents' behavior outside discipline encounters and their explanations for it provide prosocial models that can reinforce children's empathic proclivity, encourage causal attributions that foster empathic anger and feelings of injustice, and legitimize helping. Examples are empathizing with people in difficult straits (e.g., homeless persons), linking a television protagonist's feeling or situation with the child's own experience, and pointing up similarities among all humans (e.g., feeling sad due to separation and loss). Such behaviors can reinforce and broaden the scope of children's empathic dispositions, especially when someone needs help. Parent prosocial models also make children more receptive to inductions—and more receptive to the competing claims of peers, thus allowing more amicable conflict resolutions. The constructive peer interaction processes that result, as described by Piaget (1932) and others, may add a new and important dimension to the prosocial outcomes of having inductive, nurturant, prosocial models as parents.

GENDER DIFFERENCES

Girls are socialized more than boys to be kind and feel responsible for others' well-being. Girls are thus expected, increasingly with age, to be more empathic and prosocial and less likely to harm others. The research supports these expectations, but in varying degrees (Eisenberg & Fabes, 1998; Hoffman, 2001). Girls show more kindness and consideration for others, and they are more likely to help and share. They are less likely to harm others and more apt to feel guilty when they do. They also obtain higher empathy scores, but this is clearest from self-reports (especially questionnaire measures where it is obvious what is being assessed and responses are under subjects' control). It is not as clear from unobtrusive naturalistic observations or physiological indices of empathy. The empathy findings may thus reflect subjects' conceptions of what boys and girls are supposed to be like, rather than (as usually assumed in self-report research) actual memories of how they feel and behave in various situations.

The latter interpretation receives support from several findings not included in previous reviews. In an early study (Hoffman, 1975b), I found the following in three large samples of fifth and seventh graders and their parents. Girls and their mothers placed a higher value on considering others than did boys and their fathers. More important, girls' and mothers' responses to a story in which a child or an adult wins a contest by cheating and gets away with it showed more concern for the absent victim (the true winner) than did boys and fathers. This suggests that females have more "judicial empathy" (see below) than males. In studies of newborn cries in response to a newborn's cry (see the discussion of global empathic distress above), both Sagi and Hoffman (1976) and Simner (1971) found that female newborns cried more than males. Although the stimulus in both studies was a female cry, it seems unlikely that this would make a difference, given

Martin and Clark's (1982) finding that newborns do not cry more in response to the sound of their own cry. On balance, it seems reasonable to conclude that females are more empathic than males; furthermore, if the newborn-cry findings are replicated, they would suggest a possible biological basis for the difference.

EMPATHY'S LIMITATIONS

Empathy is limited by its fragility, dependence on salience of distress cues, and observers' relationship to victims (Hoffman, 1984, 2000). First, it can be trumped by egoistic motives like fear or personal ambition. Second, as discussed above, it can become so aversive (in EOA) that bystanders shift attention to their own personal distress, leave the victim, or think of other things to turn off the image of the victim. Third, though people empathize with almost anyone in distress, they empathize more with kin, friends, and their own ethnic group (ingroup or familiarity bias); this may not be a problem in small homogeneous groups, except when there are multiple victims and one must make a choice, but it could be a serious problem in complex societies when intergroup rivalry fosters intense empathic anger toward outgroups. Finally, people are far more likely to empathize with victims who are present than with those who are absent ("here-and-now" bias), probably because the preverbal empathy-arousing modes can operate only in response to victims who are present.

Here-and-now bias has been shown experimentally (Batson, Klein, Highberger, & Shaw, 1995; Batson, Batson, Todd, & Brummett, 1995). Posner (1999) views it as a manifestation of the availability heuristic in the courtroom when judges

> give too much weight to vivid immediate impressions and hence pay too much attention to the feelings, interest, and humanity of the parties in the courtroom and too little to absent persons likely to be affected by the decision. . . . You don't need much empathy to be moved by a well represented litigant pleading before you. The challenge to the empathic imagination is to be moved by thinking or reading about the consequences of the litigation for absent—often completely unknown or even unborn—others who will affected by your decision.

Posner calls this "judicial empathy."

An example of here-and-now bias is the highly publicized 1997 trial of a British nanny Louis Woodward (Hoffman, 2000). When the 8-month-old child in Woodward's care was shaken to death, there was widespread condemnation of her and sympathy for the child's parents. After her trial and conviction the empathic tide shifted in her favor (empathy can also be fickle). She became the victim and recipient of widespread empathic distress, partly because of the severe sentence. The retrial judge let her off, saying, " . . . let us bring this matter to a compassionate conclusion." The absent victim was forgotten.

Empathy is important; I view it as the bedrock of prosocial morality and the glue of society. It does have the limitations described above, however, which must be recognized and dealt with to maximize its contribution to moral behavior and social life. I have made suggestions along these lines, which I think would be out of place here (Hoffman, 1987, 2000).

NEW DIRECTIONS FOR RESEARCH

Depth of Empathic Feeling

"Depth of empathic feeling" is a concept that has been overlooked by psychology. It pertains to empathy's intensity, its duration, and the extent to which it penetrates one's motive system and changes behavior. Kaplan (2005, 2006), working on film- and TV-mediated empathic responses to trauma, has introduced two concepts at the extremes of the depth continuum: "empty empathy" and "witnessing." Empty empathy results from brief exposure to trauma images presented in rapid succession and allowing only fleeting empathic responses, each cancelled by the next and thus devoid of motivation to help the victim or victims. In witnessing, exposure to another's trauma overwhelms one with empathic distress; one experiences EOA, but, instead of turning away, is transformed in a prosocial direction—intensely motivated to help, often beyond the immediate situation and at great personal cost. Between the two is vicarious trauma, not only in clinicians but in anyone. Kaplan views all three as manifestations of living in a "trauma culture," constantly bombarded with media images of people worldwide being traumatized by wars and natural disasters (e.g., any night's news on CNN).

Kaplan's witnessing exemplar is Susan Sontag's self-described experience of shock, numbness, and "being changed forever" by images of atrocity at age 12 when first exposed to Holocaust photos. It affected her life work, which often focused on mass suffering, culminating in her last book *Regarding the Pain of Others* (Sontag, 2003). As a second exemplar, I add Harriet Beecher Stowe, cited earlier. Her big change came when her favorite son died:

> It was at his dying bed and at his grave when I learned what a poor slave mother may feel when her child is torn away from her. In those depths of sorrow which seemed to me immeasurable, it was my only prayer to God that such anguish might not be suffered in vain. . . . I felt I could never be consoled for it unless this crushing of my own heart might enable me to work out some great good to others. I allude to this here because I have often felt that much that is in that book [*Uncle Tom's Cabin*] had its roots in the bitter sorrow of that summer. It has left now, I trust, no trace on my mind except a deep compassion for the sorrowful, especially mothers who are separated from their children. (Stowe, 1852)

A third exemplar is Lyndon B. Johnson, who had "deeply felt empathy for the plight of African-Americans since emancipation and continuing through World War II into the 1950s," and for poor "dark-skinned" people in general; his empathy came from personal experience with them (Caro, 2002). At 21, he spent a year teaching Mexican children in South Texas brush country. He visited their homes, saw their poverty, and learned that their fathers were paid slave wages by Anglo farmers.

> "I saw hunger in their eyes and pain in their bodies. Those little brown bodies had so little and needed so much. . . . I could never forget the disappointment in their eyes and the quizzical expression on their faces . . . they seemed to be asking why don't people like me? Why do they hate me because I am brown?" (Quoted in Caro, 2002, p. 720)

Besides teaching, he tried to help them (getting the school board to buy play equipment, arranging games with other schools), but their life circumstances interfered. Johnson's empathic anger and feelings of injustice combined to fuel a promise of future action on their behalf: "I swore then and there that if I ever had a chance to help those underprivileged kids I was going to do it." That, he said later, was

where his dream began of an America "where race, religion, color, and language didn't count against you"—long before he was in a position to act on it.

As a U.S. Senator, Johnson's empathy (plus, of course, his drive, extraordinary persuasive skills, and personal ambition) enabled him, against relentless opposition from Southern colleagues, to get America's first civil rights legislation passed. He later backtracked when his strong civil rights stand conflicted with his goal to become President. But even as President he appointed the first African American to the Supreme Court and won a major addition to the civil rights laws he had obtained in Congress—the Fair Housing Act, which he hoped would supplement school desegregation and end ghettoization of African Americans. His domestic programs were, of course, underfunded because of the Vietnam War. Still, his accomplishments illustrate empathy's potential impact on law (and society) when it is deeply and enduringly felt and allied with the egoistic motives of a person in power, as well as its fragility when it conflicts with those same motives and is opposed by powerful social and political forces.

Although empty empathy may be a strictly film- and TV-mediated phenomenon, witnessing and depth of feeling in general, in real as well as mediated contexts, are worth intensive study by psychologists because of their potential influence on law, society, and history. Laub (1995) has made a start. Due to space limitations, I can only refer you to Laub's and Kaplan's interesting analyses of circumstances favorable to witnessing. As for witnessing's place in empathy theory, it can easily be incorporated into the most advanced stage of empathy development: empathy with a distressed group; or added as a seventh stage. And depth of feeling should perhaps be incorporated into the definition of empathy.

Empathy and Legal Judgment

For decades, legal scholars and philosophers from Kant to Rawls assumed that the law and its underlying justice principles are, and should be, cleansed of emotion so that reason and logic can prevail. Recently, however, legal scholars have acknowledged that emotions inevitably influence not only legal judgments and decisions by jurors and judges, but at times law's very substance. This literature revolves heavily around empathy—for plaintiffs or defendants, individuals or groups. Some, including long-time Supreme Court Justice Blackmun, support empathy's role in law because it takes people's needs into account and provides a humane counterpoint to cold, abstract argumentation; furthermore, it can fill gaps and provide information needed to carry out the full intent and spirit of the law (Greenhouse, 2005; Zipursky, 1990). Others disagree and argue forcefully that except under certain unusual circumstances, reasonable, just, and predictable law cannot tolerate empathy (Bandes, 1996).

I have contributed to this literature and have attempted to broaden empathy's scope by situating the law in an empathy framework; suggesting an empathic base for a sense of justice; giving examples of empathy's contribution to making and changing laws, as well as to judgment and decision making in applying laws; and describing individuals who helped pave the way for repealing unjust laws and initiating fairer ones (Hoffman, 2006). Some of this work has been covered in the earlier discussions of empathy for distressed groups, empathy over injustice, empathy's here-and-now bias in courtrooms, and witnesses who helped prepare the country for passing and changing laws. I now add a discussion of some empathy-related issues and concepts in Supreme Court deliberations.

Empathy Narratives

Empathy contributed importantly to the Court's unanimous 1954 decision in *Brown v. Board of Education*, which overturned separate-but-equal doctrine and made desegregation of public schools the law. Some writers (Henderson, 1985) see the *Brown* decision as "traditional legality" clashing with and ultimately being transformed by empathy. Here's what happened in *Brown* (which, as heard before the Supreme Court, combined cases from South Carolina, Virginia, Delaware, and Washington, D.C. with the actual *Brown* case from Kansas). First, the National Association for the Advancement of Colored People (NAACP) relied less on conventional legal argumentation than on empathy narratives to show how South Carolina's school segregation policy in particular destroyed black children's self-respect, "stamped them with a badge of inferiority . . .

put up road blocks in their minds." The NAACP also employed expert social science testimony, including the famous study of black children who preferred white dolls and labeled black dolls as "bad," to describe the nature of the humiliation and self-hatred caused by segregation. South Carolina's main argument, on separate-but-equal legal grounds, was that the state had made every effort and successfully "wiped out all inequalities between its white and colored schools (equal funding, class size, etc) . . . and this ended the matter under the law" (Henderson, 1985, p. 1598). Their response to the empathy narratives was essentially to blame the victim: If segregation stamped blacks with feeling of inferiority, that was because they chose to construe it that way, and the state lacked the power to deal with psychological reactions to segregation.

The Court's opinion is another example of empathy over injustice—empathy in this case linked to the Constitution's equal protection clause and to the segregation law's having the effect of intensifying harm to victims. Empathy narratives helped the judges clarify a legal concept—namely, showing that the prior, accepted separate-but-equal principle was actually violated. Regarding long-term impact, the image of children in segregated schools preferring white dolls to black dolls still resonates as a lasting symbol of the opinion, despite evidence that black children in Northern states did the same thing. This and other challenges have not diminished the doll study's powerful imagery (see Rich, 2004–2005).

The role of empathy gets more complex when there are conflicting claimants, as in the 1973 case of *Roe v. Wade*. Amicus briefs and oral arguments were loaded with empathy narratives of the horrible effects of unwanted pregnancies not only on women, but also on fetuses, whom antiabortion lawyers humanized by calling them "unborn children, human beings, the true silent majority that needs someone to speak for them and protect their rights." The Justices voted to allow abortion; however, most of them framed the legal issue in terms not of empathy, but of women's broad constitutional rights and the rights and expertise of medical professionals. Subsequent majority opinions undermined *Roe* in bits and pieces (e.g., abolishing federal funding for abortions except when a woman's life was in danger).

Finally, in *Thornburg v. American College of*

Obstretions (1986), a bare majority staved off an amicus attempt by President Reagan to have *Roe* overturned. The Justices were influenced by a National Abortion Rights Action League brief made up largely of letters by women who anonymously told stories of their own abortion experiences, including horror tales of abortions before *Roe* and narratives of women having to leave jobs, quit school, or marry. These were empathy narratives, but with a legal equal protection dimension: The right to choose abortion would enable women to enjoy, like men, the right to fully use the powers of their minds and bodies. The Court's majority opinion acknowledged some of these empathy narratives, and its conclusion linked empathy to legal concepts:

> . . . the Constitution embodies a promise that a certain private sphere of individual liberty will be kept largely beyond the reach of government. That promise extends to women as well as men. Few decisions are more personal and intimate, more properly private, or more basic to individual dignity and autonomy, than a woman's decision—with the guidance of her physician and within the limits specified in *Roe*—whether to end her pregnancy. A woman's right to make that decision freely is fundamental. Any other result . . . would protect inadequately a central part of the sphere of liberty that our law guarantees equally to all. (Henderson, 1985, pp. 1634–1635)

Empathy narratives may thus have contributed to saving abortion rights.

Victim Impact Statements

Lawyers use victim impact statements in criminal trials to call attention to victims' suffering. I have noted earlier how Yale Kamisar's empathy helped criminally accused persons in police interrogations. Empathy also helps criminally accused individuals in court when evidence is presented for their good character and unfortunate life circumstances. Arousing empathy for the *victim*, however, can do the accused great harm. Consider this statement by a woman whose daughter and granddaughter were murdered: "He cries for his mom. He doesn't understand why she doesn't come home. And he cries for his sister Lacie. He comes to me many times during the week and asks, Grandma, do you miss my Lacie. I tell him yes. He says I'm worried about my Lacie" (quoted in Bandes, 1996, p. 361).

Should jurors be allowed to hear such empathy-arousing testimony? The Supreme Court in 1991 ruled that they should. Some legal scholars weigh the pros and cons, and say on balance, yes, mainly to counter "the parade of witnesses who testify to the defendant's character or pressures beyond normal experience that drove him to commit his crime" (Bandes, 1996)—by allowing victims or their families to present the full reality of human suffering the defendant has produced. Others say no, because victim impact statements may appeal to hatred, vengeance, or even bigotry, or may diminish juries' ability to process evidence bearing on defendants' guilt or innocence, and are unnecessary because juries naturally empathize with victims. For a discussion of the issues, see Blume (2003).

Clearly, there is important work to be done regarding empathy and the law. Moreover, if empathy has played a role in emancipation, desegregation, civil rights, and abortion laws, then it surely has something to say about history, culture, and public policy. Not the last word, of course—empathy can't override powerful economic and political forces, ethnic divisions, natural disasters, or personal ambition—but Harriet Beecher Stowe's empathy may have advanced emancipation of slaves by months, and Lyndon B. Johnson's empathy may have advanced civil rights legislation by years. Legal scholarship now recognizes empathy's importance; shouldn't psychology research get on board?

NOTES

1. Tatiana Freedman helped construct the measures and collect the data.
2. Clinicians may hide empathic grief to allow patients to express negative feelings toward the deceased.
3. In multicultural contexts, however, empathic anger may add fuel to interethnic rivalry and contribute to violence.

REFERENCES

Bandes, S. (1996). Empathy, narrative, and victim impact statements. *University of Chicago Law Review, 63,* 361–379.

Bandes, S. A. (1999). *The passions of law.* New York: New York University Press.

Bandura, A., & Rosenthal, T. L. (1966). Vicarious classical conditioning as a function of arousal level. *Journal of Personality and Social Psychology, 3,* 54–62.

Batson, C. D., Batson, J. G., Todd, R. M., & Brummett, B. H. (1995). Empathy and the collective good: Caring for one of the others in a social dilemma. *Journal of Personality and Social Psychology, 68,* 619–631.

Batson, C. D., Early, S., & Salvarani, G. (1997). Perspective taking: Imagining how another feels versus imagining how you would feel. *Personality and Social Psychology Bulletin, 23,* 751–758.

Batson, C. D., Klein, T. R., Highberger, L., & Shaw, L. L. (1995). Immorality from empathy-induced altruism. *Journal of Personality and Social Psychology, 68,* 1042–1054.

Batson, C. D., & Weeks, J. L. (1996). Mood effects of unsuccessful helping: Another test of the empathy–altruism hypothesis. *Personality and Social Psychology Bulletin, 22,* 148–157.

Bischof-Köhler, D. (1991). The development of empathy in infants. In M. Lamb & M. Keller (Eds.), *Infant development: Perspectives from German-speaking countries* (pp. 245–273). Hillsdale, NJ: Erlbaum.

Blass, E. M., Ganchrow, J. R., & Steiner, J. E. (1984). Classical conditioning in newborn humans 2–48 hours of age. *Infant Behavior and Development, 7,* 223–235.

Blum, L. A. (1987). In J. Kagan & S. Lamb (Eds.), *The emergence of morality in young children.* Chicago: University of Chicago Press.

Blume, J. H. (2003). Ten years of *Payne*: Victim impact evidence in capital cases. *Cornell Law Review, 88,* 257–281.

Brothers, L. (1989). A biological perspective on empathy. *American Journal of Psychiatry, 146*(1), 10–19.

Caro, R. A. (2002). *Master of the Senate.* New York: Knopf/Random House.

Eisenberg, N., & Fabes, R. A. (1998). Prosocial development. In W. Damon (Series Ed.) & N. Eisenberg (Vol. Ed.), *Handbook of child psychology: Vol. 3. Social, emotional, and personality development* (5th ed., pp. 701–778). New York: Wiley.

Eisenberg, N., Fabes, R. A., Schaller, M., Carlo, G., & Miller, P. A. (1991). Parental characteristics and practices, and children's emotional responding. *Child Development, 62,* 1393–1408.

Eisenberg, N., & Miller, P. (1987). Relation of empathy to prosocial behavior. *Psychological Bulletin, 101,* 91–119.

Fabes, R. A., Eisenberg, E., Karbon, M., Troyer, D., & Switzer, G. (1994). The relations of children's emotion regulation to their vicarious emotional responses and comforting behaviors. *Child Development, 65,* 1678–1693.

Figley, C. R. (1995). *Coping with secondary traumatic stress disorder in those who treat the traumatized.* New York: Brunner/Mazel.

Gallese, V. (2003). The roots of empathy: The shared manifold hypothesis and the neural basis of intersubjectivity. *Psychopathology, 36,* 171–180.

Gnepp, J. C., & Gould, M. E. (1985). The development

of personalized inferences: Understanding other people's emotional reactions in light of their prior experiences. *Child Development, 56,* 1455–1464.

Greenhouse, L. (2005). *Becoming Justice Blackmun.* New York: Times Books.

Hareli, S., & Weiner, B. (2002). Dislike and envy as antecedents of pleasure at another's misfortune. *Motivation and Emotion, 26,* 257–277.

Hay, D. F., Nash, A., & Pedersen, J. (1981). Responses of six-month-olds to the distress of their peers. *Child Development, 52,* 1071–1075.

Henderson, L. N. (1985). Legality and empathy. *Michigan Law Review, 85,* 1574–1653.

Hickling, A. K., & Wellman, H. M. (2001). Emergence of children's causal explanations and theories: Evidence from everyday conversation. *Developmental Psychology, 37,* 668–683.

Hoffman, M. L. (1975a). Developmental synthesis of affect and cognition and its implications for altruistic motivation. *Developmental Psychology, 11,* 607–622.

Hoffman, M. L. (1975b). Sex differences in moral internalization and values. *Journal of Personality and Social Psychology, 32,* 720–729.

Hoffman, M. L. (1976). Empathy, role-taking, guilt, and the development of altruism. In T. Lickona (Ed.), *Morality: Theory, research, and social issues* (pp. 124–143). New York: Holt, Rinehart & Winston.

Hoffman, M. L. (1978). Empathy: Its development and prosocial implications. In C. B. Keasey (Ed.), *Nebraska Symposium on Motivation* (Vol. 25, pp. 169–218). Lincoln: University of Nebraska Press.

Hoffman, M. L. (1981). Is altruism part of human nature? *Journal of Personality and Social Psychology, 40,* 121–137.

Hoffman, M. L. (1984). Empathy, its limitations, and its role in a comprehensive moral theory. In J. Gewirtz & W. Kurtines (Eds.). *Morality, moral development, and moral behavior* (pp. 283–302). New York: Wiley.

Hoffman, M. L. (1987). The contribution of empathy to justice and moral judgment. In N. Eisenberg & J. Strayer (Eds.), *Empathy and its development* (pp. 47–80). New York: Cambridge University Press.

Hoffman, M. L. (2000). *Empathy and moral development: Implications for caring and justice.* New York: Cambridge University Press.

Hoffman, M. L. (2001). Prosocial behavior and empathy: Developmental processes. In N. Smelser & P. Baltes (Eds.). *International encyclopedia of the social and behavioral sciences* (pp. 12230–12233). Amsterdam: Elsevier.

Hoffman, M. L. (2002). *Empathy and vicarious traumatization in clinicians.* Unpublished manuscript, presented in part to Psychology Department, Simon Fraser University.

Hoffman, M. L. (2006). *Empathy, justice, and the law.* Unpublished manuscript, presented in part at the

Fullerton State University conference on empathy, June 2006.

Hoffman, M. L. (2007). The origins of empathic morality in toddlerhood. In C. A. Brownell & C. B. Kopp (Eds.), *Socioemotional development in the toddler years* (pp. 132–148). New York: Guilford Press.

Hume, D. (1957). *An inquiry concerning the principle of morals.* New York: Liberal Arts Press. (Original work published 1751)

Iacoboni, M., & Lenzi, G. L. (2002). Mirror neurons, the insula, and empathy. *Behavioral and Brain Sciences, 25,* 39–40.

Iacoboni, M., Molnar-Szakacs, I., Gallese, V., Buccino, G., Mazziotta, J. C., & Rizzolatti, G. (2005). Grasping the intentions of others with one's own mirror neuron system. *Public Library of Science Biology, 3,* 529–535.

Jaffe, J., Beebe, B., Feldstein, S., Crown, C. L., & Jasnow, M. D. (2001). Rhythms of dialogue in infancy. *Monographs of the Society for Research in Child Development, 66.*

Johnson, D. B. (1992). Altruistic behavior and the development of the self in infants. *Merrill–Palmer Quarterly, 28,* 379–388.

Kamisar, Y. (2000). Can (did) Congress override Miranda? *Cornell Law Review, 85,* 883–955.

Kaplan, E. A. (2005). *Trauma culture: The politics of terror and loss in media and literature.* New Brunswick, NJ: Rutgers University Press.

Kaplan, E. A. (2006). *Empathy, global trauma, and public feeling: Viewing images of catastrophe.* Unpublished manuscript, presented in part at the Fullerton State University conference on empathy, June 2006.

Keniston, K. (1968). *Young radicals.* New York: Harcourt.

Kluger, R. (1977). *Simple justice: The history of Brown v. Board of Education and Black America's struggle for equality.* New York: Vintage Books.

Laub, D. (1995). Truth and testimony: The process and the struggle. In C. Caruth (Ed.), *Trauma explorations in memory* (pp. 61–75). Baltimore: Johns Hopkins University Press.

Lewis, M., & Brooks-Gunn, J. (1979). *Social cognition and acquisition of self.* New York: Plenum Press.

Lipps, T. (1906). Das wissen von fremden Ichen. *PsycholUntersuch, 1,* 694–722.

Martin, G. B., & Clark, R. D. (1982). Distress crying in neonates: Species and peer specificity. *Developmental Psychology, 18,* 3–9.

Mill, J. S. (1952). Utilitarianism. In R. M. Hutchins (Ed.), *American state papers* (Vol. 43, pp.445–476). Chicago: University of Chicago Press. (Original work published 1861)

Neuberg, S. L., Cialdini, R. B., Brown, S. L., Luce, C., Sagarin, B. J., & Lewis, B. P. (1997). Does empathy lead to anything more than superficial helping? *Journal of Personality and Social Psychology, 73,* 310–316.

Oliner, S. P., & Oliner, P. M. (1988). *The altruistic personality.* New York: Free Press.

Pasupathi, M., Staudinger, U. M., & Baltes, P. B. (2001). Seeds of wisdom: Adolescents' knowledge and judgment about difficult life problems. *Developmental Psychology, 37,* 351–361.

Pearlman, L. A., & Saakvitne, K. W. (1995). *Trauma and the therapist.* New York: Norton.

Peterson, J. M., & Cary, J. (2002). Organizational justice, change anxiety, and acceptance of downsizing. *Motivation and Emotion, 26,* 83–103.

Piaget, J. (1932). *The moral judgment of the child.* New York: Harcourt.

Posner, R. A. (1999). Emotion vs. emotionalism in law. In S. Bandes (Ed.), *The passions of law* (pp. 309–329). New York: New York University Press.

Radke-Yarrow, M., & Zahn-Waxler, C. (1984). Roots, motives, and patterns in children's prosocial behavior. In E. Staub, D. Bar-Tal, J. Karylowski, & J. Reykowski (Eds.), *Development and maintenance of prosocial behavior* (pp. 81–99). New York: Plenum Press.

Rich, W. J. (2004–2005). Betrayal of the children with dolls: The broken promise of constitutional protection for victims of race discrimination. *Cornell Law Review, 90,* 419–442.

Ruble, D. N., & Martin, C. L. (1998). Gender development. In W. Damon (Series Ed.) & N. Eisenberg (Vol. Ed.), *Handbook of child psychology: Vol. 3. Social, emotional, and personality development* (5th ed., pp. 933–1016). New York: Wiley.

Sagi, A., & Hoffman, M. L. (1976). Empathic distress in the newborn. *Developmental Psychology, 12,* 175–176.

Simner, M. L. (1971). Newborn's response to the cry of another infant. *Developmental Psychology, 5,* 136–150.

Smith, A. (1976). *The theory of moral sentiments.* Oxford, UK: Clarendon Press. (Original work published 1759)

Sontag, S. (2003). *Regarding the pain of others.* New York: Farrar, Straus & Giroux.

Stern, D. N., Hofer, L., Haft, W., & Dore, J. (1985). Affect attunement: The sharing of feeling states between mother and infant by means of inter-modal fluency. In T. M. Fields & N. A. Fox (Eds.), *Social perception in infants* (pp. 249–268). Norwood, NJ: Ablex.

Stowe, H. B. (1852, December 16). Letter to Eliza Cabot Follen. Quote in *Harriet Beecher Stowe—mother, reformer.* Retrieved from *xroads.virginia.edu/~ma97/riedy/hbs.html*

Stowe, H. B. (1938). *Uncle Tom's cabin.* New York: Modern Library. (Original work published 1852)

Strayer, J. (1993). Children's concordant emotions and cognitions in response to observed emotions. *Child Development, 64,* 166–201.

Szporn, A. (2001). *The impact of life condition informa-*

tion on empathy. PhD dissertation, New York University.

Valiente, C., Eisenberg, N., Fabes, R. A., Shepard, S., Cumberland, A., & Losoya, S. H. (2004). Prediction of children's empathy-related responding from their effortful control and parents' expressivity. *Developmental Psychology, 40*, 911–926.

Ward, J. H. (1896, August 1). Instant power of *Uncle Tom's Cabin*. *The Washington Post*.

Weiner, B. (1985). "Spontaneous" causal thinking. *Psychological Bulletin, 97*, 74–84.

Weiner, B., Graham, S., Stern, P., & Lawson, M. E. (1982). Using affective cues to infer causal thoughts. *Developmental Psychology, 18*, 278–286.

Williams, C. (1989). Empathy and burnout in male and female helping professionals. *Research in Nursing and Health, 12*, 169–178.

Zahn-Waxler, C., Radke-Yarrow, M., & King, R. (1979). Childrearing and children's prosocial initiations toward victims of distress. *Child Development, 50*, 319–330.

Zahn-Waxler, C., Robinson, J. L., Emde, N. E., & Plomin, R. (1992). The development of empathy in twins. *Developmental Psychology, 28*, 1038–1047.

Zipursky, B. (1990). *Deshaney* and the jurisprudence of compassion. *New York University Law Review, 65*, 1101–1147.

CHAPTER 28

Social Functions of Emotion

AGNETA H. FISCHER and ANTONY S. R. MANSTEAD

The classic perspective on the functionality of emotions is that they increase the probability of an individual's survival and/or reproductive success. The general argument is that emotions are functional in the sense that they help the individual to address or overcome problems (e.g., Frijda, 1986; Lazarus, 1991; Levenson, 1999; Tooby & Cosmides, Chapter 8, this volume). Fear is an obvious example. Fear of predators or enemies is clearly adaptive in the sense that individuals who have the capacity to experience such fear are more likely to be vigilant and avoidant, and thereby to escape the threat of predation or attack (e.g., Tooby & Cosmides, Chapter 8, this volume; Öhman, Chapter 44, this volume).

In this chapter, we shift the attentional focus to functional analyses of emotion that emphasize "social survival"—that is, our human capacity to build social bonds and to address and overcome social problems such as social exclusion or loss of power (see, e.g., Barrett, 1995; Fridlund, 1994; Griffiths & Scarantino, in press; Keltner & Haidt, 1999). The central argument we advance in this chapter is that emo-

tions are important to social survival because the emotions we experience and express help us (1) to form and maintain social relationships, and (2) to establish or maintain a social position relative to others. In developing this argument, we discuss these social functions of emotions at two levels: interpersonal and group (cf. Keltner & Haidt, 1999).

The idea that emotions serve social functions assumes that emotions evolved in a social context and should therefore be beneficial for social survival. Social survival is a complex endeavor because it requires a balance between cooperation on the one hand, and competition on the other. We humans are social creatures who need social bonds in order to thrive (Baumeister & Leary, 1995): We affiliate with others; work together with others; and seek harmony, closeness, and love. The importance of social bonds is illustrated by research on social isolation, showing that this leads not only to poorer health and well-being, but also to inhibited development of various social, emotional, and cognitive skills (Williams, 2001). However, we also set ourselves goals other than

456

being accepted and liked by others: We want to avoid others who pose a threat to us, to win at the expense of others, to exert control over others, or to enhance our social power or social standing. These social goals are achieved not merely by cooperation and affiliation; they typically require distancing ourselves from others, or even competing with others or other groups.

Emotions play an important role in realizing these two types of goals, and we therefore draw a broad distinction between two general social functions of emotion. The first is helping an individual or group to establish or maintain cooperative and harmonious relations with other individuals or other social groups. We refer to this as the "affiliation function" of emotion. The second social function of emotions is helping the individual or group to differentiate the self or group from others and to compete with these others for social status or power. We refer to this second function as the "social distancing function" of emotion. Each of these general social functions of emotion operates at both the interpersonal and group levels.

Perhaps unsurprisingly, an analysis of emotion's social functions encounters many of the same conceptual problems as does an account of its general functions (Gross & John, 2002; Oatley & Jenkins, 1992; Parrott, 2001, 2002). Emotions generally have social effects (e.g., Fischer, Manstead, & Zaalberg, 2003; Fridlund, 1994; Philippot, Feldman, & Coats, 1999; Tiedens & Leach, 2004), whether or not these effects are intended. However, these social effects are not equivalent to social functions. We argue that the social functions of emotion should be inferred from the social-relational goals inherent in the prototypical appraisals and action tendencies of a given emotion (e.g., Roseman, Wiest, & Swartz, 1994). For example, the social distancing function can be observed in anger (seeking to change another person), contempt (seeking to exclude another person), or social fear (seeking distance from another person); embarrassment (admitting that one has transgressed), love (wanting to be close to the loved one), happiness (sharing positive experiences with others), or sadness (seeking help and support from others) serve the affiliation function.

Whereas social functions derive from these social-relational goals, the social effects of an emotion may vary with the specific features of the social and cultural context (e.g., Fischer et al., 2003; Parkinson, 2005; Parkinson, Fischer, & Manstead, 2005). Let us take anger as an example. The social function of anger is to impose change upon another person and this can be achieved through a variety of expressions, such as beating, scolding, threatening, or criticizing. The effects of any given expression of anger may vary, however, depending on the object of or the reason for one's anger. For example, whereas scolding a friend because he or she forgot an appointment might elicit an apology on the part of the friend, the selfsame expression of anger toward a superior who forgot an appointment might evoke an aggressive response. This does not mean that the social function of anger is to elicit an apology in the first case and an aggressive response in the second, but that the wish to impose change has different effects in different social contexts. In the same vein, the effects of emotion may differ with cultural contexts, depending on what is considered a typical or appropriate expression in a specific situation. A further complication is that the short-term effects of an emotion expression may differ from its long-term effects. The superior who failed to keep an appointment may become aggressive as an initial reaction to one's anger, but may later regret this reaction and acknowledge that he or she was at fault. Thus the anger may serve its social function of effecting change in the other person in the long run, even if it does not have this effect in the short run (see Fischer & Roseman, 2007).

Finally, the idea that emotions have social functions does not imply that emotions are always socially functional—that is, that they always have the social effects that would be predicted on the basis of their relational goals. Anger, jealousy, and contempt can clearly be socially dysfunctional: Rather than changing others' behaviors, they may irreparably damage the relationship between individuals or between groups, without achieving anything in terms of social control or social standing. The same applies to positive emotions such as pride, happiness, or love: Rather than strengthening social bonds, they may cause others to take exception to what they regard as inappropriate in the circumstances. Social dysfunctionality is especially likely to occur if the social impact of one's emotions is not taken into account or if inappropriate appraisals of the social context are made (e.g., Evers, Fischer, Rodriguez Mosquera, & Manstead, 2004; Manstead & Fischer, 2001; Parrott, 2001).

This is supported by research on emotion regulation and emotional intelligence (e.g., Lopes, Salovey, Coté, & Beers, 2005), which has shown an association between the ability to regulate one's emotions and the quality of social interactions, as rated by individuals and their peers. In other words, the social functionality of emotion in a particular set of circumstances is not a given, but rather depends on the way in which the person assesses his or her concerns or goals in relation to others' concerns or goals, and regulates his or her emotions accordingly. Becoming too jealous, getting angry too often, or feeling contempt for many people is unlikely to be socially functional. Below we further explore the social functions of emotion at the interpersonal and group levels.

INTERPERSONAL RELATIONS

The Affiliation Function of Emotions

Social relations vary in emotional tone from love affairs to work relations, but any relationship between two persons involves a degree of emotion. The amount of emotion that is experienced and expressed, however, is closely related to the nature of the relationship, reflecting an important function of emotions at the interpersonal level: Emotions enable us to form and maintain long-term and intimate relationships by promoting closeness and harmony, and thus avoiding social isolation. This function can be inferred from the social consequences or effects of emotions on the development of a relationship.

There are various lines of research providing evidence for this function. Research by Clark and colleagues (see Clark, Fitness, & Brissette, 2004, for an overview) has shown that emotions are more often experienced and expressed in communal or intimate relations than in other type of relations. In the same vein, Gottman and Levenson (2002) found in their analysis of marital conflicts that an absence of affect during such conflicts is a predictor of subsequent divorce. Emotional involvement is characteristic not only of marital or romantic relationships, but of intimate or communal relations in general. For example, Barrett, Robin, Pietromonaco, and Eyssell (1998) found that the degree of expression of specific emotions, as reported in a diary, was highly correlated with the closeness of the interaction partner.

Research on social sharing has also repeatedly shown that people share their emotions mostly with family and friends (Rimé, Philippot, Boca, & Mesquita, 1992). From this we can conclude that the experience, expression, and sharing of emotion are important ingredients in the development of intimate relations, although the evidence to date does not warrant any conclusions about the causal direction of this relationship.

The idea that intimate or communal relations are characterized by positive and negative emotions can be taken a step further by arguing that in the context of intimate relations one might start experiencing emotions similar to one's partner's emotions, because one shares the emotional perspective of the other and appraises the emotional situation in the same way. This is nicely demonstrated by Anderson, Keltner, and John (2003), who found that dating partners and college roommates became emotionally more similar over the course of a year. This emotional convergence effect applied to both positive and negative emotional reactions to events and could not be explained by increased similarity in personality variables.

Emotional convergence can also be observed at the micro level, as reported in studies of mimicry and emotional contagion (e.g., Chartrand & Bargh, 1999; Bavelas, Black, Lemery, & Mullett, 1986; Dimberg, 1982; Hatfield, Cacioppo, & Rapson, 1992; Lunquist & Dimberg, 1995; Provine, 1992). "Mimicry" refers to the automatic processing of others' nonverbal displays, resulting in similar nonverbal displays by oneself, whereas "emotional contagion" refers to a tendency for emotional experience to be influenced by others' emotions. Hatfield et al. (1992) have suggested that the function of mimicry is to synchronize and coordinate the interaction, and thereby to facilitate mutual involvement and emotional closeness. Indeed, both mimicry and emotional contagion can be seen as reflecting the affiliation function of emotions in relations, especially in view of the fact that both increase when individuals identify with another person, or when they feel more empathy toward that person (Eisenberg, 2000; Fischer, Rotteveel, Evers, & Manstead, 2004; Sonnby-Borgström, 2002).

It should be noted that the results of these various studies suggest not only that positive emotions serve a "social glue" function, but also that negative emotions can reflect and possibly contribute to the intimacy of the relationship. Studies of crying, for example, have shown that people cry more often in the company of partners or intimates than in the company of strangers (Vingerhoets & Becht, 1997). These data are consistent with the idea that the social function of sadness (i.e., crying) is a display of powerlessness and a call for support, because such support is most likely to be forthcoming in relations with intimates. Moreover, studies of anger and aggression have shown that people, especially women, are most often angry with intimates (Fischer, Rodriguez, van Vianen, & Manstead, 2004; Kring, 2000), and that physical aggression also occurs more often within intimate relationships, especially on the part of women (Archer, 2000). Also relevant is the fact that studies of guilt (Baumeister, Stillwell, & Heatherton, 1994; Tangney, Miller, Flicker, & Barlow, 1996) have shown that this emotion is mostly expressed within valued relationships in which people have high respect for the other. Similarly, research on regret shows that interpersonal regret motivates efforts to undo the harm done in the context of a relationship (Zeelenberg, Van der Pligt, & Manstead, 1998).

Collectively, this research shows that communal relations are characterized by the experience and expression of positive and negative emotions, often leading to emotional convergence, which further contributes to the intimacy of and harmony within the relationship. This is consistent with Reis and Shaver's (1988) intimacy model, in which intimacy is seen as being enhanced by reciprocal self-disclosure and partner responsiveness (see Laurenceau, Barrett, & Pietromonaco, 1998). Again, this does not imply that there are no limits to the intensity or frequency with which some negative emotions can be expressed. For example, whereas Gottman and Levenson (2002) have shown that an absence of affect predicts divorce in the longer term, they have also found that the expression of negative emotions between marital partners during conflict is predictive of divorce in the shorter term. Marriages characterized by conflicts in which one partner expresses contempt for the other are also likely to lead to a divorce. Clearly, emotions such as hatred and contempt do not serve an affiliation function.

Although emotions generally serve affiliation goals in the context of intimate relations, the promotion of these goals can also be observed in emotional interactions between strangers. Smiling people, for example, are

more likely to be ascribed positive traits, such as kindness, humor, intelligence, or honesty, than are their nonsmiling counterparts (Hess, Beaupré, & Cheung, 2002; Reis et al., 1990). Krumhuber and colleagues (Krumhuber & Kappas, 2005; Krumhuber, Manstead, & Kappas, 2007) have shown that these positive effects of smiling are moderated by the perceived genuineness of the smile. Self-conscious emotions, like guilt, have also been shown to result in more cooperation on the part of the guilty participant in interactions between strangers. Displays of embarrassment, guilt, shame, and regret serve to show and acknowledge that one has acted stupidly, transgressed a rule, hurt another person, or made a mistake. Such displays have been shown to evoke sympathy, positive evaluations, or helpful behavior in others (Keltner & Buswell, 1976, 1997; Ketelaar & Au, 2003; Miller, 2004), but also increased perceptions of trustworthiness and conscientiousness—as, for example in studies on blushing, a typical signal of embarrassment (de Jong, 1999). Interestingly, embarrassment displays tend to elicit more positive evaluations on a "warmth" dimension, but not on a "competence" dimension (Semin & Manstead, 1981), consistent with the notion that this emotion serves an affiliation function.

Another way in which emotions are socially functional in the context of interpersonal relations is that the communication of emotions can direct the behavior of others, by warning them of impending danger or reassuring them that the environment is safe. A classic example of this function is provided by research on social referencing (e.g., Sorce, Emde, Campos, & Klinnert, 1985), showing that 12-month-olds are less likely to proceed in an uncertain and possibly unsafe situation when their mothers display a negative expression, and more likely to proceed when the mothers display a positive expression. Thus emotions have informational value for others, in that they communicate our concerns and our appraisals of the current situation. However, we suggest that both the extent to which these signals are sent and the extent to which they are acted on by receivers is a function of their relational closeness, and that a key outcome of this emotional signaling is to strengthen the trust and bond between signaler and receiver.

In summary, there is abundant evidence that the more intimate a relationship is, the more the partners feel, express, and share a variety of emotions. This evidence also suggests that this emotional disclosure is not simply due to the amount of time spent together or to similarities between individuals, but rather that expressing and sharing emotions help to increase intimacy in interpersonal relations. This is because one is more likely to express emotions to a target who is expected to be able to respond appropriately to one's needs. The sharing of such intimate information through the expression of emotions is likely to result in a motivation to maintain or increase the social bond with that person (see also Clark et al., 2004). Furthermore, expressing an emotion not only conveys intimacy, because it reveals one's concerns, beliefs, and desires, but may also convey an appraisal of the situation. Thus, in addition to promoting intimacy, emotions may also serve affiliation functions, because they enhance positive interactions, cooperation, and trust.

The Social Distancing Function of Emotion

Emotions do not always fuel emotional closeness and identification. Various social-relational goals of emotions imply the reverse relational movement—namely, increasing distance from others, as in anger, contempt, disgust, or fear of another person (e.g., Fridlund, 1994; Oatley & Jenkins, 1992). Thus, alongside the affiliation function, we propose a social distancing function. Markus and Kitayama (1991) alluded to a similar notion when they distinguished between "socially engaging" and "socially disengaging" emotions. The latter are more socially desirable in cultures where an independent rather than an interdependent self is promoted. The emotions of anger, contempt, sociomoral disgust, and also pride are assumed to serve this function. We now consider examples of these emotions, and their effects on others and the self.

Anger is a prime example of an emotion that serves this function. If directly expressed to the object of the anger, this emotion confronts the other person with the fact that the angry persons wants to change the target's behavior and exert some control over the target (Fischer & Roseman, 2007; Timmers, Fischer, & Manstead, 1998). This implies that the target of the anger should apologize, yield, show submissiveness, or simply stop doing whatever he or she was doing. Studies by Van Kleef and colleagues have shown that the verbalization of anger in a negotiation context leads to more

yielding on the part of the other person (e.g., Van Kleef, De Dreu, & Manstead, 2004a, 2004b). Studies of mimicry have also shown that although angry faces sometimes lead to angry expressions (e.g., Dimberg & Lunquist, 1990), they can also give rise to fear and disgust displays (Lunquist & Dimberg, 1995). These studies suggest that anger is related to the exercise of power or influence over another person. In line with this idea that direct anger expression is an attempt to regain or maintain status or power, or simply to control the other, research by Tiedens (2001) confirms that high-status persons are expected to respond with anger (rather than sadness or guilt) to negative outcomes, and with pride (rather than appreciation) to positive outcomes (see also Kuppens, Van Mechelen, & Meulders, 2004). Moreover, when people show anger and pride they are thought of as being high in status, but when they show sadness, guilt, or appreciation they are thought of as low in status. The underlying explanation for these differences, according to Tiedens (2001), lies in the appraisals of agency that are implied by the expression of each of these emotions. An expression of anger is seen as reflecting the appraisal of other-blame and controllability; by contrast, an expression of guilt or sadness reflects appraisals of self-blame and uncontrollability. We suggest that these results also support the idea that anger and pride serve a social distancing function, in that they typically result in greater social distance between the self and the other.

A more extreme example of a social distancing function can be identified in the case of contempt. The expression of this emotion, typically in the form of derogation and rejection, often results in the social exclusion of the object (Fischer & Roseman, 2007). The aim is to make it clear that the other person is inferior and worthless, which is a way of boosting one's own social position or status, either as an individual or as a group member. Contempt may be elicited in addition to anger if alternative ways of changing others are expected to fail.

Thus anger and contempt typically serve a social distancing function by blaming another person for a negative outcome and either pressuring this person into yielding or doing what one wants (anger), or subjecting him or her to social exclusion (contempt). It is worth noting that although both emotions serve a social distancing function, they differ in the extent to which they are able also to serve an affiliation function: Whereas contempt is highly unlikely to give rise to any improvement in a social relationship, anger often does so, certainly in the longer term (Fischer & Roseman, 2007). This suggests that anger can serve both an affiliation and a social distancing function, but that these functions may be served at different points in time.

To summarize, we have described evidence showing that emotions sometimes have the effect of creating distance between oneself and others in a way that enhances one's own social standing. Expression of the emotion implies movement away from, but also above, the other person. Although one could argue that this social distancing function is less social in nature than is the affiliation function described earlier, because it appears to serve the self rather than one's relations with others, we argue that the protection or enhancement of social standing *is* a social function. Most obviously, the capacity to constrain the antisocial or dysfunctional behaviors of others by expressing anger and contempt toward them can be said to serve the function of protecting the individual or group from the harmful or dysfunctional behavior of others. Likewise, it is sometimes functional for individuals and groups to set themselves apart from or to cut themselves off from other individuals or groups. Anger felt toward an ex-partner can be helpful in detaching oneself from the relationship. Contempt expressed toward others who fail to endorse or live up to key norms and values can be beneficial in protecting those norms and values. Furthermore, the success of groups, organizations, and societies can be said to depend to some degree on the presence within them of individuals who strive to achieve more than their peers, thereby driving themselves and the groups to which they belong to better material outcomes. Thus pride in individual or collective achievements may serve a social function, not simply an individual one.

GROUP AND INTERGROUP RELATIONS

Affiliation and social distancing functions can also be applied to group emotions. The notion that groups can "have" emotions may initially seem puzzling. Common sense and emotion theory share the assumption that emotions are states experienced by individuals. We use the term "group-based emotion" here to refer to the fact that members of social groups have more similar concerns, make more similar appraisals, and therefore experience more similar emotions (Smith, 1993) than would be expected by chance (see also Smith & Mackie, Chapter 26, this volume). This idea is based on self-categorization theory (SCT; Turner, Hogg, Oakes, Reicher, & Wetherell, 1987). According to SCT, the salience of one's social identity should promote the experience of emotions that are driven by appraisals and concerns that are *group*-based rather than *individual*-based. For example, if your personal identity is salient, the success or failure of a given soccer team is likely to have little impact on your emotion; however, if your social identity as a supporter of that soccer team is salient, the selfsame success or failure of that team may lead to exhilaration or crushing disappointment (Cialdini et al., 1976; see Parkinson et al., 2005, for a review).

This idea of group-based emotions does not necessarily imply that group members need to be present, because it is the group-based concern that makes the emotion a group emotion. However, if others are present, this may exert influence on how one feels and expresses this feeling, in which case we refer to "collective emotions." A good illustration of this phenomenon is provided by Totterdell (2000), who assessed the moods of members of two professional sports teams three times a day for 4 days during a competitive match. Individual players' moods were more strongly correlated with the current aggregate mood of their own team than with the current aggregate mood of the other team or with the aggregate mood of their own team at other times. These correlations between player mood and team mood were also found to be independent of various factors, including the match situation between the two teams, effectively ruling out an explanation in terms of shared exposure to common situations.

One process that might account for collective emotions is contagion (Hatfield et al., 1992). This phenomenon occurs during face-to-face interaction. If group members engage in more frequent face-to-face interaction with each other than with nonmembers, contagion should be greater among group members than among nonmembers. Moreover, if emotion spreads from person to person in this way, the resulting shared behaviors and experiences should encourage the perception that the affected people constitute a group.

Functions of Emotion in Intragroup Relations

The functions of emotion in group settings parallel those in interpersonal contexts. First, consistent with the affiliation function, emotions can strengthen relations within a social group, enhancing a sense of commitment and belonging. The experience of shared emotion in groups strengthens bonds between group members and sharpens group boundaries, thereby enhancing loyalty to the group (see also Keltner & Haidt, 1999). In addition, the communication of emotion within a group provides group members with rapid information about group structure and the environment (Spoor & Kelly, 2004).

The function of emotions in the development and constitution of groups may be found in all types of groups. For example, emotions in sport or work teams may help to create a team spirit and strengthen the motivation to win as a team (e.g., Totterdell, 2000). Emotions in work teams may also enhance cooperation by group members (Barsade, 2002; Bartel & Saavedra, 2000). Not only do members of work groups experience "group moods," but the extent to which group members "catch" another person's mood seems to determine levels of cooperation and conflict (Barsade, 2002). In particular, dispersion of positive emotion leads to greater cooperation and reduces conflict in the group, whereas dispersion of negative emotion is associated with the opposite outcomes. George and her colleagues have also shown that group affective tone is related to prosocial behavior toward customers (see George, 1990).

Research by Kessler and Hollbach (2005) has also shown that *group-based* emotions influence ingroup identification. The context of this research was the relationship between East and West Germans. The East German participants were asked to recall an instance when they as East Germans felt either anger or happiness toward their own national subgroup or toward West Germans. A measure of identification as East Germans was taken before and after this procedure. It was found that recalled happiness toward the ingroup and anger toward the outgroup both increased ingroup identification, whereas anger toward the ingroup and happiness toward the outgroup

both decreased ingroup identification. This research provides an insight into the emotional dynamics that may underpin the "basking in reflected glory" phenomenon (Cialdini et al., 1976). The positive affect that supporters presumably experience as a result of their team's success on the football field should increase their ingroup identification. Likewise, Kessler and Hollbach's (2005) findings provide a possible emotion-based account for the related phenomenon of "cutting off reflected failure" (Snyder, Lassegard, & Ford, 1986), whereby group failure leads individuals to distance themselves from the ingroup in question.

The affiliation function of emotions in groups can also be illustrated by considering the effects of *differences* in appraisal and emotion. Sani and his associates (e.g., Sani, 2005; Sani & Reicher, 1999) have shown that schisms develop from perceptions that the positions taken by other ingroup members undermine or change in some fundamental way the shared identity of the group. Because this shared identity is a core value of the group, any serious threat to it is likely to evoke negative emotions such as dejection and agitation, and to result in decreased identification with the group and lower perceived cohesiveness. In a field study of the secession of a subgroup from the Church of England, Sani (2005) showed that strong negative emotion aroused by a perceived threat to group identity was a positive predictor of intentions to secede from the group.

In summary, emotions experienced in group settings have a number of beneficial effects on group functioning. To the extent that emotions are seen to be shared, they help to promote group cohesiveness and ingroup cooperation by providing group members with tangible evidence of their similarities. The reverse side of this coin is that when group members find themselves in disagreement about issues that in the eyes of some members threaten the integrity of the group, emotions can play a destructive role, making it more likely that the group will splinter into two or more factions.

Functions of Emotion in Intergroup Relations

Emotions not only serve to strengthen the bonds *within* one's group, but may also help to improve or worsen relations *between* social groups. One of the emotions that may serve the intergroup affiliation function is group-based guilt (Branscombe, Doosje, & McGarty, 2002; Doosje, Branscombe, Spears, & Manstead, 1998). Several studies have shown that individuals may feel guilty about past behavior of their ingroup toward an outgroup, as in the case of how the Dutch treated Indonesians during the colonial era (Doosje et al., 1998) or how European Americans have historically treated African Americans (Iyer, Leach, & Crosby, 2003). Group-based guilt implies that members of one group are perceived as responsible for disadvantages experienced by an outgroup. Doosje et al. (1998) found that levels of group-based guilt among Dutch participants were higher when past behavior of their national group toward Indonesians during the colonial era was presented in negative terms, rather than in positive or mixed terms. Moreover, they also showed that participants' levels of Dutch national identification was associated with the intensity of group-based guilt: Because high levels of identification are likely to lead to defensive denial that any wrong has been perpetrated, high identifiers were less willing to accept group-based guilt than were low identifiers, at least when the evidence concerning treatment of the outgroup was mixed.

Although these studies seem to show the beneficial effects of group-based guilt, there are alternative accounts of what follows from group-based guilt. In a study on European Americans' "white guilt" with respect to African Americans, Iyer et al. (2003) suggested that group-based guilt may involve a focus on the ingroup, implying a desire to offer an apology or engage in reparation with a view to alleviating ingroup distress, rather than a more *other-focused* desire to offer practical help to members of the disadvantaged group through programs such as affirmative action. Indeed, Iyer et al.'s studies showed that focusing on European American perpetration led to greater feelings of guilt, whereas a focus on African American suffering led to greater feelings of sympathy. Guilt predicted support for compensatory affirmative action, but not equal opportunity affirmative action, whereas sympathy predicted support for equal opportunity affirmative action and was a marginal predictor of support for compensatory affirmative action. This suggests that although both guilt and sympathy serve affiliation functions at the group level, there may be subtle differences in this function that can be inferred from the duration or size of the beneficial effects: Guilt may serve

bonding in order to alleviate the bad conscience of ingroup members, whereas sympathy improves bonding in order to help the other group.

Whereas group-based guilt or sympathy may lead to an improvement in relations with disadvantaged outgroups, other group-based emotions may function to strengthen the disadvantaged position of one's own group and thereby to enhance the social standing of the ingroup relative to other groups. A study by Gordijn, Yzerbyt, Wigboldus, and Dumont (2006), for example, shows how a perceiver's degree of identification with the victims of an injustice affects not just level of group-based anger, but also willingness to engage in collective action to redress the wrong. Here group-based anger has the effect of mobilizing people who are not themselves directly affected by the perceived injustice. In a similar vein, Van Zomeren, Spears, Fischer, and Leach (2004) sought to understand why collective disadvantage sometimes does and sometimes does not lead to collective action, and hypothesized that this was due to different expectations about the type of support that members would receive from their group. These researchers drew a distinction between "instrumental support" (support for action) and "emotional support" (sharing opinions). They found that if members anticipated instrumental support, this was enough to predict collective action in the absence of anger; however, if members anticipated emotional support, this led to more group-based anger and thereby to collective action. So here anger serves a function of motivating group members to engage in collective action.

Emotions may also serve a social distancing function, because certain emotions can also help to sharpen group boundaries by stressing dissimilarities with the outgroup, or even by promoting prejudice. DeSteno, Dasgupta, Bartlett, and Cajdric (2004) have shown that emotional states are capable of creating automatic prejudice toward outgroups. Specifically, anger was shown to influence automatic negative evaluations of outgroups, supposedly because of its functional relevance to intergroup conflict and competition. Moreover, studies on intergroup *Schadenfreude* (Leach, Spears, Branscombe, & Doosje, 2003; Spears & Leach, 2004) have shown that its intensity is, among other things, associated with feelings of inferiority with respect to the outgroup, suggesting that intergroup *Schadenfreude* can be seen as a way of coping with the lower social status of one's own group.

In summary, group-based emotions have powerful effects on both ingroup and intergroup relations. The emotions that have attracted most research attention to date, and the ones we have focused on here, are guilt and anger. There is consistent evidence that group-based guilt promotes tendencies to apologize and make reparation, just as personal guilt does in the context of interpersonal relations. On the other hand, group-based anger concerning the maltreatment of a group is more likely to result in effective political action on behalf of the disadvantaged group.

CONCLUSION

Emotions are elicited and evolve in social contexts, and they help us to deal with the challenges posed by our social environment. We have distinguished two general social functions of emotion: affiliation, which entails the promotion of interpersonal and intergroup relationships, on the one hand; and social distancing, which entails separation from and even control or power over others, on the other. Thus emotions can have the effect of reducing or increasing the distance between self and others, or between one's own group and other groups. It should be clear from our discussion that the social functions of emotion should not be equated with the social effects of expressing that emotion in a given setting. The social function of the emotion is relatively independent of social context, and intrinsic to the social-relational goals and prototypical features of the specific emotional reaction, whereas social effects are contingent upon the way in which the emotion is expressed and upon the specifics of the social context. For example, the social function of sadness is to elicit support and consolation from others, yet the consequence of crying in a given situation might be ridicule rather than comfort. This also shows that the notion that emotions serve social functions is not equivalent to the idea that emotions are always socially functional. Social functionality depends on emotional intelligence (e.g., Salovey & Mayer, 1990), and on striking an appropriate balance between affiliation and cooperation on the one hand, and social distancing and competition on the other. Social survival and social success involve a compromise between these elementary social goals.

There is a pressing need for more systematic research on these issues. Although it is clear that positive emotions foster positive social interactions between individuals, within groups, and between groups, resulting in greater cooperation and more positive outcomes, the evidence concerning negative emotions is less clear-cut—especially the circumstances under which these emotions are less socially functional. At the interpersonal level, negative emotions are more often expressed in intimate relations. Most of these emotions, like regret, embarrassment, sadness, fear, shame, or guilt, seem to serve an affiliation function, which leads us to argue that the expression of these emotions should benefit the relationship. It is obvious, however, that the expression of some negative emotions will not always improve the intimacy and quality of a relationship. Hatred and contempt seem to serve an individual's striving for social distance and social standing, rather than a desire to connect to connect with others. These emotions appear not to serve any affiliation function in an interpersonal setting.

Interestingly, *shared* hatred and contempt, along with other negative emotions directed at third persons or outgroups, *can* serve an affiliation function. When negative emotions are shared and expressed toward a third party, this results in a stronger tie with the person or group with which this negative emotion is shared. When people feel threatened by an outgroup, for example, one way to control their fear is by developing a hatred of the outgroup and perceiving its members as fundamentally bad. This strengthens bonds within the group and increases the distance between one's own group and other groups, as has been witnessed in the aftermath of the 9/11 attacks. Thus the expression of shared fear serves more of a social distancing function with respect to the object of one's fear (moving the group away from the threatening group), but more of an affiliation function with respect to ingroup members who face the same threat but who also provide a resource for dealing with the threat (fellow Americans). Thus the social function of emotions is dependent on the target of the emotion. In cases where emotions are shared with ingroup members, they are likely to serve an affiliation function.

At the intergroup level, the affiliation and social distancing functions of emotion seem to parallel those at the interpersonal level, but relatively few emotions have been studied in intergroup contexts. The affiliation function of negative emotions has most frequently been examined in the context of group-based guilt, which can lead to the tendency to repair the damage done to an outgroup. Yet some have argued that there may be limits to how beneficial group-based guilt really is, perhaps because of a tendency on the part of the advantaged group to focus on making itself feel better rather than on helping the outgroup, and partly because highly identified members of advantaged groups may be reluctant to acknowledge the harm done to an outgroup. A similar argument may apply to guilt at the interpersonal level.

When considering other emotions, such as fear and sadness, we can conclude that the consequences of groups expressing emotions like fear and sadness may depend on the status or power relations between the groups involved. For example, the obvious fear and distress of a low-power group (e.g., the refugees in the Darfur region of Sudan) may elicit empathy and help from members of other more powerful groups. By contrast, the equally obvious fear and distress of a high-power group (e.g., Americans in the aftermath of 9/11) may be less likely to arouse compassionate reactions on the part of members of other groups, unless they perceive a shared identity with the victim group.

Much the same applies at the interpersonal level, in that it seems plausible to suggest that we respond differently to fear expressed by a young child than to fear expressed by an adult who is a rival. Here again, it is clear that the social effects of specific emotions depend on the social context—that is, on the relationship between the individuals (e.g., communal, exchange) or groups (e.g., relative power and status)—but that the social function of the emotion, signaling the need for help, is relatively independent of this context. It is evident that an emotion may serve a single social function, yet have different social effects in different social settings.

A final point that bears repetition is that although we firmly believe that emotions serve social functions, this does not mean that emotions are always socially functional. The potential social functionality of emotions can be inferred from their social-relational goals and typical features. In practice, their functionality depends on how the individuals or social groups involved appraise the social context, and how they regulate their emotions and expressions in a way that is consistent with those social appraisals. Perhaps the ultimate social function of emotions is to persuade others to accept (at least to some degree) the validity of one's own or one's group's appraisals.

ACKNOWLEDGMENTS

We thank Lisa Feldman Barrett, Keith Oatley, Brian Parkinson, and Jerry Parrott for their helpful comments on a previous version of this chapter.

REFERENCES

Anderson, C., Keltner, D., & John, O. P. (2003). Emotional convergence between people over time. *Journal of Personality and Social Psychology, 84,* 1054–1068.

Archer, J. (2000). Sex differences in aggression between heterosexual partners: A meta-analytic review. *Psychological Bulletin, 126,* 651–680.

Barrett, K. C. (1995). A functionalist approach to shame and guilt. In J. P. Tangney & K. W. Fischer (Eds.), *Self-conscious emotions: The psychology of shame, guilt, embarrassment, and pride* (pp. 25–64). New York: Guilford Press.

Barrett, L. F., Robin, L., Pietromonaco, P. R., & Eyssell, K. (1998). Are women the more emotional sex?: Evidence from emotional experiences in social interactions. *Cognition and Emotion, 12,* 555–578.

Barsade, S. G. (2002). The ripple effect: Emotional contagion in groups. *Administrative Science Quarterly, 47,* 644–677.

Bartel, C. A., & Saavedra, R. (2000). The collective construction of work group moods. *Administrative Science Quarterly, 45,* 197–231.

Baumeister, R. F., & Leary, M. R. (1995). The need to belong: Desire for interpersonal attachments as a fundamental human motivation. *Psychological Bulletin, 117,* 497–529.

Baumeister, R. F., Stillwell, A. M., & Heatherton, T. F. (1994). Guilt: An interpersonal approach. *Psychological Bulletin, 115,* 243–267.

Bavelas, J. B., Black, A., Lemery, C. R., & Mullett, J. (1986). "I show how you feel": Motor mimicry as a communicative act. *Journal of Personality and Social Psychology, 50,* 322–329.

Branscombe, N. R., Doosje, B., & McGarty, C. (2002). Antecedents and consequences of collective guilt. In D. M. Mackie & E. R. Smith (Eds.), *From prejudice to intergroup emotions: Differentiated reactions to social groups* (pp. 49–66). New York: Psychology Press.

Chartrand, T. L., & Bargh, J. A. (1999). The chameleon

effect: The perception–behavior link and social interaction. *Journal of Personality and Social Psychology*, 76, 893–910.

Cialdini, R. B., Borden, R. J., Thorne, A., Walker, M. R., Freeman, S., & Sloan, L. R. (1976). Basking in reflected glory: Three (football) field studies. *Journal of Personality and Social Psychology*, 34, 366–375.

Clark, M. S., Fitness, J., & Brissette, I. (2004). Understanding people's perceptions of relationships is crucial to understanding their emotional lives. In M. B. Brewer & M. Hewstone (Eds.), *Emotion and motivation* (pp. 21–47). Malden, MA: Blackwell.

de Jong, P. J. (1999). Communicative and remedial effects of social blushing. *Journal of Nonverbal Behavior*, 23, 197–217.

DeSteno, D., Dasgupta, N., Bartlett, M. Y., & Cajdric, A. (2004). Prejudice from thin air: The effect of emotion on automatic intergroup attitudes. *Psychological Science*, 15, 319–324.

Dimberg, U. (1982). Facial reactions to facial expressions. *Psychophysiology*, 19, 643–647.

Dimberg, U., & Lunquist, L.-O. (1990). Gender differences in facial reactions to facial expressions. *Biological Psychology*, 30, 151–159.

Doosje, B., Branscombe, N. R., Spears, R., & Manstead, A. S. R. (1998). Guilty by association. When one's group has a negative history. *Journal of Personality and Social Psychology*, 75, 872–886.

Eisenberg, N. (2000). Empathy and sympathy. In M. Lewis & J. M. Haviland-Jones (Eds.), *Handbook of emotions* (2nd ed., pp. 677–691). New York: Guilford Press.

Evers, C., Fischer, A. H., Rodriguez Mosquera, P. M., & Manstead, A. S. R. (2004). Anger and social appraisal: A "spicy" sex difference? *Emotion*, 5, 258–266.

Fischer, A. H., Manstead, A. S. R., & Zaalberg, R. (2003). Social influences on the emotion process. In W. Stroebe & M. Hewstone (Eds.), *European review of social psychology* (Vol. 14, pp. 171–203). Hove, UK: Psychology Press.

Fischer, A. H., Rodriguez Mosquera, P. M., van Vianen, E. A. M., & Manstead, A. S. R. (2004). Gender and culture differences in emotion. *Emotion*, 4, 87–94.

Fischer, A. H., & Roseman, I. J. (2007). Beat them or ban them: The characteristics and social functions of anger and concept. *Journal of Personality and Social Psychology*, 93, 103–115.

Fischer, A. H., Rotteveel, M., Evers, C., & Manstead, A. S. R. (2004). Emotional assimilation: How we are influenced by others' emotions. *Cahiers de Psychologie Cognitive*, 22, 223–245.

Fridlund, A. J. (1994). *Human facial expression: An evolutionary view*. San Diego, CA: Academic Press.

Frijda, N. H. (1986). *The emotions*. Cambridge, UK: Cambridge University Press.

George, J. M. (1990). Personality, affect, and behavior in groups. *Journal of Applied Psychology*, 75, 107–116.

Gottman, J. M., & Levenson, R. W. (2002). A two-factor model for predicting when a couple will divorce: Exploratory analyses using 14-year longitudinal data. *Family Process*, 41, 83–96.

Gordijn, E., Yzerbyt, V. Y., Wigboldus, D., & Dumont, M. (2006). Emotional reactions to harmful intergroup behavior: The impact of being associated with the victims or the perpetrators. *European Journal of Social Psychology*, 36, 15–30.

Griffiths, P., & Scarantino, A. (in press). Emotions in the wild: The situated perspective on emotion. In P. Robbins & M. Aydele (Eds.), *Cambridge handbook of situated cognition*. New York: Cambridge University Press.

Gross, J., & John, O. P. (2002). Wise emotion regulation. In L. F. Barrett & P. Salovey (Eds.), *The wisdom in feeling: Psychological processes in emotional intelligence* (pp. 297–319). New York: Guilford Press.

Hatfield, E., Cacioppo, J. T., & Rapson, R. L. (1992). Primitive emotional contagion. In M. S. Clark (Ed), *Review of personality and social psychology: Vol. 14. Emotion and social behavior* (pp. 151–177). Thousand Oaks, CA: Sage.

Hess, U., Beaupré, M. G., & Cheung, N. (2002). Who, to whom, and why: Cultural differences and similarities in the function of smiles. In M. H. Abel (Ed.), *An empirical reflection on the smile* (pp. 187–216). Lewiston, NY: Edwin Mellen Press.

Iyer, A., Leach, C. W., & Crosby, F. J. (2003). White guilt and racial compensation: The benefits and limits of self-focus. *Personality and Social Psychology Bulletin*, 29, 117–129.

Keltner, D., & Buswell, B. N. (1976). Evidence for the distinctness of embarrassment, shame, and guilt: A study of recalled antecedents and facial expressions of emotion. *Cognition and Emotion*, 10, 155–171.

Keltner, D., & Buswell, B. N. (1997). Embarrassment: Its distinct form and appeasement function. *Psychological Bulletin*, 122, 250–270.

Keltner, D., & Haidt, J. (1999). Social functions of emotions at four levels of analysis. *Cognition and Emotion*, 13, 505–521.

Kessler, T., & Hollbach, S. (2005). Group based emotion as determinants of ingroup identification. *Journal of Experimental Social Psychology*, 41, 677–685.

Ketelaar, T., & Au, W. T. (2002). The effects of feelings of guilt on the behavior of uncooperative individuals in repeated social bargaining games: An affect-as-information interpretation of the role of emotion in social interaction. *Cognition and Emotion*, 17, 429–455.

Kring, A. M. (2000). Gender and anger. In A. H. Fischer (Ed.), *Gender and emotion: Social psychological perspectives* (pp. 211–232). Cambridge, UK: Cambridge University Press.

Krumhuber, E., & Kappas, A. (2005). Moving smiles: The role of dynamic components for the perception of the genuineness of smiles. *Journal of Nonverbal Behavior*, 29, 3–24.

Krumhuber, E., Manstead, A. S. R., & Kappas, A. (2007). Temporal aspects of facial displays in person and expression perception: The effects of smile dynamics, head-tilt, and gender. *Journal of Nonverbal Behavior, 31,* 39–56.

Kuppens, P., Van Mechelen, I., & Meulders, M. (2004). Every cloud has a silver lining: Interpersonal and individual differences determinants of anger-related behavior. *Personality and Social Psychology Bulletin, 30,* 1550–1564.

Laurenceau, J. P., Barrett, L. F., & Pietromonaco, P. R. (1998). Intimacy as an interpersonal process: The importance of self-disclosure, partner disclosure, and perceived partner responsiveness in interpersonal exchanges. *Journal of Personality and Social Psychology, 74,* 1238–1251.

Lazarus, R. S. (1991). *Emotion and adaptation.* New York: Oxford University Press.

Leach, C. W., Spears, R., Branscombe, N. R., & Doosje, E. J. (2003). Malicious pleasure: Schadenfreude at the suffering of another group. *Personality and Social Psychology, 84,* 932–943.

Levenson, R. W. (1999). Intrapersonal functions of emotion. *Cognition and Emotion, 13,* 481–504.

Lopes, P. N., Salovey, P., Coté, S., & Beers, M. (2005). Emotion regulation abilities and the quality of social interaction. *Emotion, 5,* 113–118.

Lunquist, L.-O., & Dimberg, U. (1995). Facial expressions are contagious. *Journal of Psychophysiology, 9,* 203–211.

Manstead, A. S. R., & Fischer, A. H. (2001). Social appraisal: The social world as object of and influence on appraisal processes. In K. R. Scherer, A. Schorr, & T. Johnstone (Eds.), *Appraisal processes in emotion: Theory, methods, research* (pp. 221–232). New York: Oxford University Press.

Markus, H. R., & Kitayama, S. (1991). Culture and the self: Implications for cognition, emotion, and motivation. *Psychological Review, 98,* 224–253.

Miller, R. S. (2004). Emotion as adaptive interpersonal communication: The case of embarrassment. In L. Z. Tiedens & C. W. Leach (Eds.), *The social life of emotions* (pp. 87–105). Cambridge, UK: Cambridge University Press.

Oatley, K., & Jenkins, J. M. (1992). Human emotions: Function and dysfunction. *Annual Review of Psychology, 43,* 55–85.

Parkinson, B. (2005). Do facial movements express emotions or communicate motives? *Personality and Social Psychology Review, 9,* 278–311.

Parkinson, B., Fischer, A. H., & Manstead, A. S. R. (2005). *Emotions in social relations: Cultural, group, and interpersonal processes.* New York: Psychology Press.

Parrott, W. G. (2001). Implications of dysfunctional emotions for understanding how emotions function. *Review of General Psychology, 5,* 180–186.

Parrott, W. G. (2002). The functional utility of negative emotions. In L. F. Barrett & P. Salovey (Eds.), *The wisdom in feeling: Psychological processes in emotional intelligence* (pp. 341–362). New York: Guilford Press.

Philippot, P., Feldman, R. S., & Coats, E. J. (Eds.).

(1999). *The social context of nonverbal behavior.* New York: Cambridge University Press.

Provine, R. R. (1992). Contagious laughter: Laughter is a sufficient stimulus for laughs and smiles. *Bulletin of the Psychonomic Society, 30,* 1–4.

Reis, H. T., McDougal Wilson, I., Monestere, C., Bernstein, S., Clark, K., Seidl, E., et al. (1990). What is smiling is beautiful and good. *European Journal of Social Psychology, 20,* 259–267.

Reis, H. T., & Shaver, P. R. (1988). Intimacy as an interpersonal process. In S. Duck, D. F. Hay, S. E. Hobfoll, W. Ickes, & B. M. Montgomery (Eds.), *Handbook of personal relationships: Theory, research, and interventions* (pp. 367–389). Chichester, UK: Wiley.

Rimé, B., Philippot, P., Boca, S., & Mesquita, B. (1992). Long-lasting cognitive and social consequences of emotion: Social sharing and rumination. In W. Stroebe & M. Hewstone (Eds.), *European review of social psychology* (Vol. 3, pp. 225–258). Chichester, UK: Wiley.

Roseman, I. J., Wiest, C., & Swartz, T. S. (1994). Phenomenology, behaviors and goals differentiate discrete emotions. *Journal of Personality and Social Psychology, 67,* 206–221.

Salovey, P., & Mayer, J. D. (1990). Emotional intelligence. *Imagination, Cognition, and Personality, 9,* 185–211.

Sani, F. (2005). When subgroups secede: Extending and refining the social psychological model of schisms in groups. *Personality and Social Psychology Bulletin, 31,* 1074–1086.

Sani, F., & Reicher, S. (1999). Identity, argument and schism: Two longitudinal studies of the split in the Church of England over the ordination of women to the priesthood. *Group Processes and Intergroup Relations, 2,* 279–300.

Semin, G. R., & Manstead, A. S. R. (1981). The social implications of embarrassment displays and restitution behaviour. *European Journal of Social Psychology, 12,* 367–377

Smith, E. R. (1993). Social identity and social emotions: Toward new conceptualizations of prejudice. In D. M. Mackie, D. Hamilton, & D. Lewis (Eds.), *Affect, cognition, and stereotyping: Interactive processes in group perception* (pp. 297–315). San Diego: Academic Press.

Sonnby-Borgström, M. (2002). Automatic mimicry reactions as related to differences in emotional empathy. *Scandinavian Journal of Psychology, 43,* 433–443.

Snyder, C. R., Lassegard, M., & Ford, C. E. (1986). Distancing after group success and failure: Basking in reflected glory and cutting off reflected failure. *Journal of Personality and Social Psychology, 51,* 382–388.

Sorce, J. F., Emde, R. N., Campos, J. J., & Klinnert, M. D. (1985). Maternal emotional signaling: Its effect on the visual cliff behavior of 1-year-olds. *Developmental Psychology, 21,* 195–200.

Spears, R., & Leach, C. W. (2004). Intergroup schadenfreude: Conditions and consequences. In L.

Z. Tiedens & C. W. Leach (Eds.), *The social life of emotions* (pp. 336–355). New York: Cambridge University Press.

Spoor, J. R., & Kelly, J. R. (2004). The evolutionary significance of affect in groups: Communication and group bonding. *Group Processes and Intergroup Relations, 7,* 401–415.

Tangney, J. P., Miller, R. S., Flicker, L., & Barlow, D. H. (1996). Are shame, guilt, and embarrassment distinct emotions? *Journal of Personality and Social Psychology, 70,* 1256–1264.

Tiedens, L. Z. (2001). Anger and advancement versus sadness and subjugation: The effect of negative emotion expressions on social status conferral. *Journal of Personality and Social Psychology, 80,* 86–94.

Tiedens, L. Z., & Leach, C. W. (Eds.). (2004). *The social life of emotions.* New York: Cambridge University Press.

Timmers, M., Fischer, A. H., & Manstead, A. S. R. (1998). Emotion expression as a function of gender and social context. *Personality and Social Psychology Bulletin, 24,* 974–985.

Totterdell, P. (2000). Catching moods and hitting runs: Mood linkage and subjective performance in professional sports teams. *Journal of Applied Psychology, 85,* 848–859.

Turner, J. C., Hogg, M. A., Oakes, P. J., Reicher, S. D., & Wetherell, M. S. (1987). *Rediscovering the social group: A self-categorization theory.* Oxford: Blackwell.

Van Kleef, G. A., De Dreu, C. K. W., & Manstead, A. S. R. (2004a). The interpersonal effects of anger and happiness in negotiations. *Journal of Personality and Social Psychology, 86,* 57–76.

Van Kleef, G. A., De Dreu, C. K. W., & Manstead, A. S. R. (2004b). The interpersonal effects of emotions in negotiations: A motivated information processing approach. *Journal of Personality and Social Psychology, 87,* 510–528.

Van Zomeren, M., Spears, R., Fischer, A. H., & Leach, C. W. (2004). Put your money where your mouth is!: Explaining collective action tendencies through group-based anger and group efficacy. *Journal of Personality and Social Psychology, 87,* 649–664.

Vingerhoets, A. J. J. M., & Becht, M. C. (1997). *The ISAC study: Some preliminary findings.* Poster presented at the annual meeting of the American Psychosomatic Society, Santa Fe, NM.

Williams, K. D. (2001). *Ostracism: The power of silence.* New York: Guilford Press.

Zeelenberg, M., Van der Pligt, J., & Manstead, A. S. R. (1998). Undoing regret on Dutch television: Apologizing for interpersonal regrets involving actions or inactions. *Personality and Social Psychology Bulletin, 24,* 1113–1119.

PART V

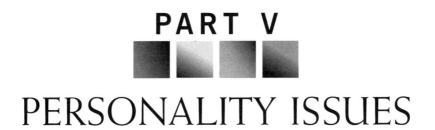

PERSONALITY ISSUES

CHAPTER 29

Subjective Well-Being

RICHARD E. LUCAS and ED DIENER

Psychological health, like physical health, can be judged on a variety of dimensions. Yet in both realms, it is difficult to say which of these dimensions are essential for overall well-being. Can a woman say that she is in good physical shape because she is free from disease, or must she also have an abundance of energy and a great deal of strength? Does a man have *psychological* well-being if he is free from depression, or must he have a positive opinion of himself and his life? Throughout the history of the field, psychologists have tended to focus on the negative end of the psychological spectrum, while often ignoring the positive (Myers & Diener, 1995). Partly in response to this unbalanced focus, researchers have become increasingly interested in positive psychological outcomes. One area where this shifting focus is very salient is the field of "subjective well-being" (SWB).

As its name implies, the field of SWB focuses on people's *own* evaluations of their lives. Although measures such as crime statistics, health indices, and indicators of wealth are surely related to quality of life, these external indicators cannot capture what it means to have a subjective sense that one's life is good. An activist for society's downtrodden, for example, may thrive in a high-crime, low-income neighborhood. The sense of meaning and personal satisfaction this individual gains from helping others may not be reflected in traditional social indicators. People evaluate conditions differently, depending on their expectations, values, and previous experiences. SWB researchers assign importance to this subjective element and assess individuals' thoughts and feelings about their lives.

DEFINING SWB

There are numerous ways in which an individual can evaluate the quality of his or her life. Perhaps the most basic of these relates to the moment-to-moment affect that a person feels over time. Emotions and moods are ubiquitous phenomena; they give a subjective feeling to virtually all of one's waking moments. In an experience-sampling study of emotional experience, Diener, Sandvik, and Pavot (1991) found that people reported some affect virtually all of the time. Furthermore, emotional experiences have valence. One of the most basic features of these experiences is that a person can easily tell whether they are positive or negative (Kahneman, 1999). Given the ubiquity of emotion and its valenced nature, it is not surprising that when people evaluate their own well-being, the pleasantness of their affect appears to play a central role. Larsen (1989) found that scores on self-report SWB scales fall at the end of the pleasantness dimension of the emotion circumplex. Thus we begin by suggesting that the experience of SWB reflects a preponderance of pleasant rather than unpleasant affect in one's life over time.

It is important to realize, however, that this relatively simple starting point belies the considerable complexity that is involved in defining and measuring SWB. First, although it is tempting to group all affective experience together, research shows that pleasant and unpleasant affect are not polar opposites. In perhaps the first investigation of this issue, Bradburn (1969) reported that pleasant and unpleasant affect were empirically separable, and that each correlated with a distinct set of personality traits. Watson and his colleagues (e.g., Watson, Clark, & Tellegen, 1988; Watson & Tellegen, 1985) showed that positive and negative affect formed distinct and orthogonal factors, and the two-factor structure that they identified has been replicated often (Diener & Emmons, 1985; Warr, Barter, & Brownbridge, 1983; Zevon & Tellegen, 1982).

Theorists on the other side of the independence debate suggest that pleasant and unpleasant affect are really two poles of a single dimension, and that empirical evidence for their independence results from a variety of artifacts. Green, Goldman, and Salovey (1993), for example, suggested that when measurement error is controlled via structural equation modeling, the correlation between pleasant and unpleasant affect becomes much stronger than it is when single-method observed variables are assessed. Similarly, Russell (1980) proposed a circumplex model of affect in which emotions can be described in terms of their pleasantness–unpleasantness and in terms of their level of arousal. According to this model, if arousal is held constant, pleasant and unpleasant affect will exhibit strong negative correlations.

Schimmack (2008) has provided a comprehensive review that addresses most of the issues surrounding the independence debate. He notes that confusion about independence often arises because multiple types of independence are sometimes discussed as if they were the same thing. Citing Bradburn's (1969) initial work in this area, Schimmack distinguishes "structural independence," "momentary independence," and "causal independence." Structural independence refers to the extent to which long-term levels of positive affect are independent from long-term levels of negative affect. Schimmack's review shows that even when the best multimethod techniques are used, and even when positive and negative affect items are matched for levels of arousal, the correlation between positive and negative affect is much lower than 1.00. Thus there is support for the idea that there is some degree of structural independence.

Momentary independence refers to the question of whether people can experience positive and negative affect simultaneously. In contrast to the question of structural independence, it appears that there is quite a bit of support for momentary independence (Schimmack, 2008). Although people can experience low levels of positive affect at the same time they experience low levels of negative affect, the simultaneous experience of more intense positive and negative affect is rare (Diener & Iran-Nejad, 1986; Schimmack, 2001). Thus people's intuition that positive and negative affect cannot be independent may be due to the fact that they are thinking about momentary independence rather than structural independence.

Causal independence refers to the question of whether positive and negative affect result from different underlying causal processes (Schimmack, 2008). Interestingly, it is possible that even if positive and negative affect show strong momentary correlations, they may still be causally independent (Larsen, McGraw, & Cacioppo, 2001). For instance, if independent underlying systems are mutually inhibitory, this may result in strong negative correlations at the level of a person's experience. Personality researchers have often emphasized the fact that different personality traits are differentially associated with positive and negative affect (e.g., Carver, Sutton, & Scheier, 2000; Elliot & Thrash, 2002; Tellegen, 1985). This provides some initial evidence for causal independence of these two affective dimensions (see Schimmack, 2008, for a more detailed review).

Finally, it is important to point out that the evaluation of one's life does not end with emotional experience itself. As Kahneman and Riis (2005) put it, in addition to living their lives, people can also think about their lives. And these retrospective, cognitive evaluations can differ from the average emotions that the persons experience over time. It is likely that people use their affective experiences as one source of information about their overall well-being. However, other sources will also play a role. For instance, it is possible that people may be willing to endure high levels of negative affect if the situational factors leading to these affective experiences ultimately contribute to the attainment of important life goals. Thus the associations between affective and cognitive components may vary across individuals. In fact, Suh, Diener, Oishi, and Triandis (1998) showed that different cultures use affective information differently when judging overall life satisfaction. Among participants from individualist nations, affective experience is strongly correlated with life satisfaction, whereas among participants from collectivist nations, the associations are somewhat weaker. Thus, although some people have suggested that psychologists place too much emphasis on hedonism by focusing on SWB, the separability of life satisfaction from affective feelings allows for a variety of paths to the subjectively good life. SWB does not result solely or inevitably from hedonistic pleasures.

Because the various components of SWB are only moderately intercorrelated (and because the size of these correlations may vary across different populations), SWB researchers recommend assessing at least four different constructs to get a relatively complete view of a person's subjective quality of life. Specifically, we (Diener, Suh, Lucas, & Smith, 1999) have recommended assessing positive affect, negative affect, life satisfaction, and satisfaction with specific life domains (e.g., one's health, one's romantic partner, and one's job). Although the various affective and cognitive components are separable (Lucas, Diener, & Suh, 1996), they are often interrelated, suggesting the existence of a higher-order construct of SWB.

MEASURING SWB

SWB has often been measured by means of simple one-time self-reports. These self-reports may consist of single-item or multiple-item scales that ask respondents to reflect on how happy they are or how happy they have been over a circumscribed period of time. The evidence to date indicates that such self-reports of happiness are reliable and valid: Most instruments show impressive internal consistency, temporal stability, convergence with non-self-report measures of well-being, and acceptable levels of criterion validity.

For instance, Fujita and Diener (2005) used data from a 17-year nationally representative panel study from Germany to show that year-to-year stabilities of a single-item life satisfaction measure averaged about .55. Schimmack and Oishi (2005) conducted a meta-analysis of stability coefficients for life satisfaction measures; they arrived at similar 1-year stabilities for single-item measures and somewhat higher estimates (~.65) for multiple-item measures. Lucas and Donnellan (2007) analyzed two nationally representative longitudinal datasets (including the one that Fujita and Diener analyzed), using latent state–trait models. These models allowed them to estimate the extent to which stable trait and transient state variance affected life satisfaction judgments. Lucas and Donnellan found that approximately 30–37% of the variance was unchanging trait variance that was stable across all waves of the study. An additional 30–33% of the variance was accounted for by a moderately stable autoregressive component that led to increased stability from one year to the next and reduced stability over time. Importantly, across the two studies, only about 35% of the variance in these single-item life satisfaction measures could be accounted for by an occasion-specific state component. Because this state component included both random measurement error and true occasion-specific variance, this figure provides a lower-bound estimate of the reliability of single-item measure of life satisfaction. These studies show that at least 65% (and probably more) of the variance in these simple measures is reliable.

Evidence for the validity of these measures is also strong. In a study examining the convergent validity of well-being measures, Sandvik, Diener, and Seidlitz (1993) found strong evidence of convergence between self-reports of SWB on the one hand, and interview ratings, peer reports, the average daily ratio of pleasant to unpleasant moods, and memory for pleasant minus unpleasant events on the other. Similarly, we (Lucas et al., 1996) showed that when multiple measures of various well-being constructs were assessed, different measures of the same construct tended to correlate more strongly than did different constructs assessed with the same method. This evidence of convergent and discriminant validity shows that SWB measures assess valid variance, and that they do not simply reflect social desirability or other irrelevant response styles and response sets.

Evidence of convergent and discriminant validity is encouraging because it suggests that existing measures tap into something real. However, to be sure that these measures assess what psychologists think they measure, it is also important to determine whether they behave in ways that SWB theories would suggest. Measures of SWB tend to be sensitive to external conditions and responsive to changing life circumstances. For instance, Dijkers (1997) showed that individuals with spinal cord injuries tend to have lower levels of subjective quality of life (see also Putzke, Richards, Hicken, & DeVivo, 2002). In addition, in a 6-year longitudinal study, Headey and Wearing (1989) found that positive and negative life events led to concomitant increases and decreases in SWB. More recently, we have used nationally representative panel studies to show that when major life events such as marriage, divorce, widowhood, and unemployment occur, life satisfaction scores change in response (Lucas, Clark, Georgellis, & Diener, 2003, 2004; Lucas, 2005). Similar results have also been found in national surveys: Reports from nations in turmoil show low well-being (e.g., Europe after World War II, Eastern Europe in 1991), suggesting that the measures are sensitive to external conditions in theoretically meaningful ways (Veenhoven, 1994).

Although these studies show that SWB measures have some degree of validity, other researchers have suggested that they are also susceptible to the influence of irrelevant contextual factors. In the most programmatic series of studies, Schwarz, Strack, and their colleagues found that the type of response scale used, the response options, and the order and presentation of questions can all influence the levels of SWB that individuals report (see Schwarz & Strack, 1999, for a review). For instance, in one of the most famous studies, Schwarz and Clore (1983) showed that people reported greater life satisfaction on sunny days than on cold rainy days. Presumably, the weather influenced mood, and people simply relied on their mood when constructing a life satisfaction judgment.

Although mood and other context effects surely occur, research shows that these contextual factors often have only small effects on the validity of SWB measures. For instance, one famous context effect that Schwarz and Strack (1999) reviewed concerned the order in which specific items were presented. Strack, Martin, and Schwarz (1988) found that participants who were asked about their satisfaction with dating before being asked about their satisfaction with life showed stronger correlations between the two questions than did participants who received the questions in the reverse order. Presumably, the experimenters made participants' satisfaction with dating salient by asking about this domain, and this increased salience led participants to incorporate this information into their overall judgments of life satisfaction. Although such context effects may influence well-being judgments, Schimmack and Oishi (2005) showed that chronically accessible factors tend to have a much larger impact on life satisfaction judgments than do transient factors made salient by situational manipulations. The fact that people tend to rely on the same information when making their satisfaction judgments results in considerable stability over time.

Similarly, Eid and Diener (2004) showed that mood effects on SWB ratings are often weak, and these transient factors tend to be overwhelmed by stable variance. To demonstrate this, Eid and Diener assessed global SWB, along with current mood, three times over the course of a 3-month period. They used structural equation modeling techniques to determine how much variability in SWB could be explained by stable trait factors versus transient state factors. They showed that the majority of the SWB variance was stable over time. Perhaps more importantly, the occasion-specific associations between current mood and global SWB were weak and inconsistent. Thus mood appears to play a small role in global SWB judgments.

Nonetheless, Diener (1994) recommends that multimethod batteries be used to assess emotional well-being (see also Eid & Diener, 2004, for a full discussion of multimethod techniques). A major limitation of self-report is that it relies exclusively on people's cognitive labels of their feelings. But the affective experience that forms one major part of SWB is recognized to be a multichannel phenomenon that includes physiological, facial, nonverbal, cognitive, behavioral, and experiential components. In addition, there may be individual- or group-level differences in self-presentational style, and these differences may affect self-reports of well-being. In order to obtain a complete picture of a person's SWB, it is desirable to use informant reports, coding of nonverbal behavior, and other techniques in order to assess the full range of cognitive and affective responses about the person's life. When the measures converge, one will obtain greater confidence in the results. When the measures diverge, one will gain more complex knowledge of the emotional well-being of the individuals or groups being compared.

CAN HAPPINESS CHANGE?

When evaluating the quality of SWB measures, psychologists often point to their stability as evidence that they have some degree of reliability and validity. As discussed above, this piece of evidence shows that contextual factors do not completely overwhelm these measures. Furthermore, because external circumstances are not expected to change that frequently, the stability of SWB measures also agrees with intuitive theories about the way external circumstances affect well-being. However, the stability of SWB measures also raises questions about the extent to which happiness can change. Do external circumstances matter, or do SWB judgments reflect an unchanging and perhaps biologically determined outlook on life?

One important piece of evidence concerning this question comes from studies that attempt to estimate the heritability of SWB by comparing the similarity of identical twins to that of fraternal twins. In perhaps the first such study, Tellegen et al. (1988) used a separated-twin design to assess the heritability of various well-being measures (all of which were derived from the Multidimensional Personality Questionnaire). They showed that these heritabilities ranged from .40 (for global positive emotionality) to .55 (for global negative emotionality). Thus about half of the variance could be accounted for by one's genes. In addition, growing up in the same household played almost no role in the similarity of twins; those who were raised together were no more similar than those who were raised apart. These broad heritability estimates have been replicated often by researchers using a variety of samples

and different measures of SWB (e.g., Nes, Roysamb, Tambs, Harris, & Reichborn-Kjennerud, 2006; Roysamb, Harris, Magnus, Vitterso, & Tambs, 2002; Roysamb, Tambs, Reichborn-Kjennerud, Neale, & Harris, 2003; Stubbe, Posthuma, Boomsma, & De Geus, 2005).

Although the broad heritability of single-occasion measures of SWB is no longer controversial, some of the implications and extensions of this research can be. For instance, in an extension of the basic twin study design, Lykken and Tellegen (1996) examined the extent to which SWB is stable over time and the extent to which the stable component is heritable. Consistent with previous studies, Lykken and Tellegen found stability estimates near .50. In addition, they showed that the cross-twin, cross-time correlations were approximately .40. This means that about 80% of the stable variance can be accounted for by genes. The authors concluded from this finding that "trying to be happier [may be] as futile as trying to be taller" (p. 189). Although at first glance this pessimistic perspective appears to be supported by Lykken and Tellegen's data, there are three reasons why psychologists should hold out hope that happiness can in fact change.

First, it is true that strong heritability estimates suggest that inborn biological factors play a role in SWB. Yet, until the precise process is understood, it cannot be determined whether happiness is changeable or not. For instance, inborn traits could affect specific behaviors, which in turn could affect happiness. If so, then interventions could be designed to change the behaviors that people with these personality traits tend to exhibit.

Second, Lykken and Tellegen's (1996) study was based on a relatively small sample of relatively young twins. Although the estimates from this study have been replicated with one larger sample of young twins from Norway (Nes et al., 2006), a separate study that assessed an older sample found much lower estimates for the heritability of the stable component of SWB (Johnson, McGue, & Krueger, 2005). Thus it is unclear whether additional factors such as the age of the participants can moderate the effects that Lykken and Tellegen reported.

Finally, additional research that directly examines the effect of major life events shows that external circumstances can have lasting effects on SWB. For instance, we (Lucas et al.,

2003) found that although people eventually adapted to the death of a spouse, this adaptation process took approximately 8 years—a substantial proportion of the respondents' lives. Other events, such as divorce (Lucas, 2005), unemployment (Lucas et al., 2004), and the onset of a long-term disability (Lucas, 2007), had even stronger and longer-lasting effects. For example, the onset of a serious disability was associated with more than a full standard deviation's drop in life satisfaction (Lucas, 2007). Importantly, this longitudinal study showed that very little adaptation occurred following this important life event. Finally, all of these studies showed considerable individual differences in reaction and adaptation to life events. Even where participants adapted to events on average, some participants experienced lasting changes from their own personal baseline. Thus studies of life events show that life circumstances can have an important impact on SWB.

CORRELATES OF SWB

In 1967 Wilson reviewed the limited empirical evidence regarding the "correlates of avowed happiness." He concluded that the happy person is a "young, healthy, well-educated, well-paid, extroverted, optimistic, worry-free, religious, married person with high self-esteem, job morale, modest aspirations, of either sex, and of a wide range of intelligence" (p. 294). In the 40 years since Wilson's review, thousands of studies have been conducted, and we now know much more about the correlates of SWB (see Diener et al., 1999, for a comprehensive review).

A number of Wilson's conclusions have stood the test of time. Most significantly, Wilson was correct about (and probably underestimated the importance of) personality. Researchers consistently find that the personality traits of extraversion, neuroticism, optimism, and self-esteem correlate with measures of emotional well-being (Diener & Lucas, 1999). However, we must caution that the pattern of relations may vary across cultures. Diener and Diener (1995) found that the size of the correlation between self-esteem and life satisfaction was greater in individualistic nations than in collectivistic nations, perhaps because the former place greater emphasis on autonomy and internal feelings. Another study (Lucas, Diener,

Grob, Suh, & Shao, 1999) found that extraversion was correlated less strongly with pleasant affect in collectivistic nations than in individualistic nations (though the correlation was strong in both). A third study (Oishi, Diener, Suh, & Lucas, 1999) suggested that values and goals may mediate the relations among personality traits and well-being constructs. Although the exact cause for the relations between personality and SWB is unclear, the relation itself is robust.

Wilson (1967) was also correct that income plays a role in SWB, though this relation is more complex than Wilson could have known. Studies of personal wealth, income change, national wealth (i.e., gross national product), and studies of very wealthy individuals consistently find significant positive correlations between wealth and SWB (Diener & Biswas-Diener, 2002). These correlations are much larger at the national level than at the individual level. However, even the relatively small effects that are found at the individual level can have practical importance. Furthermore, the relation is often larger among those at the lowest levels of income (Diener, Sandvik, Seidlitz, & Diener, 1993), and even very small differences in absolute wealth can have important implications for happiness among those with very few resources (Biswas-Diener & Diener, 2001).

Marriage and religion also show consistent correlations with SWB. A number of studies in the United States (e.g., Glenn, 1975; Gove & Shin, 1989) and other countries (e.g., Mastekaasa, 1995; White, 1992) support Wilson's (1967) conclusion that married individuals tend to be happier than divorced or unmarried individuals. However, this association may not be due to the causal effect of marriage on happiness. Although divorce is associated with lasting changes in happiness (Lucas, 2005), marriage is not (Lucas et al., 2003). Instead, it appears that single people who will eventually marry are actually happier than average, even before the marriage occurs.

Studies on religion show that religious people are often happier than nonreligious individuals. More specifically, SWB correlates with religious certainty (Ellison, 1991), strength of one's relationship with the divine (Pollner, 1989), prayer experiences (Poloma & Pendleton, 1991), and participation in religious activities (Ellison, Gay, & Glass, 1989; Gartner, Larson, & Allen, 1991). This effect holds even after other demographic factors (such as age, income, and education) are controlled for (Diener et al., 1999).

Although Wilson's (1967) description of the happy individual was accurate in a number of respects, a few of Wilson's conclusions have been overturned by subsequent research. Most significantly, SWB researchers now question the popular notion that people become more unhappy as they age. In a study that examined national probability samples from 40 nations, Diener and Suh (1998) found that although pleasant affect tended to decline with age, there were no significant trends in life satisfaction or unpleasant affect. Furthermore, decreases in positive affect may be due to the fact that most studies measure aroused types of pleasant emotions. If less aroused emotions such as "contentment" and "affection" are examined, age declines may not be found (Diener & Suh, 1998). Of course, the precise patterns of change that are found within a single study depend somewhat on the age range examined and the type of design used (Pinquart, 2001). For instance, Mroczek and Spiro (2005) found that life satisfaction increased from age 40 to 65, but then declined after that (particularly as respondents approached death).

Recent research also suggests that the association between health and SWB may be more complicated than Wilson realized. Although health is positively associated with well-being, this relation holds tends to be stronger for self-reports than for more objective measures of health (e.g., George & Landerman, 1984; Larson, 1978; Okun, Stock, Haring, & Witter, 1984). When more objective health data (e.g., physicians' ratings) are examined, the correlation sometimes weakens considerably or even disappears (e.g., Watten, Vassend, Myhrer, & Syversen, 1997).

One possible explanation for this discrepancy is that self-reports of health reflect one's level of emotional adjustment as well as one's objective physical condition (Hooker & Siegler, 1992; Watson & Pennebaker, 1989). Therefore, the relation between health and SWB may be artificially inflated by this emotional component. However, an alternative explanation is that objective measures of health are themselves flawed. Nelson et al. (1983), for example, examined the correspondence between patients' and doctors' reports of health. There were numerous disagreements between the reports, and when Nelson et al. asked doctors about the reasons for these discrepancies, the

doctors admitted that 44% of the disagreements were due to clinician error. An additional 12% were due to insufficient knowledge of the patients. This study demonstrates that "objective" reports can be wrong, and that patients' subjective ratings may actually be more valid. In fact, a number of studies have now shown that subjective reports of health can predict outcomes such as longevity, even after objective reports of health are controlled for (Ganz, Lee, & Siau, 1990; McClellan, Anson, Birkeli, & Tuttle, 1991; Mossey & Shapiro, 1982; Rumsfeld et al., 1999). Thus the association between subjective ratings of health and SWB may reflect more than just shared method variance.

THEORIES OF THE CAUSES OF SWB

Much of the research summarized above answers the question "What external conditions are necessary for happiness to ensue?" Do people need to have a lot of money to be happy, or can they have a modest income? Do they need to be married, or can they be single? These questions reflect the underlying theoretical assumption that people have universal needs, and that the degree to which these needs are met by external circumstances and personal resources determines happiness (Wilson, 1967). Unfortunately, the effects of these variables are often small, leading some researchers to complain of a lack of theoretical progress in the field (e.g., Ryff, 1989; Wilson, 1967). Fortunately, researchers have attempted to balance this emphasis on external factors and demographics with a greater focus on the psychological variables that moderate the effects of life circumstances. People's needs and resources must be examined in the context of individual lives, goals, values, and personalities. Although no complete theoretical formulation is available, we (Diener et al., 1999) have suggested some components that such a theory must include.

Dispositional Influences

One important moderator of situational effects on happiness is personality. We (Diener & Lucas, 1999) have reviewed findings from temperament studies, heritability studies, longitudinal studies, and cross-situational consistency studies that suggest the existence of stable emotional styles of responding to events and circumstances. Although people may often respond similarly to similar events, the intensity and duration of those responses are likely to be influenced by people's personality. Although a number of traits exhibit reliable correlations with SWB (including self-esteem, optimism, agreeableness, and conscientiousness), researchers often focus on the widely replicated associations between extraversion and positive affect on the one hand, and neuroticism and negative affect on the other (Diener & Lucas, 1999).

McCrae and Costa (1991) suggested that there are at least two general classes of explanations for the associations between traits like extraversion and neuroticism and SWB variables like positive and negative affect. According to instrumental explanations, personality affects well-being indirectly through choice of situations or through differential propensities to experience positive and negative life events. For instance, extraverts may be happier than introverts because they spend more time in social situations, and this increased social activity may lead to greater positive affect. Support for such instrumental models comes from studies showing that extraversion and neuroticism prospectively predict positive and negative life events, respectively (e.g., Headey & Wearing, 1989; Magnus, Diener, Fujnita, & Pavot, 1996).

In contrast to these instrumental theories, temperament theorists posit that there is a direct path from personality traits to affective experience. For instance, Gray (1981) proposed that much of the variability in personality can be traced to three fundamental systems that regulate reactions to signals of conditioned reward (the "behavioral activation system" or BAS), signals of conditioned punishment (the "behavioral inhibition system" or BIS), and signals of unconditioned punishment (the "fight–flight system" or FFS). Extraversion appears to be linked to individual differences in the BAS, whereas neuroticism appears to be linked to individual differences in the BIS (Tellegen, 1985). Thus extraverts should be more sensitive to signals of reward than are introverts, and this reward sensitivity should take the form of enhanced information processing and increased positive emotions when extraverts are exposed to rewarding stimuli. Similarly, individuals who are high in neuroticism should be more sensitive to signals of punishment than are more stable individuals. Re-

searchers have tested these theories by examining individual differences in attention to (e.g., Derryberry & Reed, 1994), memory for (e.g., Rusting, 1998), and reaction to positive and negative stimuli (e.g., Canli et al., 2001; Larsen & Ketelaar, 1991; Lucas & Baird, 2004).

It is important to note that these explanations of the personality–SWB association are not mutually exclusive. Extraverts may attend more and respond more strongly to rewarding stimuli, while simultaneously engaging in behaviors that make rewarding circumstances more likely to occur. A theory of SWB must take these dispositional influences into consideration when evaluating the effects of external influences on well-being. Although the loss of a loved one may cause sadness and grief in most individuals, the intensity, duration, and means of coping with this tragedy may all be influenced by one's personality.

Goals

A number of theoretical approaches to SWB can be grouped together as "telic theories" (Diener, 1984). These approaches posit that happiness occurs when a person arrives at some end state. The end state may be set by innate biological drives, as in some need theories (e.g., Maslow, 1954); by psychological needs or motives (Murray, 1938); or by conscious goals (Emmons, 1986). These models are similar to the dispositional explanation of well-being, in that they recognize that different events and circumstances affect individuals differently, depending on the context of their lives. Because needs and goals depend on learning, life cycle, and biological factors, SWB may result from quite different telic states for different people at different times in their lives.

At their simplest, goal theories suggest that progress toward goals and attainment of goals lead to increased positive affect (e.g., Brunstein, 1993; Emmons, 1986). However, more complex theories of the relations between goals and SWB have been proposed. Emmons (1986), for example, finds evidence that certain characteristics of goals (rather than progress toward goals) affect happiness. The value that one places on goals and the degree of effort that the goal requires tend to be associated with positive affect, whereas conflict between goals and ambivalence toward goals tends to be associated with negative affect. Other researchers (e.g., Ryan,

Sheldon, Kasser, & Deci, 1996) argue that certain types of goals are more likely to foster well-being than are others. More specifically, Kasser and Ryan (1993) found that self-acceptance, affiliation, and community goals were positively associated with higher SWB, whereas financial success, social recognition, and physical attractiveness goals were associated with lower SWB. Kasser and Ryan argue that the former goals reflect intrinsic needs such as autonomy, relatedness, and competence, and that the fulfillment of these needs is most important for SWB.

Many goal theories have the ability to explain the small effects of resources and other bottom-up factors: Only those factors that relate to one's goals (which can vary across individuals) should influence well-being. Cantor and Sanderson (1999), for example, have argued that the importance of certain goals changes across individuals, cultures, and developmental phases. According to their theory, SWB when an individual chooses and is able to attain goals that are valued by the individual and culture, and that are appropriate to the individual's developmental phase. We (Oishi et al., 1999) found that achievement in certain domains influenced overall well-being only when those domains were related to respondents' goals. Thus goals provide an important context for the events and circumstances that individuals experience. We must understand this individual context before we can understand the impact of events.

Culture

An additional contextual factor that is related to theories of goals and SWB is the culture in which individuals are immersed. Although goals can vary among individuals within a culture, certain goals may be more prevalent in certain cultures. These differences may result in differential levels of happiness in different cultures. However, the impact of culture on individuals' well-being extends beyond the goals that they hold. Culture also affects the weighting of different sources of pleasure and pain. Thus SWB may mean different things in different places.

For example, Suh et al.'s (1998) research on cross-cultural variation in the determinants of life satisfaction suggests that cultural differences in one's outlook can have important implications for theories of SWB. Considerable

research suggests that people living in individualist cultures tend to view the self as an autonomous, self-sufficient entity (Markus & Kitayama, 1991). Consequently, feelings and emotions weigh heavily as determinants of behavior. Individuals living within collectivist cultures, on the other hand, stress harmony with family and friends rather than stressing one's autonomy from these people. Feelings about the self weigh less heavily in these cultures. This difference in outlook can explain why emotions were a stronger determinant of global life satisfaction in individualist cultures than they were in collectivist cultures in Suh et al.'s study. Similarly, Diener and Diener (1995) found that feelings about the self (i.e., self-esteem) were more highly related to life satisfaction in individualist nations than in collectivist nations. Just as individuals may have different goals across cultures, they may have different ideas of what it means to be happy.

Social Comparison

It has been hypothesized that a person's level of SWB is in part determined by comparisons he or she makes with standards (Michalos, 1985). Often people's standards come from observing people around them or from remembering what they themselves were like in the past. If people exceed these standards, they should be happy and satisfied, but if they fall short of their standards, they might experience low levels of well-being. Although this process seems straightforward, the process of making social comparisons is more subtle than originally believed (Diener & Fujita, 1997). People do not simply look around and judge their happiness by their distance above or below their friends and neighbors on relevant domains. Instead, people choose their targets for comparison, the information to which they attend, and the way they use this information in complex ways.

Wood (1996) stated that social comparison is simply "the process of thinking about information about one or more other people in relation to the self" (p. 520). The targets for comparison can be proximate individuals, individuals people see on television, or even individuals that people construct in their minds (Wood, Taylor, & Lichtman, 1985). People can pay attention to similarities, dissimilarities, or both when comparing themselves to a target. And, finally, people do not always contrast themselves with the target (i.e., they do not always feel unhappy when they are worse off, and they do not always feel happy when they are better off). Some people may find comparisons with more successful individuals motivating, while others may simply be reminded of their own lack of success. Diener and Fujita (1997) suggested that social comparison may actually be used as a coping strategy and may be influenced by personality and SWB. The choice of comparison target, the type of information to which an individual attends, and the way he or she uses this information may be a result rather than a cause of SWB.

Adaptation, Adjustment, and Coping

Just as certain events may affect people differently, depending on their goals and personalities, reactions to events are markedly different, depending on the amount of time that has progressed since the event occurred. The processes that can account for these differences are an important part of theories of SWB. However, theories of adaptation have changed considerably in recent years. Adaptation effects were once thought to be so strong that some suggested that people were stuck on a "hedonic treadmill" (Brickman & Campbell, 1971). Although the treadmill theory allowed for short-lived reactions to events, many psychologists believed that emotional reactions would eventually subside and that people would inevitably return to hedonic neutrality. Although this theory has played an important role in SWB research, more recent evidence shows that adaptation processes are not as strong as once thought.

For instance, we (Diener, Lucas, & Scollon, 2006) have recently reviewed the evidence for adaptation and developed five important revisions to the treadmill theory. First, although some adaptation occurs, it does not bring people back to hedonic neutrality. Instead, most people are happy most of the time (Diener & Diener, 1996). Second, if SWB set points exist, they vary across individuals. Personality research shows that there are considerable individual differences in long-term levels of happiness. Third, adaptation occurs in different ways for different components of SWB. Although one's affective experiences may return to baseline levels after an important event has occurred, it is possible that levels of life satisfaction will not (see, e.g., Lucas, 2007). Fourth, adaptation does not inevitably occur. As re-

viewed above, some life events do seem to affect SWB permanently. Finally, there are important individual differences in adaptation, with some people quickly returning to baseline levels and others experiencing permanent effects.

Although psychologists know much more about adaptation than they used to know, a number of important questions remain. For example, it is unclear how the nature of the event affects adaptation. Do people adapt to worsening conditions, or only to stable conditions or one-time events? Do unexpected events lead to less adaptation than predictable events do (Frederick & Loewenstein, 1999)? Similarly, it is unclear what individual-difference variables predict adaptation to life events (though see Bonanno, 2004, for a discussion of some possibilities). Finally, it is unclear whether adaptation represents a decrease in emotional response, an adjustment in goals and strategies for coping with the event, or both. A theory of subjective SWB must more clearly explain the processes responsible for adaptation: When does it occur, what processes are responsible for adaptation, and what are the limits to individuals' abilities to adapt?

THE EFFECTS OF HAPPINESS

Although people tend to think about happiness as an end state that results from the accomplishment of desired goals, psychologists have begun to ask whether happiness itself can play a role in helping people attain those goals. For instance, Fredrickson (1998) developed one well-known model of the function of positive emotions. She suggested that joy and other pleasant emotions broaden one's thinking and help to build resources. The evidence she reviewed shows that positive emotions can foster creativity and can lead people to try new things. This broadened approach to the world allows happy people to develop new strategies for overcoming challenges, new social skills, and even new physical resources. Together, these resources can lead to positive outcomes in people's lives.

More recently, Lyubomirsky, King, and Diener (2005) have compiled an extensive list of domains in which happier people do better than less happy people. Their meta-analytic review (which covered both correlational and experimental research) showed that happy people are more likely to get married, to have more friends, to make more money in the future, to perform better at work, to have better health, and perhaps even to live longer than unhappy people. Thus, although the stereotype of the happy person is someone who is somewhat lazy and unthinking, a growing body of evidence suggests that happiness can be functional and may promote positive outcomes in people's lives.

FUTURE DIRECTIONS
FOR SWB RESEARCH

SWB reflects the extent to which people think and feel that their lives are going well. In the future, psychologists will need to continue to identify the processes that promote high levels of this values characteristic. However, some of the most exciting developments are taking place outside the traditional boundaries of the field. Because subjective measures capture aspects of the good life that cannot be assessed via traditional social indicators, psychologists and economists have increasingly called for national and local governments to track the SWB of populations over time (Diener & Seligman, 2004; Kahneman, Kruger, Schkade, Schwartz, & Stone, 2003). If environmental factors and policy decisions reliably affect the SWB of these populations, then this information could be used to guide future policy decisions. Ultimately, this would allow governments to use the results of SWB research to increase overall quality of life. Thus, although SWB research was initially developed within the context of existing psychological theory, it has important implications for research, theory, and application in a wide variety of domains.

REFERENCES

Biswas-Diener, R., & Diener, E. (2001). Making the best of a bad situation: Satisfaction in the slums of Calcutta. *Social Indicators Research, 55*, 329–352.

Bonanno, G. A. (2004). Loss, trauma, and human resilience: Have we underestimated the human capacity to thrive after extremely aversive events? *American Psychologist, 59*, 20–28.

Bradburn, N. M. (1969). *The structure of psychological well-being*. Chicago: Aldine.

Brickman, P., & Campbell, D. T. (1971). Hedonic relativism and planning the good society. In M. H. Appley (Ed.), *Adaptation level theory: A symposium* (pp. 287–302). New York: Academic Press.

Brunstein, J. C. (1993). Personal goals and subjective well-being: A longitudinal study. *Journal of Personality and Social Psychology, 65*, 1061–1070.

Canli, T., Zhao, Z., Desmond, J. E., Kang, E., Gross, J., & Gabrieli, J. D. E. (2001). An fMRI study of personality influences on brain reactivity to emotional stimuli. *Behavioral Neuroscience, 115*, 33–42.

Cantor, N., & Sanderson, C. A. (1999). Life task participation and well-being: The importance of taking part in daily life. In D. Kahneman, E. Diener, & N. Schwarz (Eds.), *Well-being: The foundations of hedonic psychology* (pp. 230–243). New York: Russell Sage Foundation.

Carver, C. S., Sutton, S. K., & Scheier, M. F. (2000). Action, emotion, and personality: Emerging conceptual integration. *Personality and Social Psychology Bulletin, 26*, 741–751.

Derryberry, D., & Reed, M. A. (1994). Temperament and attention: Orienting toward and away from positive and negative signals. *Journal of Personality and Social Psychology, 66*, 1128–1139.

Diener, E. (1984). Subjective well-being. *Psychological Bulletin, 95*, 542–575.

Diener, E. (1994). Assessing subjective well-being: Progress and opportunities. *Social Indicators Research, 31*, 103–157.

Diener, E., & Biswas-Diener, R. (2002). Will money increase subjective well-being?: A literature review and guide to needed research. *Social Indicators Research, 57*, 119–169.

Diener, E., & Diener, C. (1996). Most people are happy. *Psychological Science, 7*, 181–185.

Diener, E., & Diener, M. (1995). Cross-cultural correlates of life satisfaction and self-esteem. *Journal of Personality and Social Psychology, 68*, 653–663.

Diener, E., & Emmons, R. A. (1985). The independence of positive and negative affect. *Journal of Personality and Social Psychology, 47*, 1105–1117.

Diener, E., & Fujita, F. (1997). Social comparisons and subjective well-being. In B. Buunk & R. Gibbons (Eds.), *Health, coping, and social comparison* (pp. 329–357). Mahwah, NJ: Erlbaum.

Diener, E., & Iran-Nejad, A. (1986). The relationship in experience between various types of affect. *Journal of Personality and Social Psychology, 50*, 1031–1038.

Diener, E., & Lucas, R. E. (1999). Personality and subjective well-being. In D. Kahneman, E. Diener, & N. Schwarz (Eds.), *Well-being: The foundations of hedonic psychology* (pp. 213–229). New York: Russell Sage Foundation.

Diener, E., Lucas, R. E., & Scollon, C. N. (2006). Beyond the hedonic treadmill: Revisions to the adaptation theory of well-being. *American Psychologist, 61*, 305–314.

Diener, E., Sandvik, E., & Pavot, W. (1991). Happiness is the frequency, not the intensity, of positive versus negative affect. In F. Strack, M. Argyle, & N. Schwarz (Eds.), *Subjective well-being: An interdisciplinary perspective* (pp. 119–139). Elmsford, NY: Pergamon Press.

Diener, E., Sandvik, E., Seidlitz, L., & Diener, M. (1993). The relationship between income and subjective well-being: Relative or absolute. *Social Indicators Research, 28,* 195–223.

Diener, E., & Seligman, M. E. P. (2004). Beyond money: Toward an economy of well-being. *Psychological Science in the Public Interest, 5,* 1–31.

Diener, E., & Suh, E. M. (1998). Subjective well-being and age: An international analysis. *Annual Review of Gerontology and Geriatrics, 17,* 304–324.

Diener, E., Suh, E. M., Lucas, R. E., & Smith, H. (1999). Subjective well-being: Three decades of progress. *Psychological Bulletin, 125,* 276–302.

Dijkers, M. (1997). Quality of life after spinal cord injury: A meta analysis of the effects of disablement components. *Spinal Cord, 35,* 829–840.

Eid, M., & Diener, E. (2004). Global judgments of subjective well-being: Situational variability and long-term stability. *Social Indicators Research, 65,* 245–277.

Elliot, A. J., & Thrash, T. M. (2002). Approach–avoidance motivation in personality: Approach and avoidance temperaments and goals. *Journal of Personality and Social Psychology, 82,* 804–818.

Ellison, C. G. (1991). Religious involvement and subjective well-being. *Journal of Health and Social Behavior, 32,* 80–99.

Ellison, C. G., Gay, D. A., & Glass, T. A. (1989). Does religious commitment contribute to individual life satisfaction? *Social Forces, 68,* 100–123.

Emmons, R. A. (1986). Personal strivings: An approach to personality and subjective well-being. *Journal of Personality and Social Psychology, 51,* 1058–1068.

Frederick, S., & Loewenstein, G. (1999). Hedonic adaptation. In D. Kahneman, E. Diener, & N. Schwarz (Eds.), *Well-being: The foundations of hedonic psychology* (pp. 302–329). New York: Russell Sage Foundation.

Fredrickson, B. L. (1998). What good are positive emotions? *Review of General Psychology, 2*(3), 300–319.

Fujita, F., & Diener, E. (2005). Life satisfaction set point: Stability and change. *Journal of Personality and Social Psychology, 88,* 158–164.

Ganz, P. A., Lee, J. J., & Siau, J. (1991). Quality of life assessment: An independent prognostic variable for survival in lung cancer. *Cancer, 67,* 3131–3135.

Gartner, J., Larson, D. B., & Allen, G. D. (1991). Religious commitment and mental health: A review of the empirical literature. *Journal of Psychology and Religion, 19,* 6–25.

George, L. K., & Landerman, R. (1984). Health and subjective well-being: A replicated secondary analysis. *International Journal of Aging and Human Development, 19,* 133–156.

Glenn, N. D. (1975). The contribution of marriage to the psychological well-being of males and females. *Journal of Marriage and Family Relations, 37,* 594–600.

Gove, W. R., & Shin, H. (1989). The psychological well-being of divorced and widowed men and women. *Journal of Family Issues, 10,* 122–144.

Gray, J. A. (1981). A critique of Eysenck's theory of personality. In H. J. Eysenck (Ed.), *A model for personality* (pp. 246–276). New York: Springer-Verlag.

Green, D. F., Goldman, S., & Salovey, P. (1993). Measurement error masks bipolarity in affect ratings. *Journal of Personality and Social Psychology, 64,* 1029–1041.

Headey, B., & Wearing, A. (1989). Personality, life events, and subjective well-being: Toward a dynamic equilibrium model. *Journal of Personality and Social Psychology, 57,* 731–739.

Hooker, K., & Siegler, I. C. (1992). Separating apples from oranges in health ratings: Perceived health includes psychological well-being. *Behavior, Health, and Aging, 2,* 81–92.

Johnson, W., McGue, M., & Krueger, R. F. (2005). Personality stability in late adulthood: A behavioral genetic analysis. *Journal of Personality, 73*(2), 523–551.

Kahneman, D. (1999). Objective happiness. In D. Kahneman, E. Diener, & N. Schwarz (Eds.), *Well-being: The foundations of hedonic psychology* (pp. 3–25). New York: Russell Sage Foundation.

Kahneman, D., Krueger, A. B., Schkade, D., Schwarz, N., & Stone, A. (2003). Toward national well-being accounts. *American Economic Review, 94,* 429–434.

Kahneman, D., & Riis, J. (2005). Living and thinking about it: Two perspectives on life. In F. A. Huppert, N. Baylis, & B. Keverne (Eds.), *The science of well-being* (pp. 285–304). New York: Oxford University Press.

Kasser, T., & Ryan, R. M. (1993). A dark side of the American dream: Correlates of financial success as a central life aspiration. *Journal of Personality and Social Psychology, 65,* 410–422.

Larsen, J. T., McGraw, A. P., & Cacioppo, J. T. (2001). Can people feel happy and sad at the same time? *Journal of Personality and Social Psychology, 81,* 684–696.

Larsen, R. J. (1989, August). Personality as an affect dispositional system. In L. A. Clark & D. Watson (Chairs), *Emotional bases of personality.* Symposium conducted at the meeting of the American Psychological Association, New Orleans.

Larsen, R. J., & Ketelaar, T. (1991). Personality and susceptibility to positive and negative emotional states. *Journal of Personality and Social Psychology, 61,* 132–140.

Larson, R. (1978). Thirty years of research on the subjective well-being of older Americans. *Journal of Gerontology, 33,* 109–125.

Lucas, R. E. (2005). Time does not heal all wounds: A longitudinal study of reaction and adaptation to divorce. *Psychological Science, 16,* 945–950.

Lucas, R. E. (2007). Long-term disability is associated with lasting changes in subjective well-being: Evidence from the two nationally representative longitudinal studies. *Journal of Personality and Social Psychology, 92,* 717–730.

Lucas, R. E., & Baird, B. M. (2004). Extraversion and emotional reactivity. *Journal of Personality and Social Psychology, 86,* 473–485.

Lucas, R. E., Clark, A. E., Georgellis, Y., & Diener, E. (2003). Re-examining adaptation and the set point model of happiness: Reactions to changes in marital status. *Journal of Personality and Social Psychology, 84,* 527–539.

Lucas, R. E., Clark, A. E., Georgellis, Y., & Diener, E. (2004). Unemployment alters the set-point for life satisfaction. *Psychological Science, 15,* 8–13.

Lucas, R. E., Diener, E., Grob, A., Suh, E. M., & Shao, L. (2000). Cross-cultural evidence for the fundamental features of extraversion. *Journal of Personality and Social Psychology, 79,* 452–468.

Lucas, R. E., Diener, E., & Suh, E. M. (1996). Discriminant validity of well-being measures. *Journal of Personality and Social Psychology, 71,* 616–628.

Lucas, R. E., & Donnellan, M. B. (2006). How stable is happiness?: Using the STARTS model to estimate the stability of life satisfaction. *Journal of Research in Personality, 41,* 1091–1098.

Lykken, D., & Tellegen, A. (1996). Happiness is a stochastic phenomenon. *Psychological Science, 7,* 186–189.

Lyobomirsky, S., King, L., & Diener, E. (2005). The benefits of frequent positive affect: Does happiness lead to success? *Psychological Bulletin, 131,* 803–855.

Magnus, K. B., Diener, E., Fujita, F., & Pavot, W. (1993). Extraversion and neuroticism as predictors of objective life events: A longitudinal analysis. *Journal of Personality and Social Psychology, 65,* 316–330.

Markus, H. R., & Kitayama, S. (1991). Culture and the self: Implications for cognition, emotion, and motivation. *Psychological Review, 98,* 224–253.

Maslow, A. H. (1954). *Motivation and personality.* New York: Harper.

Mastekaasa, A. (1995). Age variations in the suicide rates and self-reported subjective well-being of married and never-married persons. *Journal of community and Applied Social Psychology, 5,* 21–39.

McClellan, W. M., Anson, C., Birkeli, K., & Tuttle, E. (1991). Functional status and quality of life: Predictors of early mortality among patients entering treatment for end stage renal disease. *Journal of Clinical Epidemiology, 44,* 83–89.

McCrae, R. R., & Costa, P. T. (1991). Adding *Liebe und Arbeit:* The full five-factor model and well-being. *Personality and Social Psychology Bulletin, 17,* 227–232.

Michalos, A. C. (1985). Multiple discrepancies theory (MDT). *Social Indicators Research, 16,* 347–413.

Mossey, J. M., & Shapiro, E. (1982). Self-rated health: A predictor of mortality among the elderly. *American Journal of Public Health, 72,* 800–808.

Mroczek, D. K., & Spiro, A. (2005). Change in life satisfaction during adulthood: Findings from the Veterans Affairs Normative Aging Study. *Journal of Personality and Social Psychology, 88,* 189–202.

Murray, H. A. (1938). *Explorations in personality.* New York: Oxford University Press.

Myers, D. G., & Diener, E. (1995). Who is happy? *Psychological Science, 6,* 10–19.

Nelson, E., Conger, B., Douglass, R., Gephart, D., Kirk, J., Page, R., et al. (1983). Functional health status levels of primary care patients. *Journal of the American Medical Association, 249,* 3331–3338.

Nes, R. B., Roysamb, E., Tambs, K., Harris, J. R., & Reichborn-Kjennerud, T. (2006). Subjective well-being: Genetic and environmental contributions to stability and change. *Psychological Medicine, 36*(7), 1033–1042.

Oishi, S., Diener, E., Suh, E. M., & Lucas, R. E. (1999). Values as a moderator in subjective well-being. *Journal of Personality, 67,* 157–184.

Okun, M. A., Stock, W. A., Haring, M. J., & Witter, R. A. (1984). Health and subjective well-being: A meta-analysis. *International Journal of Aging and Human Development, 19,* 111–132.

Pinquart, M. (2001). Age differences in perceived positive affect, negative affect, and affect balance in middle and old age. *Journal of Happiness Studies, 2,* 375–405.

Pollner, M. (1989). Divine relations, social relations, and well-being. *Journal of Health and Social Behavior, 30,* 92–104.

Poloma, M. M., & Pendleton, B. F. (1991). The effects of prayer and prayer experiences on measures of general well-being. *Journal of Psychology and Theology, 29,* 71–83.

Putzke, J. D., Richards, J. S., Hicken, B. L., & DeVivo, M. J. (2002). Predictors of life satisfaction: A spinal cord injury cohort study. *Archives of Physical Medicine and Rehabilitation, 83,* 555–561.

Roysamb, E., Harris, J. R., Magnus, P., Vitterso, J., & Tambs, K. (2002). Subjective well-being: Sex-specific effects of genetic and environmental factors. *Personality and Individual Differences, 32*(2), 211–223.

Roysamb, E., Tambs, K., Reichborn-Kjennerud, T., Neale, M. C., & Harris, J. R. (2003). Happiness and health: Environmental and genetic contributions to the relationship between subjective well-being, perceived health, and somatic illness. *Journal of Personality and Social Psychology, 85*(6), 1136–1146.

Rumsfeld, J. S., MaWhinney, S., McCarthy, M., Jr., Shroyer, A. L. W., VillaNueva, C. B., O'Brien, M., et al. (1999). Health-related quality of life as a predictor of mortality following coronary artery bypass graft surgery. *Journal of the American Medical Association, 281,* 1298–1303.

Russell, J. A. (1980). A circumplex model of affect. *Journal of Personality and Social Psychology, 39,* 1161–1178.

Rusting, C. L. (1998). Personality, mood, and cognitive processing of emotional information: Three conceptual frameworks. *Psychological Bulletin, 124,* 165–196.

Ryan, R. M., Sheldon, K. M, Kasser, T., & Deci, E. L. (1996). All goals are not created equal: An organismic perspective on the nature of goals and their regulation. In P. M. Gollwitzer & J. A. Bargh (Eds.), *The psychology of action: Linking cognition and motivation to behavior* (pp. 7–26). New York: Guilford Press.

Ryff, C. D. (1989). Happiness is everything, or is it?: Explorations on the meaning of psychological well-being. *Journal of Personality and Social Psychology, 57*, 1069–1081.

Sandvik, E., Diener, E., & Seidlitz, L. (1993). Subjective well-being: The convergence and stability of self-report and non-self-report strategies. *Journal of Personality, 61*, 317–342.

Schimmack, U. (2001). Pleasure, displeasure, and mixed feelings?: Are semantic opposites mutually exclusive? *Cognition and Emotion, 15*, 81–97.

Schimmack, U. (2008). The structure of subjective well-being. In M. Eid & R. J. Larsen (Eds.), *The science of subjective well-being* (pp. 97–123). New York: Guilford Press.

Schimmack U., & Oishi, S. (2005). Chronically accessible versus temporarily accessible sources of life satisfaction judgments. *Journal of Personality and Social Psychology, 89*, 395–406.

Schwarz, N., & Clore, G. L. (1983). Mood, misattribution, and judgments of well-being: Informative and directive functions of affective states. *Journal of Personality and Social Psychology, 45*, 513–523.

Schwarz, N., & Strack, F. (1999). Reports of subjective well-being: Judgmental processes and their methodological implications. In D. Kahneman, E. Diener, & N. Schwarz (Eds.), *Well-being: The foundations of hedonic psychology* (pp. 61–84). New York: Russell Sage Foundation.

Strack, F., Martin, L. L., & Schwarz, N. (1988). Priming and communication: Social determinants of information use in judgments of life satisfaction. *European Journal of Social Psychology, 18*, 429–442.

Stubbe, J. H., Posthuma, D., Boomsma, D. I., & De Geus, E. J. C. (2005). Heritability of life satisfaction in adults: A twin–family study. *Psychological Medicine, 35*(11), 1581–1588.

Suh, E. M., Diener, E., Oishi, S., & Triandis, H. (1998). The shifting basis of life satisfaction judgments across cultures. *Journal of Personality and Social Psychology, 70*, 1091–1102.

Tellegen, A. (1985). Structures of mood and personality and their relevance to assessing anxiety, with an emphasis on self-report. In A. H. Tuma & J. D. Maser (Eds.), *Anxiety and the anxiety disorders* (pp. 681–706). Hillsdale, NJ: Erlbaum.

Tellegen, A., Lykken, D. T., Bouchard, T. J., Wilcox, K. J., Segal, N. L., & Rich, S. (1988). Personality similarity in twins reared apart and together. *Journal of Personality and Social Psychology, 54*(6), 1031–1039.

Veenhoven, R. (1994). *Correlates of happiness: 7836 findings from 603 studies in 69 nations: 1911–1994.* Unpublished manuscript, Erasmus University, Rotterdam, The Netherlands.

Warr, P., Barter, J., & Brownbridge, G. (1983). On the independence of positive and negative affect. *Journal of Personality and Social Psychology, 44*, 644–651.

Watson, D., Clark, L. A., & Tellegen, A. (1988). Development and validation of brief measures of positive and negative affect: The PANAS scales. *Journal of Personality and Social Psychology, 54*, 1063–1070.

Watson, D., & Pennebaker, J. W. (1989). Health complaints, stress, and distress: Exploring the central role of negative affectivity. *Psychological Review, 96*, 234–254.

Watson, D., & Tellegen, A. (1985). Towards a consensual structure of mood. *Psychological Bulletin, 98*, 219–235.

Watten, R. G., Vassend, D., Myhrer, T., & Syversen, J. L. (1997). Personality factors and somatic symptoms. *European Journal of Personality, 11*, 57–68.

White, J. M. (1992). Marital status and well-being in Canada. *Journal of Family Issues, 13*, 390–409.

Wilson, W. (1967). Correlates of avowed happiness. *Psychological Bulletin, 67*, 294–306.

Wood, J. V. (1996). What is social comparison and how should we study it? *Personality and Social Psychology Bulletin, 22*, 520–537.

Wood, J. V., Taylor, S. E., & Lichtman, R. R. (1985). Social comparison in adjustment to breast cancer. *Journal of Personality and Social Psychology, 49*, 1169–1183.

Zevon, M. A., & Tellegen, A. (1982). The structure of mood change: An idiographic/nomothetic analysis. *Journal of Personality and Social Psychology, 43*, 111–112.

CHAPTER 30

Temperament and Emotion

JOHN E. BATES, JACKSON A. GOODNIGHT, and JENNIFER E. FITE

Temperament provides ways to talk about individual differences in emotion and how they develop. Temperament and emotion can be separated for the sake of theoretical analysis, but they correspond in so many ways that it is clear that they are part of the same whole (an impression supported by the 1,680,000 Google listings for the phrase "temperament and emotion" and 4,548 published sources identified by PsycINFO). As theory about emotion advances, theory about temperament advances in the same directions.

Since the chapter on temperament in the second edition of this handbook (Bates, 2000) appeared, the literature on emotion has grown, especially on the topic of self-regulation; correspondingly, this has been an especially important theme of work on temperament in that time (Rothbart & Bates, 2006). Conversely, individual differences and their development are crucial parts of emotional phenomena. Closely connected to interest in individual differences and development, and also providing a framework for understanding the basic phenomena of emotions, is interest in social adaptation. Emotions serve crucial functions in social adaptation, and individuals' characteristic pat-

terns of emotions influence and are influenced by variations in social adaptations. Variations in social adaptations are of interest in both basic and applied research.

There are direct linkages between temperament dimensions and social adjustment. A number of studies show that early childhood tendencies to be distressed by novelty predict later internalizing behaviors, that tendencies to be impulsive or unmanageable predict externalizing behaviors, and that tendencies to be high in negative emotionality predict both internalizing and externalizing behaviors (Bates, 1989; Rothbart & Bates, 2006). However, the predictive links between temperament and adjustment are of a moderate size, even if we allow for attenuated relations due to error of measurement. This suggests that a given temperament does not by itself produce adjustment. Developmental-systems theories propose many other causal factors. The most prominent kinds of additional factors are family characteristics, such as parenting style. One would expect that temperament and family qualities might additively predict child adjustment outcomes. Empirical findings in support of this expectation are surprisingly sparse (Bates & Pettit, 2007). This may be because relatively few studies have evaluated such additive models of social development. However, it may also be due to unreported failures to find such effects. If the latter is true, it could be due to overlap in variance between child temperament and parenting, due to common measurement sources (often parent report) or due to shared genetic roots for both child and parent traits. Another possible explanation is that temperament and family environment interact in shaping social development (Chess & Thomas, 1984; Wachs, 2000). A temperament trait becomes a behavior problem only in some kinds of families, or a parenting characteristic promotes behavior problems only for children with certain temperaments. Since the second edition of this handbook (Lewis & Haviland-Jones, 2000) was published, there has been remarkable growth in the literature on how temperament and environmental characteristics interact with one another in shaping social adaptations. This chapter considers temperament, emotion, and the development of social adaptations, with special emphases on self-regulation and the interaction between emotional dispositions and environmental qualities in shaping social development.

CONCEPTS OF EMOTION AND TEMPERAMENT

Emotion Concepts

We think of "emotion" as a set of hypothetical constructs representing processes that range across all levels of psychological theory—including genetics, biochemistry, neural systems, perceptual and cognitive processes (both conscious and nonconscious), motivation, affective displays, behavior, and social systems. We are most interested in the aspects of emotion constructs that help to describe social transactions. Although emotion constructs share properties that tie them to the general concept of emotion, specific emotions (such as joy, interest, fear, or anger) are the main foci of scientific study, not emotion as an umbrella concept. More detailed consideration of the basic emotion constructs guiding the present chapter can be found in Bates (2000). Recent writings have further refined appreciation of the neural and cognitive underpinnings of regulation of emotion (e.g., Lewis, 2005).

Temperament Concepts

We think of "temperament" as a set of hypothetical constructs describing individual differences in reactivity and self-regulation (Rothbart & Bates, 2006). One kind of reactivity dimension includes negative reactions, such as general distress and more specific fear and frustration. For example, some infants become angry faster and more intensely than other infants when their arms are held down, preventing them from reaching an attractive toy. Another kind of reactivity includes positive reactions, such as interest and joy. For example, some infants show more excitement when they see a toy and are more eager to reach it than other infants. An emotion in one such situation does not define a temperament trait. Temperament is the pattern of responses in a given type of incentive condition across many occasions.

Such behavior patterns are rooted in biological traits, at both genetic and neural levels. They appear relatively early, befitting a concept of core personality, but they are not fully formed at birth. As brain and behavioral repertoire develop, temperamental traits emerge and stabilize. The key example of this is effortful control of attention, which depends on maturation of the relevant frontal lobe structures of the infant's brain, beginning late in the first year and continuing throughout childhood (Reuda, Posner, & Rothbart, 2004; Rothbart, Derryberry, & Posner, 1994). Any personality trait is by definition stable, and it would be fitting for temperament traits, since they are core in personality, to be highly stable. However, measures of temperament are typically found to be only moderately stable.

Part of the limitation in stability of temperament traits is theoretically appropriate, and part is due to error of measurement of the temperament phenotype. The theoretically appropriate part of the limited stability concerns the fundamental nature of temperament and how this might be measured. Temperament can be conceived at three different levels: genetic, neural, and behavioral. One might presuppose that the action of genes underlying temperament would be highly stable, but in theory it should only be relatively stable. We may eventually have specific genetic configurations that underlie temperament. This seems possible as a product of today's extremely vigorous efforts to use molecular genetics tools in developmental science. For example, genes coding for dopamine functions may influence attraction to novelty, and genes controlling for serotonin functions may influence distress tendencies (Auerbach, Faroy, Ebstein, Kahana, & Levine, 2001; Lakatos et al., 2003; Rothbart & Bates, 2006). However, even as we look forward to such markers, it is important to keep in mind that genes do not operate like a fixed program. Multiple genes interact with one another and with other factors in the biological environment, and thus there still may be some instability in the functioning of genes that code for temperament-relevant processes. Likewise, although there has been enormous progress in describing the anatomy and functioning of the nervous system, we do not have measures of the neural patterns that constitute temperament. And even when such markers are defined, we would expect that individuals would show changes in neural patterns, reflecting both experience and maturation. For example, a child might develop new emotional appraisals of situations by forming new associations via synaptic changes in structures such as the amygdala and hippocampus (Lewis, 2005; Posner & Rothbart, 2000). Finally, to consider observable behavior (the top level of a temperament construct), all measures of behavior patterns—whether based on self-report, caregiver report, or direct observation—have limitations in reliability and validity (Rothbart & Bates, 1998). However, even if ideal measures were possible, there would still be changes in the behavior patterns due to changes in individuals' life circumstances and the corresponding changes in the incentive conditions for activating motivations and emotions. Nevertheless, despite these considerations, temperament measures do show sufficient levels of stability, even across many years of development, to retain their usefulness as markers of traits (Caspi, 1998; Kagan, 1998; Rothbart & Bates, 2006).

Emotion versus Emotion Regulation

A particularly interesting discussion has concerned the distinction between "emotion" and "emotion regulation." This conceptual distinction echoes the distinction between reactive and regulatory aspects of temperament. Campos, Frankel, and Camras (2004) argue that emotion and emotion regulation are functionally inseparable. There is no "pure" emotion, in the sense of an event that exists in a measurable way separate from regulation. Emotion

and emotion regulation are concurrent processes, and an emotional response to a given incentive stimulus depends on preexisting regulatory processes, such as cortical inhibition or the way the stimulus is interpreted. Nevertheless, although Campos and his colleagues do see emotion and emotion regulation as inextricably part of the same whole and reject a formulation in which an emotion occurs and is subsequently regulated, they also admit to a conceptual, analytical distinction between the two intimately related concepts. In a somewhat different view, Cole, Martin, and Dennis (2004) argue that emotion regulation can be conceptually defined as separate from the emotions that are regulated and empirically defined by systematically measuring changes in emotions, even though they also agree that "emotions are inherently regulatory" (p. 319). Cole et al. review several areas of research that can be interpreted as showing the emotion–regulation distinction, such as studies in which high levels of regulatory responses—both at the level of directly observable behavior and at the level of psychophysiological indices such as vagal tone—are associated with low levels of negative affect. In summary, although it seems that emotion and emotion regulation are conceptually part of the same set of processes, there are also theoretical reasons to distinguish the two separate components in at least some concrete ways.

Related to the issue of how to distinguish between emotion and emotion regulation is the issue of how to distinguish between reactive and effortful or executive forms of regulation (Nigg, 2000). It is likely that regulatory behavior differences often involve components of both reactive and effortful control (Eisenberg, Spinrad, & Smith, 2004). Nevertheless, the theoretical distinction can be useful. Gray (1993) has described two neural systems. The behavioral inhibition system (BIS) processes stimuli that may signify danger or loss, such as novelty, and produces inhibition as a primary motor output. Fear and anxiety are the emotional products of activity in these circuits. The behavioral activation system (BAS) processes stimuli that may signify potential rewards, and produces approach actions as a primary motor output. Interest, excitement, and joy are the emotional products. Suppose that it is the beginning of the year in a preschool class, and the teacher has asked the children to stand in a line. Most of the children will comply, but there may be different temperamental–emotional bases for their compliance. Some will be very interested in the room, and would otherwise be exploring; however, the teacher's command cues their effortful self-regulation, and they focus their attention away from the exciting toys and onto the markers on the floor that the teacher has asked them to stand next to. Some—discomfited by the general novelty of the situation, and thus reactively or fearfully inhibited—are predisposed to stand still anyway. Some will comply with difficulty because they are so positively aroused by the situation, and others will comply with ease because they are relatively uninterested. Among the few who have to be helped to comply, there will be at least one who is joyfully pursuing fun (e.g., showing a new friend how he or she can jump, or trying to look more closely at the collection of toy cars). And there may even be one who has reacted with anger to the restriction. Empirical measurement of effortful control separate from reactive control is difficult. Casual observation may not reveal the components of the behavior, but detailed and extensive observation of the children may help in distinguishing the underlying systems. The distinctions may not matter for some purposes, but may ultimately be important in understanding development of individual differences in social adaptation (Eisenberg, Spinrad, et al., 2004; Fox & Calkins, 2003; Stifter, Spinrad, & Braungart-Rieker, 1999). In addition to having measures of behavior patterns across different kinds of incentive conditions and at different stages of development, it will also be useful to have measures that can more clearly refer to the effortful forms of emotion regulation.

Emotion Regulation and Social Adaptation

Promising measures of core emotion regulation processes are being developed. Some of these measures have implications for the study of individual differences in social development, and we mention several examples here. Lewis and Steiben (2004) argue that emotion regulation can be measured via event-related potentials in the prefrontal cortex. They review past findings on two event-related potentials that are thought to reflect the activity of the anterior cingulate cortex. The inhibitory N2 response, occurring between 200 and 350 milliseconds following a challenging stimulus, and the error-related negativity (ERN) response, occurring about 80 milliseconds after an error such as

pushing the wrong button, both reflect aspects of cognitive control. Individuals low on N2 and ERN responses have been found to be relatively high on impulsivity and aggression. Lewis and Steiben (2004) also report an intriguing preliminary result from a study of children in a go/no-go task. In a go/no-go task, a prepotent "go" response (typically pushing a button upon seeing a particular symbol on the computer screen) is established via rewards, but also, less frequently, a stimulus calls for a nondominant nonresponse, which requires effortful control. The Lewis and Steiben version of the task included a block of trials in which the experimenter increased the rate of errors via faster presentation of stimuli, thereby creating a failure experience. Lewis and Steiben found that children who were high on internalizing problems showed bigger N2 and ERN responses than other children, and in the block of failure trials showed a significant increase in size of the ERN, which the other children did not. This suggests that tendencies to be highly prepared to detect and regulate errors at speeds faster than conscious processing are associated with symptoms of anxiety and depression.

A second possible index of emotional self-regulation ability is the time it takes to stop a response that has been triggered by a stimulus—an executive ability that is mediated by the orbito-frontal region of the prefrontal cortex. The stop signal reaction time measure of response inhibition has been previously used for understanding adaptive difficulties such as attention-deficit/hyperactivity disorder (Logan, Schachar, & Tannock, 1997). In a small experience-sampling study with preadolescent children, Hoeksma, Osterlaan, and Schipper (2004) found that variability of anger over the period of self-observation was positively correlated with stop signal reaction time. The longer it took a child to inhibit a motor response in a laboratory test, the more variability the child showed in naturally occurring levels of anger. Basing their argument on the assumptions that feelings of anger reflect emotional process and are cues for cognitive regulation (because unregulated anger is maladaptive), Hoeksma et al. interpreted their obtained correlation as showing that the capacity for quick response inhibition leads to more effective anger regulation.

Attentional measures, such as sustained attention and tendency to direct attention away from frustrating objects, are associated with tendencies to modulate negative emotions and ultimately with social adjustment (Hill & Braungart-Rieker, 2002; Stifter & Spinrad, 2002). An interesting index of an attention-related regulatory process is the suppression of heart rate variability associated with breathing (respiratory sinus arrhythmia). For example, in one study, infants who showed lower levels of suppression of respiratory sinus arrhythmia in an attention task (they were given a block to examine) showed higher levels of frustration in tasks where they were prevented from reaching goals (Calkins, Dedmon, Gill, Lomax, & Johnson, 2002). It appears that the angry infants were less able to focus their attention on nonfrustrating aspects of a situation. Similar patterns of association between ability to focus attention and lower tendencies to express negative affect have been found in a number of other studies (Eisenberg, Smith, Sadovsky, & Spinrad, 2004).

Finally, more traditional measures of early childhood effortful control are found in numerous response inhibition measures, based on laboratory tasks in which a child is asked to do such things as walk a line slowly or delay before consuming a piece of candy, and in questionnaires asking caregivers about children's ability to focus and shift attention and to inhibit responses where appropriate (Rothbart & Bates, 2006). Such measures are successful in forecasting children's adjustment in later childhood, even after early childhood adjustment is controlled for. Children who are more successful on response inhibition tasks are less aggressive, are less noncompliant, and show more positive social qualities in childhood and adolescence than children who are less successful at inhibiting behaviors on demand (Denham et al., 2003; Eisenberg, Smith, et al., 2004; Eisenberg et al., 2005; Olson, Sameroff, Kerr, Lopez, & Wellman, 2005; Olson, Schilling, & Bates, 1999; Rothbart & Bates, 2006). There are also a few studies that show that children who are very high on regulation in laboratory tasks show correspondingly high levels of internalizing problems (e.g., Murray & Kochanska, 2002). However, it seems likely that such patterns reflect overcontrol that is based in reactive, anxious inhibition rather than effortful, executive control (Rothbart & Bates, 2006).

In summary, the distinctions between reactive and regulatory aspects of temperament closely parallel similar distinctions between emotion and emotion regulation. It is likely that in nature, emotion and its regulation and their corresponding personality traits constitute parts of the same complex processes. Nevertheless, at this time, it does seem theoretically helpful to keep them as separate concepts. It is possible that the distinction will help describe important details in how children attain their unique social adaptations. At this point, a fair amount of research has suggested that a temperamental tendency toward wariness forecasts later, conceptually analogous internalizing problems. The same tendency also sometimes serves to retard the growth of conduct problems, which can be seen as a function of sensitivity to the punishment that externalizing behavior often brings (Bates, Pettit, & Dodge, 1995; Keiley, Lofthouse, Bates, Dodge, & Pettit, 2003). Other kinds of reactive regulation, such as the quick detection of errors (Lewis & Steiben, 2004), could also play a role in the development of anxiety and prevention of aggression. Research has also suggested that temperamental tendencies toward unmanageability or impulsivity, including low effortful control, forecast conceptually analogous tendencies toward externalizing behavior. And temperamental negative emotionality—which can reflect irritability due to sensitivity to unpleasant stimuli, sensitivity to frustration of efforts to approach or control, and weak ability to divert attention from such stimuli—turns out to predict both internalizing and externalizing problems. This differential pattern of linkage between temperament and adjustment provides a basis for appreciating the complex but theoretically important recent trend in research to explore how children's adjustment outcomes develop as an interactive function of both temperament and environmental characteristics.

ADJUSTMENT AS THE INTERACTIVE PRODUCT OF TEMPERAMENT AND ENVIRONMENT

Developmental theory has for a long time emphasized complex relations between child and environment as determinants of adjustment differences between children. A given environment may have different implications for children with different temperament or other characteristics, such as intelligence; or a given child characteristic may have different implications, depending on the environment within which it is expressed (Collins, Maccoby, Steinberg, Hetherington, & Bornstein, 2000; Wachs,

2000). As recently as 10 years ago, there was barely a smattering of studies showing temperament–environment interaction effects. Theory expected interaction effects, but few had been found. As we have discussed in previous reviews of this topic (e.g., Rothbart & Bates, 2006), this might have been a function of the methodological difficulties of finding such interaction effects (McClelland & Judd, 1993). However, temperament–environment interaction effects have been reported at such an accelerating rate in recent years that we now entertain the possibility that the previous paucity of findings was due less to methodological obstacles than to the research *Zeitgeist* in that era.

The emerging research, despite being quite encouraging, still has methodological shortcomings. For example, not all interaction effect findings adequately control for main effects, and not all findings fully evaluate the effects of different distributions of predictor and outcome variables at the contrasting levels of the moderator variable (Bates & McFadyen-Ketchum, 2000). Nor are we totally sanguine about the adequacy of measurement of any of the key constructs. The temperament measures in most of the relevant studies are behavioral, which in effect means that it is often difficult to distinguish between emotional reactivity and emotion regulation traits. For example, high levels of frustration reactivity could reflect temperament substrates of strong tendencies to approach, weak ability to turn attention away from a frustrating stimulus, or both. However, the overall pattern of results allows us to see the glass as half full. We believe that the temperament constructs do have some meaning. As mentioned earlier, there is a differential pattern of linkages between temperament and adjustment dimensions, with a temperament low in regulation predicting high levels of externalizing problems and a temperament high in novelty distress predicting high levels of internalizing problems. Furthermore, there are emerging patterns of temperament–environment interaction effects in the development of children's adjustment. There is a substantial pattern of temperament–environment interaction results for three categories of temperament: novelty distress, negative emotionality, and impulsivity–effortful control (Bates & Pettit, 2007).

In the novelty distress category, two patterns stand out, each with some but not yet adequate replication. First, for young children with high

novelty distress, gentle maternal control appears to promote the development of prosocial behavior better than harsh control does, whereas for low-fear children the harshness of maternal control does not seem related to development of prosocial behavior (Kochanska, 1997). Second, children who are reactive in ways that predispose them to novelty distress are less likely to develop full-blown behavioral inhibition and anxiety problems if they are handled in more directive and challenging ways (e.g., curtly or even in an irritated way) than if they are handled in less directive and challenging ways (Arcus, 2001; Bates & Pettit, 2007).

In the negative emotionality category, there is a pattern in which negative parenting appears to amplify the links between child negative emotionality and the development of externalizing behavior problems—or the converse, in which child negative emotionality amplifies the links between negative parenting and behavior problems (Bates & Pettit, 2007). And there is also the pattern referred to in connection with novelty distress: Young infants who are negatively emotional in a challenging laboratory situation are at risk for the behavioral inhibition pattern, but they appear to be less likely to develop this pattern if treated in more rather than less challenging ways (Arcus, 2001; Bates & Pettit, 2007). Negative emotionality, especially when assessed in younger infants, may signify tendencies toward frustration and anger, or it may signify tendencies toward fearful distress. These are not well differentiated until later in infancy. In any event, the patterns are at this point suggestive, rather than fully established.

In the impulsivity–effortful control category, there are suggestions (again needing further replication), for two kinds of patterns. First, children who are low in self-regulation—that is, children high in unmanageability or impulsivity, and low in effortful control of attention—are more likely to develop externalizing problems if their parents are negative and lacking in warmth and responsiveness, whereas parenting does not matter so much for children who are high in self-regulation (Bates & Pettit, 2007). The second pattern is that children's early unmanageability tendencies are more likely to become externalizing behavior problems when mothers are less rather than more controlling of the children's misbehavior (Bates & Pettit, 2007; Bates, Pettit, Dodge, & Ridge, 1998). Because our emphasis here is on advances in understanding self-regulation, the remainder of this chapter expands on the role of children's self-regulatory characteristics in interaction with characteristics of their environments.

Developmental Process and Self-Regulation

Consistent with the preceding paragraph's summary of some relevant studies, we assume that children who are well regulated—that is, able to control their attention and to inhibit dominant responses for the sake of performing subdominant responses—will be less likely than poorly self-regulated children to behave in disruptive ways when attracted to potential rewards in a situation where approach or dominance behaviors are not appropriate. We also assume that they will be less likely to behave in neurotic ways when frightened by potential punishers in a situation where pursuit of rewards is more appropriate than withdrawal. These assumptions are essentially definitional, however. They do not explain how behavioral adjustment develops. What happens as a result of a child's successful adaptation in a particular situation? What happens in instances where the adaptation is unsuccessful? How are these experiences in some way carried forward? In modern, systems-based theories, it is assumed that the child learns something or fails to learn something, but that in addition, the child's transactions in some way transform the environment. Over many iterations, tendencies may become increasingly solidified.

Initial probabilities of well-regulated children's self-regulative responses should not have to be markedly higher than those of poorly regulated children for them to contribute eventually to a substantial difference in adaptive outcomes. Over the multiple steps of a real-life event, a well-regulated child will experience a success that may condition, in some small way, dispositions to expect good results. And then in the future, the child will be a little more likely to approach a similar task with positive emotion or a minimum of negative emotion. If we assume that caregivers will feel similarly and will be more likely to provide more advanced opportunities, the child will take further steps toward competence. Repeated over many such occasions, small initial differences between a well-regulated child and a less well-regulated young child may grow to socially significant differences in the developmental trajectories of these children.

A recent model of such processes builds on the widely used and well-supported coercive

family process model of Patterson and his colleagues (e.g., Patterson, Reid, & Dishion, 1992): In this new model, Granic and Patterson (2006) provide a nonlinear dynamic-systems account of how children and their social systems may develop toward clinically significant antisocial behavior problems. For example, to consider one kind of situation, a boy at risk for conduct problems and his parent experience cognitive–emotional–behavioral feedback processes that frequently resolve toward an "attractor state" of mutual hostility. Essentially, the probability that a hostile act by one party will be followed by a hostile act by the other party increases in a nonlinear way, and this state, among all the other possible ones, comes to be especially likely. Alternatively, sometimes the same system resolves toward a child's being sullen or defiant and the parent's being permissive or even submissive toward the child; and sometimes it resolves toward fun and mutually satisfying states. As the transactions of a given event proceed, small factors (e.g., the actors' initial moods and motives, their skills for self-regulation, or the presence of other actors) may probabilistically influence the dyad's movements through the various mutual state possibilities, shaping the likelihood that one attractor state, such as repeated hostile exchanges, will dominate. After many such experiences, such a coercive state may be achieved in just an exchange or two, and from there hostility may escalate even to violence. Over time, these experiences shape development. In a cascading series, initial constraints on the phase transitions and attractors of the system, such as child temperament or parent stress, produce further constraints, such as rigid patterns of coercive parent–child interaction and rigid patterns of child approach to various opportunities (e.g., learning and peer interaction opportunities in preschool); these patterns lead to key conflicts and, fairly abruptly, to aggressive behavior. These difficulties are constraints that in turn create further constraints, such as peer rejection, teacher negativity, and so on.

The emerging findings on how temperament and environment moderate one another's influence in shaping social development are interesting from a number of perspectives, but most particularly in the context of the Granic and Patterson (2006) formulation, because they can provide plausible leads in the search for control parameters that explain how a developmental system may turn one way versus another. It is important to learn about moderators of risk conditions, such as child temperament—both for the sake of further development of theories such as Granic and Patterson's, and for the guidance of practical experiments, such as improved treatments for child behavior problems. Self-regulation differences may be particularly critical parameters in the developmental system, and ones whose implications influence the implications of other parameters and vice versa. We therefore now turn to a discussion of a handful of recent studies of regulation × environment interactions in the development of children's adjustment.

Recent Examples of Self-Regulation × Environment Interactions

Decades of research have firmly established an association of generally moderate strength between negative parenting (or the absence of positive parenting) and child behavior problems (Rothbaum & Weisz, 1994). This negative parenting risk factor also interacts, it now appears, with child temperament in the production of behavior problems. As mentioned, one pattern in the recent literature is that children with tendencies to be dysregulated are more likely to have concurrent or future conduct problems when they experience hostile or otherwise dysregulated parenting. One good example of this is the study by Rubin, Burgess, Dwyer, and Hastings (2003), which predicted later adjustment from a composite of laboratory and mother-rated measures of child self-regulation of frustration and inhibition of prohibited behavior at age 2, and from a composite of lab observations and self-report measures of intrusive and hostile parenting, also at age 2. The study showed a stronger prediction from children's poor self-regulation of frustration and poor inhibition of prohibited behavior at age 2 to mother-rated externalizing problems at age 4 when their mothers were highly intrusive and hostile at age 2 than when they were low on negative parenting. In other words, toddlers' emotional and behavioral self-regulation deficits were less likely to become conduct problems if their mothers were measured and positive in their dealings with the children, presumably not building a mutual hostility "attractor." Thus, we can speculate, a more benign system allowed the children to learn more adaptive, less rigid patterns of conflict resolution and to develop more positive expectancies about social interactions in general. A mother

characteristic moderated the developmental implications of a toddler characteristic. In a conceptually related way, but from another perspective, Rubin et al. (2003) also found a stronger relation between children's aggressiveness observed in play with a peer at age 2 and mother-rated externalizing problems at age 4 when the children were low on the self-regulation index than when they were high on it. In other words, children's self-regulation characteristics moderated the developmental implications of their early aggressiveness. Perhaps the children's ability to regulate frustration and restrain actions in the face of a prohibition allowed adaptive responses to the negative feedback that often follows aggressive acts, and thus the children learned socially acceptable ways to express assertive (or low-level aggressive) motives.

Aside from negative parenting, another well-established risk factor for child behavior problems is a family's socioeconomic status (SES) (e.g., Dodge, Pettit, & Bates, 1994). Of course, SES sums a wide variety of differences in the experiences of children, including multiple qualities of parenting (Dodge et al., 1994); neighborhood qualities (Beyers, Bates, Pettit, & Dodge, 2003); and major stressors and daily hassles, including poverty (McLeod & Shanahan, 1996). In a recent, large-scale, cross-sectional study, Veenstra, Lindenberg, Oldehinkel, DeWinter, and Ormel (2006) found that the predictable relation of SES to preadolescents' antisocial behavior (a composite of parent and youth report) held only for youths who were described as high on frustration and low on effortful control (also measured by both parent and youth report). These findings suggest that child emotional and behavioral self-regulation may be important in determining whether negative experiences in the family and neighborhood cascade toward stable patterns of externalizing behavior.

Similar processes may influence the development of internalizing problems. A study by Crockenberg and Leerkes (2006) illustrates this in a particularly important way. Not only does this study consider a temperament–environment interaction; it also considers an interaction between two temperament characteristics, one concerning reactivity and the other concerning regulation. Recall that distress to novelty has been theoretically and empirically linked to later anxiety behaviors, and that looking away from something that might cause distress is viewed as an early marker of self-regulation ability (Rothbart & Bates, 2006). Infants who were described by their mothers as high in distress to novelty at 6 months, but who also were observed to look away from a novel toy presented to them (and look at something else), showed less mother-reported anxiety at 30 months than those who did not show this attention-regulating ability. Importantly, however, this effect was found when mothers were observed at 6 months to be low in sensitivity and engagement (in situations away from the novel toy presentation), and not when they were high in sensitivity and engagement. It appears that sensitive, engaged mothers may have been able to provide a compensating form of regulation to prevent experiences of novelty distress from growing into more generalized anxious behavior. This illustrates a theoretical point often made in developmental psychopathology (e.g., Cummings, Davies, & Campbell, 2000): Developmental systems typically allow more than one way to reach a socially important outcome. If one mechanism is lacking, such as early-developing self-regulation ability, another mechanism, such as appropriately supportive parenting, can help maintain adaptive development.

Two recent studies from our own lab provide further examples of ways in which self-regulatory tendencies may interact with environment and other characteristics of youths to shape the development of externalizing behaviors. We (Goodnight, Bates, Newman, Dodge, & Pettit, 2006) found that adolescents' performance in a laboratory game (the Card Playing Task; Newman, Patterson, & Kosson, 1987) moderated the often-observed association between their friends' deviance and their own externalizing behaviors. Youths who continued to pursue rewards in the Card Playing Task, despite experiencing an increasingly higher ratio of punishment to reward, showed a stronger association between their friends' and their own externalizing behaviors 2 years later. This was so even when their own, earlier levels of externalizing behavior were controlled for. Friends' deviance may reflect the degree to which youths' peer groups provide positive reinforcement for antisocial behavior (Dishion, Spracklen, Andrews, & Patterson, 1996). It is also important to note that the findings indicate that high-impulsivity, reward-dominant youths who had nondeviant peers showed *re-duced* development of conduct problems relative to other youths, perhaps because their peer groups provided reinforcement for normative and achievement-related behavior rather than antisocial behavior. In other words, youths' strong response to rewarding events or failure to modulate their pursuit of rewards in the face of punishment was found to predict higher-than-typical growth of conduct problems when their friends engaged in antisocial activities, but lower-than-typical growth of conduct problems when their friends were not antisocial. Thus the same temperamental, regulatory characteristic could be either a risk factor for antisocial or an aid to prosocial development, depending on qualities of the peers.

In a second study (Fite, Goodnight, Bates, Dodge, & Pettit, in press), we have found that a temperament-like tendency toward impulsive action can moderate the extent to which one's style of social information processing, as measured by responses to hypothetical vignettes (Crick & Dodge, 1994), predicts actual behavior. We think of social information processing as potentially influenced by self-regulation abilities. For example, highly regulated children may tell themselves to stop and think before responding to some ambiguous provocation (e.g., someone's cutting in line), thus allowing them to fully process the relevant details of the situation and to generate multiple response options. However, impulsivity is not the same as social information processing, so we were able to ask whether the two kinds of tendency might interact in predicting adaptive behavior. We reasoned that highly impulsive youths might be more likely to act without fully processing real-world social situations, making them more likely to display their default or most characteristic patterns of social information processing, rather than to let the actual situations guide their behavior. We found for highly impulsive youths, as rated by their teachers at ages 11–13, that the youths' endorsement of aggressive responses in a social information-processing assessment at age 13 was significantly predictive of their later, parent-reported aggressive behavior at ages 14–17, even when earlier levels of aggression were controlled for; however, the hypothetical endorsement of aggression did not predict behavior for low-impulsivity youths. Thus adolescents' impulsivity increased the likelihood that a cognitive processing default would be translated into behavior in real life.

CONCLUSION

Temperament concepts are a subset of emotion concepts that aid in thinking about individual differences in emotion and how they develop. This chapter has summarized ways in which temperament accounts for individual differences in social development. Self-regulation has been of increasing interest in the area of temperament, in the same way as in the broader area of emotion, so the chapter has emphasized regulatory traits and how they pertain to social development. The conceptual distinction between emotion and emotion regulation appears somewhat useful, even though it also seems clear that in terms of psychological process they are closely intertwined elements of a larger phenomenon. The same may be true of the conceptual distinction between temperamental reactivity and self-regulation. Nevertheless, there have been some interesting empirical efforts to highlight regulatory processes against a backdrop of other emotion processes—for instance, careful descriptions of changes in emotion following regulatory responses such as attention and the activity of brain centers such as the anterior cingulate gyrus. Although there have been some direct links between regulatory traits and behavioral adjustment outcomes, the links are of moderate size. Theorists in developmental psychopathology have long argued that individual child characteristics should affect outcomes to a large extent in interaction with characteristics of the environment. However, until very recently, there was almost no empirical evidence of such processes. In the years since the second edition of this handbook appeared, there has been an explosion of research that shows temperament–environment interaction effects upon social development outcomes. As exciting as this emerging research has been, further research is needed. Methodological advances will be important. For example, one methodological issue is how to measure the different emotional components of a temperament trait separately. It is often hard to know to what extent a measure of a youth's impulsive, reward-seeking behavior reflects a strong positive emotion/approach system, a weak fear/inhibition system, or a poor executive self-control system. One promising avenue is cognitive modeling of individuals' trial-by-trial decision making in a task such as a go/no-go task, as in another study from our lab (Yechiam et al., 2006). This study derived parameters for sensitivity to reward versus pun-ishment, attention to feedback from the most recent trials versus earlier trials, and rate of improvement in performance on the task.

As the work on temperament–environment interaction effects proceeds, we will also want to begin learning how the moderator effects occur. That is, what mediates the moderator effects? Perhaps they are mediated by observable transactions, as in models like that of Granic and Patterson (2006). For example, the parent's irritability exacerbates the child's irritability, and the product of mutual irritability creates obstacles to learning crucial self-regulatory skills. Or perhaps they are mediated by genetic factors. For example, if parental responsiveness moderates the relation between child frustration and later behavior problems, perhaps the parental responsiveness may mark a trait also inherited by the child that comes online later in development and that allows for improved child self-regulation. Obviously, these are advanced questions requiring new methodologies, such as detailed observations over critical periods of development; perhaps these should include observations of not only parent–child interactions, but also brain functioning, along with precisely targeted measurements of configurations of genetic polymorphisms whose emotional functions will have become well described. However, technologies are advancing rapidly, so we can envision efforts to address such questions. In the meanwhile, we are pleased and encouraged by the advances in developmental research, including sharper concepts of emotion and regulation traits, and the beginnings of richer empirical models of how these traits act in developmental systems to shape children's social adaptations.

REFERENCES

Arcus, D. (2001). Inhibited and uninhibited children: Biology in the social context. In T. D. Wachs & G. A. Kohnstamm (Ed.), *Temperament in context* (pp. 43–60). Mahwah, NJ: Erlbaum.

Auerbach, J. G., Faroy, M., Ebstein, R., Kahana, M., & Levine, J. (2001). The association of the dopamine D4 receptor gene (DRD4) and the serotonin transporter promoter gene (5-HTTLPR) with temperament in 12-month-old infants. *Journal of Child Psychology and Psychiatry, 42*(6) 772–783.

Bates, J. E. (1989). Applications of temperament concepts. In G. A. Kohnstamm, J. E. Bates, & M. K. Rothbart (Eds.), *Temperament in childhood* (pp. 321–355). Chichester, UK: Wiley.

Bates, J. E. (2000). Temperament as an emotion construct: Theoretical and practical issues. In M. Lewis

& J. M. Haviland-Jones (Eds.), *Handbook of emotions* (2nd ed., pp. 382–396). New York: Guilford Press.

Bates, J. E., & McFadyen-Ketchum, S. (2000). Temperament and parent–child relations as interacting factors in children's behavioral adjustment. In V. J. Molfese & D. L. Molfese (Eds.), *Temperament and personality across the life span* (pp. 141–176). Mahwah, NJ: Erlbaum.

Bates, J. E., & Pettit, G. S. (2007). Temperament, parenting, and socialization. In J. Grusec & P. Hastings (Eds.), *Handbook of socialization* (pp. 153–177). New York: Guilford Press.

Bates, J. E., Pettit, G. S., & Dodge, K. A. (1995). Family and child factors in stability and change in children's aggressiveness in elementary school. In J. McCord (Ed.), *Coercion and punishment in long-term perspectives* (pp. 124–137). New York: Cambridge University Press.

Bates, J. E., Pettit, G. S., Dodge, K. A., & Ridge, B. (1998). Interaction of temperamental resistance to control and restrictive parenting in the development of externalizing behavior. *Developmental Psychology, 34*(5), 982–995.

Beyers, J. M., Bates, J. E., Pettit, G. S., & Dodge, K. A. (2003). Neighborhood structure, parenting processes, and the development of youths' externalizing behaviors: A multilevel analysis. *American Journal of Community Psychology, 31*(1–2), 35–53.

Calkins, S. D., Dedmon, S. E., Gill, K. L., Lomax, L. E., & Johnson, L. M. (2002). Frustration in infancy: Implications for emotion regulation, physiological processes, and temperament. *Infancy, 3*(2), 175–197.

Campos, J. J., Frankel, C. B., & Camras, L. (2004). On the nature of emotion regulation. *Child Development, 75*(2), 377–394.

Caspi, A. (1998). Personality development across the life course. In W. Damon (Series Ed.) & N. Eisenberg (Vol. Ed.), *Handbook of child psychology: Vol. 3. Social, emotional, and personality development* (5th ed., pp. 311–388.). New York: Wiley.

Chess, S., & Thomas, A. (1984). *Origins and evolution of behavior disorders: From infancy to early adult life.* New York: Brunner/Mazel.

Cole, P. M., Martin, S. E., & Dennis, T. A. (2004). Emotion regulation as a scientific construct: Methodological challenges and directions for child development research. *Child Development, 75*(2), 317–333.

Collins, W. A., Maccoby, E. E., Steinberg, L., Hetherington, E. M., & Bornstein, M. H. (2000). Contemporary research on parenting: The case for nature and nurture. *American Psychologist, 55*(2), 218–232.

Crick, N. R., & Dodge, K. A. (1994). A review and reformulation of social information-processing mechanisms in children's social adjustment. *Psychological Bulletin, 115*, 74–101.

Crockenberg, S. C., & Leerkes, E. M. (2006). Infant and maternal behavior moderate reactivity to novelty to predict anxious behavior at 2.5 years. *Development and Psychopathology, 18*, 17–34.

Cummings, E. M., Davies, P. T., & Campbell, S. B. (2000). *Developmental psychopathology and family process: Theory, research, and clinical implications.* New York: Guilford Press.

Denham, S. A., Blair, K. A., DeMulder, E., Levitas, J., Sawyer, K., Auerbach-Major, S., et al. (2003). Preschool emotional competence: Pathway to social competence? *Child Development, 74*(1), 238–256.

Dishion, T. J., Spracklen, K. M., Andrews, D. W., & Patterson, G. R. (1996). Deviancy training in male adolescent friendships. *Behavior Therapy, 27*, 373–390.

Dodge, K. A., Pettit, G. S., & Bates, J. E. (1994). Socialization mediators of the relation between socioeconomic status and child conduct problems. *Child Development, 65*, 649–665.

Eisenberg, N., Sadovsky, A., Spinrad, T., Fabes, R. A., Losoya, S. H., Valiente, C., et al. (2005). The relations of problem behavior status to children's negative emotionality, effortful control, and impulsivity: Concurrent relations and prediction of change. *Developmental Psychology, 41*(1), 193–211.

Eisenberg, N., Smith, C. L., Sadovsky, A., & Spinrad, T. L. (2004). Effortful control: Relations with emotion regulation, adjustment, and socialization in childhood. In R. F. Baumeister & K. D. Vohs (Eds.), *Handbook of self-regulation: Research, theory, and applications* (pp. 259–282). New York: Guilford Press.

Eisenberg, N., Spinrad, T. L., & Smith, C. L. (2004) Emotion-related regulation: Its conceptualization, relations to social functioning, and socialization. In P. Philippot, & R. S. Feldman (Eds.), *The regulation of emotion* (pp. 277–306). Mahwah, NJ: Erlbaum.

Fite, J. E., Goodnight, J. A., Bates, J. E., Dodge, K. A., & Pettit, G. S. (in press). Adolescent aggression and social cognition in context: Impulsivity as a moderator of predictions from social information processing. *Aggressive Behavior.*

Fox, N. A., & Calkins, S. D. (2003). The development of self-control of emotion: Instrinsic and extrinsic influences. *Motivation and Emotion, 27*(1), 7–26.

Goodnight, J. A., Bates, J. E., Newman, J. P., Dodge, K. A., & Pettit, G. S. (2006). The interactive influences of friend deviance and reward dominance on the development of externalizing behavior during middle adolescence. *Journal of Abnormal Child Psychology, 34*, 573–583.

Granic, I., & Patterson, G. R. (2006). Toward a comprehensive model of antisocial development: A dynamic systems approach. *Psychological Review, 113*(1), 101–131.

Gray, J. A. (1993). The neuropsychology of temperament. In J. Strelau & A. Angleitner (Eds.), *Explorations in temperament: International perspectives on theory and measurement* (pp. 105–128). New York: Plenum Press.

Hill, A. L., & Braungart-Rieker, J. M. (2002). Four-month attentional regulation and its prediction of three-year compliance. *Infancy, 3*(2), 261–273.

Hoeksma, J. B., Oosterlaan, J., & Schipper, E. M. (2004). Emotion regulation and the dynamics of feelings: A conceptual and methodological framework. *Child Development*, 75(2), 354–360.

Kagan, J. (1998). Biology and the child. In W. Damon (Series Ed.) & N. Eisenberg (Vol. Ed.), *Handbook of child psychology: Vol. 3. Social, emotional, and personality development* (5th ed., pp. 177–235). New York: Wiley.

Keiley, M. K., Lofthouse, N., Bates, J. E., Dodge, K. A., & Pettit, G. S. (2003). Differential risks of covarying and pure components in mother and teacher reports of externalizing and internalizing behavior across ages 5 to 14. *Journal of Abnormal Child Psychology*, 31, 267–283.

Lakatos, K., Nemoda, Z., Birkas, E., Ronai, Z., Kovacs, E., Ney, K., et al. (2003). Association of D4 dopamine receptor gene and serotonin transporter promoter polymorphisms with infants' response to novelty. *Molecular Psychiatry*, 8, 90–97.

Kochanska, G. (1997). Multiple pathways to conscience for children with different temperaments: From toddlerhood to age 5. *Developmental Psychology*, 33(2), 228–240.

Lewis, M., & Haviland-Jones, J. M. (Eds.). *Handbook of emotions* (2nd ed.). New York: Guilford Press.

Lewis, M. D. (2005). Bridging emotion theory and neurobiology through dynamic systems modeling. *Behavioral and Brain Sciences*, 28, 169–245.

Lewis, M. D., & Stieben, J. (2004). Emotion regulation in the brain: Conceptual issues and directions for developmental research. *Child Development*, 75(2), 371–376.

Logan, G. D., Schachar, R. J., & Tannock, R. (1997). Impulsivity and inhibitory control. *Psychological Science*, 8, 60–64.

McClelland, G. H., & Judd, C. M. (1993). Statistical difficulties of detecting interactions and moderator effects. *Psychological Bulletin*, 114, 376–390.

McLeod, J. D., & Shanahan, M. J. (1996). Trajectories of poverty and children's mental health. *Journal of Health and Social Behavior*, 37, 207–220.

Murray, K. T., & Kochanska, G. (2002). Effortful control: Factor structure and relation to externalizing and internalizing behaviors. *Journal of Abnormal Child Psychology*, 30(5), 503–514.

Newman, J. P., Patterson, C. M., & Kosson, D. S. (1987). Response perseveration in psychopaths. *Journal of Abnormal Psychology*, 96, 145–148.

Nigg, J. T. (2000). On inhibition/disinhibition in developmental psychopathology: Views from cognitive and personality psychology and a working inhibition taxonomy. *Psychological Bulletin*, 126(2), 220–246.

Olson, S. L., Sameroff, A. J., Kerr, D. C. R., Lopez, N. L., & Wellman, H. M. (2005). Developmental foundations of externalizing problems in young children: The role of effortful control. *Development and Psychopathology*, 17, 23–45.

Olson, S. L., Schilling, E. M., & Bates, J. E. (1999). Measurement of impulsivity: Construct coherence, longitudinal stability, and relationship with externalizing problems in middle childhood and adolescence. *Journal of Abnormal Child Psychology*, 27(2), 151–165.

Patterson, G. R., Reid, J. B., & Dishion, T. J. (1992). *Antisocial boys*. Eugene, OR: Castalia.

Posner, M. I., & Rothbart, M. K. (2000). Developing mechanisms of self-regulation. *Development and Psychopathology*, 12, 427–441.

Reuda, M. R., Posner, M. I., & Rothbart, M. K. (2004). Attentional control and self-regulation. In R. F. Baumeister & K. D. Vohs (Eds.), *Handbook of self-regulation: Research, theory, and applications* (pp. 283–300). New York: Guilford Press.

Rothbart, M. K., & Bates, J. E. (1998). Temperament. In W. Damon (Series Ed.) & N. Eisenberg (Vol. Ed.), *Handbook of child psychology: Vol. 3. Social, emotional, and personality development* (5th ed., pp. 105–176). New York: Wiley.

Rothbart, M. K., & Bates, J. E. (2006). Temperament. In W. Damon (Series Eds.) & N. Eisenberg (Vol. Ed.), *Handbook of child psychology: Vol. 3. Social, emotional, and personality development* (6th ed., pp. 99–166). Hoboken, NJ: Wiley.

Rothbart, M. K., Derryberry, D., & Posner, M. I. (1994). A psychobiological approach to the development of temperament. In J. E. Bates & T. D. Wachs (Eds.), *Temperament: Individual differences at the interface of biology and behavior* (pp. 83–116). Washington, DC: American Psychological Association.

Rothbaum, F., & Weisz, J. R. (1994). Parental caregiving and child externalizing behavior in nonclinical samples: A meta-analysis. *Psychological Bulletin*, 116, 55–74.

Rubin, K. H., Burgess, K. B., Dwyer, K. M., & Hastings, P. D. (2003). Predicting preschoolers' externalizing behaviors from toddler temperament, conflict, and maternal negativity. *Developmental Psychology*, 39(1), 164–176.

Stifter, C. A., & Spinrad, T. L. (2002). The effect of excessive crying on the development of emotion regulation. *Infancy*, 3(2), 133–152.

Stifter, C. A., Spinrad, T. L., & Braungart-Rieker, J. M. (1999). Toward a developmental model of child compliance: The role of emotion regulation in infancy. *Child Development*, 70(1), 21–32.

Veenstra, R., Lindenberg, S., Oldehinkel, A. J., DeWinter, A. F., & Ormel, J. (2006). Temperament, environment, and antisocial behavior in a population sample of preadolescent boys and girls. *International Journal of Behavioral Development*, 30(5), 422–432.

Wachs, T. D. (2000). *Necessary but not sufficient: The respective roles of single and multiple influences on individual development*. Washington, DC: American Psychological Association.

Yechiam, E., Goodnight, J. A., Bates, J. E., Busemeyer, J. R., Dodge, K. A., Pettit, G. S., et al. (2006). A formal cognitive model of the go/no-go discrimination task: Evaluation and implications. *Psychological Assessment*, 18(3), 239–249.

CHAPTER 31

Emotion Regulation

JAMES J. GROSS

Have you ever gotten so angry that you've done something really spiteful? Or felt so much love for your child that you've bored someone to tears by recounting your child's exploits? Or been so sad that life has temporarily lost its meaning? If your answer to any of these questions is "yes"—or if anyone you care about would answer "yes"—then this chapter is for you.

The focus of this chapter is *emotion regulation*, which refers to how we try to influence which emotions we have, when we have them, and how we experience and express these emotions (Gross, 1998b). Although the topic of emotion regulation is a relatively late addition to the field of emotion, a concern with emotion regulation is anything but new. Emotion regulation has been a focus in the study of psychological defenses (Freud, 1926/1959), stress and coping (Lazarus, 1966), attachment (Bowlby, 1969), and self-regulation (Mischel, Shoda, & Rodriguez, 1989).

What is new are the theoretical and empirical advances that have been made in recent years, thanks to a dramatic increase in atten-

tion to this topic (Gross, 2007). Until the early 1990s, there were just a few citations a year containing the phrase "emotion regulation." For example, in 1990, PsycINFO listed 4 citations containing the phrase "emotion regulation." Since this time, there has been an astonishing increase in citations: In 2005, for instance, the PsycINFO citation count was 671. Although citation counts are an imperfect metric, the 150-fold-plus increase in citations over this 15-year period clearly reflects the growing popularity of this topic.

Popularity is a wonderful thing, but despite this increased attention, there remains an unfortunate degree of confusion about what emotion regulation is (and isn't), and what effects (if any) emotion regulation has on important outcomes. My goal in this chapter is to provide a conceptual map and readable introduction useful to anyone who is interested in emotion regulation. In the first section, I provide an orientation to emotion and emotion regulation, and sketch a process model of emotion regulation that my colleagues and I have found useful in our work. In the second section, I describe the five major families of processes that populate our conception of emotion regulation. In the third section, I consider three exciting growth points for the field: (1) an emerging understanding of the way particular beliefs encourage or discourage specific forms of emotion regulation; (2) an increasing appreciation of automatic (as opposed to effortful) forms of emotion regulation; and (3) a growing sense of the implications the field of emotion regulation has for the diagnosis and treatment of psychopathology.

EMOTION AND EMOTION REGULATION

Contemporary emotion theories emphasize the ways emotions facilitate adaptation by readying behavioral responses (Tooby & Cosmides, Chapter 8, this volume), enhancing memory for important events (Phelps, 2006), and guiding interpersonal interactions (Keltner & Kring, 1998). However, emotions are by no means always helpful. They can hurt us as well as help us (Parrott, 1993). They do so when they are of the wrong type, when they come at the wrong time, or when they occur at the wrong intensity level. At times such as these, we may be highly motivated to try to regulate our emotions. To understand how emotions are regulated (or become dysregulated), we first must consider the target of emotion regulation—namely, emotion itself.

What Is Emotion?

As with many of the terms we use in psychology, "emotion" was lifted from everyday discourse. For this reason, it has fuzzy boundaries rather than classical edges, and it refers to an astonishing array of happenings—from the mild to the intense, the brief to the extended, the simple to the complex, and the private to the public. Irritation when a shoelace breaks counts. So do amusement at a joke, anger at political oppression, surprise at a friend's new "look," grief at the death of a parent, and guilt over a moral lapse. This incredible diversity has led many theorists to despair of ever deriving a tidy classical definition of emotion—one that lists the necessary and sufficient conditions for something to qualify as a "real" emotion. Instead, they have begun to think of emotion in

prototype terms, and have identified three key features.

One commonly described feature has to do with what gives rise to emotions. Emotions are thought to arise when an individual attends to a situation and understands it as being relevant to his or her current goals (Lazarus, 1991a). It's important to appreciate that these goals may be enduring and central to the person's self-concept (wanting to be trustworthy) or transient and peripheral (wanting the last slice of cake). They may be conscious and complicated (wanting to survive the rigors of graduate school) or unconscious and simple (wanting to distance oneself from a snake). They may be widely shared and understood in a given culture (wanting to be a good son/daughter) or idiosyncratic and somewhat mysterious to others (wanting to travel on a UFO). Whatever the goal, and whatever meaning a situation has for the individual, it is this meaning that gives rise to emotion. As either the goal or meaning change over time (due to a change in the person, the situation, or the meaning the situation holds for an individual), the emotion will also change.

A second commonly described feature of emotion has to do with its constituent elements. Emotions are generally conceptualized as multifaceted, embodied phenomena that involve loosely coupled changes in the domains of *subjective experience*, *behavior*, and *peripheral physiology* (Mauss, Levenson, McCarter, Wilhelm, & Gross, 2005). The experiential aspect of emotion—or what it feels like when we have an emotion—is so tightly bound up with what we mean by emotion that in everyday speech, the terms "emotion" and "feeling" are often used interchangeably. However, surprisingly little is known about the psychological and biological underpinnings of emotion experience (Barrett, Mesquita, Ochsner, & Gross, 2007), and there are many contexts in which there are dissociations between emotion experience and other aspects of an emotion (e.g., Bonanno, Keltner, Holen, & Horowitz, 1995). In addition to giving rise to subjective feelings, emotions also often make us more likely to do something (e.g., approach others, say something mean, cry) than we otherwise would have been (Frijda, 1986). These impulses to act in certain ways (and not to act in others) are associated with autonomic and neuroendocrine changes that both anticipate the associated behavioral responses (thereby providing metabolic support for the action) and follow it, often as a consequence of the motor activity associated with the emotional response. As the many chapters of this volume attest, there remains considerable debate about which of these aspects of emotion should be prioritized, and how these aspects of emotion co-occur during emotion. For our purposes, it is enough to note that emotions often involve changes in each of these response domains.

A third commonly described feature of emotion has to do with its malleability. Emotions possess an imperative quality, in that they can interrupt what we are doing and force themselves upon our awareness (Frijda, 1988). However, emotions must compete with other responses occasioned by the situations we are in, and therefore do not automatically trump other possible responses to the situation. The malleability of emotion has been emphasized since William James (1884), who viewed emotions as response tendencies that may be modulated in a large number of ways. It is this third aspect of emotion that is most crucial for an analysis of emotion regulation, because it is this feature that gives rise to the possibility for regulation.

The "Modal Model" of Emotion

Because these three core features of emotion are emphasized in many different theories of emotion, I have found it useful to refer to them as constituting a consensual model or "modal model" of emotion (Barrett, Ochsner, & Gross, 2007; Gross, 1998a). According to this model, emotion arises in the context of a person–situation transaction that compels attention, has a particular meaning to an individual, and gives rise to a coordinated yet malleable multisystem response to the ongoing person–situation transaction. I believe that it is no accident that this heuristic "modal model" underlies lay intuitions about emotion, and also represents crucial points of convergence among researchers and theoreticians concerned with emotion.

In Figure 31.1, I present in schematic form the situation–attention–appraisal–response sequence specified by the modal model of emotion (with the organismal "black box" interposed between situation and response). This sequence begins with a psychologically relevant

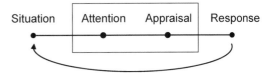

FIGURE 31.1. The "modal model" of emotion. From Gross and Thompson (2007). Copyright 2007 by The Guilford Press. Reprinted by permission.

situation, which is often external and hence physically specifiable. This situation is attended to in various ways, giving rise to appraisals that constitute the individual's assessment of—among other things—the situation's familiarity, valence, and value relevance (Ellsworth & Scherer, 2003). As noted above, the emotional responses generated by appraisals are thought to involve changes in experiential, behavioral, and physiological response systems. It is important to keep in mind that these responses often change the situation that gave rise to the response in the first place. For example, when someone appears embarrassed after committing a faux pas, others see this embarrassment, and are then more likely to forgive the social lapse (Keltner, 1995). One way to depict this recursive aspect of emotion is by an arrow that shows the response feeding back to (and modifying) the situation. The key idea here is that emotions can and often do change the environment, thereby altering the probability of subsequent instances of emotion.

What Is Emotion Regulation?

With this schematic conception of emotion in view, we are ready to turn to emotion regulation. It will come as no great surprise that like "emotion," the concept of "emotion regulation" is a slippery one. This is partly because the concept inherits all of the complexities that are inherent in the term "emotion." But the construct is confusing in a second way, in that it isn't clear whether it refers to how emotions regulate something else, such as blood pressure, memory, or parent–child interactions (regulation *by* emotions) or to how emotions are themselves regulated (regulation *of* emotions). Both usages have currency, but the problem with the first usage (regulation *by* emotions) is that one of the functions of emotion is the coordination of diverse response systems

(Levenson, 1999). Thus emotion regulation in this first sense is redundant with emotion, in that *all* instances of emotion would constitute emotion regulation. I therefore find the second usage more sensible (regulation *of* emotions), in which emotion regulation refers to the heterogeneous set of processes by which emotions are themselves regulated.

Another point of confusion is whether emotion regulation refers to intrinsic processes (Amy regulates her own emotions: regulation *in self*), to extrinsic processes (Amy regulates baby Bob's emotions: regulation *in other*), or to both. In general, researchers in the adult literature typically focus on intrinsic processes, whereas researchers in the developmental literature focus more on extrinsic processes (Gross & Thompson, 2007). In my view, it makes sense to include both forms of regulation, and to use the qualifiers "intrinsic" and "extrinsic" whenever clarification is needed, such as when Amy helps Bob to regulate his anger (extrinsic emotion regulation) in order to be able to calm down herself (intrinsic emotion regulation).

Putting aside for a moment the complexity associated with intrinsic versus extrinsic emotion regulation, what are people trying to accomplish when they regulate emotions? When we think of emotion regulation, many of the instances that leap to mind—at least in a Western cultural context—involve turning down (decreasing) the experiential and/or behavioral aspects of negative emotions such as anger, fear, and sadness (Gross, Richards, & John, 2006). This is not to say that positive emotions aren't regulated; they certainly are, as when we try to look less happy than we are about winning a hard-fought tennis game, or when we try to decrease feelings of attraction that (for whatever reason) we find objectionable. It's also important to note that emotion regulation needn't involve down-regulation. It can also involve maintaining or increasing emotion, as when we share good news with others, thereby prolonging its effects (Langston, 1994), or even—in the context of negative emotion—when bill collectors try to increase their anger to help collect delinquent accounts (Sutton, 1991).

Many of these emotion regulation goals are readily understood in hedonistic terms: People are motivated to avoid pain and seek pleasure. But if emotion regulation involves increasing/initiating and decreasing/stopping negative or positive emotions, it is not clear how we can explain the "odd" cells (increasing negative

emotion and decreasing positive emotion) on the basis of short-term hedonic considerations. Tamir (2005) has argued that hedonic considerations can sometimes be trumped by other considerations, such as whether a given emotion will help a person achieve his or her immediate objectives. One example is when individuals high (vs. low) in neuroticism try to increase their levels of negative emotion in order to maximize their performance on a demanding cognitive task. This finding suggests that emotions are regulated with a view to both how they feel and what they help us to do.

EMOTION REGULATION STRATEGIES

If "emotion regulation" refers to the processes by which we influence which emotions we have, when we have them, and how we experience and express these emotions, we face an embarrassment of riches. Many processes are involved in decreasing, maintaining, or increasing one or more aspects of emotion. Indeed, relevant processes range from changing one's job to calling one's mother to keeping a stiff upper lip. How should we conceptualize the potentially overwhelming number of processes involved in regulating our own or others' emotions?

My approach has been to undertake a conceptual analysis of the processes underlying diverse emotion regulatory acts. Using the modal model of emotion shown in Figure 31.1 as a starting point, I have argued that emotion regulatory acts may be seen as having their primary impact at different points in the emotion generative process (Gross, 2001). In particular, I have suggested that the modal model specifies a sequence of processes involved in emotion generation, each of which is a potential target for regulation. In Figure 31.2, I have redrawn the modal model, highlighting five points at which individuals can regulate their emotions. These five points represent five families of emotion regulation processes: situation selection, situation modification, attentional deployment, cognitive change, and response modulation.

Two complementary points should be made about this process model of emotion regulation. First, although this model makes a five-way distinction among emotion regulation processes, there are higher-order commonalities. For example, for some purposes, the first four emotion regulation families may be considered

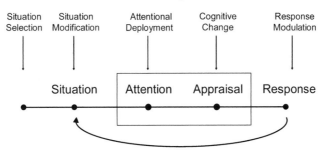

FIGURE 31.2. A process model of emotion regulation that highlights five families of emotion regulation strategies. From Gross and Thompson (2007). Copyright 2007 by The Guilford Press. Reprinted by permission.

"antecedent-focused," in that they occur before appraisals give rise to full-blown emotional responses. These may be contrasted with "response-focused" emotion regulation, which occurs after the responses are generated (Gross & Munoz, 1995; Gross & Thompson, 2007). The second point about these distinctions is that what someone does in everyday life to regulate emotions—such as going fishing with a buddy to cool down after a big fight with a spouse—often involves multiple regulatory processes. Nonetheless, I believe that this process model provides a conceptual framework useful for understanding the causes, consequences, and mechanisms underlying various forms of emotion regulation.

In the following sections, I selectively review research relevant to each of the five families of emotion regulation processes. My focus is on emotion regulation processes in adults (for considerations of developmental issues, see Charles & Carstensen, 2007; Eisenberg & Morris, 2002; Gross & Thompson, 2007; Thompson, 1994; for considerations of individual differences in emotion regulation, see John & Gross, 2004, 2007).

Situation Selection

The first type of emotion regulation we'll consider is *situation selection*, which I've placed at the leftmost point in Figure 31.2 because it affects the situation to which a person is exposed, and thus shapes the emotion trajectory from the earliest possible point. Situation selection involves taking actions to make it more likely that we'll be in a situation we expect will give rise to the emotions we'd like to have (or less likely that we'll be in a situation that will give rise to emotions we'd prefer not to have).

Of course, many of our decisions about which appointments to keep, where to go to lunch, whom to spend time with, and what to do after work have implications for how we'll later feel, but these decisions are not always shaped by our estimates of which emotions these situations will engender. "Situation selection" refers to the subset of these choices that are taken with a view, at least in part, to the future consequences of our actions for our emotional responses. Often we are aware of the trajectory our emotions are likely to take during a given period of time (e.g., a day) if we don't take steps to influence our emotions. This awareness may motivate us to take steps to alter the default emotional trajectory via situation selection. Thus we may try hard to avoid situations we know will bring us face to face with an ex-spouse or ex-lover, or we may actively seek out situations that will provide us with contact with friends when we need a chance to vent and/or share positive emotions.

These examples make situation selection sound like a rather simple calculus. It is not. Indeed, there is a growing appreciation of just how difficult it is either to remember how we used to feel, or to predict how we will feel. When we look backward in time, there is a profound gap between what might be called the "experiencing self" and the "remembering self" (Kahneman, 2000). In one of the more colorful illustrations of this gap, Redelmeier and Kahneman (1996) studied patients who were undergoing colonoscopies (a decidedly unpleasant procedure in which a probe is inserted into one's innermost recesses) and provided pain ratings at regular intervals throughout the procedure. They found that even when the procedure was longer (and thus gave rise to more "units" of experienced pain), participants later expressed a preference for the longer procedure when it ended with lower levels of pain.

This "duration neglect" is also evident in affective forecasting, when we look forward rather than backward in time. In one illustration of this phenomenon, Gilbert, Pinel, Wilson, Blumberg, and Wheatley (1998) asked participants how they would feel if they broke up with a partner or were denied academic tenure. They found that participants did a good job of figuring out *what* they would feel. Where participants miscalculated was in figuring out how long they would feel that way. In particular, participants dramatically overestimated how long their negative responses would last. These backward- and forward-looking biases hint at the complexity and the fallibility of the judgments involved in using situation selection.

Even if we had perfect information regarding past and future emotional responses to situations, there would remain the thorny issue of how to appropriately weigh short-term benefits of emotion regulation versus longer-term costs. For example, take Harold, a mild-mannered person who hates angry confrontations. If he is interested in maximizing short-term psychological comfort, it seems obvious that he should avoid situations in which angry confrontations will occur. But is this the best long-term strategy? What if his avoidance of conflict is giving implicit permission to others to bully him, and to behave in generally unreasonable and toxic ways to him? For his long-term (rather than short-term) happiness, it might be better to seek out an opportunity for a confrontation—even an angry one—if this meant that his work situation were changed in ways that made it a better place for him. Because of the complexity of these tradeoffs, situation selection often requires the perspective of others, whether parents, friends, or therapists.

Situation Modification

Potentially upsetting situations—such as making a social gaffe or seeing the family television go dead just before a favorite show is to start—do not inevitably lead to negative emotional responses. After all, one can always make a joke of one's social lapse or play a family game instead of watching television. Such efforts to modify the situation directly so as to alter its emotional impact constitute a second form of

emotion regulation, shown next in line in Figure 31.2. In the stress and coping tradition, this type of emotion regulation is referred to as "problem-focused coping" (Lazarus & Folkman, 1984) or "primary control" (Rothbaum, Weisz, & Snyder, 1982).

What forms may situation modification take? When a romantic interest comes over for dinner, it may take the form of mood lighting, music, and the strategic excision of unflattering memorabilia. Situation modification may also take the form (with children) of laying out games in a way that will ensure a smooth play date, helping with scaffolding that will allow them to solve a difficult problem, (partially) absenting oneself when their friends come over, or reinforcing one's limits via clear emotion expressions. The last case is particularly interesting theoretically, because it's a case in which emotion expressions themselves can be a potent extrinsic form of emotion regulation. This is because emotional expressions have important social consequences: If one's partner suddenly looks sad, this can shift the trajectory of an angry interaction as one pauses to express concern, apologize, or offer support.

Given the vagueness of the term "situation," it is sometimes difficult to draw a bright line between situation selection and situation modification. This is because efforts to modify a situation may effectively call a new situation into being. Also, although I have previously emphasized that situations can be external or internal, situation modification (as I mean it here) has to do with modifying external physical environments. I consider efforts at modifying "internal" environments (i.e., cognitions) in the section on cognitive change below.

Attentional Deployment

The first two forms of emotion regulation—situation selection and situation modification—both help to shape the situation to which an individual will be exposed. However, it is also possible to regulate emotions without actually changing the environment. Situations have many aspects, and *attentional deployment* refers to influencing emotional responding by redirecting attention within a given situation. Attentional deployment is thus an internal version of situation selection, in that attention is used to select which of many possible "internal situations" are active for an individual at any point in time. In Figure 31.2, attentional deployment comes after situation modification in the emotion trajectory.

In one form or another, attentional deployment is used from infancy through adulthood, particularly when it is not possible to change or modify one's situation (Rothbart, Ziaie, & O'Boyle, 1992). It is used, for example, by children who are waiting for delayed rewards, and spontaneous use of attentional deployment powerfully affects success during delay of gratification (Mischel et al., 1989). Attentional deployment may also include physical withdrawal of attention (e.g., covering the eyes or ears), internal redirection of attention (e.g., through distraction), and responding to external redirection of attention (e.g., a parent's redirection of a hungry child by telling the child an interesting story). Two of the best-researched forms of attentional deployment are distraction and rumination.

"Distraction" involves a shift in attention either away from emotional aspects of the situation or away from the situation altogether, such as when an infant shifts its gaze during an overly intense emotional interaction (Stifter & Moyer, 1991). Distraction may also involve a change in internal focus, such as when an individual invokes thoughts or memories that are inconsistent with the undesirable emotional state. Distraction has often been studied in the context of pain, where it leads to increased activation of brain regions associated with cognitive control (such as lateral prefrontal cortical regions) and diminished activation of brain regions associated with pain generation (such as the insula) (Ochsner & Gross, 2005).

"Rumination" refers to a perseverative focus on thoughts and feelings associated with an emotion-eliciting event. Rumination on sad or angry events increases the duration and intensity of negative emotion (Bushman, 2002; Morrow & Nolen-Hoeksema, 1990; Ray, Wilhelm, & Gross, in press) and is associated with greater levels of depressive symptoms (Nolen-Hoeksema, Morrow, & Fredrickson, 1993; Spasojevic & Alloy, 2001). Unlike distraction, rumination involves a sustained focus on emotion-eliciting stimuli. Another point of difference is that while distraction can take the form of attention directed outwards, to competing stimuli, or inwards, to thoughts, rumination typically involves an inflexibility in inner-directed attention.

Cognitive Change

Even after a potentially emotion-eliciting situation has arisen and been attended to, emotion does not necessarily follow. This is because an emotion further requires that the individual imbue the situation with a certain kind of meaning. As noted above, emotion theorists have delineated the different appraisals that are thought to lead to different emotions (Scherer, Schorr, & Johnstone, 2001). *Cognitive change* (shown fourth in line in Figure 31.2) refers to changing one or more of these appraisals in a way that alters the situation's emotional significance, by changing how one thinks either about the situation itself or about one's capacity to manage the demands it poses.

One form of cognitive change that has received particular attention is reappraisal (Gross, 2002). "Reappraisal" involves changing a situation's meaning in such a way that there is a change in the person's emotional response to that situation. For example, take a situation in which an acquaintance breezes by us in the hall and seems to ignore our smile and wave of greeting. For many, a natural response in such a situation is to feel hurt or angry at this perceived snub. In this case, cognitive change may take the form of thinking about the acquaintance as distracted, or perhaps preoccupied with his or her own problems. Such an interpretation of the situation—whether objectively correct or not—can profoundly affect the quality (which emotion) as well as the quantity or intensity (how much emotion) of the subsequent emotional response.

To date, studies of reappraisal have focused on quantitative changes in emotion, particularly decreases in negative emotion. These studies have provided evidence that reappraisal leads to decreased negative emotion experience and expressive behavior (Dandoy & Goldstein, 1990; Gross, 1998a). Reappraisal has also been shown to lead to decreased startle responses (Dillon & LaBar, 2005; Jackson, Malmstadt, Larson, & Davidson, 2000), decreased neuroendocrine responses (Abelson, Liberzon, Young, & Khan, 2005), and decreased autonomic responses (Stemmler, 1997; but see Gross, 1998a). Importantly, comparable effects have been observed when research participants spontaneously use reappraisal, either in a negative-emotion-eliciting situation in the lab (Egloff, Schmukle, Burns, &

Schwerdtfeger, 2006), or in everyday life (Gross & John, 2003). These findings suggest that studies manipulating emotion regulation have ecological validity: They provide insights into reappraisal as it naturally occurs in everyday life.

Consistent with these behavioral and physiological findings, reappraisal in the service of emotion down-regulation is associated with decreased activation in subcortical emotion-generative regions (such as the insula and amygdala), as well as increased activation in dorsolateral and medial prefrontal regions associated with cognitive control (Levesque et al., 2003; Ochsner, Bunge, Gross, & Gabrieli, 2002; Ochsner et al., 2004). When reappraisal is used in the service of emotion up-regulation, similar prefrontal regions are activated, but in this context (as one might expect), there are increases rather than decreases in activation of emotion-generative structures such as the amygdala (Ochsner & Gross, 2004; Schaefer et al., 2002). As our process model would predict, activations in prefrontal regions associated with the top-down control of emotion seem to occur relatively early (in the first few seconds), whereas the downstream consequences of decreased experience and behavior seem to last considerably longer (Goldin, McRae, Ramel, & Gross, in press).

If reappraisal occurs relatively early in the emotion-generative process, we might expect that using reappraisal would not interfere with other ongoing cognitive processes. This is just what we've found in a series of studies that have tested whether reappraisal impairs subsequent memory for information presented during the reappraisal period (Richards & Gross, 1999, 2000, 2006). Findings from these studies, which have used slides or films to elicit emotion, and have used a variety of techniques to probe incidental memory, show that reappraisal does not compromise later memory for material presented while a participant was engaging in reappraisal (relative to not using reappraisal). We have also found that when unacquainted pairs of participants interacted socially, there are no signs of social disruption when one member of a dyad is covertly instructed to engage in cognitive reappraisal during the interaction (Butler et al., 2003). Taken together, these findings suggest that reappraisal intervenes early in the emotion-generative process, and alters the experiential, behavioral,

and physiological components of the emotional response without incurring any appreciable costs.

Response Modulation

Response modulation, the last of the emotion regulation families, is shown on the right side of Figure 31.2. As this placement indicates, it occurs late in the emotion-generative process, after response tendencies have been initiated. "Response modulation" refers to influencing physiological, experiential, or behavioral responses relatively directly. For example, exercise and relaxation may be used to decrease physiological and experiential aspects of negative emotions.

One of the best-researched forms of response modulation is "expressive suppression," which refers to attempts to decrease ongoing emotion-expressive behavior (Gross, 2002). Examples of suppression abound, including our efforts to hide the anger we feel toward a boss, the anxiety we feel during an interview, or the amusement we feel at a coworker's decidedly politically incorrect joke. One reason suppression has attracted interest is that there are two opposing ideas about what happens when emotions are suppressed (Gross & Levenson, 1993). One idea is that behavioral expressions of emotion constitute a channel for discharging emotion. According to this "hydraulic" model, if emotions are denied expression, they will leak out elsewhere—for example, as increased physiological responses. A second idea, however, leads to opposite conclusions about the effects of suppression. According to this "facial feedback" model, behavioral expressions of emotion (such as facial expressions) actually serve to amplify the emotional response; thus if they are inhibited, the emotion itself will be muted.

Empirical studies of expressive suppression have yielded findings that conform neatly to neither of these two models. On the one hand, participants who have been instructed to suppress their emotions (during emotion-eliciting slides, films, or conversations) have shown increases in sympathetic activation of the cardiovascular system, as indexed, for example, by measures that reflect blood pressure (Demaree et al., 2006; Gross, 1998a; Gross & Levenson, 1993, 1997; Harris, 2001). On the other hand, when asked to suppress their emotions, participants report feeling either comparable or decreased levels of emotion (with decreases occurring more commonly for positive emotion) (Goldin et al., in press; Gross, 1998a; Gross & Levenson, 1993, 1997; McCanne & Anderson, 1987; Stepper & Strack, 1993; Strack, Martin, & Stepper, 1988).

Neurally, only one study to date has been conducted on expressive suppression (Goldin et al., in press). In this study, participants were asked to suppress their ongoing emotion-expressive behavior in the scanner during 15-second film segments that elicited intense levels of disgust. Findings indicated that suppression led to robust increases in the activation of dorsal and medial prefrontal regions associated with cognitive control, as well as to increased activation in emotion-generative regions such as the amygdala. Importantly, as the process model of emotion regulation would predict, these activations were evident late in the induction period, suggesting that suppression was associated with ongoing cognitive activity as the participants effortfully tried to manage each emotional impulse as it arose throughout the course of each film.

If this conception of expressive suppression is correct, we might expect that unlike reappraisal, suppression should have clear cognitive and social costs. In a series of studies, this is precisely what we have found. In studies of memory, we have repeatedly found that suppression (compared to no emotion regulation) leads to worse memory for material presented during the suppression period (Richards & Gross, 1999, 2000). Indeed, the degree of memory impairment associated with suppression was as large as when we instructed participants to distract themselves as much as possible during the presentation of information (Richards & Gross, 2006). In studies of social interactions in the laboratory, we have similarly found that suppression is associated with significant social costs: Partners of suppressors report less comfort and ease with their interaction partners (Butler et al., 2003). As with the reappraisal findings, we would note that the costs that have been associated with instructed suppression in the laboratory also seem to be evident when suppression is used spontaneously in the laboratory (Egloff et al., 2006; Richards & Gross, 2006); during an important life transition, the transition to college (Srivastava, Tamir, McGonigal, John, & Gross, 2008); and in everyday life (Gross & John, 2003).

EMERGING DIRECTIONS IN THE STUDY OF EMOTION REGULATION

Now that we have reviewed the emotion-regulation processes shown in Figure 31.2, we can step back and take stock of where this field is now and where it is going. Clearly, this is a time of unmatched excitement for the field of emotion regulation. There has never before been such a focused scientific effort to examine emotion regulation processes, nor has there been such a variety of perspectives brought to bear. Because emotion regulation lies at the intersection of the major subareas of psychology, it benefits from—and contributes to—developments in biological, cognitive, developmental, personality, social, and clinical areas (Gross, 1998b, 2007).

In the following sections, I consider three promising new directions for research in emotion regulation, each of which seems likely to broaden and extend the way we think about emotion regulation. The first concerns the cognitive antecedents of emotion regulation; the second concerns the boundaries of emotion regulation; the third concerns the implications emotion regulation research may have for understanding psychopathology. Although by no means exhaustive, these three selections exemplify the promise of emotion regulation research.

Beliefs and Emotion Regulation

One intriguing puzzle is *why* people use one emotion regulation strategy rather than another. If some strategies are associated with generally beneficial consequences (such as reappraisal), while others are associated with generally harmful consequences (such as suppression), why doesn't everyone use reappraisal and not suppression? One possibility, of course, is that people differ in their emotion regulation goals. Thus some people may want to increase high-arousal positive emotions, whereas others may want to decrease these emotions. This possibility is consistent with growing evidence of cultural differences in emotion regulation goals (Mesquita & Albert, 2007). For example, in individualistic cultural contexts, people generally seek out high-arousal positive emotional states; in collectivistic cultural contexts, people generally seek out low-arousal positive emotional states (Tsai, Knutson, & Fung, 2006).

But what about when emotion regulation goals are shared (e.g., when people wish to decrease their sadness)? How can we explain why people differ even when they are pursuing the same emotion regulation goal? One interesting possibility is that people may differ in their *beliefs* regarding emotion and emotion regulation, and these differences may in turn shape whether people try to regulate their emotions, and (when they do so) which emotion regulation strategies they employ. This idea derives from the "lay theories" perspective, a perspective that draws inspiration from the social-cognitive approach to personality (Molden & Dweck, 2006). The lay theories perspective holds that people differ in the assumptions they make about themselves and the social world (these constitute their "lay theories"), and it seeks to determine whether and how such lay theories influence important life outcomes.

One particular focus of the work on lay or implicit theories has been the distinction between "entity theories" (which hold that attributes such as personality and intelligence are fixed and stable) and "incremental theories" (which hold that such attributes are dynamic and malleable) (Dweck, 1986, 1999; Dweck, Chiu, & Hong, 1995). Individuals who hold incremental beliefs make flexible, contextual interpretations of events; when challenged, they make assertive attempts at self-regulation, increasing the chances of successful behavior. In contrast, individuals who hold entity beliefs view attributes as fixed and impossible to control; when challenged, they make fewer attempts at self-regulation, leading to self-regulation failure.

Prior work on lay theories has focused on intelligence, but we (Tamir, John, Srivastava, & Gross, 2007) wondered whether extending this work to the domain of emotion might help to unravel the mystery of why people differ so dramatically in their use of successful emotion regulation strategies. We (1) hypothesized that people differ in whether they believe emotions are generally malleable (incremental theorists) or fixed (entity theorists), and (2) suggested that incremental theorists should be more likely than entity theorists to use antecedent-focused emotion regulation strategies such as reappraisal. To test these hypotheses, we devised a measure of implicit beliefs regarding emotion, and administered it to students facing a crucial life transition—namely, the transition to college.

Findings revealed that participants did differ in their beliefs about emotion, and that participants with incremental as opposed to entity views of emotion reported greater emotion regulation self-efficacy and greater use of reappraisal. By the end of freshman year, participants with incremental views of emotion reported greater levels of positive emotions, lesser levels of negative emotions, higher levels of well-being, and lower levels of depression. Incremental participants also had higher levels of social adjustment and lower levels of loneliness.

These findings indicate that participants' naïve beliefs concerning their emotions—as either fixed or malleable—influenced how they regulated their emotions, and how they fared in an important life transition. Although this finding clearly must be replicated in other samples and in the context of other transitions, one important emerging direction for research in this area is the study of the role played by beliefs about emotion and emotion regulation in shaping emotion regulation choices and success.

Automatic versus Effortful Emotion Regulation

Many of the examples of emotion regulation that come to mind—and the majority of examples offered so far in this chapter—involve effortful and conscious attempts to down-regulate negative emotion. As we have discussed, however, emotion regulation can occur anywhere in the 2 × 2 matrix formed by crossing negative and positive emotion (say, as columns) with up- and down-regulation (say, as rows). Each of these dimensions can be further fleshed out, too. Additional columns can be added for those who prefer to think in discrete-emotion terms (e.g., pride, amusement, sadness, disgust), and additional rows for those wanting to do fuller justice to the complexities of the temporal dynamics of emotion (e.g., maintaining emotion). This sounds complicated enough—even before we recall the many families of regulation strategies that are used to achieve each of these types of change in emotion described by our 2 (or more) × 2 (or more) matrix—and we may be tempted to stop here. But one other dimension of variation has recently begun to be explored systematically, and this concerns variation in whether a given episode of emotion regulation is relatively effortful and conscious or relatively automatic and unconscious (Bargh & Williams, 2007; Mauss, Bunge, & Gross, 2007).

Just what does "automatic" mean in this context? Contemporary dual-process models contrast "automatic" (also called "nonconscious," "implicit," or "impulsive") processes with "deliberate" (also called "controlled," "conscious," "explicit," or "reflective") processes (e.g., Strack & Deutsch, 2004). Whereas deliberate processes require attentional resources, are volitional and conscious, and are goal-driven, automatic processes require neither attention nor intention, occur outside of awareness, and are stimulus-driven. Although often framed as clear opposites, many researchers think that these processes are located on a continuum from conscious, effortful, and controlled regulation to unconscious, effortless, and automatic regulation (Shiffrin & Schneider, 1977).

The notion that relatively high-level self-regulatory processes such as emotion regulation can be performed automatically may seem counterintuitive (Bargh, 2004). However, research on automatic goal pursuit has challenged the notion that "higher-level" processes can only take place in a deliberate fashion, and it appears that the full sequence of goal pursuit—from goal setting to the completion of the goal—can proceed outside of conscious awareness. In a series of studies, Bargh and colleagues have shown that goals can indeed be activated and executed without the intervention of conscious awareness. For example, they implicitly primed goals such as the intention to cooperate with others or to perform well on a cognitive task, and found that subsequently participants behaved in agreement with these goals, without knowing *why* or even *that* they were acting this way (Bargh, Gollwitzer, Lee-Chai, Barndollar, & Trötschel, 2001).

To see whether emotion regulation could also operate automatically, we (Mauss, Cook, & Gross, 2007) manipulated automatic emotion regulation by priming emotion control versus emotion expression with an adaptation of the Sentence Unscrambling Task (e.g., Bargh, Chen, & Burrows, 1996; Bargh et al., 2001; Srull & Wyer, 1979). This task unobtrusively exposed participants to words relating to emotion control or expression, thereby *implicitly* activating (priming) related concepts and goals. Participants were then instructed by an "unfriendly" and "arrogant" experimenter to repeatedly perform a boring yet cognitively straining task.

As expected, most participants became angry during the task. Of particular interest, however, was the finding that participants primed with emotion control reported less anger than did participants primed with emotion expression. These results have been corroborated by an individual-difference study that employed an emotion regulation implicit association test; this study showed that participants with positive implicit associations with emotional control felt less angry when provoked, and exhibited an adaptive challenge response (rather than a maladaptive threat response), characterized by greater sympathetic activation, greater cardiac output, and lower total peripheral resistance (Mauss, Evers, Wilhelm, & Gross, 2006).

Although these initial studies are promising, it's important to note that it is too early to conclude that all forms of automatic emotion regulation are benign or helpful. The venerable clinical literature on repression (e.g., Freud, 1936) has long cautioned that certain forms of automatic emotion regulation—such as when someone struggles to keep anxiety out of awareness—may have maladaptive consequences ranging from personality disturbances to psychosomatic illnesses. One of the challenges we face in understanding automatic emotion regulation is developing methods for assessing and manipulating different automatic emotion regulation processes. Difficult as this challenge is, work in this area is badly needed to clarify the types and timing of automatic emotion regulation processes that are helpful versus unhelpful.

Emotion Regulation and Psychopathology

Inappropriate emotional responses are implicated in a large number of forms of psychopathology (Gross & Levenson, 1997; Thoits, 1985). Indeed, more than half of the Axis I clinical disorders (such as the anxiety disorders and mood disorders), and all of the Axis II personality disorders (such as borderline personality disorder), involve problematic emotional responses (American Psychiatric Association, 2000). What's proven more difficult than one might expect, however, has been moving from broad statements such as these to specific empirically grounded insights concerning how differences in emotional reactivity and/or emotion regulation contribute to different forms of psychopathology (Rottenberg & Gross, 2003; Rottenberg & Johnson, 2007), and how therapeutic interventions might be used to correct dysregulated emotion (Moses & Barlow, 2006).

Take major depressive disorder. This disorder is a devastating psychiatric condition whose definition includes increased negative affect and anhedonia (diminished positive affect). From this definition, it might seem obvious that depression leads to disrupted emotion regulation (Gross & Munoz, 1995). However, there are no fewer than three competing views of how depression disrupts emotional responding, and without clarity about the nature of the problematic emotions, it is very difficult to draw conclusions about the role of emotion regulation (Rottenberg, Gross, & Gotlib, 2005). The first view is that depression involves diminished emotional reactivity to positive situations. In support of this "positive attenuation" view, convincing evidence from a variety of induction contexts suggests that individuals who are depressed respond with less positive emotion than individuals who are not depressed. The second view is that depression involves increased negative emotional reactivity. Like the positive attenuation hypothesis, the "negative potentiation" view seems to follow directly from the very definition of depression, as well as from major theories of depression (e.g., Beck, Rush, Shaw, & Emery, 1979). However, the preponderance of empirical evidence actually suggests that individuals who are depressed show lesser rather than greater emotional reactivity.

These findings suggest a third view—namely, the "emotion context insensitivity" view (Rottenberg et al., 2005). This view derives from evolutionary accounts of depression as characterized by disengagement (Nesse, 2000), and sees emotional responses (whether negative or positive) as involving energetic engagement with the environment. In this view, depression leads to pervasive disengagement, and hence to diminished levels of both positive and negative emotional reactivity. Consistent with this third view, Rottenberg and colleagues (Rottenberg, Kasch, Gross, & Gotlib, 2002; Rottenberg & Johnson, 2007) have presented studies showing that relative to either formerly depressed or never-depressed participants, depressed individuals showed less reactivity to happy and sad stimuli.

Are the challenges associated with specifying precise emotion and emotion regulation deficits unique to depression? It appears that they are not. Take social anxiety disorder (social phobia), another common and debilitating psychiatric condition, which by definition includes high levels of anxiety in social contexts. Given this definition, it seems obvious that social anxiety involves heightened levels of experiential, behavioral, and physiological responses in social contexts. To test this hypothesis, individuals who were either high or low in social anxiety were asked to give a speech on a difficult topic. Participants rated how anxious they felt at several points during the session. They also rated their physiological responses (e.g., how much their hearts were racing), and objective physiological measures were taken throughout the study (Mauss, Wilhelm, & Gross, 2004).

As might be expected, compared to low-trait-anxiety participants, high-trait-anxiety participants said that they were feeling more anxious, and that their bodies were responding much more violently. Intriguingly, however, there were no differences in the observed physiological responses between the high- and low-anxiety participants. Participants in both groups showed expected increases in various indicators of sympathetic nervous system responding, but there was no difference between the groups, either in the magnitude of their responses to the initial speech or in their responses to a second speech (Mauss, Wilhelm, & Gross, 2003). Although it is possible that these findings are specific to nonclinical samples, the available evidence does not suggest this is so. Like the findings from major depressive disorder, these findings from social anxiety hint at the complexities that lie ahead as we try to discern the ways in which emotion and emotion regulation are disrupted in various forms of psychopathology.

SUMMARY

Emotions have been said to represent the "wisdom of the ages" (Lazarus, 1991b, p. 820), and functionalist approaches to emotion have rightly emphasized the many adaptive benefits of emotion. But even the wisest guides have their limits, and since the early 1990s there has been a dramatic increase in research attention to how emotions can be regulated so as to help people benefit from what is useful about them, but avoid what is not useful.

In this chapter, I have used the "modal model" of emotion to highlight the idea that emotions arise in the context of person–situation transactions that compel attention, have particular meaning to an individual, and give rise to coordinated yet flexible sets of experiential, behavioral, and physiological responses to the ongoing person–situation transactions. Using the modal model as a jumping-off point, I have described a process model of emotion regulation that my colleagues and I have found useful, and have argued that this model provides a valuable conceptual framework for organizing and directing research on emotion regulation processes. Within this framework, I have distinguished five families of emotion regulation processes that have their primary impact at different points in the emotion-generative process. For each of these families of processes, I have selectively sampled recent research findings. Taken together, these findings suggest that different emotion regulation processes have different consequences; what seems crucial, therefore, is using a strategy that matches one's goals.

One reason why research in this area is so compelling is that we all come face to face with emotion regulation issues in our lives—whether in handling our own emotions or those of family members, friends, or work associates. Emotions matter, and when emotions go wrong, we want to do something about it. Another reason why emotion regulation research is attracting so much attention is that it is a "poster child" for two broad scientific trends: multilevel/multispecialty collaboration, and the bidirectional interplay between basic research and clinical application. Of the many growth points in this field, I have identified three as particularly exciting: (1) the role of beliefs in shaping when and how we try to regulate our emotions; (2) the largely unexplored realm of automatic emotion regulation processes; and (3) the bridges that are beginning to be built between basic research on emotion and emotion regulation on the one hand, and clinical science and practice on the other. Findings from these research areas, and others, promise to transform how we think about the intricate dance in which we at once regulate and are regulated by our emotions.

ACKNOWLEDGMENTS

I would like to thank Lisa Feldman Barrett, Iris Mauss, Kateri McRae, Jon Rottenberg, and Maya Tamir for their helpful comments on this chapter. Work on this chapter was supported by National Institutes of Health Grants R01 MH66957, R01 MH58147, and R01 MH76074.

REFERENCES

Abelson, J. L., Liberzon, I., Young, E. A., & Khan, S. (2005). Cognitive modulation of the endocrine stress response to a pharmacological challenge in normal and panic disorder subjects. *Archives of General Psychiatry, 62,* 668–675.

American Psychiatric Association. (2000). *Diagnostic and statistical manual of mental disorders* (4th ed., text rev.). Washington, DC: Author.

Bargh, J. A. (2004). Being here now: Is consciousness necessary for human freedom? In J. Greenberg, S. L. Koole, & T. Pyszczynski (Eds.), *Handbook of experimental existential psychology* (pp. 385–397). New York: Guilford Press.

Bargh, J. A., Chen, M., & Burrows, L. (1996). Automaticity of social behavior: Direct effects of trait construct and stereotype activation on action. *Journal of Personality and Social Psychology, 71,* 230–244.

Bargh, J. A., Gollwitzer, P. M., Lee-Chai, A., Barndollar, K., & Trötschel, R. (2001). The automated will: Nonconscious activation and pursuit of behavioral goals. *Journal of Personality and Social Psychology, 81,* 1014–1027.

Bargh, J. A., & Williams, L. E. (2007). The nonconscious regulation of emotion. In J. J. Gross (Ed.), *Handbook of emotion regulation* (pp. 429–445). New York: Guilford Press.

Barrett, L. F., Mesquita, B., Ochsner, K. N., & Gross, J. J. (2007). The experience of emotion. *Annual Review of Psychology, 58,* 373–403.

Barrett, L. F., Ochsner, K. N., & Gross, J. J. (2007). On the automaticity of emotion. In J. Bargh (Ed.), *Social psychology and the unconscious: The automaticity of higher mental processes* (pp. 173–217). New York: Psychology Press.

Beck, A. T., Rush, A. J., Shaw, B. F., & Emery, G. (1979). *Cognitive therapy of depression.* New York: Guilford Press.

Bonanno, G. A., Keltner, D., Holen, A., & Horowitz, M. J. (1995). When avoiding unpleasant emotions might not be such a bad thing: Verbal–autonomic response dissociation and midlife conjugal bereavement. *Journal of Personality and Social Psychology, 69,* 975–989.

Bowlby, J. (1969). *Attachment and loss: Vol. 1. Attachment.* New York: Basic Books.

Bushman, B. J. (2002). Does venting anger feed or extinguish the flame?: Catharsis, rumination, distraction, anger and aggressive responding. *Personality and Social Psychology Bulletin, 28,* 724–731.

Butler, E. A., Egloff, B., Wilhelm, F. W., Smith, N. C., Erickson, E. A., & Gross, J. J. (2003). The social consequences of expressive suppression. *Emotion, 3,* 48–67.

Charles, S. T., & Carstensen, L. L. (2007). Emotion regulation and aging. In J. J. Gross (Ed.), *Handbook of emotion regulation* (pp. 307–327). New York: Guilford Press.

Dandoy, A. C., & Goldstein, A. G. (1990). The use of cognitive appraisal to reduce stress reactions: A replication. *Journal of Social Behavior and Personality, 5,* 275–285.

Demaree, H. A., Schmeichel, B. J., Robinson, J. L., Pu, J., Everhart, D. E., & Berntson, G. G. (2006). Up- and down-regulating facial disgust: Affective, vagal, sympathetic, and respiratory consequences. *Biological Psychology, 71,* 90–99.

Dillon, D. G., & LaBar, K. S. (2005). Startle modulation during conscious emotion regulation is arousal-dependent. *Behavioral Neuroscience, 119,* 1118–1124.

Dweck, C. S. (1986). Motivational processes affecting learning. *American Psychologist, 41,* 1040–1048.

Dweck, C. S. (1999). *Self-theories: Their role in motivation, personality, and development.* New York: Psychology Press.

Dweck, C. S., Chiu, C. Y., & Hong, Y. Y. (1995). Implicit theories and their role in judgments and reactions: A world from two perspectives. *Psychological Inquiry, 6,* 267–285.

Egloff, B., Schmukle, S. C., Burns, L. R., & Schwerdtfeger, A. (2006). Spontaneous emotion regulation during evaluated speech tasks: Associations with negative affect, anxiety expression, memory, and physiological responding. *Emotion, 6,* 356–366.

Eisenberg, N., & Morris, A. S. (2002). Children's emotion-related regulation. *Advances in Child Development, 30,* 189–229.

Ellsworth, P. C., & Scherer, K. R. (2003). Appraisal processes in emotion. In R. J. Davidson, K. R. Scherer, & H. H. Goldsmith (Eds.), *Handbook of affective sciences* (pp. 572–595). New York: Oxford University Press.

Freud, A. (1936). *The ego and the mechanisms of defense.* New York: International Universities Press.

Freud, S. (1959). *Inhibitions, symptoms and anxiety* (A. Strachey, Trans., & J. Strachey, Ed.). New York: Norton. (Original work published 1926)

Frijda, N. H. (1986). *The emotions.* Cambridge, UK: Cambridge University Press.

Frijda, N. H. (1988). The laws of emotion. *American Psychologist, 43,* 349–358.

Gilbert, D. T., Pinel, E. C., Wilson, T. D., Blumberg, S. J., & Wheatley, T. P. (1998). Immune neglect: A source of durability bias in affective forecasting. *Journal of Personality and Social Psychology, 75,* 617–638.

Goldin, P. R., McRae, K., Ramel, W., & Gross, J. J. (in press). The neural bases of emotion regulation during reappraisal and suppression of negative emotion. *Biological Psychiatry.*

Gross, J. J. (1998a). Antecedent- and response-focused emotion regulation: Divergent consequences for experience, expression, and physiology. *Journal of Personality and Social Psychology, 74,* 224–237.

Gross, J. J. (1998b). The emerging field of emotion regulation: An integrative review. *Review of General Psychology, 2,* 271–299.

Gross, J. J. (2001). Emotion regulation in adulthood: Timing is everything. *Current Directions in Psychological Science, 10,* 214–219.

Gross, J. J. (2002). Emotion regulation: Affective, cognitive, and social consequences. *Psychophysiology, 39,* 281–291.

Gross, J. J. (Ed.). (2007). *Handbook of emotion regulation.* New York: Guilford Press.

Gross, J. J., & John, O. P. (2003). Individual differences in two emotion regulation processes: Implications for affect, relationships, and well-being. *Journal of Personality and Social Psychology, 85,* 348–362.

Gross, J. J., & Levenson, R. W. (1993). Emotional suppression: Physiology, self-report, and expressive behavior. *Journal of Personality and Social Psychology, 64,* 970–986.

Gross, J. J., & Levenson, R. W. (1997). Hiding feelings: The acute effects of inhibiting positive and negative emotions. *Journal of Abnormal Psychology, 106,* 95–103.

Gross, J. J., & Munoz, R. F. (1995). Emotion regulation and mental health. *Clinical Psychology: Science and Practice, 2,* 151–164.

Gross, J. J., Richards, J. M., & John, O. P. (2006). Emotion regulation in everyday life. In D. K. Snyder, J. A. Simpson, & J. N. Hughes (Eds.), *Emotion regulation in couples and families: Pathways to dysfunction and health* (pp. 13–35). Washington, DC: American Psychological Association.

Gross, J. J., & Thompson, R. A. (2007). Emotion regulation: Conceptual foundations. In J. J. Gross (Ed.), *Handbook of emotion regulation* (pp. 3–24). New York: Guilford Press.

Harris, C. R. (2001). Cardiovascular responses of embarrassment and effects of emotional suppression in a social setting. *Journal of Personality and Social Psychology, 81,* 886–897.

Jackson, D. C., Malmstadt, J. R., Larson, C. L., & Davidson, R. J. (2000). Suppression and enhancement of emotional responses to unpleasant pictures. *Psychophysiology, 37,* 515–522.

James, W. (1884). What is an emotion? *Mind, 9,* 188–205.

John, O. P., & Gross, J. J. (2004). Healthy and unhealthy emotion regulation: Personality processes, individual differences, and lifespan development. *Journal of Personality, 72,* 1301–1334.

John, O. P., & Gross, J. J. (2007). Individual differences

in emotion regulation. In J. J. Gross (Ed.), *Handbook of emotion regulation* (pp. 351–372). New York: Guilford Press.

Kahneman, D. (2000). Experienced utility and objective happiness: A moment-based approach. In D. Kahneman & A. Tversky (Eds.), *Choices, values, and frames* (pp. 673–692). Cambridge, UK: Cambridge University Press.

Keltner, D. (1995). Signs of appeasement: Evidence for the distinct displays of embarrassment, amusement, and shame. *Journal of Personality and Social Psychology, 68,* 441–454.

Keltner, D., & Kring, A. (1998). Emotion, social function, and psychopathology. *Review of General Psychology, 2,* 320–342.

Langston, C. A. (1994). Capitalizing on and coping with daily-life events: Expressive responses to positive events. *Journal of Personality and Social Psychology, 67,* 1112–1125.

Lazarus, R. S. (1966). *Psychological stress and the coping process.* New York: McGraw-Hill.

Lazarus, R. S. (1991a). *Emotion and adaptation.* Oxford: Oxford University Press.

Lazarus, R. S. (1991b). Progress on a cognitive–motivational–relational theory of emotion. *American Psychologist, 46,* 819–834.

Lazarus, R. S., & Folkman, S. (1984). *Stress, appraisal and coping.* New York: Springer.

Levenson, R. W. (1999). The intrapersonal functions of emotion. *Cognition and Emotion, 13,* 481–504.

Levesque, J., Fanny, E., Joanette, Y., Paquette, V., Mensour, B., Beaudoin, G., et al. (2003). Neural circuitry underlying voluntary suppression of sadness. *Biological Psychiatry, 53,* 502–510.

Mauss, I. B., Bunge, S. A., & Gross, J. J. (2007). Automatic emotion regulation. *Socil and Personality Psychology Compass, 1,* 146–167.

Mauss, I. B., Cook, C. L., & Gross, J. J. (2007). Automatic emotion regulation during an anger provocation. *Journal of Experimental Social Psychology, 43,* 698–711.

Mauss, I. B., Evers, C., Wilhelm, F. H., & Gross, J.J. (2006). How to bite your tongue without blowing your top: Implicit evaluation of emotion regulation predicts affective responding to anger provocation. *Personality and Social Psychology Bulletin, 32,* 589–602.

Mauss, I. B., Levenson, R. W., McCarter, L., Wilhelm, F. H., & Gross, J. J. (2005). The tie that binds?: Coherence among emotion experience, behavior, and physiology. *Emotion, 5,* 175–190.

Mauss, I. B., Wilhelm, F. H., & Gross, J. J. (2003). Autonomic recovery and habituation in social anxiety. *Psychophysiology, 40,* 648–653.

Mauss, I. B., Wilhelm, F. W., & Gross, J. J. (2004). Is there less to social anxiety than meets the eye? Emotion experience, expression, and bodily responding. *Cognition and Emotion, 18,* 631–662.

McCanne, T. R., & Anderson, J. A. (1987). Emotional responding following experimental manipulation of

facial electromyographic activity. *Journal of Personality and Social Psychology, 52,* 759–768.

Mesquita, B., & Albert, D. (2007). The cultural regulation of emotions. In J.J. Gross (Ed.), *Handbook of emotion regulation* (pp. 486–503). New York: Guilford Press.

Mischel, W., Shoda, Y., & Rodriguez, M. L. (1989). Delay of gratification in children. *Science, 244,* 933–938.

Molden, D. C., & Dweck, C. S. (2006). Finding "meaning" in psychology: A lay theories approach to self-regulation, social perception, and social development. *American Psychologist, 61,* 192–203.

Morrow, J., & Nolen-Hoeksema, S. (1990). Effects of responses to depression on the remediation of depressive affect. *Journal of Personality and Social Psychology, 58,* 519–527.

Moses, E. B., & Barlow, D. H. (2006). A new unified treatment approach for emotional disorders based on emotion science. *Current Directions in Psychological Science, 15,* 146–150.

Nesse, R. M. (2000). Is depression an adaptation? *Archives of General Psychiatry, 57,* 14–20.

Nolen-Hoeksema, S., Morrow, J., & Fredrickson, B. L. (1993). Response styles and the duration of episodes of depressed mood. *Journal of Abnormal Psychology, 102,* 20–28.

Ochsner, K. N., Bunge, S. A., Gross, J. J., & Gabrieli, J. D. E. (2002). Rethinking feelings: An fMRI study of the cognitive regulation of emotion. *Journal of Cognitive Neuroscience, 14,* 1215–1229.

Ochsner, K. N., & Gross, J. J. (2004). Thinking makes it so: A social cognitive neuroscience approach to emotion regulation. In R. F. Baumeister & K. D. Vohs (Eds.), *Handbook of self regulation: Research, theory, and applications* (pp. 229–255). New York: Guilford Press.

Ochsner, K. N., & Gross, J. J. (2005). The cognitive control of emotion. *Trends in Cognitive Sciences, 9,* 242–249.

Ochsner, K. N., Ray, R. R., Cooper, J. C., Robertson, E. R., Chopra, S., Gabrieli, J. D. E., & Gross, J. J. (2004). For better or for worse: Neural systems supporting the cognitive down- and up-regulation of negative emotion. *NeuroImage, 23,* 483–499.

Parrott, W. G. (1993). Beyond hedonism: Motives for inhibiting good moods and for maintaining bad moods. In D. M. Wegner & J. W. Pennebaker (Eds.), *Handbook of mental control* (pp. 278–305). Englewood Cliffs, NJ: Prentice-Hall.

Phelps, E. A. (2006). Emotion and cognition: Insights from studies of the human amygdala. *Annual Review of Psychology, 57,* 27–53.

Ray, R. D., Wilhelm, F. H., & Gross, J. J. (in press). All in the mind's eye?: Anger rumination and reappraisal. *Journal of Personality and Social Psychology.*

Redelmeier, D. A., & Kahneman, D. (1996). Patients' memories of painful medical treatments: Real-time and retrospective evaluations of two minimally invasive procedures. *Pain, 66,* 3–8.

Richards, J. M., & Gross, J. J. (1999). Composure at any cost?: The cognitive consequences of emotion suppression. *Personality and Social Psychology Bulletin, 25,* 1033–1044.

Richards, J. M., & Gross, J. J. (2000). Emotion regulation and memory: The cognitive costs of keeping one's cool. *Journal of Personality and Social Psychology, 79,* 410–424.

Richards, J. M., & Gross, J. J. (2006). Personality and emotional memory: How regulating emotion impairs memory for emotional events. *Journal of Research in Personality, 40,* 631–651.

Rothbart, M. K., Ziaie, H., & O'Boyle, C. G. (1992). Self-regulation and emotion in infancy. In N. Eisenberg & R. A. Fabes (Eds.), *Emotion and its regulation in early development* (pp. 7–23). San Francisco: Jossey-Bass.

Rothbaum, F., Weisz, J. R., & Snyder, S. S. (1982). Changing the world and changing the self: A two-process model of perceived control. *Journal of Personality and Social Psychology, 42,* 5–37.

Rottenberg, J., & Gross, J. J. (2003). When emotion goes wrong: Realizing the promise of affective science. *Clinical Psychology: Science and Practice, 10,* 227–232.

Rottenberg, J., Gross, J. J., & Gotlib, I. H. (2005). Emotion context insensitivity in major depressive disorder. *Journal of Abnormal Psychology, 114,* 627–639.

Rottenberg, J., & Johnson, S. L. (2006). *Emotion and psychopathology: Bridging affective and clinical science.* Washington, DC: American Psychological Association.

Rottenberg, J., Kasch, K. L., Gross, J. J., & Gotlib, I. H. (2002). Sadness and amusement reactivity differentially predict concurrent and prospective functioning in major depressive disorder. *Emotion, 2,* 135–146.

Schaefer, S. M., Jackson, D. C., Davidson, R. J., Aguirre, G. K., Kimberg, D. Y., & Thompson-Schill, S. L. (2002). Modulation of amygdalar activity by the conscious regulation of negative emotion. *Journal of Cognitive Neuroscience, 14,* 913–921.

Scherer, K. R., Schorr, A., & Johnstone, T. (Eds.). (2001). *Appraisal processes in emotion: Theory, methods, research.* New York: Oxford University Press.

Shiffrin, R. M., & Schneider, W. (1977). Controlled and automatic human information processing: II. Perceptual learning, automatic attending, and a general theory. *Psychological Review, 84,* 127–190.

Spasojevic, J., & Alloy, L. B. (2001). Rumination as a common mechanism relating depressive risk factors to depression. *Emotion, 1,* 25–37.

Srivastava, S., Tamir, M., McGonigal, K. M., John, O. P., & Gross, J. J. (2008). *The social consequences of emotional suppression: A prospective study of the transition to college.* Manuscript submitted for publication.

Srull, T. K., & Wyer, R. S. (1979). The role of category accessibility in the interpretation of information about persons: Some determinants and implications. *Journal of Personality and Social Psychology, 37,* 1660–1672.

Stemmler, G. (1997). Selective activation of traits: Boundary conditions for the activation of anger. *Personality and Individual Differences, 22,* 213–233.

Stepper, S., & Strack, F. (1993). Proprioceptive determinants of emotional and nonemotional feelings. *Journal of Personality and Social Psychology, 64,* 211–220.

Stifter, C. A., & Moyer, D. (1991). The regulation of positive affect: Gaze aversion activity during mother–infant interaction. *Infant Behavior and Development, 14,* 111–123.

Strack, F., & Deutsch, R. (2004). Reflective and impulsive determinants of social behavior. *Personality and Social Psychology Review, 8,* 220–247.

Strack, F., Martin, L. L., & Stepper, S. (1988). Inhibiting and facilitating conditions of the human smile: A nonobtrusive test of the facial feedback hypothesis. *Journal of Personality and Social Psychology, 54,* 768–777.

Sutton, R. I. (1991). Maintaining norms about expressed emotions: The case of bill collectors. *Administrative Science Quarterly, 36,* 245–268.

Tamir, M. (2005). Don't worry, be happy?: Neuroticism, trait-consistent affect regulation, and performance. *Journal of Personality and Social Psychology, 89,* 449–461.

Tamir, M., John, O. P., Srivastava, S., & Gross, J. J. (2007). Implicit theories of emotion: Affective and social outcomes across a major life transition. *Journal of Personality and Social Psychology, 92,* 731–744.

Thoits, P. A. (1985). Self-labeling processes in mental illness: The role of emotional deviance. *American Journal of Sociology, 91,* 221–249.

Thompson, R. A. (1994). Emotion regulation: A theme in search of definition. In N. A. Fox (Ed.), The development of emotion regulation: Biological and behavioral considerations. *Monographs of the Society for Research in Child Development, 59*(2–3, Serial No. 240), 25–52).

Tsai, J. L., Knutson, B., & Fung, H. H. (2006). Cultural variation in affect valuation. *Journal of Personality and Social Psychology, 90,* 288–307.

CHAPTER 32

Emotional Complexity

KRISTEN A. LINDQUIST and LISA FELDMAN BARRETT

Imagine someone who is "emotionally complex," and a number of characteristics might come to mind: the ability to see the good and the bad in all things; the ability to describe feelings with detail and precision; the ability to specifically and reliably anticipate which feelings will arise in a given situation; or the tendency to remember experiencing many emotions at once. You might also imagine someone who tends to characterize himself or herself as an emotionally complex person. It appears that there are myriad ways in which a person can be considered "emotionally complex." In fact, the concept of emotional complexity is similarly varied in the psychological literature. In this chapter, we review this literature with a focus on three main formulations of emotional complexity as (1) dialecticism and precision in people's self-reports of emotion experiences; (2) explicit, propositional knowledge about emotion in situations; and (3) people's self-characterizations of their degree of complexity.

Before we begin our review of the emotional complexity literature, it seems apropos to clearly define just *what* we think people are be-

ing complex about. There are two general approaches to defining the nature of emotion. A "natural-kinds" perspective (e.g., Ekman, 1972; Izard, 1994; Tomkins, 1962; Panksepp, 2000; Roseman, 1984) views a select set of emotions (e.g., anger, sadness, fear, anger, disgust, and happiness) as biologically given and fixed categories (for recent reviews of the natural-kinds perspective, see Barrett, 2006a; Barrett, Lindquist, et al., 2007). In this perspective, complexity in self-reports of online experiences of emotion results when more than one emotion circuit fires at a given point in time, or is caused by variations in the accuracy with which people translate experience into words. In this sense, emotion categories are perceptual categories that are either hard-coded into the brain at birth or learned by inducing statistical regularities in the environment. According to this perspective, people gain complexity in propositional knowledge of emotion when they learn to associate the consequences of the firing of a given emotion circuit with certain environmental conditions. Complexity in self-characterizations of experience derives from differences in people's ability to characterize their experiences as complex. In this sense, complexity in self-characterizations of experience exists because some people merely overlay complexity onto what is really a fixed and stable system.

The second approach to the nature of emotion takes a "psychological constructionist" perspective (e.g., Barrett, 2006b; Barrett, Lindquist, et al., 2007; Russell, 2003; Mandler, 1975; Schacter & Singer, 1962). In this view, complexity is not a conceptual overlay; it is intrinsic to the neurobiological and psychological systems that constitute emotional experience. From this point of view, a discrete emotional event emerges in consciousness (i.e., a person "has an emotion") when an instance of a more basic core affective state is automatically and implicitly categorized as having emotional meaning. *Core affect* is an ongoing, ever-changing psychologically primitive state that has both valenced, and to some extent, arousal-based properties (see Barrett, 2004; Russell, 2003; Russell & Barrett, 1999). The events that people call (in English) anger, sadness, fear, and so on, result when core affect is categorized using the "conceptual system for emotion." This term refers to what people know about emotion and how that knowledge is represented in emotion categories (see Barrett, 2006b). Categorizing an instance of core affect proceeds efficiently and automatically to produce a state that is at once affective and conceptual, where internal sensory information from the body and external sensory information from the world are bound together in a moment in time. A person experiences an emotion like anger, for example, when a state of unpleasant affect is categorized as having been caused by an event that blocked a person's goals. Categorizing core affect bounds it as a discrete experience: it allows core affective experience to pop out in consciousness and gives it meaning. Categorization transforms core affect into an intensional state, allowing a person to make inferences about what caused the affective change, what to do next, and to communicate that state to others in an effective and efficient manner. From this perspective, emotional complexity is the direct result of the conceptual system for emotion.

In the context of this review, we explore how various forms of emotional complexity result from the form and function of the conceptual system for emotion. The idea that emotional and conceptual complexity are related is not new. Lane and colleagues have proposed a cognitive-developmental model of emotional awareness (e.g., Lane & Garfield, 2005; Lane & Pollermann, 2002) that argues for conceptual development as the core determinant of emotional complexity. The view that we propose in this chapter is distinct from the cognitive-developmental model on several points. First, we propose that emotional complexity is grounded in a highly flexible, context-dependent conceptual system of situated representations of emotion (see Niedenthal, Chapter 36, this volume), rather than a system composed of schemas or fixed prototypic or script-like concepts. Second, we emphasize the possibility that conceptual complexity has a hand in psychologically constructing each episode that we call "emotion" during the online categorization of affective (pleasant or unpleasant) events (cf. Barrett, 2006b). Finally, our perspective assumes that complexity in the conceptual system derives not only from *which* categories of emotion populate a person's conceptual system (i.e., whether or not a person possesses categories such as "sad," "happy," "fear," etc.), but also from idiographic variations in the *content* of category knowledge (e.g., what exactly a person knows about happiness, sadness, or fear), in the *representational format* of category knowledge (i.e., how that category knowledge is constituted in memory and during online use of category information), and in the resources to *use* category knowledge to construct the experience of emotion (i.e., whether people can readily access and manipulate what they know during online experience). In this chapter, we argue that greater complexity in the structure, content, and representational format of the conceptual system, and deftness in wielding such knowledge, contribute to greater complexity in the psychological events that we call "emotion." The conceptual system for emotion is a unifying factor in producing emotional complexity in its various forms.

COMPLEXITY IN SELF-REPORTED EXPERIENCES OF EMOTION

The best way to assess the properties of an experience (such as its complexity) is to ask people how they feel and to examine the content of what they answer. Although self-report methods have obvious drawbacks for assessing the processes that might produce emotional complexity, they can tell scientists a good deal about the contents of what people feel (cf. Barrett, 2004; Barrett, Mesquita, Ochsner, & Gross, 2007; Conner, Barrett, Bliss-Moreau, Lebo, & Kashub, 2003). "Emotional complexity" refers to two types of contents in emotion self-reports: dialecticism and granularity in the experience of emotion. Implicit in both is the idea that self-reports are verbal behaviors that can be analyzed in a way that unearths the structure of emotion experience.

Dialecticism in Self-Reported Experience of Emotion

As a form of emotional complexity, "dialecticism" refers to the experience of pleasant and unpleasant states in a coincidental or temporally related fashion (Bagozzi, Wong, & Yi, 1999). The term is derived from Confucian philosophy (see Peng & Nisbett, 1999) and was first used in the context of cross-cultural research (Bagozzi et al., 1999). In the context of this chapter, "dialecticism" refers to all studies assessing the relation in reported experiences of positive and negative emotions.

Cross-Cultural Variation in Dialectic Experience of Emotion

There appears to be general scientific consensus that individuals from Eastern cultures such as China, Korea, or Japan are more likely to have dialectic experiences of emotion than people from Western cultures such as the United States or Europe are (Bagozzi et al., 1999; Kitayama, Markus, & Kurokawa, 2000; Scollon, Oishi, Diener, & Biswas-Diener, 2005; Shimmack, Oishi, & Diener, 2002). There is also some evidence for a Yiddish form of dialecticism (see Peng & Nisbett, 1999), but most research focuses on the East–West dichotomy. The psychological dimensions typically used to describe the difference between Eastern and Western cultures (e.g., individualism–collectivism) fail to account for the cross-cultural variance in the dialectic experience of emotions, however (cf. Shimmack et al., 2002). Instead, differences in dialecticism are thought to derive from emotion regulation strategies that are promoted by the philosophical traditions within each culture. Eastern dialecticism has been linked to a philosophical tradition that promotes balance and the acceptance of contradiction (Peng & Nisbett, 1999, although see Lee, 2000), where opposites are conceptualized as being intrinsically related to one another. In this tradition, the concept "good" overlaps with "bad" such that something can be both good and bad at the same time. This orientation leads people to enlist in strategies that promote more affectively balanced lives. In contrast, Western experience is grounded in Aristotelian philosophy that favors an "either–or" type of reasoning, where opposites are bipolar. In this tradition, the concept "good" is the antithesis of "bad," so something can never be both at the same time. This orientation leads people to enlist in strategies that promote maximally pleasant (at the expense of unpleasant) experience (Heine, Lehman, Markus, & Kitayama, 1999). The philosophical differences that characterize the East–West divide translate into different conceptions of what constitutes "ideal affect" (the affective states that people deem most valuable and desire to feel most; Tsai, 2007). What may lie at the heart of the cross-cultural differences in the dialectic experience of emotion is a difference in the value that cultures place on the experience of unpleasant emotion.

The claims for broad cross-cultural variation in dialecticism may hide individual variability in dialectic experience within each cultural tradition, however. "Dialecticism" is sometimes operationally defined as a negative correlation between reported pleasant and unpleasant emotions (e.g., Bagozzi et al., 1999), but it has also been defined as a zero correlation (e.g., Diener & Emmons, 1985) or any decrease in the magnitude of negative correlation between the two (Shimmack et al., 2002; Carstensen, Pasupathi, Mayr, & Nesselroade, 2000).[1] In cross-sectional studies, the presence of a near-zero correlation between reports of pleasant and unpleasant experience indicates that there is no systematic covariation between reports of these states within a group of people. Whereas some respondents report feeling both more pleasant and more unpleasant emotion when compared to each respective group mean, other individuals report greater pleasant emotion with an absence of negative emotion (i.e., pleasant scores fall above the group mean for pleasure, but unpleasant scores fall below the mean for displeasure), or vice versa. In reality, then, correlations near zero mask individual differences in the dialectic experience of emotion that appear to be present in both Eastern and Western contexts, although perhaps at different base rates.

Individual Variation in Dialectic Experience of Emotion

Several lines of research point to individual differences in the dialectic experience of emotion. As people age, their experience becomes more dialectic. In an experience-sampling study of American participants ranging in age from 18 to 94, younger participants experienced pleasant and unpleasant emotions as inversely related, but this correlation diminished with age (Carstensen et al., 2000). Greater cognitive complexity promotes dialectic thought (i.e., the ability to conceptualize contradiction), thereby producing more dialectic experience. Individuals greater in cognitive complexity did not demonstrate a systematic relationship between pleasant and unpleasant experiences, as compared to individuals low in complexity, whose pleasant and unpleasant experiences were inversely related (Davis, Zautra, & Smith, 2004; Reich, Zautra, & Potter, 2001).

Women demonstrate exaggerated versions of the dialecticism patterns associated with their culture (e.g., Bagozzi et al., 1999; Shimmack et al., 2002). In one cross-cultural study, American women had less dialectic experience (i.e., larger negative correlations between experience of pleasant and unpleasant emotions), but Chinese women had more dialectic experience (i.e., larger positive correlations between experiences of pleasant and unpleasant emotions), than their respective male counterparts (Bagozzi et al., 1999). These findings stand in contrast to the stereotype that women are the more emotionally complex sex (for a discussion, see Barrett, Robin, Pietromonaco, & Eyssell, 1998), and call into question the generalizability of findings that Western women have more complex emotional awareness than Western men do (Barrett, Lane, Sechrest, & Schwartz, 2000).

Sources of Knowledge Sampled

The strongest evidence for dialecticism comes from responses that are more likely to be infused with culturally embedded beliefs, such as judging how a hypothetical scenario might feel (e.g., Leu et al., 2007), recalling prior experiences (e.g., Kitayama et al., 2000; Reich et al.,

2001; Oishi, 2002; Ong & Bergeman, 2004; Carstensen et al., 2000), or summarizing experiences across a period of time to produce a response (e.g., Larsen, McGraw, & Cacioppo, 2001; Larsen, McGraw, Mellers, & Cacioppo, 2004; for discussions, see Barrett, 1997; Robinson & Clore, 2002; Ross, 1989). Momentary experiences of emotion ("How happy are you right now?") are less belief-based and correspondingly fail to yield evidence for dialecticism (e.g., Vansteelandt, Van Mechelen, & Nezlek, 2005), even in cultures typically characterized as more prone to dialectic experiences of emotion (e.g., Chinese culture; Scollon et al., 2005).

Granularity in Self-Reported Experience of Emotion

A second form of complexity in self-reports of emotion experience is the ability to verbally characterize such experiences with precision, referred to as "emotional granularity" (Barrett, 1998, 2004; Barrett, Gross, Christensen, & Benvenuto, 2001; Feldman, 1995; Tugade, Barrett, & Gross, 2007).[2] Individuals who are emotionally granular use emotion adjectives (such as "sad," "contented," "angry," "afraid," "joyful," etc.) to represent discrete and qualitatively different experiences. Those lower in granularity use these same words in a less precise way to represent broad, global affective states, such as pleasantness–unpleasantness or arousal–quiescence.

Determining Emotional Granularity

Emotional granularity is determined by assessing the relatedness in emotion experiences as they are represented through people's endorsement of emotion adjectives during the self-report process. Typically, participants are given a set of adjectives ("happy," "anxious," "annoyed," etc.) and rate, on a Likert scale, how closely each adjective described their emotional state at a given measurement moment; this is done across a series of measurement instances (e.g., in an experience-sampling paradigm). The relatedness between ratings is then calculated by using person-correlations (e.g., Barrett, 1998; Barrett et al., 2001; Feldman, 1995) or intraclass correlations (Tugade et al., 2007). A strong positive correlation between two such ratings is evidence for low granularity, meaning that an individual uses emotion words (e.g., "angry" and "sad") in a nonspecific fashion to represent what those two feeling states have in common (e.g., displeasure). A weak (or zero) correlation, or a strong negative correlation, indicates high granularity, meaning that an individual uses two emotion words to represent two qualitatively different states (e.g., "angry" as a different feeling from "sad"). (A correlation of zero between ratings of "angry" and "sad" indicates high granularity, because it reflects the fact that a person uses the words differently across measurement occasions. In some instances, "angry" and "sad" are rated above a person's own mean [indicating that both intense anger and sadness are being felt], whereas in other instances, "angry" is rated higher and "sad" rated lower, or vice versa [indicating that one is being felt in the absence of the other].)

Individuals from the United States vary tremendously in their degree of emotional granularity, even when verbal ability is controlled for. Estimates from one study (Barrett, 1998) put the granularity for unpleasant experiences between .16 and .89 ($M = .52$, $SD = .24$). The granularity for pleasant experiences ranged between .51 and .96 ($M = .77$, $SD = .28$). People who represent their negative states in a granular way also typically report their positive states in a granular way (Barrett, 1998).

Processes Underlying Emotional Granularity

THE CONCEPTUAL SYSTEM FOR EMOTION

When people report on their experiences, they must represent and communicate those experiences in words. Differences in the structure of the conceptual system for emotion may be one source of variation in how people describe their experiences of emotion, leading to variation in emotional granularity. For example, the words that correspond to basic-level categories may influence how people use emotion words to represent experience during the self-report process. Categories for emotion can be thought of as hierarchically organized, ranging from categories that represent the most general feelings to categories that represent the most specific feelings (e.g., "pleasant" and "unpleasant") (e.g., "frustration," "aggravation," "irritation," etc., for the category of "anger"). Basic-level categories represent the level of conceptualization that people prefer when parsing a domain (Murphy, 2002; Rosch, Mervis, Gray, Johnson, & Boyes-

Braem, 1976), and words that correspond to basic-level categories are used most frequently by parents when naming objects and events for their children (Brown, 1957). Most researchers assume that the categories corresponding to the words "anger," "sadness," "fear," and so forth are basic-level, and cross-sectional research bears this out (e.g., Alonso-Arbiol et al., 2006; Fehr & Russell, 1984; Shaver, Schwartz, Kirson, & O'Connor, 1987; Shaver, Murdaya, & Fraley, 2001). It is possible, however, that significant and important individual differences exist in which categories are used as basic. We propose that individuals lower in granularity use nomothetically superordinate category knowledge as the modal means of categorizing their experiences (e.g., they categorize as "unpleasant" those feelings that might normatively be categorized as "sadness," "anger," or "fear," and categorize as "pleasant" those feelings that would normatively be categorized as "joy," "happiness," or "interest"). Categorizing an affective state gives it meaning, so that a person can communicate it to others, make inferences about it, and make predictions about how to act (cf. Barrett, 2006b). If a person uses superordinate categories of emotion (e.g., "pleasant" and "unpleasant") as the modal means of categorization, then that person not only will communicate affective experience in a broad manner, but may also experience those states as broad and undifferentiated. Alternately, individuals higher in granularity may be experts in emotion and use subordinate categories as basic (e.g., they may use "frustration," "annoyance," and "rage" as basic, rather than "anger"). These individuals may report and experience affect as discrete and nuanced emotional events, much in the same way that experts in reading X-rays (Christensen et al., 1981), sexing chickens (Biederman & Shiffrar, 1987), and judging wine (Solomon, 1990, 1997), can perceive important differences that novices cannot (for a similar point, see Lane, 2000, p. 348).

Although no studies have yet explicitly examined the relation between conceptual basicness and emotional granularity, existing findings suggest the plausibility of such a link. Two-year-old children typically use the word "sad" to refer to anything unpleasant (such as faces depicting "anger," "sadness," and "fear"), and the word "happy" to refer to anything pleasant (see Widen & Russell, Chapter 21, this volume); that is, their basic level of categorization is "pleasant–unpleasant." This pattern of response is very similar to how low-granularity adults use emotion adjectives to communicate only the most global or general affective states (Barrett, 1998, 2004; Feldman, 1995). As children's conceptual systems become more differentiated, they learn to distinguish reliably between exemplars of other emotion categories (e.g., "anger," "fear," and "sadness"). As children develop, their ability to correctly identify faces depicting these emotions begins to mirror that of adults high in granularity, and who use emotion words in a precise way to represent emotional experience. We would expect, then, that a child's experience of emotion becomes more granular as his or her conceptual system becomes more differentiated. Even more tempting are the implications for emotional complexity in adulthood. Complexity in the content of a person's conceptual system for emotion might intrinsically shape the complexity of emotion experience in much the same way that conceptual complexity shapes children's perceptions of emotion across early stages of development.

In addition to variation in structure, the content of the conceptual system for emotion may be linked to emotional granularity. Typically, emotion concepts (e.g., the concept for "anger") have been conceived of as single, stable representations of information that are organized classically (e.g., Johnson-Laird & Oatley, 1989; Ortony, Clore, & Foss, 1987), as prototypes (Russell, 1991), as schemas (Lane & Pollermann, 2002), or as theories (Clore & Ortony, 1991) that can be retrieved from long-term memory when needed. More recently, emotion concepts have been understood as flexible constructions deriving from a more generative system of heterogeneous and varied situated conceptualizations (see Niedenthal, Chapter 36, this volume). From the vantage point of this more recent view, emotion concepts are examples of what Edelman (1989) has termed the "remembered present," where neural representations of an emotion exemplar combines information from the current situation with information stored from previous experience. The result contributes to the representational structure that is utilized during later online categorizations of percepts from that domain.

To date, no studies have examined idiographic variability in the richness of conceptual content. Studies assessing the conceptual system for emotion primarily ask individuals to

list words for emotion categories (e.g., Fehr & Russell, 1984, Study 1), to rate the similarity between words (e.g., Alonso-Arbiol et al., 2006, Study 2; Barrett, 2004; Shaver et al., 1987, Study 1), or to rate the prototypicality of emotion words (e.g., Alonso-Arbiol et al., 2006, Study 1; Fehr & Russell, 1984, Study 3; Shaver et al., 1987, Study 1). Emotion words are not synonymous with emotion concepts, however, so tests of how people use and think about emotion words may not sufficiently map the variability and detail in what people know about emotion. Words can be processed by using shallow, quick, associative methods that fail to activate deeper representations of category information (Barsalou, Santos, Simmons, & Wilson, in press). Even studies that ask participants to write narratives for episodes of "anger," "sadness," and "fear," and then code those narratives for their prototypical features (Shaver et al., 1987, Study 2), may not be suitably sensitive to capture individual differences, because people can construct a prototype of a category even if conceptual knowledge is not stored that way.

There is some evidence to suggest that socialization contributes to variability in the conceptual system for emotion. People may have a richer conceptual base for emotion available to them if they are exposed to a wider range of emotion categories, are taught a more varied emotion vocabulary, and learn to represent their experiences with greater detail and complexity. Children learn about emotion categories through formal, rule-based instruction, where parents make explicit links among affective feelings, a situational context, and emotion words (e.g., when a child throws a toy at Jimmy, a parent might say, "You're feeling *angry* right now, because Jimmy grabbed your toy without asking"). Parents also reminisce about emotional memories in a way that helps children learn about a particular emotion category—by discussing the feelings that were involved during the experience of that emotion, the interpersonal consequences of expressing that emotion, or coping strategies relevant to that emotion (e.g., Fivush, Berlin, Sales, Mennuti-Washburn, & Cassidy, 2003; Miller & Sperry, 1988). Indeed, children whose parents speak to them about emotion know more about emotion (e.g., Harris, 2006a, 2006b; Harris, de Rosnay, & Pons, 2005; de Rosnay, Pons, Harris, & Morell, 2004).

Children may also acquire emotion concepts via inductive, associative learning, such as when an emotion word is used (but not explicitly paired) with features of an emotional episode (e.g., a child hears a parent refer to feeling depressed while the parent is slumped at the table with a defeated expression, discussing a recent job loss). The role of associative learning in the acquisition of emotion category knowledge remains to be empirically tested, however.

COGNITIVE RESOURCES

Differences in granularity may stem not only from what people know about emotion, but also from how well they use what they know. For example, a person's working memory capacity (WMC) probably shapes his or her ability to attend to affective states and to access and efficiently wield conceptual knowledge during emotion representation. WMC is the ability to control attention for the purposes of processing information in contexts where there are competing demands (Barrett, Tugade, & Engle, 2004). Working memory is required during the self-report process, where respondents must hold an experience in mind as they describe that feeling, using emotion adjectives presented to them in a serial format. With effortful, controlled processing, people can reject adjectives that are not characteristic of the current state: The resulting correlations between emotion adjectives will be substantially lower, resulting in high emotional granularity. WMC may also have an impact on emotional experience itself, because people higher in WMC will be able to hold more information about the current affective state in mind as conceptual knowledge about emotion (i.e., content specific to a certain emotion category such as contextual information, arousal content, linguistic representations) is retrieved to aid in online categorization that feeling. This should result not only in the report of more discrete emotional experiences, but also in the experience of more discrete emotional states.

Summary

In this section, we have discussed how emotional complexity is observed in verbal representations of experience. In studies of both dialecticism and emotional granularity, evidence of emotional complexity is derived from the structure of people's self-reports of emotion experience; self-reports are treated as verbal behaviors, and the degree of complexity in the structure of those behaviors is examined. We have suggested that conceptual knowledge about emotion seems to play a role in both forms of complexity, but not merely because self-reports require language. Rather, there is good reason to hypothesize that conceptual knowledge about emotion plays an intrinsic role in the complexity of emotions as they are experienced. Individual differences in the content of the conceptual system for emotion and in executive function, as well as the ways in which these differences shape experience, have yet to be explored and constitute a new frontier of research in emotional complexity. In the next section, we examine what is known about complexity in a particular form of conceptual knowledge: propositional knowledge for emotion. We then explore the experiential ramifications of deficits in this type of knowledge, to shed further light on the potential mechanisms underlying emotional complexity.

COMPLEXITY IN PROPOSITIONAL KNOWLEDGE OF EMOTION

The Levels of Emotional Awareness Scale

To date, complexity in conceptual knowledge of emotion has been assessed with measures that ask individuals to make explicit, propositional statements about emotion experience (e.g., "If I didn't win a contest, then I would feel disappointed"). The Levels of Emotional Awareness Scale (LEAS; Lane, Quinlan, Schwartz, Walker, & Zeinlin, 1990) is the most frequently used measure and is based on the assumption that emotion experience occurs when feelings of emotional arousal are conceptualized using knowledge about emotion. Individual differences in emotional complexity, as measured by the LEAS, reflect variations in the degree of differentiation and integration of a person's "emotional schemas" (Lane & Pollermann, 2002; Lane & Schwartz, 1987; Lane et al., 1990). According to Lane and colleagues, the development of emotional schemas is facilitated both by language and by individuals' ability to encode and represent past experiences of emotional arousal. Individuals who focus on proprioceptive information during emotional arousal will be more likely to encode and later represent emotion knowledge in visceral or action-oriented terms. Individuals who abstract relational meaning from feelings of emotional arousal (such as how different feelings relate, how they are coordinated, etc.) will be more likely to encode and later represent emotion knowledge in a nuanced and differentiated fashion.

The LEAS measures the complexity of propositional knowledge of emotion by asking individuals to describe the types of emotional experiences that would occur during hypothetical emotion-eliciting situations (e.g., "You and your friend are competing for a prize and your friend wins. How would you feel? How would your friend feel?"). Responses are coded for the extent to which they make reference to bodily sensations, specific behavioral responses or action tendencies, or discrete-emotion words, each of which is taken as evidence of increasing emotional complexity (see, Lane et al., 1990). LEAS scoring criteria can be used on any narrative of emotional experience, whether it describes a current experience or a prior, remembered experience (e.g., Bliss-Moreau, Barrett, Connor, & McCarthy, 2007). In such cases, the scoring represents a person's tendency to represent his or her experience as emotional (rather than somatic or affective), and to characterize that experience by using multiple emotion concepts (rather than reflecting anything about the detail and situated nature of the conceptual content).

Complexity in propositional knowledge for emotion predicts more normative identification of emotion cues in others and the surrounding context. People who score higher on the LEAS are better able to identify emotional content in other people's facial behaviors and in the environment, using Rau's (1993) Perception of Affect Test (Lane, Sechrest, Riedel, Shapiro, & Kazniak, 2000; Lane et al., 1996). Higher LEAS scores are also associated with greater right cerebral hemisphere dominance during perception of emotional face stimuli (Lane, Kivley, Du Bois, Shamasundara, & Schwartz, 1995)—a phenomenon that is thought to index heightened sensitivity to external emotion cues (see Lane et al., 1995).

Sex Differences in Propositional Knowledge of Emotion

There are robust and consistent sex differences in complexity of propositional knowledge for emotion. Women from Western contexts routinely outperform men on the LEAS (e.g.,

Conway, 2000; Bliss-Moreau et al., 2007), even when factors such as verbal intelligence, language of origin, or socioeconomic status (SES) are controlled for (Barrett et al., 2000). These sex differences are even present in children: Girls outperform boys on the children's version of the LEAS (LEAS-C; Bajgar, Ciarrochi, Lane, & Deane, 2005). At face value, these findings suggest that males and females routinely differ in their use of emotion knowledge, but this may not actually reflect differences in emotional aptitude. Sex differences in LEAS performance disappear when items on the LEAS are made particularly self-relevant (Bliss-Moreau et al., 2007), suggesting that men and women may possess the same range of knowledge, but use it differently under the testing circumstances imposed by the standard LEAS administration (i.e., a controlled lab situation with few contextual or social cues). Under such circumstances, responses to hypothetical scenarios (as in the LEAS) are very likely to draw on culturally infused gendered beliefs about emotion. Consistent with this idea is the finding that both male and female respondents who describe themselves as more masculine perform more poorly on the LEAS than do those who describe themselves as less masculine (Conway, 2000).

Cultural stereotypes about emotion will have both distal and proximal effects on LEAS responses. The distal effects of stereotypes begin in childhood, where parents transmit stereotypes about sex roles to children via implicit means (talking about emotion differently with boys and girls) or explicit means (teaching boys and girls to behave in different ways during emotional situations). For example, middle-class European American mothers elaborate and evaluate emotional memories more and are more likely to discuss the interpersonal contexts of those memories, when speaking to their daughters as opposed to their sons (Fivush et al., 2003). Proximally, stereotypes may have an impact on LEAS performance because they affect the motivation to respond in a complex manner, or because they act as a filter through which participants retrieve conceptual knowledge about emotion.

Developmental Differences in Propositional Knowledge of Emotion

Individual differences in propositional knowledge for emotion also exist among children with the LEAS-C (Bajgar et al., 2005). Consistent with research using the LEAS in some adult samples (e.g., Lane et al., 1990), performance on the LEAS-C was associated with increased verbal skill and vocabulary. Although linguistic and cognitive capacity may drive LEAS-C performance, the evidence is also consistent with the idea that children with greater language skills have a better understanding of emotion (e.g., de Rosnay & Harris, 2002; Pons & Harris, 2005; Pons, Lawson, Harris, & de Rosnay, 2003; Widen & Russell, Chapter 21, this volume). LEAS-C scores increase with age (Bajgar et al., 2005), suggesting that propositional knowledge about emotion increases in complexity as people learn about emotion.

Alexithymia: An Absence of Conceptual Knowledge of Emotion

Deficits in propositional knowledge of emotion characterize an emotional disturbance known as "alexithymia." The term "alexithymia" (literally meaning "absence of words for emotion") was first coined by Sifneos (1973) to describe patients who appeared to lack conceptual knowledge of emotion, resulting in an impaired ability to symbolically represent their affective feelings as emotional. Alexithymic individuals' apparent lack of conceptual knowledge results in difficulties expressing emotion, imagining, and socializing, and increases the likelihood that emotion will be experienced as somatic symptoms (Haviland & Reise, 1996; Rieffe, Oosterveld, & Meerum Terwogt, 2006; see Lane, Ahern, Schwartz, & Kazniak, 1997, for a discussion of the alexithymia construct). As might be expected, individuals high in alexithymia consistently perform poorly on the LEAS (e.g., Lane et al., 1996) and on measures of emotional intelligence (e.g., Lumley, Gustavson, Partridge, & Labouvie-Vief, 2005; Parker, Taylor, & Bagby, 2001). Alexithymia occurs most frequently in older individuals (although see Rieffe et al., 2006), men, individuals of lower SES, and persons with fewer years of education (Lane, Sechrest, & Riedel, 1998). Alexithymia is also seen in patients with various psychological and somatic disorders.

It is widely believed that alexithymia results when individuals fail to develop the cognitive resources needed to consciously represent emotional states (Berenbaum & James, 1994; Frawley & Smith, 2001; Lane & Schwartz, 1987; Taylor, 2000; Taylor, Bagby, & Parker, 1997). This rudimentary conceptual system for emotion results in a form of "affective blindsight," where individuals experience subjective bodily sensations or "background feelings" but fail to experience them as emotional (Lane et al., 1997; Lane & Garfield, 2005); the analogy is to patients with classic blindsight, who have behavioral awareness of visual objects in the absence of the conscious experience of seeing those objects (e.g., de Gelder, Vroomen, Pourtois, & Weiskrantz, 1999).

Deficits in Emotion Experience Associated with Alexithymia

Alexithymic individuals report less intense experience of emotion (e.g., Luminet, Rimé, Bagby, & Taylor, 2004; Mantani, Okomoto, Shirao, Okada, & Yamawaki, 2005; Stone & Nielson, 2001), and use fewer emotion words to describe their emotional states (e.g., Luminet et al., 2004; Roedema & Simons, 1991) than do their nonalexithymic counterparts. Alexithymic individuals also demonstrate decreased capacity for coping with emotion (Parker, Taylor, & Bagby, 1998), supporting the idea that such individuals lack the complex conceptual system that contributes to successful regulatory strategies.

Even as the experience of emotion is disrupted, the experience of core affect (i.e., psychologically primitive states of pleasure and displeasure; see discussion on p. 514) is not. Alexithymic and non-alexithymic individuals make similar ratings when they report pleasure and displeasure in response to stimuli (Aftanas, Varlamov, Reva, & Pavlov, 2003; Berthoz et al., 2002; McDonald & Prkachin, 1990). Alexithymic persons have difficulty describing their affective states as discrete instances of emotion, but report experiencing many somatic symptoms (e.g., Joergen Grabe, Spitzer, & Juergen Freyberger, 2004), consistent with reporting a basic experience of feeling "good" or "bad." Some studies find that alexithymic individuals actually experience more intense negative affect (e.g., Friedlander, Lumley, Farchione, & Doyal, 1997), and enlist more behaviors designed to reduce the experience of negative affect (e.g., Troisi et al., 2000), than do their nonalexithymic counterparts; these findings suggest that alexithymic individuals do in fact have preserved experience of core affect.

Alexithymic individuals also have preserved (and sometimes greater) physiological arousal to evocative stimuli when compared to those without alexithymia. For example, individuals with and without alexithymia did not differ in skin conductance rate or heart rate while watching an unpleasant, highly arousing video (Stone & Nielson, 2001). Although they had intact physiological reactions to the movie, the alexithymic participants reported less intense feelings (disgust, concern, depression, surprise, fear, etc.) than the nonalexithymic participants did (Stone & Nielson, 2001). In some studies, individuals with alexithymia actually experience greater physiological arousal in reaction to emotionally evocative stimuli (Byrne & Ditto, 2005; Infrasca, 1997; Luminet et al., 2004; Martínez-Sánchez, Ortiz-Soria, & Ato-García, 2001; Wehmer, Brejnak, Lumley, & Stettner, 1995).

Taken together, these findings suggest that people with alexithymia *feel* core affect (again, defined as psychologically primitive pleasant and unpleasant states; Barrett, 2006a; Russell, 2003), perhaps as somatic symptoms, but that they fail to translate this core affective state into a mental representation of emotion (i.e., the experience of "having" an emotion) (see Barrett, 2006b; Barrett, Mesquita, et al., 2007). Existing neuroscientific evidence is consistent with the idea that alexithymic individuals suffer from a deficit in the ability to experience their affective states as emotional. Studies find that during emotional experience, individuals with alexithymia show less activation in several areas within medial prefrontal cortex (MPFC) (e.g., Berthoz et al., 2002) and within anterior cingulate cortex (ACC) (Berthoz et al., 2002; Lane et al., 1998) than individuals without alexithymia do. These areas seem to play an important function in representing core affective states as experiences of emotion (see Barrett, Mesquita, et al., 2007; Wager et al., Chapter 15, this volume).

Although the majority of studies find deficits in alexithymic persons' tendency to report discrete experiences of emotion, those that do not are particularly illuminating. Studies that use more complex cues to induce emotion, such as video clips or imagery, tend to find evidence of emotion experience deficits in alexithymic participants (e.g., Luminet et al., 2004; Mantani et al., 2005; Stone & Nielson, 2001; although see Aftanas & Varlamov, 2004), whereas studies that use less complex cues, such as pictures

(e.g., International Affective Picture System), do not (e.g., Aftanas et al., 2003; McDonald & Prkachin, 1990). Sufficiently simple cues may facilitate alexithymic individuals' ability to access a rudimentary cache of emotion knowledge, and to make "normal" reports about emotion experience.

Deficits in Emotion Expression Associated with Alexithymia

People who suffer from alexithymia not only have deficits in the experience of emotion, but also exhibit low levels of spontaneous expressive behavior. Alexithymic individuals are typically rated as less expressive during social interactions (e.g., Luminet et al., 2004) and more humorless during clinical interviews (Lumley et al., 2005) than their nonalexithymic counterparts are. In one study, individuals with alexithymia produced significantly less intense and more ambiguous spontaneous emotional facial behaviors when viewing unpleasant stimuli than those without alexithymia did, although both groups were equally capable of posing emotional expressions when prompted (McDonald & Prkachin, 1990).

This decrease in emotional expressivity occurs alongside greater somatic manifestations of emotion. Alexithymic persons report greater bodily concerns and somatic complaints (e.g., Nakao, Barsky, Kumano, & Kuboki, 2002; Taylor, Parker, Bagby, & Acklin, 1992; for a meta-analytic review, see de Gucht & Heiser, 2003). They have also been found to have more tension headaches (e.g., Yücel et al., 2002), and to demonstrate higher levels of hypertension (e.g., Todarello, Taylor, Parker, & Fanelli, 1995) and cortisol reactivity during stress (e.g., Lindholm, Lehtinen, Hyyppa, & Puukka, 1990). With an impoverished conceptual system for emotion, alexithymic individuals may be more likely to experience free-floating affect as somatic. This would explain why the link between alexithymia and somatic complaints disappears when factors such as trait anxiety, depression, or experience of negative affect are controlled for (de Gucht, Fischler, & Heiser, 2004; Lundh & Simonsson-Sarnecki, 2001).

Deficits in Emotion Perception Associated with Alexithymia

Individuals suffering from alexithymia have difficulty not only with perceiving their own affective states as emotion, but also with perceiving emotion depicted in other people's faces (e.g., Lane et al., 1995, 1996, 2000; Parker, Taylor, & Bagby, 1993; Vermeulen, Luminet, & Corneille, 2006). This effect extends to processing emotional content in other stimuli, such as sentences about emotion, pictures depicting emotional situations (Lane et al., 1996, 2000), and words that are emotional in content (Luminet, Vermeulen, Demaret, Taylor, & Bagby, 2006; Suslow & Junghanns, 2002). Neuroscientific evidence supports the idea that alexithymic individuals have difficulty conceptualizing external cues such as faces and words as emotional. Alexithymic as compared to nonalexithymic individuals exhibited decreases in brain activity in a number of brain regions—such as right inferior frontal gyrus (IFG) (Brodmann's area [BA] 44–45), orbito-frontal cortex (OFC) (BA 11), middle frontal gyrus (MFG) (BA 9), anterior cingulate cortex (ACC) (BA 24), and cerebellum—while viewing emotional facial behaviors (Kano et al., 2003). Meta-analyses of the imaging literature suggest that these regions are consistently implicated in tasks involving the perception and categorization of emotion (see Wager et al., Chapter 15, this volume).

SELF-CHARACTERIZATIONS OF COMPLEXITY

Thus far, we have examined emotional complexity as displayed in self-report behaviors (where individuals verbally represent their experiences of emotion) and in propositional conceptual knowledge of emotion (where individuals make explicit, propositional statements about emotion). In both domains, complexity is assessed using performance measures: scientists abstract information about a person's emotional complexity from patterns of responses or the ability to perform emotionally complex operations. The third and final way of conceptualizing emotional complexity is as self-characterization, where respondents are asked to describe their own degree of emotional complexity.

A number of existing scales tap an individual's beliefs about his or her own emotional complexity. Scales typically ask individuals to characterize how aware they are of their own affective states (e.g., the Mood Awareness Scale; Swinkels & Giuliano, 1995), as well as

the degree to which they attend to, can distinguish between, and are capable of repairing those states (e.g., the Trait Meta-Mood Scale; Mayer & Stevens, 1994). Perhaps the best example of a self-characterization measure of complexity is the Range and Differentiation of Emotional Experience Scale (RDEES; Kang & Shaver, 2005), which assesses the degree to which people believe that they experience a broad range of emotional states with subtle distinctions between them. Recently, self-characterization scales of emotional complexity have been developed for use in child samples (e.g., the Emotion Awareness Questionnaire; Rieffe et al., 2007; the Alexithymia Questionnaire for children; Rieffe et al., 2006). The various self-characterization measures sometimes correlate strongly with one another (e.g., Gohm & Clore, 2000), but often do not (e.g., Kang & Shaver, 2005).

More importantly, studies comparing self-characterizations and performance measures of emotional complexity reveal a disconnection between the two. For example, the RDEES is only moderately correlated with the LEAS ($r = .30$) and the Toronto Alexithymia Scale (Bagby, Parker, & Taylor, 1994) (r's ranged from .36 to .38 across three studies; Kang & Shaver, 2005). The RDEES also failed to correlate with indices of emotional granularity computed over a 1-month period (Barrett, unpublished data). It would be tempting to assume that people's beliefs about themselves do not match their behavior, were it not for the fact that the performance measures themselves often fail to correlate. Granularity is essentially unrelated to performance on the LEAS (Barrett, 2001). Taken together, these findings suggest that emotional complexity may not be a single, homogeneous construct, but rather a heterogeneous construct encompassing many different aspects of complexity.

The link between greater conceptual complexity and complexity in people's self-characterizations of emotion experience is at present speculative, but we suggest that there is good reason to assume the existence of such a link. When people complete self-characterization scales of emotional complexity, they are typically asked to rate the frequency, intensity, or differentiation with which they typically experience discrete emotions. To describe themselves on such questionnaires, respondents must remember, summarize, and integrate their past experiences into a consistent set of responses to the questionnaire items. Recalling information is a reconstructive process, however. Those people who have a greater store of emotion knowledge to draw from may find it easier to construct a response during the self-report process. In essence, people who possess more complex conceptual systems for emotion should exhibit greater fluency of emotion knowledge during the self-characterization process, resulting in a higher degree of self-characterized complexity.

OUTSTANDING ISSUES

Measurement and Conceptualization of Emotional Complexity

Emotional complexity is a broad and varied construct. In this review, we have seen that emotional complexity has been conceptualized as dialecticism or emotional granularity in the experience of emotion, as the ability to use multiple emotion adjectives in propositional responses to emotion-evoking scenarios, and as self-characterizations of complexity. If these different forms of complexity really tap a common construct, then we would expect them to be strongly correlated, such that one type of complexity could stand in for another. Yet this type of coherence does not describe the state of the literature. One possibility is that the various forms of complexity fail to cohere as a single construct because the measures that have been used to assess them are flawed.

A second, perhaps more likely possibility is that the measures are *causal indicators* of emotional complexity, so that complexity is a construct that emerges from its measured parts. In causal indicator models, a latent construct (in this case, emotional complexity) is a linear combination of its essentially uncorrelated causes (or measures) (Bollen & Lennox, 1991). The validity of the emergent construct cannot be judged on the basis of covariation among its indicators, but is instead determined by its ability to predict an externally measured criterion—such as well-being, interpersonal adaptability, emotion regulation, prosocial behavior, or perhaps another person's perception of the target person's emotional complexity in a given instant.

A third possibility is that various conceptualizations of complexity are causally related under certain (but perhaps not all) conditions.

We have suggested that richness and detail in the conceptual system for emotion may serve a common function in the various forms of emotional complexity. This perspective calls for a more detailed, idiographically sensitive mapping of the conceptual system for emotion. Studies assessing the nature of the conceptual system for emotion would determine which emotion categories people know and use, what the content of those categories are, and how that content is represented.

Variability in Emotional Complexity

A more comprehensive examination of sex and developmental differences in the various facets of emotion complexity is warranted. Clear sex differences exist in LEAS performance (Barrett et al., 2000) and in self-characterizations of complexity (see Gohm & Clore, 2000, for a review), but there are no consistent sex differences in emotional granularity. To gain an understanding of sex differences in complexity, future research must flesh out when and why sex differences appear. Mothers make more frequent references to emotion when discussing emotional memories with their daughters than they do with their sons (Adams, Keubli, Boyle, & Fivush, 1995), and they also discuss the interpersonal content and connotations of negative emotional memories more with daughters (Fivush et al., 2003). This socialization process should have implications for the richness of children's conceptual systems for emotion. There are also developmental changes in emotional complexity (indicated by age differences in LEAS-C performance, differences in self-reported complexity in children, and implied by observed increases in facility with emotion perception in early childhood). Little is known however, about how these differences might extend to the experience of emotion. Children's ability to precisely identify other people's emotional behavior mirrors the stages of conceptual development (see Widen & Russell, Chapter 21, this volume), and as we have noted previously, it is possible that those with more well-defined conceptual systems may more precisely represent their own experiences of emotion. At the other end of the lifespan, developmental differences also exist. Dialecticism increases in old age, and more recent work demonstrates age differences in the organization of positive and negative information in memory, indicating that older adults organize and represent emotional memories in a more dialectic fashion than younger adults do (Ready, Robinson, & Weinberger, 2006). There may also be age-related increases in granularity, although this hypothesis has not been explicitly tested. Carstensen et al. (2000) found that older adults used emotion words in a more differentiated manner to represent online experience, whereas younger adults used emotion words in a less differentiated manner.

Finally, person factors such as WMC may influence emotional complexity, because greater WMC facilitates the creation of a complex conceptual system for emotion and allows for more efficient use of that system. WMC influences the construction of mental representations that support new learning (Cantor & Engle, 1993) and shapes how individuals use already existing information to support the encoding of new knowledge (Daily, Lovett, & Reder, 2001; Hambrick & Engle, 2002; but for evidence of additive effects, see Rukavina & Daneman, 1996). Thus, all other factors being equal, individuals higher in WMC may have more complex or idiographic detail in their conceptual systems for emotion, merely because they are better at learning and storing category content. During online experience, WMC may affect how individuals wield conceptual knowledge because it facilitates easier, more efficient access to conceptual knowledge of emotion (see Barrett et al., 2004), allowing individuals to make more specific, situationally tuned categorizations of their affective experiences as they occur.

CONCLUSION

Regardless of how emotional complexity is conceptualized, one thing is clear: Emotional complexity is advantageous. Greater dialecticism, for example, is associated with greater resilience and lower stress in Western contexts (Davis et al., 2004; Ong & Bergeman, 2004), particularly in older individuals (Carstensen et al., 2000; Charles, 2005). Greater emotional granularity confers more frequent and flexible emotion regulation (Barrett et al., 2001; Tugade, Fredrickson, & Barrett, 2004; Tugade et al., 2007). Complexity in propositional knowledge of emotion is also loosely associated with greater psychological well-being, as indicated by the fact that complexity in propositional knowledge of emotion increases after

psychodynamic treatment in a patient population (Subic-Wrana, Bruder, Thomas, Lane, & Köehle, 2005). Children who are better at identifying and verbalizing their emotions experience less worry and depression than those children who have difficulty distinguishing or communicating their emotions (e.g., Rieffe et al., 2007). Finally, self-characterized complexity is related to greater interpersonal adaptability (e.g., Kang & Shaver, 2005). It would appear that greater emotional complexity confers greater capacity to navigate and cope with the emotional world.

ACKNOWLEDGMENTS

This work was supported by a National Science Foundation (NSF) Graduate Research Fellowship to Kristen A. Lindquist; by NSF Grants (No. BCS 9727896 and No. SES 0074688); and by a National Institute of Mental Health Independent Scientist Research Award (K02 MH001981) to Lisa Feldman Barrett.

NOTES

1. The *absence* of dialecticism has also been defined as a zero correlation (e.g., Scollon et al., 2005).
2. Emotional granularity is not defined in terms of validity, because it is currently not possible to verify objectively that a certain emotional event is present or absent (i.e., there is no empirically justifiable accuracy criterion that is independent of an observer; Barrett, 2006b). It might be possible to examine whether observers' perceptions of emotion agree with persons' ratings of their own experiences, but estimates of self–other agreement address a different question.

REFERENCES

Adams, S., Keubli, J., Boyle, P. A. & Fivush, R. (1995). Gender differences in parent–child conversations about past emotions: A longitudinal investigation. *Sex Roles, 33,* 309–324.

Aftanas, L. I., & Varlamov, A. A. (2004). Associations of alexithymia with anterior and posterior activation asymmetries during evoked emotions: EEG evidence of right hemisphere "electrocortical effort." *International Journal of Neuroscience, 114,* 1443–1462.

Aftanas, L. I., Varlamov, A. A., Reva, N. V., & Pavlov, S. V. (2003). Disruption of early event-related theta synchronization of human EEG in alexithymics viewing affective pictures. *Neuroscience Letters, 340,* 57–60.

Alonso-Arbiol, I., Shaver, P. R., Fraley, C., Oronoz, B.,

Unzurrunzaga, E., Ruben, U. (2006). Structure of the Basque emotion lexicon. *Cognition and Emotion, 20*, 836–865.

Bagby, R. M., Parker, J. D. A., & Taylor, G. J. (1994). The twenty-item Toronto Alexithymia Scale: I. Item selection and cross-validation of the factor structure. *Journal of Psychosomatic Research, 38*, 23–32.

Bagozzi, R. P., Wong, N., & Yi, Y. (1999). The role of culture and gender in the relationship between positive and negative affect. *Cognition and Emotion, 13*, 641–672.

Bajgar, J., Ciarrochi, J., Lane, R., & Deane, F. P. (2005). Development of the Levels of Emotional Awareness Scale for Children (LEAS-C). *British Journal of Developmental Psychology, 3*, 569–586.

Barrett, L. F. (1997). The relationship among momentary emotion experiences, personality descriptions and retrospective ratings of emotion. *Personality and Social Psychology Bulletin, 23*, 1100–1114.

Barrett, L. F. (1998). Discrete emotions or dimensions?: The role of valence focus and arousal focus. *Cognition and Emotion, 12*(4), 579–599.

Barrett, L. F. (2001). [Granularity and Emotional Complexity]. Unpublished raw data.

Barrett, L. F. (2004). Feelings or words?: Understanding the content in self-report ratings of experienced emotion. *Journal of Personality and Social Psychology, 87*, 266–281.

Barrett, L. F. (2006a). Emotions as natural kinds? *Perspectives on Psychological Science, 1*, 28–58.

Barrett, L. F. (2006b). Solving the emotion paradox: Categorization and the experience of emotion. *Personality and Social Psychology Review, 10*, 20–46.

Barrett, L. F., Gross, J., Christensen, T. C., & Benvenuto, M. (2001). Knowing what you're feeling and knowing what to do about it: Mapping the relation between emotion differentiation and emotion regulation. *Cognition and Emotion, 15*(6), 713–724.

Barrett, L. F., Lane, R., Sechrest, L., & Schwartz, G. (2000). Sex differences in emotional awareness. *Personality and Social Psychology Bulletin, 26*, 1027–1035.

Barrett, L. F., Lindquist, K. A., Bliss-Moreau, E., Duncan, S., Gendron, M., Mize, J., et al. (2007). Of mice and men: Natural kinds of emotions in the mammalian brain? A response to Panksepp and Izard. *Perspectives on Psychological Science, 2*, 297–312.

Barrett, L. F., Mesquita, B., Ochsner, K. N., & Gross, J. J. (2007). The experience of emotion. *Annual Review of Psychology, 58*, 373–403.

Barrett, L. F., Robin, L., Pietromonaco, P. R., & Eyssell, K. M. (1998). Are women the "more emotional sex"?: Evidence from emotional experiences in social context. *Cognition and Emotion, 12*, 555–578.

Barrett, L. F., Tugade, M. M., & Engle, R. W. (2004). Individual differences in working memory capacity and dual-process theories of the mind. *Psychological Bulletin, 130*, 553–573.

Barsalou, L. W., Santos, A., Simmons, W. K., & Wilson, C. D. (in press). Language and simulation in conceptual processing. In M. de Vega, A. M. Glenberg, & A. C. Graesser (Eds.), *Symbols, embodiment, and meaning.* Oxford: Oxford University Press.

Berenbaum, H. H., & James, T. T. (1994). Correlates and retrospectively reported antecedents of alexithymia. *Psychosomatic Medicine, 56*, 353–359.

Berthoz, S., Artiges, E., Van De Moortele, P. F., Poline, J. B., Rouquette, S., Consoli, S. M., et al. (2002). Effect of impaired recognition and expression of emotions on frontocingulate cortices: An fMRI study of men with alexithymia. *The American Journal of Psychiatry, 159*, 961–967.

Biederman, I., & Shiffrar, M. M. (1987). Sexing day-old chicks: A case study and expert systems analysis of a difficult perceptual-learning task. *Journal of Experimental Psychology: Learning, Memory and Cognition, 13*, 640–645.

Bliss-Moreau, E., Barrett, L., Connor, T., & McCarthy, K. (2007). *Are men really from Mars? Understanding sex differences in emotional awareness.* Manuscript in preparation.

Bollen, K., & Lennox, R. (1991). Conventional wisdom on measurement: A structural equation perspective. *Psychological Bulletin, 110*, 305–314.

Brown, R. W. (1957). Linguistic determinism and the part of speech. *Journal of Abnormal and Social Psychology, 55*, 1–5.

Byrne, N., & Ditto, B.. (2005). Alexithymia, cardiovascular reactivity, and symptom reporting during blood donation. *Psychosomatic Medicine, 67*, 471–475.

Cantor, J. J., & Engle, R. W. (1993). Working-memory capacity as long-term memory activation: An individual-differences approach. *Journal of Experimental Psychology: Learning, Memory, and Cognition, 19*, 1101–1014.

Carstensen, L. L., Pasupathi, M., Mayr, U., & Nesselroade, J. R. (2000). Emotional experience in everyday life across the adult life span. *Journal of Personality and Social Psychology, 79*, 644–655.

Charles, S. T. (2005). Viewing injustice: Age differences in emotional experience. *Psychology and Aging, 20*, 159–164.

Christensen, E. E., Murry, R. C., Holland, K., Reynolds, J., Landay, M. J., & Moore, J. G. (1981). The effect of search time on perception. *Radiology, 138*, 361–365.

Clore, G. L., & Ortony, A. (1991). What more is there to emotion concepts than prototypes? *Journal of Personality and Social Psychology, 60*, 48–50.

Conner, T., Barrett, L. F., Bliss-Moreau, E., Lebo, K., & Kashub, C. (2003). A practical guide to experience-sampling procedures. *Journal of Happiness Studies, 4*, 53–78.

Conway, M. (2000). On sex roles and representations of emotional experience: Masculinity, femininity, and emotional awareness. *Sex Roles, 43*, 687–698.

Daily, L. Z., Lovett, M. C., & Reder, L. M. (2001).

Modeling individual differences in working memory performance: A source activation account. *Cognitive Sciences, 25*, 315–353.

Davis, M. C., Zautra, A. J., & Smith, B. W. (2004). Chronic pain, stress, and the dynamics of affective differentiation. *Journal of Personality, 72*, 133–1159.

de Gelder, B., Vroomen, J., Pourtois, G., & Weiskrantz, L. (1999). Non-conscious recognition of affect in the absence of striate cortex. *NeuroReport, 10*, 3759–3763.

de Gucht, V., Fischler, B., & Heiser, W. (2004). Neuroticism, alexithymia, negative affect, and positive affect as determinants of medically unexplained symptoms. *Personality and Individual Differences, 36*, 1655–1667.

de Gucht, V., & Heiser, W. (2003). Alexithymia and somatisation: quantitative review of the literature. *Journal of Psychosomatic Research, 54*, 425–434.

de Rosnay, M., & Harris, P. L. (2002). Individual differences in children's understanding of emotion: The roles of attachment and language. *Attachment and Human Development, 4*, 39–54.

de Rosnay, M., Pons, F., Harris, P., & Morrell, J. (2004). A lag between understanding false belief and emotion attribution in young children: Relationships with linguistic ability and mothers' mental-state language *British Journal of Developmental Psychology, 22*, 197–218.

Diener, E., & Emmons, R. A. (1985). The independence of positive and negative affect. *Journal of Personality and Social Psychology, 47*, 1105–1117.

Edelman, G. M. (1989). *The remembered present: A biological theory of consciousness.* New York: Basic Books.

Ekman, P. (1972). Universals and cultural differences in facial expressions of emotion. 1971. In J. R. Cole (Ed.), *Nebraska Symposium on Motivation* (Vol. 19, pp. 207–283). Lincoln: University of Nebraska Press.

Fehr, B., & Russell, J. A. (1984). Concept of emotion viewed from a prototype perspective. *Journal of Experimental Psychology: General, 113*, 464–486.

Feldman, L. A. (1995). Valence focus and arousal focus: Individual differences in the structure of affective experience. *Journal of Personality and Social Psychology, 69*, 153–166.

Fivush, R., Berlin, L. J., Sales, J. M., Mennuti-Washburn, J., & Cassidy, J. (2003). Functions of parent–child reminiscing about emotionally negative events. *Memory, 11*, 179–192.

Frawley, W., & Smith, R. N. (2001). A processing theory of alexithymia. *Journal of Cognitive Systems Research, 2*, 189–206.

Friedlander, L., Lumley, M. A., Farchione, T., & Doyal, G. (1997). Testing the alexithymia hypothesis: Physiological and subjective responses during relaxation and stress. *Journal of Nervous and Mental Disorders, 185*, 233–239.

Gohm, C. L., & Clore, G. L. (2000). Individual differences in emotional experience: Mapping available scales to processes. *Personality and Social Psychology Bulletin, 26*, 679–697.

Hambrick, D. Z., & Engle, R. W. (2002). Effects of domain knowledge, working memory capacity, and age on cognitive performance: An investigation of the knowledge-is-power hypothesis. *Cognitive Psychology, 44*, 339–387.

Harris, P. L. (2006a). Use your words. *British Journal of Developmental Psychology, 24*, 253–261.

Harris, P. L. (2006b). It's probably good to talk. *Merrill–Palmer Quarterly, 52*, 158–169.

Harris, P. L., de Rosnay, M., & Pons, F. (2005). Language and children's understanding of mental states. *Current Directions in Psychological Science, 14*, 69–73.

Haviland, M. G., & Reise, S. P. (1996). A California Q-set alexithymia prototype and its relationship to ego-control and ego-resiliency. *Journal of Psychosomatic Research, 41*, 597–407.

Heine, S. J., Lehman, D. R., Markus, H. R., & Kitayama, S. (1999). Is there a universal need for positive self-regard? *Psychological Review, 106*, 766–794.

Infrasca, R. R. (1997). Alexithymia, neurovegetative arousal and neuroticism: An experimental study. *Psychotherapy and Psychosomatics, 66*, 276–280.

Izard, C. E. (1994). Innate and universal facial expressions: Evidence from developmental and cross-cultural research. *Psychological Bulletin, 115*, 288–299.

Joergen Grabe, H., Spitzer, C., & Juergen Freyberger, H. (2004). Alexithymia and personality in relation to dimensions of psychopathology. *American Journal of Psychiatry, 161*, 1299–1301.

Johnson-Laird, P. N., & Oatley, K. (1989). The language of emotions: An analysis of a semantic field. *Cognition and Emotion, 3*, 81–123.

Kang, S., & Shaver, P. R. (2005). Individual differences in emotional complexity: Their psychological implications. *Journal of Personality, 72*, 687–726.

Kano, M., Fukudo, S., Gyoba, J., Kamachi, M., Tagawa, M., Mochizuki, H., et al. (2003). Specific brain processing of facial expressions in people with alexithymia: An H2 15O-PET study. *Brain, 126*, 1474–1484.

Kitayama, S., Markus, H. R., & Kurokawa, M. (2000). Culture, emotion, and well-being: Good feelings in Japan and the United States. *Cognition & Emotion, 14*, 93–124.

Lane, R. D. (2000). Neural correlates of conscious emotional experience. In R. D. Lane & L. Nadel (Eds.), *Cognitive neuroscience of emotion* (pp. 345–370). New York: Oxford University Press.

Lane, R. D., Ahern, G. L., Schwartz, G. E., & Kaszniak, A. W. (1997). Is alexithymia the emotional equivalent of blindsight? *Biological Psychiatry, 42*, 834–844.

Lane, R. D., & Garfield, D. A. S. (2005). Becoming

aware of feelings: Integration of cognitive-developmental, neuroscientific, and psychoanalytic perspectives. *Neuro-Psychoanalysis*, 7, 5–30.

Lane, R. D., Kivley, L. S., Du Bois, M. A., Shamasundara, P., & Schwartz, G. E. (1995). Levels of emotional awareness and the degree of right hemispheric dominance in the perception of facial emotion. *Neuropsychologia*, 33, 525–538.

Lane, R. D., & Pollermann, B. Z. (2002). Complexity of emotion representations. In L. F. Barrett & P. Salovey (Eds.), *The wisdom in feeling: Psychological processes in emotional intelligence* (pp. 271–293). New York: Guilford Press.

Lane, R. D., Quinlan, D. M., Schwartz, G. E., Walker, P. A., & Zeitlin, S. B. (1990). The Levels of Emotional Awareness Scale: A cognitive-developmental measure of emotion. *Journal of Personality Assessment*, 55, 124–134.

Lane, R. D., & Schwartz, G. E. (1987). Levels of emotional awareness: A cognitive-developmental theory and its application to psychopathology. *American Journal of Psychiatry*, 144, 133–143.

Lane, R. D., Sechrest, L., & Riedel, R. (1998). Sociodemographic correlates of alexithymia. *Comparative Psychiatry*, 39, 377–385.

Lane, R. D., Sechrest, L., Riedel, R., Shapiro, D. E., & Kaszniak, A. W. (2000). Pervasive emotion recognition deficit common to alexithymia and the repressive coping style. *Psychosomatic Medicine*, 62(4), 492–501.

Lane, R. D., Sechrest, L., Reidel, R. G., Weldon, V., Kaszniak, A. W., & Schwartz, G. E. (1996). Impaired verbal and nonverbal emotion recognition in alexithymia. *Psychosomatic Medicine*, 58, 203–210.

Larsen, J. T., McGraw, A. P., & Cacioppo, J. T. (2001). Can people feel happy and sad at the same time? *Journal of Personality and Social Psychology*, 81, 684–696.

Larsen, J. T., McGraw, A. P., Mellers, B. A., & Cacioppo, J. T. (2004). The agony of victory and thrill of defeat: Mixed emotional reactions to disappointing wins and relieving losses. *Psychological Science*, 15, 325–330.

Lee, Y. (2000). What is missing in Chinese–Western dialectical reasoning? *American Psychologist*, 55, 1065–1067.

Leu, J., Mesquita, B., Ellsworth, P. C., Zhiyong, Z., Huijian, Y., Buchtel, E., et al. (2007). *Cultural models of emotion regulation in the East and West: "Dialectical" emotions vs. the pursuit of pleasantness.* Manuscript in preparation.

Lindholm, T., Lehtinen, V., Hyyppa, M. T., & Puukka, P. (1990). Alexithymic features in relation to the dexamethasone suppression test in a Finnish population sample. *American Journal of Psychiatry*, 147, 1216–1219.

Luminet, O., Rimé, B., Bagby, R. M., & Taylor, G. J. (2004). A multimodal investigation of emotional responding in alexithymia. *Cognition and Emotion*, 18, 741–766.

Luminet, O., Vermeulen, N., Demaret, C., Taylor, G. J., & Bagby, R. M. (2006). Alexithymia and levels of processing: Evidence for an overall deficit in remembering emotion words. *Journal of Research in Personality*, 40, 713–733.

Lumley, M. A., Gustavson, B. J., Partridge, R. T., & Labouvie-Vief, G. (2005). Assessing alexithymia and related emotional ability constructs using multiple methods: Interrelationships among measures. *Emotion*, 5, 329–342.

Lundh, L., & Simonsson-Sarnecki, M. M. (2001). Alexithymia, emotion, and somatic complaints. *Journal of Personality*, 69, 483–510.

Mandler, G. (1975). *Mind and emotion*. New York: Wiley

Mantani, T., Okamoto, Y., Shirao, N., Okada, G., & Yamawaki, S. (2005). Reduced activation of posterior cingulate cortex during imagery in subjects with high degrees of alexithymia: A functional magnetic resonance imaging study. *Biological Psychiatry*, 57, 982–990.

Martínez-Sánchez, F., Ortiz-Soria, B., & Ato-García, M. (2001). Subjective and autonomic stress responses in alexithymia. *Psicothema*, 13, 57–62.

Mayer, J. D., & Stevens, A. A. (1994). An emerging understanding of the reflective (meta-)experience of mood. *Journal of Research in Personality*, 28, 351–373.

McDonald, P. W., & Prkachin, K. M. (1990). The expression and perception of facial emotion in alexithymia: A pilot study. *Psychosomatic Medicine*, 52, 199–210.

Miller, P. J., & Sperry, L. L. (1988). Early talk about the past: The origins of conversational stories of personal experience. *Journal of Child Language*, 15, 293–315.

Murphy, G. L. (2002). *The big book of concepts*. Cambridge, MA: MIT Press.

Nakao, M., Barsky, A. J., Kumano, H., & Kuboki, T. (2002). Relationship between somatosensory amplification and alexithymia in a Japanese psychosomatic clinic. *Psychosomatics*, 43, 55–60.

Oishi, S. (2002). The experiencing and remembering of well-being: A cross-cultural analysis. *Personality and Social Psychology Bulletin*, 28, 1398–1406.

Ong, A. D., & Bergeman, C. S. (2004). The complexity of emotions in later life. *Journals of Gerontology: Series B: Psychological Sciences and Social Sciences*, 59, 117–122.

Ortony, A., Clore, G. L., & Foss, M. A. (1987). The psychological foundations of the affective lexicon. *Journal of Personality and Social Psychology*, 53, 751–766.

Panksepp, J. (2000). Emotions as natural kinds within the mammalian brain. In M. Lewis & J. M. Haviland-Jones (Eds.), *Handbook of emotions* (2nd ed., pp. 137–156)). New York: Guilford Press.

Parker, J. D., Taylor, G. J., & Bagby, R. M. (1993).

Alexithymia and the recognition of facial expressions of emotion. *Psychotherapy and Psychosomatics, 59*, 197–202.

Parker, J. D., Taylor, G. J., & Bagby, R. M. (1998). Alexithymia: Relationship with ego defense and coping styles. *Comprehensive Psychiatry, 39*, 91–98.

Parker, J. D., Taylor, G. J., & Bagby, R. M. (2001). The relationship between emotional intelligence and alexithymia. *Personality and Individual Differences, 30*, 107–115.

Peng, K., & Nisbett, R. E. (1999). Culture, dialectics and reasoning about contradiction. *American Psychologist, 54*, 741–754.

Pons, F., & Harris, P. L. (2005). Longitudinal change and longitudinal stability of individual differences in children's emotion understanding. *Cognition and Emotion, 19*, 1158–1174.

Pons, F., Lawson, J., Harris, P. L., & de Rosnay, M. (2003). Individual differences in children's emotion understanding: Effects of age and language. *Scandinavian Journal of Psychology, 44*, 347–353.

Rau, J. C. (1993). Perception of verbal and nonverbal affective stimuli in complex partial seizure disorder. *Dissertation Abstracts International, 54*, 506B.

Ready, R. E., Robinson, M. D., & Weinberger, M. (2006). Age differences in the organization of emotion knowledge: Effects involving valence and time frame. *Psychology and Aging, 21*, 726–736.

Reich, J. W., Zautra, A. J., & Potter, P. T. (2001). Cognitive structure and the independence of positive and negative affect. *Journal of Social and Clinical Psychology, 20*, 99–115.

Rieffe, C., Meerum Terwogt, M., Petrides, K. V., Cowan, R., Miers, A. C., & Tolland, A. (2007). Psychometric properties of the Emotion Awareness Questionnaire for children. *Personality and Individual Differences, 43*, 95–105.

Rieffe, C., Oosterveld, P., & Meerum Terwogt, M. (2006). An Alexithymia Questionnaire for children: Factorial and concurrent validation results. *Personality and Individual Differences, 40*, 123–133.

Robinson, M. D., & Clore, G. L. (2002). Belief and feeling: Evidence for an accessibility model of emotional self-report. *Psychological Bulletin, 128*, 934–960.

Roedema, T. M., & Simons, R. F. (1999). Emotion-processing deficit in alexithymia. *Psychophysiology, 36*, 379–387.

Rosch, E., Mervis, C. B., Gray, W. D., Johnson, D. M., & Boyes-Braem, P. (1976). Basic objects in natural categories. *Cognitive Psychology, 8*, 382–439.

Roseman, I. J. (1984). Cognitive determinants of emotion: A structural theory. *Review of Personality and Social Psychology, 5*, 11–36.

Ross, M. (1989). Relation of implicit theories to the construction of personal histories. *Psychological Review, 96*, 341–357.

Rukavina, I., & Daneman, M. (1996). Integration and its effect on acquiring knowledge about competing

scientific theories for text. *Journal of Educational Psychology, 88*, 272–287.

Russell, J. A. (1991). Culture and the categorization of emotions. *Psychological Bulletin, 110*, 426–450.

Russell, J. A. (2003). Core affect and the psychological construction of emotion. *Psychological Review, 110*, 145–172.

Russell, J. A., & Barrett, L. F. (1999). Core affect, prototypical emotional episodes, and other things called emotion: Dissecting the elephant. *Journal of Personality and Social Psychology, 76*, 805–819.

Schachter, S., & Singer, J. E. (1962). Cognitive, social, and physiological determinants of emotional state. *Psychological Review, 69*, 379–399.

Scollon, N. C. Diener, E., Oishi, S., & Biswas-Diener, R. (2005). An experience sampling and cross cultural investigation of the relation between pleasant and unpleasant affect. *Cognition and Emotion, 19*, 27–52.

Shaver, P. R., Murdaya, U., & Fraley, C. (2001). Structure of the Indonesian emotion lexicon. *Asian Journal of Social Psychology, 4*, 201–224.

Shaver, P. R., Schwartz, J., Kirson, D., & O'Connor, C. (1987). Emotion knowledge: Further exploration of a prototype approach. *Journal of Personality and Social Psychology, 52*, 1061–1086.

Shimmack, U., Oishi, S., & Diener, E. (2002). Cultural influences on the relation between pleasant emotions and unpleasant emotions: Asian dialectic philosophies or individualism–collectivism? *Cognition and Emotion, 16*, 705–719.

Sifneos, P. E. (1973). The prevalence of 'alexithymic' characteristics in psychosomatic patients. *Psychtherapy and Psychosomatics, 22*, 255–262.

Solomon, G. E. A. (1990). Psychology of novice and expert wine talk. *American Journal of Psychology, 103*, 495–517.

Solomon, G. E. A. (1997). Conceptual change and wine expertise. *Journal of the Learning Sciences, 6*, 41–60.

Stone, L. A., & Nielson, K. A. (2001). Intact physiological response to arousal with impaired emotional recognition in alexithymia. *Pscyhotherapy and Psychosomatics, 70*, 92–102.

Subic-Wrana, C., Bruder, S., Thomas, W., Lane, R. D., & Köhle, K. (2005). Emotional awareness deficits in inpatients of a psychosomatic ward: a comparison of two different measures of alexithymia. *Psychosomatic Medicine, 67*, 483–489.

Suslow, T., & Junghanns, K. (2002). Impairments of emotion situation priming in alexithymia. *Personality and Individual Differences, 32*, 541–550.

Swinkels, A., & Guiliano, T. A. (1995). The measurement and conceptualization of mood awareness: Monitoring and labeling one's mood states. *Personality and Social Psychology Bulletin, 21*, 934–949.

Taylor, G. J. (2000). Recent developments in alexithymia theory and research. *Canadian Journal of Psychiatry, 45*, 134–142.

Taylor, G. J., Bagby, R. M., & Parker, J. D. (1997). *Disorders of affect regulation: Alexithymia in medical and psychiatric illness.* Cambridge, UK: Cambridge University Press.

Taylor, G., Bagby, R. M., Ryan, D. P., Parker, J. D., Doody, K. F., & Keefe, P. P. (1988). Criterion validity of the Toronto Alexithymia Scale. *Psychosomatic Medicine, 50,* 500–509.

Taylor, G. J., Parker, J. D., Bagby, R. M., & Acklin, M. W. (1992). Alexithymia and somatic complaints in psychiatric out-patients. *Journal of Psychosomatic Research, 36,* 417–424.

Todarello, O. O., Taylor, G. J., Parker, J. D., & Fanelli, M. M. (1995). Alexithymia in essential hypertensive and psychiatric outpatients: A comparative study. *Journal of Psychosomatic Research, 39,* 987–994.

Tomkins, S. S. (1962). *Affect, imagery, consciousness: Vol. 1. The positive affects.* New York: Springer.

Troisi, A., Belsanti, S., Bucci, A. R. Mosco, C., Sinti, F., & Verucci, M. (2000). Affect regulation in alexithymia: An ethological study of displacement behavior during psychiatric interviews. *Journal of Nervous and Mental Disease, 188,* 13–18.

Tsai, J. L. (2007). Ideal affect: Cultural causes and behavioral consequences. *Perspectives on Psychological Science, 2,* 242–259.

Tugade, M., Barrett, L. F., & Gross, J. (2007). *Distinctions that matter: Emotional granularity and emotion regulation profiles.* Manuscript submitted for publication.

Tugade, M. M., Fredrickson, B. L., & Barrett, L. F. (2004). Psychological resilience and emotional granularity: Examining the benefits of positive emotions on emotion regulation and health. *Journal of Personality, 72,* 1161–1190.

Vansteelandt, K., Van Mechelen, I., & Nezlek, J. B. (2005). The co-occurrence of emotions in daily life: A multilevel approach. *Journal of Research in Personality, 39,* 325–335.

Vermeulen, N., Luminet, O., & Corneille, O. (2006). Alexithymia and the automatic processing of affective information: Evidence from the affective priming paradigm. *Cognition and Emotion, 20,* 64–91.

Wehmer, F., Brejnak, C., Lumley, M., & Stettner, L. (1995). Alexithymia and physiological reactivity to emotion-provoking visual scenes. *Journal of Nervous and Mental Disease, 183,* 351–357.

Yücel, B., Kora, K., Ozyalçín, S., Alçalar, N., Ozdemir, O., & Yücel, A. (2002). Depression, automatic thoughts, alexithymia, and assertiveness in patients with tension-type headache. *Headache, 42,* 194–199.

PART VI

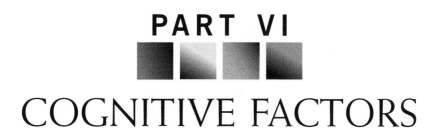

COGNITIVE FACTORS

CHAPTER 33

Emotional Intelligence

PETER SALOVEY, BRIAN T. DETWEILER-BEDELL, JERUSHA B.
DETWEILER-BEDELL, and JOHN D. MAYER

Basic research in emotion has proliferated over the past few decades, and although there is still a great deal to be learned, a consistent view of emotion has begun to emerge. Affective phenomena constitute a unique source of information for individuals about their surrounding environment and prospects, and this information informs their thoughts, actions, and subsequent feelings. The essential assumption in our work has been that individuals differ in how skilled they are at perceiving, understanding, regulating, and utilizing this emotional information, and that a person's level of "emotional intelligence" contributes substantially to his or her intellectual and emotional well-being and growth. In this chapter, we review our model of emotional intelligence and the competencies it highlights, including a discussion of measurement issues. We then describe how emotional intelligence influences important psychological phenomena.

Personality psychology most often emphasizes differences in the way people typically think, feel, and act. However, as Mischel (1990) has pointed out, people relate to the world in a manner that is much more flexible than the terms "dispositions" and "styles" might alone suggest. According to Mischel, cognitive psychology's essential lesson for personality psychologists is that individuals selectively construct their experiences of reality, and that the result of this process depends heavily on individuals' construction competencies (i.e., information-processing abilities that determine the range of potential thoughts, feelings, and behaviors the individual can enlist within and across situations). To understand the person, we must augment our study of dispositions with an appreciation for these competencies. The investigation of such competencies, aside from general intelligence, has focused largely on social problem-solving skills and other practical abilities and has been referred to as "social intelligence," among other labels (Cantor & Kihlstrom, 1985, 1987; Gardner, 1983; Sternberg, 1985, 1988; Sternberg & Smith, 1985; Thorndike, 1920; Thorndike & Stein, 1937; Wagner & Sternberg, 1985).

We believe that emotional competencies are fundamental to social intelligence (Mayer,

Caruso, & Salovey, 2004; Salovey & Mayer, 1990). This is because social problems and situations are laden with affective information. Moreover, emotional competencies apply not only to social experiences, but also to experiences within the individual. Indeed, some investigators have argued that self-knowledge and the individual's inner life are characterized most saliently by emotional experiences (e.g., Showers & Kling, 1996). Thus emotional intelligence is more focused than social intelligence, in that it pertains specifically to emotional phenomena; yet it can be applied directly to a broad range of emotional problems embedded in both interpersonal *and* intrapersonal experience (Epstein, 1998; Mayer & Salovey, 1997; Saarni, 1990, 1997; Salovey & Mayer, 1990). It is this efficient, parsimonious nature of the emotional intelligence framework that we find so compelling. Indeed, we find it puzzling that psychology has taken so long to recognize the importance of emotional competencies.

EMOTION: FROM DISINFORMATION TO INFORMATION

Emotion, historically, has taken a back seat to cognition. Philosophers and scientists (psychologists included) have relied on and glorified analytic intelligence throughout much of Western history. Aristotle (384–322 B.C.E.), for example, argued that the human intellect is "the highest thing in us, and the objects that it apprehends are the highest things that can be known" (1976, p. 328; see also Aristotle, 1947). At the same time, emotion has been regarded as an inferior, often disruptive element of human nature. The passions are fallible guides for action. Anger often leads to unjust acts of violence; fear often leads to debilitating cowardice. This sentiment toward feeling was the impetus for Malebranche's unequivocal prescription: "Impose silence on your senses, your imagination, and your passions, and you will hear the pure voice of inner truth" (quoted in James, 1890/1950, p. 10).

As a result of the historic mistrust of emotion, many psychologists have taken the position that the intellect and passions are at cross-purposes (e.g., Schaffer, Gilmer, & Schoen, 1940; Woodworth, 1940). In this view, the intellect provides accurate information, whereas emotion clouds our minds with disinformation. Young (1936) even went so far as to say that emotions have no conscious purpose and cause "a complete loss of cerebral control" (pp. 457–458). It is quite understandable, then, that early conceptions of intelligence in the field of psychology were decidedly rational. Terman stated, "An individual is intelligent in proportion as he is able to carry on abstract thinking" (1921, p. 128). Being emotional was not considered smart.

Contemporary psychology has moved away from this view that reason is superior to emotion, and toward an emphasis on the functionality of emotions. This shift originated in the philosophy of David Hume and the ethological observations of Charles Darwin. Hume (1739/1948), an early 18th-century empiricist philosopher, argued that emotional impulses motivate all action. He believed that reason does nothing more than consider facts and generate inferences about the world relevant to achieving and prioritizing the agendas set by the passions. Freud (1923/1962) held a somewhat similar position. He emphasized the primacy of the id—the seat of the self's emotionality and psychic energy—and maintained that the other aspects of the self are derivative. Freud, much like Hume, put reason in the service of emotion.

Although Hume challenged the position that reason is superior to emotion, it was not until Darwin published *The Expression of the Emotions in Man and Animals* (1872/1965) that the functional purpose of emotion was established. Through his intensive ethological observations of animal life, Darwin revealed that emotion serves at least two highly advantageous functions. First, emotion energizes adaptive behaviors such as flight (fear) and procreation (love or lust). Second, emotion gives rise to a signaling and communication system that confers a significant survival advantage on entire species as well as individual organisms (e.g., a single deer's fear response upon seeing a predator quickly informs other deer of the threat). By attributing these functions to emotion, Darwin brought attention to the adaptive, seemingly intelligent nature of emotional expression.

Today great emphasis is placed on the psychological importance of emotion, and it is generally accepted that emotions augment rather than interfere with other cognitive capacities. Emotions certainly have the signaling function identified by Darwin (e.g., Ekman, 1984). Moreover, there is wide agreement that emotions are the primary sources of motivation: They arouse, sustain, and direct human action (e.g., Izard, 1971; Frijda, 1986; Leeper, 1948; Tomkins, 1962). Finally, many emotion researchers have adopted a broad affect-as-information view, according to which internal emotional experiences provide individuals with important information about their environment and situation. This information shapes the individual's judgments, decisions, priorities, and actions (e.g., Schwarz, 1990; Schwarz & Clore, 1983, 2003).

A FRAMEWORK

When we first began developing the concept of emotional intelligence (e.g., Salovey & Mayer, 1990), our intention was to draw closer attention to the cooperative relationship between emotion and reason (Mayer, Caruso, & Salovey, 1999). Humans are not, in any practical sense, predominantly rational beings, nor are they predominantly emotional beings. They are both. Thus people's abilities to adapt and cope in life depend on the integrated functioning of their emotional and rational capacities. As Tomkins has said, "Out of the marriage of reason with affect there issues clarity with passion. Reason without affect would be impotent, affect without reason would be blind" (1962, p. 112). Success in life depends on one's ability to reason about emotional experiences and other affect-laden information, and to respond in emotionally adaptive ways to the inferences drawn by reason about one's situation, prospects, and past.

Generally, we have described emotional intelligence as the ability to perceive and express emotions, to understand and use them, and to manage emotions so as to foster personal growth (Mayer & Salovey, 1997; Mayer et al., 2001, 2004; Salovey & Grewal, 2005; Salovey & Mayer, 1990). More formally, however, we define emotional intelligence by the specific competencies it encompasses, including the ability to perceive emotion accurately; the ability to access and generate feelings when they facilitate cognition; the ability to understand affect-laden information and make use of emotional knowledge; and the ability to manage or regulate emotions in oneself and others to promote emotional and intellectual growth and well-being. Our model of emotional intelligence is presented in Figure 33.1. The model is composed of four branches, each of which rep-

Perception, Appraisal, and Expression of Emotion
- Ability to identify emotion in one's physical and psychological states.
- Ability to identify emotion in other people and objects.
- Ability to express emotions accurately, and to express needs related to those feelings.
- Ability to discriminate between accurate and inaccurate, or honest and dishonest, expressions of feelings.

Emotional Facilitation of Thinking
- Ability to redirect and prioritize one's thinking based on the feelings associated with objects, events, and other people.
- Ability to generate or emulate vivid emotions to facilitate judgments and memories concerning feelings.
- Ability to capitalize on mood swings to take advantage of multiple points of view; ability to integrate these mood-induced perspectives.
- Ability to use emotional states to facilitate problem solving and creativity.

Understanding and Analyzing Emotional Information
- Ability to understand how different emotions are related.
- Ability to perceive the causes and consequences of feelings.
- Ability to interpret complex feelings, such as emotional blends and contradictory feeling states.
- Ability to understand and predict likely transitions between emotions.

Regulation of Emotion
- Ability to be open to feelings, both those that are pleasant and those that are unpleasant.
- Ability to monitor and reflect on emotions.
- Ability to engage, prolong, or detach from an emotional state depending upon its judged informativeness or utility.
- Ability to manage emotion in oneself and others.

FIGURE 33.1. The emotional intelligence framework. Adapted from Mayer and Salovey (1997). Copyright 1997 by Peter Salovey and David J. Sluyter. Adapted by permission of Basic Books, a member of Perseus Books, L.L.C.

resents a class of skills. The subskills of each branch are organized according to their complexity, such that the more sophisticated subskills of each branch are more likely to depend on skills from the other branches of the model (Mayer & Salovey, 1997).

Perceiving Emotions

The first branch of emotional intelligence, "perceiving emotions," is the ability to detect and decipher emotions in faces, pictures, voices, and cultural artifacts. It also includes the ability to identify one's own emotions. Perceiving emotions may represent the most basic aspect of emotional intelligence, as it makes all other processing of emotional information possible.

Individuals can be more or less skilled at attending to, appraising, and expressing their own emotional states. These competencies are basic information-processing skills in which the relevant information consists of feelings and mood states. For example, some individuals are unable to express their emotions verbally, presumably because they have difficulty identifying their feelings; this condition is called "alexithymia" (Apfel & Sifneos, 1979; Lumley, Stettner, & Wehmer, 1996). These basic emotional competencies are important, because those who can quickly and accurately appraise and express their emotions are better able to respond to their environment and to others. There is some evidence, for instance, that individuals who can communicate their emotions skillfully are more empathic and less depressed than those who are unable to do so (Mayer, DiPaolo, & Salovey, 1990; Notarius & Levenson, 1979; Prkachin, Craig, Papageorgis, & Reith, 1977).

Individuals also must appraise the emotions of others. Again, there are individual differences in people's ability to perceive accurately, understand, and empathize with others' emotions (reviewed in Buck, 1984; Barrett & Salovey, 2002), and individuals who are best able to do so may be better able to respond to their social environment and build a supportive social network (Salovey, Bedell, Detweiler, & Mayer, 1999).

Using Emotions to Facilitate Thinking

The second branch of emotional intelligence, "using emotions," is the ability to harness emo-

tions to facilitate various cognitive activities, such as thinking and problem solving. Emotional states and their effects can be harnessed by individuals toward a number of ends. For example, positive moods make positive outcomes appear more likely, whereas negative moods make negative outcomes appear more likely (Johnson & Tversky, 1983; Mayer, Gaschke, Braverman, & Evans, 1992). Thus addressing a problem while in different moods may enable individuals to consider a wider range of possible actions and outcomes (Mayer & Hanson, 1995).

Likewise, a number of investigators (e.g., Isen, 1987; Magai & Havliand-Jones, 2002; Palfai & Salovey, 1993; Schwarz, 1990) have argued that emotions create different mental sets that are more or less adaptive for solving certain kinds of problems. That is, different emotions create different information-processing styles. Happy moods facilitate a mental set that is useful for creative tasks in which one must think intuitively or expansively in order to make novel associations (e.g., Isen, Daubman, & Nowicki, 1987). Sad moods generate a mental set in which problems are solved more slowly, with particular attention to detail, and via more focused and deliberate strategies. Palfai and Salovey (1993) argued that these two different information-processing styles (i.e., intuitive and expansive vs. focused and deliberate) should be effective for two different kinds of problem-solving tasks: inductive problems like analogical reasoning, and deductive logical tasks, respectively.

Emotionally intelligent individuals may also be able to harness the motivational qualities of emotion. For example, a student may focus purposefully on the negative consequences of failing to submit a term paper on time, in order to self-induce a state of fear that will spur him to get an early start on the paper. Another student may remind herself of all her successes before sitting down to write the paper. The self-induced positive mood that results bolsters her confidence in writing the paper, and she may be more likely to persevere when faced with a particularly challenging section of it.

Understanding Emotional Information

A third branch of emotional intelligence concerns essential knowledge about the emotional system. "Understanding emotions" is the ability to comprehend emotion language and to appreciate complicated relationships between emotions. The most fundamental competencies at this level are the abilities to label emotions with words and to recognize the relationships among exemplars of the affective lexicon. The emotionally intelligent individual is able to recognize that the terms used to describe emotions are arranged into families, and that groups of emotion terms form fuzzy sets (see Ortony, Clore, & Collins, 1988). For instance, individuals learn that words such as "rage," "irritation," and "annoyance" can be grouped together as terms associated with anger. Perhaps more importantly, the relations among these terms are deduced—that annoyance and irritation can lead to rage if the provocative stimulus is not eliminated; or that envy is often experienced in contexts that evoke jealousy, but jealousy is less likely to be part of envy-provoking situations (Salovey & Rodin, 1986, 1989).

To understand the emotions, individuals must learn what emotions convey about relationships. Lazarus (1991), for example, describes how core relational themes—the central harm or benefit in adaptational encounters that underlies each emotion—are associated with different kinds of feelings. Anger results from a demeaning offense against the self, guilt from transgressing a moral imperative, and hope from facing the worst but yearning for better (see Table 3.4 in Lazarus, 1991).

Increased complexity in this domain of emotional intelligence is represented by knowledge that emotions can combine in interesting and subtle ways. At a high school reunion, nostalgic conversation can give rise to wistfulness, a blend of both joy and sorrow. Startled surprise at the wonders of the universe combined with fear about one's insignificant place in it may give rise to awe.

Finally, understanding and analyzing emotions include the ability to recognize transitions among emotions. For example, Tangney and her colleagues have written extensively about how shame but not guilt can turn quickly to rage. Individuals can literally be shamed into anger (Tangney, Wagner, Fletcher, & Gramzow, 1992; Tangney & Salovey, 1999).

Managing Emotion

Emotional knowledge also contributes to the fourth component of emotional intelligence,

"emotion regulation." However, individuals must develop further competencies in order to put their knowledge into action. They must first be open to the experience of mood and emotion, and then practice and become adept at engaging in behaviors that bring about desired feelings in themselves and others. These emotion regulation skills enable individuals to engage in mood maintenance and mood repair strategies, such as avoiding unpleasant activities or seeking out activities that they typically find rewarding. Individuals who are unable to manage their emotions are more likely to experience negative affect and remain in poor spirits (Erber, 1996).

Through the self-reflective experience of emotion, individuals acquire knowledge of the correlates and causes of their emotional experiences. Knowledge of emotion thus enables individuals to form theories of how and why emotions are elicited by different situations. This ability to understand and analyze emotional experiences translates into the ability to understand oneself and one's relation to the environment better, which may foster effective emotional regulation and greater well-being. In the psychotherapy literature, this has been termed "emotional literacy" (Steiner & Perry, 1997; see also Maurer & Brackett, 2004, for an application to education).

Although our work has focused primarily on reflective metamood abilities (i.e., thoughts about moods; see Mayer & Gaschke, 1988), it is worth noting that emotional intelligence may manifest itself in a second way. Individuals often react emotionally toward their direct experiences of emotion, and these metaemotional experiences can either facilitate or impede functioning (Gottman, 1997). For example, a person can feel ashamed for having felt or expressed anger toward a loved one. The metaemotion in this case is shame, which takes as its object the individual's direct experience of anger, and it may motivate the individual to inhibit anger or at least suppress angry behavior in the future. This type of learned emotional restraint can be highly advantageous between parents and children, between lovers, and in most other social relationships. To date, there have been very few investigations of metaemotion (although see Gottman, 1997), in part because studying emotional responses to direct emotional experiences is a complex affair. However, metaemotion is a fascinating instance of how humans take themselves and their experiences as objects and respond to these objects in a higher-order manner.

The ability to help others enhance or repair their moods is also an important skill. Individuals often rely on their social networks to provide not just a practical but an emotional buffer against negative life events (for a review, see Stroebe & Stroebe, 1996). Moreover, individuals appear to derive a sense of efficacy and social worth from helping others feel better and from contributing to the joy of their loved ones. The ability to manage others' emotional experiences also plays a significant role in impression management and persuasion. Although this skill is sometimes employed unscrupulously by sociopaths, cult leaders, and some advertisers, impression management and persuasion are often employed prosocially as well. Thus individuals who are effective at regulating the emotions of others are better able to act prosocially and to build and maintain solid social networks.

One might wonder what skills, beyond emotional knowledge, undergird competence at emotion regulation. We cannot answer this question definitively, because very little research has explored the distinction between emotional knowledge and emotion regulation. However, this distinction can be illustrated quite easily. Consider the embarrassment many of us experience while dancing. Those of us who enjoy dancing are able to lose ourselves in the music and motion of dance. Unfortunately, this delightful state is elusive when we are anxious about being evaluated by others. The reality, however, is that few others typically care how we dance. Other dancers are either too engrossed or, ironically, too embarrassed themselves to notice us; spectators pass over those of us whose dancing is at worst a little boring, and are attracted instead to those whose dancing is marked by skill and elegance. Interestingly, those of us who find dancing embarrassing are often aware that no one else is paying attention to our dancing. We even understand that our fear of being evaluated is itself our greatest impediment on the dance floor. This is metaemotional knowledge. However enlightening this knowledge is, it enables only a few of us to actually overcome our embarrassment. This is because emotional regulation is distinct from the metaemotional knowledge it presupposes. That is, regulatory skills are needed in order to put metaemotional knowledge into action.

Summary

Much remains to be learned about each of the components of emotional intelligence. As a result, our conception of emotional intelligence is still evolving. Nonetheless, our understanding of emotional intelligence has already translated into some research fundings. We next turn to measures of emotional intelligence, after which we discuss some of the findings and implications that have stemmed from the use of these measures and the theory more generally.

MEASURING EMOTIONAL INTELLIGENCE

The introduction of the concept of emotional intelligence (Salovey & Mayer, 1990) had immediate intuitive and popular appeal (e.g., Goleman, 1995a; Segal, 1997), and this idea has been used to organize much past and contemporary research. Attempts to operationalize and directly measure this construct were inevitable. Guided by the original framework of emotional intelligence, Mayer and Salovey initially examined the metaexperience, or reflective experience, of mood (e.g., Mayer & Gaschke, 1988; Salovey, Mayer, Goldman, Turvey, & Palfai, 1995). Two self-report scales to assess metamood cognitions have been employed: a trait scale (Salovey et al., 1995) and a state scale (Mayer & Stevens, 1994). The former, for example, is the Trait Meta-Mood Scale (TMMS), which taps into people's beliefs about their propensity to attend with clarity to their own mood states and to engage in mood repair. The items of this measure are straightforward—for instance, "I pay a lot of attention to how I feel" (Attention), "I can never tell how I feel" (Clarity, reverse-scored), and "I try to think good thoughts no matter how badly I feel" (Repair). The psychometric properties of the TMMS are quite good, and some empirical findings have been generated from its use (Goldman, Kraemer, & Salovey, 1996; Salovey et al., 1995; Salovey, Stroud, Woolery, & Epel, 2002). Nevertheless, this trait scale has its limitations. First, its factor structure consists of only three dimensions (i.e., Attention, Clarity, and Repair), representing only a few of the emotional competencies outlined in our framework. Moreover, the TMMS, like other self-report measures (see, e.g., Bar-On, 1997), essentially asks individuals whether or not they are emotionally intelligent; it does not require individuals to demonstrate their emotional competencies. We believe that a more valid measure of core emotional intelligence requires a test that relies on tasks and exercises rather than on self-report.

More recent task-based attempts to measure emotional intelligence have focused on comprehensive aptitude-type tests that rely on the assessment of relevant skills. The Multifactor Emotional Intelligence Scale can be administered with pencil and paper or on a computer (Mayer, Caruso, & Salovey, 1998). It is organized into four main branches, reflecting our current framework for understanding emotional intelligence: perceiving emotions, using emotions, understanding emotions, and managing emotions. Within each of these four branches, we designed a series of subtests to assess various competencies.

More recently, we have published a shorter and better-normed ability-based test of emotional intelligence, called the Mayer–Salovey–Caruso Emotional Intelligence Test (MSCEIT; Mayer, Salovey, & Caruso, 2002). The MSCEIT is a 40-minute battery that may be completed either on paper or on a computer. By testing a person's abilities on each of the four branches of emotional intelligence, it generates five scores: one for each of the four branches as well as a total score. Central to the four-branch model is the idea that emotional intelligence requires attunement to social norms. Therefore, the scoring of the MSCEIT is based on consensual norms, with higher scores indicating the amount of overlap between an individual's answers and those provided by a broad sample of thousands of respondents. In addition, the MSCEIT can be expert-scored, so that the amount of overlap is calculated between an individual's answers and those provided by a group of 21 emotion researchers. Importantly, both methods are reliable and yield similar scores, indicating that both laypeople and experts possess shared social knowledge about emotions (Mayer, Salovey, Caruso, & Sitarenios, 2003).

Creating an assessment battery that successfully tests a construct as broad as emotional intelligence is challenging, but it appears that the MSCEIT is an appropriate starting point. Scores on each of the four branches (perceiving, using, understanding, and managing emotions) correlate modestly with one another, and the subscales and overall measure are reliable

(Mayer et al., 2003). Lopes et al. (2003) found small positive correlations between scores on the MSCEIT and the traits of agreeableness and conscientiousness. The MSCEIT appears to test emotional abilities rather than personality traits, however, and does not correlate with social desirability scales.

Although the construct of emotional intelligence and its measurement have generated considerable interest, validity data are only beginning to appear. There is a converging sense among researchers, although not necessarily among those working in more applied settings, of what emotional intelligence is (a set of competencies concerning the appraisal and expression of feelings, the use of emotions to facilitate cognitive activities, knowledge about emotions, and the regulation of emotion) and what emotional intelligence is not (good character, optimism, delay of gratification, or persistence; see Mayer, Salovey, & Caruso, 2000, for a comparison of our model of emotional intelligence to those popularized by others). Yet there is considerably less consensus on how best to measure emotional intelligence. Although we have argued for the advantages of task-based and behavioral assessment (Mayer et al., 1990, 2000), various self-assessments have also appeared that may measure important aspects of individuals' perceptions of their competencies in this and related domains (e.g., Bar-On, 1996, 1997; Petrides & Furnham, 2003; Schutte et al., 1998; Tett, Fox, & Wang, 2005). There is a concern, however, that such self-report tests correlate quite highly with traditional measures of personality and well-being (Brackett & Mayer, 2003; Brackett, Rivers, Shiffman, Lerner, & Salovey, 2006). Other self-report tests that have been repackaged under the emotional intelligence rubric appear to have little to do with this construct (e.g., Simmons & Simmons, 1997).

Findings concerning the correlates of emotional intelligence as operationalized by the MSCEIT are now being reported. Emotional intelligence is negatively associated with deviant behavior in male adolescents (Brackett, Mayer, & Warner, 2004). College-age males who scored lower on the MSCEIT reported engaging in more recreational drug use and greater alcohol consumption. In addition, these participants reported having more unsatisfying relationships with their friends. Even when the effects of participants' personality and analytic intelligence were controlled, the findings involving emotional intelligence remained significant. Similarly, Lopes, Salovey, and Straus (2003) administered the MSCEIT to a sample of college students, along with questionnaires that assessed self-reported satisfaction with social relationships. Participants who scored higher on the MSCEIT were more likely to report having positive relationships with others, including greater perceived support from their parents and fewer negative interactions with their close friends.

A limitation of the two studies described above is that they used the MSCEIT to predict the self-reported quality of social relationships. Lopes et al. (2004), however, examined the relationship between emotional intelligence and peer reports of one's attributes. American college students took the MSCEIT and were asked to have two of their close friends rate their personal qualities. The students who scored higher on the MSCEIT received more positive ratings from their friends. The friends also reported that students high in emotional intelligence were more likely to provide them with emotional support in times of need. In another study, German students were asked to keep diaries of their daily social interactions. Those students who scored higher on the MSCEIT reported greater success in their social interactions with members of the opposite sex. For example, they were more likely to report that they had come across in a competent/attractive manner and that their opposite-sex partners perceived them as having desirable qualities, such as intelligence and friendliness.

Emotional intelligence may also help people in relationships with their partners and spouses. One study examined the emotional intelligence of 180 college-age couples (Brackett, Cox, Gaines, & Salovey, 2005). They completed the MSCEIT and then answered questions about the quality of their relationships. The couples were classified by how well matched the partners were in emotional intelligence. The couples in which both individuals scored low on the MSCEIT reported the greatest unhappiness with their relationship, as compared to the happiness ratings of the other two groups. The couples in which both partners were emotionally intelligent were very happy. Furthermore, couples in which only one partner had high emotional intelligence tended to fall in between the other groups in happiness.

Emotional intelligence also may matter at work. A sample of employees of a Fortune 500 insurance company, who worked in small teams each headed by a supervisor, completed the MSCEIT. All employees were asked to rate each other on the qualities they displayed at work, such as handling stress and conflict well and displaying leadership potential. Supervisors were also asked to rate their employees. Employees with higher scores on the MSCEIT were rated by their colleagues as easier to deal with and more responsible for creating a positive work environment. Their supervisors rated them as more interpersonally sensitive, more tolerant of stress, more sociable, and having greater potential for leadership. Moreover, higher scores on the MSCEIT were related to higher salaries and larger annual raises (Lopes, Grewal, Kadis, Gall, & Salovey, 2006).

Despite what has been learned about the measurement of emotional intelligence over the past few years, research on the validity, in particular, of most emotional intelligence tests is still in its adolescence. Thus Boring's (1923) suggestion that "intelligence is what the tests test" (p. 35) is especially misleading in this area of study. Nonetheless, we are excited that emotional intelligence as measured with the MSCEIT seems to moderate robust (and what have been thought to be relatively universal) psychological phenomena, such as biases in affective forecasting (Dunn, Brackett, Ashton-James, Schneiderman, & Salovey, 2007). As we settle on a clear conceptual understanding of emotional intelligence, we will continue to refine and expand measures of emotional intelligence to reflect this understanding, and especially to look for ways to measure emotional intelligence with information-processing tasks. With this in mind, we now turn our attention toward promising findings pertaining to emotional intelligence and what these findings suggest with respect to particularly relevant domains—coping with stressors and other aspects of self-regulation.

EMOTIONALLY INTELLIGENT COPING AND SELF-REGULATION

We believe, with others (e.g., Izard, 1971; Tomkins, 1962), that emotion is the wellspring of human motivation, the "primary provider of blueprints for cognition, decision and action" (Tomkins, 1962, p. 22). This view implies that emotional intelligence amounts to motivational or self-regulatory intelligence. To the extent that one has highly developed emotional knowledge and competencies, successful and efficient self-regulation toward desired ends should be facilitated.

Because past events cannot be changed, coping with a previous traumatic experience is a matter of understanding the event and reinterpreting it in a more meaningful way. The importance of emotional competencies is perhaps most evident in these cases, in that individuals are forced to respond to the powerful emotions elicited by memories of past events. Elsewhere, we have argued that successful coping depends on the integrated operation of many emotional competencies, and we have suggested that deficiencies in such basic emotional competencies as emotion perception and expression will interfere with the development and implementation of more complex coping skills, such as emotion regulation (Salovey, Bedell, Detweiler, & Mayer, 1999). The relevance of the emotional intelligence framework to specific methods of coping such as rumination, disclosure, and distraction is reviewed below.

"Rumination" is defined as "passively and repetitively focusing on one's symptoms of distress and the circumstances surrounding those symptoms" (Nolen-Hoeksema, McBride, & Larson, 1997, p. 855). Nolen-Hoeksema (1991; Treynor, Gonzalez, & Nolen-Hoeksema, 2003), who has investigated rumination extensively, regards it as a particular style of responding to stressful events that tends to intensify and lengthen periods of depressed mood. Following the 1989 Loma Prieta earthquake in California, for example, Nolen-Hoeksema and Morrow (1991) found that people who had a more ruminative response style before the earthquake exhibited higher levels of depression 10 days after the event. Similarly, newly bereaved men identified as ruminators prior to their loss experienced longer and more severe periods of depression after their partners' deaths (Nolen-Hoeksema et al., 1997). The deleterious effects of ruminative coping have been corroborated in a number of laboratory studies as well (e.g., Nolen-Hoeksema & Morrow, 1993).

Although ruminating about a negative experience exacerbates one's negative mood, Pennebaker has demonstrated that disclosing emotional traumas in writing, even anonymously, has numerous beneficial effects (see Pennebaker, 1997, for a review). In general, we believe that individuals who can identify how they are feeling, understand the implications of these feelings, and effectively regulate their emotional experiences will cope more successfully with negative experiences than less emotionally intelligent individuals will. At a basic level, those who are unable to perceive and appraise their own emotional states accurately may fail to recognize the origin of their troubles. If so, the coping process will stall, precluding effective emotional disclosure. In previous work from our own lab, individuals open to emotional experience (even when this was negative) reported lower levels of depression than those who claimed to fight the feeling or asserted that everything is okay (Mayer, Salovey, Gomberg-Kaufman, & Blainey, 1991).

In addition, emotionally intelligent individuals should be able to recognize and pursue the most effective means of coping. For instance, Nolen-Hoeksema and colleagues have argued that one of the most effective approaches for disengaging from a ruminative coping cycle is distraction (Morrow & Nolen-Hoeksema, 1990; Nolen-Hoeksema & Morrow, 1993). When people use pleasant activities to relieve their moods, they show better problem-solving skills and fewer negative thoughts (Lyubomirsky & Nolen-Hoeksema, 1995). One of the most advanced skills within the reflective regulation of emotion is the ability to ameliorate negative emotions and promote pleasant emotions (Mayer & Salovey, 1997). Thus we would argue that individuals who are skilled at regulating emotions should be better able to move to repair their emotional states by using pleasant activities as a distraction from negative affect.

Engaging in distraction is different, however, from avoiding negative affect altogether. Wegner's work on ironic processes (e.g., Wegner, Erber, & Zanakos, 1993) has demonstrated that attempts to avoid negative thoughts and feelings altogether are doomed to fail. The failure of sheer mental willpower occurs because the suppressed thoughts and feelings are maintained as markers of how successfully the person has avoided them. This work is consistent with the model of cognitive changes, suggesting that a negative experience will continue to challenge one's thoughts and feelings until it is resolved and is thus no longer something that needs to be avoided. A further component of reflective regulation is the ability to understand emotions without exaggerating or minimizing their importance (Mayer &

Salovey, 1997). As a result, emotionally intelligent individuals should be able to strike a healthy balance between pleasant distractions and coming to terms with their feelings. Some types of distractions may even facilitate active coping. For instance, we would expect emotionally intelligent individuals to seek out the company of others in an effort to be reminded by them that life is good. Individuals naturally turn to others in order to discuss and make sense of negative life events (Pennebaker & Harber, 1993), and the availability of high-quality social support may prevent individuals from ruminating (Nolen-Hoeksema, 1991).

Emotionally intelligent individuals should disclose their emotional experiences more often, because they are more apt to recognize that sharing is an efficient means of organizing and thus regulating one's emotions. Moreover, the linguistic features characterizing effective emotional disclosure (i.e., insight, causal thinking, and a balance of emotion) reflect one's ability to understand, analyze, and actively regulate emotion. Thus individuals with strong emotional competencies should be able to (1) recognize their emotional responses to a trauma as natural, (2) see the trauma and their emotions in the broader context of their lives, and (3) make positive attributions about the trauma and their emotions.

Emotional intelligence should also lead to more adaptive coping when goals are blocked. Obviously, failing to attain a goal is unpleasant. Even moving more slowly than expected toward a goal can be aversive (Carver & Scheier, 1990; Hsee & Abelson, 1991). However, not everyone reacts similarly when a goal is blocked. Some people are able to disengage gracefully when they realize a goal is out of reach. Others react more negatively, ruminating about their failure and its broader implications.

McIntosh (1996) has proposed a model explaining why certain individuals react strongly to goal nonattainment. The model begins with the observation that goals are structured hierarchically, which restates the notion that proximal day-to-day goals (such as going for a run) are instrumental in achieving more general, distal strivings (such as being healthy or slim). Occasionally a particular lower-order goal must be achieved in order to reach a higher-order goal, but typically there are a number of ways to accomplish goals higher up the goal hierarchy (e.g., eating properly also promotes health

and weight control). Nonetheless, some individuals tend to view particular lower-order goals as necessary even when they are not. McIntosh refers to these individuals as "linkers," because they interpret failure to attain lower-order goals as failure to attain their more distal goals. Linkers believe more strongly than others that their happiness depends on the accomplishment of goals, both big and small, proximal and distal. When a proximal goal is linked to an intermediate goal in the hierarchy, the person may become distressed if the initial goal is blocked. For instance, not running today may be taken as evidence that one will never routinely exercise, which may be disheartening. More dramatically, the proximal goal may be linked to a goal at the very top of the hierarchy. Not running today may be taken as evidence that one will never be healthy, slim, attractive, happy, or a good person. In this way, a minor failure can lead to a depressed or even hopeless state.

In support of the linking model, McIntosh has shown that linkers are more likely than nonlinkers to ruminate about a current unrealized goal (Martin, Tesser, & McIntosh, 1993), and linkers report less happiness and more negative feelings as a result of their propensity to ruminate (McIntosh, 1996). In a short-term prospective study, McIntosh, Harlow, and Martin (1995) asked college students to complete measures of linking, stress, rumination, depression, and physical symptoms at an initial session and then again after a 2-week interval. Students who tend to link the attainment of lower-order goals to the attainment of higher-order goals reported more rumination, depression, and physical symptoms overall than their nonlinking peers did. Moreover, linkers who reported experiencing stressful events at the time of the first session were the most likely to report depression and physical symptoms at the second session. In contrast, high stress at the first session failed to predict later depression and physical symptoms among nonlinkers. This parallels Nolen-Hoeksema's (e.g., Nolen-Hoeksema, 2000; Nolen-Hoeksema & Morrow, 1991, 1993) finding that ruminators report elevated levels of depression after experiencing stress, whereas individuals who do not ruminate are more resilient. Indeed, McIntosh's studies may explain in part why some people ruminate whereas others do not. People who link lower-order goals to higher-order goals appear to ruminate more when they experience stress or failure, and rumination mediates the influence of goal linking on subsequent dissatisfaction and negative affect.

Emotional intelligence may make it easier to take stock of various goals; it enables the individual to sense the personal importance of each goal and to use this information in reasoning about competing goals as well as alternate means of achieving long-term pursuits. This analysis enables emotionally intelligent individuals to invest themselves wisely in specific activities. If a setback or failure occurs, these individuals experience a loss, but the loss is well defined and assessable with respect to other means of moving forward. This stabilizes self-regulation in much the same way that effective emotional disclosures facilitate coping: by clarifying the individual's situation and averting ruminative thinking and paralysis.

FINAL THOUGHTS ON EMOTIONAL INTELLIGENCE

Most constructs in personality and social psychology mature for decades before they find a popular audience. The fate of emotional intelligence, however, was quite different. Some time after our initial work on the subject was published (e.g., Mayer et al., 1990; Mayer & Salovey, 1993; Salovey & Mayer, 1990), a popular book on emotional intelligence appeared and skyrocketed up the best-seller list (Goleman, 1995a). With this book, emotional competencies went almost overnight from a set of abilities worthy of further study (our view) to a wealth of personal assets capable of determining a person's character, life achievements, and health (Goleman's view). Truly extraordinary claims on behalf of emotional intelligence became commonplace—for instance, "Having great intellectual abilities may make you a superb fiscal analyst or legal scholar, but a highly developed emotional intelligence will make you a candidate for CEO or a brilliant lawyer" (Goleman, 1995b, p. 76). In proposing the framework of emotional intelligence, it would seem that we stumbled upon a panacea for individual and society alike without even knowing it!

Despite the popularization of the construct in the 1990s, serious empirical research on emotional intelligence has begun to emerge in the present decade. The problematic issues in this area of work are not surprising, given the relative immaturity of this research domain (see, e.g., Matthews, Roberts, & Zeidner, 2004; Matthews, Zeidner, & Roberts, 2003). For one thing, the term "emotional intelligence" is used to represent various aspects of the human condition. We prefer to focus narrowly on specific abilities and competencies concerned with appraising, understanding, and regulating emotions, and using them to facilitate cognitive activities. However, others have defined emotional intelligence in terms of motivation (persistence, zeal), cognitive strategies (delay of gratification), and even character (being a good person). Emotional intelligence may contribute to persistence, delay, and character, but they are not one and the same thing. A con artist may be especially skilled at reading and regulating the emotions of other people, but may have little of what is commonly thought to be good character.

Second, this area of research will not prove to be productive unless the abilities that make up emotional intelligence can be measured reliably, and unless these abilities are related to important, real-world outcomes. We think less attention should be focused on the issue of whether a monolithic "emotional intelligence quotient" has utility, or on gathering together various measures of social competence and calling them "emotional intelligence," and more on the development of tasks that can be used to assess actual emotion-related skills. We are not confident that self-reported abilities in this domain will prove any more useful than they have in the measurement of traditional, analytic intelligence. Finally, we urge educators and business managers to maintain their present interest in emotional intelligence, but to be skeptical of "quick-fix" programs. Although emotional intelligence research may challenge us to reconsider our notions of what it means to be smart (and what it means to be in touch with feelings), it will not, at the end of the day, be the key to reducing international conflict, fighting the war on drugs, or terminating the global plague of AIDS. Grandiose claims to the contrary serve only as palliatives to the public and as suppressors of scientific inquiry.

ACKNOWLEDGMENTS

Preparation of this chapter was facilitated by grants from the National Cancer Institute (No. R01-CA68427) and the National Institute of Mental Health (No. P01-MH/DA56826).

REFERENCES

Apfel, R. J., & Sifneos, P. E. (1979). Alexithymia: Concept and measurement. *Psychotherapy and Psychosomatics, 3,* 180–190.

Aristotle. (1947). On the soul (J. A. Smith, Trans.). In R. McKeon (Ed.), *Introduction to Aristotle* (pp. 145–235). New York: Random House.

Aristotle. (1976). *Ethics* (J. A. K. Thomson, Trans.). London: Penguin Books.

Bar-On, R. (1996, August). *The era of the EQ: Defining and assessing emotional intelligence.* Paper presented at the 104th Annual Convention of the American Psychological Association, Toronto.

Bar-On, R. (1997). *EQ-I: Bar-On Emotional Quotient Inventory.* Toronto: Multi-Health Systems.

Barrett, L. F., & Salovey, P. (Eds.). (2002). *The wisdom in feeling: Psychological processes in emotional intelligence.* New York: Guilford Press.

Boring, E. G. (1923, June 6). Intelligence as the tests test it. *New Republic,* pp. 35–37.

Brackett, M. A., Cox, A., Gaines, S. O., & Salovey, P. (2005). *Emotional intelligence and relationship quality among heterosexual couples.* Manuscript submitted for publication.

Brackett, M. A., & Mayer, J. D. (2003). Convergent, discriminant, and incremental validity of competing measures of emotional intelligence. *Personality and Social Psychology Bulletin, 29,* 1147–1158.

Brackett, M. A., Mayer, J. D., & Warner, R. M. (2004). Emotional intelligence and the prediction of behavior. *Personality and Individual Differences, 36,* 1387–1402.

Brackett, M. A., Rivers, S. E., Shiffman, S., Lerner, N., & Salovey, P. (2006). Relating emotional abilities to social functioning: A comparison of self-report and performance measures of emotional intelligence. *Journal of Personality and Social Psychology, 91,* 780–795.

Buck, R. (1984). *The communication of emotion.* New York: Guilford Press.

Cantor, N., & Kihlstrom, J. F. (1985). Social intelligence: The cognitive basis of personality. *Review of Personality and Social Psychology, 6,* 15–33.

Cantor, N., & Kihlstrom, J. F. (1987). *Personality and social intelligence.* Englewood Cliffs, NJ: Prentice Hall.

Carver, C. S., & Scheier, M. F. (1990). Origins and functions of positive and negative affect: A control-process view. *Psychological Review, 97,* 19–35.

Darwin, C. (1965). *The expression of the emotions in man and animals.* Chicago: University of Chicago Press. (Original work published 1872)

Dunn, E. W., Brackett, M. A., Ashton-James, C., Schneiderman, E., & Salovey, P. (2007). On emotionally intelligent time travel: Individual differences in affective forecasting ability. *Personality and Social Psychology Bulletin, 33,* 85–93.

Ekman, P. (1984). Expression and the nature of emotion. In K. Scherer & P. Ekman (Eds.), *Approaches to emotion* (pp. 319–344). Hillsdale, NJ: Erlbaum.

Epstein, S. (1998). *Constructive thinking: The key to emotional intelligence.* New York: Praeger.

Erber, R. (1996). The self-regulation of moods. In L. L. Martin & A. Tesser (Eds.), *Striving and feeling: Interactions among goals, affect, and self-regulation* (pp. 251–275). Mahwah, NJ: Erlbaum.

Freud, S. (1962). *The ego and the id* (J. Strachey, Ed., & J. Riviere, Trans.). New York: Norton. (Original work published 1923)

Frijda, N. (1986). *The emotions.* Cambridge, UK: Cambridge University Press.

Gardner, H. (1983). *Frames of mind: The theory of multiple intelligences.* New York: Basic Books.

Goldman, S. L., Kraemer, D. T., & Salovey, P. (1996). Beliefs about mood moderate the relationship of stress to illness and symptom reporting. *Journal of Psychosomatic Research, 41,* 115–128.

Goleman, D. (1995a). *Emotional intelligence.* New York: Bantam.

Goleman, D. (1995b). EQ: What's your emotional intelligence quotient? *The Utne Reader, 72,* 74–76.

Gottman, J. M. (1997). *Meta-emotion: How families communicate emotionally.* Mahwah, NJ: Erlbaum.

Hsee, C. K., & Abelson, R. P. (1991). Velocity relation: Satisfaction as a function of the first derivative of outcome over time. *Journal of Personality and Social Psychology, 41,* 1–15.

Hume, D. (1948). A treatise of human nature. In H. D. Aiken (Ed.), *Hume: Moral and political philosophy* (pp. 1–169). New York: Hafner Press. (Original work published 1739)

Isen, A. M. (1987). Positive affect, cognitive processes, and social behavior. In L. Berkowitz (Ed.), *Advances in experimental social psychology* (Vol. 20, pp. 203–253). New York: Academic Press.

Isen, A. M., Daubman, K. A., & Nowicki, G. P. (1987). Positive affect facilitates creative problem solving. *Journal of Personality and Social Psychology, 52,* 1122–1131.

Izard, C. E. (1971). *The face of emotion.* New York: Appleton-Century-Crofts.

James, W. (1950). *The principles of psychology* (Vol. 2). New York: Dover. (Original work published 1890)

Johnson, E. J., & Tversky, A. (1983). Affect, generalization, and the perception of risk. *Journal of Personality and Social Psychology, 15,* 294–301.

Lazarus, R. S. (1991). *Emotion and adaptation.* New York: Oxford University Press.

Leeper, R. W. (1948). A motivational theory of emotions to replace "emotions as disorganized response." *Psychological Review, 55,* 5–21.

Lopes, P. N., Brackett, M. A., Nezlek, J. B., Schütz, A., Sellin, I., & Salovey, P. (2004). Emotional intelligence and social interaction. *Personality and Social Psychology Bulletin, 30,* 1018–1034.

Lopes, P. N., Grewal, D., Kadis, J., Gall, M., & Salovey, P. (2006). Evidence that emotional intelligence is related to job performance and affect and attitudes at work. *Psicothema, 18*, 132–138.

Lopes, P. N., Salovey, P., & Straus, R. (2003). Emotional intelligence, personality, and the perceived quality of social relationships. *Personality and Individual Differences, 35*, 641–658.

Lumley, M. A., Stettner, L., & Wehmer, F. (1996). How are alexithymia and physical illness linked?: A review and critique of pathways. *Journal of Psychosomatic Research, 41*, 505–518.

Lyubomirsky, S., & Nolen-Hoeksema, S. (1995). Effects of self-focused rumination on negative thinking and interpersonal problem solving. *Journal of Personality and Social Psychology, 69*, 176–190.

Magai, C., & Haviland-Jones, J. (2002). *The hidden genius of emotion.* New York: Cambridge University Press.

Martin, L. L., Tesser, A., & McIntosh, W. D. (1993). Wanting but not having: The effects of unattained goals on thoughts and feelings. In D. M. Wegner & J. W. Pennebaker (Eds.), *Handbook of mental control* (pp. 552–572). Englewood Cliffs, NJ: Prentice Hall.

Matthews, G., Roberts, R. D., & Zeidner, M. (2004). Seven myths about emotional intelligence. *Psychological Inquiry, 15*, 179–196.

Matthews, G., Zeidner, M., & Roberts, R. D. (2003). *Emotional intelligence: Science and myth.* Cambridge, MA: MIT Press.

Maurer, M., & Brackett, M. A. (2004). *Emotional literacy in the middle school.* Port Chester, NY: Dude.

Mayer, J. D., Caruso, D., & Salovey, P. (1998). *The Multifactor Emotional Intelligence Scale: MEIS.* (Unpublished manual available from John D. Mayer, Department of Psychology, University of New Hampshire, Conant Hall, Durham, NH 03824).

Mayer, J. D., Caruso, D., & Salovey, P. (1999). Emotional intelligence meets traditional standards for an intelligence. *Intelligence, 27*, 267–298.

Mayer, J. D., DiPaolo, M., & Salovey, P. (1990). Perceiving the affective content in ambiguous visual stimuli: A component of emotional intelligence. *Journal of Personality Assessment, 54*, 772–781.

Mayer, J. D., & Gaschke, Y. N. (1988). The experience and meta-experience of mood. *Journal of Personality and Social Psychology, 55*, 102–111.

Mayer, J. D., Gaschke, Y. N., Braverman, D. L., & Evans, T. W. (1992). Mood-congruent judgment is a general effect. *Journal of Personality and Social Psychology, 63*, 119–132.

Mayer, J. D., & Hanson, E. (1995). Mood-congruent judgment over time. *Personality and Social Psychology Bulletin, 21*, 237–244.

Mayer, J. D., & Salovey, P. (1993). The intelligence of emotional intelligence. *Intelligence, 17*, 433–442.

Mayer, J. D., & Salovey, P. (1997). What is emotional intelligence? In P. Salovey & D. J. Sluyter (Eds.), *Emotional development and emotional intelligence* (pp. 3–31). New York: Basic Books.

Mayer, J. D., Salovey, P., & Caruso, D. (2000). Models of emotional intelligence. In R. J. Sternberg (Ed.), *Handbook of human intelligence* (2nd ed., pp. 396–420). New York: Cambridge University Press.

Mayer, J. D., Salovey, P., & Caruso, D. (2002). *The Mayer–Salovey–Caruso Emotional Intelligence Test (MSCEIT).* Toronto: Multi-Health Systems.

Mayer, J. D., Salovey, P., & Caruso, D. (2004). Emotional intelligence: Theory, findings, and implications. *Psychological Inquiry, 15*, 197–215.

Mayer, J. D., Salovey, P., Caruso, D., & Sitarenios, G. (2001). Emotional intelligence as a standard intelligence. *Emotion, 1*, 232–242.

Mayer, J. D., Salovey, P., Caruso, D., & Sitarenios, G. (2003). Measuring emotional intelligence with the MSCEIT V2.0. *Emotion, 3*, 97–105.

Mayer, J. D., Salovey, P., Gomberg-Kaufman, S., & Blainey, K. (1991). A broader conception of mood experience. *Journal of Personality and Social Psychology, 60*, 100–111.

Mayer, J. D., & Stevens, A. (1994). An emerging understanding of the reflective (meta-)experience of mood. *Journal of Research in Personality, 60*, 100–111.

McIntosh, W. D. (1996). When does goal nonattainment lead to negative emotional reactions, and when doesn't it?: The role of linking and rumination. In L. L. Martin & A. Tesser (Eds.), *Striving and feeling: Interactions among goals, affect, and self-regulation* (pp. 53–77). Mahwah, NJ: Erlbaum.

McIntosh, W. D., Harlow, T. F., & Martin, L. L. (1995). Linkers and nonlinkers: Goal beliefs as a moderator of the effects of everyday hassles on rumination, depression, and physical complaints. *Journal of Applied Social Psychology, 25*, 1231–1244.

Mischel, W. (1990). Personality dispositions revisited and revised: A view after three decades. In L. A. Pervin (Ed.), *Handbook of personality: Theory and research* (pp. 111–134). New York: Guilford Press.

Morrow, J., & Nolen-Hoeksema, S. (1990). Effects of responses to depression on the remediation of depressive affect. *Journal of Personality and Social Psychology, 58*, 519–527.

Nolen-Hoeksema, S. (1991). Responses to depression and their effects on the duration of depressive episodes. *Journal of Abnormal Psychology, 100*, 569–582.

Nolen-Hoeksema, S. (2000). The role of rumination in depressive disorders and mixed anxiety/depressive symptoms. *Journal of Abnormal Psychology, 109*, 504–511.

Nolen-Hoeksema, S., McBride, A., & Larson, J. (1997). Rumination and psychological distress among bereaved partners. *Journal of Personality and Social Psychology, 72*, 855–862.

Nolen-Hoeksema, S., & Morrow, J. (1991). A prospective study of depression and posttraumatic stress symptoms after a natural disaster: The 1989 Loma Prieta earthquake. *Journal of Personality and Social Psychology, 61*, 115–121.

Nolen-Hoeksema, S., & Morrow, J. (1993). Effects of

rumination and distraction on naturally occurring depressed mood. *Cognition and Emotion, 7,* 561–570.

Notarius, C. I., & Levenson, R. W. (1979). Expressive tendencies and physiological response to stress. *Journal of Personality and Social Psychology, 37,* 1201–1204.

Ortony, A., Clore, G. L., & Collins, A. (1988). *The cognitive structure of emotions.* Cambridge, UK: Cambridge University Press.

Palfai, T. P., & Salovey, P. (1993). The influence of depressed and elated mood on deductive and inductive reasoning. *Imagination, Cognition, and Personality, 13,* 57–71.

Pennebaker, J. W. (1997). Writing about emotional experiences as a therapeutic process. *Psychological Science, 8,* 162–166.

Pennebaker, J. W., & Harber, K. D. (1993). A social stage model of collective coping: The Loma Prieta earthquake and the Persian Gulf War. *Journal of Social Issues, 49,* 125–145.

Petrides, K. V., & Furnham, A. (2003). Trait emotional intelligence: Behavioural validation in two studies of emotion recognition and reactivity to mood induction. *European Journal of Personality, 17,* 39–57.

Prkachin, K. N., Craig, K. B., Papageorgis, D., & Reith, G. (1977). Nonverbal communication deficits and response to performance feedback in depression. *Journal of Abnormal Psychology, 86,* 224–234.

Saarni, C. (1990). Emotional competence: How emotions and relationships become integrated. In R. A. Thompson (Ed.), *Nebraska Symposium on Motivation* (Vol. 36, pp. 115–182). Lincoln: University of Nebraska Press.

Saarni, C. (1997). Emotional competence and self-regulation in childhood. In P. Salovey & D. J. Sluyter (Eds.), *Emotional development and emotional intelligence: Educational implications* (pp. 35–66). New York: Basic Books.

Salovey, P., Bedell, B. T., Detweiler, J. B., & Mayer, J. D. (1999). Coping intelligently: Emotional intelligence and the coping process. In C. R. Snyder (Ed.), *Coping: The psychology of what works* (pp. 141–164). New York: Oxford University Press.

Salovey, P., & Grewal, D. (2005). The science of emotional intelligence. *Current Directions in Psychological Science, 14,* 281–285.

Salovey, P., & Mayer, J. D. (1990). Emotional intelligence. *Imagination, Cognition and Personality, 9,* 185–211.

Salovey, P., Mayer, J. D., Goldman, S. L., Turvey, C., & Palfai, T. P. (1995). Emotional attention, clarity, and repair: Exploring emotional intelligence using the Trait Meta-Mood Scale. In J. W. Pennebaker (Ed.), *Emotion, disclosure, and health* (pp. 125–154). Washington, DC: American Psychological Association.

Salovey, P., & Rodin, J. (1986). Differentiation of social-comparison jealousy and romantic jealousy.

Journal of Personality and Social Psychology, 50, 1100–1112.

Salovey, P., & Rodin, J. (1989). Envy and jealousy in close relationships. *Review of Personality and Social Psychology, 10,* 221–246.

Salovey, P., Stroud, L. R., Woolery, A., & Epel, E. S. (2002). Perceived emotional intelligence, stress reactivity, and symptom reports: Further explorations using the Trait Meta-Mood Scale. *Psychology and Health, 17,* 611–627.

Schaffer, L. F., Gilmer, B., & Schoen, M. (1940). *Psychology.* New York: Harper.

Schutte, N. S., Malouff, J. M., Hall, L. E., Haggerty, D., Cooper, J. T., Golden, C. J., et al. (1998). Development and validation of a measure of emotional intelligence. *Personality and Individual Differences, 25,* 167–177.

Schwarz, N. (1990). Feelings as information: Informational and motivational functions of affective states. In E. T. Higgins & E. M. Sorrentino (Eds.), *Handbook of motivation and cognition* (Vol. 2, pp. 527–561). New York: Guilford Press.

Schwarz, N., & Clore, G. L. (1983). Mood, misattribution, and judgments of well-being: Informative and directive functions of affective states. *Journal of Personality and Social Psychology, 45,* 513–523.

Schwarz, N., & Clore, G. L. (2003). Mood as information: Twenty years later. *Psychological Inquiry, 14,* 294–301.

Segal, J. (1997). *Raising your emotional intelligence: A practical guide.* New York: Holt.

Showers, C. J., & Kling, K. C. (1996). The organization of self-knowledge: Implications for mood regulation. In L. L. Martin & A. Tesser (Eds.), *Striving and feeling: Interactions among goals, affect, and self-regulation* (pp. 151–173). Mahwah, NJ: Erlbaum.

Simmons, S., & Simmons, J. C. (1997). *Measuring emotional intelligence.* Arlington, TX: Summit.

Steiner, C., & Perry, P. (1997). *Achieving emotional literacy: A personal program to increase your emotional intelligence.* New York: Avon.

Sternberg, R. J. (1985). *Beyond IQ: A triarchic theory of human intelligence.* Cambridge, UK: Cambridge University Press.

Sternberg, R. J. (1988). *The triarchic mind: A new theory of human intelligence.* New York: Viking.

Sternberg, R. J., & Smith, C. A. (1985). Social intelligence and decoding skills in nonverbal communication. *Social Cognition, 3,* 168–192.

Stroebe, W., & Stroebe, M. (1996). The social psychology of social support. In E. T. Higgins & A. W. Kruglanski (Eds.), *Social psychology: Handbook of basic principles* (pp. 597–621). New York: Guilford Press.

Tangney, J. P., & Salovey, P. (1999). Problematic social emotions: Shame, guilt, jealousy, and envy. In R. M. Kowalski & M. R. Leary (Eds.), *The social psychol-*

ogy of emotional and behavioral problems: Interfaces of social and clinical psychology (pp. 167–195). Washington, DC: American Psychological Association.

Tangney, J. P., Wagner, P. E., Fletcher, C., & Gramzow, R. (1992). Shamed into anger?: The relation of shame and guilt to anger and self-reported aggression. Journal of Personality and Social Psychology, 62, 669–675.

Terman, L. M. (1921). Second contribution to "Intelligence and its measurement: A symposium." Journal of Educational Psychology, 12, 127–133.

Tett, R. P., Fox, K. E., & Wang, A. (2005). Development and validation of a self-report measure of emotional intelligence as a multidimensional trait domain. Personality and Social Psychology Bulletin, 31, 859–888.

Thorndike, E. L. (1920). Intelligence and its uses. Harper's Magazine, 140, 227–235.

Thorndike, R. L., & Stein, S. (1937). An evaluation of the attempts to measure social intelligence. Psychological Bulletin, 34, 275–284.

Tomkins, S. S. (1962). Affect, imagery, and consciousness: Vol. 1. The positive affects. New York: Springer.

Treynor, W., Gonzalez, R., & Nolen-Hoeksma, S. (2003). Rumination reconsidered: A psychometric analysis. Cognitive Therapy and Research, 27, 247–259.

Wagner, R. K., & Sternberg, R. J. (1985). Practical intelligence in real-world pursuits: The role of tacit knowledge. Journal of Personality and Social Psychology, 50, 737–743.

Wegner, D. M., Erber, R., & Zanakos, S. (1993). Ironic processes in the mental control of mood and mood-related thought. Journal of Personality and Social Psychology, 65, 1093–1104.

Woodworth, R. S. (1940). Psychology (4th ed.). New York: Holt.

Young, P. T. (1936). Motivation of behavior. New York: Wiley.

CHAPTER 34

Some Ways in Which Positive Affect Influences Decision Making and Problem Solving

ALICE M. ISEN

In the years since the publication of the second edition of this *handbook*, interest in the topic of affect or emotion has grown tremendously, both among researchers and in the popular press. Not only has this growth been evident in several subareas of psychology, and in related applied domains such as consumer behavior and organizational behavior; it has also captured attention in fields such as economics and finance.

Still, it remains true that, with a few notable exceptions, understanding of emotion and the role that common, everyday mild affect (feelings, emotion) plays in people's thinking and behavior is still relatively rudimentary. Most people seem to have a sense that affect can influence their decisions and thought processes, but it is still usually assumed that affect's influence is something irregular or unusual; that only strong and infrequent feelings will have such influence; and that most often only basic negative feelings (such as anger, sadness, or fear) will have an impact on thinking processes. Furthermore, most people assume that when affect—even positive affect—plays a role in

their decision processes, such influences are disruptive and tend to make their decisions "irrational" and less appropriate than otherwise.

The research that has been carried out, however, indicates that even mild and even positive affect can markedly influence everyday thought processes, and does so regularly. Some of the earliest work in the field showed that mild positive feelings cue positive material in memory, making access to such thoughts easier, and thus making it more likely that positive material will "come to mind," while at the same time not impairing access to negative material when that is relevant (e.g., Isen, Shalker, Clark, & Karp, 1978; Teasdale & Fogarty, 1979).

This effect on memory reflects the fact that material in mind is organized and accessible in terms of its positive affective tone, and that people spontaneously use positive affect as a way to organize their thoughts (Isen, 1987). The same is not true for negative affect such as sadness, though, and I will say more about the asymmetry later in this chapter. Thus the evidence indicates that, far from being an infrequent influence on thought processes, common positive feelings are fundamentally involved in cognitive organization and cognitive processing.

However, mild positive affect has even more far-reaching effects on thinking and decision making than are implied by its effects on memory, and even beyond its effects on cognitive organization. Positive affect has also been found to promote flexibility in thinking—which in turn has been shown to facilitate problem solving (including creative problem solving) and innovation, as well as both efficiency and thoroughness in decision making, and to enable improved thinking, especially where tasks are complex (e.g., Carnevale & Isen, 1986; Derryberry, 1993; Estrada, Isen, & Young, 1997; Greene & Noice, 1988; Fredrickson, 2001; Isen, Daubman, & Nowicki, 1987; Isen, Rosenzweig, & Young, 1991; Kazen & Kuhl, 2005; Kuhl & Kazen, 1999; Roehm & Sternthal, 2001; Staw & Barsade, 1993). These effects have been found in a wide range of settings and populations, ranging from young adolescents (e.g., Greene & Noice, 1988) to practicing physicians engaging in diagnostic reasoning (Estrada et al., 1997), and in the literature on consumer behavior (e.g., Barone, Miniard, & Romeo, 2000; Roehm & Sternthal, 2001) and on behavior in organizations (e.g., Amabile, Barsade, Mueller, & Staw, 2005; Staw & Barsade, 1993). Furthermore, recent studies in the coping literature are finding that even when people must cope with adverse events, positive affect is helpful, facilitating effective coping and reducing defensiveness (e.g., Aspinwall & MacNamara, 2005; Aspinwall & Taylor, 1997; Fredrickson, 2001; Trope & Pomerantz, 1998).

Thus the influence of mild positive feelings on thinking and decision making has been found to be not only substantial but facilitative under many circumstances, leading to improved decision making and problem solving. How can these two views—people's intuitions and the findings of such studies—be reconciled?

First, it is likely that when people typically think about the effects of emotion, they tend not to pay a lot of attention to mild affect, and therefore are less likely to attribute influence to it. Second, they may be especially unlikely to pay attention to common, mild *positive* feelings. Third, the influence of positive affect is usually facilitative, but we often take positive outcomes of everyday processes more or less

for granted, not searching for causes or connections unless things go wrong or performance is impaired (e.g., Weiner, 1985). Thus we may not notice facilitative effects of positive feelings, but may pay more attention when we have reason to think that happy feelings have impaired people's judgment or problem solving.

All of these phenomena most probably contribute to people's underestimation of positive affect as a facilitating factor in decision making and problem solving. In addition, results of some studies have also indicated that there are times when positive affect actually does at least appear to impair or interfere with problem solving or thinking (e.g., Bless, Bohner, Schwarz, & Strack, 1990; Bodenhausen, Kramer, & Susser, 1994; Mackie & Worth, 1989; Melton, 1995). However, most studies reporting such effects find specific conditions under which impairment is observed, rather than general impairment; they also tend to involve situations in which participants may not be engaging in the task, or not fully engaging in it, on account of aspects of the task and the way it is presented. For example, Bodenhausen et al. (1994) reported that people in whom positive affect had been induced were more likely to use a stereotype—a process assumed to imply superficial processing—in making judgments about another person, but only when the task was not relevant to them. By contrast, in Bodenhausen et al.'s Study 4, when people knew that they would have to account for their judgment, those in positive affect did not engage in more stereotyping than controls, and even tended to stereotype less than controls.

Similarly, the majority of studies addressing positive affect's influence on thinking do not report impaired performance, but rather indicate more flexibility in information-processing strategies, and generally enhanced thinking and problem solving whenever a person has reason to engage a problem fully. This point was more recently noted by Bodenhausen, Mussweiler, Gabriel, and Moreno (2001), in their summary of the influence of positive affect on stereotyping, when they concluded, "Claims that happy people are generally unable or unwilling to engage in systematic thinking appear to be inaccurate. Rather, happy people appear to be flexible in their information-processing strategies (cf. Isen, 1993)" (Bodenhausen et al., 2001, p. 334). Thus one important question will be to try to understand what factors play a role in determining the influence of positive affect on performance in different situations, and, more importantly, what processes underlie these influences. This chapter argues that flexibility, rather than superficiality or "playfulness" (both of which have been suggested in the literature), is a better way to characterize the effect of positive affect on thinking and decision making.

In order to understand affect's influence on decisions, it is necessary to consider its impact on processes underlying decision making, such as cognitive organization (the way material is thought about and related to other material), cognitive flexibility (the ability to think about material in multiple ways or to change the way one is thinking about the material as needed), focus of attention, and motivation. This is because organization, context, and motivation, including a person's goals and the way he or she is thinking about the situation, play crucial roles in decision making (e.g., Simonson, 1989; Tversky & Kahneman, 1981). In fact, as was evident in considering the findings reported by Bodenhausen et al. (1994) some of the reasons for the discrepancy among the studies, mentioned above, may lie in these other effects of positive feelings, such as motivation and sense of freedom to behave as one thinks appropriate or to pursue one's goals. In addition, many other effects of positive affect—including some relating to expectancy motivation, intrinsic motivation, self-control, integration of context, and aspects of cognitive flexibility such as flexibility in focus of attention, are being found to have basic influences on thinking and behavior, and need to be integrated into consideration of the decision-making process. Finally, the chapter briefly mentions a theoretical account at the neurological level (the dopamine hypothesis; Ashby, Isen, & Turken, 1999) that sheds light on why and how positive affect may have its effects on thinking and decision making, as well as on cognitive flexibility, the process that is so central to its influence on thinking and behavior.

To address all of these topics in this single chapter, consideration of each must be brief. I hope that the chapter will serve as a springboard for thought, even though it cannot be exhaustive or provide a detailed review of all of the literature in this rapidly growing field. I begin, then, by considering the influence of positive affect on cognitive flexibility and organization.

POSITIVE AFFECT, COGNITIVE FLEXIBILITY, AND COGNITIVE ORGANIZATION

The Flexibility Hypothesis

There is growing evidence that positive affect leads people to be more flexible thinkers and decision makers—able to consider multiple aspects of situations and switch attention among them, and thus to respond effectively to complex or changing circumstances. This evidence comes from studies showing that positive affect promotes such processes as elaboration, responsiveness to context, creative problem solving, and flexible focus of attention, all of which result in changes in cognitive organization and the ability to see things in new or multiple ways without losing sight of the usual ways. Note that "flexible" does not mean unconstrained or loose, and is not a synonym for "creative" or "easygoing"; even though flexibility can lead to innovation, it is based on assessment of the situation, responsiveness to the context, and thus appropriateness and effectiveness in the situation. Theoretical support for the idea that this kind of flexibility results from positive affect comes from the dopamine hypothesis, noted above; this hypothesis suggests that positive affect involves release of dopamine in the brain, activating brain regions that include frontal areas responsible for high-level thinking, executive processes such as working memory, and processes such as ability to switch attention and resolve conflicting stimuli. This increased flexibility seems responsible for many of the effects of positive affect, including improved problem solving and decision making.

Elaboration

Considerable research indicates that positive affect influences cognitive organization—the way in which stimuli or ideas are thought about or related to other ideas in mind. The effects are thought to occur through processes of elaboration and ability to switch flexibly among elaborated ideas. But this process of elaboration has been found to depend on the nature of the materials.

Range of Associations, Categorization, and Similarity–Difference Judgment

Studies have shown that people in whom positive affect has been induced in any of several simple ways—such as watching 5 minutes of a nonsexual, nonaggressive comedy film; receiving (not eating) a cute, small bag of 10 wrapped pieces of hard candy, given as a token of appreciation; or responding with word associations to positive words—have a broader range of word associates, and more diverse associates, to neutral material (Isen, Johnson, Mertz, & Robinson, 1985). Similarly, people in such conditions are able to categorize material more flexibly, seeing ways in which nontypical members of categories can fit into or be viewed as members of these categories, while not losing the understanding that typical members of the categories are better exemplars of them (Isen & Daubman, 1984; Isen, Niedenthal, & Cantor, 1992; Kahn & Isen, 1993). This has been found for items in natural categories, for products in the mildly pleasant class of snack foods, and for person types in positive—but not in negative—person categories. Thus positive affect enables people to see more similarities or connections among items (and they have also been found to see more differences, if looking for differences; e.g., Murray, Sujan, Hirt, & Sujan, 1990).

The process that underlies these effects, as suggested by the word association findings, may be that people experiencing positive affect engage in greater elaboration about the material and reason flexibly about it, seeing both similarities and differences. Thus they see more aspects of the items and have more thoughts about them and associations to them. Then, as explained by Tversky and Gati (1978) for knowledge about material in general (not affective material or induced affect specifically), the context supplied by the task (looking for similarities vs. differences) determines whether this greater elaboration (greater knowledge, in the work by Tversky & Gati) results in a judgment of greater similarity or greater difference.

Context: Nature of the Materials, Importance of the Task, Potential Benefit–Cost

Valence of the Materials

One aspect of the context that is critically important in determining the impact of positive affect is the nature, including the valence, of the materials being considered. In accord with results of studies showing that positive affect cues positive material in memory and enables readier access to such material and a broader range of associates, presumably people in positive affect will see more positive aspects of relatively neutral material, and will rate such material more positively than at another time. But nothing in their positive state would be expected to prompt their rating negative stimuli (about which there are few if any positive aspects to be cued) more positively. Similarly, they would not be expected to rate mildly negative material as more negative, as if just judging everything as more extreme. Likewise, with already positive material, one would not expect positive affect to lead to higher evaluation (because the positives are already clear to people in all conditions of the experiment).

These expectations have been upheld in several studies. One study, for example, showed that positive affect influenced the categorization of relatively neutral person types into positive categories, but did not change the perceived category fit of neutral types into negative categories (Isen et al., 1992). For another example, a study of the impact of positive affect on job perceptions and satisfaction found that people in whom positive affect had been induced perceived an interesting task that they had been assigned, but not a meaningless one, as richer and more satisfying (Kraiger, Billings, & Isen, 1989). Again, this can be seen as reflecting an ability of those experiencing positive affect to see additional associations and aspects of interesting things, not a global effect on ratings. Another paper reporting results supportive of this point (Isen & Reeve, 2005) investigated the influence of positive affect on intrinsic motivation and self-control. In two experiments, induced positive affect led to increased liking for an enjoyable task, but did not affect liking for a dull, routine work task. Finally, in two studies looking at the influence of positive affect on components of expectancy motivation, results showed that people in positive affect rated the attractiveness of moderately attractive, but not unattractive or extremely attractive, outcomes as more positive (Erez & Isen, 2002). Thus both theory and empirical evidence suggest that one cannot expect positive affect to influence the rating, the categorization, or the perceived similarity (or difference) of *all* stimuli in the same way, regardless of the valence of the materials and the situation. Although an underlying process (increased elaboration) is postulated to occur, this process is expected to have different effects on different kinds of material.

Importance or Usefulness of the Task

Besides valence, other aspects of the situation play a role in the specific effect that positive affect will have. As discussed in the context of the work by Bodenhausen et al. (1994) on stereotype use, the importance or relevance of the task has been shown to play a role in the impact of positive affect on judgment and decisions. However, beyond that, this aspect of the situation has even been found to influence the effect that valence itself will have. For example, whether the context is one of danger versus enjoyment, and whether the task is or is not important or useful, both influence the way people in positive affect respond to negative material. If the task to be done, or material to be evaluated, is boring or negative, *and if there is no purpose or benefit to paying attention to it*, then positive affect may result in people's not dealing with the material or not dealing with it carefully. This tendency may be more notable among people in positive affect because—all else being equal—they may be seeking to maintain that positive state (e.g., Isen & Simmonds, 1978; Wegener, Petty, & Smith, 1995), and they may feel freer to behave as they think appropriate (Forest, Clark, Mills, & Isen, 1979). Whether such a reaction occurs, however, will depend on the importance of the task. Where the task is important, but requires people to focus on possible meaningful loss or to cope with difficult situations, the evidence shows that people in positive affect face the situation directly and deal with it. For example, in a high-risk situation, those in positive affect have been found to have more thoughts about losing than do controls, and to behave more conservatively so as to protect themselves from the loss (e.g., Isen & Geva, 1987; Isen, Nygren, & Ashby, 1988). This is also compatible with data showing that positive affect promotes effective coping in negative or stressful situations that have to be dealt with or in which there is some benefit to be obtained from attending to the task (e.g., Aspinwall & MacNamara, 2005; Aspinwall & Taylor, 1997), and that positive affect also reduces "defensiveness" (e.g., Aspinwall, 1998; Trope & Pomerantz, 1998). The way positive affect influences response to negative material, then, depends on other aspects of the context and situation.

One point illustrated in this discussion is that although people in positive affect may be found to ignore negative material if there is no reason in the situation to attend to it, positive affect does not lead to distortion of negative material, and it does not lead to ignoring of negative material if attending to that material can benefit the person in either the long term or short term. In addition, the interactions between positive affect and type of task or situation illustrate that a substantive process related to elaboration and flexible thinking characterizes the influence of positive affect and underlies the observed effects—not an artifact such as response bias, "seeing things through rose-colored glasses," over-inclusiveness in categorization, or generally poor (nonsystematic, impaired, or sloppy) processing. Another point illustrated here is that use of negative material in studies of the influence of positive affect (such as occurred in attitude change studies) can make for complexity in formulating predictions.

Creative Problem Solving

An ability that is greatly desired by most people, organizations, and society at large is creativity—and especially the capacity for innovation or creative problem solving. This is a set of skills that evidence shows is fostered by mild, everyday positive affect. As we have seen, positive affect facilitates innovative but sensible responding in measures of word association, and in categorization of plausible category members that are typically not seen as members of the category (e.g., "elevator" in the category "vehicle"). Such responding can be seen as involving cognitive flexibility or the ability to put ideas together in new ways, and perhaps it reflects not only a change in cognitive organization but also in creativity. Compatibly with that suggestion, another series of studies (e.g., Isen, Daubman, & Nowicki, 1987) indicates more specifically that positive affect does enable creative problem solving, as measured by performance on tasks such as Duncker's (1945) candle problem and items of the Remote Associates Test (RAT; Mednick, Mednick, & Mednick, 1964).

It is important to note that these tasks—the Duncker task and the RAT, which are usually considered to require innovative responding and to reflect creativity—are not simply measures of fluency or expansive thinking, but require specific answers to specific, difficult problems. In the Duncker task, the participant is given a book of matches, a box of tacks, and a candle, and is told to affix the candle to the wall (a cork board) so that the candle can be lit and will not drip wax on the table or floor. The problem can be solved if the tacks are removed from the box and the box is then tacked to the wall and used as a holder for the candle. In the RAT, which involves word problems in each item, the person is given three words and needs to think of a fourth word that fits with each of the other three (e.g., for the stem "mower, atomic, foreign," the correct answer is "power"). These tasks are very difficult: For example, on the candle task, the rate of correct solution in the control conditions is about only 11–16%; that rate rises to about 58–75% in the positive affect conditions.

Thus it is not correct to think of creative problem solving as involving only divergent, expansive thinking or unconstrained, loose thinking. Some authors have done that, and thus have dismissed the importance of success on these tasks as shedding light on the basic effect that positive affect has on thinking and decision making. Those authors maintain that positive affect, when it affects thinking and behavior, reduces thinking to superficial, careless, non-detail-oriented, schematic thought, and they argue that the findings with regard to creative problem solving can be explained as involving only playfulness and superficial thinking (e.g., Forgas, 2002; Schwarz, 2002; Schwarz & Bless, 1991). In actuality, successful solutions to these kinds of problems require not only inventiveness in coming up with possible solutions, but also convergent, focused thinking, to bring the new ideas to bear accurately on the task that needs to be accomplished. If expansive thinking is required, so also are inhibition of that process and constrained thinking, in a reciprocal process that applies the novel ideas to the current situation and utilizes them to solve the specific problem. Neither is there reason to interpret performance on either of these tasks (or others shown to be facilitated by positive affect, such as effective negotiation between parties with conflicting interests; e.g., Carnevale & Isen, 1986) as evidence of having taken a "playful" approach (e.g., Schwarz, 2002).

It should also be noted that in the work showing that positive affect facilitates creative problem solving, the effects have been found with both verbal (e.g., the RAT items) and spatial (the candle problem) tasks as assessments of creative problem solving. This, then, is not compatible with the hypothesis put forth by Gray (2001) that positive affect facilitates performance on verbal tasks but impairs performance on spatial tasks. The reasons for the discrepancy between Gray's finding and that of the work on creative problem solving are not clear at present, but perhaps they will become so in the near future.

Focus of Attention

Recently there has been increased interest in the influence of affect on focus of attention—particularly on the ability to switch among relevant stimuli, and on broad versus narrow focus, or focus on global versus local aspects of the context (e.g., Baumann & Kuhl, 2005; Derryberry, 1993; Fredrickson, 2001; Friedman & Forster, 2005; Gasper & Clore, 2002; Isen & Shmidt, 2007). This topic is relevant to decision making because it deals not only with the aspects of stimuli or situations that people notice first in a situation (which could influence their decisions), but also with whether people can consider multiple aspects of situations as they proceed in decision making.

It has been known for a long time that negative affect in the form of anxiety or arousal (sometimes referred to as "emotion"), or "high drive" (in the language of the learning theories of the 1940s and 1950s), narrows the focus of attention, impairs cue utilization, and can impair performance as a result (e.g., see Easterbrook, 1959; Isen, 2008). More recently, affect, arousal, and motivation have been distinguished and studied separately, as have specific emotions and positive and negative affect (although there continues to be some confusion among them). Some models of emotion distinguish between affect and arousal (see, e.g., Russell & Carroll, 1999; Watson & Tellegen, 1999, for discussions of these models), and some research has investigated valence and arousal separately (e.g., Mano, 1994; Sanbonmatsu & Kardes, 1988). Similarly, some work has contrasted effects of positive and negative affect and affectless arousal (induced by simple physical activity; e.g., Isen, Daubman, & Nowicki, 1987).

Thus, as positive and negative affect have been distinguished and studied independently, there have been new investigations of the influence of positive and negative affect on focus of attention, to see whether positive affect (in contrast with negative) might actually broaden focus. The idea that positive affect might result in the ability to broaden attention was suggested in an early study of affect's influence on helping behavior (see Isen, 2008, for a discussion). Participants were asked a set of questions about a person and activities that had unexpectedly occurred in the room where they were waiting for the experimenter to return. Not only did people experiencing negative affect (created by report of failure on a task) perform significantly more poorly on the surprise question about the surroundings; those in whom positive affect had been induced (by report of success on the task) did not have narrowed attention, as people in the negative affect condition did, but actually reported significantly more correct information about what had happened around them.

Results compatible with these were reported by Derryberry (1993), using a different task and materials. He found that success resulted in the ability to attend to low-value targets without missing high-value targets, whereas failure reduced the ability to attend to the low-value targets while the person was attending to the high-value targets. Thus it appears that positive affect (success) facilitates broader deployment of attention with no loss of accuracy or speed of processing, and that negative affect (failure) reduces breadth of attention in order to remain accurate on a subset of the items. Derryberry (1993, p. 84) summarized the work on this effect as best described as showing that stressful states "narrow" focus rather than "concentrating" it, because they impaired performance on the secondary information *without improving performance on the primary targets*. With regard to positive affect, he concluded that attention broadens, but that this broadening is not accompanied by dilution of resources devoted to the primary focus.

More recently, authors have begun to investigate the question of focus of attention during positive and negative affect in a different way—by looking at matters such as, literally, whether people, when shown a display, tend to use its broad features ("global focus") or its more narrowly focused features ("local focus") to understand what they are seeing (e.g., Gasper & Clore, 2002). For example, some studies use a task similar to the one developed by Navon (1977) or Kimchi and Palmer (1982), in which a stimulus is presented to participants that is a shape constructed out of smaller building blocks of another shape. In these studies, people are asked to identify the shape that is presented, and responding in terms of the superordinate shape is taken as evidence of having a global focus; responding in terms of the building-block shape is regarded as reflecting a local focus. According to those authors, most people respond based on the broader focus, indicating a hierarchical organization of perception. But the point of the research on affect and focus has been to see how positive and negative affect influence focus of attention. This research has reported that people in negative affect tend more to process the narrow dimension initially, and that people in positive affect tend to use the global dimension initially, just as controls do (Gasper & Clore, 2002). Some researchers assume that this means that people in positive affect can *only* process broadly, that they cannot focus narrowly, or that they will have difficulty (or show impaired processing and distractibility) when required to focus narrowly.

Baumann and Kuhl (2005) addressed this question specifically, by having the experimental participants solve a problem that required using both the broader dimension and the narrower dimension in order to obtain the correct solutions. Their data show that when a focus on the narrow dimension was necessary in order to solve the problem, people in positive affect opted for that focus and performed well, as reflected by both reaction time and error rates. These findings then, support the view that positive affect enables flexible deployment of attention, rather than merely broadening attention or limiting people to the one perspective. They are thus also compatible with the work reported by Derryberry (1993), showing that positive affect leads to broad or narrow focus as needed (attention to secondary targets without cost in terms of the processing of primary targets)—that is, to more flexible processing.

It must be noted that what Gasper and Clore (2002) actually found was that the positive affect condition and the control condition did not differ, and that the participants experiencing negative affect were more narrowly focused than the controls. The normal focus for people is the broader one, and, as noted above, it is thought to reflect the normal hierarchical organization of perception. Although in places Gasper and Clore (2002) are careful to refer to the difference between the positive and negative conditions in terms of negative affect's causing a narrower focus, they do imply that their results indicate that positive mood fosters a global focus—which they did not actually find. Furthermore, they assert the points, made in more detail elsewhere (e.g., Bless et al., 1996; Schwarz, 2002), that positive affect can be assumed to prompt less careful or less detailed processing (less detailed processing, they believe, would correspond to the more typical global focus), and that negative affect can be assumed to foster more intensive processing (which they argue would correspond to the more local focus). Gasper and Clore acknowledge that their findings are not supportive of such views: They did *not* find, for example, evidence that negative affect increased processing or facilitated performance of any kind; nor did they find that positive affect led to less careful processing. However, these authors invite confusion by their repeated statements of those unsupported hypotheses, as if their findings had confirmed them.

Flexibility in Focus of Attention

Consequently, it is useful to consider the findings of other authors, such as those presented above—Baumann and Kuhl (2005), Derryberry (1993), and others—to provide more context for the paper by Gasper and Clore (2002). As suggested by Derryberry and colleagues, narrow focus may not indicate more extensive or detailed processing, and the broad focus shown by the positive feedback group in his studies corresponds to more (not less) extensive, detailed, and effective processing. This interpretation fits with the flexibility hypothesis—which predicts improved ability to change focus as appropriate and switch among stimuli, as a result of positive affect, and which is also compatible with the data described earlier showing that positive affect broadens the range of material *thought about*, resulting in more diverse associations, flexible categorization, and more effective ways of solving problems.

Another program of research dealing with the question of focus, but in a different way, is that of Fredrickson, who postulates that people in positive affect "broaden and build" their skills, knowledge, and resources and then can use them in multiple ways, and who describes "upward spirals" of well-being as resulting from positive feelings (e.g., Fredrickson, 2001; Fredrickson & Branigan, 2005; Fredrickson & Joiner, 2002). That is, not only do people in positive affect look at the bigger picture, but

they develop broader thought–action repertoires and build their resources as they do so. Although Fredrickson and her colleagues do not address flexibility directly, this work would be compatible with the interpretation (and findings described above) that people in positive affect are flexible and not *limited* to the wider perspective, even though they may be able to access it and use it more readily than those in comparison affect states.

Applications of Broadened Perspective

Another study that may relate to positive affect's broadening of focus or perspective is one mentioned earlier, showing that positive affect can facilitate the process of negotiation and result in improved outcomes in an integrative bargaining situation (Carnevale & Isen, 1986). This may be an application of the broaden-and-build hypothesis, and an example of the integration of context into a situation, because it shows that the broadened perspective is *used* to put information together to solve a problem and come up with an integrative solution. It is certainly an example of the flexibility that accompanies positive affect, because people experiencing positive affect, in contrast with controls, were better able to figure out the other person's payoff matrix and integrate information to come up with good solutions for the problem (see Isen, 2000, for a discussion).

Does Broadened Focus Imply Increase in Distractibility?

A related topic is whether this broadened focus, or increased ability to switch among aspects of a stimulus display or tasks, implies decreased ability to remain focused on a focal task that one is trying to perform. Some authors (e.g., Dreisbach & Goschke, 2004) have hypothesized, and found, that positive affect reduces perseveration (i.e., increases ability to switch when the context calls for it), but that it also increases distractibility (i.e., reduces ability to stay on target on a focal task when there are potentially distracting stimuli present). In contrast, work by others indicates no such loss of ability to perform well on the main targets (e.g., Derryberry, 1993; Friedman & Forster, 2005; Isen & Shmidt, 2007; Kazen & Kuhl, 2005; Kuhl & Kazen, 1999). In addition, the flexibility hypothesis proposes that people experiencing positive affect should not become stuck on a broadened perspective, or unable to focus on the task they are trying to perform; rather, they should be able to switch attention flexibly between the broad and the narrow, as needed in the situation. This also would be more compatible with Fredrickson's (e.g., 2001) broaden-and-build hypothesis, because in that view one uses the information from the broadened perspective to build something. Some additional evidence on this point may also be available in the experiments on creative problem solving, where the innovative or broadened responses were successfully applied to specific problems that needed to be solved. Thus the topic of affect and distractibility is likely to attract continuing research interest.

Affect and False Memory?

Still another question possibly related to breadth of focus is whether positive affect may lead to an increase in false memory. A full consideration of this topic is beyond the scope of this chapter, but a few words on the subject seem appropriate (see Roediger, McDermott, & Robinson, 1998, for a review, and Isen, 2008, for a fuller discussion of this topic in the context of affect). False memory is studied in experimental psychology with a procedure in which participants are presented with multiple lists of semantically associated words (e.g., "snow," "winter," "ice") that are also related to a critical item (e.g., "cold") that is not presented. Then they are given a recognition test that presents words that were previously presented and words that were not previously presented, including the critical word (the one that is related to the theme of the presented words but was not itself presented), and asks participants to say whether each word in the test was presented before or not. The test for false memory is whether the critical word is erroneously identified as having been presented previously. Results in the cognitive psychology literature indicate that false memory measured in this way is very common, with people generally making this error as often as they correctly identify words that had been presented (see Roediger et al., 1998).

It is easy to see how this task might be thought to relate to the effects of positive affect—either from the point of view of the flexibility hypothesis (which would expect no increase in false memory from positive affect, and possibly even a decrease, if something in the situation led people to realize the potential for such errors); or from the point of view of the researchers who believe that positive affect leads to superficial reliance on schematic processing, dependence on habitual or routine concepts/structures that come to mind most easily, and failure to attend to detail. Those researchers presumably would expect increased false memory with positive affect.

In fact, there have recently been some attempts to address this question, but thus far positive affect has not been found to increase false memory (e.g., Storbeck & Clore, 2005, despite the title of their paper; Yang, Ceci, & Isen, 2006). In fact, one series of studies has found that when participants were told ahead of time about the possibility of such errors, people experiencing positive affect made *fewer* false-memory judgments than controls (Yang et al., 2006).

Summary

Thus, to summarize this section on positive affect, cognitive flexibility, and cognitive organization, positive affect appears to influence the way in which cognitive material is organized—how ideas are related to one another in the mind. In particular, positive affect has been found, in most situations, to give rise to greater elaboration in response to neutral or positive stimulus material (but not negative or tedious material unless there is a reason to engage it) and to a richer cognitive context, which in turn promotes flexibility in thinking.

This means that in a task dealing with material of neutral to positive valence, and undertaken while a person is feeling happy, one should expect unusual and innovative (though reasonable and logical) thoughts and responses. It is a mistake to assume that people experiencing positive affect will think only those arguments and thoughts about the experimental materials suggested by the experimenters. Based on the research reviewed here, we should expect people in positive affect to think about the materials in a more elaborated, extensive, flexible, responsible way—provided that the materials are not negative or boring, or provided that there is sufficient reason for these people to consider the materials carefully, even if they *are* negative or boring.

In the case of negative material, it is more difficult to predict the behavior of people in positive affect. If there is not a clear reason to focus on the negative material, we would not expect these people to elaborate the negative material more than controls do. On some tasks (e.g., categorization, word association), this will result in their responses' not differing from those of control subjects (e.g., Isen et al., 1985, 1992); on other tasks, we would expect participants in positive affect to avoid or show caution with the materials, if either is possible in the situation. This might mean that they would be slower to engage in the task, or appear to be impaired in ability to perform the task, compared with controls (e.g., Melton, 1995). However, in situations where people need to deal with the negative material, or where it would be to the persons' benefit (immediate or long-term) to do so, the research indicates that people in positive affect will show greater elaboration and enhanced coping even with negative materials or problematic situations (e.g., Aspinwall & Taylor, 1997; Isen & Geva, 1987; Trope & Pomerantz, 1998).

We have also seen that positive affect leads to more flexibility in focus of attention, as well as to broader thinking and ability to process and integrate more aspects of situations and stimuli. For now, the evidence is mixed with regard to whether there is a cost for the ability to engage this broader focus: Some authors report that positive affect does lead people to be more easily distracted, but others indicate that people in positive affect do not suffer increased distractibility (as would be reflected by impaired performance on the focal task when participants are asked to perform a second task simultaneously). Regarding the related hypothesis that positive affect may lead to more false memory, there is no evidence supporting this as yet, despite repeated attempts to find it; there is also some evidence that positive affect improves monitoring and avoidance of such errors when people are made aware of the possibility of them.

POSITIVE AFFECT AND MOTIVATION

The basic principle to be kept in mind in considering motivation is that behavior is multidetermined and results from the resolution of many motives and factors, all potentially operative at the same time. A person's choice of action depends on how he or she resolves all of the competing influences, in the context of his or her goals, strategies, concerns,

and constraints in the given situation. Positive affect has several potential influences on motivation, not just one, and the motives that will govern behavior, decisions, and choice in any given situation will depend on what the person believes is the most appropriate behavior under those circumstances. It is not appropriate to isolate one motive that is engendered by positive affect and assume that it, above all others, will necessarily determine behavior when a person is feeling happy.

For example, some authors, based on a limited reading of the affect literature, single out maintenance of positive affect as the primary (or only) motive of people in positive affect, and assume that the desire to stay happy will always govern behavior and choice when someone is feeling happy. What the research shows, however, is that this is far from true. As we have seen, people in positive affect are more likely than controls to pay attention to negative or threatening material if it is useful in either the long term or short term, or if there is another reason to attend to it (e.g., Aspinwall, 1998; Aspinwall & Taylor, 1997; Isen & Geva, 1987; Isen & Reeve, 2005; Trope & Pomerantz, 1998; see Isen, 2003, for a discussion). Thus a better way to think about the affect maintenance motive in positive affect is that it will be considered, and, *all else being equal*, people who are feeling happy will behave in such a way as to remain so.

Not only do the various motivations associated with positive affect need to be integrated in order to predict resultant behavior, but the effects of positive affect on cognitive processing also must be taken into account at the same time. For example, positive affect leads to more likely integration of context, and greater flexibility in focus and interpretation of contextual factors; these processes and interpretations may also influence what the person is motivated to do, or what strategies seem appropriate, in a situation. Flexibility seems a key to understanding how the various motives activated by positive affect will be integrated and/or resolved.

Regarding a Global Increase or a Global Decrease in Motivation

Two kinds of possible effects of feelings on global motivation have been suggested in the literature: trying harder (as would follow from the view of emotion as arousal), and, ironically, trying less hard (as would follow from the mood-as-information or "cognitive tuning" view).

Global Increase in Motivation

The suggestion that positive affect will increase motivation in general, or will lead a person to try harder, seems intuitively correct to many people. All of the work that indicates that positive affect promotes enjoyment and enrichment of potentially enjoyable, though work-related, tasks suggests that positive affect may influence task motivation (because richer tasks and task enjoyment are also more motivating; e.g., Kanfer, 1990). However, no evidence as yet suggests that positive affect simply raises effort on all tasks, as the concept of arousal has been thought to do. Rather, it has been found that positive affect leads people to try harder on some tasks or in some situations—those in which there is a reason to try or it seems that their effort will make a difference—but not on other tasks or situations in which there is no point in trying (e.g., Erez & Isen, 2002; Isen & Reeve, 2005).

General Decrease in Motivation

Another possibility that has been suggested is that positive affect will lead people to try *less* hard—an implication of the mood-as-information or cognitive tuning view that positive affect reduces motivation and leads to less effort and/or care, because it signals that all is well (e.g., Schwarz, 2002; Schwarz & Bless, 1991). This effect on motivation seems unlikely, in view of the evidence (summarized in this chapter and elsewhere) showing that people in positive affect often do voluntarily try hard and perform well, when the task is either interesting or important, with no sign that such performance has taken special effort and exhausted them, required a sense of ill ease, or spoiled their mood (Ashby et al., 1999; Bodenhausen et al., 1994, 2001; Erez & Isen, 2002; Isen, 1993). Given the lack of evidence for either type of global effect of positive affect on motivation, it seems more promising to ask about specific aspects of tasks and task motivations that seem to result from positive feelings.

Helping

One of the first effects of positive affect discovered has been an increased tendency, under normal circumstances, to be helpful, generous, socially responsible, friendly, and kind (e.g., Cunningham, 1979; Isen & Levin, 1972; see Isen, 1987, for a review and discussion). The evidence suggests that these effects are not the result of simple compliance or giving in to others' wishes or demands, but rather result from a person's flexibility in thinking and his or her resultant decision in the situation. For example, these effects include helping others and donating to charity, all else being equal—but not when the helping task would cause discomfort to a third party (e.g., Isen & Levin, 1972), not when it would threaten the helper's affective state (and the other's need is not pressing; Isen & Simmonds, 1978), and not when the cause to be helped would benefit a disliked group (Forest et al., 1979). In those situations, people in positive affect were *less* likely than controls to help. Moreover, these effects may themselves depend on such factors as the amount of harm that might come to the person in need if the potential helper did not help, and so on (see Isen, 1987, for a discussion).

The point here is that in general, positive affect promotes not selfishness and not compliance—but a tendency to be kind and fair to both self and others, social connectedness, responsibility, the ability to see situations from another person's perspective as well as one's own, and the ability to navigate among the conflicting needs and goals to reach a satisfying solution to the dilemma. Thus the evidence shows that people who are feeling happy are more motivated to be helpful and socially responsible, and they are also more flexible in their thinking with the result that they can adopt a problem-solving approach where there are conflicting needs of people with differing concerns, in a way that is appropriately responsive to the situation.

Maintenance of Positive Affect

There is evidence that a motive to maintain the positive state is one of the motives engendered by positive affect. For example, as noted in the discussion of affect's influence on helping, people in positive affect were less likely than controls to help a stranger when the helping task was portrayed as virtually certain to make the participants feel depressed, and when the other person's need was not pressing (Isen & Simmonds, 1978). The results of that study were interpreted as indicating that, at least under some circumstances, positive affect engenders a motive to avoid loss of the positive state. Such a motive has also been theorized to relate to positive affect subjects' relative risk aversion, which has been observed under certain circumstances, and which is discussed further in the section on decision making. In addition, work by Petty and colleagues is compatible with the idea that positive affect fosters an affect maintenance motive, which then also plays a role in other choices and behavior (e.g., Wegener et al., 1995).

Besides these effects, this preference to avoid loss of the positive state may cause people who are feeling happy to tend to leave more negative topics for another time, or at least to consider doing so, when that is possible. Consequently, positive affect may influence responses, performance, or latency of responding on tasks involving negative material. Thus positive affect maintenance will be a factor when all else is equal, or when the situation is such that attention to one's own affect maintenance is the most appropriate focus. However, as noted earlier, research has shown that it will not be the only, or even the primary, concern of a person who is feeling happy.

To some extent, then, this motive has been overemphasized in the literature on positive affect, with some authors assuming that maintaining positive affect will be the only or the primary motive engendered by such affect, and will govern behavior and style of cognitive processing—causing not only "defensive" blind spots, but also avoidance of careful, effortful thought (e.g., Erber & Erber, 2000; Loewenstein & Lerner, 2002; Schwarz, 2003; see Isen, 2003, for a discussion). As noted above, the evidence does not actually support such assumptions.

Thus the motive to maintain positive affect should not be expected to be absolute in its effects; it has not been found to result in blind, irrational bias, or in distortion of negative stimuli or tasks. In fact, far from leading people to ignore or distort needed negative information, positive affect has been shown to enable effective coping and reduce "defensiveness" in problematic situations that must be dealt with. Thus it appears that positive affect promotes effective thinking about even negative material, if doing so is useful or necessary, even though it leads people to sidestep unnecessary consideration of unpleasant material when that is appropriate.

Expectancy Motivation

Although I have noted that positive affect does not simply raise general motivation or effort on all tasks, through something akin to general "arousal" or activation, recent work suggests that it may influence the cognitive processes related to expectancy motivation, which is thought to underlie motivation in specific circumstances. Thus positive affect may increase motivation through cognitive processes in certain situations.

The theory of expectancy motivation proposes that work motivation is a function of the connection a person sees among his or her effort, performance, and the outcomes he or she receives, as well as the desirability of those outcomes (see Kanfer, 1990, for a fuller description). Basically, if a person sees relatedness between his or her effort and performance, *and* between his or her successful performance and the ultimate obtaining of a desired reward, *and* if the reward is seen as desirable, the person will be motivated to try; if one of those components is missing or low, the person will not be motivated to work or try.

This theory is especially relevant to the role of positive affect in motivation, because positive affect is known to have the potential to influence the perceived desirability of desirable rewards, as well as to influence the ability to see connections or relationships among components of situations. Thus positive affect may increase motivation through raising the expectation that one's effort will lead to good performance, and that good performance will result in obtaining a desirable reward. However, if all of the details proposed regarding positive affect are correct, then this effect of positive affect should be true primarily within certain ranges of valence, performance, and effort, and it should hold only where outcome is not chance-dependent. That is, for very high or very low levels of effort, positive affect should not increase one's expectation that one will perform well; and for very high or very low levels of performance, positive affect should not increase the sense that one will get the reward. Only in the moderate range of effort, and performance, should positive affect have an influence. Regarding the desirability of the reward, as noted in the context of affect's influence on evaluation of other stimuli, positive affect should increase the perceived desirability of moderately attractive outcomes, but not extremely attractive or extremely unattractive outcomes. Finally, if these effects result from a rational decision by a person in positive affect, as held in this chapter, then positive affect should not have an effect when the results are described as dependent on chance.

This is exactly what was found in two studies investigating these possibilities (Erez & Isen, 2002). Positive affect, induced in either of two ways, increased each of the components of expectancy motivation, but only in the moderate ranges, and only when the outcome was not dependent on chance. In a moderate range of expected performance (but not at extremely high or extremely low expected performance levels), people in positive affect saw more connection between how hard they tried and how well they would do; this resulted in greater motivation, more actual task persistence, and improved actual performance (see Erez & Isen, 2002, for more details). This is not just a matter of affect's influencing motivation globally in the sense of "trying harder." It reflects how effective a person expects to be (and is) if he or she tries moderately hard in a situation where effort can have influence.

These findings provide strong additional evidence that people in positive affect do not lose or lack motivation, provided that it makes sense to try in the situation. Furthermore, they are not superficial in their processing or consideration of the task, and they pay careful attention to the details and make fine distinctions among the characteristics of the situations. The findings also add support to the point raised earlier that positive affect does not function as a lens or filter—that is, does not improve the estimates of all concepts or stimuli considered while people are feeling happy.

Intrinsic Motivation and Variety Seeking

Intrinsic Motivation

In one series of studies, it was found that people in whom positive affect had been induced showed more intrinsic motivation than controls, but also responded well to extrinsic motivation when there was a work task that needed to be done (Isen & Reeve, 2005). Intrinsic motivation was measured, as is standard in that literature (e.g., Deci & Ryan, 1985), in a free-choice situation by (1) choice of a more interesting task over a dull task (which, in this case, had a very small chance of paying a small amount of money; and (2) reported enjoyment of the pleasant task while engaging in it. However, when participants were informed that there was some work that needed to be done, and again had the choice of activity during the time period, they chose to do the work that needed to be done (thus significantly reducing the amount of time they spent on the enjoyable task)—but they spent the rest of the time with the more enjoyable task, and thus still spent more time than controls on the liked task (even though they got the work done with few errors, just as the control group did). They again liked the enjoyable task more than controls (but did not differ from controls in evaluation of the tedious work task). Thus they displayed self-control in the sense in which that term is normally used: They did not like the work task as much as the puzzle, but voluntarily engaged in it to complete it well. Furthermore, there was no evidence of any kind of superficial processing or ignoring of details, and this was true even though they were deferring playing with the puzzle in favor of the work that needed to be done.

These results show that people in positive affect are more intrinsically motivated, but at the same time show that positive affect will not cause people to avoid work tasks or more boring or unpleasant or difficult tasks, if it is clear that those tasks need to be done, or if there is some potential benefit in doing them. People who feel good prefer pleasant things, and enjoy them more when they do them; however, relative to control subjects, they do not shirk, irrationally "defend against," or irresponsibly refuse to engage in, less pleasant tasks. Moreover, they do not rate the tedious work task as more pleasant, showing again that the influence of positive affect is not like a lens or filter, coloring all stimuli. It is also of interest, in view of attribution theory or other type of "signaling" theory, that when the people in positive affect worked on the tedious task (which they did voluntarily in both of these studies), they did not inflate their evaluation of that task.

Variety Seeking

Another type of motive that appears to be induced by positive affect is variety seeking among safe, enjoyable options (Kahn & Isen, 1993). Three studies reported that when people in whom positive affect had been induced were given the opportunity to make several choices in a food category such as snacks, they showed more switching among alternatives than controls did and included a broader range of items in their choice sets, as long as unpleasant or negative potential features of the items were not salient. In contrast, when a negative but not risky feature (such as the possibility that a low-salt product would taste less good than the regular) was salient, there was no difference between the groups in variety seeking. Thus there is evidence that positive affect promotes preference for variety and a wider range of options considered. This can be seen as safe stimulation seeking, but it is not risk seeking. The empirical difference in affect's influence on variety seeking and risk seeking will become clear when we discuss the results of studies on positive affect's influence on risk taking.

The observed effects of positive affect on intrinsic motivation and variety seeking relate to a developing area of decision making focused on what has been called the "demotivating" effects of "too much" variety on choosing and on satisfaction with the choice (e.g., Iyengar & Lepper, 2000). Several studies show that having a large variety can result in people's deferring the choice or feeling less satisfied with their ultimate choice. Space limitations preclude detailed consideration of this topic here, but of interest in the present context is that positive affect has been found to counter the effects of this "choice overload" (Isen & Spassova, 2008), leading to more satisfaction with both the choice process and the item selected from the very large variety.

Summary

Thus, in summary, positive affect appears to produce behavior that may be seen as resulting not only from the cognitive effects that have been discussed (such as increased flexibility, elaboration and access to positive material in memory, increased integration of concepts and ability to see connections among ideas, etc.), but also from apparent motivational changes. The work on expectancy motivation shows that people in positive affect work diligently on tasks, if there is reason to believe that doing so makes sense; indeed, they may be even more motivated than people in neutral affect, because they are more likely to see a connection between how hard they try and the outcomes they achieve. As has been found in many other experiments reviewed in this chapter, there is

no evidence in these studies that people in positive affect typically ignore or miss details. In fact, they persist longer and perform better than controls, as long as the goal is at least moderately desirable and achievable through their effort.

Similarly, the work on intrinsic motivation and self-control indicates that people in positive affect show more intrinsic motivation and enjoy pleasant tasks more than controls, but that they voluntarily readily and accurately perform work tasks that need to be done, even if doing so requires reducing time on a pleasurable task. As illustrated, the desire to maintain the pleasant affective state—one of the motives engendered by positive affect that was identified several years ago—does not necessarily take precedence over other motives fostered by happy feelings, other motives in the situation, or other effects of positive affect such as carefulness and flexibility in thinking.

POSITIVE AFFECT
AND DECISION MAKING

In the years since the second edition of this handbook was published, interest in the role of emotion has increased notably within the field of cognitive psychology and decision making, as it also has in some related fields such as economics and finance (e.g., Hirshleifer & Shumway, 2003; Lerner, Small, & Loewenstein, 2004; Slovic, Finucane, Peters, & MacGregor, 2004, just to name a few of the many, many papers appearing in the past several years from these and related domains). Some of these papers still focus on negative affect and still retain the assumption that affect, when it has influence on thinking, disrupts systematic thinking. But some, like those mentioned above, are reaching beyond those positions.

A few representative examples of the various approaches that now characterize the treatment of affect in these various fields related to decision making include the following: Hirshleifer and Shumway (2003) looked at the effect of sunshine, which is known to be related to positive affect and to produce some of the same effects as positive affect (e.g., Cunningham, 1979), on stock market investment decisions; they reported that when other variables were controlled, sunshine was related to better stock returns. Djamasbi (2007) examined the role of positive affect in utilization of a decision support system, and found positive affect to increase the number of cues used and the accuracy of the judgment made.

Lerner et al. (2004) looked at the effects of two different negative affects, disgust and sadness, and reported different effects on the sales prices and buying prices found acceptable under those conditions in an "endowment effect" paradigm taken from the behavioral economics literature. Those authors argued for the importance of considering the effects of individual emotions, rather than just considering the general valence of the emotion. This suggestion comes out of the discrete-emotions tradition, but it happens to be also compatible with the view that the influence of affect depends on what the affect leads the person to think about in the situation (e.g., Isen, 1987, 2000)—which can be different not only for discrete emotions, but also for any given emotion in different situations, or when the person has different goals. Unlike negative affect, positive affect of many different kinds has been found to have similar effects on such behaviors as helping, problem solving, and so on (e.g., Isen, 1987). However, the point here may still apply to positive affect, in that it would mean that one might expect different effects of such affect in different situations or with differing goals of the person as well—which, of course, is what has been found in many studies, as noted throughout this chapter.

Slovic et al. (2004) discuss what has been called a "two-systems" approach: They propose that decision making can take place both by calculation and by intuitive reaction, and that the two may often have something to contribute to one another. They do assume that the intuitive system will be the one that involves affect, and that the rational system does not involve affect (assumptions that may not be supported), but they allow for the integration of the two by the means just described.

Other scholars in decision making have proposed models by which the affect is a part of the decision-making model itself, in that the expected enjoyment or pleasure at the outcome is considered part of the calculus by which a rational decision is reached (e.g., Mellers, 2000). This idea is compatible with other work that also views affect as part of a rational decision-making process, in the sense that affect's influence on the processes that are involved in the calculation, or on thoughts about the situation, plays a role in the ways the components are

viewed and weighted (see Isen, 2003, for a discussion). Hermalin and Isen (in press) have also proposed an economic model of some of the effects of affect in which the influence of affect is represented as part of the model. These are just a few of the initiatives that have begun in the past few years to integrate affect into decision making from the decision-making or economic side, and it seems likely that these and others will be developed further in the near future.

It should be clear by now that considering the influence of affect on decision making involves recognizing the interacting roles of affect, the valence or interestingness of the task, the importance or utility of the task, the framing of the situation, the person's goals and motives in the situation, and other aspects of the context. Furthermore, the processes described are seen as depending on people's interpretations of the situation. This suggests that processes such as decision making and problem solving may be hierarchically organized: Before the problem is actually addressed, some command or executive decisions (attention deployment decisions) or evaluations may be made regarding how important the task is, what its utility might be, how dangerous or safe the situation is, or whether the person has any control over its eventual outcome, as well as what its hedonic consequences might be, and other possible interpretations of the situation (e.g., Martin, Ward, Achee, & Wyer, 1993). These decisions may influence the way in which the problem is framed or addressed. Furthermore, the person may also reevaluate such decisions while solving the task, using incoming information as he or she proceeds.

That is, perhaps the person makes a series of decisions in deciding or solving a problem, and perhaps an early one relates to the domain of the task, with regard to both valence and importance. A helpful way of viewing this first level of decision may be in terms of the framing of the problem. The person may derive a sense of whether this is a situation that he or she can enjoy (gain something, share, etc.) or a situation in which he or she must be concerned not to be harmed (not to lose what he or she already has or needs), and a sense of what his or her options are.

A conceptualization in terms of the framing of the situation has been useful in the decision-making and risk-taking literature, where differences have been found in people's decisions, depending on whether a problem was framed as a potential gain or as a potential loss (e.g., Tversky & Kahneman, 1981). The parallel to this work is not exact, because, in the well-known Asian disease problem, for example, the situation still involves danger and death, whether it is framed negatively (percentage of lives to be lost) or positively (percentage of lives to be saved). However, framing as studied previously in this literature may nonetheless bear some relevance to the two types of motives and actions (exploration vs. self-protection) resulting from positive affect that are under discussion here. Issues related to the framing of the experimental situation, and to the possibility of a kind of hierarchical evaluation or decision process (especially as this interacts with affect), may be explored more fully in the years to come.

Risk Preference

One kind of decision that has been studied as a function of positive affect is risk preference. In these studies on positive affect and risk, people experiencing positive affect were more risk-averse than controls, but only when the risk situation about which they were reasoning was a realistic one, involving potential for a real, substantial, meaningful loss.

For example, when betting chips representing their credit for participating in the study, those in positive affect bet less (Isen & Patrick, 1983), and required a higher probability of winning before agreeing to a substantial bet (but not a trivial bet), and also showed more thoughts about losing in a thought-listing task following this assessment (Isen & Geva, 1987). However, when asked about taking a chance on a hypothetical risk, without having to risk their own resources, people in positive affect responded as if they would be more willing to take this chance (Isen & Patrick, 1983). Similarly, when people were asked, without an affect induction, to estimate what effect they *thought* positive affect would have on their risk preference, they intuited that it would increase their willingness to take the risk. This suggests that it may not be wise to rely on people's hypothetical estimates of preferences and choices in assessing the influence of positive affect on risk.

The relative risk aversion observed in positive affect subjects considering real risks may relate to affect maintenance: People who are feeling happy risk losing that state, as well as

any tangible stake, if they lose the gamble. Therefore, perhaps because they have more to lose if facing a consequential risk, they are risk-averse relative to controls. This interpretation is supported by results of a study that examined the utility associated with various outcomes and found that people in positive affect displayed a greater negative utility for a substantial loss than did controls (Isen et al., 1988). That is, the same potential loss seemed worse to people in positive affect—and this may reflect a motive to maintain the positive state.

Some authors have assumed that affect maintenance, when it plays a role in a situation such as risk preference, influences decisions and behavior by causing a person to ignore details of the situation. For example, Loewenstein and Lerner (2003) assume that affect maintenance implies that people in positive affect will not pay attention to details and will oversimplify tasks. Furthermore, some researchers—also thinking that affect maintenance dominates all the effects of positive affect—may misunderstand the effects of positive affect more broadly, assuming that in order to maintain positive affect, a person in a positive state will always engage in superficial cognitive processing. The context of this work on risk perception and risk-related behavior, then, is a good place to point out once again that positive affect maintenance does not imply either that people in positive affect will not pay attention to details, or that they will oversimplify the task or perform poorly on it. The details of the risk studies show instead that people in positive affect consider the options in detail and quite carefully; for example, they differentiate among gambles and even have significantly more thoughts than controls do about a potential substantial loss. Desire for affect maintenance, then, when it is a factor in determining behavior in these risk situations, is theorized to play a role—not through careless information processing—but through avoiding the possibility of loss by reducing betting or risky behavior.

The results described above indicate that positive affect increases the negative utility of a real, meaningful potential loss. At the same time, positive affect has been found to increase the subjective probability of success in situations of risk assessment (e.g., Johnson & Tversky, 1983; Nygren, Isen, Taylor, & Dulin, 1996). Thus it seems that the two components of risk assessment, probability and utility, are influenced in functionally opposite ways by positive affect: Although the subjective probability of winning is increased, the negative utility or perceived danger of the potential loss is also increased. And the resultant behavior—relative risk avoidance by people in positive affect—suggests that the utility information is more influential in such people's decisions than the probability information (Nygren et al., 1996). These findings regarding positive affect and risk illustrate, as noted in other contexts, that the influence of positive affect on risk perception is not simple; it depends on, and interacts with, task and setting conditions.

Complex Decision Making

Another type of decision making that has been studied as a function of positive affect is what might be called "complex decision making," in which people are asked to choose the best item from among several alternatives varying on a number of dimensions, or to solve a complex problem (e.g., making a medical diagnosis). Research has shown that positive affect, induced by either an unrelated success or a small bag of candy, leads to decision making that is both more efficient and more thorough, if the task lends itself to increased effort or care.

For example, in one study (Isen et al., 1991), the participants were advanced medical students whose task was to choose, from among six descriptions of patients varying with regard to each of nine health-relevant factors, the patient most likely to have lung cancer. Results showed that people in positive affect solved (correctly) the assigned task more efficiently than controls, but then went on to do more than was required, such as suggesting treatments or offering diagnoses for the other patients. Thus they were both more efficient and more thorough than controls. In addition, the people in positive affect showed significantly less confusion and a significantly greater tendency to integrate the material with which they were working.

The results of this study are compatible with those of other research on affect and decision making, such as research on hypothetical car choice; however, particular measures (such as total amount of time and amount of redundancy in looking at the materials) produced different results, because of the contextual differences that made continuing to work with the materials after the assigned task was completed

sensible and appropriate (see Isen, 2000, for a discussion).

Another study, examining physicians' diagnostic processes, reported that doctors in whom positive affect had been induced (this time by receipt of a small bag of candy) identified the domain of the medical problem significantly earlier in their protocols and were more open to information, being significantly less likely than physicians in a control group to distort or ignore information that did not fit with a diagnostic hypothesis they were considering (Estrada at al., 1997). Thus this study confirms that positive affect does facilitate integration of information for decision making, and also fosters openness to information. At the same time, this study found no evidence that positive affect promotes premature closure, superficial thinking, jumping to conclusion without sufficient evidence, or any other indication of any impairment or carelessness in thinking. There was also no evidence of increased reliance on established schemas in preference to incoming new information; in fact, just the opposite was found.

The findings of the studies on medical decision making suggest that positive affect may promote not only more efficiency but also more thoroughness, as well as openness to information and the tendency to check hypotheses and tentative answers against additional information. It is likely that such an effect may be observed only where the materials allow for that possibility, and only where there is some reason to engage the task. It is clear, however, that such tasks include ones requiring complex consideration of serious topics of interest to the subjects; they are not limited to stereotypically "positive" or fun topics, and not to so-called "insight" or creativity problems. Moreover, the fact that people in positive affect were open to information disconfirming their initial hypotheses, and checked their work carefully, speaks against the hypothesis that positive affect leads to a careless, superficial, or "playful" approach, or to reliance on a person's established mental schemas rather than incoming new information.

Positive Affect and Use of Heuristics

Does Positive Affect Lead to Careless Thinking?

Several studies have addressed the issue of whether positive affect, rather than facilitating careful thinking and performance, impairs careful thinking because it takes up cognitive capacity (e.g., Mackie & Worth, 1989, 1991) and/or undermines the motivation to think carefully (e.g., Bless et al., 1990; Schwarz, 2002; Schwarz & Bless, 1991). The theoretical positions underlying the latter work hold that positive affect, by its nature, provides a "signal" that leads to careless, superficial thinking and use of heuristics, as contrasted with systematic cognitive processing (and thus often results in impaired processing). As we have seen in the preceding discussion of the decision-making studies, however, there are also findings that are not compatible with such formulations. How can the differences be understood? Perhaps specific methods are playing a role.

One approach to demonstrating the view that positive affect typically promotes use of heuristics uses an attitude change paradigm and infers nonsystematic processing from the patterns of arguments that are successful in bringing about attitude change. For example, attitude change in response to relatively weak (though not irrational) arguments is taken as indication of nonsystematic processing; therefore, if people in positive affect show as much attitude change when weaker arguments are presented as they do when strong arguments are presented, the conclusion is that positive affect interferes with systematic processing (e.g., Mackie & Worth, 1989).

As suggested in the earlier editions of this chapter, one problem with this inference, however, is that attitude change could be reported for reasons unrelated to processing of the message: People in positive affect may want to be more agreeable (which is known from the social psychology literature to be associated with positive affect, all else being equal). Or they may think of additional good arguments of their own, and this may lead them to display more change in attitude, independent of the strength of the arguments presented in the task.

The need for alternative interpretations such as these is also suggested by the fact that participants experiencing positive affect did not differ from other participants in their recognition that the "weak" arguments were weaker than the "strong" arguments, or in their ability to recall the message content, when that was measured directly (Bless et al., 1990; Mackie & Worth, 1989). In addition, in some instances the materials used in the studies focused on

negative, upsetting topics, and the situation did not provide much justification for working on the task. As noted earlier, it is becoming apparent that without a reason to work on an unpleasant task—that is, if the task is both unpleasant and unimportant—people in positive affect may not engage the task. Thus it is far from clear, from such studies, that lack of either cognitive capacity or motivation to "think straight" is what causes any difference between groups in reported attitude change.

In another approach that has been taken, researchers reasoned that use of stereotypes could be employed as an indication of heuristic or nonsystematic processing, and on this basis positive affect was investigated as a determinant of stereotype use (e.g., Bodenhausen et al., 1994, to mention one of several). The paper by Bodenhausen et al. (1994) illustrates the complexity of the findings in that area: Although three of four studies in that paper indicated that positive affect did result in increased use of a stereotype, the fourth study showed that this difference was not found—and the results even exhibited a marginally significant tendency toward the reverse, if participants were given a reason to pay more attention to the task (e.g., if they were to be accountable for their decision). The fact that the effect disappeared when the importance of the task was increased undermines the suggestion that, as a rule, positive affect leads to use of stereotypes and to nonsystematic processing generally; moreover, the fact that the people in positive affect responded appropriately to the different condition in Study 4 indicates their flexibility, rather than inability or unwillingness to process more carefully and individually. As mentioned earlier, these points were noted by Bodenhausen et al. (2001) in their more recent summary of the influence of positive affect on stereotyping, when they pointed out that happy people are flexible in their information-processing strategies, rather than *either* unable or unwilling to engage in systematic thinking.

Recent evidence reported by Johnson and Fredrickson (2005) runs counter to the interpretation that any increased use of stereotypes that is observed occurs because positive affect impairs the ability or motivation to process details, or promotes use of established schemas. These authors found that positive affect, relative to neutral affect and to fear, significantly improved white people's ability to recognize individual black persons' faces, and reduced the "own-race-bias effect" (the relative inability to distinguish among faces of individuals of a race other than one's own), which is usually taken to be part of the tendency to stereotype. These results, then, add to the evidence that positive affect does not necessarily promote use of stereotypes. More importantly in the present context, they suggest that people in positive affect can and do, pay close attention and process detail rather than relying on their established schemas.

Finally with regard to stereotype use, as is evident from the examples here, any evidence that studies of this type might provide for the suggestion that positive affect interferes with systematic processing is not compelling, because it would be indirect and open to alternative interpretation. This is similar to the point made with regard to using the attitude change paradigm to try to show that positive affect impairs systematic thinking: Stereotype use could occur for reasons other than nonsystematic thinking, impaired processing, or desire for noneffortful thinking.

In another approach to the question of whether positive affect impairs systematic processing, one paper has reported impaired reasoning performance among people in whom positive affect was induced (e.g., Melton, 1995). As noted above, in the context of the attitude change studies, it is possible that findings of seemingly impaired processing may result from the materials and context of the particular experiments that show the findings. This may be the case in the paper by Melton (1995) as well. A recent preliminary study has found that materials like those used in that paper are actually tedious and annoying to experimental participants, and it is known that use of this kind of material can lead—especially among participants in positive affect—to less engagement with the task unless there is a reason for the participants to engage the task carefully (e.g., Isen & Reeve, 2005). Preliminary results indicate that equally difficult material of the same kind (logical reasoning), but more interestingly formatted, actually reveals improved rather than impaired performance among participants in positive affect (Isen, Erez, Nester, & Shmidt, 2007). In addition, it has recently been proposed that positive affect may give rise to people's being able to notice that information needed for drawing a conclusion or making a decision is actually missing (Mantel et al., 2007).

Thus the evidence that positive affect per se promotes superficial processing per se is not as clear as is often assumed. In cases where it appears to do so, this may result from a lack of motivation for, or interest in, *the task presented*; however, this kind of motivational effect is different from one that postulates general interference with motivation overall, or with motivation to process carefully or to pay attention to detail. On the contrary, as shown in the section on motivation, the evidence suggests that positive affect can facilitate motivation by increasing the perceived link between effort and outcome, and there is much evidence that people in positive affect regularly pay attention to detail.

Use of Established Cognitive Structures

In addition, Schwarz, Clore, Bless, and their colleagues—long-time proponents of the view that positive affect interferes with systematic processing because it undermines the motivation to think carefully—have reported results incompatible with that view, and have promoted an alternative but similar view (Bless et al., 1996). In the 1996 paper, they acknowledge that "the evidence that heuristic processing is due to the hypothesized motivational or capacity deficits is less conclusive than is often assumed" (p. 665). They report results of studies showing that although people in positive affect demonstrated a greater tendency, relative to controls, to use a script to organize their learning and memory of a story, those participants also performed better than controls on a secondary task that had to be performed simultaneously. In the words of those authors, this finding "is incompatible with the assumption that happy moods decrease either cognitive capacity or processing motivation in general, which would predict impaired secondary-task performance" (Bless et al., 1996, p. 665).

As an outgrowth of that thinking, those researchers have proposed that positive affect leads to reliance on established cognitive structures (such as schemas or scripts) and habitual routines, but they still propose that positive affect leads to heuristic, superficial, nonsystematic cognitive processing (e.g., Bless et al., 1996; Gasper & Clore, 2002; Schwarz, 2002; Storbeck & Clore, 2005). In some places, there is fleeting acknowledgment that use of established schemas and routines says nothing about systematic processing, that it may even free up capacity, and/or that positive affect may enable flexibility and enhanced overall performance. Nevertheless, their primary argument is still that positive affect is expected to lead to overreliance on global, general knowledge structures, and to discourage careful processing or attention to detail, often to the detriment of performance. Thus this position still promotes the view that positive affect will result in superficial, careless cognitive processing, with lack of attention to detail (and that negative affect will promote careful, detailed processing)—even though their own data often do not confirm those predictions (e.g., Gasper & Clore, 2002, pp. 37, 39; Storbeck & Clore, 2005).

They maintain this stance even though it also ignores the fact that, as pointed out in this chapter, a great many data show that positive affect is compatible with careful, detailed thinking under most conditions. In addition, the position that positive affect will lead to reliance on one's "usual routines" that come to mind most easily (e.g., Schwarz, 2002) is at variance with the wide range of findings in the literature for quite some time, showing that positive affect increases the innovativeness of people's responses and thinking, their openness and flexibility in thinking, and their preference for variety (as well as their careful attention to detail and their improved performance in a wide range of tasks and problems). These findings regarding creative problem solving and variety seeking do not fit with the notion that positive affect promotes only (or even primarily) use of existing general knowledge structures and old, "routine," or habitual ways of looking at things.

Flexibility as an Alternative Interpretation

Those authors contrast the process of using general knowledge structures with that of relying on data and engaging in learning, as if these two processes will not occur together. In contrast, the flexibility hypothesis suggests that people in positive affect should be able to utilize both kinds of information—information that is new in the situation, and information from established schemas, past experiences, and past learning—and that they should be better at switching among these various sources and integrating them and the information available from them. These approaches (flexibility vs. schema-based) differ in many predictions that would follow from them. It is

also worth noting that the kind of integration proposed by the flexibility hypothesis—integration of new and established material through processes of assimilation (of new material into existing schemas) and accommodation (change of existing schemas in response to the new material)—is at the heart of the process of learning, according to several theories of education (e.g., see Isen, Daubman, & Gorgoglione, 1987, for consideration of the potential role of positive affect in this and related processes of learning).

The findings reviewed in the present chapter also support the suggestion made in the earlier editions of this handbook chapter that heuristic and systematic cognitive processes may not necessarily be alternatives to one another (as is often assumed), but may occur together. Perhaps, also, chunking, integration, or some other method of simplifying or organizing of a complex set of data actually frees up capacity or resources for use on other tasks. Thus processing in positive affect that appears "simplified" may actually result from more elaborated, differentiated thinking and from better understanding of the issues (see, e.g., Isen, 1993, for a fuller discussion).

Summary

The evidence that as a rule mild positive affect disrupts systematic thinking or leads to superficial processing is actually not compelling. This is because the studies attempting to show this are difficult to interpret—either because several layers of inference are required in order to reach that conclusion (as in the attitude-change and stereotyping studies); because they did not include a control group (positive affect and negative affect were contrasted); or because they used materials or tasks allowing for alternative interpretation, such as ones involving unimportant/tedious tasks, negative topics, or topics over which participants had no control.

In contrast, for more than a decade now, studies have been confirming that positive affect enables improved performance, even when simplifying devices are also used. In addition, people in positive affect seem to be able to use simplifying devices and systematic processing together, rendering their processing both more efficient and more thorough. These findings suggest that the consequence of positive affect is *flexibility* in modes of thinking and decision making—attention to new data and detail, integrated with existing knowledge structures, rather than exclusive reliance on existing knowledge structures and inability or reluctance to attend to detail.

A NEUROPSYCHOLOGICAL THEORY OF POSITIVE AFFECT'S INFLUENCE ON COGNITION

As noted at the outset of this chapter, research on the neuropsychology of emotion is growing at a rapid pace. Because of space limitations, I can only touch the surface of this topic, briefly mentioning one theory that may help to understand how positive affect has its effects on flexibility, thinking, and behavior—the dopamine hypothesis (Ashby et al., 1999). This theory focuses on the role of the neurotransmitter dopamine and proposes that many of the observed effects of positive affect on cognition may result from increased levels of dopamine in certain brain regions. Noting that dopamine is known to be associated with reward, this theory proposes that it is also present at increased levels during positive affect situations. Although other neurotransmitters no doubt play a role as well (see, e.g., Katz, 1999), and may even act in concert with dopamine to determine specific nuances of behavior, the evidence is strong that brain levels of dopamine play an important role in mediating many of the cognitive effects of positive affect that have been observed.

For example, because dopamine release into portions of the anterior cingulate region of the brain is thought to be involved in flexible selection of cognitive perspective and switching among alternative perspectives, it is likely that release of dopamine in such frontal brain areas mediates the increased flexibility observed under conditions of positive affect. This, then, would implicate dopamine in many of the effects of positive feelings that have been observed: creative problem solving, openness to information, exploration, integration of ideas, ability to focus on important negative information when that is needed, and ability to keep others' perspectives as well as one's own in mind (which may also play a role in many of the social effects of positive affect that have been established over the years, such as cooperativeness, social responsibility, improved negotiation skills, and generosity to both self and others), just to name a few.

In addition, because there are many excitatory dopamine receptors in frontal brain areas and prefrontal cortex, this theory also predicts that positive affect will facilitate processes influenced by those brain regions, such as attention deployment, working memory, and memory consolidation. Evidence is accumulating that supports this theory (e.g., Isen & Shmidt, 2007; Kazen & Kuhl, 2005; Kuhl & Kazen, 1999), although it is too soon to draw firm conclusions. Much remains to be explored relating to the dopamine hypothesis, but its predictions provide more specific targets than we have had in the past, and ideally these will add to our understanding.

This neurological theory adds to our tools for studying the impact of affect; however, it cannot replace studies conducted on the cognitive and behavioral levels. Rather than viewing these levels of analysis (e.g., neurological vs. behavioral) as opposing ways to advance understanding, it is possible instead to attempt to bring them together and integrate work from these multiple levels of analysis. Insights from the neurological level can help to inform and guide our search for effects and determinants of feelings on the behavioral and cognitive levels as well. Similarly, research on the behavioral and cognitive levels can point to neurological processes that may be critical. Indeed, studies on the behavioral and cognitive levels of analysis led to our understanding that positive affect promotes flexibility, problem solving, innovation, and improved attention deployment, and thus to the hypothesis that dopamine might mediate some of the cognitive and behavioral effects of positive affect.

CONCLUSION

In summary of the work presented in this chapter, it seems appropriate to emphasize once again that the influence of affect depends on what it makes the person think about, and that this is determined not by the affective state alone, but by this state in conjunction with several aspects of the situation that together influence the person's motives or goals, judgments, expectations, and choices. Brain regions activated by neurotransmitters (particularly dopamine) associated with positive affect play a role in the effects of feelings, but this is only one of several influences that together determine cognitive processes and behavior.

Despite the complex interaction of factors that determines affect's ultimate impact on thought processes, decision making, and behavior, a few general conclusions can be offered. All else being equal, mild positive affect tends to promote exploration and enjoyment of new ideas and possibilities, and new ways of looking at things, especially in safe, enjoyable situations. Thus people in positive affect may be alert to possibilities and may solve problems both more efficiently and more thoroughly than controls. However, in situations of potential harm, people who are feeling good respond appropriately cautiously and are not likely to take chances. Nonetheless, where there is a reason to think about possible losses or difficulties, they will elaborate and consider the negative possibilities thoroughly and effectively. Thus positive affect facilitates coping and focus on long-term welfare as well.

The majority of existing data, then, suggest that mild positive affect enables cognitive flexibility and thus fosters improved consideration of situations and problems, and improved performance on a wide range of tasks, as long as there is reason for the person to engage the task. People who are feeling mildly happy are better able to think about multiple aspects of situations and to see situations and stimuli in multiple ways, seemingly simultaneously.

Compatibly with both the neurological interpretation of the underpinnings of these findings, and the cognitive interpretation (in terms of range of concepts activated), there is no reason to expect the influence of positive affect to be linear, or to think that more intense positive affect will generate more (or even as much) or better problem solving. Everything that has been said in this chapter applies to *mild* positive affect, and there is no reason to think that it would also be true of intense positive affect. That is, once dopamine is released or extensive cognitive context is cued, the effects are enabled, and more intense affect would not necessarily cause more of those effects. In fact, intense positive feelings or very good news may even interfere with performance rather than facilitating it. But the reason may be that the news changes what people want to think about—not that positive affect itself drains their capacity, distracts them, or signals them not to process carefully. In other words, in this regard, the positive event would not be different from any other interesting topic that causes people to refocus their attention.

Regarding positive affect's influence on systematic thinking, the popular idea that positive affect undermines the ability or motivation to think carefully, pay attention to detail, or take in new information fails to account for a very large and growing literature examining the performance of people in positive affect. Many researchers have now concluded that that idea is not correct. Similarly, the suggestion that positive affect leads people to use their established cognitive structures *rather than* taking in new information—which, again, is proposed to be caused by and/or to result in lack of attention to detail—is not itself well supported by data and also fails to account for many of the other existing data. Therefore, the "signaling" and speculative "cognitive tuning" metaphor described by Schmarz (2002) as applying to positive and negative emotion seem overused and misleading in the context of positive affect.

This chapter has examined some of the evidence regarding ways in which positive affect influences decision making, including some cognitive and motivational processes involved. However, more work is needed to explore these relationships, the circumstances under which they occur, and the processes that are involved in producing them. Simple answers seem not to be supported; for example, positive affect has been found to give rise to elaboration and a wide range of cognitive associations in response to neutral stimulus material, while not reducing association or thought about other material, and not reducing the ability to stay focused on a task a person is trying to perform. Feeling happy does not function as a lens or filter, improving evaluation of everything in the person's line of vision or thought, but instead increases liking only for likable things. It increases preference for variety and acceptance of a broader range of options into people's choice sets, when the choice is among safe, enjoyable alternatives, but it does not promote risk taking in situations of genuine risk. Happy feeling can lead to efficient and thorough decision making; it stimulates enjoyment of enjoyable tasks and perception of interesting tasks as even more enriched (but not at the cost of working on less interesting things if they need to be done). When less interesting, or annoying, tasks are presented, those things may be deferred if deferring them is an option, but will be addressed effectively if it is not. Positive feelings seem to promote activities that foster enjoyment and maintenance of those feelings, but in rational, responsible, adaptive ways—not as if affect maintenance were of primary or singular importance. Socially, of course, positive affect is known to promote the very important processes of generosity, helpfulness, responsibility, and taking the perspective of another person as well as one's own, under most circumstances, but it does not lead to mere compliance. Thus happy feelings provide many benefits, but the processes involved are complex. Given the importance of positive affect in our lives, and the great advantages to social behavior and problem solving that result from feeling happy, positive affect seems an important topic for continued investigation.

REFERENCES

Amabile, T. M., Barsade, S. G., Mueller, J. S., & Staw, B. M. (2005). Affect and creativity at work. *Administrative Science Quarterly*, 50, 367–403.

Ashby, F. G., Isen, A. M., & Turken, A. U. (1999). A neuropsychological theory of positive affect and its influence on cognition. *Psychological Review*, 106, 529–550.

Aspinwall, L. G. (1998). Rethinking the role of positive affect and self-regulation. *Motivation and Emotion*, 22(1), 1–32.

Aspinwall, L. G., & MacNamara, A. (2005). Taking positive changes seriously: Toward a positive psychology of cancer survivorship and resilience. *Cancer*, 104(11, Suppl.), 2549–2556.

Aspinwall, L. G., & Taylor, S. E. (1997). A stitch in time: Self-regulation and proactive coping. *Psychological Bulletin*, 121, 417–436.

Barone, M. J., Miniard, P. W., & Romeo, J. B. (2000). The influence of positive mood on brand extension evaluations. *Journal of Consumer Research*, 26, 386–400.

Baumann, N., & Kuhl, J. (2005). Positive affect and flexibility: Overcoming the precedence of global over local processing of visual information. *Motivation and Emotion*, 29, 123–134.

Bless, H., Bohner, G., Schwarz, N., & Strack, F. (1990). Mood and persuasion: A cognitive response analysis. *Personality and Social Psychology Bulletin*, 16, 331–345.

Bless, H., Clore, G. L., Schwarz, N., Golisano, V., Rabe, C., & Wolk, M. (1996). Mood and the use of scripts: Does a happy mood really lead to mindlessness? *Journal of Personality and Social Psychology*, 71, 665–679.

Bodenhausen, G. V., Kramer, G. P., & Susser, K. (1994). Happiness and stereotypic thinking in social judgment. *Journal of Personality and Social Psychology*, 66, 621–632.

Bodenhausen, G. V., Mussweiler, T., Gabriel, S., &

Moreno, K. N. (2001). Affective influences on stereotyping and intergroup relations. In J. P. Forgas (Ed.), *Handbook of affect and social cognition* (pp. 319–343). Mahwah, NJ: Erlbaum.

Carnevale, P. J. D., & Isen, A. M. (1986). The influence of positive affect and visual access on the discovery of integrative solutions in bilateral negotiation. *Organizational Behavior and Human Decision Processes*, 37, 1–13.

Cunningham, M. R. (1979). Weather, mood, and helping behavior: Quasi-experiments in the sunshine Samaritan. *Journal of Personality and Social Psychology*, 37, 1947–1956.

Deci, E. L., & Ryan, R. M. (1985). *Intrinsic motivation and self-determination in human behavior.* New York: Plenum Press.

Derryberry, D. (1993). Attentional consequences of outcome-related motivational states: Congruent, incongruent, and focusing effects. *Motivation and Emotion*, 17, 65–89.

Djamasbi, J. (2007). Does positive affect influence the effective usage of a decision support system? *Decision Support Systems*, 43, 1707–1717.

Dreisbach, G., & Goschke, T. (2004). How positive affect modulates cognitive control: Reduced perseveration at the cost of increased distractibility. *Journal of Experimental Psychology: Learning, Memory, and Cognition*, 30, 343–353.

Duncker, K. (1945). On problem-solving. *Psychological Monographs*, 58(Whole No. 5).

Easterbrook, J. A. (1959). The effect of emotion on cue utilization and the organization of behavior. *Psychological Review*, 66, 183–201.

Erber, R., & Erber, M. W. (2000). The self-regulation of moods: Second thoughts on the importance of happiness in everyday life. *Psychological Inquiry*, 11, 142–148.

Erez, A., & Isen, A. M. (2002). The influence of positive affect on components of expectancy motivation. *Journal of Applied Psychology*, 89, 1055–1067.

Estrada, C. A., Isen, A. M., & Young, M. J. (1997). Positive affect facilitates integration of information and decreases anchoring in reasoning among physicians. *Organizational Behavior and Human Decision Processes*, 72, 117–135.

Forest, D., Clark, M., Mills, J., & Isen, A. M. (1979). Helping as a function of feeling state and nature of the helping behavior. *Motivation and Emotion*, 3, 161–169.

Forgas, J. P. (2002). Feeling and doing: Affective influences on interpersonal behavior. *Psychological Inquiry*, 13, 1–29.

Fredrickson, B. L. (2001). The role of positive emotions in positive psychology: The broaden-and-build theory of positive emotions. *American Psychologist*, 56, 218–226.

Fredrickson, B. L., & Branigan, C. (2005). Positive emotions broaden the scope of attention and thought–action repertoires. *Cognition and Emotion*, 19, 313–332.

Fredrickson, B. L., & Joiner, T. (2002). Positive emotions trigger upward spirals toward emotional well-being. *Psychological Science, 13,* 172–175.

Friedman, R. S., & Forster, J. (2005). The influence of approach and avoidance cues on attentional flexibility. *Motivation and Emotion, 29,* 69–81.

Gasper, K., & Clore, G. L. (2002). Attending to the big picture: Mood and global versus local processing of visual information. *Psychological Science, 13,* 34–40.

Gray, J. R. (2001). Emotion modulation of cognitive control: Approach–withdrawal states double-dissociate spatial from verbal two-back task performance. *Journal of Experimental Psychology: General, 130,* 436–452.

Greene, T. R., & Noice, H. (1988). Influence of positive affect upon creative thinking and problem solving in children. *Psychological Reports, 63,* 895–898.

Hermalin, B. E., & Isen, A. M. (in press). A model of the effect of affect on economic decision making. *Quantitative Marketing and Economics.*

Hirshleifer, D., & Shumway, T. (2003). Good day sunshine: Stock returns and the weather. *Journal of Finance, 58,* 1009–1032.

Isen, A. M. (1987). Positive affect, cognitive processes, and social behavior. In L. Berkowitz (Ed.), *Advances in experimental social psychology* (Vol. 20, pp. 203–253). New York: Academic Press.

Isen, A. M. (1993). Positive affect and decision making. In M. Lewis & J. M. Haviland (Eds.), *Handbook of emotion* (pp. 261–277). New York: Guilford Press.

Isen, A. M. (2000). Positive affect and decision making. In M. Lewis & J. M. Haviland-Jones (Eds.), *Handbook of emotions* (2nd ed., pp. 417–435). New York: Guilford Press.

Isen, A. M. (2003). Positive affect as a source of human strength. In L. G. Aspinwall & U. Staudinger (Eds.), *A psychology of human strengths* (pp. 179–195). Washington, DC: American Psychological Association.

Isen, A. M. (2008). Positive affect and decision processes: Some recent theoretical developments with practical implications. In C. Haugdvedt, P. M. Herr, & F. R. Kardes (Eds.), *Handbook of consumer psychology* (pp. 273–296). New York: Psychology Press.

Isen, A. M., & Daubman, K. A. (1984). The influence of affect on categorization. *Journal of Personality and Social Psychology, 47,* 1206–1217.

Isen, A. M., Daubman, K. A., & Gorgoglione, J. M. (1987). The influence of positive affect on cognitive organization: Implications for education. In R. E. Snow & J. M. Farr (Eds.), *Aptitude, learning, and instruction* (Vol. 3, pp. 143–164). Hillsdale, NJ: Erlbaum.

Isen, A. M., Daubman, K. A., & Nowicki, G. P. (1987). Positive affect facilitates creative problem solving. *Journal of Personality and Social Psychology, 52,* 1122–1131.

Isen, A. M., Erez, A., Nester, M. A., & Schmidt, E. (2007). *Positive affect facilitates recognition of insufficient information in logical reasoning.* Unpublished manuscript, Cornell University.

Isen, A. M., & Geva, N. (1987). The influence of positive affect on acceptable level of risk: The person with a large canoe has a large worry. *Organizational Behavior and Human Decision Processes, 39,* 145–154.

Isen, A. M., Johnson, M. M. S., Mertz, E., & Robinson, G. F. (1985). The influence of positive affect on the unusualness of word associations. *Journal of Personality and Social Psychology, 48,* 1413–1426.

Isen, A. M., & Levin, P. F. (1972). Effect of feeling good on helping: Cookies and kindness. *Journal of Personality and Social Psychology, 21,* 384–388.

Isen, A. M., Niedenthal, P., & Cantor, N. (1992). An influence of positive affect on social categorization. *Motivation and Emotion, 16,* 65–78.

Isen, A. M., Nygren, T. E., & Ashby, F. G. (1988). The influence of positive affect on the subjective utility of gains and losses: It is just not worth the risk. *Journal of Personality and Social Psychology, 55,* 710–717.

Isen, A. M., & Patrick, R. (1983). The effect of positive feelings on risk-taking: When the chips are down. *Organizational Behavior and Human Performance, 31,* 194–202.

Isen, A. M., & Reeve, J. (2005). The influence of positive affect on intrinsic and extrinsic motivation: Facilitating enjoyment of play, responsible work behavior, and self-control. *Motivation and Emotion, 29,* 297–325.

Isen, A. M., Rosenzweig, A. S., & Young, M. J. (1991). The influence of positive affect on clinical problem solving. *Medical Decision Making, 11,* 221–227.

Isen, A. M., Shalker, T., Clark, M. S., & Karp, L. (1978). Affect, accessibility of material and behavior: A cognitive loop? *Journal of Personality and Social Psychology, 36,* 1–12.

Isen, A. M., & Shmidt, E. (2007, January). *Positive affect: Broadened focus without increased distractibility.* Paper presented at the Emotions preconference to the annual meeting of the Society for Personality and Social Psychology, Memphis, TN.

Isen, A. M., & Simmonds, S. F. (1978). The effect of feeling good on a helping task that is incompatible with good mood. *Social Psychology Quarterly, 41,* 345–349.

Isen, A. M., & Spassova, G. (2008, February). *Positive affect reduces the demotivating effects of choice overload.* Paper presented at the annual meeting of the Society for Personality and Social Psychology, Albuquerque, NM.

Iyengar, S. S., & Lepper, M. R. (2000). When choice is demotivating: Can one desire too much of a good thing? *Journal of Personality and Social Psychology, 79,* 995–1006.

Johnson, E., & Tversky, A. (1983). Affect, generalization and the perception of risk. *Journal of Personality and Social Psychology, 45,* 20–31.

Johnson, K. J., & Fredrickson, B. L. (2005). "We all look the same to me": Positive emotions eliminate the own-race bias in face recognition. *Psychological Science*, 16, 875–881.

Kahn, B. E., & Isen, A. M. (1993). The influence of positive affect on variety-seeking among safe, enjoyable products. *Journal of Consumer Research*, 20, 257–270.

Kanfer, R. (1990). Motivation theory and industrial and organizational psychology. In M. D. Dunnette & L. M. Hough (Eds.), *Handbook of industrial and organizational psychology* (Vol. 1, pp. 75–170). Palo Alto, CA: Consulting Psychologists Press.

Katz, L. D. (1999). Dopamine and serotonin: Integrating current affective engagement with longer-term goals. *Behavioral and Brain Sciences*, 22, 527.

Kazen, M., & Kuhl, J. (2005). Intention memory and achievement motivation: Volitional facilitation and inhibition as a function of affective contents of need-related stimuli. *Journal of Personality and Social Psychology*, 89, 426–448.

Kimchi, R., & Palmer, S. E. (1982). Form and texture in hierarchically constructed patterns. *Journal of Experimental Psychology*, 8, 521–535.

Kraiger, K., Billings, R. S., & Isen, A. M. (1989). The influence of positive affective states on task perceptions and satisfaction. *Organizational Behavior and Human Decision Processes*, 44, 12–25.

Kuhl, J., & Kazen, M. (1999). Volitional facilitation of difficult intentions: Joint activation of intention memory and positive affect removes Stroop interference. *Journal of Experimental Psychology: General*, 128, 382–399.

Lerner, J., Small, D. A., & Loewenstein, G. (2004). Heart strings and purse strings: Carryover effects of emotions on economic decisions. *Psychological Science*, 15, 337–341.

Loewenstein, G., & Lerner, J. S. (2003). The role of affect in decision making. In R. J. Davidson, K. R. Scherer, & H. H. Goldsmith (Eds.), *Handbook of affective sciences* (pp. 619–642). New York: Oxford University Press.

Mackie, D. M., & Worth, L. T. (1989). Processing deficits and the mediation of positive affect in persuasion. *Journal of Personality and Social Psychology*, 57, 27–40.

Mackie, D. M., & Worth, L. T. (1991). Feeling good but not thinking straight: The impact of positive mood on persuasion. In J. P. Forgas (Ed.), *Emotion and social judgment* (pp. 201–220). Oxford: Pergamon Press.

Mano, H. (1994). Risk taking, framing effects, and affect. *Organizational Behavior and Human Decision Processes*, 57, 38–58.

Mantel, S. P., Kardes, F. R., & Isen, A. M. (2007). *Effects of positive affect on omission detection in the multiattribute evaluation and Ellsberg Paradigms*. Unpublished manuscript, Indiana University.

Martin, L. M., Ward, D. W., Achee, J. W., & Wyer, R. A. (1993). Mood as input: People have to interpret the motivational implications of their moods. *Journal of Personality and Social Psychology*, 64, 317–326.

Mednick, M. T., Mednick, S. A., & Mednick, E. V. (1964). Incubation of creative performance and specific associative priming. *Journal of Abnormal and Social Psychology*, 69, 84–88.

Mellers, B. A. (2000). Choice and the relative pleasure of consequences. *Psychological Bulletin*, 126, 910–924.

Melton, R. J. (1995). The role of positive affect in syllogism performance. *Personality and Social Psychology Bulletin*, 21, 788–794.

Murray, N., Sujan, H., Hirt, E. R., & Sujan, M. (1990). The influence of mood on categorization: A cognitive flexibility interpretation. *Journal of Personality and Social Psychology*, 59, 411–425.

Navon, D. (1977). Forest before trees: The precedence of global features in visual perception. *Cognitive Psychology*, 9, 353–383.

Nygren, T. E., Isen, A. M., Taylor, P. J., & Dulin, J. (1996). The influence of positive affect on the decision rule in risk situations: Focus on outcome (especially avoidance of loss) rather than probability. *Organizational Behavior and Human Decision Processes*, 66, 59–72.

Roediger, H. L., III, McDermott, K. B., & Robinson, K. J. (1998). The role of associative process in creating false memories. In M. A. Conway, S. E. Gathercole, & C. Cornoldi (Eds.), *Theories of memory II* (pp. 187–245). Hove, UK: Psychological Press.

Roehm, M., & Sternthal, B. (2001). The moderating effects of knowledge and resources on the persuasive impact of analogies. *Journal of Consumer Research*, 28, 257–272.

Russell, J. A., & Carroll, J. M. (1999). On the bipolarity of positive and negative affect. *Psychological Bulletin*, 125, 3–30.

Sanbonmatsu, D. M., & Kardes, F. R. (1988). The effects of physiological arousal on information processing and persuasion. *Journal of Consumer Research*, 15, 379–385.

Schwarz, N. (2002). Situated cognition and the wisdom of feelings: Cognitive tuning. In L. F. Barrett & P. Salovey (Eds.), *The wisdom in feeling* (pp. 144–166). New York: Guilford Press.

Schwarz, N., & Bless, H. (1991). Happy and mindless, but sad and smart? The impact of affective states on analytic reasoning. In J. P. Forgas (Ed.), *Emotion and social judgment* (pp. 55–71). Oxford: Pergamon Press.

Simonson, I. (1989). Choice based on reasons: The case of attraction and compromise effects. *Journal of Consumer Research*, 16, 158–174.

Slovic, P., Finucane, M. L., Peters, E., & MacGregor, D. G. (2004). Risk as analysis and risk as feelings. *Risk Analysis*, 24, 311–322.

Staw, B. M., & Barsade, S. G. (1993). Affect and managerial performance: A test of the sadder-but-wiser vs. happier-and-smarter hypotheses. *Administrative Science Quarterly*, 38, 304–331.

Storbeck, J., & Clore, G. L. (2005). With sadness comes accuracy, with happiness, false memory: Mood and the false memory effect. *Psychological Science*, *16*, 785–791.

Teasdale, J. D., & Fogarty, S. J. (1979). Differential effects of induced mood on retrieval of pleasant and unpleasant events from episodic memory. *Journal of Abnormal Psychology*, *88*, 248–257.

Trope, Y., & Pomerantz, E. M. (1998). Resolving conflicts among self-evaluative motives: Positive experiences as a resource for overcoming defensiveness. *Motivation and Emotion*, *22*, 53–72.

Tversky, A., & Gati, I. (1978). Studies of similarity. In E. Rosch & B. B. Lloyd (Eds.), *Cognition and categorization* (pp. 79–98). Hillsdale, NJ: Erlbaum.

Tversky, A., & Kahneman, D. (1981). The framing of decisions. *Science*, *211*, 453–458.

Watson, D., & Tellegen, A. (1999). Issues in the dimensional structure of affect: Effects of descriptors, measurement error, and response formats-Comment on Russell and Carroll (1999). *Psychological Bulletin*, *125*, 601–610.

Wegener, D. T., Petty, R. E., & Smith, S. E. (1995). Positive mood can increase or decrease message scrutiny: The hedonic contingency view of mood and message processing. *Journal of Personality and Social Psychology*, *69*, 5–15.

Weiner, B. (1985). "Spontaneous" causal thinking. *Psychological Bulletin*, *97*, 74–84.

Yang, H., Ceci, S., & Isen, A. M. (2006, January). *Positive affect increases monitoring and does not increase false memory*. Poster presented at the annual meeting of the Society for Personality and Social Psychology, Palm Springs, CA.

CHAPTER 35

Advances in Modeling Emotion and Thought

The Importance of Developmental, Online, and Multilevel Analyses

NANCY L. STEIN, MARC W. HERNANDEZ, and TOM TRABASSO

How do we process, represent, and understand emotional experience? How can we best describe the memory, thinking, and evaluation processes that continually accompany the experience of emotion? How do memory and thinking processes interleave with the physiological and neurophysiological processes of emotion? What are the developmental origins of this representational process? Do the representation and expression of emotional experience change as a function of development, or are stable representational structures present at birth, only to be fine-tuned by environmental and physiological factors? These are the questions that motivate the theoretical overview presented in this chapter.

In the last 20 years, serious attempts have been made to describe the thinking and physiological processes that accompany emotional experience. These theoretical approaches (Frijda, 1987, 1988, 2005; Lazarus, 1982, 1984, 1991; Oatley & Johnson-Laird, 1987;

Sandler, Grandjean, & Scherer, 2005; Scherer, 1984; Roseman, 1991; Stein & Jewett, 1986; Stein & Levine, 1987; Stein, Trabasso, & Liwag, 1993, 2000; Zajonc, 1980), despite their different perspectives, derive from an effort to describe the ways in which thinking, planning, and action interact with the physiological and neurological processes that occur when an emotion is experienced. The goal of this chapter is to discuss some of the difficulties associated with modeling emotion and thought, and to bring evidence to bear on a set of issues that has influenced our models and understanding of emotion and thought.

One feature that distinguishes our approach from other models of emotion and thought is that we study emotion and thought in children as well as adults. Our approach is further differentiated from others because we examine the online thinking and appraisal processes that precede, accompany, and follow the experience of emotion. Thus we focus on the entire *emotion episode*, not just individual components of an emotion episode (such as physical emotion expression, physiological change, or verbal reports). Our analysis is grounded in a theory of goal-based action that elucidates the attention, thinking, and appraisal processes occurring during the course of emotional experience and intentional action (Stein et al., 1993, 2000; Stein & Hernandez, 2007). We also examine the physiological processes that accompany goal-based action, especially those that precede, accompany, and follow emotional experience. Heart rate, blood pressure, the activation of the autonomic nervous system (ANS), changes in galvanic skin response, and changes in cortisol levels are all physiological measures that we consider (Stein & Boyce, 2005).

Goals are central to our theory of emotion, because the monitoring of personally significant goals, in terms of their failure and success, set the conditions for the experience and evocation of emotion. The evocation and experience of emotion occur when unexpected changes in personally significant goals are perceived. The episode that surrounds an emotion begins when a precipitating event occurs and alerts a person to some type of change in a personally significant goal. Once a person perceives this change, all cognitive effort is focused on determining the nature of the change and the impact the change will have on personally relevant goals. We define an "emotion episode" as a sequence of events that includes the precipitating event; appraisals of the change in the status of a goal; the physiological and neurophysiological reactions that occur in relation to the change; the emotional reaction itself; and subsequent appraisal, planning, and behavior sequences carried out to cope with the impact of the goal change.

An emotion is said to occur when four dimensions are present: (1) when unexpected changes occur in personal goal states; (2) when subsequent changes occur in the ANS to shift attention to the changes in goal states; (3) when cognitive evaluations have been carried out to assess the impact of these changes on the person's well-being; and (4) when beliefs about the probability of attaining, maintaining, avoiding, or preventing a goal state are activated.

"Beliefs" are organized forms of knowledge that carry expectations about the state of some aspect of the world. They often carry a value judgment (e.g., good or bad) or a preference (e.g., like or dislike) for the aspect of the object being evaluated. Beliefs reflect what people think is, was, or could be true about their world (Folkman & Stein, 1997; Stein & Hernandez, 2007; Stein & Levine, 1987, 1990, 1999; Stein et al., 1993, 2000). Prior knowledge in the form of organized belief systems is activated to evaluate and understand the personal impact of an event on well-being. In activating belief systems, people are able to generate precise inferences about how an event has already affected them and how it will affect them in the future.

The ways in which goal appraisal processes operate during emotion understanding and remembering correspond to a series of five questions: (1) What happened? (2) How do I feel about it? (3) What can I do about it? (4) What did I do about it? and (5) What were the consequences of carrying out a plan of action? (Stein & Hernandez, 2007). Each question reflects a class of inferences made in relation to evaluating the status of a goal that has been affected by a precipitating event. We use these five questions as a pedagogical device to organize our inquiry into the sequences of goal appraisal processes that occur online during an emotional episode. The questions correspond to the temporal and causal unfolding of an emotional episode and allow us to specify the exact nature of goal appraisal processes involved in understanding and remembering emotional events.

The questions were derived by describing *in toto* all of the information contained in over 1,000 different narratives generated as children and adults actually experienced an emotion (Stein & Hernandez, 2007; Stein, Trabasso, & Albro, 2001) or recalled a past experience and attempted to reenact the scenario (Liwag & Stein, 1995; Stein & Albro, 2001). Using these online procedures enables us to describe and unfold the dynamic properties and sequence of behavioral, cognitive, and physiological processes that interleave as emotions are experienced, expressed, and enacted. The language, emotion expressions, and emotional behaviors are videotaped before, during, and after the online experience of emotion, enabling us to determine subjects' focus of attention when emotions are experienced and expressed (Ross, Ross, Stein, & Trabasso, 2007; Stein & Boyce, 2005; Stein & Hernandez, 2007; Stein, Sheldrick, & Broaders, 1999).

Using all of these techniques, we are able to document the content and natural language used during and after an emotion episode. We determine whether it matches the emotion expression on the face, test how it corresponds to changes in heart rate and blood pressure, judge the accuracy of the memory for the emotion episode, and assess how aware family members are of each other's emotions. Finally, we discuss data that show how emotions, appraisals, and plans affect and predict psychological well-being.

We have found that the talk accompanying emotional experience is so constrained that we have created a computer program that encodes and analyzes much of the online talk of emotion and coping (Stein & Hernandez, 2007). Although some researchers are wary of the infinite variation in and unreliability of talk surrounding emotion (see LeDoux, 2002; Mandler, 1975, 1984, for examples), we have found just the opposite to be the case. The constraints on the talk of emotional understanding occur over development and across cultures. Describing the online thinking, planning, and talk about emotion has allowed us to outline the temporal and causal sequences accompanying emotional experience.

The ability to outline the temporal and causal sequences of the cognitive processing associated with emotion experience is a unique advantage of our methodology. We fully support and use physiological measures and neuroscience technology to advance our theory of emotion, but we are also aware of the limitations that the technology of neuroscience places on the temporal description of emotion processes. Thus we use those modalities in conjunction with paradigms that allow us to probe more deeply into the processes of emotion experience, and we then try to map the thinking, talk, and behaviors of emotion onto the physiology and neurophysiology of emotion.

When researchers fail to unfold the thinking processes involved in emotion experience, serious theoretical errors are made. Specifically, the amount and type of thinking and decision making that occur during emotional experience are underestimated. Descriptions of the organization of the temporal and causal sequence of emotional experience are incorrect. The speed with which cognitive processes are carried out is sorely underestimated. Finally, descriptions of unconscious and conscious processing are lacking in accuracy, in terms of when people are consciously aware of the events surrounding emotion and when they use unconscious processing to encode and interpret the meaning of an event.

MODELING EMOTION AND THOUGHT

Throughout this chapter, we argue that both children and adults use conscious and unconscious cognitive processes to understand, evaluate, plan, and respond to events that provoke emotion. From the very beginning of life, experiencing and expressing emotion are goal-based, expressive, and action-oriented. Experiencing emotion involves continual monitoring of personally relevant goals, and involves a constant appraisal of the value and worth of events, people, objects, activities, ideas, internal states, and anything else that impinges on the psychological and physical well-being of the person involved. The monitoring of goals requires both unconscious and conscious processing, and the evocation of emotion is the result of both types of processing. One of the main questions surrounding the description of the thinking that accompanies emotion is when and under what conditions emotional processing results in conscious awareness, as opposed to remaining an unconscious process.

As we have shown in almost all of our work on children and adults over the last 25-plus years, everyone, including 3-year-old children, is highly aware of the causes and consequences of emotional experience (Stein & Albro, 2001; Stein & Levine, 1989, 1999; Trabasso, Stein, & Johnson, 1981). In talking about the causes of their emotions, people can verbalize the goals that have changed, those that are at stake, and those that have failed. They can distinguish between their desires for action and the actions that actually get carried out, and they are keenly aware of the consequences of their actions. Although many current lines of research are aimed at studying the unconscious processes involved in the experience of emotion, it is important that we describe the conscious processes as well as the unconscious processes.

The same should hold for the study of developmental processes. Although the emphasis in development is on the nature and type of change that occur over the lifespan, similarities in functioning and understanding must also be considered. The fact that emotion is central to survival and is central to a theory of evolution suggests that the very young may experience rapid growth and understanding of emotion and its impact on behavior.

The belief that goal-directed action is central to emotional processing is not a new idea. Almost all current theories of emotion speak to the necessity of goals, values, desires, concerns, or motives as one of the critical components "driving" appraisal processes, which interact with and regulate emotional experience. The words that theorists use for goals are different, but the concepts and final results are the same. Much of the goal-based theory used in models of emotion theory derives from Miller, Galanter, and Pribram's (1960) seminal work on the importance of goals and planning in all of human action and interaction.

Magda Arnold (1960a, 1960b) influenced many emotion researchers (see Frijda, 1987, 1988; Lazarus, 1991; Stein & Oatley, 1992; Scherer, 1984) because of her sensitivity to and necessity for characterizing the importance of appraisal and evaluation. However, in order to advance such a theory, a model of the online temporal and causal properties of emotion needs to be formulated. The necessary step in building a theory of emotion and thinking, especially one that focuses on the dynamic unfolding and expression of emotion and behavior, is to describe the content and organization of the appraisal and goal-based thinking processes that occur from the beginning to the end of an emotion episode (Stein & Hernandez, 2007; Stein et al., 1993; Trabasso & Stein, 1993). The theory of Miller et al. (1960) has been critical in this endeavor. These researchers modeled the ways in which goals regulate the planning process and constrain the actions that are undertaken, as well as the outcomes associated with goal attainment. Our theory builds on this model and so do other appraisal theories, especially those of Frijda (1987), Oatley and Johnson-Laird (1987), Scherer (1984), and Roseman (1984, 1991).

Constraints on the outcomes of goals are important in mapping patterns of appraisal processes onto emotions. The pursuit of a goal can end in only three ways: People can be successful in achieving a goal; they can fail at achieving a goal; or the attainment of a goal can remain uncertain, with neither success nor failure occurring. The limited number of possible goal outcomes constrains the experience of emotion, even across development and culture. The achievement of goals is responsible for positive emotion, while the failure or blockage of goals is responsible for negative emotion. These outcomes result in the familiar valenced nature of emotion. Despite the frustration of philosophers in terms of using valence to classify emotion (Charland, 2005), the specific combina-

tions of goals and outcomes associated with each of the five basic emotions remain constant across situations and people. Thus understanding the definition of a goal and the ways goals constrain outcomes is essential for understanding emotion and testing an appraisal theory of emotion and goal-directed action.

In our theory of emotion, a "goal" is defined as a desire to go from one state to another or as a desire to maintain a specific state. A goal may involve any valued object, activity, or state that a person wants to attain or maintain. Goals often occur in conjunction with statements of preference, which almost always include some reference to liking, loving, missing, hating, avoiding, or disliking: "I really like it when we can just spend some quiet time without fighting," " I really hate the way he leaves his room a mess in the morning." A preference may imply a goal, but preference by itself is not a goal. Preferences encode an evaluation of the positive or negative value of something, but need not include the desire to change from one state to another. Preferences reflect the pleasure and displeasure associated with anything of value, but do not necessitate a desire to change from one state to another. Appraising the value of something is necessary but not sufficient for the emergence and pursuit of a goal. People need to decide, either consciously or unconsciously, to pursue a goal that would result in a state concordant with a given preference.

Linguistically, goals can be identified by verbs such as "wish," "want," "decide," "going to do," "try to do," or "must do": "I really wish she didn't interfere so much," "I wish I could make him understand what I want," "I really don't want her to eat so much junk food after school," "I wish he would have a more positive attitude toward helping around the house." Goals can also be identified as the stated reasons or purposes for actions that were taken. Goals or reasons motivate action and are often connected to them by words or phrases such as "to," "for," "so that," or "in order to": For example, "I read some of her favorite books so that she would go to sleep at her proper bedtime."

Even in infancy, at least from the age of 3 months on, children understand emotion-laden events in an organized and systematic way, much as adults do. The basis of their understanding, like that of adults, is dependent upon a continual evaluation and appraisal of incoming information, especially information that is related to personally meaningful goals and to the success or failure of a goal. The critical task is to show that monitoring of a goal occurs very early in infancy, and that emotions occur because of perceived changes in important goals. The use of the word "goal" has been problematic for many researchers, because they envision a goal as something abstract and inaccessible to an infant. However, goals can be very concrete and very simple. The desire to eliminate noxious stimulation (e.g., the desire to stop someone who is restraining an infant's movement), the desire to get out of a state of hunger, the desire to get out of a state of wetness, and the desire for stimulation all have very concrete aspects of goal-directed action attached to them.

The work of Stenberg and Campos (1990), Willatts (1990), and Woodward (1998) all show strong support for infants' sensitivity to goals. Furthermore, the work of Lewis (1990) and his colleagues (Alessandri et al., 1990) shows that very young infants can and do habituate to incoming information, that they are quite good at detecting novelty and discrepancies, and that they respond differently to the onset of different events. As both Sroufe (1979) and Emde (1980) have noted, if we take the time to watch and film infants in dynamic action, infants engage in quite a bit of looking, gaze shifting, and eye contact before they respond emotionally and with action. Their emotional responses do not occur spontaneously or automatically in response to most stimuli. Many emotion expressions occur after prolonged looking or after a switch of attention and more looking. Stenberg and Campos (1990) showed that this is the case when infants express anger at being physically constrained. Thus, in describing the unfolding of action over time, characterizing the looking, attention, and shifts in gaze is critical to determining the nature and sequence of thoughts and actions during the experience of emotion.

EMOTIONAL VERSUS AFFECTIVE RESPONSES

Both infants and adults respond automatically and affectively to certain types of stimuli. Automatic physical responses are generated in a fixed action pattern, without evaluating information. The startle response is one such example. The eye-blinking response is another. These types of responses are seen frequently in children and to some extent less frequently in adults, due to adults' ability to cognitively dampen or inhibit these responses. Affective responses can also include feelings of general distress and are evoked when the speed, intensity, and duration of the stimulus (usually sensory stimulation) are at a high level. Affective responses are evolutionary primitive signals that communicate a state of change in physiological reactivity. The ANS is aroused, with little cognitive activity preceding the arousal.

The important point we wish to make is that automatic responses to sensory input require little or no cognitive evaluation. They are reflexive in nature. Affective feelings require little cognitive evaluation and play an important informational role in indicating the changes that occur either in the environment or in the body. In our theory, however, emotional responses are distinct from automatic, affective, and physical responses, in that emotions require higher-order cognitive processes and encode a plan of action. Affective responses do not require higher-order cognitive responses and do not encode a plan of action.

In our online studies, affective responses precede emotional responses, with the affective responses occurring rapidly in response to an initiating event and resulting in a "stunned" demeanor, followed by evaluation of the incoming information, an emotional response, and a plan of action. A pause almost always occurs between the affective and emotional responses. Appraisals and planning occur after as well as during the experience of emotion (Stein & Boyce, 2005).

Failure to distinguish between affective and emotional responses is one of the most frequent reasons for different stances on the relationship between emotion and thought. A failure to understand how thought gets carried out over the course of emotional experience, where talk is interleaved with nonverbal components of emotional experience, is a second difference in the various emotion and appraisal theories that exist. Researchers like LeDoux (2002) interpret the freezing response that goes along with intense stimulation or the introduction of novelty as an innate action that gets carried out in the service of protecting an animal or human being.

In our theory, freezing is a response that automatically occurs without cognitive evaluation or planning. Freezing may occur because the incoming stimulation has triggered an intense ANS response that momentarily inhibits access to any thinking and planning. As the intensity of the physiological response declines, however, access to planning and thinking is reinstated. If animals and humans engage in behaviors such as "flight or fight," we posit that some form of evaluation or goal-directed planning precedes the flight or fight response of an animal. The timing and unfolding of the flight or fight response are critical, as is the measurement of thinking.

Despite the fact that many situations engender very rapid action responses in animals and humans, rapid cognitive evaluations can precede almost any directed action pattern. The speed with which cognitive processes get carried out is extremely fast—just as fast as, or faster than, access to a motor plan of action. Many cognitive processes are parallel in nature, and are in part unconscious and automatic. To withdraw from a painful stimulus requires the retrieval of a plan of action for withdrawal. Without the plan, extreme distress occurs in reaction to pain, along with body writhing, but no withdrawal action will be carried out. Similarly, approaching something requires an evaluation of the object being approached, as well as a plan of action. The focus of attention needs to be shifted toward the object being approached, and the object needs to be constantly monitored in order to keep the target on the path of approach. Gaze behavior, a shift in attention, and the speed of attack all suggest that rapid evaluation of the situation has been carried out. The important point is to acknowledge the speed with which cognitive processes get carried out, especially since many of the cognitive processes are automatic and unconscious.

To determine whether emotion precedes thinking and evaluation in any critical fashion, we need to focus on unfolding in a dynamic fashion all of the behaviors that get carried out in reaction to an initiating event that begins the sequence of emotional experience. We must also determine whether distinctions between emotional and affective responding are valid. Distress, startle, surprise, and stun responses are not considered emotions in our theory, because a plan of action is not encoded in any of these responses. As we have illustrated in both our nonverbal and verbal data, distress responses almost always precede emotional responses and goal-directed action. Furthermore, the expression of startle or surprise always pre-

cedes the expression of fear (Stein & Boyce, 2005), if startle and surprise occur in the same emotion sequence.

When children experienced a fire alarm going off, Stein and Boyce (2005) were able to monitor talk, emotion experience, and expression, as well as heart rate and blood pressure, throughout a 10-minute session. They were also able to collect retrospective memory accounts of the fire alarm experience, so that accuracy for emotion experience and the events surrounding the fire alarm could be evaluated. Stein and Boyce found that of the 24 children participating in their study, 22 expressed some type of emotion in reaction to the fire alarm's going off. Of those children who expressed an emotion, 8 out of 22 expressed the affective state of surprise, followed by either fear or happiness. Surprise was always followed by the expression of an emotional state.

Furthermore, children who were classified as "low reactors" (i.e., their heart rate and blood pressure decreased as a function of the fire alarm's going off) were more likely to be the ones who experienced an affective state coupled with an emotion. Seventy-five percent of the low reactors expressed startle, compared to 25% of the "high reactors." A second difference between the high and low reactors was in the length of time that affective states and emotions were expressed. The average length of time that an affective or emotion state was expressed by low reactors was 5 seconds, compared to 11.5 seconds for high reactors. Thus the expressive time for high reactors was twice as long as that for low reactors. After the fire alarm was turned off, significant differences between high and low reactors were still apparent. Over half of the low reactors expressed no emotion after the alarm went off, whereas 84% of the high reactors continued to express an emotion state and did not return to a neutral stance.

The affective response of startle was always followed by more scanning of the environment, and then fear responses were expressed. The fixed nature of this sequence suggests strongly that affective responses are mechanisms that further alert the cognitive and physiological systems that something has changed. However, further appraisal and scanning were necessary to encode exactly what had changed, after which an emotion was expressed. The length of time varied in terms of the duration of emotion, and half of the children had difficulty returning to a baseline stance.

These findings underscore the fact the significant individual differences are expressed in the ability to think and plan during emotional experience. Although emotions do encode plans of action, and very rapid action can be taken when emotions are experienced, the person experiencing the emotion may not be able to solve the problem or cope with the emotion situation in a constructive fashion. The fact that arousal remained high for half of the children in the fire alarm study, especially for high reactors, suggests that more reflective planning may not be available until arousal returns to normal.

UNFOLDING APPRAISAL PROCESSES FOR EMOTIONS

Since all current models of emotion (see Frijda, 2005, and Sandler et al., 2005, for examples of other appraisal models) argue for the use of an appraisal system that regulates emotional responses, it becomes imperative that appraisals be clearly defined, described, and identified, so that tests of an appraisal theory can be made and compared to theories that do not posit the necessity of appraisals. As we discuss our model of the appraisal process, we highlight the differences between our model and those of other researchers.

Our model includes descriptions of the content of appraisals, as well as descriptions of how children and adults are similar to and different from one another. We require that processes of emotion be described as they unfold over time, in real situations. We need to determine the sequence of processes that get carried out, which ones occur in parallel with others, and which ones occur in a temporal sequence. Without these data, we cannot test the crucial hypotheses associated with different theories of emotion and appraisal.

Elsewhere, we and our associates have described the appraisal and planning processes that evoke emotions such as happiness, sadness, anger, fear, and disgust (Stein & Hernandez, 2007; Stein & Jewett, 1986; Stein & Levine, 1987, 1989, 1990; Stein & Trabasso, 1992; Stein et al., 1993, 2000). The specific content of the appraisal process that leads to different emotional experiences indicates how appraisals of each emotion are unique in relation to other emotions. Unlike Ortony and Turner (1990) and Johnson-Laird and Oatley (1989, 1992), who believe that single components of the appraisal process can elicit an emotion, we believe that at least three goal outcome evaluations must be inferred and necessary for any one specific emotion to be experienced. First, an evaluation must be made about the certainty or uncertainty of goal attainment (did a goal fail, succeed, or remain uncertain/threatened?). Second, an evaluation must be made about whether a goal state can be reinstated, maintained, avoided, or protected. Third, an evaluation of the outcome and of the future possibilities for goal success or failure is crucial for the experience of an emotion.

The presence of a novel or unexpected element in an event must also be detected. Novelty signals that some component of the emotion situation is unexpected and requires immediate attention and immediate processing. The necessity of novelty or an unexpected element in an ongoing event was seminal to both Mandler's (1975, 1984) and Gray's (1971; 1990) descriptions of emotion processing. Scherer (1984) picked up on the importance of novelty in emotion processes, but never gave an explanatory analysis of why he chose to incorporate novelty into his theory of appraisals. Frijda (1988) argued for the necessity of considering habituation (repeated processing of the same event) in relation to emotion and novelty, but never provided empirical evidence to answer his question of what happens to thinking and emotion when an event is repeated over time. Frijda concluded that one habituates to events that cause joy and pleasure, but does not get used to aversive events, harassment, or humiliation (i.e., the law of hedonic asymmetry).

The data from our repeated-event study (Stein & Trabasso, 1989) showed that some children habituated to both painful and pleasant events. The repetition of a painful event allows an increase in tolerance for a particular type of stimulation, so that the meaning and seriousness of the painful event change. Training soldiers for war is a good example of people's becoming habituated to events that are initially painful, aversive, and noxious, but over time become less painful, even when intense horror and pain are initially perceived. The key to whether habituation or nonhabituation occurs lies in the meaning given to an event, the context in which the event is interpreted, and the intensity of pain that the event causes.

During habituation, events that were initially interpreted as horrific can be appraised as acceptable and necessary to the final achievement of an important goal. The dropping of a nuclear bomb is a good example. So is killing a person at short range. Indeed, a major problem that the armed forces of any country must confront is the challenge of debriefing soldiers and providing them with the necessary psychological and physical training to desist in the use of certain appraisal strategies that are appropriate for coping with harm on the battlefield, but do not work in civil society.

In terms of testing whether the perception of novelty is required for an emotion to be experienced, however, a repeated-event paradigm is an excellent way to assess how thought relates to emotion. Emotions do not occur without some type of internal or external event's impinging on an organism, both psychologically and physiologically. If novelty is a necessary component of emotion, then over time, as a person gets used to and encodes the basic structure of a presented event, one of two things should happen. If the person adds no new meaning to the incoming information from a repeated event, then the person should desist from responding emotionally as the event is presented repeatedly. A neutral stance should emerge without any emotion. If, however, new meaning is inferred from observing a repeated event, so that the event is now connected to new information not accessed previously, an emotional response should continue to be experienced and expressed.

This is exactly what happened in the Stein and Trabasso (1989) study. When repeatedly presented with an event that ended in a positive or negative outcome, some children gave emotional responses of lessening intensity, while other children stopped expressing emotion altogether. Some children, however, continued to give emotional responses that were as strong as, or stronger than, their reaction the first time the event was presented. When asked why they responded with such strength, all children mentioned the focus of attention on a novel element that for them was unexpected. That is, they linked the information from the focal event to new information that had consequences for personally relevant goals, *not previously noted on their first exposure to the event*. Thus new appraisals were made about an event despite the repeated nature of the event. Whether or not habituation occurred depended upon the interpretation of the event and the goals the perceiver brought to the situation. Furthermore, it was possible to habituate to negative events as well as positive events, and it was also possible to interpret a repeated positive or negative event in a new light, despite the frequency of presentation. The crucial element was the meaning attributed to an event.

Although emotions such as happiness, anger, sadness, and fear by no means encompass the spectrum of possible emotions, we have used them as examples because, along with disgust, these five emotions represent a set of emotions found in some form in every known culture. Each of these emotions corresponds to a particular goal–outcome combination in terms of whether or not valued goals have failed or been fulfilled (Stein et al., 1993, 2000). Although the exact label given to each of these five emotion states may vary across development and culture (e.g., "angry," "mad," "furious"), the goal outcomes, initial desires, and types of appraisals associated with each of the five emotions do not vary.

CONSTRAINTS ON THE MENTAL REPRESENTATIONS AND LANGUAGE OF EMOTION

The mapping of specific types of goal outcomes onto each emotion is hard and fast. Emotion categories do not have fuzzy boundaries, as initially suggested by Shaver, Schwartz, O'Connor, and Kirson (1987). When anger is experienced, the event under consideration has to have led to the failure of an important goal or the inability to avoid an aversive state. Furthermore, the person experiencing anger has to believe that the focal goal can somehow be reinstated, that an aversive state can be removed, or that the source of goal failure can be removed. These types of inferences remain necessary over age and culture, despite variation in the specific events under consideration or the society's approval or disapproval in regard to the actions carried out in the service of a goal.

The language associated with emotional experience is also highly constrained. We (Stein & Hernandez, 2007) have illustrated that people use a very restricted range of emotion terminology when they freely narrate a past event. The constraints hold for adults (Stein et al., 2001) as well as for children (Stein & Hernandez, 2007). In analyzing over 1,000 narrative accounts from both adults and children, we found that the range and frequency of negative emotions were focused on 12 specific emotion states. Four emotion terms and their variants ("sad," "angry," "afraid," "anxious") accounted for 95% of all expressed negative emotions during talk about stressful, traumatic, or unexpected events. Similarly, three emotion terms and their variants ("happy," "hopeful," "relieved") accounted for over 97% of all expressed positive emotions during such talk. These data provide strong evidence that a small set of emotion terms is used to describe all types of stressful experiences.

Most of the time, the emotional terminology of adults in describing ongoing or past events is highly similar to the language of children. Adults produce more mental state and emotion language than children do, but the same categories of words are used. Adults' and children's emotion narratives, in terms of the presence of mental state beliefs, are also similar. Three-year-old children produced statements in every mental and internal state category that was proposed in the Stein and Hernandez (2007) study. Thus, before we conclude that emotional experience is infinitely varied over development and time, we need data from real-world experiences, where adults and children actually use emotion and mental state language that has not been constrained by any particular instrument or theory.

Finally, the analysis of children's emotional accounts elicited during an ongoing event (Stein & Hernandez, 2007), or told retrospectively right after the event has occurred (Stein & Boyce, 2005), show that 3-year-old children have a far greater understanding of events than has been evident in more experimental studies, where children are presented with events that are somewhat unfamiliar to them or events that they have not actually experienced. When very young children talk about events they have actually experienced (Levine, Stein, & Liwag, 1999; Stein & Albro, 2001), they narrate with the precision and complexity of older children, and sometimes with far more detail than their parents do. Furthermore, when children are in conflict with their parents, and are asked to give both their account as well as their parents' account of the conflict, children are often more accurate about their parents' emotions and mental states than parents are about their children's mental states (Stein & Hernandez, 2007).

The rapid development of emotional understanding, in terms of the mental representations used to understand and respond to emotion events (Stein & Albro, 1997), strongly suggests that much of the structure needed to understand emotional interaction is well in place by late infancy, before children are using language freely to communicate what they want and know about emotion situations. The data also suggest that theories of emotion formulated by testing only adults will need testing on children to determine whether the processes of emotion posited in the theory also hold for children.

Learning and Emotional Experience

As a function of attending to novel information, learning almost always results during emotional experience. Some type of violation of expectation always occurs before the experience of emotion, and the violation signals that currently held beliefs are incorrect (Stein & Jewett, 1986; Stein & Levine, 1987, 1989). In an effort to understand the consequences of succeeding or failing to attain their goals, people are forced to revise and update their beliefs about two dimensions: (1) what the probability is of maintaining their goals under a new set of circumstances; and (2) whether or not they can generate a plan that will lead to successful goal maintenance, reinstatement, or revision. For example, when people fail to maintain or attain a desired goal state, they attend to the conditions that prevented them from being successful, the consequences of their failure, and the probability of generating a plan of action to overcome goal failure. This sequence characterizes both adults' and children's emotional responses (Capatides, 1989; Stein & Levine, 1989; Stein & Hernandez, 2007), as well as parents' descriptions and responses to their children's emotional behaviors (Capatides, 1989; Levine et al., 1999).

In updating knowledge about viable conditions that lead to goal success or failure, people may change the value they have imputed to a particular set of goals. That is, when a person attains or fails to attain a goal, the value associated with that and other goals may increase or decrease in strength. As a result, people often forfeit their goals, or they may intensify their efforts to achieve them, depending on the new value that these goals now possess.

In privileging intentional action as a core part of our theory, we are assuming that people have a built-in mechanism that allows them to represent goal–action–outcome sequences in relationship to the maintenance of goals

(Gallistel, 1985; Piaget, 1981; Stein & Levine, 1987, 1990; Stein et al., 1993, 2000). Even infants are able to infer and represent the causal conditions that produce actions resulting in certain outcomes, and they are able to use this knowledge to achieve goals (Woodward, 1998). Thus, when a change in goal status occurs and emotions are experienced, a revised goal is accessed and a plan is developed. Creating or accessing a plan that specifies the conditions necessary to achieve a goal provides an opportunity for coping with goal failure. Similarly, constructing and carrying out a plan enable the maintenance of a goal, once the goal has been achieved.

There are situations, however, where little planning occurs or where plans are not easily available and retrieved. Intense emotional experience often precludes access to certain types of information (Stein & Boyce, 1997, 2005). Under these conditions, critical inferences about the emotion situation are not made. Thus the intensity of an emotional experience and the associated sensory and physiological feedback become important variables in predicting the thinking, decision making, and quality of planning that take place during an emotional experience.

MEMORY FOR EMOTIONAL EVENTS

Although there are reports that emotional involvement enhances the accuracy of memory for events (Burke, Heuer, & Reisberg, 1992; Goodman, 1991), this is not always the case (Peters, 1991; Rachman, 1978). Depending upon the intensity of the emotional response and the necessity to take action, memory for the external events surrounding the emotion can be diminished or facilitated. The relationship among memory, thinking, and emotion, then, must be stipulated according to the specific circumstances that constrain the experience.

Stein and Boyce (1997, 2005) reported that memory for a stressful event (a real-life fire alarm experience) is regulated in part by the physiological reactivity of the individual child involved. Those children who responded to the stressful event with an increase in heart rate and blood pressure had poorer memories for the event than those children who responded with a decrease in heart rate and blood pressure. Children's attention and emotional re-

sponses, as well as their memory, were also a function of whether their heart rate and blood pressure increased or decreased in response to a stressful event. Children whose heart rate increased as a function of the fire alarm had less accurate memory for their emotional response and less accurate memory for the events that occurred before and after the fire alarm went off.

Three types of memory were evaluated: the number of clauses occurring in free recall, the number of clauses occurring in probed recall, and the number of explanatory statements given throughout the recall of the fire alarm experience. Children who were identified as low reactors recalled more clauses in both spontaneous and probed recall, compared to children labeled as high reactors. Furthermore, children labeled as low reactors also gave more explanations or sought more explanations throughout the fire alarm experience than children labeled as high reactors.

The fact that low- and high-reacting children had different quantities of memory, and the fact that these two groups of children also experienced emotions for different lengths of time, serve as evidence for the absolute necessity of beginning to link physiological and neurological processes to cognitive activity during the experience of an emotion. The fact that low-reacting children rarely lost sight of new incoming information, compared to high-reacting children (who were often stunned and experienced a startle response), may indicate that emotional events are processed differently as a function of reactivity, right from the beginning of an event. Stein and Boyce found that once heart rate and blood pressure were raised, they stayed raised for about 45 minutes and did not decrease or increase quickly. These changes indicate that an intense emotional experience may regulate behavior far in advance.

CONCLUSION

The appraisal model that we advocate requires that we try to unfold the temporal properties of thinking and emotion as they occur in real time throughout an emotional experience. The failure to use and present online data for psychological, physiological, and neurological processes severely limits the accuracy of what is said about the relationship between emotion and thought, as well as our ability to link the psychological, physiological, and neurological processes that get carried out during emotional experience. The fact that the experience of emotion is not recognized as a basic component associated with learning also limits how much we understand about the function of emotion. If belief violations occur every time an emotion is experienced (current data on emotion strongly supports this viewpoint), then we need to be focused on ways in which emotion regulates and affects learning and the ability to change.

The data that we have presented in this chapter show that the thinking and learning processes, as well as the affective and physiological processes surrounding emotion experience, are far more complex than most emotion researchers have described. Cognitive processing occurs much more rapidly than many researchers think, and the temporality of cognitive and physiological processes has yet to be elucidated in the necessary depth. Unfolding the timing of cognitive and affective variables further shows the need to acknowledge the multilayered properties of both processes. What we have argued for is the existence of two very different types of affective processes. The first occurs in an automatic fashion, as a function of incoming information and a change in ANS levels. These responses need little or no cortical input, and are not considered emotional responses. They have no plans of action attached to them. Emotional responses include affective responses, but they occur because of the appraisal of personally meaningful goals. They also encode a plan of action.

We have further shown that despite the variation in the language used to verbally express different emotions, everyday emotion language used to describe personally meaningful events is constrained to the five basic emotions plus or minus a few others. These constraints are important, because they reflect the constraints put on problem solving, planning, and behavior. Certain types of appraisals and plans will occur only with certain types of emotions, and this specificity is seen in children as young as 3 years, as well as in mature adults.

Finally, the link between physiological indicators of reactivity (heart rate and blood pressure) and memory has been shown to be significant. Although most researchers would predict that the experience of emotion is always correlated with a rise in blood pressure and heart rate, this is not the case. Bauer, Quas, and Boyce (2002)

and Jacobson and Gottman (1998) have shown that both increases and decreases in heart rate occur in response to emotion-eliciting information. The Stein and Boyce (1997) data further indicate that the control of attention and subsequent encoding processes are affected by whether an increase or decrease occurs in heart rate and blood pressure. Linking these different physiological responses to brain activity during the experience of emotion would allow us to understand better the variation in responses to emotion-eliciting stimuli. It may be that planning and thinking are not as greatly disrupted during emotional experience in low reactors as they are in high reactors. This would explain the different reports and beliefs about the salience of emotion-laden memories in terms of their accuracy. It would also allow us to better understand the connection between thought and emotion, in terms of how emotion regulates thought and vice versa.

REFERENCES

Alessandri, S. M., Sullivan, M. W., & Lewis, M. (1990). Violation of expectancy and frustration in early infancy. *Developmental Psychology, 26*(5), 738–744.

Arnold, M. B. (1960a). *Emotions and personality: Vol. 1. Psychological aspects.* New York: Columbia University Press.

Arnold, M. B. (1960b). *Emotions and personality: Vol. 2. Neurological and physiological aspects.* New York: Columbia University Press.

Bauer, A. M., Quas, J. A., & Boyce, W. T. (2002). Associations between physiological reactivity and children's behavior: Advantages of a multisystem approach. *Journal of Developmental and Behavioral Pediatrics, 23*(2), 102–113.

Burke, A., Heuer, F., & Reisberg, D. (1992). Remembering emotional events. *Memory and Cognition, 20*(3), 277–290.

Capatides, J. (1989). *Mothers' socialization of children's affect expression.* Unpublished doctoral dissertation, Columbia University, New York.

Charland, L. C. (2005). The heat of emotion: Valence and the demarcation problem. *Journal of Consciousness Studies, 12*(8–10), 82–102.

Emde, R. (1980). Levels of meaning in infant development. In W. A. Collins (Ed.), *Minnesota Symposium on Child Psychology* (Vol. 13, pp. 1–38). Hillsdale, NJ: Erlbaum.

Folkman, S., & Stein, N. L. (1997). The analysis of belief and goal processes during reports of stressful events by caregivers of men with AIDS. In N. L. Stein, P. A. Ornstein, B. Tversky, & C. Brainerd (Eds.), *Memory for everyday and emotional events* (pp. 113–138). Hillsdale, NJ: Erlbaum.

Frijda, N. H. (1987). Emotion, cognitive structure, and action tendency. *Cognition and Emotion, 1,* 115–143.

Frijda, N. (1988). The laws of emotion. *American Psychologist, 43*(5), 349–358.

Frijda, N. (2005). Emotion experience. *Cognition and Emotion, 19*(4), 473–497.

Gallistel, C. R. (1985). Motivation, intention, and emotion: Goal-directed behavior froma cognitive neuroethological perspective. In M. Frese & J. Sabini (Eds.), *Goal-directed behavior: The concept of action in psychology* (pp. 48–66). Hillsdale, NJ: Erlbaum.

Goodman, G. S. (1991). Commentary: On stress and accuracy in research in children's testimony. In J. Doris (Ed.), *The suggestibility of children's recollections* (pp. 77–82). Washington, DC: American Psychological Association.

Gray, J. A. (1971). *The psychology of fear and stress.* London: Weidenfeld & Nicolson.

Gray, J. A. (1990). Psychobiological aspects of relationships between emotions and cognition [Special issue]. *Cognition and Emotion, 4.*

Jacobson, N., & Gottman, J. (1998). *When men batter women.* New York: Simon & Schuster.

Johnson-Laird, P. N., & Oatley, K. (1989). The language of emotions: An analysis of a semantic field. *Cognition and Emotion, 3*(2), 81–123.

Johnson-Laird, P. N., & Oatley, K. (1992). Basic emotions, rationality, and folk theory. *Cognition and Emotion, 6*(3–4), 201–223.

Lazarus, R. S. (1982). Thoughts on the relations between emotion and cognition. *American Psychologist, 37,* 1019–1024.

Lazarus, R. S. (1984). On the primacy of cognition. *American Psychologist, 39*(2), 124–129.

Lazarus, R. S. (1991). *Emotion and adaptation.* New York: Oxford University Press.

LeDoux, J. (2002). *Synaptic self.* New York: Viking.

Levine, L., Stein, N. L., & Liwag, M. (1999). Remembering children's emotions: Sources of concordant and discordant accounts between parents and children. *Developmental Psychology, 5*(3), 210–230.

Lewis, M. (1990). The development of intentionality and the role of consciousness. *Psychological Inquiry, 1*(3), 231–247.

Liwag, M. D., & Stein, N. L. (1995). Children's memory for emotion episodes: The importance of emotion enactment cues. *Journal of Experimental Child Psychology, 60,* 2–31.

Mandler, G. (1975). *Mind and emotion.* New York: Wiley.

Mandler, G. (1984). *Mind and body: Psychology of emotion and stress.* New York: Norton.

Miller, G. A., Galanter, E., & Pribram, K. H. (1960). *Plans and the structure of behavior.* New York: Holt, Rinehart & Winston.

Oatley, K., & Johnson-Laird, P. N. (1987). Towards a cognitive theory of emotions. *Cognition and Emotion, 1*(1), 29–50.

Ortony, A., & Turner, T. J. (1990). What's basic about basic emotion? *Psychological Review, 97,* 315–331.

Peters, D. (1991). The influence of stress and arousal on the child witness. In J. Doris (Ed.), *The suggestibility of children's recollections* (pp. 60–76). Washington, DC: American Psychological Association.

Piaget, J. (1981). *Intelligence and affectivity.* Palo Alto, CA: Annual Reviews.

Rachman, S. J. (1978). *Fear and courage.* San Francisco: Freeman.

Roseman, I. (1984). Cognitive determinants of emotion: A structural theory. *Review of Personality and Social Psychology,* 11–36.

Roseman, I. (1991). Appraisal determinants of discrete emotions. *Cognition and Emotion, 5*(3), 161–200.

Ross, H., Ross, M., Stein, N. L., & Trabasso, T. (2007). How siblings negotiate and resolve their conflicts. *Child Development, 77*(6), 1730–1745.

Sandler, D., Grandjean, D., & Scherer, K. R. (2005). A systems approach to appraisal mechanisms in emotion. *Neural Networks, 18,* 317–352.

Scherer, K. R. (1984). On the nature and function of emotion: A component process approach. In K. R. Scherer & P. Ekman (Eds.), *Approaches to emotion* (pp. 293–318). Hillsdale, NJ: Erlbaum.

Shaver, P., Schwartz, J., O'Connor, C., & Kirson, D. (1987). Emotion knowledge: Further explanations of a prototype approach. *Journal of Personality and Social Psychology, 52,* 1016–1086.

Sroufe, A. (1979). Socioemotional development. In J. Osofsky (Ed.), *Handbook of infant development* (pp. 462–516). New York: Wiley.

Stein, N. L., & Albro, E. R. (1997). The emergence of narrative understanding: Evidence for rapid learning in personally relevant contexts. *Contemporary Issues in Education, 60,* 83–98.

Stein, N. L., & Albro, E. R. (2001). The origins and nature of arguments: Studies in conflict understanding, emotion, and negotiation. *Discourse Processes, 32*(2&3), 113–133.

Stein, N. L., & Boyce, W. T. (1997). *The role of individual differences in reactivity and attention in accounting for on-line and retrospective memory.* Paper presented at the biennial meeting of the Society for Research in Child Development, Washington, DC.

Stein, N. L., & Boyce, W. T. (2005). *The unfolding of children's emotional experience in response to a stressful event: How reactivity influences emotion.* Unpublished manuscript, University of Chicago.

Stein, N. L., & Hernandez, M. W. (2007). Assessing emotional understanding in narrative on-line interviews: The use of the Narcoder. In J. A. Coan & J. J. B. Allen (Eds.), *Handbook of emotion elicitation and assessment* (pp. 298–317). New York: Oxford University Press.

Stein, N. L., & Jewett, J. (1986). A conceptual analysis of the meaning of negative emotions: Implications for a theory of development. In C. Izard & P. Read (Eds.), *Measuring emotions in infants and children* (Vol. 2, pp. 238–267). Cambridge, UK: Cambridge University Press.

Stein, N. L., & Levine, L. (1987). Thinking about feelings: The development and organization of emotional knowledge. In R. Snow & M. Farr (Eds.), *Aptitude, learning, and instruction* (Vol. 3, pp. 165–197). Hillsdale, NJ: Erlbaum.

Stein, N. L., & Levine, L. (1989). The causal organization of emotional knowledge: A developmental study. *Cognition and Emotion, 3*(4), 343–378.

Stein, N. L., & Levine, L. (1990). Making sense out of emotion: The representation and use of goal structured knowledge. In N. L. Stein, B. Leventhal, & T. Trabasso (Eds.), *Psychological and biological approaches to emotion* (pp. 45–73). Hillsdale, NJ: Erlbaum.

Stein, N. L., & Levine, L. J. (1999). The early emergence of emotional understanding and appraisal. Implications for theories of development. In T. Dalgleish & M. Power (Eds.), *Handbook of cognition and emotion* (pp. 383–410). Chicester: Wiley.

Stein, N. L., & Oatley, K. (1992). Basic emotions: Theory and measurement. *Cognition and Emotion, 6*(3–4), 161–168.

Stein, N. L., Sheldrick, R., & Broaders, S. (1999). Predicting psychological well-being from beliefs and goal appraisal processes during the experience of emotional events. In S. Goldman, P. L. Van den Broek, & A. Graesser (Eds.), *Essays in honor of Tom Trabasso* (pp. 279–302). Mahwah, NJ: Erlbaum.

Stein, N. L., & Trabasso, T. (1989). Children's understanding of changing emotion states. In C. Saarni & P. L. Harris (Eds.), *Children's understanding of emotion* (pp. 50–77). New York: Cambridge University Press.

Stein, N. L., & Trabasso, T. (1992). The organization of emotional experience: Creating links among emotion, thinking and intentional action. *Cognition and Emotion, 6*(3–4), 225–244.

Stein, N. L., Trabasso, T., & Albro, E. R. (2001). Understanding and organizing emotional experience: Auto-biographical accounts of traumatic events. *English Studies of America, 19*(1), 111–130.

Stein, N. L., Trabasso, T., & Liwag, M. (1993). The representation and organization of emotional experience. Unfolding the emotional episode. In M. Lewis & J. Haviland (Eds.), *Handbook of emotions* (pp. 279–300). New York: Guilford Press.

Stein, N. L., Trabasso, T., & Liwag, M. D. (2000). A goal appraisal theory of emotional understanding: Implications for development and learning. In M. Lewis & J. M. Haviland-Jones (Eds.), *Handbook of emotions* (2nd ed., pp. 436–457). New York: Guilford Press.

Stenberg, C. R., & Campos, J. J. (1990). The development of anger expressions in infancy. In N. L. Stein, B. Leventhal, & T. Trabasso (Eds.), *Psychological and biological approaches to emotion* (pp. 247–282). Hillsdale, NJ: Erlbaum.

Trabasso, T., & Stein, N. L. (1993). How do we represent both emotional experience and meaning?: A review of Richard Lazarus' *Emotion and Adaptation,* New York: Oxford University Press, 1991. *Psychological Inquiry, 41*(4), 326–333.

Trabasso, T., Stein, N. L., & Johnson, L. R. (1981). Children's knowledge of events: A causal analysis of story structure. In G. Bower (Ed.), *Learning and motivation* (Vol. 15, pp. 237–282). New York: Academic Press.

Willatts, P. (1990). The development of problem-solving strategies in infancy. In D. Bjorklund (Ed.), *Children's strategies: Contemporary views of cognitive development* (pp. 23–66). Hillsdale, NJ: Erlbaum.

Woodward, A. (1998). Infants selectively code the goal object of an actor's reach. *Cognition, 69,* 1–34.

Zajonc, R. (1980). Feeling and thinking: Preferences need no inferences. *American Psychologist, 35,* 151–175.

CHAPTER 36

Emotion Concepts

PAULA M. NIEDENTHAL

"Concepts" are mental representations of categories of entities (natural and artifactual), situations, experience, and action. Cognitive scientists study concepts because they are used in most acts of cognition—including high-level processes such as thinking, reasoning, and language use, and also lower-level processes such as perception, attention, and recognition. Supporting the vast literature in cognitive psychology, the social-psychological literature reports evidence that concepts facilitate encoding, memory retrieval processes (e.g., Cohen, 1981), and the ability to make inferences about never-before-seen entities (e.g., Cantor & Mischel, 1977). When, in a crowded train station, I suddenly "see" my husband carrying our child, I am relying on my concepts of my husband and child to categorize the input as these particular people. Other experiences with the social world also involve concept use. Understanding another person's emotions and knowing how the emotions have come about and what we might do to alter or celebrate them also involves the use of concepts. So does perceiving a facial display as an expression of dis-

gust or contempt. These phenomena are supported by emotion concepts—the topic of interest in the present chapter.

Emotion concepts are not only fundamental for an understanding of the social world; they are fundamental to the development of an individual's behavioral repertoire. One of the most compelling examples of this (an example to which I will return) is that of instructed fear learning. If I tell my son that a certain object or event would be painful or frightening to encounter, he can, even at a relatively early point in cognitive development, avoid that object or event without ever having to experience the pain or fear with which it is (held to be) associated. The example of instructed fear learning is noteworthy, because it demonstrates that individuals' concepts of "fear" or "pain" are sufficiently powerful to determine future behavior. This observation suggests that the understanding of emotion concepts is vital for a full account of human behavior.

It should be noted in starting that in order to study emotion concepts at all, theorists have had to decide on the set of categories that they are working with. What are the categories of emotion? How can we specify the "natural kinds" to which emotion concepts refer? Or can we (Barrett, 2006)? Because scientists are able to point to cats and trees and furniture in the perceivable world, and even to measure their physical properties, they can be in reasonable agreement about the existence of and labels for these and many other natural-kind and artifactual categories (within a culture). They can then ask in experimental research: What are the properties of such categories that are preserved in individuals' concepts; how are the properties and related concepts structured in memory; and how are the concepts used to understand newly encountered category instances (e.g., Lamberts & Shanks, 1997)? The same is not true of emotions. Some parts of an emotion can be seen, such as a facial expression or a posture, but others cannot. Theorists and laypeople disagree about the categories that accurately cut emotional experience at its joints. So how do scientists proceed in the study of emotion concepts when there is no a priori agreement about the categories that constitute the domain of interest?

There are two ways in which this decision has been made by scientists interested in emotion concepts. One is an empirical method. In this case, many things that could be "an emotion" are studied (usually represented by words), and then the underlying conceptual structure is empirically derived (e.g., Ortony, Clore, & Foss, 1987; Shaver, Schwartz, Kirson, & O'Connor, 1987). The most fully developed account of emotion concepts that relies on this method is the dimensional approach, in which, as we shall see, the underlying structure is derived by the application of various scaling methods to judgments about emotional states and emotional objects. Other approaches, such as semantic-primitives and the semantic-network accounts, rely on evidence in favor of the existence of certain irreducible, perhaps biologically basic emotions (evidence concerned with possible structures for the set of emotion concepts is reviewed in Barrett, 2006, and Niedenthal, Krauth-Gruber, & Ric, 2006, as well as in several chapters of the present handbook). These approaches then try to define the conceptual content for what people appear to explicitly "know" about a set of categories so chosen, rather than what they apparently know, as revealed by scaling studies.

In their explicit knowledge about emotion, individuals seem to know about at least three classes of information. First, people's concepts contain information about the situational antecedents or elicitors of emotions. Individuals know that seeing an oncoming car lose control and head directly at one's own car most often elicits fear (though it can also elicit exhilaration, for example). Second, such concepts contain information about the actions that are likely to be taken when a given emotion is experienced. Thus people know that fear in humans is often associated with an avoidance or a flight response from the situation. Third, concepts contain information about the introspective states that constitute the "hot" component of emotions. So people know, for instance, that fear is associated with very negative and highly aroused feelings, with a high heart rate, and often with sweating and trembling (Rimé, Philippot, & Cisamolo, 1990). A complete model of emotion concepts must be able to account for the representation of all three types of knowledge (most desirably in a parsimonious way), as well as for the differences between what people say they know about emotion and what is revealed by objective measures of parts of emotional experience (Philippot, 1991).

To preview what follows, the first part of this chapter reviews ways in which emotion concepts have been characterized in the literature. These approaches include dimensional, semantic-primitive, prototype, and semantic-network models. After briefly describing these accounts, I discuss some of the assumptions about representation upon which they are more or less explicitly based. By and large, these accounts view the conceptual system as encapsulated from perceptual (input) and motor (output) systems, and thus as a disembodied system of amodal, abstract symbols. An alternative account, an "embodied-simulation" account, is then presented. Evidence in favor of the idea that concepts in general and emotion concepts in particular are embodied (and what that means) is discussed in greater detail.

EMOTION CONCEPTS AS COMPOSED OF IRREDUCIBLE DIMENSIONS OF MEANING

As mentioned, one way to determine how emotions are conceptualized is to find the basic dimensions underlying the ways in which individuals make judgments about different aspects of emotions, including the co-occurrences of emotions and the perceived similarity in their various components. This approach does not deny that emotion concepts can be more nuanced and contain further information (as in the prototype account discussed later). But the concern is to uncover the fundamental or irreducible features of emotion concepts. Such dimensions have been referred to as the "primary dimensions of meaning," and they were originally thought to include "evaluation," "activity," and "potency" (Osgood & Suci, 1955).

More recently, researchers taking this approach have endorsed a two-dimensional account of emotion knowledge (e.g., Barrett & Russell, 1999; Larsen & Diener, 1992; Mayer & Gaschke, 1988; Russell & Barrett, 1999; Watson & Tellegen, 1985). The two dimensions, with some differences in how they are believed to be related to each other, correspond to the degree to which a state is "pleasant" versus "unpleasant" and the degree to which a state is experienced as "activated" versus "deactivated." The evidence in favor of a two-dimensional structure of emotion concepts is interpreted as meaning that states that are labeled as "fear" and "anger" are understood in terms of the degree of pleasure and activation that typically characterize them. For example, "anger" is conceptualized as highly unpleasant and moderately activated. And many states of "fear" are conceptualized as moderately unpleasant and highly activated (see, e.g., Russell & Barrett, 1999, and Russell & Mehrabian, 1977, for specific empirical demonstrations of these descriptions).

Although relevant research has repeatedly revealed a two-dimensional structure, the meaning of the dimensions and the relationships between them have not been interpreted in precisely the same way by different theorists. Figure 36.1 depicts the ways that the two dimensions have been interpreted in three theories. As the figure illustrates, although the terms that have been employed differ somewhat, Russell (1980; Barrett & Russell, 1999) and Larsen and Diener (1992) both consider the two underlying dimensions of emotion to be something akin to "pleasantness" and "activation." In contrast, although Watson and Tellegen (1985) also find a two-dimensional structure, these researchers propose that a rotation of the axis of the observed factors by 45 degrees constitutes the best characterization of it. Specifically, while two dimensions—"pleas-

antness" versus "unpleasantness" and what they call "engagement" versus "disengagement" (which can be considered a reinterpretation of the activation dimension)—emerge from their data, they hold that the dimensions of theoretical interest lie 45 degrees between those axes, and should be labeled "negative activation" (high to low) and "positive activation" (high to low) (Watson, Wiese, Vaidya, & Tellegen, 1999). In the original Watson and Tellegen paper, these dimensions were called "positive affect" and "negative affect." In this view, fundamental emotion concepts contain the notion of being engaged in an experience while feeling unpleasant and highly activated ("negative activation") and the notion of being engaged in an experience and feeling pleasant and highly activated ("positive activation").

In support of their interpretation, Tellegen, Watson, and their colleagues note that most of the terms that individuals use in daily life to label their emotions seem to cluster in the parts of the dimensional space corresponding to the 45-degree rotation, so that characterizing emotion structure with a focus on these parts of the space is important. Furthermore, they are most interested in *high* negative activation and *high* positive activation, in part because they do not believe that words such as "sleepy" that anchor the low-activation ends of the dimensions necessarily refer to actual emotional states.

The type of methodological and analytic strategy applied to judgments of and perceptions of the subjective experience of emotion and emotional objects tells us something about the concepts that underlie individuals' perception of the subjective experience of emotion. It does not reveal or account for the antecedent and situational knowledge about emotion that individuals apparently possess. The next two approaches, the semantic-primitives and the prototype approaches, try to readdress these shortcomings.

DEFINING EMOTION CONCEPTS WITH SEMANTIC PRIMITIVES

There is debate about the meaning of the structure revealed by multidimensional and factor analyses of individuals' perceptions of the relations between emotional states. According to some theorists, the resulting dimensional structures reveal the dimensions that are most important for building emotion concepts, but do

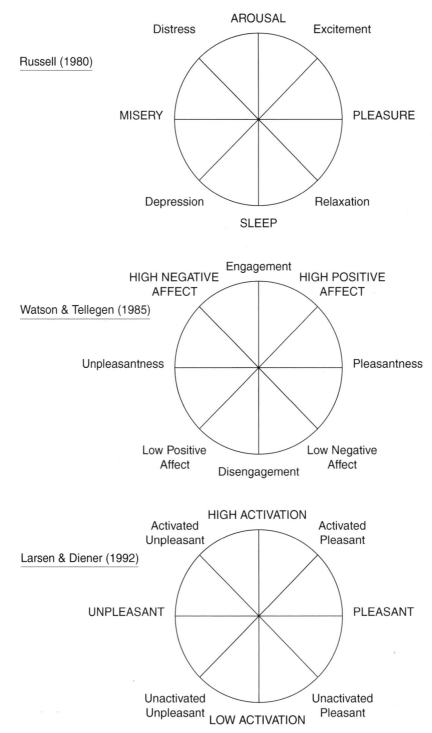

FIGURE 36.1. Three descriptive models of experienced affect. Dimensions of theoretical interest are given in capital letters. From Russell and Barrett (1999). Copyright 1999 by the American Psychological Association. Reprinted by permission.

not solve the problem of characterizing the content of emotion concepts. Wierzbicka (1992), for instance, suggests that the concept "pleasant," while perhaps more inclusive and even basic than the concept "happy," is not in any way better defined; it is probably as complex an abstract concept as "happy." Therefore, while "pleasantness" may be a more fundamental component of experience, this only pushes the need to define emotion concepts to a different level. Now we have to ask what constitutes the concept "pleasant."

One possibility is that emotions, perhaps some set of biologically basic ones, possess classical definitions. Classical theories of concepts call for sets of necessary and sufficient features that characterize all members of a class. A number of arguments can and have been leveled against the classical view as useful to define emotion concepts (Russell, 1991). Because concepts appear to vary across individuals and even within individuals across situations (Barsalou, 2005), it seems that the possibility of deriving classical definitions for any natural kind is unlikely. An alternative approach to defining emotion concepts has been to isolate a set of "semantic primitives" and then to examine the possibility that such concepts can be constructed from this limited set. The construction of lists of semantic primitives is a bootstrapping, bottom-up activity that involves the generation of possibilities and the attempt to define as many concepts as possible, independent of

a specific language, and without adding more. Thus, according to proponents of this approach, while the words "anger" and "sadness" are culture-bound and language-specific, semantic primitives such as "good" and "bad," and "want" and "happen," are not. Wierzbicka (1992) proposed the primitives listed in Table 36.1.

These primitives can describe some of the basic themes that characterize emotion (Johnson-Laird & Oatley, 1989). For example, it has been noted that emotions involve good and bad things that happen to ourselves and other people, and that we ourselves and other people do. They also involve other people's and our own evaluations of ourselves and our actions, and the relationships that can be constructed on the bases of these evaluations and reactions. When semantic primitives are used to build these themes, they seem to provide enough nuances to characterize many different emotions. For example, the emotions "happiness" and "fear" can be defined as follows:

Happiness
X feels happy.
X feels something.
Sometimes a person thinks something like this:
    Something good happened to me.
    I wanted this.
    I don't want other things.
Because of this, this person feels something good.
X feels like this.

TABLE 36.1. A List of Semantic Primitives Proposed by Wierzbicka (1992)

Category	Item
Substantives	I, you, someone, something, people
Determiners and qualifiers	this, the same, other, one, two, many/much, all
Mental predicates	thinking (about), say, know (about), feel, want (to)
Actions and events	do, happen (to)
Evaluative	good, bad
Descriptive	big, small
Time and place	when, where, after/before, under/above
Metapredicates	no/negation, because, if/would, can/may
Intensifier	very
Taxonomy/partonomy	kind of, part of
Hedge/prototype	like

Note. From Wierzbicka (1992). Copyright 1992 by the Cognitive Science Society, Inc. Reprinted by permission.

Fear

X feels frightened.

Sometimes a person thinks something like this:

Something bad can happen.

I don't want this.

Because of this, I would want to do something.

I don't know what I can do.

Because of this, this person feels something bad.

X feels like this.

Despite its appeal, the semantic-primitives approach also has some shortcomings. Although the definitions seem to contain information about the antecedents of and situations for emotions, the "hot" or bodily aspect of the emotion, except for its being good or bad, is not contained in the definition. Presumably the bodily experience can be derived from locating a good or bad feeling in the specific semantic context, but it is not clear just how. Some of these problems could be handled by the proposition made by Johnson-Laird and Oatley (1989) that a set of what might be called basic emotions—fear, anger, happiness, sadness, and disgust—are themselves semantic primitives. Then all of the information is consolidated into one symbol for a complex state involving perception, interoception, and action. However, neither use of the semantic-primitives approach addresses the way in which semantic primitives are represented and processed. Although the assumption must be that the primitives are innate, it is still not clear what is being used when they are activated. By default to what has been called "first-generation" representational models in cognitive science (Gallese & Lakoff, 2005), the primitives may be abstract symbols built into the system.

EMOTION CONCEPTS AS PROTOTYPES

As with the search for semantic primitives, the proposal that emotion concepts are defined in terms of probabilistic features was motivated by opposition to classical theories of concepts. Rosch (1973) was an early proponent of two important features of conceptual structure. One is that concepts are organized hierarchically—that is, people know about the features of abstract categories, such as "furniture"; their more specific exemplars, such as "chair"; and even more specific categories, such as "kitchen chair"—and the hierarchies possess certain structural properties, such as nested features and graded structure. Another important idea was that at any given level of abstraction, the represented category (the concept) is a fuzzy one defined by a set of probable features, but not necessary and sufficient ones, that overlap with closely related categories. Thus the boundaries between concepts representing related categories are not strict or impenetrable.

Several researchers have tested the applicability of Rosch's theory of conceptual structure in the domain of emotion knowledge, in order to learn more about how individuals use their knowledge of categories of emotion (e.g., Fehr & Russell, 1984; Shaver et al., 1987). For instance, in Shaver et al.'s (1987) work, experimental participants were supplied with 135 cards, each containing the English name of one emotion or affective state. The participants sorted the cards into piles that represented, for them, groups of words whose meanings went together or were similar. The card sorts were analyzed with another statistical technique—hierarchical cluster analysis, which identifies clusters of variables (emotion words, in this case) and provides information about their hierarchical relations.

Consistent with the work of Rosch, the findings revealed three levels in the structure. The most abstract contained the categories of "negative" and "positive" emotions. The next level contained what appeared to be five or six basic categories. Shaver and colleagues labeled these "love," "joy," "anger," "sadness," and "fear." Although they also found a possible "surprise" category, they were not in favor of allocating it the status of a basic-emotion category. Finally, there were many subordinate categories that reflected fine gradations of the five or six basic categories. For example, the category "fear" could be further broken down into something like "horror/panic" and "nervousness/dread." The authors noted that the five basic categories revealed by the hierarchical cluster analysis are the same as those shown by Bretherton and Beeghly (1982) in their study of emotion terms learned in early childhood. In addition, these five basic categories correspond to the emotions most often proposed to be biologically basic ones in the various lists of basic emotions (e.g., Ekman, 1984). Additional analyses of language report similar findings (e.g., Conway

& Bekerian, 1987; Johnson-Laird & Oatley, 1989; Russell & Bullock, 1986).

Analyses of the explicit content of emotion concepts, as revealed by property generation tasks, have also provided support for Rosch's prototype theory of natural concepts (e.g., Fehr & Russell, 1984; Keltner & Haidt, 2003; Shaver et al., 1987). Knowledge about the basic-emotion categories appears to contain the three types of features described previously (i.e., knowledge of antecedents, situations, and the bodily characteristics of the emotion). Russell (1991) further characterizes the prototypes as scripts (e.g., Abelson, 1981), arguing that prototypes are to objects what scripts are to events. For Russell, emotions are events having a causal and temporal structure, and not objects, and so the notion of a temporally structured script best captures the representation of an emotion (see Table 36.2 for a possible script for anger, based on Lakoff's [1987] analysis). Consistent with prototype theory, moreover, the script contains features that are probabilistic and not "all or none" in nature. Russell (1991) notes that "the features that constitute emotion concepts describe the subevents that make up the emotion: causes, beliefs, feelings, physiological changes, desires, overt actions, and vocal and facial expressions. . . . To know the sense of a term like anger, fear, or jealousy is to know the script for that emotion" (p. 39).

The prototype account of emotion concepts can show and has shown how the three types of information are contained and fit together in an emotion concept. The notion of a prototype, or a script, largely makes claims about how

something emotional (a facial expression, a subjective experience, a situation, or a behavior) is classified as constituting an instance of a particular emotion. Or, as Clore and Ortony (1991) have noted, "Prototypes seem, therefore, not to be concerned with the function of 'defining the concept' but with the function of identifying instances" (p. 50). The semantic-network models, discussed last, represent perhaps the only approach to modeling concepts that is not agnostic to the representation and processing of emotional information.

SEMANTIC-NETWORK MODELS OF EMOTION CONCEPTS

The single explicit class of representational models of emotion concepts in the literature to date consists of the semantic-network models of emotion (Bower, 1981, 1991; Ingram, 1984; Lang, 1984; Teasdale, 1983). The variations on these models hold that knowledge is represented in a semantic network of units of representation sometimes called "nodes," or alternatively "concepts," "categories," "traces," "processors," or "units" (Collins & Loftus, 1975; Anderson & Bower, 1973). Nodes store and transform information in propositional form. They are linked by connecting pathways that reflect the strength of semantic associations among them. A particular idea comes to mind, or enters consciousness, when its node is activated above some critical threshold. A node can be excited by the spread of activation from neighboring nodes, or through direct sensory stimulation.

The semantic-network models of emotion all propose that emotions impose a fundamental organizational structure on information stored in the semantic network. Each emotion or affective state is conceptualized as a central, organizing node. Nodes that represent beliefs, antecedents, and physiological patterns associated with given emotions are linked to the nodes corresponding to those nodes in memory. Of course, one has to ask this question: Which emotions impose a fundamental organization? Bower (1981) proposed that the set of so-called "basic emotions" imposed such organization, although his later writings suggested that the network was organized according to valence (e.g., Bower, 1991). Research and theoretical considerations (see Niedenthal, Setterlund, & Jones, 1994, for a discussion)

TABLE 36.2. An Anger Script

Step	Subevent
1	The person is offended. The offense is intentional and harmful. The person is innocent. An injustice has been done.
2	The person glares and scowls at the offender
3	The person feels internal tension and agitation, as if heat and pressure were rapidly mounting inside. He feels his heart pounding and his muscles tightening.
4	The person desires retribution.
5	The person loses control and strikes out, harming the offender.

Note. From Russell (1991). Copyright 1991 by the American Psychological Association. Reprinted by permission.

provide strong arguments in favor of the 1981 model.

A categorical or discrete-emotions version of the model makes the straightforward prediction that when an emotion unit (e.g., the unit that represents "sadness") is activated above some threshold, activation spreads throughout the network to associated information. Autonomic reactions, expressive behaviors, emotion-related events, and personal memories are thereby excited and may enter consciousness. For instance, when one is feeling happy, the material in memory related to happiness becomes activated. As a consequence, one may experience an increase in heart rate and in blood pressure, an activation of the zygomaticus major muscle, and a heightened accessibility to the words and memories associated with happiness. In some versions of this model, the nodes that represent "opposite" states (e.g., perhaps happiness and sadness) are connected by inhibitory links, such that the activation of one emotion node leads to the inhibition of the other one (Bower, 1981). For instance, activating happiness is expected to inhibit the activation of sadness.

This model has been applied to account for "emotion congruence" and to generate other predictions about emotion and information processing. The emotion congruence hypothesis states that the processing of emotional information that has an emotional quality congruent with the quality of the emotional state experienced by the individual/perceiver will be more efficient than the processing the processing of information that has an incongruent emotional quality. For example, when applied to perception, the emotion congruence hypothesis states that objects and events that have the same emotion significance as the individual's current affective state are perceived by that individual with greater efficiency than other stimuli, such as neutral or emotion-incongruent stimuli. Findings supportive of this hypothesis have been reported (e.g., Niedenthal, Halberstadt, & Setterlund, 1997; Niedenthal & Setterlund, 1994; see Niedenthal et al., 1994, for a discussion). Other demonstrations of an emotion congruence effect as predicted by a semantic-network model have been reported for retrieval from long-term memory (e.g., Bower, Gilligan, & Monteiro, 1981; Eich, Macaulay, & Ryan, 1994; Ehrlichman & Halpern, 1988; Fiedler & Stroehm, 1986;

Mayer, McCormick, & Strong, 1995) and judgment (e.g., Abele & Petzold, 1994; DeSteno, Petty, Wegener, & Rucker, 2000; Forgas, 1992, 1993, 1995; Lerner & Keltner, 2001).

The semantic-network models are powerful for accounting for and generating some hypotheses regarding the structure and content of emotion concepts (see Niedenthal et al., 1994, for a discussion). However, in these models, each node is connected to many other nodes, and each node is itself defined entirely in terms of its relation to the other nodes. The problem, then, is that tracing out relations between undefined nodes does not result in meaning. Therefore, as in the other models described thus far, it is not clear what grounds emotion concepts. Some underlying assumptions of the approaches described thus far are considered explicitly in the next section.

FIRST-GENERATION MODELS OF EMOTION REPRESENTATION

Although their purposes were not always to test this assumption, or even to be explicit about it, all the accounts of emotion concepts described thus far represent concepts as redescriptions of the input from the sensory system into an abstract language (Barsalou, 1999; Gallese & Lakoff, 2005). Thus extant and explicit representational models of emotion are based on a general view of cognition in which higher-order mental content is represented in an abstract, language-like code (e.g., Fodor, 1975), and the symbols used in higher-level cognitive processes are "amodal." An amodal representation does not preserve anything analogical about the perceptual experience of the object, event, or state, but is abstracted and abstract in format (e.g., Ortony, Clore, & Collins, 1988).

Whether the resulting representation takes a form something like a word, a feature list, or vectors on which different values can be positioned, the assumption is that the representation and the initial perception do not take place in the same system. The dominant approach to representing emotion knowledge thus rests on the "transduction" principle (Bower, 1981; Johnson-Laird & Oatley, 1989; Ortony et al., 1987). According to this principle, knowledge structures are taken from emotional experience and then redescribed to represent emotion concepts. Furthermore, representing knowledge of an emotion in the absence of experiencing it involves activating the appropriate amodal representation (e.g., in the case of the semantic-network models, an emotion node). Because it describes different parts of the events and experiences relevant to the emotion, when activated the knowledge structure can support inferences about it.

In evaluating the strength of such models, we (Niedenthal et al., 1994) noted:

> [Although] some emotion theorists view propositional codes as sufficient for representing emotional stimuli, meaning, and responses[,] it is possible that other types of code preserve the visual, motor, and somatovisceral aspects of such experience. That we recognize a subjective feeling as "what it is like to be in love" is neither cold nor trivial. Rather, this fact means that there exists a memory of the bodily feeling of an emotion that has been associated with a verbal label. Thus, the general idea that emotions are stored in and organize memory in an associative way does not have to do away with the "hot" aspects of emotion; an exclusive focus on propositional representation may do so. (p. 106)

EMBODIED-SIMULATION THEORY

The social psychology and emotion literatures are filled with evidence (see a review in Niedenthal, Barsalou, Ric, & Krauth-Gruber, 2005), now supported also by findings from neuroimaging studies, that there is a different way to model emotion concepts—one that follows from the concerns cited in the quotation above (Barsalou, 1999; Gallese & Lakoff, 2005). In theories of "embodied cognition," the modality-specific states that represent perception, action, and introception when one is actually in interaction with a particular entity, or having a particular subjective experience, *represent* these same stimuli and events when the original entity or experience is not actually present. Put otherwise, in this view, using knowledge involves simulations that are reactivations in the sensorimotor system. For example, retrieving the memory of a landscape involves reactivating parts of the visual states that were active while the person was originally perceiving it. In the same manner, thinking about the movements involved in riding a bi-

cycle involves partially activating the motor states that support the activity.

What having a concept is, then, is having the ability to reenact being with an instance of a category, or having the ability to simulate it. Concepts in this approach are therefore also called "simulators" (Barsalou, 2003) or "embodied simulations" (Gallese & Lakoff, 2005). According to Barsalou's account, a simulator develops for any object, event, or aspect of experience that has been repeatedly attended to. Due to its exquisite flexibility, attention can be allocated to different parts of our overall experience. Across development, a number of simulators are established in long-term memory to represent these different experiences. After a simulator is established, it can be used to reenact aspects of experience, thus supporting the capacity to perform conceptual tasks.

Representing Emotion Concepts Modally

Extending the embodied-simulation account to emotion knowledge holds that modality-specific states represent the content of concepts of emotion. In considering the three domains of emotion knowledge mentioned earlier—antecedent situations, actions or action tendencies, and introceptive states—the embodied-simulation account says that reenactments of modality-specific states, rather than amodal symbols, represent the conceptual content in these domains. So reenactments of visually perceiving smiles on other people's faces belong to the situational knowledge that triggers "happiness," as do the motor and somatosensory experiences of smiling oneself. Similarly, reenactments of valence and arousal states represent these introspective aspects of emotion concepts, rather than amodal symbols that stand in for them.

In such a view, then, knowledge of an emotion concept is not a separate description of the respective emotion. Instead, knowledge of the emotion is grounded in actual emotional states, some conscious and some unconscious. Although these states may not constitute full-blown emotions, they may usually contain enough information about the original states to function as representations of them conceptually. Importantly, these partial reenactments constitute the core knowledge of emotional concepts. Embodied states are not merely peripheral events that trigger emotion concepts, or that result from the activation of such concepts. (This latter description does characterize accurately how a semantic-network model would link conceptual knowledge and bodily manifestations of emotion.) Instead, embodied states represent the core conceptual content of an emotion.

Empirical Support
for Embodied-Emotion Concepts

Evidence in favor of simulation in the conceptual processing of emotion was recently demonstrated in two studies (Mondillon, Niedenthal, Vermeulen, & Winkielman, 2007). In the first of those studies, individuals had to make judgments about whether words referring to concrete objects (e.g., "vomit") were associated with an emotion (they did not have to say which emotion; they provided simply a "yes" or "no" response). The list of concepts to which the experimental participants were exposed included concepts that were associated with joy, disgust, and anger, as well as no particular emotion. While the participants were exposed to the concepts and making their judgments, the activation of four facial muscles was measured with electromyographic recording. Two of the muscles, the orbicularis (around the eyes) and the zygomaticus major (around the mouth) muscles, are typically activated when an individual is smiling with happiness. The corrugator (over the eyebrows) is typically activated when an individual is frowning with anger. And the levator muscle is activated when an individual makes the grimace of disgust.

According to the amodal representational models, the judgment that, for example, the word "slug" is associated with disgust does not require the simulation of being there with a slug. That it engenders disgust is another feature of slugs that is represented in a feature list by an amodal representation. It can be accessed without recourse to the emotion itself. On the other hand, the embodied-simulation model predicts that the judgment is based on a simulation of being there with a slug. Consequently, the amodal models do not predict that judgments about whether an object is associated with an emotion are accompanied by the specific emotional experience (a simulation, which can be detected by activation of facial muscles), whereas the embodied-simulation model does predict this.

The results of the study just described, as well as a second study in which the words to be judged were abstract emotion words (e.g., "enraged," "delighted," and "disgusted"), supported predictions of a modal account of representation. Specifically, in both studies, judgments about words that refer to objects eliciting joy or that are synonyms for "joy" were accompanied by specific activation of the orbicularis and the zygomaticus major muscles; judgments about words that refer to objects eliciting anger or that are synonyms for "anger" were accompanied by specific activation of the corrugator muscle; and judgments about words that refer to objects eliciting disgust or that are synonyms for "disgust" were accompanied by activation of the levator muscle. Thus the findings support a proposed process by which conceptual processing involves simulation of the concept in sensorimotor systems.

Another type of specific evidence comes from an extension of research on "switching costs" to the area of emotion. Researchers in perception have known for a while that shifting attention from processing in one sensory modality, such as vision, to another, such as audition, involves temporal processing costs (e.g., Posner & DiGirolamo, 2000; Spence, Nicholls, & Driver, 2000). Interestingly, similar costs are also found when participants engage in a purely conceptual task. For example, Pecher, Zeelenberg, and Barsalou (2003) found that participants were slower in verifying properties of a concept from one modality after they had just verified a concept from another modality (e.g., "bomb–loud" followed by "lemon–tart"), once again suggesting involvement of perceptual processes in conceptual representation (see also Kan, Barsalou, Solomon, Minor, & Thompson-Schill, 2003, for neuroimaging evidence).

We (Vermeulen, Niedenthal, & Luminet, 2007) examined switching costs in verifying properties of positive and negative concepts such as "triumph" and "victim." Properties of these concepts were taken from vision, audition, and the affective system. Parallel to the switching costs observed for neutral concepts, the study showed that for positive and negative concepts, verifying properties from different modalities produced costs, such that reaction times were longer and error rates were higher than if no modality switching was required. Importantly, this effect was observed when participants had to switch from the affective system to sensory modalities, and vice versa. In other words, verifying that a "victim" can be "stricken" was slower and less accurate if the previous trial involved verifying that a "spider" can be "black" than if the previous trial involved verifying that an "orphan" can be "hopeless." And verifying that a "spider" can be "black" was less efficient when preceded by the judgment that an "orphan" can be "hopeless" than that a "wound" can be "open." This research provides evidence that affective properties of concepts are simulated in the emotional system when the properties are the subject of active thought.

Recently, we (Niedenthal, Barsalou, Ric, & Krauth-Gruber, 2005) reviewed many additional findings from the emotion literature to further reinforce this view of how emotion concepts are grounded. The additional findings indicate that individuals embody other people's emotional gestures and postures; that embodied emotional gestures and postures can produce corresponding emotional states in an individual; that imagining other people and events also produces embodied emotions and corresponding feelings; and that embodied emotions mediate cognitive responses. Taken together, then, the logical and experimental data in favor of this modal account of emotion concepts are very strong and motivate many important questions for the field.

EMOTION CATEGORIES AND CONCEPTUAL CONTENT

If knowledge acquisition occurs through embodiment (Niedenthal, Barsalou, Winkielman, Krauth-Gruber, & Ric, 2005), then this account suggests ways to address two important concerns that have been raised in this chapter. One concerns what emotion concepts really correspond to. In the embodied-simulation account of emotion, concepts are simulations that are used online for the purposes of performing conceptual tasks. So, as we have seen, in order to know that a "slug" is associated with an emotion, we simulate the sight of a slug and our affective response (if any) to it. Or, if we need to list (for Shaver et al. or for Russell) the typical features of a state of anger, we can simulate it and describe that (re)experience in words. This means that there is little difference

between what we know about emotion and the process of having an emotion. The situated nature of knowledge about emotion, moreover, makes the link between a concept and a specific "natural-kind" (or other) category a moot point (Barrett, 2006).

Thus the account can address a second concern—namely, individual and cultural differences in emotion concepts. As we have learned, acquiring emotion knowledge is in part determined by the allocation of selective attention to parts of experience or incoming information (such as facial expressions or other emotional gestures). That is, even if many processes operate automatically when an emotion is evoked and experienced, this does not mean that a residue of all such processes is present in a representation in long-term memory of the antecedent events or of the experience of the emotion. Over different experiences with an emotional state, selective attention can be allocated to different aspects of the embodied emotion (because much of it is potentially available to consciousness, including changes in heart rate, breathing, and muscular tension), and this supports nuanced individual and cultural differences in the content of emotion concepts.

Strategies for characterizing these differences are already established. Neuroimaging studies of the brain subsystems that support conditioned learning (e.g., conditioned fear learning), observational learning, and instructed learning can help us better understand the differences in the role of experience versus concepts in knowledge about emotional events. Suggestive evidence shows that there are important similarities, and fewer but also important differences, in neural activation during these three types of fear learning (e.g., Phelps et al., 2001). Future studies will be able to link the role of attention to specific features of the initial experienced situation that are simulated in concept use.

CONCLUSION

In this chapter, I have reviewed some of the dominant models of emotion concepts. I have noted that the models are not competing with each other, as they actually attempt to do quite different things. Dimensional analyses try to define the irreducible structure and content for emotion concepts. A semantic-primitives approach has a similar aim for defining the content, although not the structure, of emotion concepts. A prototype approach says quite a bit about the content of emotion concepts and how it is used to identity instances. And only the semantic-network models address representation and process. Recent findings in the cognitive, social, and emotion psychology literatures indicate that there is a closer relationship between sensorimotor experience of and with entities in the world and the knowledge we possess about them than the semantic-network models would suggest. In the present chapter, therefore, I have tried to summarize the principles of and the utility of the more recent theory that the conceptual content for emotion knowledge is grounded in the sensorimotor states occurring in interaction with emotional stimuli and in the experience of emotional states. This model will not suffice for accounting for all cognitive phenomena that we observe, and I do not make that argument here (see Solomon & Barsalou, 2004). I believe, however, that this theory should be viewed as providing a priori accounts of embodied phenomena that traditionally have been difficult to explain. I believe that an embodied-simulation account of emotion concepts can provide emotion psychologists with powerful new ways of theorizing about representations and the mechanisms that process emotions.

REFERENCES

Abele, A., & Petzold, P. (1994). How does mood operate in an impression formation task?: An information integration approach. *European Journal of Social Psychology, 24*, 173–184.

Abelson, R. P. (1981). Psychological status of the script concept. *American Psychologist, 36*, 715–729.

Anderson, J. R., & Bower, G. H. (1973). *Human associative memory.* Washington, DC: Winston.

Barrett, L. F. (2006). Emotions as natural kinds? *Perspectives on Psychological Science, 1*, 28–58.

Barrett, L. F., & Russell, J. A. (1999). Structure of current affect. *Current Directions in Psychological Science, 8*, 10–14.

Barsalou, L. W. (1999). Perceptual symbol system. *Behavioral and Brain Sciences, 22*, 577–660.

Barsalou, L. W. (2003). Situated simulation in the human conceptual system. *Language and Cognitive Processes, 18*, 513–562.

Barsalou, L. W. (2005). Situated conceptualization. In H. Cohen & C. Lefebvre (Eds.), *Handbook of cate-*

gorization in cognitive science (pp. 619–650). Amsterdam: Elsevier.

Bower, G. H. (1981). Mood and memory. *American Psychologist, 36*, 129–148.

Bower, G. H. (1991). Mood congruity in social judgments. In J. P. Forgas (Ed.), *Emotion and social judgments* (pp. 31–53). Oxford: Pergamon Press.

Bower, G. H., Gilligan, S. G., & Monteiro, K. P. (1981). Selectivity of learning caused by affective states. *Journal of Experimental Psychology: General, 110*, 451–473.

Bretherton, I., & Beeghly, M. (1982). Talking about internal states: The acquisition of an explicit theory of mind. *Developmental Psychology, 18*, 906–912.

Cantor, N., & Mischel, W. (1977) Traits as prototypes: Effects on recognition memory. *Journal of Personality and Social Psychology, 35*, 38–48.

Clore, G. L., & Ortony, A. (1991). What more is there to emotion concepts than prototypes? *Journal of Personality and Social Psychology, 60*, 48–50.

Cohen, C. E. (1981). Person categories and social perception: Testing some boundaries of the processing effects of prior knowledge. *Journal of Personality and Social Psychology, 40*, 441–452.

Collins, A. M., & Loftus, E. F. (1975). A spreading-activation theory of semantic processing. *Psychological Review, 82*, 407–428.

Conway, M. A., & Bekerian, D. A. (1987). Situational knowledge and emotions. *Cognition and Emotion, 1*, 145–191.

DeSteno, D., Petty, R. E., Wegener, D. T., & Rucker, D. D. (2000). Beyond valence in the perception of likelihood: The role of emotion specificity. *Journal of Personality and Social Psychology, 78*, 397–416.

Ehrlichman, H., & Halpern, J. N. (1988). Affect and memory: Effects of pleasant and unpleasant odors on retrieval of happy and unhappy memories. *Journal of Personality and Social Psychology, 55*, 769–779.

Eich, E., Macaulay, D., & Ryan, L. (1994). Mood-dependent memory for events of the personal past. *Journal of Experimental Psychology: General, 123*, 201–215.

Ekman, P. (1984). Expression and the nature of emotion. In P. Ekman & K. Scherer (Eds.), *Approaches to emotion* (pp. 319–343). Hillsdale, NJ: Erlbaum.

Fehr, B., & Russell, J. A. (1984). Concept of emotion viewed from a prototype perspective. *Journal of Experimental Psychology: General, 113*, 464–486.

Fiedler, K., & Stroehm, W. (1986). What kind of mood influences what kind of memory? *Memory and Cognition, 14*, 181–188.

Fodor, J. (1975). *The language of thought.* Cambridge, MA: Harvard University Press.

Forgas, J. P. (1992). On mood and peculiar people: Affect and person typicality in impression formation. *Journal of Personality and Social Psychology, 62*, 863–875.

Forgas, J. P. (1993). On making sense of odd couples:

Mood effects on the perception of mismatched relationships. *Personality and Social Psychology Bulletin, 19,* 59–71.

Forgas, J. P. (1995). Strange couples: Mood effects on judgments and memory about prototypical and atypical targets. *Personality and Social Psychology Bulletin, 21,* 747–765.

Gallese, V., & Lakoff, G. (2005). The brain's concepts: The role of the sensory–motor system in reason and language. *Cognitive Neuropsychology, 22,* 455–479.

Ingram, R. E. (1984). Toward an information processing analysis of depression. *Cognitive Therapy and Research, 8,* 443–478.

Johnson-Laird, P. N., & Oatley, K. (1989). The meaning of emotions: Analysis of a semantic field. *Cognition and Emotion, 3,* 81–123.

Kan, I. P., Barsalou, L. W., Solomon, K. O., Minor, J. K., & Thompson-Schill, S. L. (2003). Role of mental imagery in a property verification task: fMRI evidence for perceptual representations of conceptual knowledge. *Cognitive Neuropsychology, 20,* 525–540.

Keltner, D., & Haidt, J. (2003). Approaching awe, a moral, spiritual, and aesthetic emotion. *Cognition and Emotion, 17,* 297–314.

Lakoff, G. (1987). *Women, fire, and dangerous things: What categories reveal about the mind.* Chicago: University of Chicago Press.

Lamberts, K., & Shanks, D. (Eds.). (1997). *Knowledge, concepts and categories.* Cambridge, MA: MIT Press.

Lang, P. J. (1984). Cognition in emotion: Cognition in action. In C. E. Izard, J. Kagan, & R. B. Zajonc (Eds.), *Emotions, cognition, and behavior* (pp. 192–226). New York: Cambridge University Press.

Larsen, R. J., & Diener, E. (1992). Promises and problems with the circumplex model of emotion. *Review of Personality and Social Psychology, 13,* 25–59.

Lerner, J. S., & Keltner, D. (2000). Beyond valence: Toward a model of emotion specific influences on judgment and choice. *Cognition and Emotion, 14,* 473–493.

Mayer, J. D., & Gaschke, Y. N. (1988). The experience and meta-experience of mood. *Journal of Personality and Social Psychology, 55,* 102–111.

Mayer, J. D., McCormick, L. J., & Strong, S. E. (1995). Mood-congruent memory and natural mood: New evidence. *Personality and Social Psychology Bulletin, 21,* 736–746.

Mondillon, L., Niedenthal, P. M., Winkielman, P., & Vermeulen, N. (2007). *Embodiment of emotion concepts: Evidence from EMG measures.* Manuscript submitted for publication.

Niedenthal, P. M., Barsalou, L. W., Ric, F., & Krauth-Gruber, S. (2005). Embodiment in the acquisition and use of emotion knowledge. In L. F. Barrett, P. M. Niedenthal, & P. Winkielman (Eds.), *Emotion and consciousness* (pp. 21–50). New York: Guilford Press.

Niedenthal, P. M., Barsalou, L. W., Winkielman, P., Krauth-Gruber, S., & Ric, F. (2005). Embodiment in

attitudes, social perception, and emotion. *Personality and Social Psychology Review, 9,* 184–211.

Niedenthal, P. M., Halberstadt, J. B., & Setterlund, M. B. (1997). Being happy and seeing "happy": Emotional state mediates visual word recognition. *Cognition and Emotion, 11,* 403–432.

Niedenthal, P. M., Krauth-Gruber, S., & Ric, F. (2006). *Psychology of emotion: Interpersonal, experiential, and cognitive approaches.* New York: Psychology Press.

Niedenthal, P. M., & Setterlund, M. B. (1994). Emotion congruence in perception. *Personality and Social Psychology Bulletin, 20,* 401–411.

Niedenthal, P. M., Setterlund, M. B., & Jones, D. E. (1994). Emotional organization of perceptual memory. In P. M. Niedenthal & S. Kitayama (Eds.), *The heart's eye: Emotional influences in perception and attention* (pp. 87–113). San Diego, CA: Academic Press.

Ortony, A., Clore, G. L., & Collins, A. (1988). *The cognitive structure of emotions.* Cambridge, UK: Cambridge University Press.

Ortony, A., Clore, G. L., & Foss, M. A. (1987). The referential structure of the affective lexicon. *Cognitive Science, 11,* 341–364.

Osgood, C. E., & Suci, G. J. (1955). Factor analysis of meaning. *Journal of Experimental Psychology, 50,* 25–338.

Pecher, D., Zeelenberg, R., & Barsalou, L. W. (2003). Verifying different-modality properties for concepts produces switching costs. *Psychological Science, 14*(2), 119–124.

Phelps, E. A., O'Connor, K. J., Gateby, J. J., Grillon, C., Gore, J. C., & Davis, M. (2001). Activation of the amygdala by cognitive representations of fear. *Nature Neuroscience, 4,* 437–441.

Philippot, P. (1991). Reported and actual physiological changes in emotion. In A. J. W. Boelhouwer & C. H. M. Brunia (Eds.), *Proceedings of the First European Physiological Conference* (p. 132). Tilburg, The Netherlands: Tilburg Press.

Posner, M. I., & DiGirolamo, G. J. (2000). Cognitive neuroscience: Origins and promise. *Psychological Bulletin, 126,* 873–889.

Rimé, B., Philippot, P., & Cisamolo, D. (1990). Social schemata of peripheral changes in emotion. *Journal of Personality and Social Psychology, 59,* 38–49.

Rosch, E. H. (1973). Natural categories. *Cognitive Psychology, 4,* 328–350.

Russell, J. A. (1980). A circumplex model of affect. *Journal of Personality and Social Psychology, 39,* 1161–1178.

Russell, J. A. (1991). In defense of a prototype approach to emotion concepts. *Journal of Personality and Social Psychology, 60,* 37–47.

Russell, J. A., & Barrett, L. F. (1999). Core affect, prototypical emotional episodes, and other things called emotion: Dissecting the elephant. *Journal of Personality and Social Psychology, 76,* 805–819.

Russell, J. A., & Bullock, M. (1986). Fuzzy concepts and the perception of emotion in facial expressions. *Social Cognition, 4,* 309–341.

Russell, J. A., & Mehrabian, A. (1977). Evidence for a three-factor theory of emotions. *Journal of Research in Personality, 11,* 273–294.

Shaver, P., Schwartz, J., Kirson, D., & O'Connor, C. (1987). Emotion knowledge: Further exploration of a prototype approach. *Journal of Personality and Social Psychology, 52,* 1061–1086.

Solomon, K. O., & Barsalou, L. W. (2004). Perceptual simulation in property verification. *Memory and Cognition, 32,* 244–259.

Spence, C., Nicholls, M. E., & Driver, J. (2001). The cost of expecting events in the wrong sensory modality. *Perception and Psychophysics, 63*(2), 330–336.

Teasdale, J. D. (1983). Negative thinking in depression: Cause, effect or reciprocal thinking? *Advances in Behaviour Research and Therapy, 5,* 3–25.

Vermeulen, N., Niedenthal, P. M., & Luminet, O. (2007). Switching between sensory and affective systems incurs processing costs. *Cognitive Science, 31,* 183–192.

Watson, D., & Tellegen, A. (1985). Toward a consensual structure of mood. *Psychological Bulletin, 98,* 219–235.

Watson, D., Wiese, D., Vaidya, J., & Tellegen, A. (1999). The two general activation systems of affect: Structural findings, evolutionary considerations, and psychobiological evidence. *Journal of Personality and Social Psychology, 76,* 820–838.

Wierzbicka, A. (1992). Defining emotion concepts. *Cognitive Science, 16,* 539–581.

CHAPTER 37

Memory and Emotion

ELIZABETH A. KENSINGER and DANIEL L. SCHACTER

Although the concept of memory has existed for thousands of years, its systematic study was launched in the 1880s by the seminal experiments of the German philosopher Hermann Ebbinghaus. Through careful assessments of his own memory, Ebbinghaus forged the way for the field of memory research by demonstrating that humans' ability to retain information over time could be studied scientifically. It is telling that Ebbinghaus's studies involved the intentional memorization of nonsense syllables: He believed that to understand memory processes, one should study retention of information that is void of meaning or personal importance. Although memory researchers seemed to embrace Ebbinghaus's views on this issue for nearly a century, over the past couple of decades there has been increased emphasis on examining memory for personally important experiences and for events that evoke emotional reactions.

Throughout this chapter, we use terms like "emotional stimuli" as shorthand to denote information in the environment that elicits a change in the internal affective state of the organism. The focus of this chapter is on how these internal changes affect memory. Behavioral examinations of explicit (conscious) memory for emotional experiences have revealed three broad influences of emotion on memory: on the number (quantity) of events remembered, on the subjective vividness (quality) of the remembered events, and on the amount of accurate detail remembered about prior experiences. This chapter explores these three lines of investigation, highlighting both the general conclusions that have emerged from the research and the open questions that remain. We conclude with a brief discussion of recent research suggesting an effect of emotion on implicit (unconscious) memory. In addition to presenting the behavioral data and cognitive

601

theories of emotional memory, this chapter includes discussion of relevant neuroimaging and neuropsychological research that has been influential in examining the extent to which memory for emotional experiences is supported by processes distinct from those supporting memory for nonemotional events.

EMOTION'S INFLUENCE ON THE QUANTITY OF REMEMBERED INFORMATION

Individuals often remember more emotional events than nonemotional ones. Within the laboratory, recall rates are higher for positive and negative stimuli than for neutral stimuli (reviewed by Buchanan & Adolphs, 2002; Hamann, 2001). This finding has been documented with a variety of stimuli, including words, sentences, pictures, and narrated slide shows (e.g., Bradley, Greenwald, Petry, & Lang, 1992; Cahill & McGaugh, 1995; Kensinger, Brierly, Medford, Growdon, & Corkin, 2002). Similar effects have been noted within the autobiographical memory literature. For example, when individuals are asked to generate memories in response to cue words, the retrieved memories are often rated as personally significant and emotional (e.g., Conway, 1990; Rubin & Kozin, 1984). There are also many instances in which positive and negative events are more likely to be recognized than neutral ones, although the recognition memory advantage is seen less consistently than the recall advantage (reviewed by Christianson, 1992)—a finding that we will return to later in this chapter.

A topic of ongoing investigation is the extent to which the "valence" of an event (i.e., whether it elicits positive or negative affect) influences the likelihood that the event is remembered, and virtually every conceivable outcome has been observed. Often the boost in recall or recognition is comparable for positive and negative stimuli (e.g., Bradley et al., 1992; Kensinger et al., 2002). However, in some studies, particularly those assessing memory for verbal or pictorial stimuli presented within a laboratory setting, negative items are more likely to be recalled than positive ones (e.g., Charles, Mather, & Carstensen, 2003; Ortony, Turner, & Antos, 1983). Yet other studies, generally those assessing memory for autobiographical experiences or information encoded

in reference to the self, have revealed the opposite pattern: a greater tendency to recall positive events than negative ones (e.g., D'Argembeau, Comblain, & van der Linden, 2005; Linton, 1975; Matt, Vasquez, & Campbell, 1992; White, 2002).

Some of these conflicting findings with regard to the effect of valence on the likelihood of remembering information may be explained by the proposal that memory mechanisms have evolved to facilitate the encoding and retrieval of the affective information that is most relevant to one's goals (Lazarus, 1991; LeDoux, 1996). Remembering a negative experience often may be relevant to survival or well-being, because reexperiencing the event will help a person plan for (or avoid) its future recurrence (LeDoux, 1996). In these instances, more attention may be paid to the negative item, thereby enhancing memory for this negative information. However, there are probably instances in which positive events are just as relevant, or more relevant, to one's goals as negative events. Indeed, when positive and negative stimuli are equally related to one's current concerns, they show similar capture of attention (Riemann & McNally, 1995). Furthermore, there is some evidence that individuals (e.g., older adults) who seek positive goal states show enhanced memory for positive as compared to negative events (reviewed by Mather & Carstensen, 2005).

Researchers have focused intensively on whether this mnemonic benefit for personally relevant and emotional information results from the engagement of processes that are related specifically to the processing of emotional information, or whether the memory boost stems from engagement of the same processes that allow accurate remembering of neutral information. Although parsimony favors the hypothesis that the same processes are recruited to remember emotional and neutral information, lesion and neuroimaging studies suggest that the amygdala (an almond-shaped region of the medial temporal lobe) is specifically related to memory for emotional, but not for neutral, information. Patients with damage to the amygdala do not show a memory boost for emotional information: They are no more likely to remember positive or negative events than they are to remember neutral ones. The absence of the emotional memory enhancement has been reported in patients with focal amygdala damage (e.g., Adolphs, Cahill, Schul,

& Babinsky, 1997; Brierley, Medford, Shaw, & David, 2004; Cahill, Babinsky, Markowitsch, & McGaugh, 1995; Markowitsch et al., 1994) and in individuals with amygdala atrophy caused by Alzheimer's disease (e.g., Abrisqueta-Gomez, Bueno, Oliveira, & Bertolucci, 2002; Kensinger et al., 2002; Kensinger, Anderson, Growdon, & Corkin, 2004). In these latter individuals, the amount of the amygdala damage corresponds with the degree of blunted emotional memory enhancement (Mori et al., 1999).

Although these neuropsychological studies have demonstrated the necessary contribution of the amygdala to emotion-mediated memory enhancements, they do not allow investigation of the memory stage(s) during which the amygdala exerts its influence. Neuroimaging methods provide a way to address this issue. Researchers can examine the neural processes associated with the successful encoding of emotional information (by comparing brain activity while participants are encoding items that will later be remembered vs. items that will later be forgotten) or with the successful retrieval of emotional information (by comparing brain activity associated with correct endorsements vs. misses). These neuroimaging studies have demonstrated that the amygdala plays a fundamental role during the encoding of emotional information. Individuals who show the greatest amygdala activity during the viewing of emotional items are those who show the greatest emotional memory enhancement (Cahill et al., 1996). Moreover, for a particular individual, those emotional items that elicit the greatest amygdala activity during encoding are those that are most likely to be remembered (reviewed by Hamann, 2001; Phelps, 2004; Kensinger, in press). Although the vast majority of neuroimaging studies have examined the amygdala's role in encoding *negative* information, a recent neuroimaging study indicated that the amygdala was equally active during the successful encoding of positive and negative high-arousal items (Kensinger & Schacter, 2006a). This finding is consistent with research demonstrating that the amygdala is important for processing reward-related information as well as threat-related information (see Davidson & Irwin, 1999; Baas, Aleman, & Kahn, 2004), and that it may primarily respond based on the arousal, and not the valence, of information (Anders, Lotze, Erb, Grodd, & Girbaumer, 2004; Anderson et al.,

2003; Garavan, Pendergrass, Ross, Stein, & Risinger, 2001; Hamann, Ely, Hoffman, & Kilts, 2002; Kensinger & Schacter, 2006c; Royet et al., 2000; Small et al., 2003; however, see Buchanan, Tranel, & Adolphs, 2006, for evidence that the right amygdala may be more involved in memory for negatively valenced than positively valenced information).

The amygdala, of course, does not act in isolation. It has been proposed that once the amygdala is activated during the processing of emotional information, it can modulate the functioning of sensory cortices to assure that the information is attended to (reviewed by Dolan & Vuilleumier, 2003), and to enhance mnemonic consolidation processes in the hippocampal formation to increase the likelihood that emotional information is retained in a stable memory trace (reviewed by McGaugh, 2004; Phelps, 2004). The amygdala is well suited for these modulatory functions, as it is one of the most extensively connected subcortical regions of the brain, with links to numerous cortical and subcortical regions (Amaral, Price, Pitkanen, & Carmichael, 1992; Amaral, 2003).

Recent neuroimaging studies have provided strong evidence for these modulatory effects of the amygdala. In one study investigating the links between amygdala activity and visual attention, patients with varying amounts of amygdala damage were scanned while they performed a task in which they had to attend to fearful or neutral faces (Vuilleumier, Richardson, Armony, Driver, & Dolan, 2004). Individuals with intact amygdalas showed enhanced activity in the fusiform gyrus (a visual processing region) when they attended to fearful faces as compared to neutral faces. Patients with extensive amygdala damage did not show this pattern: They showed equivalent fusiform activity for neutral and fearful faces. Moreover, the amount of amygdala preservation corresponded with the amount of fusiform modulation based on the emotional content of the attended faces. These results suggest that the amygdala can modulate visual processing in humans, increasing the likelihood that an emotional item in the environment is detected and attended to.

In addition to these influences on sensory processes, a number of neuroimaging studies have provided evidence for amygdalar modulation of mnemonic processes, suggesting that interactions between the amygdala and the hippocampus serve a critical role in modulating the memory enhancement for emotional information in humans (reviewed by McGaugh, 2004). In healthy individuals, there are strong correlations between the amount of activity in the amygdala and in the hippocampus during the encoding of emotional information (e.g., Dolcos, LaBar, & Cabeza, 2004; Hamann, Ely, Grafton, & Kilts, 1999; Kensinger & Corkin, 2004; Kensinger & Schacter, 2005a). Although these correlations cannot speak to the direction of modulation, a neuroimaging study of encoding-related neural activity in patients with varying amounts of amygdala and hippocampal damage provided evidence for the importance of reciprocal connections. While in the scanner, patients were asked to encode a series of emotionally aversive and neutral words. Outside the scanner, they performed a recognition task, and the encoding trials were sorted on a post hoc basis into those words that were later remembered and those that were later forgotten. The critical findings from the study were that the extent of amygdala atrophy correlated negatively with the magnitude of activity in the hippocampus during the encoding of emotional information, and that the amount of hippocampal atrophy was also inversely related to amygdala activity (Richardson, Strange, & Dolan, 2004). Thus bidirectional connections between the amygdala and the hippocampus may be important for modulating the encoding of emotional information (see also Kilpatrick & Cahill, 2003).

In contrast to the extensive literature examining the amygdala's role during encoding, relatively few studies have considered its role during episodic retrieval. It is clear that the amygdala is engaged during retrieval of emotional items (e.g., Dolan, Lane, Chua, & Fletcher, 2000; Taylor et al., 1998) and is more active during retrieval of information learned in emotional contexts compared to nonemotional ones (e.g., Maratos, Dolan, Morris, Henson, & Rugg, 2001; Smith, Henson, Dolan, & Rugg, 2004; Sterpenich et al., 2006). The strongest test for the role of the amygdala in retrieval, however, is a demonstration of an interaction between emotional content and successful retrieval—that is, a stronger relation to successful retrieval (as compared to retrieval failures) for emotional items than for neutral items. Some recent studies have provided evidence for such an interaction, underscoring the

potential importance of amygdala engagement during the retrieval process (Dolcos, LaBar, & Cabeza, 2005; Kensinger & Schacter, 2005b; Sergerie, Lepage, & Armony, 2006).

As this section has highlighted, a tremendous amount has been learned about the effects of emotion on memory by focusing on emotion-induced enhancements in the likelihood of remembering information. These studies have demonstrated that positive and negative events often are more likely to be remembered than nonemotional ones are, and that the amygdala appears to be critical for this quantitative memory boost. Through its interactions with other cortical and subcortical regions, the amygdala can modulate sensory and mnemonic functions, increasing the likelihood that emotional information is perceived and retained in a stable memory trace.

QUALITY-BASED INFLUENCES

Although quantitative assessments of memory have been instrumental in laying the groundwork for investigations of emotion–memory interactions, they may underestimate the influence of emotion. Not all remembrances are created equal. Sometimes we feel transported in time as we reexperience a prior event, and our memory seems to include a tremendous amount of detail about where and when the event occurred. Other times we recognize that we've seen something before, but our memory does not include information about the context of the prior encounter: We recognize an individual in the airport but do not know where we met this person, or we recognize a stretch of road without knowing when we have driven it before (reviewed by Gardiner & Java, 1993; Yonelinas, 2002).

Many of emotion's effects on memory become apparent only when the quality of a memory is considered. As noted in the section above, there are many instances in which individuals are no more likely to correctly recognize an emotional item than a nonemotional one. One potential reason for this null effect of emotion is that successful recognition performance does not require a vivid memory: Although we can recognize an item because we vividly remember its prior presentation, simply knowing that we've seen something before is sufficient. Indeed, effects of emotion are more likely to occur when the vividness of a memory is considered. For example, when individuals are asked not only whether they recognize an item but also whether they vividly "remember" the item's prior presentation, rates of "remembering" tend to be much higher for emotional pictures or words than for nonemotional ones (Dewhurst & Parry, 2000; Kensinger & Corkin, 2003; Ochsner, 2000; Sharot, Delgado, & Phelps, 2004). This boost in the ability to vividly remember emotional information often occurs even when overall recognition rates are equivalent for emotional and neutral information (e.g., Ochsner, 2000; Sharot et al., 2004).

In many instances, enhanced vividness defines an emotional memory. An extreme example is a "flashbulb memory": As the term implies, individuals sometimes believe that they have maintained an almost photographic-quality memory of a highly emotional and consequential event (Brown & Kulik, 1977). For example, people claim to remember where they were and what they were doing when they learned of the assassination of President John F. Kennedy (Brown & Kulik, 1977; Christianson, 1989; Winograd & Killinger, 1983); the September 11, 2001, terrorist attacks (Budson et al., 2004; Paradis, Solomon, Florer, & Thompson, 2004; Pezdek, 2003; Smith, Bibi, & Sheard, 2003); or the explosions of the space shuttles *Challenger* and *Columbia* (Bohannon, 1988; Kensinger, Krendl, & Corkin, 2006; Neisser & Harsch, 1986). Although such extremely vivid memories are formed only rarely, studies of autobiographical memory have confirmed that individuals often remember emotional experiences in a particularly vivid manner (e.g., Conway, 1990; Rubin & Kozin, 1984; Schaefer & Philippot, 2005). In all of these examples, what is noteworthy about the memories is not that the individuals remember the experience, but rather that they reexperience it with tremendous vividness.

In this section, we examine whether the emotional qualities of events can affect how vividly they are remembered. In particular, we will discuss whether the arousal (the degree of excitation or pacification) or valence (the degree of displeasure or contentment; e.g., Russell, 1980; Lang, Greenwald, Bradley, & Hamm, 1993) elicited by an event influences the vividness with which a person remembers those experiences.

Effects of Arousal on Memory's Vividness

The vast majority of studies examining the effects of emotion on memory's vividness have focused on stimuli that elicit high arousal. For these stimuli, mnemonic influences appear to occur via interactions between the amygdala and the hippocampus. For example, Kensinger and Corkin (2004) compared encoding-related activity for words that participants later vividly remembered and for words that participants later forgot. For the arousing words, interactions between the amygdala and the hippocampus were found to be critical: Activity in both of these regions corresponded with the likelihood that a participant would later vividly remember a negative arousing word, and the amount of activity in the two regions was correlated strongly. For nonarousing words, hippocampal activity predicted the vividness of a memory, but amygdala activity did not. Thus amygdala activity during encoding relates not only to an increased likelihood of remembering an emotional item (as discussed in the prior section), but also to an increased likelihood of remembering such an item vividly (see also Dolcos et al., 2004, for evidence that amygdala activity during encoding leads to vivid memories of emotionally arousing information).

These mnemonic influences appear to occur relatively automatically. Kensinger and Corkin (2004) asked participants to study words either with full attention devoted toward the encoding task, or with attention divided between the encoding task and a secondary (sound discrimination) task. The addition of the secondary task impaired the vividness with which the nonarousing words were remembered, whereas it did not have a large effect on the vividness of memories for the arousing words (see also Bush & Geer, 2001). This finding is consistent with proposals that emotional information is privy to prioritized or relatively automatic processing (reviewed by Dolan & Vuilleumier, 2003; Pessoa, Kastner, & Ungerleider, 2003).

Although these studies demonstrate that emotional arousal can be a critical factor contributing to the emotional memory enhancement effect (see also Cahill & McGaugh, 1995; McGaugh, 2004), an arousal response is not required for emotional modulation of memory's vividness. Items that evoke changes in valence, but not changes in arousal, also can be remembered with enhanced vividness

(Kensinger & Corkin, 2003; Ochsner, 2000). The processes that lead to the mnemonic enhancements for nonarousing items, however, seem to be distinct from those mechanisms engaged for arousing information. In particular, the mnemonic boost for nonarousing stimuli appears to stem from controlled and elaborative processing of the stimuli (see Kensinger, 2004, for further discussion). Thus, in contrast to the minimal effect of divided attention on participants' memories for arousing items (Bush & Geer, 2001; Kensinger & Corkin, 2004), divided attention has a large detrimental effect on the likelihood that participants will vividly remember negative nonarousing items. In fact, when participants' attention is divided during encoding, the mnemonic enhancement for negative nonarousing words disappears (Kensinger & Corkin, 2004).

There also are distinct neural signatures associated with the successful encoding of arousing and nonarousing words (Kensinger & Corkin, 2004). In contrast to arousing items, which appear to be vividly remembered due to amygdala engagement, successful encoding of nonarousing items is associated with increased activity in the prefrontal cortex and hippocampus (and see LaBar & Phelps, 1998, for evidence that memory for negative nonarousing stimuli was not impaired in a patient with amygdala damage). The prefrontal cortex and hippocampus support later memory for neutral items as well, but the strength of their correspondence with later memory is greater for the negative nonarousing items (Kensinger & Corkin, 2004). This overlap in the neural processes engaged to remember neutral and negative nonarousing words is consistent with the conclusion that participants are remembering the negative nonarousing words because of increased engagement of the same types of cognitive and neural processes that lead to a vivid memory for nonemotional information. This finding emphasizes that simply showing a memory benefit for emotional stimuli does not necessitate that a distinct mnemonic mechanism be postulated (and see Talmi & Moscovitch, 2004).

Thus, although many researchers have focused on amygdala-mediated effects of emotion on memory (thought to arise due to the action of stress hormones; McGaugh, 2000; McGaugh & Roozendaal, 2002), emotional information that does not elicit amygdalar modulation of memory can also be more vividly remembered than neutral information. These

effects may arise because individuals are more likely to elaborate on the material during encoding or to rehearse the information (for discussions of effects of elaboration and rehearsal on memory for emotional information, see Bohannon, 1988; Brown & Kulik, 1977; Christianson & Engelberg, 1999; Isen, 1999).

Effects of Valence on the Quality of a Memory

To assess the effects of valence on memory, researchers have contrasted memory for positive arousing and negative arousing stimuli. If highly arousing positive and negative experiences have different memory characteristics, then it cannot be only the arousal of the events that influences memory quality. A number of studies have suggested that the valence elicited by the event does influence the subjective vividness of the memory. Within the laboratory, negative events are often remembered with a greater sense of vividness than positive events are (e.g., Ochsner, 2000; Dewhurst & Parry, 2000). Positive stimuli, in contrast, are often remembered with only a feeling of familiarity, or with general (nonspecific) information (e.g., Ochsner, 2000; Bless & Schwarz, 1999). This effect of valence on memory for detail can hold even in individuals (e.g., older adults) who tend to focus more on positive information than on negative, and it can exist even when overall recognition rates are equated for negative and positive information (Kensinger, O'Brien, Swanberg, Garoff-Eaton, & Schacter, in press; Kensinger, Garoff-Eaton, & Schacter, 2007). Positive mood also has been associated with more memory reconstruction errors than negative mood has, probably because individuals in a happy mood rely on gist-based information or on heuristics, while individuals in a negative mood are more likely to focus on the specific details of information (e.g., Bless et al., 1996; Storbeck & Clore, 2005).

It has been unclear to what extent these laboratory findings extend to real-life events infused with emotional importance. Research on autobiographical memory has often supported the opposite conclusion from laboratory research: that positive memories are more vivid than negative ones (e.g., D'Argembeau, Comblain, & van der Linden, 2003; Schaefer & Philippot, 2005). For example, Schaefer and Philippot (2005) asked participants to recall positive, negative, and neutral events, and for each one to rate the number of sensory, semantic, temporal, and contextual associations retrieved about the memory (using the Memory Characteristics Questionnaire; Johnson, Foley, Suengas, & Raye, 1988). They found that participants' ratings were higher for positive than for negative memories, indicating greater retrieval of contextual detail for positive events. However, some studies suggest little effect of valence on memory vividness, and instead have found intensity to be the primary predictor of autobiographical memory characteristics (e.g., Talarico, LaBar, & Rubin, 2004).

A difficulty in these studies is finding positive and negative events that are comparable across a range of dimensions (e.g., duration of event, public or private nature of event, amount of media coverage or rehearsal). Two prior studies have attempted to circumvent many of these difficulties by examining whether a person's response to an event outcome (finding it positive or negative) affects what the person remembers about the event (Levine & Bluck, 2004; Kensinger & Schacter, 2006e). Levine and Bluck (2004) asked participants to indicate whether particular events had occurred during the verdict decision in the O. J. Simpson trial. We (Kensinger & Schacter, 2006e) examined what Red Sox fans and Yankees fans remembered about the final game of the 2004 American League Championship Series, in which the Red Sox overcame a surprising 0–3 setback in the series to win the championship. Consistent with Talarico et al. (2004), both studies found that the overall amount of detail remembered about the event was not influenced by the event's valence. Valence did, however, affect some memory characteristics: Levine and Bluck (2004) found that individuals who were happy about the Simpson verdict remembered the event more vividly and were more liberal in accepting that something had occurred. Similarly, we (Kensinger & Schacter, 2006e) found that Red Sox fans, who found the outcome positive, showed more memory inconsistencies and were more likely to be overconfident in their memories than were Yankees fans. In both studies valence did not affect the quantity of remembered information, but it did influence the qualitative nature of the retrieved memories. These results emphasize the need to examine the effects of emotion not only on the likelihood of remembering information, but also on the quality of remembered information.

EFFECTS OF EMOTION ON MEMORY FOR DETAIL

The prior section emphasizes that emotion can affect not only the likelihood of remembering an event, but also the subjective vividness with which it is remembered. Individuals can say that they vividly remember an item for a variety of reasons, however. They may remember specific perceptual details of the event; they may recollect specific contextual details, such as something they thought of during the event; or they may be biased to say that they remember the prior experience vividly. In this section we first examine whether emotion primarily inflates people's confidence in their memories, or whether it also has beneficial effects on memory for detail. We then discuss the neural processes that mediate the effects of emotion on memory for detail, as well as the types of details that are most likely to be remembered about an emotional event.

Inflated Confidence or Enhanced Detail?

When Brown and Kulik (1977) coined the term "flashbulb memory" to refer to the vivid recollection of a surprising and consequential event, they believed that it reflected a separate memory mechanism, immune to memory distortion or disruption. Numerous studies have now demonstrated that these memories are in fact prone to significant distortions over time. Individuals often report high confidence in so-called flashbulb memories despite low consistency in their reports over time, and there is often little or no correlation between how confident individuals are about their memories and how accurate or consistent their memories are (Neisser & Harsch, 1992; Schmidt, 2004; Schmolck, Buffalo, & Squire, 2000; Talarico & Rubin, 2003). Clearly, emotional events do not leave indelible traces. Nevertheless, the question remains of whether enhanced confidence in memories of emotional experiences is justified: Are individuals just biased to believe that they have retained a detailed memory of an emotional experience, or are these events retrieved with more accurate detail than nonemotional events are?

On the one hand there is some evidence that emotion may primarily bias people to believe that they remember a prior experience: Across a number of recognition paradigms, emotional items (and particularly negative ones) have been more likely to be falsely recognized than nonemotional ones (Budson et al., 2006; Ehlers et al., 1988; Windmann & Kruger, 1998; Windmann & Kutas, 2001). Because the increased false alarms occur not only for related lures but also for unrelated emotional words, these results suggest that individuals may be biased to believe that they have encountered an emotional item previously. One likely contributor to this bias is the fact that emotional items (and negative ones in particular) tend to be processed more fluently than neutral items (Bargh, Chaiken, Govender, & Pratto, 1992; Kitayama, 1990; Öhman, 1988). Because items that have been studied recently tend to be processed more fluently than items that have not been encountered recently (Whittlesea, 1993; Whittlesea & Williams, 2000), participants may misinterpret the fluid processing of an emotional item on a recognition task as evidence that they have recently studied the item. Thus enhanced fluency could lead individuals to falsely endorse more nonpresented negative items than nonpresented neutral items. Another possible contributor to the bias is the semantic relatedness of most emotional items (see Talmi & Moscovitch, 2004). Because thematically associated lures tend to be falsely endorsed more often than unrelated lures (Roediger, Watson, McDermott, & Gallo, 2001; Stradler, Roediger, & McDermott, 1999), emotional items may be falsely recognized more frequently because of their semantic cohesion.

Sharot et al. (2004) have suggested that amygdala activity at retrieval may primarily serve to inflate a person's estimate of a memory's vividness and level of detail. They found that amygdala activity at retrieval corresponded with an individual's belief that an emotional item was vividly remembered (see also Dolcos et al., 2005), whereas activity in the parahippocampal gyrus (associated with visual memory) corresponded with vivid remembering of neutral information. Because the enhancement in subjective vividness for the emotional items occurred in the absence of an emotion-related boost in the ability to discriminate "old" from "new" items, Sharot et al. interpreted their findings as indicating that amygdala engagement at retrieval leads individuals to feel that they have a vivid memory not because they remember perceptual detail (as is the case with neutral items), but rather because of the feeling of arousal and perceptual

fluency that accompanies the remembrance of emotional items.

On the other hand, however, there are instances in which emotion can increase the likelihood that details are remembered about an item. In a couple of studies (Kensinger, Garoff-Eaton, & Schacter, 2006; Kensinger et al., 2007), participants were shown a series of negative and neutral objects (e.g., a spider, a blender) and later were asked to distinguish "same" objects (those that were identical to a studied item) from "similar" objects (those that had the same verbal label as a studied item, but that differed in any number of visual details). Individuals were more accurate at discriminating "same" from "similar" negative items than they were at distinguishing "same" from "similar" neutral items. Importantly, this enhancement in memory specificity occurred even when the ability to recognize that a particular item type had been presented (e.g., to remember that a snake or a blender had been studied) was not influenced by emotion. These results parallel the self-report data (Ochsner, 2000; Sharot et al., 2004), with negative emotional content enhancing not the ability to recognize an item from a study episode, but rather the ability to vividly remember its presentation. According to our results (Kensinger, Garoff-Eaton, & Schacter, 2006), the pattern of self-report data does not necessitate that individuals are biased to believe that they vividly remember an emotional item. Rather, emotion can affect the amount of detail remembered about a studied item, while not affecting the overall proportion of items remembered.

Although these studies focused on memory for perceptual detail, emotion may have a broader effect on the ability to remember contextual (or "source") information. "Source memory" is frequently defined as any contextual aspect (e.g., perceptual, spatiotemporal, affective) present when an encoding event occurred (Johnson, Hashtroudi, & Lindsay, 1993). Source memory can be contrasted with "item memory"—the ability to recall or recognize that an item was previously encountered, without the ability to retrieve details about its encoding context. In a number of paradigms emotion has been found to enhance memory for such details as the color in which a word was presented (Doerksen & Shimamura, 2001; Kensinger & Corkin, 2003; D'Argembeau & van der Linden, 2004; MacKay et al., 2004), the spatial location of a word (D'Argembeau

& van der Linden, 2004; MacKay & Ahmet-zanov, 2005), or whether words or objects were imagined or visually presented (Kensinger & Schacter, 2006d). Contextual information presented in a sentence may also be more likely to be remembered if the sentence is emotionally negative than if it is neutral (Kensinger et al., 2002, 2004). These results indicate that events with emotional meaning are often more likely to be remembered with detail than are events void of emotional importance.

Moreover, amygdala activity at retrieval can correspond with retrieval of accurate detail. We (Kensinger & Schacter, 2005b) asked participants to view photographs of some objects, but only to imagine viewing others. At retrieval, participants were required to indicate which items they had imagined viewing and which ones they had actually seen (i.e., to make a reality-monitoring decision). The critical finding was that activity in the orbito-frontal cortex, amygdala, and hippocampus, was greater for emotional items accurately attributed to presentation or to imagination than for emotional items misattributed. Convergent findings were revealed in an elegant study by Smith, Stephan, Rugg, and Dolan (2006). Participants studied neutral objects in either neutral or emotional scenes. Some of the neutral and emotional scenes contained people, while others did not. Participants were then asked to report the context in which objects had been studied. In one condition, the options were "emotional context" or "neutral context"; in another condition, the options were "context with people" or "context without people." The data revealed enhanced hippocampus–amygdala connectivity whenever individuals retrieved information studied in an emotional context, regardless of whether the task required reporting of the emotional context (i.e., in both the "emotional" vs. "neutral" and "people" vs. "no-people" conditions). When the retrieval of the emotional information was critical to successful memory performance (i.e., in the "emotional" vs. "neutral" condition), hippocampus–amygdala connectivity increased bidirectionally, modulated by the orbitofrontal cortex. Taken together, these two studies provide strong evidence that limbic engagement during memory retrieval does not relate only to an inflated confidence in the subjective richness of a memory; rather, increased limbic activity can correspond with the retrieval of details regarding an item's presentation.

How Emotion Influences Memory for Detail

Although these studies indicate that at least some details are more likely to be remembered for items with negative emotional content than for items with neutral content, they do not clarify whether this increased memory accuracy for the negative arousing information is specifically related to the processing of the emotional information, or whether it stems from engagement of the same processes that lead to accurate memory for neutral information. The increased memory accuracy for negative arousing information could result from domain-general factors, such as the greater semantic relatedness (Talmi & Moscovitch, 2004) or the greater distinctiveness of emotional items (Schmidt, 2002); or the enhanced accuracy could stem from processes specific to emotional processing.

To adjudicate between these alternatives, we conducted a series of studies to examine the effect of emotion on reality-monitoring ability (the ability to distinguish what has been perceived from what has been imagined; Johnson & Raye, 1981). Accurate reality-monitoring attributions are thought to rely on an individual's ability to encode, and later to retrieve, details of the encoding episode. Memories for perceived events typically include more sensory and contextual information, whereas memories for imagined events often include more information about the cognitive operations that supported the internal generation of information (Johnson & Raye, 1981). Thus retrieval of perceptual information will tend to correspond with attribution of a memory to a presented source, whereas retrieval of information linked to self-referential processing is related to an attribution of a memory to an internal source (Gonsalves & Paller, 2000; Kensinger & Schacter, 2006b).

We demonstrated that negative arousing items were more often accurately attributed than were neutral items (Kensinger & Schacter, 2006d). This enhanced discrimination occurred both when encoding was incidental and when it was intentional, and the effect was present both for verbal stimuli and for single objects. Using functional magnetic resonance imaging, we investigated the neural processes that led to accurate memory attributions (Kensinger & Schacter, 2005a). Most notably, whereas enhanced encoding-related activity in the posterior hippocampus was related to accurate memory attributions for all items (negative arousing and nonemotional), enhanced encoding-related activity in the amygdala and the orbito-frontal cortex corresponded with a reduction in the likelihood of memory misattributions specifically for the negative arousing items. Activity in these limbic regions, often engaged during the processing of emotional information (e.g., Bechara, Damasio, & Damasio, 2000; Phan et al., 2005; Zald, 2003), showed no correspondence to memory accuracy for the neutral items. Thus the enhanced accuracy for negative arousing items did not stem solely from the additional engagement of domain-general processes that enhanced accuracy for all items. Rather, domain-specific processes (processing of emotional information in the amygdala and orbito-frontal cortex) increased the likelihood of accurate memory attributions for the emotional items.

It is important to note, however, that part of the effect of these emotion-specific processes appeared to have been exerted via their interactions with regions that promote accurate encoding of both emotional and nonemotional items. In particular, activity in the amygdala was highly correlated with activity in the hippocampus during the encoding of negative arousing items that were accurately attributed later. Many studies have demonstrated the critical role of the hippocampus in binding together a nonemotional item and its context: Patients with hippocampal lesions have difficulties remembering the context in which an item was studied (Giovanello, Verfaellie, & Keane, 2003; Shoqeirat & Mayes, 1991); older adults who exhibit medial temporal lobe dysfunction have deficits on these types of binding tasks as well (Chalfonte & Johnson, 1996; Collie, Myers, Schnirman, Wood, & Maruff, 2002); and neuroimaging studies have implicated the hippocampus specifically in the ability to learn associative information, as compared to nonassociative information (e.g., Davachi & Wagner, 2002; Giovanello, Schnyer, & Verfaellie, 2004; Jackson & Schacter, 2004; but see Stark & Squire, 2001). Thus it appears that memory for the details of an emotional event can be enhanced not because individuals bring online an entirely distinct set of processes to help them remember the information, but rather because of limbic modulation of the same processes (e.g., hippocampal binding mechanisms) that are typically recruited to remember the details of nonemotional information.

In this reality-monitoring paradigm, memory accuracy was higher for items with negative content. However, not all types of contextual details seem to be enhanced by emotional content. For example, emotion conferred no advantage when individuals were asked to remember whether they rated an item as animate–inanimate or as common–uncommon (Kensinger & Schacter, 2006a). Importantly, in this paradigm, amygdala activity corresponded only with memory for the item (i.e., knowing whether something was "old" or "new"), but not with memory for the task performed with the item (i.e., the "source"). A related finding has been reported by Adolphs and colleagues (reviewed by Buchanan & Adolphs, 2002): They have found that although emotion enhances the ability to remember the "gist" (general semantic theme) of scenes or stories, it can reduce memory for specific details. They have also provided evidence that this emotion-related effect on memory may be mediated by the amygdala: Patients with damage to the amygdala do not show the enhanced memory for gist or the impaired memory for detail (Adolphs, Tranel, & Buchanan, 2005).

These results highlight the fact that the role of the amygdala during encoding of event details may depend on the particular type of detail that is assessed. Emotion does not enhance memory for all aspects of an encoding episode, and amygdala engagement at encoding does not ensure that all details will be accurately remembered. Although additional research will be needed to clarify the circumstances in which amygdala activity does or does not relate to the encoding of event details, one possible explanation is that amygdala activity guides encoding of details that are intrinsic to an item (e.g., its physical appearance or its gist), but does not enhance encoding of attributes that are extrinsic to an item (e.g., the task performed with the item; and see Mather et al., 2006, for evidence that the neural processes supporting working memory for spatial location are disrupted for items that elicit an arousal response). Thus recall of such details as a word's font may be enhanced by emotion (Doerksen & Shimamura, 2001; Kensinger & Corkin, 2003; MacKay et al., 2004) because those details are processed as intrinsic item attributes: A vivid memory of a word's presentation is likely to include the color or location of the word. Similarly, individuals may be more likely to remember neutral words occurring in an emotional sentence (Kensinger et al., 2002, 2004) because individuals process the entire sentence as a single stimulus rather than as a series of individual words. In contrast, focusing on the emotional item may actually preclude the processing of details extrinsic to that item. This hypothesis would be consistent with the proposal that the effects of emotion on memory may best be characterized as tradeoffs: Some aspects of an event are better remembered because of the event's emotional salience, whereas other aspects are more likely to be forgotten (see reviews by Buchanan & Adolphs, 2002, and Reisberg & Heuer, 2004). Of course this proposal leaves open a number of questions, including how the amygdala can exert these selective effects on memory. One possibility is that, just as amygdala–hippocampus interactions at retrieval are guided by the orbito-frontal cortex (Smith et al., 2006), so does orbito-frontal activity during encoding guide the stimulus attributes that are attended and remembered.

EMOTION'S EFFECTS ON IMPLICIT MEMORY

Although we have focused exclusively on emotion's influence on conscious retrieval of previously learned information, emotion also modulates implicit memory, altering how recent experiences for which we do not have conscious memory affect our behavior (but see Steidl, Mohiuddin, & Anderson, 2006, for evidence that emotion can have dissociable effects on some forms of implicit memory compared to explicit memory). Implicit memory can take many forms, but here we focus on emotion's effects on "priming"—changes in a person's perception or response to a stimulus due to its prior exposure (for a recent review on priming, see Schacter, Dobbins, & Schnyer, 2004; for reviews of emotion's effects on other forms of implicit memory, such as fear conditioning, see Maren, 2001; Lavond, Kim, & Thompson, 1993; LeDoux, 1996). A tremendous amount of research has indicated that prior exposure to a stimulus can influence people's affective response toward it: Even when individuals are not aware that they have encountered a stimulus previously, they often will have a preference for the previously seen item as compared to a novel one (the "mere-exposure effect"; for reviews, see Bornstein, 1989; Harrison, 1977; Zajonc, 2001).

Although this research has focused on how unconscious processing of information can influence a person's affective response to a stimulus, more recent research has begun to address whether emotional content of information influences responses within nonaffective domains (see Butler & Berry, 2004, for discussion of similarities and differences between the mere-exposure effect and repetition priming). For example, are individuals faster to perceptually identify or to make decisions about previously encountered information with emotional content, as compared to previously encountered information lacking emotional meaning? The literature in this area is relatively sparse, but the studies to date suggest that emotional content of information confers an advantage on priming tasks, just as it does on tasks of explicit memory: Emotional stimuli show larger enhancements on perceptual and conceptual priming tasks than do nonemotional stimuli (Burton et al., 2004; Collins & Cooke, 2005; LaBar et al., 2005; Michael, Ehlers, & Halligan, 2005). Future studies will be required to elucidate the range of tasks for which emotion confers these priming benefits; the extent to which emotional stimuli are sensitive to manipulations that alter the magnitude of priming for nonemotional information (e.g., changes in modality of presentation, of stimulus appearance, or of task instructions); and the degree to which the affective quality of the stimuli (e.g., the valence or arousal elicited, or the discrete emotion evoked; see Burton et al., 2005) influences the strength of the priming. Future studies would also do well to investigate the neural correlates of emotional influences on priming. Neuroimaging studies of nonemotional information have consistently revealed that priming is accompanied by decreased activity in a number of cortical regions (for reviews, see Grill-Spector, Henson, & Martin, 2006; Schacter & Buckner, 1998; Wiggs & Martin, 1998). Initial neuroimaging evidence suggests that emotion can modulate the magnitude of such decreases (Ishai, Pessoa, Bikle, & Ungerleider, 2004), but further studies of the issue are required.

CONCLUSIONS

In this chapter, we have reviewed three approaches to examining the effects of emotion on memory: those focused on understanding what makes individuals more likely to remember emotional experiences than nonemotional ones; those examining why emotional memories often are reexperienced with tremendous vividness; and those investigating the types of details that are more likely to be remembered about emotional experiences than about nonemotional ones. Each of these lines of research has provided behavioral evidence of emotion–memory interactions, and neuroimaging and neuropsychological studies have demonstrated that the effects of emotion are not due to domain-general processes that boost memory for all information, but rather stem from engagement of emotion-specific processing (particularly in the amygdala and the orbito-frontal cortex). The modulatory influence of these regions is apparent during memory encoding, consolidation, and retrieval; during each of these memory phases, limbic activity serves to modulate perceptual and mnemonic function to increase the likelihood that information is attended to and that at least some details are retained. Thus, at least in part, emotional information is remembered better than nonemotional information not because of the engagement of processes unique to memory for emotional information, but rather because of limbic modulation of the same processes that are typically recruited to remember nonemotional information. Although increasing behavioral evidence indicates that this limbic modulation does not boost memory for all details of an encoding episode, future studies will be required to delineate the types of details that are better remembered for emotional than for neutral information, as well as the neural mechanisms that allow emotion to exert selective effects on memory for some item attributes but not for others.

REFERENCES

Abrisqueta-Gomez, J., Bueno, O. F., Oliveira, M. G., & Bertolucci, P. H. (2002). Recognition memory for emotional pictures in Alzheimer's disease. *Acta Neurologica Scandinavica, 105,* 51–54.

Adolphs, R., Cahill, L., Schul, R., & Babinsky, R. (1997). Impaired declarative memory for emotional material following bilateral amygdala damage in humans. *Learning and Memory, 4,* 291–300.

Adolphs, R., Tranel, D., & Buchanan, T. W. (2005). Amygdala damage impairs emotional memory for gist but not details of complex stimuli. *Nature Neuroscience, 8,* 512–518.

Amaral, D., Price, J., Pitkanen, A., & Carmichael, S. (1992). Anatomical organization of the primate amygdaloid complex. In J. Aggleton (Ed.), *The amygdala: Neurobiological aspects of emotion, memory, and mental dysfunction* (pp. 1–67). New York: Wiley-Liss.

Amaral, D. G. (2003). The amygdala, social behavior, and danger detection. *Annals of the New York Academy of Sciences, 1000,* 337–347.

Anders, S., Lotze, M., Erb, M., Grodd, W., & Girbaumer, N. (2004). Brain activity underlying emotional valence and arousal: A response-related fMRI study. *Human Brain Mapping, 23,* 200–209.

Anderson, A. K., Christoff, K., Stappen, I., Panitz, D., Ghahremani, D. G., Glover, G., et al. (2003). Dissociated neural representations of intensity and valence in human olfaction. *Nature Neuroscience, 6,* 196–202.

Baas, D., Aleman, A., & Kahn, R. S. (2004). Lateralization of amygdala activation: A systematic review of functional neuroimaging studies. *Brain Research Reviews, 45,* 96–103.

Bargh, J. A., Chaiken, S., Govender, R., & Pratto, F. (1992). The generality of the attitude activation effect. *Journal of Personality and Social Psychology, 62,* 893–912.

Bechara, A., Damasio, H., & Damasio, A. R. (2000). Emotion, decision making and the orbitofrontal cortex. *Cerebral Cortex, 10,* 295–307.

Bless, H., Clore, G. L., Schwarz, N., Golisano, V., Rabe, C., & Wolk, M. (1996). Mood and the use of scripts: Does a happy mood really lead to mindlessness? *Journal of Personality and Social Psychology, 71,* 665–679.

Bless, H., & Schwarz, N. (1999). Sufficient and necessary conditions in dual-process models: The case of mood and information processing. In S. Chaiken & Y. Trope (Eds.), *Dual-process theories in social psychology* (pp. 423–440). New York: Guilford Press.

Bohannon, J. N. (1988). Flashbulb memories for the space shuttle disaster: A tale of two theories. *Cognition, 29,* 179–196.

Bornstein, R. F. (1989). Exposure and affect: Overview and meta-analysis of research, 1968–1987. *Psychological Bulletin, 106,* 265–289.

Bradley, M. M., Greenwald, M. K., Petry, M. C., & Lang, P. J. (1992). Remembering pictures: pleasure and arousal in memory. *Journal of Experimental Psychology: Learning, Memory, and Cognition, 18,* 379–390.

Brierley, B., Medford, N., Shaw, P., & David, A. S. (2004). Emotional memory and perception in temporal lobectomy patients with amygdala damage. *Journal of Neurology, Neurosurgery and Psychiatry, 75,* 593–599.

Brown, R., & Kulik, J. (1977). Flashbulb memories. *Cognition, 5,* 73–99.

Buchanan, T. W., & Adolphs, R. (2002). The role of the human amygdala in emotional modulation of long-term declarative memory. In S. Moore & M. Oaksford (Eds.), *Emotional cognition: From brain to behavior* (pp. 9–34). Amsterdam: Benjamins.

Buchanan, T. W., Tranel, D., & Adolphs, R. (2006). Memories for emotional autobiographical events following unilateral damage to medial temporal lobe. *Brain, 129,* 115–127.

Budson, A. E., Simons, J. S., Sullivan, A. L., Beier, J. S., Solomon, P. R., Scinto, L. F., et al. (2004). Memory and emotions for the 9/11/01 terrorist attacks in patients with Alzheimer's disease, mild cognitive impairment, and healthy older adults. *Neuropsychology, 18,* 315–327.

Budson, A. E., Todman, R. W., Chong, H., Adams, E. H., Kensinger, E. A., Krandel, T. S., et al. (2006). False recognition of emotional word lists in aging and Alzheimer's disease. *Cognitive and Behavioral Neurology, 19,* 71–78.

Burton, L. A., Rabin, L., Vardy, S. B., Frohlich, J., Wyatt, G., Dimitri, D., et al. (2004). Gender differences in implicit and explicit memory for affective passages. *Brain and Cognition, 54,* 218–224.

Burton, L. A., Rabin, L., Wyatt, G., Frohlich, J., Bernstein Vardy, S., & Dimitri, D. (2005). Priming effects for affective vs. neutral faces. *Brain and Cognition, 59,* 322–329.

Bush, S. I., & Geer, J. H. (2001). Implicit and explicit memory of neutral, negative emotional, and sexual information. *Archives of Sexual Behavior, 30,* 615–631.

Butler, L. T., & Berry, D. C. (2004). Understanding the relationship between repetition priming and mere exposure. *British Journal of Psychology, 95,* 467–487.

Cahill, L., Babinsky, R., Markowitsch, H. J., & McGaugh, J. L. (1995). The amygdala and emotional memory. *Nature, 377,* 295–296.

Cahill, L., Haier, R. J., Fallon, J., Alkire, M. T., Tang, C., Keator, D., et al. (1996). Amygdala activity at encoding correlated with long-term, free recall of emotional information. *Proceedings of the National Academy of Sciences USA, 93,* 8016–8021.

Cahill, L., & McGaugh, J. L. (1995). A novel demonstration of enhanced memory associated with emotional arousal. *Consciousness and Cognition, 4,* 410–421.

Chalfonte, B. L., & Johnson, M. K. (1996). Feature memory and binding in young and older adults. *Memory and Cognition, 24,* 403–416.

Charles, S. T., Mather, M., & Carstensen, L. L. (2003). Aging and emotional memory: The forgettable nature of negative images for older adults. *Journal of Experimental Psychology: General, 132,* 310–324.

Christianson, S.-A. (1989). Flashbulb memories: special, but not so special. *Memory and Cognition, 17,* 435–443.

Christianson, S.-A. (1992). Emotional stress and eyewitness testimony: A critical review. *Psychological Bulletin, 112,* 284–309.

Christianson, S.-A., & Engelberg, E. (1999). Organization of emotional memories. In T. Dalgleish & M. Power (Eds.), *Handbook of cognition and emotion* (pp. 211–227). Chichester, UK: Wiley.

Collie, A., Myers, C., Schnirman, G., Wood, S., & Maruff, P. (2002). Selectively impaired associative learning in older people with cognitive decline. *Journal of Cognitive Neuroscience, 14,* 484–492.

Collins, M. A., & Cooke, A. (2005). A transfer appropriate processing approach to investigating implicit memory for emotional words in the cerebral hemispheres. *Neuropsychologia, 43,* 1529–1545.

Conway, M. A. (1990). Conceptual representation of emotions: The role of autobiographical memories. In K. J. Gilhooly, M. T. G. Keane, R. H. Logie, & G. Erdos (Eds.), *Lines of thinking: Reflections on the psychology of thought. Vol. 2. Skills, emotion, creative processes, individual differences and teaching thinking* (pp. 133–143). Chichester, UK: Wiley.

D'Argembeau, A., Comblain, C., & van der Linden, M. (2003). Phenomenal characteristics of autobiographical memories for positive, negative, and neutral events. *Applied Cognitive Psychology, 17,* 281–294.

D'Argembeau, A., Comblain, C., & van der Linden, M. (2005). Affective valence and the self-reference effect: Influence of retrieval conditions. *British Journal of Psychology, 96,* 457–466.

D'Argembeau, A., & van der Linden, M. (2004). Influence of affective meaning on memory for contextual information. *Emotion, 4,* 173–188.

Davachi, L., & Wagner, A. D. (2002). Hippocampal contributions to episodic encoding: Insights from relational and item-based learning. *Journal of Neurophysiology, 88,* 982–990.

Davidson, R. J., & Irwin, W. (1999). The functional neuroanatomy of emotion and affective style. *Trends in Cognitive Sciences, 3,* 11–20.

Dewhurst, S. A., & Parry, L. A. (2000). Emotionality, distinctiveness, and recollective experience. *European Journal of Cognitive Psychology, 12,* 541–551.

Doerksen, S., & Shimamura, A. (2001). Source memory enhancement for emotional words. *Emotion, 1,* 5–11.

Dolan, R. J., Lane, R., Chua, P., & Fletcher, P. (2000). Dissociable temporal lobe activations during emotional episodic memory retrieval. *NeuroImage, 11,* 203–209.

Dolan, R. J., & Vuilleumier, P. (2003). Amygdala automaticity in emotional processing. *Annals of the New York Academy of Sciences, 985,* 348–355.

Dolcos, F., LaBar, K. S., & Cabeza, R. (2004). Interaction between the amygdala and the medial temporal lobe memory system predicts better memory for emotional events. *Neuron, 42,* 855–863.

Dolcos, F., LaBar, K. S., & Cabeza, R. (2005). Remembering one year later: Role of the amygdala and the medial temporal lobe memory system in retrieving emotional memories. *Proceedings of the National Academy of Sciences USA, 102,* 2626–2631.

Ehlers, A., Margraf, J., Davies, S., & Roth, W. T. (1988). Selective processing of threat cues in subjects with panic attacks. *Cognition and Emotion, 2,* 201–219.

Garavan, H., Pendergrass, J. C., Ross, T. J., Stein, E. A., & Risinger, R. C. (2001). Amygdala response to both positively and negatively valenced stimuli. *Neuro-Report, 12,* 2779–2783.

Gardiner, I. M., & Java, R. I. (1993). Recognizing and remembering. In A. F. Collins, S. E. Gathercole, M. A. Conway, & P. E. Morris (Eds.), *Theories of memory* (pp. 163–188). Hove, UK: Erlbaum.

Giovanello, K. S., Schnyer, D. M., & Verfaellie, M. (2004). A critical role for the anterior hippocampus in relational memory: Evidence from an fMRI study comparing associative and item recognition. *Hippocampus, 14,* 5–8.

Giovanello, K. S., Verfaellie, M., & Keane, M. M. (2003). Disproportionate deficit in associative recognition relative to item recognition in global amnesia. *Cognitive, Affective, and Behavioral Neuroscience, 3,* 186–194.

Gonsalves, B., & Paller, K. A. (2000). Neural events that underlie remembering something that never happened. *Nature Neuroscience, 3,* 1316–1321.

Grill-Spector, K., Henson, R., & Martin, A. (2006). Repetition and the brain: Neural models of stimulus-specific effects. *Trends in Cognitive Sciences, 10,* 14–23.

Hamann, S. (2001). Cognitive and neural mechanisms of emotional memory. *Trends in Cognitive Sciences, 5,* 394–400.

Hamann, S. B., Ely, T. D., Grafton, S. T., & Kilts, C. D. (1999). Amygdala activity related to enhanced memory for pleasant and aversive stimuli. *Nature Neuroscience, 2,* 289–293.

Hamann, S. B., Ely, T. D., Hoffman, J. M., & Kilts, C. D. (2002). Ecstasy and agony: Activation of the human amygdala in positive and negative emotion. *Psychological Science, 13,* 135–141.

Harrison, A. A. (1977). Mere exposure. In L. Berkowitz (Ed.), *Advances in experimental social psychology* (Vol. 10, pp. 39–83). New York: Academic Press.

Isen, A. M. (1999). Positive affect. In T. Dalgleish & M. Powers (Eds.), *Handbook of cognition and emotion* (pp. 75–94). Chichester, UK: Wiley.

Ishai, A., Pessoa, L., Bikle, P. C., & Ungerleider, L. G. (2004). Repetition suppression of faces is modulated by emotion. *Proceedings of the National Academy of Sciences, 101,* 9827–9832.

Jackson, O., & Schacter, D. L. (2004). Encoding activity in anterior medial temporal lobe supports associative recognition. *NeuroImage, 21,* 456–464.

Johnson, M. K., Foley, M. A., Suengas, A. G., & Raye, C. L. (1988). Phenomenal characteristics of memories for perceived and imagined autobiographical events. *Journal of Experimental Psychology: General, 117,* 371–376.

Johnson, M. K., Hashtroudi, S., & Lindsay, D. S. (1993). Source monitoring. *Psychological Bulletin, 114,* 3–28.

Johnson, M. K., & Raye, C. L. (1981). Reality monitoring. *Psychological Review, 88,* 67–85.

Kensinger, E. A. (2004). Remembering emotional experiences: The contribution of valence and arousal. *Reviews in the Neurosciences, 15,* 241–252.

Kensinger, E. A. (in press). Neuroimaging the formation and retrieval of emotional memories. In *Brain mapping: New research.* Hauppauge, NY: Nova Science.

Kensinger, E. A., Anderson, A., Growdon, J. H., & Corkin, S. (2004). Effects of Alzheimer disease on memory for verbal emotional information. *Neuropsychologia, 42,* 791–800.

Kensinger, E. A., Brierley, B., Medford, N., Growdon, J. H., & Corkin, S. (2002) The effect of normal aging and Alzheimer's disease on emotional memory. *Emotion, 2,* 118–134.

Kensinger, E. A., & Corkin, S. (2003). Memory enhancement for emotional words: Are emotional words more vividly remembered than neutral words? *Memory and Cognition, 31,* 1169–1180.

Kensinger, E. A., & Corkin, S. (2004). Two routes to emotional memory: Distinct neural processes for valence and arousal. *Proceedings of the National Academy of Sciences of the USA, 101,* 3310–3315.

Kensinger, E. A., Garoff-Eaton, R. J., & Schacter, D. L. (2006). Memory for specific visual details can be enhanced by negative arousing content. *Journal of Memory and Language, 54,* 99–112.

Kensinger, E. A., Garoff-Eaton, R. J., & Schacter, D. L. (2007). Effects of emotion on memory specificity in young and older adults. *Journal of Gerontology, 62,* 208–215.

Kensinger, E. A., Garoff-Eaton, R. J., & Schacter, D. L. (2007). Effects of emotion on memory specificity: Memory trade-offs elicited by negative visually arousing stimuli. *Journal of Memory and Language, 56,* 575–591.

Kensinger, E. A., Krendl, A. C., & Corkin, S. (2006). Memories of an emotional and a nonemotional event: Effects of aging and delay interval. *Experimental Aging Research, 32,* 23–45.

Kensinger, E. A., O'Brien, J., Swanberg, K., Garoff-Eaton, R. J., & Schacter, D. L. (in press). The effects of emotional content on reality-monitoring performance in young and older adults. *Psychology and Aging.*

Kensinger, E. A., & Schacter, D. L. (2005a). Emotional content and reality-monitoring ability: FMRI evidence for the influence of encoding processes. *Neuropsychologia, 43,* 1429–1443.

Kensinger, E. A., & Schacter, D. L. (2005b). Retrieving accurate and distorted memories: Neuroimaging evidence for effects of emotion. *NeuroImage, 27,* 167–177.

Kensinger, E. A., & Schacter, D. L. (2006a). Amygdala activity is associated with the successful encoding of item, but not source, information for positive and negative stimuli. *Journal of Neuroscience, 26,* 2564–2570.

Kensinger, E. A., & Schacter, D. L. (2006b). Neural processes underlying memory attribution on a reality-monitoring task. *Cerebral Cortex, 16,* 1126–1133.

Kensinger, E. A., & Schacter, D. L. (2006c). Processing emotional pictures and words: Effects of valence and arousal. *Cognitive, Affective, and Behavioral Neuroscience, 6,* 110–127.

Kensinger, E. A., & Schacter, D. L. (2006d). Reality monitoring and memory distortion: Effects of negative, arousing content. *Memory and Cognition, 34,* 251–260.

Kensinger, E. A., & Schacter, D. L. (2006e). When the Red Sox shocked the Yankees: Comparing negative and positive memories. *Psychonomic Bulletin and Review, 13,* 757–763.

Kilpatrick, L., & Cahill, L. (2003). Amygdala modulation of parahippocampal and frontal regions during emotionally influenced memory storage. *NeuroImage, 20,* 2091–2099.

Kitayama, S. (1990). Interaction between affect and cognition in word perception. *Journal of Personality and Social Psychology, 58,* 209–217.

LaBar, K. S., & Phelps, E. A. (1998). Arousal-mediated memory consolidation: Role of the medial temporal lobe in humans. *Psychological Science, 9,* 490–493.

LaBar, K. S., Torpey, D. C., Cook, C. A., Johnson, S. R., Warren, L. H., Burke, J. R., et al. (2005). Emotional enhancement of perceptual priming is preserved in aging and early-stage Alzheimer's disease. *Neuropsychologia, 43,* 1824–1837.

Lang, P. J., Greenwald, M. K., Bradley, M. M., & Hamm, A. O. (1993). Looking at pictures: Affective, facial, visceral, and behavioral reactions. *Psychophysiology, 30,* 261–273.

Lavond, D. G., Kim, J. J., & Thompson, R. F. (1993). Mammalian brain substrates of aversive classical conditioning. *Annual Review of Psychology, 44,* 317–342.

Lazarus, R. S. (1991). *Emotion and adaptation.* New York: Oxford University Press.

LeDoux, J. E. (1996). *The emotional brain: The mysterious underpinnings of emotional life.* New York: Simon & Schuster.

Levine, L. J., & Bluck, S. (2004). Painting with broad strokes: Happiness and the malleability of event memory. *Cognition and Emotion, 18,* 559–574.

Linton, M. (1975). Memory for real-world events. In D. A. Norman & D. E. Rumelhart (Eds.), *Explorations in cognition* (pp. 376–404). San Francisco: Freeman.

MacKay, D. G., & Ahmetzanov, M. V. (2005). Emotion, memory and attention in the taboo Stroop paradigm: An experimental analogue of flashbulb memories. *Psychological Science, 16,* 25–32.

MacKay, D. G., Shafto, M., Taylor, J. K., Marian, D. E., Abrams, L., & Dyer, J. R. (2004). Relations between emotion, memory, and attention: Evidence from taboo Stroop, lexical decision, and immediate memory tasks. *Memory and Cognition, 32,* 474–488.

Maratos, E. J., Dolan, R. J., Morris, J. S., Henson, R. N., & Rugg, M. D. (2001). Neural activity associated with episodic memory for emotional context. *Neuropsychologia, 39,* 910–20.

Maren, S. (2001). Neurobiology of Pavlovian fear conditioning. *Annual Review of Neuroscience, 24,* 897–931.

Markowitsch, H. J., Calabrese, P., Wurker, M., Durwen, H. F., Kessler, J., Babinsky, R., et al. (1994). The amygdala's contribution to memory: A study on two patients with Urbach–Wiethe disease. *NeuroReport, 5,* 1349–1352.

Mather, M., & Carstensen, L. L. (2005). Aging and motivated cognition: The positivity effect in attention and memory. *Trends in Cognitive Sciences, 9,* 496–502.

Mather, M., Mitchell, K. J., Raye, C. L., Novak, D. L., Greene, E. J., & Johnson, M. K. (2006). Emotional arousal can impair feature binding in working memory. *Journal of Cognitive Neuroscience, 18,* 614–625.

Matt, G. E., Vazquez, C., & Campbell, W. C. (1992). Mood-congruent recall of affectively toned stimuli: A meta-analytic study. *Clinical Psychology Review, 12,* 227–255.

McGaugh, J. L. (2004). The amygdala modulates the consolidation of memories of emotionally arousing experiences. *Annual Review of Neuroscience, 27,* 1–28.

McGaugh, J. L., & Roozendaal, B. (2002). Role of adrenal stress hormones in forming lasting memories in the brain. *Current Opinion in Neurobiology, 12,* 205–210.

Michael, T., Ehlers, A., & Halligan, S. L. (2005). Enhanced priming for trauma-related material in post-traumatic stress disorder. *Emotion, 5,* 103–112.

Mori, E., Ikeda, M., Hirono, N., Kitagaki, H., Imamura, T., & Simomura, T. (1999). Amygdalar volume and emotional memory in Alzheimer's disease. *American Journal of Psychiatry, 156,* 216–222.

Neisser, U., & Harsch, N. (1992). Phantom flashbulbs: False recollections of hearing the news about *Challenger.* In E. Winograd & U. Neisser (Eds.), *Affect and accuracy in recall: Studies of 'flashbulb' memories* (pp. 9–31). Cambridge, UK: Cambridge University Press.

Ochsner, K. N. (2000). Are affective events richly "remembered" or simply familiar? The experience and process of recognizing feelings past. *Journal of Experimental Psychology: General, 129,* 242–261.

Öhman, A. (1988). Preattention processes in the generation of emotions. In V. Hamilton, G. H. Bower, & N. H. Frijda (Eds.), *Cognitive perspectives on emotion and motivation* (Vol. 44, pp. 127–143). Norwell, MA: Kluwer Academic.

Ortony, A., Turner, T. J., & Antos, S. J. (1983). A puzzle about affect and recognition memory. *Journal of Experimental Psychology: Learning, Memory, and Cognition, 9,* 725–729.

Paradis, C. M., Solomon, L. Z., Florer, F., & Thompson,

T. (2004). Flashbulb memories of personal events of 9/11 and the day after for a sample of New York City residents. *Psychological Reports*, *95*, 304–310.

Pessoa, L., Kastner, S., & Ungerleider, L. G. (2003). Neuroimaging studies of attention: From modulation of sensory processing to top-down control. *Journal of Neuroscience*, *23*, 3990–3998.

Pezdek, K. (2003). Event memory and autobiographical memory for the events of September 11, 2001. *Applied Cognitive Psychology*, *17*, 1033–1045.

Phan, K. L., Fitzgerald, D. A., Nathan, P. J., Moore, G. J., Uhde, T. W., & Tancer, M. E. (2005). Neural substrates for voluntary suppression of negative affect: A functional magnetic resonance imaging study. *Biological Psychiatry*, *57*, 210–219.

Phelps, E. A. (2004). Human emotion and memory: Interactions of the amygdala and hippocampal complex. *Current Opinion in Neurobiology*, *14*, 198–202.

Reisberg, D., & Heuer, F. (2004). Remembering emotional events. In D. Reisberg & P. Hertel (Eds.), *Memory and emotion* (pp. 3–41). New York: Oxford University Press.

Richardson, M. P., Strange, B., & Dolan, R. J. (2004). Encoding of emotional memories depends on the amygdala and hippocampus and their interactions. *Nature Neuroscience*, *7*, 278–285.

Riemann, B., & McNally, R. J. (1995). Cognitive processing of personally relevant information. *Cognition and Emotion*, *9*, 325–340.

Roediger, H. L., III, Watson, J. M., McDermott, K. B., & Gallo, D. A. (2001). Factors that determine false recall: A multiple regression analysis. *Psychonomic Bulletin and Review*, *8*, 385–407.

Royet, J.-P., Zald, D., Versace, R., Costes, N., Lavenne, F., Koenig, O., et al. (2000). Emotional responses to pleasant and unpleasant olfactory, visual, and auditory stimuli: A positron emission tomography study. *Journal of Neuroscience*, *20*, 7752–7758.

Rubin, D. C., & Kozin, M. (1984). Vivid memories. *Cognition*, *16*, 63–80.

Russell, J. A. (1980). A circumplex model of affect. *Journal of Personality and Social Psychology*, *39*, 1161–1178.

Schacter, D. L., & Buckner, R. L. (1998). Priming and the brain. *Neuron*, *20*, 185–195.

Schacter, D. L., Dobbins, I. G., & Schnyer, D. M. (2004). Specificity of priming: A cognitive neuroscience perspective. *Nature Reviews Neuroscience*, *5*, 853–862.

Schaefer, A., & Philippot, P. (2005). Selective effects of emotion on the phenomenal characteristics of autobiographical memories. *Memory*, *13*, 148–160.

Schmidt, S. R. (2002). Outstanding memories: The positive and negative effects of nudes on memory. *Journal of Experimental Psychology: Learning, Memory, and Cognition*, *28*, 353–361.

Schmidt, S. R. (2004). Autobiographical memories for the September 11th attacks: Reconstructive errors and emotional impairment of memory. *Memory and Cognition*, *32*, 443–454.

Schmolck, H., Buffalo, E. A., & Squire, L. R. (2000). Memory distortions develop over time: Recollections of the O. J. Simpson trial verdict after 15 and 32 months. *Psychological Science*, *11*, 39–45.

Sergerie, K., Lepage, M., & Armony, J. L. (2006). A process-specific functional dissociation of the amygdala in emotional memory. *Journal of Cognitive Neuroscience*, *18*, 1359–1367.

Sharot, T., Delgado, M. R., & Phelps, E. A. (2004). How emotion enhances the feeling of remembering. *Nature Neuroscience*, *12*, 1376–1380.

Shoqeirat, M. A., & Mayes, A. R. (1991). Disproportionate incidental spatial-memory and recall deficits in amnesia. *Neuropsychologia*, *29*, 749–769.

Small, D. M., Gregory, M. D., Mak, Y. E., Gitelman, D., Mesulam, M. M., & Parrish, T. (2003). Dissociation of neural representation of intensity and affective valuation in human gustation. *Neuron*, *39*, 701–711.

Smith, A. P., Henson, R. N., Dolan, R. J., & Rugg, M. D. (2004). fMRI correlates of the episodic retrieval of emotional contexts. *Neuroimage*, *22*, 868–878.

Smith, A. P., Stephan, K. E., Rugg, M. D., & Dolan, R. J. (2006). Task and content modulate amygdala-hippocampal connectivity in emotional retrieval. *Neuron*, *49*, 631–638.

Smith, M. C., Bibi, U., & Sheard, D. E. (2003). Evidence for the differential impact of time and emotion on personal and event memories for September 11, 2001. *Applied Cognitive Psychology*, *17*, 1047–1055.

Stark, C. E., & Squire, L. R. (2001). Simple and associative recognition memory in the hippocampal region. *Learning and Memory*, *8*, 190–197.

Steidl, S., Mohiuddin, S., & Anderson, A. (2006). Effects of emotional arousal on multiple memory systems: Evidence from declarative and procedural learning. *Learning and Memory*, *13*, 650–658.

Sterpenich, V., D'Argembeau, A., Desseilles, M., Balteau, E., Albouy, G., Vandewalle, G., et al. (2006). The locus ceruleus is involved in the successful retrieval of emotional memories in humans. *Journal of Neuroscience*, *26*, 7416–7423.

Storbeck, J., & Clore, G. L. (2005). With sadness comes accuracy; with happiness, false memory: Mood and the false memory effect. *Psychological Science*, *16*, 785–791.

Stradler, M. A., Roediger, H. L., III, & McDermott, K. B. (1999). Norms for word lists that create false memories. *Memory and Cognition*, *27*, 494–500.

Talarico, J. M., LaBar, K. S., & Rubin, D. C. (2004). Emotional intensity predicts autobiographical memory experience. *Memory and Cognition*, *32*, 1118–1132.

Talarico, J. M., & Rubin, D. C. (2003). Confidence, not consistency, characterizes flashbulb memories. *Psychological Science*, *14*, 455–461.

Talmi, D., & Moscovitch, M. (2004). Can semantic relatedness explain the enhancement of memory for emotional words? *Memory and Cognition, 32,* 742–751

Taylor, S. F., Liberzon, I., Fig, L. M., Decker, L. R., Minoshima, S., & Koeppe, R. A. (1998). The effect of emotional content on visual recognition memory: A PET activation study. *NeuroImage, 8,* 188–197.

Vuilleumier, P., Richardson, M. P., Armony, J. L., Driver, J., & Dolan, R. J. (2004). Distinct influences of amygdala lesion on visual cortical activation during emotional face processing. *Nature Neuroscience, 7,* 1271–1278.

White, R. T. (2002). Memory for events after twenty years. *Applied Cognitive Psychology, 16,* 603–612.

Whittlesea, B. W. A. (1993). Illusions of familiarity. *Journal of Experimental Psychology: Learning, Memory, and Cognition, 19,* 1235–1253.

Whittlesea, B. W. A., & Williams, L. D. (2000). The source of feelings of familiarity: The discrepancy-attribution hypothesis. *Journal of Experimental Psychology: Learning, Memory, and Cognition, 26,* 547–565.

Wiggs, C. L., & Martin, A. (1998). Properties and mechanisms of perceptual priming. *Current Opinion in Neurobiology, 8,* 227–233.

Windmann, S., & Kruger, T. (1998). Subconscious detection of threat as reflected by an enhanced response bias. *Consciousness and Cognition, 7,* 603–633.

Windmann, S., & Kutas, M. (2001). Electrophysiological correlates of emotion-induced recognition bias. *Journal of Cognitive Neuroscience, 13,* 577–592.

Winograd, E., & Killinger, W. A., Jr. (1983). Relating age at encoding in early childhood to adult recall: Development of flashbulb memories. *Journal of Experimental Psychology: General, 112,* 413–422.

Yonelinas, A. P. (2002). The nature of recollection and familiarity: A review of 30 years of research. *Journal of Memory and Language, 46,* 441–517.

Zajonc, R. B. (2001). Mere exposure: A gateway to the subliminal. *Current Directions in Psychological Science, 10,* 224–228.

Zald, D. H. (2003). The human amygdala and the emotional evaluation of sensory stimuli. *Brain Research: Brain Research Reviews, 41,* 88–123.

CHAPTER 38

A Framework for Representing Emotional States

MARVIN MINSKY

We often describe personalities in terms of contrasting pairs of traits (e.g., solitary vs. sociable, tranquil vs. anxious, or joyous vs. sorrowful). But sorrow is not the mere absence of joy, nor is anxiety the reverse of tranquility. Similarly, we often describe how a person is thinking in terms of opposing characteristics (e.g., rational vs. intuitive, intellectual vs. emotional, conscious vs. unconscious, or deliberate vs. spontaneous). Indeed, such pairwise divisions seem indispensable for everyday social communication, by providing us with compact expressions for depicting a person's mental condition. However, it seems to me that when we use those distinctions in psychology, this retards our technical progress by making it very difficult to see inside our mental processes. This chapter suggests a way to describe our minds in terms of larger numbers of smaller parts, which might make better ingredients for us to use to construct the kinds of theories we need.[1]

Many attempts to classify emotions begin by describing some of them as "primary"—and then try to show how these might combine to produce more complex states of mind. For example, we might start with the likes of pleasure, anger, fear, and disgust—and then combine these to represent such conditions as happiness, grief, and anxiety. This approach was successful in physical science; once we discovered the chemical elements and how these combined to form molecules, this soon led to deep understandings of the properties of common substances. So why not use the same approach to show how our high-level feelings and traits could come from combining simpler, more basic ones?

But what should we choose for those basic ingredients? It is tempting to use the familiar terms that we find in our everyday folk psychology, because the meanings of words such as "thinking," feeling," "emotion," and "consciousness" seem so natural, clear, and direct to us. But then we find it extremely hard to answer questions like these "Can you have feelings without being conscious?" or "Can you think without having emotions?" The trouble is that each of those common words refers to so many different mental processes that they simply don't serve well as "elements" for making good theories about how minds work.

What "elements" could we use instead as a basis for psychology? One answer comes from anatomy. We know, both from neuropathology and from the new scanners we use today, that each human brain has hundreds of parts, each of which does different kinds of jobs. Some of them recognize situations; others tell muscles to execute actions; and yet other regions of the brain accumulate and go on to exploit enormous bodies of common-sense knowledge. And although our present-day methods don't yet have enough resolution (in space or in time) to tell us how those processes work, they certainly show solid evidence that our present theories don't have enough parts. So now let's consider a view of the mind that does, at least in principle, provide enough room to include the many sorts of processes that support our human resourcefulness.

A METATHEORY OF EMOTIONS

What are emotions, and how do they work? Perhaps the most popular view of emotions is that they somehow add feelings, values, and other dimensions to ordinary rational thinking—just as artists add colors to black-and-white drawings. But that does not help much to explain how those processes produce their complex effects.

Another popular approach is to try to classify emotions by starting with some "primary" ones (e.g., discomfort, pleasure, anger, and joy) and using these as coordinates that generate simple two- or four-dimensional spaces; then we can try to represent higher-level emotions as regions in a metrical space. This can yield some clinically useful distinctions, but does not provide good explanations. We can't understand a complex machine just from distinguishing some of its parts; we also need ideas about how each part works and how they are all connected. Those popular diagrams and charts simply do not tell us enough.

Furthermore, it seems to me that the language of common-sense psychology makes it hard for us to formulate good theories about the great networks of processes inside our brains because, to understand that machinery, we'll need much more expressive terms than words like "feelings," "emotion," and "con-sciousness." For example, Chapter 4 of *The Emotion Machine* (Minsky, 2006) argues that "consciousness" refers to at least 20 different kinds of processes! If so, we'll need to replace each traditional term with a substantial collection of technical concepts.

At first, replacing some ideas that seem simple at first with new ones that seem much more difficult might appear to make everything worse. However, on a larger scale, this increase in complexity can actually make our job easier. For once we split each old idea into parts, we then can replace each old unsolvable mystery with several new and smaller ones—each of which still presents obstacles, but no longer seems unsolvable. So, to start dividing those old big problems into smaller ones, this new theory begins by portraying a typical brain as containing a great many parts, each of which can do some particular kind of job (see Figure 38.1). I'll use the term "resource" to refer to any such structure or function inside the brain, from the lowest-level reactions to the highest-level mental activities.[2]

We can use this image whenever we want to explain some mental condition or activity (such as anger or fear) by trying to show how that state of mind might result from activating a certain collection of mental resources. For example, the state called "anger" appears to arouse resources that make us react with unusual speed and strength, while suppressing resources that we might otherwise use to plan and act more prudently; thus anger replaces cautiousness with aggressiveness and changes sympathy into hostility. Similarly, the condition called "fear" appears to engage resources in ways that cause us to retreat.[3]

CITIZEN: I sometimes find myself in a state where everything seems cheerful and bright.

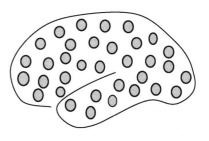

FIGURE 38.1. An image of the typical human brain containing many parts. Adapted from Minsky (2006).

At other times (although nothing has changed), all my surroundings seem dreary and dark, and my friends describe me as being "depressed." Why do I have such moods, or feelings, or dispositions—and what causes all their strange effects?

Some popular answers to this person's question are "Those states are caused by chemicals in the brain," or "They result from an excess of stress," or "They come from thinking depressing thoughts." However, such statements say little about how those processes work, whereas the idea of selecting a set of resources can suggest more specific ways in which thinking can change, as in the case of another phenomenon:

When a person has fallen in love, it's almost as though someone new has emerged—a person who thinks in other ways, with altered goals and priorities. It's almost as though a switch has been thrown and a different program has started to run.

What could happen inside a brain to make such changes in how it thinks? Here is an approach that we could take: *Each of our major "emotional states" results from turning certain resources on while turning certain others off—and thus changing some ways that our brains behave.* But what activates such sets of resources? The new theory suggests that our brains are equipped with resources that I shall call "Critics"—each of which is specialized to recognize a certain condition, and then to activate some particular set of other resources. Some of our Critics are built in from birth, to activate certain "instinctive" reactions that evolved to help our ancestors survive (see Figure 38.2). Thus anger and fear evolved for defense and protection, while hunger and thirst evolved for nutrition.

The first few chapters of *The Emotion Machine* also try to show how this kind of machinery could activate states of mind that we might identify with feelings like attachment, grief, and depression. However, as we learn and grow, we also develop new sets of higher-level resources—and this leads to the types of mental states that we regard as more "intellectual" than "emotional." For example, whenever a problem seems hard to you, your mental Critics may start to switch among different sets of resources. One such set may help you to divide the problem into smaller parts; another may start to search through your memories to find suggestive analogies; and yet another set of resources may lead you to ask some other person for help. In effect, your collection of mental Critics may switch you into many different "Ways to Think." *Each of our major Ways to Think results from turning certain resources on while turning certain others off—and thus changing some ways that our brains behave* (see Figure 38.3).

CITIZEN: It seems strange that you've given the same description both for emotions and for regular thinking. But thinking is basically rational—dry, detached, and logical—whereas emotions enliven our ways to think by adding irrational feelings and biases.

I think it's a myth that there's any such thing as purely logical, rational thinking, because our thoughts are always affected by our assumptions, biases, values, and goals. Furthermore, emotions don't always *add* features to thoughts; indeed, many so-called emotional states appear to *suppress* the use of certain resources, as in this case of infatuation:

"I've just fallen in love with a wonderful person. I scarcely can think about anything else. My sweetheart is unbelievably perfect—of indescribable beauty, flawless character, and incredible intelligence. There is nothing I would not do for her."

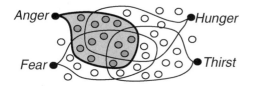

FIGURE 38.2. Examples of built-in critics. Adapted from Minsky (2006).

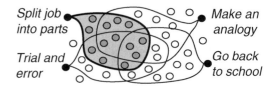

FIGURE 38.3. Examples of Ways to Think. Adapted from Minsky (2006).

This speaker sees all this as positive, and it makes him feel happy and more productive. But note that there's something strange about those superlatives: Most of those phrases of positive praise use syllables like "un-," "-less," and "in-"—which show that they really are negative statements describing the person who's saying them!

Wonderful. Indescribable.
>   (I can't figure out what attracts me to her.)
I scarcely can think about anything else.
>   (Most of my mind has stopped working.)
Unbelievably perfect. Incredible.
>   (No sensible person believes such things.)
She has a flawless character.
>   (I've abandoned my critical faculties.)
There is nothing I would not do for her.
>   (I've forsaken most of my usual goals.)

This example suggests that some of the pleasant effects of infatuation may result from suppressing some mental resources that a person otherwise uses to recognize faults and defects in somebody else. In other words, what we're seeing here is the turning off of some of this speaker's mental Critics!

CITIZEN: I still think that your view of emotions ignores too much. For example, emotional states like fear and disgust involve the body as well as the brain, as when we feel discomfort in the chest or gut, or when we sense palpitations of the heart, or when we feel faint or tremble or sweat.

We can make our model account for the ways in which emotions involve the body's condition by regarding our body parts as additional resources that our brains can use to change (or maintain) their mental states—as when we make ourselves stick to a plan by maintaining a certain facial expression.

THE "CRITIC–SELECTOR" MODEL OF MIND

Some early behaviorist theories described an animal's mind as mainly composed of a simple collection of "If → Do" rules, where each "If" describes an external situation, and its "Do" describes a way to react to it (see Figure 38.4). Now let us try to extend this idea to include

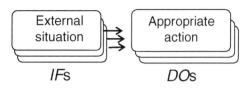

FIGURE 38.4. "If–Do" rules. Adapted from Minsky (2006).

mental reactions to *mental* situations. In this more general view of the mind, a mental Critic can react to recent mental events by making a large-scale change in how we think. It does this by changing the set of resources in use. So we'll suppose that each Critic has learned to recognize a certain type of mental situation, so that then, whenever that condition occurs, that Critic will try to activate a state of mind that has been useful in the past for dealing with that type of situation. For example, if you fail to achieve some goal—and if one of your Critics can diagnose what has gone wrong—then it can activate a different Way to Think that might help you to deal with that problem (see Figure 38.5).

Here are a few useful ways in which this could work; several chapters of *The Emotion Machine* (Minsky, 2006) describe these in much greater detail.

- *Analogy:* If a problem seems familiar, try using a method that has worked on some similar problems.
- *Reformulation:* If the problem seems unfamiliar, change how you are describing it by using a different kind of representation.
- *Planning:* If the problem seems too difficult, try to divide it into several smaller parts, which you can use as separate goals or steppingstones.
- *Simplification:* If a problem seems too complex, ignore some aspects that seem

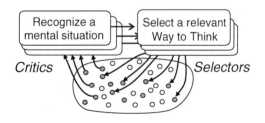

FIGURE 38.5. Selecting from a cloud of resources. Adapted from Minsky (2006).

difficult—and then try to restore them, one at a time.

- *Contradiction*: Try to prove that your problem cannot be solved, and then find a flaw in that argument.
- *Simulation to anticipate*: Mental experiments in virtual worlds can help you safely make predictions.
- *Emotion*: A flash of impatience or anger can cut what seems like a hopelessly tangled knot. Each "emotional state" is a somewhat different way to think.
- *Collaboration*: If none of your usual methods work, ask some other person to assist, in much the same way as an infant will cry for help.

To develop this view of the mind further, several chapters of *The Emotion Machine* discuss what sorts of mental resources a person might have. Some resources act as Critics that can recognize ways in which you get stuck and then act to select which other resources will be engaged next. Thus, when you have trouble with solving a problem, a Critic may turn some of your active resources off, while turning on others that may help to split that problem into parts. Other Critics may use other tricks—such as to remember a similar task from the past, or to change how you're describing that problem. Some such selections may change your mental state so much that, in effect, you'll be using a quite different Way to Think.

STUDENT: Why should you ever turn off a resource? Why not keep them all working all the time?

Indeed, certain resources are *never* switched off—such as those involved with vital functions like respiration, balance, and posture, or those that constantly keep watch for certain particular types of danger. However, if *all* your resources were active at once, they would too often get into conflicts. You can't make your body both walk and run, or move in two different directions at once. So when you have several goals that conflict (say, because they compete for the same energy, time, or space), then you need some machinery that helps to select which resources to activate, and with how much intensity or priority.

One of the functions that mental Critics could serve could be to assess progress toward one of your current goals—and if there's no

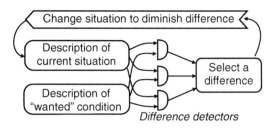

FIGURE 38.6. The process of wanting. Adapted from Minsky (2006).

movement in that direction, a Critic could try to replace it by one or more other goals. But how could you represent a goal so that it takes the form of some sort of resource? One way to do this would be to say that when you "want" a certain condition or thing, this means that you're using a mental process *that works to reduce the difference between your present situation and a condition in which you possess that thing* (Newell & Simon, 1963). Figure 38.6 is a diagram that shows a way to embody that process as a machine.

For example, every baby is born with multiple systems for maintaining normal body temperature. Such a goal is aroused when the infant is too hot, and causes it to sweat, pant, stretch out, or vasodilate. However, when the baby is too cold, this goal will cause it to curl up, shiver, vasoconstrict, or raise its metabolic rate. And whereas infants do these by using innate reactions, they eventually learn to use higher-level, more deliberate methods (see Figure 38.7).

A SIX-LEVEL MODEL OF MIND

A particular Critic might observe that two subgoals are incompatible, that the system has been repeating itself, or that some other problem needs more urgent attention. If just one of your Critics is thus aroused, then it is clear what to do next. But what happens when several Critics are aroused, but disagree about how to proceed? You could sometimes solve such conflicts by arranging for those Critics to compete in some sort of marketplace, where they each have different weights, priorities, or some other sorts of currencies. However, when simple schemes like that don't work, then you'll need higher-level Critics that can recognize this conflict itself as being another prob-

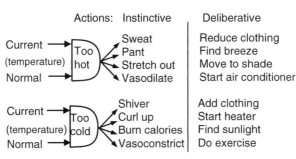

FIGURE 38.7. The process of maintaining normal body temperature. Adapted from Minsky (2006).

lem to solve. For example, if you have no simple way to choose between two conflicting alternatives (such as whether to fight or to flee), then it might make sense to "look ahead" by imagining, and then comparing, the likely consequences of both alternatives. (Note that simple "If → Do" rules cannot make such predictions; one would need more powerful "If → Do → Then" rules to envision effects of imagined actions.) This suggests that such a system would need a second layer of machinery to criticize and supervise the collection of simpler, reactive behaviors (see Figure 38.8).

To see how such a system might work, consider this pair of episodes in which a young infant got upset. At first, that change seemed as quick as the flip of a switch:

> A certain infant could not bear frustration, and would react to each setback by throwing a tantrum. He'd hold his breath and his back would contract, so that he'd fall backward on his head.

Yet several weeks later, that behavior had changed:

> No longer completely controlled by his rage, he could also add ways to protect himself, so that when he felt this coming on, he'd run to collapse on some soft, padded place.

This example suggests that the infant brain is not at first able to resolve the kinds of conflicts we face in our later lives. This led our human brains to evolve higher-level systems that made us much more able to "control ourselves." Then some instincts that formerly were distinct could now become increasingly mixed.

In adult human beings, these processes have evolved to a high degree, and *The Emotion Machine* concludes that they extend to include least six different levels (see Figure 38.9). The lowest level of this figure includes the kinds of instinctive reactions with which all mammalian brains are equipped from birth. Then, in childhood, we go on to develop several more levels of methods that we use to deal with various kinds of problems, situations, and conflicts (this includes much of what we call "common-

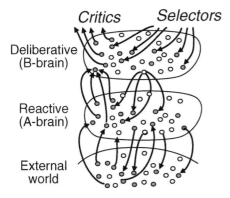

FIGURE 38.8. A system with three levels of Critics and Selectors. Adapted from Minsky (2006).

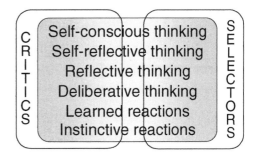

FIGURE 38.9. The six-level model of mind. Adapted from Minsky (2006).

sense thinking"), and eventually we each develop systems that support the sorts of concepts that we call by names like "ethics" or "values." (I don't mean to suggest that these levels are formed by some uniform, general-purpose learning scheme; instead, I suspect that those layers are formed by specific systems of highly evolved genetic machinery. That's why you cannot teach calculus to your cat.)

We can see some aspects of how such a system might work in this example of an everyday human event:

> Joan is starting to cross the street on the way to deliver a finished report. While thinking about what to say at the meeting, she hears a sound and turns her head —and sees a quickly oncoming car. Uncertain whether to cross or retreat, but uneasy about arriving late, Joan decides to sprint across the road. She later remembers her injured knee and reflects upon her impulsive decision: "If my knee had failed, I could have been killed—and what would my friends have thought of me?"

Let's try to describe the events in Joan's mind in relation to the six levels of activities, ranging from her simplest instinctive reactions up to the processes that engage her highest ideals and personal goals:

• *Innate reactions*: Joan hears a sound and turns her head. Some reactions evolved to help us to survive, by responding in particular ways to certain kinds of events in the world, in the body, or inside the mind.

• *Learned reactions*: Joan sees a quickly oncoming car. She has had to learn that certain conditions demand specific new ways to react.

• *Deliberative thinking*: Joan is considering what to say at the meeting. She attempts to predict and compare the effects of some alternatives—just as an adult who encounters a threat need not just react instinctively, but instead could *deliberate* on whether to retreat or attack. Indeed, it can make sense to make oneself angry deliberately, if one believes that this will intimidate an adversary.

• *Reflective thinking*: Joan reflects on her decision. Here she reviews her recent selections of methods and actions, and wonders whether those decisions were good.

• *Self-reflective thinking*: Joan is uneasy about arriving late. Now she sees that in the

plan she made, she may not have allowed enough time to be sure she could actually carry it out.

• *Self-conscious thinking*: "What would my friends have thought of me?" Here Joan wonders how well her actions agreed with her ideals, and appraises her abilities and goals in comparison with those of other people she knows.

At the lowest levels, these Critics and Selectors are almost the same as the "Ifs" and "Thens" of simple reactions. But at the higher reflective levels, these Critics and Selectors can cause so many changes that, in effect, they switch us to different Ways to Think. I should note that this model agrees with some of Sigmund Freud's ideas, in which he recognized that human thinking does not proceed in any single, uniform way, but as a host of diverse activities that often lead to conflicts and inconsistencies (see Figure 38.10).

PSYCHOLOGIST: I do not see clear distinctions among the six levels of your model—especially among the three at the top, because they seem to use similar thinking techniques. Why do you think we should treat them as separate—and do you really need so many levels? Most physicists would be inclined to insist that we should never make more assumptions than we need.

I agree that those boundaries are indistinct. However, as Freud might suggest, we shouldn't succumb to "physics envy." It is true that the science of physics has progressed amazingly well by trying to find the simplest possible explanations. However, we already know that our brains contain hundreds of structural parts, and when we *know* that our theories are

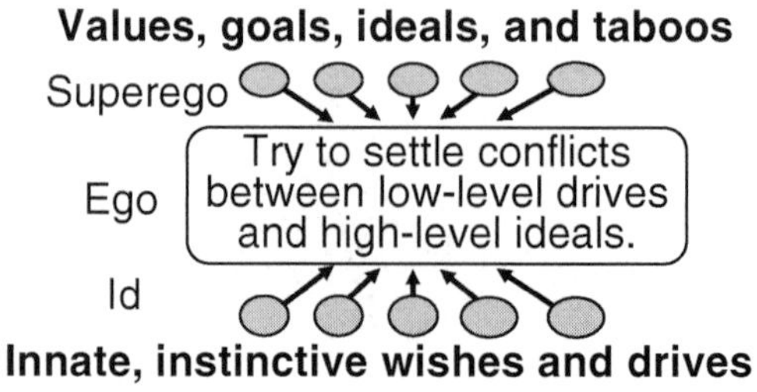

Values, goals, ideals, and taboos

Superego

Ego | Try to settle conflicts between low-level drives and high-level ideals.

Id

Innate, instinctive wishes and drives

FIGURE 38.10. A model of some Freudian concepts. Adapted from Minsky (2006).

incomplete (as is clearly the case in psychology), then it is risky to use a model that leaves no room for other ideas that we're likely to need.

Viewing the mind as a cloud of resources could be a powerful tool to help understand many kinds of mental processes. However, to develop this scheme further, we'll need many far more specific ideas about which resources are engaged for each particular mental function—along with some suggestions about how each particular such resource works, and which others it gets connected to. *The Emotion Machine* proposes several such schemes, but there is not enough space here to describe their details, so below I'll just outline a few of them (readers will find a final draft of that book at *www.emotionmachine.net*, and several related essays at *web.media.mit.edu/~minsky*).

OUTLINE OF THEORIES
IN *THE EMOTION MACHINE*

The goal of *The Emotion Machine* is to try to explain the diversity that distinguishes us humans from most other animals—and from all the machines that we've built in the past. So each chapter discusses a different collection of sources of our uniquely human resourcefulness.

Chapter 1 suggests that our mental states change when we alter our set of active resources. Such a transition may start when one resource gains enough control to turn on several more, while also suppressing a number of others. Then, if some of those newly aroused resources start to affect yet other ones, this can lead to a spreading cascade that may greatly modify the way in which we think about things. Of course, many resources will remain unchanged, so that we will still be the same in many respects. We will still be able to see, hear, and speak—but now we'll perceive things in different ways, and select different subjects to think about. We still will have access to most of our knowledge—but now we will have different attitudes. We may still hold some of the same plans and goals—but now they'll have different priorities. Yet, despite all these changes, our self-reflective processes may insist that we retain the same "identity"— a concept discussed in Chapter 9.

Chapter 2 is concerned with questions about how human children acquire their goals. Many

traditional theories of learning attribute our acquisition of knowledge to a process called "reinforcement," in which we learn from being rewarded for each successful performance. But what we perceive as a failure or success depends on the goals that we then are pursuing; for instance, food won't reward a sated animal. Each of us is born with some "basic" goals that evolved for nutrition, health, comfort, and defense; then later, we learn to connect new subgoals to these. However, this connecting does not explain how we can learn new kinds of goals (such as the ones we call "values" or "ideals") that are not connected to existing goals—so we also need some theories about how we acquire new kinds of goals. In other words, we need some ideas about how we learn what we "ought" to want.

Accordingly, this chapter conjectures that the special emotions called "pride" and "shame" may play unique and peculiar roles in how we humans develop new values, ideals, and goals. When children are praised or rejected by the persons to whom they've become attached, they don't simply just feel pleasure or dissatisfaction, which would merely reinforce or extinguish their currently active wants; instead, these would be elevated or depressed. In other words, whereas trial and error teach us new ways to achieve the goals we already maintain, attachment-related shame and praise teach us which goals we should discard or retain. If so, then we need a theory about what sorts of brain machinery could be involved with exploiting those special social relationships. To illustrate the power of such emotions, here is how Michael Lewis (1995) depicts some effects of shame:

> Shame results when an individual judges his or her actions as a failure in regard to his or her standards, rules and goals and then makes a global attribution. The person experiencing shame wishes to hide, disappear or die. It is a highly negative and painful state that also disrupts ongoing behavior and causes confusion in thought and an inability to speak. The body of the shamed person seems to shrink, as if to disappear from the eye of the self or others. Because of the intensity of this emotional state, and the global attack on the self-system, all that individuals can do when presented with such a state is to attempt to rid themselves of it. (pp. 68–78)

Chapter 3 asks how the sensation called "pain" can lead to the kinds of conditions that we describe as "hurting," "distress," and "suffering." I conjecture that prolonged or chronic pain (no matter whether mental or physical) can start to suppress so many goals and processes that we become imprisoned from having so few remaining alternatives. I also discuss what would happen when too many Critics become suppressed or aroused (which could lead to manic or depressive states), as well as the extent to which our higher levels could learn to control or exploit such conditions.

Chapter 4 discusses the extent to which various parts of a brain can know, represent, or comprehend the events in other parts of that brain. I argue that when we use terms like "conscious" or "self-aware," these do not refer to some single thing, but to some 20-odd different sorts of processes—so, naturally, their meanings will seem controversial and mysterious. I try to resolve this by observing that most mental processes work in ways that do not lead us to reflect on why and how we are doing them. However, when those processes don't function well, or when they encounter obstacles, this can cause our Critics to initiate at least four kinds of higher-level activities— which (1) make use of our most recent memories, (2) tend to be more serial and less parallel, (3) tend to use symbolic descriptions, and (4) involve the models we make of ourselves. I argue that such processes could help to account for many properties of what we like to call "conscious thought."

Chapter 5 develops more details of how the six-level model of mind can help to explain our abilities to "imagine" things—that is, how parts of our higher-level machinery can enable us to make predictions about what would happen if we were to perform some sequence of mental or physical actions. The chapter focuses mainly on visual perceptions and their internal representations.

Chapter 6 is about common-sense knowledge— the things we expect other persons to know, so that we rarely need to mention them. Consider what happens when you hear your telephone ring. When you move to pick the receiver up, at first you see only one side of it, yet you feel that you've seen the entire thing; you anticipate how it will fit in your grasp, and how it will feel when it contacts your ear; you know that you speak into the bottom of the receiver and hear answers from the top; and you know that if you dial a number, another phone will ring somewhere else—and if anyone happens to an-

swer it, then you and that person can start to converse. How does such scanty evidence make it seem that the object you're "looking at" has been transported into your mind—where you can move it and touch it and turn it around, even open it up and look inside? This chapter proposes some theories about how we acquire, represent, retrieve, and apply multiple kinds of common-sense knowledge.

Chapter 7 develops more ideas about the Critic–Selector model of mind, and makes an attempt to classify our various ways to think about things. How do we learn and organize our new collections of resources? How do we know when to quit or persist? And how do we choose what next goal to pursue? I conjecture that those strategies use mainly unconscious processes, some of which may be cyclical in character.

Chapter 8 explores the sources of the human brain's resourcefulness. My central conjecture here is that our ancestors evolved several different ways to deal with every important threat to survival. Accordingly, we have evolved many ways to represent knowledge, each with different kinds of interconnections that give us a variety of methods for retrieving records that might be relevant. For example, we can describe events in terms of lists of images, words, or story-like scripts, which in turn can be composed of pairs of "frames" that represent the situations before and after an action is taken. These in turn can be represented by using the branching web-like structures that researchers in artificial intelligence call "semantic networks." At lower levels, we also can use "connectionistic" neural or statistical networks, which often are useful for rapid reactions, but tend to be extremely opaque to more symbolic, abstract, or reflective methods. Figure 38.11 illustrates the various structures we can use to represent objects and ideas, which enable us to see each situation from many different points of view.[4] Also, we seem to have evolved special machinery that helps us to switch rapidly among those perspectives; I call those systems "panalogies" (for "parallel analogies") and would welcome future experiments to see whether those structures really exist.

Chapter 9 proposes some theories about what we refer to as our "selves" or "identities," and discusses some possible reasons for why we find feelings so hard to describe, and also why we like pleasure and dislike pain. It also considers our sense of experiencing (and

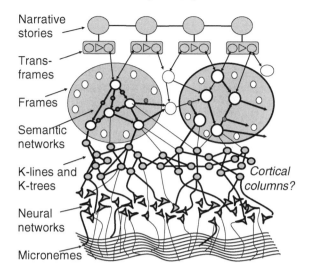

Narrative
stories

Trans-
frames

Frames

Semantic
networks

K-lines and
K-trees

*Cortical
columns?*

Neural
networks

Micronemes

FIGURE 38.11. The structures we can use at different levels to represent objects and ideas. Adapted from Minsky (2006).

why some philosophers regard this as very mysterious). The book concludes by arguing that we don't need to appeal to magical "gifts" to account for our human intelligence; the trick is that we each develop a massive collection of different ways to deal with each challenge that faces us.[5]

NOTES

1. Much of this chapter is condensed from parts of *The Emotion Machine* (Minsky, 2006), which describes more details about these ideas. Copyright 2006 by Marvin Minsky. Adapted by permission.
2. In earlier publications, I have used the term "agents" to refer to mental resources, but today that term is often used for other purposes.
3. Some resources may simply turn on or off, while others may be aroused to various degrees. Also, some may have serious conflicts with others—and this may require additional Critics to recognize and deal with these.
4. Figure 38.11 combines ideas about ways to represent knowledge that range from the low-level k-lines and micronemes of Chapters 8 and 20 of Minksy (1986) to the high-level semantic networks and narratives of Chapter 5 through 8 of Minksy (2006). The cognitive

levels of Figure 38.9 need not closely correspond to the neurological levels of Figure 38.9 because similar structures could be reused for different kinds of functions.

5. Several reviewers have complained about the lack of neurological evidence for many of these hypotheses. However, it seems to me that most such objections miss the mark, because the proposals herein are largely based on computational concepts that have not yet spread through the neuroscience community. So, naturally, we won't find many experiments relevant to these kinds of conjectures until researchers begin to think about them.

REFERENCES

Lewis, M. (1995). Self-conscious emotions. *American Scientist, 83,* 68–78.

Minsky, M. (1986). *The society of mind.* New York: Simon & Schuster.

Minsky, M. (2006). *The emotion machine: Commonsense thinking, artificial intelligence, and the future of the human mind.* New York: Simon & Schuster.

Newell, A., & Simon, H. A. (1963). GPS, a program that simulates human thought. In E. A. Feigenbaum & J. Feldman (Eds.), *Computers and thought.* New York: McGraw-Hill.

CHAPTER 39

Appraisal Theories
How Cognition Shapes Affect into Emotion

GERALD L. CLORE and ANDREW ORTONY

At dusk recently, while walking in the woods, I (G. C.) was startled by an arresting sound. It turned out to be a male deer announcing his presence with a loud snort. The realization that it was only a deer came quickly, and the whole sequence from startle to categorization took only an instant. But then I experienced a novel, surprising sensation as the hair on the back of my neck stood up. Despite the cognitive reassurance that it was only a deer, the body was apparently still preparing for a nameless threat.

What happened in this episode in the woods? Were appraisals involved? Was fear elicited? If so, did fear cause the piloerection? To this last question, William James would certainly have replied, "No," claiming that we are "afraid because we tremble" rather than the other way around (James, 1890, p. 450). In this chapter, we explore such questions, and end up agreeing both with James and with appraisal theorists.

APPRAISAL THEORY AND ITS CRITICS

Appraisal theory as we know it today is usually attributed to Magda Arnold (1960), who made an early and influential statement of the cognitive approach to emotion. She proposed that people implicitly appraise or evaluate everything they encounter, and that such evaluations occur immediately and automatically. Among others who were important in defining cognitive approaches to emotion were Schachter and Singer (1962), Lazarus (1966), and Mandler (1975). But it was not until the 1980s that the seed planted by Arnold began to take root. Following pioneering work by Roseman (1979, 1984), a number of appraisal theories appeared, including an often-cited account by Smith and Ellsworth (1985), an influential theory by Frijda (1986), and accounts by Oatley and Johnson-Laird (1987) and ourselves

(Ortony, Clore, & Collins, 1988). In addition, Scherer (1984) proposed a theory emphasizing the temporal sequence of appraisals. These theories are compared in Clore, Schwarz, and Conway (1994), and some are elaborated by their authors in a volume edited by Scherer, Schorr, and Johnstone (2001).

Despite this flowering of interest, appraisal theories turned out to be controversial. Some investigators found them implausible, because they read accounts of appraisal *structure* as though they were assertions about appraisal *process* (e.g., Prinz, 2005). Although appraisal theorists themselves often helped blur the distinction, it is an important one. The difference can perhaps be appreciated from an analogous difference between the formal rules of syntax and the processes involved in speaking. Linguists might all agree that observing the rules of syntax is important for communication, but none assume that speakers consult such rules before opening their mouths to speak. Similarly, theories of the structure of emotional appraisals do not claim that people consult such rules before feeling anything. In addition, some critics argue that emotions occur too quickly for cognitive appraisals to be possible. However, the validity of structural accounts of emotion is no more contingent on the speed of emotion than the validity of structural accounts of language is dependent on how fast people talk.

In this chapter we focus on issues relevant to theories of appraisal process rather than appraisal structure. Also, instead of focusing on what has been said in the past, we emphasize ideas that have appeared recently. We ask questions about emotion and appraisal, including what emotions are and in what sense they exist. One answer to the latter question is that emotions exist only in the sense that the Big Dipper exists—namely, in our perceptions (Russell, 2003). We also ask whether emotions cause behavior. Some investigators argue that unconscious affect causes behavior, but that full-blown emotions do not (Baumeister, Vohs, DeWall, & Zhang, 2007). We go on to ask whether appraisals are really necessary in the emotion process. The philosopher Prinz (2005) argues that appraisals are no more necessary for emotion than for pain. Finally, we ask what process theorists have in mind when they refer to "appraisals." We review both dual-process models (Clore & Ortony, 2000; C. A. Smith, Griner, Kirby, & Scott, 1996; E. R. Smith &

Neumann, 2005) and alternatives to dual process models (e.g., Barrett, 2006a; Huron, 2006; Cunningham & Zelazo, 2007).

In our own view, "emotions" are cognitively elaborated affective states (e.g., Ortony et al., 1988; Ortony, Norman, & Revelle, 2005). In this characterization, we take "affective" to mean anything evaluative, and we propose that "states" exist when multiple components represent or register the same internal or external situation in the same time frame. Thus one can think of emotions as involving multiple representations of something as good or bad in some way. Appraisal theories address the nature of such evaluations. The general view we take in this chapter is that (as in the piloerection example with which we have begun this chapter) low-level bodily, hormonal, and affective reactions often get the emotional process started, and that cognitive appraisal processes act like a sculptor, shaping general affective reactions into specific emotions. But before addressing the process, we ask about the nature of the emotions that involve such appraisals.

THE NATURE OF EMOTIONS

Are Emotions Situated Constructions?

Theorists increasingly view psychological processes as distributed across multiple sources (e.g., Clark, 1997), and behavioral and affective responses as situated or context-specific (e.g., Brown, Collins, & Duguid, 1989). Consistent with such approaches, Barrett (e.g., 2006a) has proposed that emotions are not distinct states with clear boundaries, that they are not hard-wired in the brain, and that they don't have distinctive psychophysiological signatures and facial expressions. Emotions do, of course, involve facial expressions, psychophysiology, and specialized brain areas, but the boundaries of these are not those of specific emotions such as anger, fear, and shame. Barrett suggests that emotions, rather than reflecting similar entities in the brain, involve combinations of processes with much more variability than is implied by the discrete-emotions or basic-emotions view.

The prevailing psychological picture has been that emotions are distinct entities in the body or evolved modules (e.g., Ekman, 1984). Once activated by emotional stimuli, these emotions are evident in distinctive expressions, thoughts, feelings, neurochemistry, and behavior. But for Barrett positive and negative affective reactions and arousal—the dimensions of "core affect" (Russell & Barrett, 1999)—may be the only necessary givens in the body. Specific emotions are situated instances of such affect. Thus "fear" is a label for negative affect in situations involving threat, whereas the same negative affect in situations of loss may be called "sadness," and a reaction to blameworthy behavior may be called "anger" (for a related view, see Sabini & Silver, 2005).

If Barrett (2006a) is right that the boundaries between similarly valenced emotions are not as distinct as is usually assumed, it would not necessarily make specific emotions any less important, powerful, or universal. It would simply change the locus and nature of their distinctiveness. In such a view what makes emotions universal is not their biological status, but the situations to which they are responses. If there is anything basic about fear, anger, joy, and disgust, it lies in the ubiquity of the life situations to which these emotions are responses, rather than in distinctive biological signatures, which Barrett says research does not find.

In this alternative view the experience of specific, distinct emotions arises partly from cultural knowledge about emotions. In a similar manner, experiencing colors of similar wavelengths as the same or as different depends partly on the boundaries provided by a culture's language. Members of cultures with separate concepts for blue and green may see two different colors, where those without a separate category for green may see only variants of blue. Barrett suggests that whether people experience two points along the affect dimension as two emotions, rather than as variants of one, may be similarly influenced. Thus concepts may augment sensations to create distinct emotions, as well as distinct colors.

Evidence that concepts do help create the boundaries of emotions comes from experiments inducing semantic satiation of an emotion word by multiple repetitions, which makes the word temporarily lose meaning (Lindquist, Barrett, Bliss-Moreau, & Russell, 2006). After semantic satiation of the word "anger," for example, people were no longer able to swiftly recognize that two patently angry faces were expressing the same emotion, presumably because the temporary breakdown of access to the anger concept caused by the satiation manipulation made it difficult to "see" anger in the faces.

Barrett's work appears likely to spark debate in much the same way as Mischel's (1968) book did about personality. Mischel argued that the available evidence failed to show the high degree of cross-situational consistency in behavior demanded by traditional ideas about personality. He proposed a view of personality reflecting the situated nature of individual differences in behavior potential. After 40 years of debate and revision, the field of personality study is arguably healthier, even though many personality theorists still disagree with Mischel's position. Similarly, Barrett is saying that the evidence also does not show that emotions are tightly organized, evolved modules with distinctive expressive, experiential, and neural signatures. It remains to be seen whether her claims will have a similar effect on the study of emotion.

Do Emotions Cause Expressions?[1]

Theorists have traditionally thought about emotion within a kind of latent-trait model. Thus research focuses on evidence of an unseen entity measured by indicators—expressions, physiology, behavior, and feelings that are symptoms or consequences of an emotion. An alternative approach might treat emotion not as causing these disturbances, but as emerging from them. Such a model would not include arrows going outward from emotion to its several indicators; instead, the arrows would go the other way, pointing inward from cognitions, expressions, and feelings to the emotion they constitute. The factors considered as indicators of emotion in the traditional latent-trait model can be seen instead as constituents of emotion in an emergence model. Bollen and Lennox (1991) distinguish these as "effect indicator" and "causal indicator" models (see also Barrett, 2006b).

In this view, emotions are the conjunction of expressions, physiology, behavior inclination, experience, and so on (Barrett, Ochsner, & Gross, 2006; Clore & Centerbar, 2004; Clore & Ortony, 2000). It sees emotions as affective states, in which multiple components register the same emotional significance in different ways at the same time. For example, if threat were registered simultaneously in facial expression, posture, tone of voice, thought, motivation, neurochemistry, autonomic activity, brain activation, and so on, a person would be in a state of fear. Indeed, that is what we mean by "fear"—being in a state dedicated to threat.

In the conventional latent-trait or effect indicator model, expressions in the face, voice, and posture and actions, thoughts, and desires are different indicators of an underlying emotion. In the emergence model, these things are constituents of emotions, so that an emotion exists by virtue of their co-occurrence. If one's thoughts turn elsewhere, one's physiology reverts to baseline, and one's voice, face, posture, and motivation no longer represent threat, then one is no longer afraid. Of course, in neither model is it necessary for each and every aspect to be evident. One can be afraid without gaping, opening one's eyes widely, and developing a squeaky voice. But for one to be in a genuine state of fear, threat must be multiply represented.

In summary, in this section we have compared classical views that emotions are evolved, tightly organized modules with an alternative view of emotions as loosely organized, psychologically constructed states, consisting of situated elicitations of core affect (Barrett, 2006a). We have considerable sympathy for the latter view (e.g., Ortony et al., 2005). Next, we have contrasted a model in which expressions and feelings are indicators of underlying emotion with an emergence model in which expressions and feelings are constituents rather than consequences of emotion. Our own view is compatible with an emergence variable model (e.g., Clore & Centerbar, 2004). We turn next to an examination of the process of appraisal.

THE NATURE OF APPRAISALS

Are Appraisals Cognitive or Perceptual?

Critics of appraisal theory often object not to appraisals per se, but to the idea that they are cognitive in nature. Some consider themselves appraisal theorists, but not *cognitive* appraisal theorists (J. E. LeDoux, personal communication, March 2006). In contrast to cognitive accounts of emotion elicitation, Parkinson (2007, p. 22) suggests that emotions are "direct adjustments to relational dynamics, not articulated responses to propositional representations of appraisal information." He argues that if one steps onto a bus and one's carrier bag splits apart, scattering groceries across the pavement, one feels frustrated directly in a way that does not require verification of appraisal-relevant propositions. Similarly, Parkinson (2007, p. 21) says that "the minimal precondition for anger is simply resistance stopping us from getting through," and that a person brandishing a gun can be directly perceived as scary without any need for (cognitive) appraisals by the perceivers (for a similar view, see Berkowitz, 1990).

Parkinson may be interpreting propositional accounts (e.g., Siemer & Reisenzein, 2007) of goals and goal blockage as requiring an explicit analysis of situations before emotions can arise. But we doubt that anyone holds such a position. A propositional analysis of the distress at seeing one's groceries scattered across the pavement does not imply that people explicitly entertain propositions. A propositional analysis is a *formal description* of the implicit meaning of that perception. Similarly, a parabolic equation might be a formal description of the trajectory of a ball thrown through the air. But neither the distress nor the flight of the ball requires a propositional or mathematical analysis for its occurrence. Seeing one's groceries spill out surely would produce distress directly and without thought, but a propositional analysis does not suggest otherwise. Whatever cognitive activity is involved is implicit. A number of models (described below) have addressed such issues, arguing that any requisite cognitive activity can occur exceedingly rapidly and without conscious thought.

Nevertheless, we agree that many of the criteria for emotion elicitation are as much perceptual as cognitive. Gibson (1979) challenged orthodoxy by throwing out the Cartesian idea of the mind as a separate entity that creates a perceptual model of the world from sensory inputs and guides action. Perception, he said, reflects the environment directly, and action reflects its affordances. Many appraisals may also be perceptual rather than mental products: Is an outcome my own or another's? Is it past or future? Is it human or environmentally caused? Thus some appraisals are already in the topography of psychological situations, so that explanations for emotion lie not in the mind, but in what the mind is in (Buck, March 4, 2007).

Are Appraisals Cognitive or Situational?

Thus far we have treated emotions as emergent, situated, and constructed from underlying affective dimensions. In this view, when the elements in a situation match patterns of the kind specified in appraisal theories, the corresponding emotion can result. If so, then emotion might be thought of as radically situated, so that emotional variation directly reflects situational variation.

If we think of emotions as reactions to different situational structures, then the only essence that instances of emotion share is in the situation they represent. If so, the fact that one instance of anger or fear or joy looks a lot like another is evidence not so much that a discrete emotion has been evoked, as that aspects of whatever situations elicit fear, anger, or joy have constrained affective reactions in distinctive ways. Thus the distinctiveness of an emotion may lie in the nature of the situation it represents, not in a stored pattern of latent emotional potential. In this view, emotions are not entities, any more than cognitions exist as entities. Just as chameleons cope with variations in their environment by changing color, so we cope by transforming ourselves emotionally into reflections of our environment.

Many different writers have tried to equate emotions and situations. For example, Polti (1921/1977) proposed that there are 36 basic plots in the history of drama corresponding to 36 emotions. They concern love, tragedy, hope, fear, betrayal, honor, sacrifice, passion, lust, sympathy, ambition, jealousy, shortsightedness, courage, revelation, forgiveness, deliverance, rivalry, jealousy, and more. There is no reason to assume that these categories are truly basic, or that another investigator might not find more or fewer. Moreover, each narrative situation would surely involve many emotions. But the larger point is that there are recurrent patterns of situations in human affairs, which have been the stuff of drama from the Greeks to the present. The actions depicted are energized and directed by universal human motivations, and the dramatic turning points are marked by the emotions of characters and audiences.

In summary, we have suggested that some aspects of emotional appraisals may be perceptual rather than cognitive, and that appraisals often directly reflect the structure of the situations in which they arise, with little cognitive elaboration. But cognition is involved in full-blown emotions, and a central question concerns how it is involved.

THE PROCESS OF APPRAISAL

Are Emotions Too Fast or Too Mindless for Cognitive Appraisals?

Automaticity

Reservations about cognitive appraisal theories often rest on the claim that emotions are too fast or mindless to involve cognition. In fact, mindlessness is a feature of most cognitive reactions as well. For example, many people are good at determining whether the footsteps they hear belong to a man or a woman (Huron, 2006). It turns out that the sound is different because the timing of first heel and then toe hitting the ground is shorter for small than for large shoes. People who are good at making this discrimination do it mindlessly, however. They are unaware of what cues they use, and certainly never think of foot size or shoe movements in order to decide on the sex of the person. Instead, they directly hear a man or a woman. It is a learned association, but they have no explicit knowledge of what they have learned.

In addition to being mindless, emotional reactions are often assumed to be too fast for cognitive appraisals. However, Moors (2006) has recently reported research explicitly examining appraisal time, and she concludes that there is no reason to assume that cognitive processes are too slow to produce emotion. Through clever experiments that build on prior research on automaticity and affective priming, she has shown that appraisal judgments can be rapid and automatic. Also, Moors and DeHouwer (2001) have demonstrated that stimulus valence and motivational relevance can be determined rapidly and automatically, as assumed in many appraisal theories.

Other research has shown that people may be faster to infer emotions (on the basis of brief vignettes) than to infer the appraisals on which these emotions are believed to depend (Siemer & Reisenzein, 2007). But, of course, this finding does not mean that emotions cannot be based on cognitive appraisals. Nor do these authors suggest otherwise. Categorizing a figure as a bird may also be faster than judging whether the figure has wings, even though having wings may be one of the criteria for making that categorization in the first place. Since multiple attributes contribute to birdness (or to emotion), a categorization may be made as soon as the collective activation of some of them is adequate. This may occur before any single attribute is sufficiently activated to serve as a basis by itself, and long before respondents can affirm the presence of that attribute in self-reports.

Siemer and Reisenzein (2007) adapt an existing cognitive model (Anderson, 1983) to explain why their finding does not mean that emotions precede appraisal. They argue that with experience, appraisals become automated; appraisal programs get compiled so that not only do the appraisals become rapid, but the intervening steps become inaccessible (Wegner & Vallacher, 1986). This dual-process approach assumes that with practice, emotion inferences can become faster than appraisal inferences. As in playing the piano, routines become automated as they are repeated over and over. One might think that this implies that whereas emotions might be quick to arise in adults, children might have to think before they feel. But this particular implication seems unlikely, so that dual processes reflecting the automatic–controlled distinction, in which automaticity is achieved through practice, may be less relevant than models in which one of the processes is, for example, heuristic or associative rather than simply well practiced.

Dual-Process Theories

Dual-process theories have become common in psychology as a way of handling conflicting results. Rather than having to choose whether thinking is propositional or heuristic, dual-process theorists say that both are at work. The claim is that people engage in both heuristic and systematic (Chaiken, Liberman, & Eagly, 1989) or both central and peripheral (Petty & Cacioppo, 1986) processing.

Dual-process models have similar power for handling data about emotion. A useful dual-process model of appraisal has been based on a distinction between "associative processing" and "rule-based processing" (Sloman, 1996). This approach has been developed by Craig Smith and colleagues (e.g., Smith et al., 1996; Smith & Kirby, 2001), but others have also found the idea useful (Clore & Ortony, 2000; E. R. Smith & Neumann, 2005). Associative processing is guided by subjective similarity and temporal contiguity, whereas rule-based processing involves symbolic reasoning. In ev-

eryday categorization, people appear to use both subjective similarity and rule-based reasoning.

Both kinds of reasoning have also been proposed as playing a role in emotion elicitation. In new situations, emotions may involve considerable bottom-up processing. As perceptions of a situation unfold and requirements for specific emotions are satisfied, reactions may become correspondingly differentiated. Similarly, as children develop and become capable of making relevant distinctions, their emotions may become more differentiated. Such rule-based reasoning is rarely conscious, explicit, or deliberative, and preverbal infants are already surprisingly adept at implicit rule-based processing (e.g., Kotovsky & Baillargeon, 1994; Needham & Baillargeon, 1993).

But emotions are presumably also elicited by associative processes. One may become happy, angry, or anxious simply by being in situations similar to those in which one was previously happy, angry, or anxious. And since cognitive systems capitalize on prior experience rather indiscriminately, such associative processing may be the rule rather than the exception. The meaning and significance of an event are perhaps always partly contingent on its resemblance to other situations in one's experience. LeDoux (1996) captured this idea by saying, "Emotion is memory" (p. 249). Rather than confronting each situation as a blank slate, people assume that the emotionally relevant aspects of situations recur, so that prior appraisals often get reinstated.

The kind of reinstatement mechanism we have in mind was actually proposed by Freud. In his view, "the act of birth, moreover, is the first experience attended by anxiety, and is thus, the source and model of the affect of anxiety" (Freud, 1911, p. 251). He also believed that reactions to one's father serve as a prototype for later emotional orientations to authority figures, and that falling in love is a reinstatement of a child's love for its parent. Some of Freud's examples seem bizarre and implausible, but the general mechanism of reinstatement has great explanatory power.

Bowlby's (1969) infant attachment theory also assumes that early emotional reactions of love and attachment are the basis of later emotions. He saw the emotional protests of infants separated from caregivers as evidence of an evolved tendency for children to become emotionally attached to caregivers. Later Ainsworth, Blehar, Waters, and Wall (1978) identified specific patterns of infantile attachment believed to be reinstated in later romantic attachments. The idea that early emotional patterns reappear when people fall in love and select their mates continues to be fruitful in contemporary attachment work (e.g., Morgan & Shaver, 1999; Shaver & Clark, 1994).

Although there may be more than one route to emotion elicitation, the appraisal for a given emotion remains the same. Regardless of whether fear or anger arises from computation, conditioning, imitation, or predisposition, fear is always a response to apparent threat, and anger to apparent infringement. Whereas the constituent thoughts, feelings, and physiology may differ, each instance of anger or fear involves similar perceptions. Lazarus (1994) referred to these as co-relational themes. This idea, common to all appraisal approaches, is that there is an underlying constancy in situations that makes them sources of anger, fear, or joy.

In summary, in this section, we have examined an example of a dual-process model (Clore & Ortony, 2000; see also Sloman, 1996; C. A. Smith et al., 1996). We assume that different routes to emotional appraisal serve different functions. The typically faster, associative process of emotion reinstatement is useful for preparedness, whereas the typically slower, rule-based process of computation affords flexibility. Creatures with more restricted emotional repertoires are less capable of flexible responding than creatures with more complex emotional repertoires. Presumably there is an advantage to automatic preparation for responding, as well as to flexibility in responding. As Scherer (1984) pointed out, the evolutionary advantage of emotion was that a stimulus could be registered and reacted to without the organism's being committed to behavior.

These considerations suggest that emotion allows behavior to be contingent on a stimulus without being dictated by it. There are, therefore, two fingers on the emotional trigger—one from early perceptual processes that identify the emotional value of a stimulus to prepare for action; and one from cognitive processes that verify the nature of the stimulus, situate it, and appraise it. Before discussing cognitive involvement, however, let us examine further the role of low-level, subcortical processes.

Is There a Low Route to Emotion?

Investigators of emotion have become increasingly interested in the role of subcortical processes in emotion. The work of LeDoux and colleagues (e.g., LeDoux, Romanski, & Xagoraris, 1989) in finding a subcortical "low route" to the elicitation of fear-relevant responses is well known. In studying fear conditioning in rats, LeDoux and his colleagues found a pathway from the sensory thalamus directly to the amygdala, without first going to relevant areas of the cortex to be interpreted. To the extent that the amygdala is involved in fear and other emotions, this low route appeared capable of generating emotional responses before the organism could know what it was responding to or have any experience of fear. This finding was taken to imply that cognitive appraisal is not required for emotion.

It would be difficult to overstate the impact of this discovery on thinking about emotion. It was excellent science and has been important in stimulating further research on subcortical processes. However, many criticisms of the accepted interpretation have appeared (for an accessible review, see Storbeck, Robinson, & McCourt, 2006). The work was done on rats, and it now appears that the particular pathway examined may not be functional in primates and humans. Moreover, by itself, this pathway would not be able to discriminate stimuli that had acquired emotional significance from those that had none, unless reduced to light versus dark or similarly gross kinds of stimulation. Thus the popular narrative that this pathway alone—that is, without cognitive involvement—could generate a genuine emotion of fear of a snake may be untenable. Similarly untenable is the idea that human emotions, economic decisions, and political preferences take place without cortical involvement (see Clore, Storbeck, Robinson, & Centerbar, 2005; Davidson, 2003). However, even if this particular pathway did not turn out to be as important as initially believed, and despite the fact that any subcortical process is insufficient to account for emotion, this work has stimulated important additional research and thinking about the critical role of subcortical processes in emotion.

Increasingly, it is apparent that behavior-relevant processing in the brain is highly recursive (Storbeck & Clore, 2007). Incoming sensory information is progressively refined in an iterative process (Cunningham & Zelazo, 2007). The kinds of subcortical processes that LeDoux and colleagues' work has highlighted presumably serve as early signals that something should be processed further, so that its significance can be determined. The pervasiveness and importance of these processes mean that many existing appraisal theories are incomplete. We discuss in the next section two accounts that do include low-level, reflex-like processes at the beginning of the emotion sequence.

Is Appraisal Sequential?

Charles Osgood (e.g., Osgood, Suci, & Tannebaum, 1957) proposed a theory of connotative meaning that was in many ways an affective appraisal theory. He proposed (and produced relevant evidence) that all words in all languages convey connotative meaning along three dimensions—"evaluation," "potency," and "activity" (the dimensions of E, P, and A). Osgood (1969) was interested in the origins of language and communication, and he speculated about what kinds of information prelinguistic humans would have needed most to communicate. He reasoned that the most important information for survival would have been whether something was good or bad, whether it was strong or weak, and whether its approach was fast or slow. Once one could locate something within this E-P-A space, coping behavior would be appropriately constrained. His idea was that triangulations from these connotative dimensions would have allowed people to make behavior-relevant distinctions between saber-toothed tigers and mosquitoes, and to communicate these distinctions to others.

Scherer (1984, 2001) echoes the importance of E, P, and A, and also treats them as dimensions of emotional meaning. He suggests that E is linked to appraisals of stimuli with regard to goals and needs, P to appraisals of coping potential, and A to appraisals of urgency. He has proposed a series of "stimulus evaluation checks" believed to underlie stimulus appraisal. The type and intensity of any resulting emotion, then, reflect the profile of results of the appraisal process based on these stimulus evaluation checks.

The stimulus evaluation checks proposed by Scherer begin with a (1) "novelty check," followed by (2) an "intrinsic pleasantness check,"

based on innate feature detectors and learned associations; (3) a "goal/need significance check," evaluating whether an event is relevant to goals, conducive to goals, expected, and urgent; (4) a "coping potential check," evaluating causation, coping potential, control over consequences, relative power, and options for internal adjustment; and finally (5) a "norm–self compatibility check," evaluating the compatibility of actions or events with social norms, conventions, or expectations of others, as well as with internalized norms or standards of self. Scherer assumes that the outcomes of these checks change various subsystems that serve emotion (physiology, expression, motivation, feelings), creating a telltale trace that *is* the emotion. In addition, he emphasizes that emotions are fluid, reflecting constant evaluative activity.

In a somewhat related way, the music cognition theorist David Huron (2006) has analyzed the emotion process and suggested six stages of emotion elicitation in response to auditory stimulation. He proposes that the process may start with various (1) "reflexive responses," including the orienting response, the startle reflex, defensive reflex, and reflex-like reactions based on various overlearned perceptual schemas. Thus an unexpected bang of a door is marked physiologically by flexing of the shoulder muscles and by the release of epinephrine and norepinephrine into the bloodstream, which cause increases in heart rate and respiration, sweating, pupil dilation, and so on. These reactions may facilitate perceptual intake and protective action. At the same time, (2) "denotative responses" allow stimulus identification (e.g., "slamming door") on the basis of passive associations; (3) "connotative responses" are also passively learned processes using the physical properties of timing, energy, proximity, and so on to determine what the sound is like (e.g., "forceful," "loud"). The reflexive, denotative, and connotative responses are all fast and automatic. (4) "Associative responses" are arbitrary, learned associations that may activate an emotional response on the basis of memory (e.g., "That reminds me of my dad slamming doors when he was upset"). (5) "Empathetic responses" identify whether a sound was generated by an animate agent and what state of mind is signaled by the sound (e.g., anger). Finally, (6) "critical responses" are conscious, cognitive processes that evaluate the intentions or sincerity of the agent; these may also involve self-monitoring processes concerning the appropriateness of one's own response.

These two accounts of the appraisal process (Scherer's and Huron's) have in common the idea that low-level and higher-level processes are both operative, rather than being alternatives. However, in these models reflexes, such as the orienting or startle reflex, provide the low-level impetus to emotion. Some other low-level affective or evaluative reactions are discussed in the next section.

How Basic and Broadly Distributed Is Affect?

Although appraisal theories concentrate on cognitive distinctions, emotion does not start there. The process often begins as a very low-level affective reaction—a reaction that is not yet an emotion (Barrett, 2006a; Baumeister et al., 2007; Berkowitz & Harmon-Jones, 2004; LeDoux, 1996; Ortony et al., 2005). Most cognitive appraisal theories have not included a stage for such early affective reactions.

Although full-blown emotional states involve multiple components, including cognition, what gets the emotional ball rolling is sometimes quite low-level. For example, people apparently respond more positively to smooth, curved objects than to objects with sharp-angled edges (Bar & Neta, 2006). That preference also holds for roundish as opposed to angular faces (Zebrowitz, 1997). Some have hypothesized that sharp shapes may convey threat, and round shapes warmth (Aronoff, Woike, & Hyman, 1992).

In a related vein, lightness and darkness appear to have reliable affective values that may have both universal application and ancient origins (Meier, Robinson, & Clore, 2004). High versus low physical location (Meier & Robinson, 2004) and high versus low pitch in music or speech (Huron, 2006) have a similar evaluative impact. Each of these stimulus characteristics may have an associated valence for different reasons. It seems likely, for example, that young children's preference for sweetness and aversion to bitterness may be innate, whereas some other quite common preferences may be learned.

Beyond such specific preferences, familiar stimuli generally elicit more positive reactions than do novel stimuli—a preference that appears to be a general design feature of verte-

brates. Moreover, this process is evident at the group level, and even at the cellular level.[2] The "minimal-groups" effect is a highly reliable social-psychological effect (Tajfel, Billig, Bundy, & Flament, 1971). Any distinction among a collection of individuals, no matter how arbitrary, leads to a surprising degree of ingroup favoritism and outgroup disfavor. Such a principle is presumably also at work in xenophobia, racism, and religious intolerance. However, our point is that the criterion of "like me" versus "not like me" may be a very basic principle of evaluation.

A more general statement about the lower-level nature of affective processes was recently made by Buck (March 4, 2007):

> Brains, after all, are only about 0.6 billion years old, compared to the 3.5 billion year history of life on the earth; and . . . we have about 40% of our genes in common with microbes. . . . I think it is of significance that one can find in microbes genes that encode for dopamine, serotonin, norepinephrine, ACTH [adrenocorticotropic hormone], many of the peptide neurohormones, etc. dating from long before the evolution of the brain. This suggests that prototypical motivational–emotional systems are design principles in the most elemental life forms.

What are the implications of such observations? What does it mean that processes analogous to those of social groups are already present at the cellular level, and that the neurochemistry of evaluation may be widely distributed among animate organisms down to the level of microbes? Since no one seriously champions the idea of microbe emotions, a distinction must be drawn between affective processes and emotional states.

Are Appraisals Sequential, Dual, Chaotic, or Recursive?

We have discussed one kind of dual-process model and two sequential models of emotional appraisal. We turn next to dual-process models, and alternatives to such models, that specifically distinguish affect from emotion.

Baumeister, Vohs, DeWall, and Zhang

A dual-process view proposed by Baumeister et al. (2007) not only specifies two processes, but suggests how they interact. Drawing on literature reviewed by Schwarz and Clore (2007), they note that although there is abundant evidence for the influence of emotion on cognition, there is scant evidence for a direct influence of emotion on behavior. They propose that behavior is controlled in a bottom-up way by unconscious affect, in a manner similar to that demonstrated by Winkielman, Berridge, and Wilbarger (2005) in their studies of how unconscious priming with happy faces stimulated thirsty people to drink more of a novel beverage.

Baumeister et al. suggest that full-blown, conscious emotions are re-representations or constructions of affectively significant situations for the purpose of remembering the lessons of those situations. They argue that human social life is vastly more complex than that of any other species, and that it requires a corresponding richness and variety of emotional representation. In their view, emotion is an elaborated, conscious state that is memorable and hence useful for self-instruction. This theoretical maneuver of drawing a sharp distinction between affect and emotion strikes us as a useful one. In addition, specifying emotion as a high-level state that does not drive behavior, but that provides information to the experiencer, may help resolve some of the inherent conflicts between cognitive and noncognitive approaches to affect and emotion. On the other hand, some theorists have also suggested useful alternatives to dual-process accounts, as we see next.

Barrett, Ochsner, and Gross

In some accounts, both of the processes of a dual-process model are handled in a single-network model (e.g., Barrett et al., 2006). In such a model, a psychological process may be represented by activation distributed across multiple nodes. Network models can either be "localist" (e.g., Thagard & Erb, 2002) or reflect "parallel distributed processing" (Wager & Thagard, 2004). In the former, each node may correspond to a given emotion or emotion instance; in the latter, the nodes may correspond to elements of emotion, with an emotion emerging from their joint action. Network models operate through multiple-constraint satisfaction. Each item of information in a network may constrain other items, such that the overall state of the network at any given mo-

ment is emergent from these multiple constraints. With respect to appraisal theory, the solution of the multiple constraints would be a specific emotion.

Rather than contending that such models represent a category of processing that is either automatic (associative) or controlled (rule-governed), Barrett et al. (2006) envision a continuum along which a given solution might represent a given combination or partially automated reaction. Processes combine componentially so that a given processing event is conditionally automatic (Bargh, 1997), in that it falls on the continuum from automatic to controlled. This approach is compatible with the notion of emotion emergence discussed earlier. If we think of the nodes as brain regions or perhaps as circuits corresponding to ways of representing evaluation, then a particular emotion would emerge as the best-fitting solution to the constraints of the currently active goals, attitudes, perceptions, knowledge, and situational parameters. The funneling toward a solution presumably can take place very rapidly and involves both top-down and bottom-up processing. As the bottom-up processes of constraint satisfaction take place, one may feel visited by an emotion, whereas when one engages in imaginative constructions of emotional events, one may feel more like the author of one's emotions. In this view, automatic and controlled processes have different functions within the same system, rather than being two different systems.

Ortony, Norman, and Revelle

A related view has been proposed by Ortony et al. (2005). They think of emotions similarly as interpreted affect or affect with a cognitive–perceptual frame. Their view is that feeling is undifferentiated positive or negative affect, and that specific emotions are transformations of feeling by appraisal. Appraisals, which are sometimes conscious but more often unconscious, situate and make sense of affect. Feeling is generated quite automatically, and its cognitive or perceptual framing may also generally be automatic. People are necessarily aware of feeling, in that the idea of "unfelt feeling" involves a contradiction in terms, but such awareness need not extend to the causes of feeling. Thus emotions in these views are cognitively elaborated states of affective feeling.

Cunningham and Zelazo

Finally, still another alternative to dual-process models is an approach in which levels of processing are iterative. Cunningham and Zelazo (2007) suggest that exposure to an object initiates an iterative sequence of evaluative processes—"the evaluative cycle." In this cycle, stimuli are interpreted and reinterpreted in light of an increasingly rich set of contextually meaningful representations. Evaluations based on few iterations of the cycle may be unconscious and automatic, whereas those based on additional iterations become relatively reflective. Thus implicit evaluations have fewer iterations and recruit fewer processes than explicit ones.

Cunningham and Zelazo propose that after initial affective reactions fire, sensory information may be reprocessed. Then, after more detailed stimulus identification, the information is again sent to the amygdala. One's own visceral reactions may also be reprocessed, so that the autonomic state also becomes cortically represented. At each stage, the amygdala may be used again, reacting to ever more detailed information at each iteration. In general, then, these authors view information processing as a series of recursive feedback loops that involve additional regions of the cortex as the process continues. With continual interaction of limbic and cortical areas, evaluations that start out as automatic become situated and progressively refined. In short, they become emotions.

Such an iterative model helps sharpen our notion of implicit and explicit processes. People tend to think of implicit emotional processes and attitudes as unconscious versions of what they see in conscious, explicit versions. Thus when research (Phelps et al., 2000) showed that Implicit Association Test (IAT) measures of racial attitudes were related to amygdala activation of white participants in response to black faces, people might assume that these reactions were unconscious versions of explicit and fully formed attitudes or prejudices. Indeed, in studies of racism, some writers seem to view conscious awareness solely as regulating or suppressing fully formed attitudes lurking within.

However, an iterative model suggests a different account. The amygdala is sensitive to novelty and violations of expectation. For most white research participants, black faces are non-normative. The presented image is likely to be processed and reprocessed, and each time, the amygdala receives a more and more differentiated form of the same information. Cortical processing, then, is not simply regulatory, but also helps define the reaction. The explicit, fully elaborated attitude is probably not the same as whatever is reflected in response times on the IAT, and the explicit, fully elaborated emotion is also not the same thing as initial subcortical and neurochemical reactions of affect. They are the same thing only in the sense that the block of marble that Leonardo da Vinci selected for his statue of David was the same thing as the statue that emerged from it. Both are made of the same material, but the latter has a very different form as a result of being processed and reprocessed many times. In a similar way, affect and emotion are made of the same stuff, but they have very different forms as a result of similarly iterative processing.

SUMMARY AND CONCLUSIONS

In this chapter we have focused on the process rather than the structure of emotion appraisal. We have argued that some kind of appraisal or evaluation is a necessity, since emotions are inherently about various kinds of goodness or badness. The issue of primary interest concerns how such evaluations are made. In the 1980s, Lazarus (1984) and Zajonc (1984) argued about whether affect and emotion required cognitive appraisals or not. It was an exchange that was more heated than illuminating, because critical terms were often used in different ways. In the end, both Lazarus and Zajonc were correct, but they were talking about different things. In general, cognitive theorists have focused on full-blown emotional states involving subjective experience, whereas critics have often focused on low-level, nonconscious, automatic processes. Both believe that they are explaining emotion, but it might be more accurate to say that the latter are studying undifferentiated affect (Ortony et al., 2005), whereas the former are studying emotion. If so, then an important task is to ask how these fit into a single processing model. Leading up to that task, we have asked questions about the nature of emotion as well as of appraisal and the appraisal process.

Much research has been inspired by the assumption that emotional life issues from a small number of basic emotions, which are defined by distinctive physiology and neurology, and are marked by distinctive feelings, expressions, and actions. A failure to find the kind of coherence implied by that model might imply either a limitation of method or of conceptualization. We have focused on alternative possible conceptualizations both of emotions and of the appraisal processes that differentiate them. In one model, the emotions are treated as emergent states from partially redundant affective representations across multiple components. We have contrasted this emergence model, in which physiology, expression, and cognition are constituents of emotion, with the traditional latent-trait model, in which these are indicators of an underlying emotion. Taking the view of these as constituents, we end up in agreement with William James's dictum that we are "angry because we strike" and "afraid because we tremble."

In an examination of the idea of appraisal, we have suggested that the concept of appraisal should probably be expanded to reflect the fact that appraisals are often as much perceptual as cognitive, and as much dictated by the topography of situations as by mental action. On the basis of Sloman's (1996) distinction between associative and rule-based reasoning, we have suggested that emotions can arise either from rule-based processing or by reinstatement.

We have also reviewed the impact of LeDoux's (1996) proposal of a low route to emotion without cortical involvement, and have cited critical reviews that cast doubt on the relevance of this particular pathway for human emotion. However, we have noted that the work in this area has done much to stimulate the study of subcortical contributions to emotion.

We have then reviewed two sequence models of emotional appraisal (Huron, 2006; Scherer, 2001), which propose that emotional processes are often initiated by reflexes such as the startle or orienting reflex, which activate appraisal processes. In the next section, we have reviewed low-level affective reactions, including preferences for curved versus jagged lines, and the evaluative implications of lightness and darkness and of high versus low pitch. We have also noted reactions to novelty versus identity that are present even at the cellular level, and that are perhaps continuous with behavioral reactions at the level of human groups, suggesting a surprising continuity of affective processes.

The observations of amazingly low-level affect-like processes make it clear that theorists must distinguish emotions from the affective reactions that are their seeds. Hence we have reviewed several models that make this distinction one way or another, including a dual-process model (Baumeister et al., 2007), a parallel-constraint model (Barrett et al., 2006), a sequence model (Ortony et al., 2005), and an iterative-process model (Cunningham & Zelazo, 2007).

In the end, the model of emotion and emotional appraisal that we have entertained is different in many respects from the received model. It emphasizes emotions as emergent constructions rather than as latent entities; it makes a sharp distinction between affective reactions and emotions; and it sees appraisal as an iterative process. Reflexes and low-level affective reactions often get the emotional ball rolling. These undifferentiated states are then refined, situated, further evaluated, and re-represented. The results are the rich and nuanced emotional states that mark the important occasions and turning points in people's lives, that embody people's aspirations and fears, and that are capable of motivating their best and worst actions.

ACKNOWLEDGMENTS

Support is acknowledged from National Institute of Mental Health Grant No. MH 50074 and National Science Foundation Grant No. BCS 0518835.

NOTES

1. The writing of this section benefited greatly from discussions with James Coan and Lisa Barrett.
2. Lydia Wraight (personal communication, November 2006) has pointed out that a preference for the familiar is evident in the cells of vertebrates, which express proteins that allow mutual recognition among, and preference for the cells of, a given individual.

REFERENCES

Ainsworth, M. D. S., Blehar, M. C., Waters, E., & Wall, T. (1978). *Patterns of attachment.* Hillsdale, NJ: Erlbaum.

Anderson, J. R. (1983). *The architecture of cognition.* Cambridge, MA: Harvard University Press.

Arnold, M. B. (1960). *Emotion and personality* (2 vols.). New York: Columbia University Press.

Aronoff, J., Woike, B. A., & Hyman, L. M. (1992). Which are the stimuli in facial displays of anger and happiness?: Configurational bases of emotion recognition. *Journal of Personality and Social Psychology, 62*, 1050–1066.

Bar, M., & Neta, M. (2006). Humans prefer curved visual objects. *Psychological Science, 17*, 645–648.

Bargh, J. (1997). The automaticity of everyday life: A manifesto. In R. S. Wyer (Ed.), *Advances in social cognition* (pp. 1–61). Mahwah, NJ: Erlbaum.

Barrett, L. F. (2006a). Emotions as natural kinds? *Perspectives on Psychological Science, 1*, 28–58.

Barrett, L. F. (2006b). Solving the emotion paradox: Categorization and the experience of emotion. *Personality and Social Psychology Review, 10*, 20–46.

Barrett, L. F., Ochsner, K. N., & Gross, J. J. (2006). On the automaticity of emotion. In J. Bargh (Ed.), *Social psychology and the unconscious: The automaticity of higher mental processes.* New York: Psychology Press.

Baumeister, R. F., Vohs, K. D., DeWall, C. N., & Zhang, L. (2007). How emotion shapes behavior: Feedback, anticipation, and reflection, rather than direct causation. *Personality and Social Psychology Review, 11*, 167–203.

Berkowitz, L. (1990). On the formation and regulation of anger and aggression: A cognitive–neoassociationistic analysis. *American Psychologist, 45*, 494–503.

Berkowitz, L., & Harmon-Jones, E. (2004). Toward an understanding of the determinants of anger. *Emotion, 4*, 107–130.

Bollen, K. A., & Lennox, R. (1991). Conventional wisdom on measurement: A structural equation perspective. *Psychological Bulletin, 110*, 305–314.

Bowlby, J. (1969). *Attachment and loss: Vol. 1. Attachment.* New York: Basic Books.

Brown, J. S., Collins, A., & Duguid, S. (1989). Situated cognition and the culture of learning. *Educational Researcher, 18*(1), 32–42.

Buck, R. (2007, March 4). Message posted to listserv of the International Society for Research on Emotions. Postings may be requested from *ISRE-L@lists.psu.edu*

Chaiken, S., Liberman, A., & Eagly, A. H. (1989). Heuristic and systematic processing within and beyond the persuasion context. In J. S. Uleman & J. A. Bargh (Eds.), *Affect and social behavior* (pp. 152–206). New York: Cambridge University Press.

Clark, A. (1997). *Being there: Putting brain, body, and world together again.* Cambridge, MA: MIT Press.

Clore, G. L., & Centerbar, D. (2004). Analyzing anger: How to make people mad. *Emotion, 4*, 139–144.

Clore, G. L., & Ortony, A. (2000). Cognitive in emotion: Never, sometimes, or always? In L. Nadel & R. Lane (Eds.), *The cognitive neuroscience of emotion* (pp. 24–61). New York: Oxford University Press.

Clore, G. L., Schwarz, N., & Conway, M. (1994). Affective causes and consequences of social information processing. In R. S. Wyer & T. Srull (Eds.), *Handbook of social cognition* (2nd ed., pp. 323–417). Hillsdale, NJ: Erlbaum.

Clore, G. L., Storbeck, J., Robinson, M. D., & Centerbar, D. (2005). Seven sins of research on unconscious affect. In L. F. Barrett, P. Niedenthal, & P. Winkielman (Eds.), *Emotion and consciousness* (pp. 384–408). New York: Guilford Press.

Cunningham, W. A., & Zelazo, P. D. (2007). Attitudes and evaluations: A social cognitive neuroscience perspective. *Trends in Cognitive Sciences, 11*, 97–104.

Davidson, R. J. (2003). Seven sins in the study of emotion: Correctives from affective neuroscience. *Brain and Cognition, 52*, 129–132.

Ekman, P. (1984). Expression and the nature of emotion. In K. Scherer & P. Ekman (Eds.), *Approaches to emotion* (pp. 319–343). Hillsdale, NJ: Erlbaum.

Freud, S. (1911). *The interpretation of dreams* (3rd ed., Trans A. A. Brill).New York: Macmillan.

Frijda, N. H. (1986). *The emotions.* New York: Cambridge University Press.

Gibson, J. J. (1979). *The ecological approach to visual perception.* Boston: Houghton Mifflin.

Huron, D. (2006). *Sweet anticipation: Music and the psychology of expectation.* Cambridge, MA: MIT Press.

James, W. (1890). *Principles of psychology.* New York: Holt.

Kotovsky, L., & Baillargeon, R. (1994). Calibration-based reasoning about collision events in 11-month-old infants. *Cognition, 51*, 107–129.

Lazarus, R. S. (1966). *Psychological stress and the coping process.* New York: McGraw-Hill.

Lazarus, R. S. (1984). On the primacy of cognition. *American Psychologist, 39*, 124–129.

Lazarus, R. S. (1994). Universal antecedents of the emotions. In P. Ekman & R. J. Davidson (Eds.), *The nature of emotion: Fundamental questions* (pp. 163–171). New York: Oxford University Press.

LeDoux, J. E. (1996). *The emotional brain.* New York: Simon & Schuster.

LeDoux, J. E., Romanski, L., & Xagoraris, A. (1989). Indelibility of subcortical emotional memories. *Journal of Cognitive Neuroscience, 1*, 238–243.

Lindquist, K., Barrett, L. F., Bliss-Moreau, E., & Russell, J. A. (2006). Language and the perception of emotion. *Emotion, 6*, 125–138.

Mandler, G. (1975). *Mind and emotion.* New York: Wiley.

Meier, B. P., & Robinson, M. D. (2004). Why the sunny side is up: Associations between affect and vertical position. *Psychological Science, 15*, 243–247.

Meier, B. P., Robinson, M. D., & Clore, G. L. (2004). Why good guys wear white: Automatic inferences about stimulus valence based on color. *Psychological Science, 15*, 82–87.

Mischel, W. (1968). *Personality and assessment.* New York: Wiley.

Moors, A. (2006, April 18). *Investigating the auto-maticity of constructive appraisals.* Paper presented at the 18th European Meeting on Cybernetics and Systems Research, Vienna.

Moors, A., & De Houwer, J. (2001). Automatic appraisal of motivational valence: Motivational affective priming and Simon effects. *Cognition and Emotion, 15,* 749–766.

Morgan, H. J., & Shaver, P. R. (1999). Attachment processes and commitment to romantic relationships. In J. M. Adams & W. H. Jones (Eds.), *Handbook of interpersonal commitment and relationship stability* (pp. 109–124). New York: Plenum Press.

Needham, A., & Baillargeon, R. (1993). Intuitions about support in 4.5-month-old infants. *Cognition, 47,* 121–148.

Oatley, K., & Johnson-Laird, P. N. (1987). Towards a cognitive theory of the emotions. *Cognition and Emotion, 1,* 29–50.

Ortony, A., Clore, G. L., & Collins, A. (1988). *The cognitive structure of emotions.* New York: Cambridge University Press.

Ortony, A., Norman, D. A., & Revelle, W. (2005). Affect and proto-affect in effective functioning. In J. M. Fellous & M. A. Arbib (Eds.), *Who needs emotions?: The brain meets the machine* (pp. 173–202). New York: Oxford University Press.

Osgood, C. E. (1969). On the whys and wherefores of E, P, and A. *Journal of Personality and Social Psychology, 12,* 194–199.

Osgood, C. E., Suci, G. J., & Tannenbaum, P. H. (1957). *The measurement of meaning.* Urbana: University of Illinois Press.

Parkinson, B. (2007). Getting from situations to emotions: Appraisal and other routes. *Emotion, 7,* 21–25.

Petty, R. E., & Cacioppo, J. T. (1986). The elaboration likelihood model of persuasion. In L. Berkowitz (Ed.), *Advances in experimental social psychology* (Vol. 19, pp. 123–205). New York: Academic Press.

Phelps, E. A., O'Connor, K. J., Cunningham, W. A., Funayama, E. S., Gatenby, J. C., Gore, J. C., et al. (2000). Performance on indirect measures of race evaluation predicts amygdala activation *Journal of Cognitive Neuroscience, 12,* 729–738.

Polti, G. (1977). *The thirty-six dramatic situations.* Boston: The Writer. (Original work published 1921)

Prinz, J. J. (2005). Emotions, embodiment, and awareness. In L. F. Barrett, P. M. Niedenthal, & P. Winkielman (Eds.), *Emotion and consciousness* (pp. 363–383). New York: Guilford Press.

Roseman, I. J. (1979, September). *Cognitive aspects of emotion and emotional behavior.* Paper presented at the 87th Annual Convention of the American Psychological Association, New York.

Roseman, I. J. (1984). Cognitive determinants of emotion: A structural theory. *Review of Personality and Social Psychology, 5,* pp. 11–36.

Russell, J. A. (2003). Core affect and the psychological construction of emotion. *Psychological Review, 110,* 145–172.

Russell, J. A., & Barrett, L. F. (1999). Core affect, prototypical emotional episodes, and other things called emotion: Dissecting the elephant. *Journal of Personality and Social Psychology, 76,* 805–819.

Sabini, J., & Silver, M. (2005). Why emotion names and experiences don't neatly pair. *Psychological Inquiry, 16,* 1–10.

Schachter, S., & Singer, J. E. (1962). Cognitive, social, and physiological determinants of emotional state. *Psychological Review, 69,* 379–399.

Scherer, K. R. (1984). On the nature and function of emotion: A component process approach. In K. R. Scherer & P. Ekman (Eds.), *Approaches to emotion* (pp. 293–317). Hillsdale, NJ: Erlbaum.

Scherer, K. R. (2001). Appraisal considered as a process of multilevel sequential processing. In K. R. Scherer, A. Schorr, & T. Johnstone (Eds.), *Appraisal processes in emotion: Theory, methods, research* (pp. 92–120). New York: Oxford University Press.

Scherer, K. R., Schorr, A., & Johnstone, T. (Eds.). (2001). *Appraisal processes in emotion: Theory, methods, research.* New York: Oxford University Press.

Schwarz, N., & Clore, G. L. (2007). Feelings and phenomenal experiences. In A. K. Kruglanski & E. T. Higgins (Eds.), *Social psychology: Handbook of basic principles* (2nd ed., pp. 385–407). New York: Guilford Press.

Shaver, P. R., & Clark, C. L. (1994). The psychodynamics of adult romantic attachment. In J. M. Masling & R. F. Bornstein (Eds.), *Empirical perspectives on object relations theories* (pp. 105–156). Washington, DC: American Psychological Association.

Siemer, M., & Reisenzein, R. (2007). The process of emotion inference. *Emotion, 7,* 1–20.

Sloman, S. A. (1996). The empirical case for two systems of reasoning. *Psychological Bulletin, 119,* 3–22.

Smith, C. A., & Ellsworth, P. C. (1985). Patterns of cognitive appraisal. *Journal of Personality and Social Psychology, 48,* 813–838.

Smith, C. A., Griner, L. A., Kirby, L. D., & Scott, H. S. (1996). Toward a process model of appraisal in emotion. In N. H. Frijda (Ed.), *Proceedings of the Ninth Conference of the International Society for Research on Emotion* (pp. 101–105). Toronto: International Society for Research on Emotion.

Smith, C. A., & Kirby, L. D. (2001). Toward delivering on the promise of appraisal theory. In K. R. Scherer, A. Schorr, & T. Johnstone (Eds.), *Appraisal processes in emotion: Theory, methods, research* (pp. 121–138). New York: Oxford University Press.

Smith, E. R., & Neumann, R. (2005). Emotion processes considered from the perspective of dual-process models. In L. F. Barrett, P. M. Niedenthal, & P. Winkielman (Eds.), *Emotion and consciousness* (pp. 287–311). New York: Guilford Press.

Storbeck, J., & Clore, G. L. (2007). On the interdependence of cognition and emotion. *Cognition and Emotion, 21,* 1212–1237.

Storbeck, J., Robinson, M. D., & McCourt, M. E. (2006). Semantic processing precedes affect retrieval: The neurological case for cognitive primacy in visual processing. *Review of General Psychology, 10,* 41–55.

Tajfel, H., Billig, M. G., Bundy, R. P., & Flament, C. (1971). Social categorization and intergroup behaviour. *European Journal of Social Psychology, 1,* 149–177.

Thagard, P., & Erb, J. (2002). Emotional gestalts: Appraisal, change, and the dynamics of affect. *Personality and Social Psychology Review, 6,* 274–282.

Wager, B. M., & Thagard, P. (2004). Spiking Phineas Gage: A neurocomputational theory of cognitive–affective integration in decision making. *Psychological Review, 111,* 67–79.

Wegner, D. M., & Vallacher, R. R. (1986). Action identification. In R. M. Sorrentino & E. T. Higgins (Eds.), *Handbook of motivation and cognition: Vol. 1. Foundations of social behavior* (pp. 550–582). New York: Guilford Press.

Winkielman, P., Berridge, K. C., & Wilbarger, J. (2005). Unconscious affective reactions to masked happy versus angry faces influence consumption behavior and judgments of value. *Personality and Social Psychology Bulletin, 31,* 121–135.

Zajonc, R. B. (1984). On the primacy of affect. *American Psychologist, 39,* 117–123.

Zebrowitz, L. A. (1997). *Reading faces: Window to the soul?* Boulder, CO: Westview Press.

PART VII

HEALTH AND EMOTIONS

CHAPTER 40

Emotions and Health Behavior
A Self-Regulation Perspective

MICHAEL A. DIEFENBACH, SUZANNE M. MILLER,
MATTHEW PORTER, ELLEN PETERS, MICHAEL STEFANEK,
and HOWARD LEVENTHAL

The study of emotions and health has had a long history. To begin with, research was concerned with the influence of physiological reactions (later termed "stress") to outside aversive events (Selye, 1951). Subsequent research examined the influence of experienced negative emotions on the body's ability to fight infections (Cohen & Wills, 1985). More recently, Leventhal and Patrick-Miller (2000) have argued that emotions can be causes of health states as well as outcomes, and can even be indicators of health. Such relationships usually assume a direct pathway between health and emotions. However, it is also plausible to envision indirect influences between emotions and health—for example, those in which emotions influence health behaviors (e.g., screening for cancer), which in turn might influence health states.

Traditional health behavior theories, such as the health belief model or the theory of planned behavior (Ajzen, 1985), have not been concerned with the influence of emotional states on health behavior. Such theories stand in contrast to a self-regulation perspective, as

elaborated in the parallel-processing model (Leventhal, 1970) or the cognitive–social health information processing (C-SHIP) framework (Miller, Shoda, & Hurley, 1996). In both of these latter approaches, emotional states are given equal weight to the cognitive processing of a health threat. Still, the specific roles of emotions in health cognitions and health behavior have not as yet been well described, compared to the body of literature that has concerned itself with the description and influence of health-related beliefs and illness representations (Lau & Hartman, 1983; Meyer, Leventhal, & Gutmann, 1985; Miller, Diefenbach, Krantz, Baum, & Academy of Behavioral Medicine Research, 1998).

This chapter explores the possible roles emotions may play in health cognitions and subsequent health behaviors. In our effort to address this topic, we rely on a self-regulation perspective and will also draw from other perspectives, including those from health, social, and cognitive psychology, as well as from the judgment and decision literature. The chapter is structured as follows. First, a historical perspective relating results from the early fear studies (e.g., Janis & Feshbach, 1953) to the emergence of the cognitive–affective parallel–processing framework (Leventhal, 1970) is presented. Next, studies on negative emotions and breast cancer screening are described, to illustrate the complex relationship between emotions and health behavior. This description is followed by a brief discussion of cognitive models of decision making, focusing primarily on a description of heuristics, and their relationship to cognitive and affective threat representations in a self-regulation framework (Leventhal & Diefenbach, 1991; Miller et al., 1996, 1998). Following this, we return to the example of breast cancer screening, applying theory to resolve divergent findings in that literature. We conclude with a discussion of new areas of research emanating from our review; we focus in particular on four functions of emotions derived from the decision-making literature and applied to the self-regulation framework.

EARLY STUDIES ON EMOTIONS AND BEHAVIOR

It is worthwhile to briefly review the original studies on fear communications. Fear appeals (or communications) originated from the fear-drive reduction model advanced by Dollard and Miller (1950). The central hypothesis underlying this model was that fear acts as a motivating force prompting individuals to perform recommended behaviors, which in turn reduce the unpleasant fear state. This model generally assumed that as the level of fear increases, so too does the likelihood of changes in behavior and attitude. Interventions based on this model consisted of fear-arousing messages that paired images of the undesired outcome with a recommendation for new behaviors. For example, pictures of decaying teeth were presented with the message to brush one's teeth regularly.

One of the first experimental studies to test this model was conducted by Janis and Feshbach (1953). Junior high school students received recommendations for oral hygiene (i.e., brushing one's teeth three times a day) coupled with three different fear appeals. The high-fear condition consisted of vivid pictures of decaying teeth and gums; the mild-fear condition consisted of less vivid pictures; and the no-fear condition had no pictures of decaying teeth. It was hypothesized that a positive linear

relationship between intensity of fear and a person's willingness for behavior change would be found, such that higher levels of fear would be associated with a greater likelihood of behavior change. Contrary to the researchers' expectations, students in the no-fear condition were more likely to change their dental hygiene than students in either the mild-fear or high-fear conditions. Janis and Feshbach attributed these findings to defensive avoidance aroused among students exposed to the fear messages (see also Janis, 1967).

A majority of subsequent studies, however, did not confirm these initial results or this interpretation. In studies that employed Janis and Feshbach's basic experimental design, higher levels of fear were consistently associated with stronger behavioral intentions or actual behavior changes. One such study (Dabbs & Leventhal, 1966) exposed students to three levels of fear-arousing information about the consequences of failing to obtain a tetanus shot. Both intentions and actual inoculation behavior correlated linearly with increased fear arousal; that is, students with higher fear were much more likely to obtain a tetanus shot. This basic pattern of results has been confirmed in studies using a number of paradigms, such as safe driving (Leventhal & Trembly, 1968; Rogers & Deckner, 1975), dental hygiene (Leventhal & Singer, 1966), and smoking cessation (Leventhal & Watts, 1966; Rogers & Thistlethwaite, 1970).

Another implication of these studies was the realization that the effects of fear appeals are transient and short-lived (Leventhal & Niles, 1965), and that intentions can best be translated into behavior if an individual receives an action plan. An "action plan" is a concrete set of instructions containing information about how, when, and where to execute a desired action in the context of the individual's life (e.g., getting a tetanus shot—Leventhal, Singer, & Jones, 1965; quitting smoking—Leventhal, Watts, & Pagano, 1967). Most importantly, it was found that if an action plan was provided, the attitude change and desired behaviors were sustained over weeks or months (in the case of smoking cessation) beyond the immediate effects of the fear appeal. The results suggested that neither fear (high or low) nor an action plan alone was sufficient to result in behavioral change; rather, the combination of fear and an action plan resulted in changes to individuals' cognitive and emotional representations of a threat, and these led in turn to changes in behavior (Leventhal, 1970).

THE FIRST PARALLEL-PROCESSING FORMULATION OF COGNITION AND EMOTION

The realization that individuals' threat representations are central to motivating behavior had two major implications. First, it led to research describing the content and nature of threat representations; second, it led to the development of a new theoretical framework, the parallel-processing model (Leventhal, 1970). In contrast to the fear-drive reduction model, which assumed serial processing of cognition and emotion (i.e., emotion follows cognition), this framework postulates the parallel processing of fear messages on both cognitive and emotional levels. Stimuli and potential responses are evaluated and represented simultaneously with both cognitions and emotions. The representations are situated within a processing network that is modified as new information enters.

The notion of "separate but equal" processing arms for cognition and emotion in a parallel framework raises the question of how the two arms interact to determine coping and appraisal behaviors. Much past research in this vein has assumed the existence of a processing system heavily influenced by a cognitive approach to information processing and decision making (e.g., Simon, 1967; Kahneman & Tversky, 1982). Zajonc (1984) was a strong proponent of the importance of emotion. He noted that although cognitions are traditionally viewed as the primary driver of decisions, emotions need not always be postcognitive phenomena. According to Zajonc, emotions can be quite independent of cognitive operations and can precede them in time. Indeed, some investigators have proposed that people use an emotion heuristic for decision making; this means that individuals' representations of objects or people are "tagged" with emotion (Finucane, Alhakami, Slovic, & Johnson, 2000), and that individuals access this "affective pool" in the process of making judgments. This is not unlike Damasio's (1994) hypothesis that thought is drawn largely from images consisting of symbolic representations. Individuals over time learn to "mark" these images as positive or negative, based on personal experiences.

Hence, if a negative image is linked to an image of a future outcome, it may serve as a barrier to a given action; if a positive image is associated with the outcome image, it may serve as an incentive. This is important, as we shall see when discussing further developments of the parallel-processing framework, such as the common-sense model of illness behavior and the C-SHIP model (Miller et al., 1996).

THE EXAMPLE OF FEAR AND BREAST CANCER SCREENING

Having reviewed the early literature on fear processing and the emergence of a psychological model to account for divergent experimental findings, we turn to a more recent example that illustrates the complex relationship between emotion and health behavior. We have chosen the example of how negative emotional states such as worry or fear affect breast cancer screening, because it is one of the best-developed areas within the otherwise sparse body of empirical studies on the relationship between emotions and cancer screening.

The U.S. Department of Health and Human Services (2000) report *Healthy People 2010* makes screening a cornerstone of cancer prevention and control efforts. It recognizes that one of the most important weapons in the battle against cancer is early detection through screening. Existing guidelines, endorsed by all major health institutes, recommend screening for breast, cervical, and colon cancer. Because patients' uptake of these recommendations has been variable, research on patients' decisions about screening is of paramount importance, and this is an area where emotions play a key role.

We conducted broad searches of comprehensive computerized databases (MEDLINE, PsycLIT, and CancerNet). This process identified 21 relevant, quantitative, empirical studies of breast cancer screening, published in English in peer-reviewed journals between 1990 and 2006. All studies included quantitative measures of worry or fear and actual screening behavior (not intentions to be screened).

"Cancer worry" or "cancer fear" is defined as a negative emotional state with specific reference to cancer. It is often assessed with a four-item scale developed by Lerman and colleagues (Lerman, Trock, Rimer, Boyce, et al., 1991; Lerman, Trock, Rimer, Jepson, et al., 1991).

This scale not only measures the degree of worry in response to cancer, but determines the impact such worry has on daily functioning. An alternative approach is to use a single item such as "When thinking about cancer, I am worried," which is scored on a 4- or 5-point Likert scale.

Results across the pool of 21 primary studies were mixed and are summarized in Table 40.1. Thirteen studies reported a positive association between anxiety and screening; that is, greater anxiety was associated with more screening behavior. Four studies reported a negative or inverse association; that is, greater anxiety was associated with less screening behavior. The remaining four studies reported no relationship between anxiety and screening behavior. Generally, stronger relationships with screening behavior were demonstrated for cancer-specific anxiety than for trait anxiety (see Diefenbach, Miller, & Daly, 1999). In addition, several studies suggested that the relationship between anxiety and screening may be curvilinear, taking the shape of an inverted-U curve—a relationship where moderate anxiety is associated with greater screening, but very high and very low levels of anxiety are associated with less screening (Bowen, Alfano, McGregor, & Andersen, 2004; Lerman et al., 1993; Schwartz, Taylor, & Willard, 2003). Substantiating such a pattern would require further research.

The diversity of results in part reflects methodological heterogeneity among the studies. Primary studies differed in sampling (e.g., women with or without a family history of breast cancer, women of different demographic backgrounds), construct operationalization (e.g., general vs. cancer-specific anxiety), and outcome (i.e., breast self-examination, clinical breast examination, or mammography attendance). Some of the studies used a cross-sectional/retrospective design, measuring both emotion and history of screening behavior at a single time point. Others employed a longitudinal/prospective design, measuring emotion at baseline and subsequent screening behavior at a later time point. Due to the quasi-experimental nature of all the investigations, establishing causality is difficult. However, the longitudinal studies at least establish that emotion preceded screening behavior, making a stronger argument for the hypothesized causal relationship between emotion and screening.

Based on the number and quality of studies reviewed, we can cautiously support the notion that cancer worry motivates breast cancer screening behavior. Even so, the question of how to account for the different effects of cancer worry on screening behavior remains. To explore why this may be so, we turn our attention to the role of cognitive heuristics and biases.

COGNITIVE HEURISTICS AND BIASES IN DECISION MAKING

Our knowledge of decision making and judgment under uncertainty has been heavily influenced by the study of cognitive heuristics and biases (Kahneman & Tversky, 1982). The original work by Tversky and Kahneman (1981) described 12 cognitive biases related to subjective judgment of probability, such as salience and availability. The potential influence of the most common biases listed by Kahneman and Tversky (1982) on cancer screening, prevention, or treatment decision making has not been systematically evaluated for their relevance; nor, obviously, have strategies been tested to ameliorate these biases. For example, according to the availability heuristic, knowledge that no one in one's own family has had any type of cancer associated with the human papillomavirus (HPV) could lead to a predisposition to judge HPV-related cancer as less likely for oneself (regardless of one's own exposure history), thereby decreasing screening behavior. According to the salience heuristic, knowledge of a friend or relative who endured a difficult treatment regimen for breast cancer could lead to a predisposition to judge a diagnosis of breast cancer as more likely for oneself, due simply to the greater cognitive salience of that particular information (which presumably results from its emotional impact). In both examples, screening decisions are based on cognitive biases rather than objective reality. Yet the operation of these cognitive biases in making decisions about cancer screening has not yet been systematically investigated; nor have interventions to correct them been developed or tested. The need to clarify the role of cognitive biases in screening and treatment decision making is heightened, because health care providers often provide relatively complex incidence and prevalence statistics to patients who may not be equipped to interpret them.

TABLE 40.1. Summary of Investigations of the Relationship between Anxiety and Breast Cancer Screening

Author	Design	Screening modality	Population	Affect measure
Studies reporting a positive relationship				
Diefenbach et al. (1999)	Prospective	Mammogram	FDRs of women with cancer (N = 213)	Breast cancer worry, 1 item
McCaul et al. (1998)	Prospective	BSE	Women with (n = 65) and without (n = 70) family history of breast cancer	Breast cancer worry, 4 items
McCaul et al. (1996)	Prospective	BSE, mammogram, CBE	Women from the community (N = 353)	Breast cancer concerns, 3 items
Tinley et al. (2004)	Prospective	BSE, CBE, mammogram	Women from BRCA1/2 families (N = 112)	IES Intrusion Scale
Young & Severson (2005)	Prospective	Mammogram	African American women eligible for federally funded cancer screening program (N = 405)	Cancer fear, 11 items
Andersen et al. (2003)	Retrospective	Mammogram	Population sample (N = 6,512), including some women with family history (n = 948)	Cancer worry, 5 items
Bowen et al. (2004)	Retrospective	BSE, mammogram	Population-based (N = 1,366) sample of women	Breast cancer worry, 4 items; general anxiety and depression (Brief Symptom Inventory)
Burnett et al. (1999)	Retrospective	BSE, CBE, mammogram	Women with family history (N = 139)	Breast cancer worry, 3 items
Consedine et al. (2004)	Retrospective	BSE, CBE, mammogram	Cluster sampling of older women from six ethnic groups (N = 1,364)	Cancer worry (Cancer Attitude Inventory, 4 items)
Epstein et al. (1997)	Retrospective	BSE	FDRs of women with cancer (N = 1,053); focused on 85 excessive BSE performers	Cancer worry, 3 items
Gram & Slenker (1992)	Retrospective	Mammogram	Women invited to a free mammography screening (N = 1,349) in two cities	Breast cancer anxiety, recalled 1 year later
Lauver et al. (1999)	Retrospective	BSE, CBE, mammogram	Patients at an urban hospital who had not had a mammogram in the last 13 months (N = 119)	Profile of Mood States
Stefanek & Wilcox (1991)	Retrospective	BSE, mammogram	FDRs of breast cancer patients (N = 125)	Breast cancer worry, no specific information given

(continued)

TABLE 40.1. *(continued)*

Author	Design	Screening modality	Population	Affect measure
Studies reporting a negative relationship				
Schwartz et al. (2003)	Prospective	Mammogram	FDRs of women with breast cancer (N = 159)	Breast cancer worry, 2 items; general distress mental health inventory
Lerman et al. (1993)	Retrospective	Mammogram	Women with family history (N = 140)	Breast cancer worry, 1 item; IES Intrusion Scale
Kash et al. (1992)	Retrospective	BSE, CBE, mammogram	Women enrolled in a breast protection program (N = 217)	Taylor Manifest Anxiety Scale; cancer-related anxiety and helplessness scale
Lerman et al. (1994)[a]	Retrospective	BSE, mammogram	Women < 50 years old with family history of breast cancer (N = 783) from three study sites	Breast cancer worry, 2 items; psychological distress; IES Intrusion Scale
Studies reporting a null relationship				
Aro et al. (1999)	Prospective	Mammogram	Attenders and nonattenders of a mammography screening program (n's = 946 and 641, respectively)	General anxiety and depression
Sutton et al. (1995)	Prospective	Mammogram	Community sample of women 50–64 years old (N = 1,500)	State–Trait Anxiety Inventory; General Health Questionnaire; 7-item anxiety measure
Lindberg & Wellisch (2001)	Retrospective	BSE, mammogram	Attenders and nonattenders of a mammography screening program (n's = 191 and 174, respectively)	Breast cancer worry
Drossaert et al. (1996)	Retrospective	Mammogram	Women with and without family history of breast cancer (n's = 389 and 295, respectively)	Breast cancer anxiety; investigator-developed anxiety scale

Note. FDRs, first-degree relatives; BSE, breast self-examination; CBE, clinical breast examination; BRCA1/2, breast cancer susceptibility genes 1 and 2; IES, Impact of Events Scale.
[a]This study provides inconclusive results, as they vary by study site.

Although "virtually all current theories of choice under risk or uncertainty are cognitive and consequentalist" (Loewenstein, Weber, Hsee, & Welch, 2001, p. 267), relatively few of these theories attempt to link the roles of cognition and emotion. Schwarz (1990), for example, has pointed out that the anticipation of emotion as a consequence of a decision is capable of influencing the decision, as well as the formation of attitudes. Mellers and McGraw (2001) have found that anticipated pleasure is closely connected to choice. They have proposed, as part of their theory of subjective expected pleasure, that individuals predict the pleasurable emotion that could result from each potential outcome of a particular behavioral option, weight these by the perceived chances of their occurrence, and combine them to form an average anticipated pleasure index for each behavioral option. This is done for all behavioral options under consideration, and then the option with the greatest average anticipated pleasure index is selected. A corollary of this theory is that individuals will avoid selecting any option that could make them feel worse. The theory has not yet been applied to medical decision situations, and thus it is unknown how accurate individuals are in predicting emotional consequences of future events (Loewenstein & Schkade, 1999; Ditto & Hawkins, 2005; Ubel, Loewenstein, Schwarz, & Smith, 2005).

A COMMON-SENSE MODEL OF COGNITIVE–AFFECTIVE PROCESSING

As the discussion to this point has suggested, biased cognitive processing exists within a larger cognitive–affective framework. This idea is supported by research that attempted to characterize the cognitive attributes of a threat stimulus and led to the formulation of the common-sense model of illness representations (Meyer et al., 1985). At the beginning of the threat identification and processing sequence is the individual's attempt to identify the threat, and thus to assign it a "label" (e.g., "I can feel something in my breast; is it cancer?"). The use of a label often determines subsequent attributes, such as "timeline or duration," "consequences," "cause," and "controllability" (Lau & Hartman, 1983). Each attribute answers a different question in the attempt to define the

unknown stimulus. Timeline or duration addresses the perceived temporal progression of the stimulus. It answers the question of whether the threat represents an acute condition (e.g. a benign tumor), a chronic condition (e.g., cancer), or a condition that might disappear and reappear (e.g., an allergy). The consequence attribute defines the stimulus in terms of its potential impact on the individual's overall health—whether it is minor, major, or life-threatening. The cause attribute categorizes the stimulus in terms of potential factors that might have led to the stimulus. Controllability answers the question of whether anything can be done about it. Attributes of illness representations are highly individualized and are not necessarily consistent with medical knowledge. Although there is a lack of research on the influence of cognitive biases and heuristics on the representational level, it is most likely that cognitive biases work at this initial encoding level.

The next step in the processing of the stimulus involves the selection of a coping response. Coping responses can be triggered as a result of a cognitive evaluation of the threat, as a way to deal with the emotional impact of the threat, or as the result of an interaction of the two. For example, coping with a cold will probably prompt a person to take some over-the-counter cold medication—an act that involves only minimal emotional processing. In contrast, the occurrence of a persistent stuffy nose with symptoms of achiness may lead the person to consider a more severe diagnosis, triggering feelings of worry and anxiety. In that case, the coping response may be triggered as much to allay worry about an unknown condition as it is to relieve the discomfort.

After selecting and executing a coping action, the individual next appraises the chosen coping response for its effectiveness. To continue the prior example, if the cold symptoms subside after the person ingests the medication, the coping procedure has been successful. If however, the cold symptoms persist, the individual will have to change his or her initial diagnosis to consider more severe illnesses, such as a type of flu. This leads to a revision of the relevant illness representation attributes (i.e., label, time line, consequences, cause, and controllability), triggering new negative feelings and prompting the selection of other coping procedures.

An often overlooked feature of the common-sense model is that coping requires not just the representation of the threat, but also the representation of coping procedures—the action plan. Thus this approach integrates the earlier finding from the fear communication literature that an action plan is an important addition to the cognitive and emotional threat representations. This approach leads to a coherent, action-oriented model, in which the threat is placed in an action framework. Of course, the individual must appraise the available responses as effective—and, more importantly, actions must seem necessary and feasible as a way to limit the threat. If the responses are not adequate, an individual faces a health threat without an action plan, with a likely increase in negative emotional states.

COGNITIVE–SOCIAL HEALTH INFORMATION PROCESSING

The cognitive–affective approach has been expanded and applied to coping with cancer threat and disease (Miller et al., 1996, 1998). The C-SHIP framework frees itself from a parallel-processing mechanism by postulating the existence of five main cognitive–affective mediating units that process cancer-relevant information. These units are interconnected and include many of the primary theoretical constructs from existing health behavior theories developed in the cognitive, social, and health sciences. Specifically, the units consist of (1) the individual's encoding/self-construals of the cancer threat (Champion, 1985, 1987, 1988; Lazarus & Folkman, 1984; Leventhal, 1970, 1983, 1990); (2) the individual's cancer-related self-efficacy beliefs (Bandura, 1977) and outcome expectations (Bandura, 1986; Scheier & Carver, 1985); (3) the individual's cancer-related values and goals (Lau & Hartman, 1983); (4) the individual's emotional responses to cancer threats (Horowitz, 1991; Leventhal, 1970); and (5) the individual's repertoire of self-regulatory/coping skills and strategies (Carver, Scheier, & Weintraub, 1989). Figure 40.1 displays the interconnected network of emotion and cognition at work in the example of making a decision about breast cancer screening. Specifically, a woman may react to information about breast cancer risk, the effectiveness of mammograms, and screening recommendations with increased risk perception (Path 1), a belief that mammograms will be able to detect cancer in an early stage (Path 2), or the intention to adhere to a regular screening regimen (Path 3). Beliefs of increased vulnerability to breast cancer may be followed by a related belief that a lump may be found soon (Path 4), which will be cured by treatment (Path 8). However, to take advantage of early treatment, screening is necessary (Path 10), and this realization may lead to the intention to have regular mammograms. A woman may also react to information about breast cancer with increased helplessness, anxiety, and depression (Paths 4 and 7). A belief that "a lump will be detected sooner or later" does not necessarily lead to action, as can be seen in Path 11, which points to a predominantly negative affective reaction. It is possible, however, that some women use action in the form of screening as a way to control their negative emotions. This possibility is accounted for in Paths 12 and 13.

Thus, depending on the initial encoding of an external or internal stimulus, different mediating units are activated that trigger individual beliefs, values, and goals; outcome expectations; and an emotional response to the stimulus. Ultimately, this processing will lead to the execution or inhibition of behaviors related to coping and adjustment to cancer risk and disease.

The conceptualization of information processing within C-SHIP as a model of mediating units can be compared to the excitation of nodes within the actual physiological nervous system. The mediating units, or nodes, are excited or inhibited based on the information that is processed through the connected nodes, eventually resulting in a behavioral action. Implicit in the C-SHIP framework is the development of information-processing signatures. These signatures are the result of repeated processing of similar information, resulting in similar responses. Thus the behavioral signatures reflect a system's tendency to react with similar behavioral patterns, given that similar nodes are activated. In other words, these signatures can be thought of as a sequence of "if–then" statements resulting in more or less consistent behavioral responses. The identification of such sequences or signatures will facilitate the accurate prediction of individual responses to threat messages and different health behaviors by incorporating an individual's habitual response style.

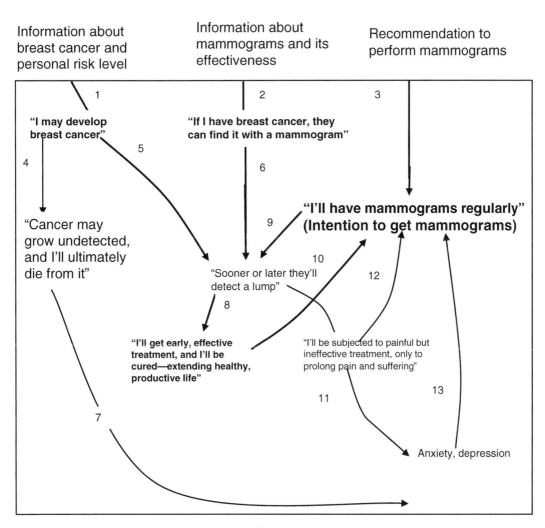

FIGURE 40.1. Example of hypothesized activation of cognition and affect in the C-SHIP model leading to mammography screening. Thick arrows are activated paths; thin arrows are possible but nonactivated paths.

COGNITIVE AND EMOTIONAL HEURISTICS WITHIN A SELF-REGULATION FRAMEWORK

The self-regulation approach sees the patient as an active protagonist who is constantly evaluating his or her internal and external environment to control health behavior. These evaluation behaviors can be executed on both an automatic and a deliberate level. Research has identified a number of such mental rules or shortcuts in somatic processing and has connected them to the basic illness representation attributes. For example, the "symmetry" rule is used to link the somatic experience to the iden-

tity attribute or label. A patient experiencing symptoms searches for a meaning-giving identity to the symptomatic process. However, in the case of an illness label, a patient is also inclined to search for symptoms in support of his or her own illness experience: symptoms are there for a reason and have a name, and illnesses are characterized by a set of symptoms (Meyer et al., 1985). Other heuristics that help patients to process somatic and experiential information include the "stress–illness" heuristic and the "age–illness" heuristic. The stress–illness heuristic categorizes general somatic events (e.g., fatigue, muscle aches, headaches) as either stress responses or, in the absence of stressful events, as symptoms of an illness (Cameron, Leventhal, & Leventhal, 1995). The age–illness heuristic similarly attributes somatic events that fit with a perceived aging model to aging and not to illness (Prochaska, Keller, Leventhal, & Leventhal, 1987; Stoller, 1984). Illness attributions are made if the somatic event significantly departs from the aging attribution—for example, if there is a sharp pain that is distinguishable from regular arthritic pain. Other heuristics are concerned with the "duration" of a somatic event (a more enduring event is more serious and threatening) and its "prevalence." Finally, the "affect" heuristic connects negative emotions, such as anxious and depressed moods, to increased disease vulnerability (Salovey & Birnbaum, 1989).

Thus the self-regulation framework not only allows for the processing of the threat stimulus on the cognitive and emotional level, but also permits the formulation of some rules that govern the emotional and cognitive processing of health-threatening events. In addition, as in any complex regulatory system that strives for equilibrium, it provides for a feedback loop with the potential to revise the underlying cognitive and emotional representations, heuristics, and subsequent selection of coping procedures (see Figure 40.2). Such a feedback mechanism increases the complexity of the model—a cost that is offset by improved explanatory power for the processes hypothe-

sized to underlie health behaviors. Thus we argue that comprehensive models of health behavior need to include constructs of emotions as well as cognitive representations. Models such as the theory of planned behavior (Ajzen, 1985) and the health belief model, which lack such components, consequently have limited explanatory utility, even though they address cognitive factors as well as external societal factors. Similarly, single-variable models, such as the focus on self-efficacy (Bandura, 1977), have limited utility in predicting health behavior.

FUNCTIONS OF AFFECT[1] AND THEIR ROLE IN DECISION MAKING

Although the role of emotion in decision making has received renewed attention over the past several years, a formal description of the specific roles of emotionally based heuristics is lacking. A recent paper by Peters, Lipkus, and Diefenbach (2006) has begun to address this point by focusing on the functions of affect, a concept closely related to emotion. Peters et al. argue that affect has four separable roles important to health decision-making processes. First, affect can act as "information." This function is best exemplified by the affect heuristic (Slovic, Peters, Finucane, & MacGregor, 2005). That is, affect may serve as a cue for

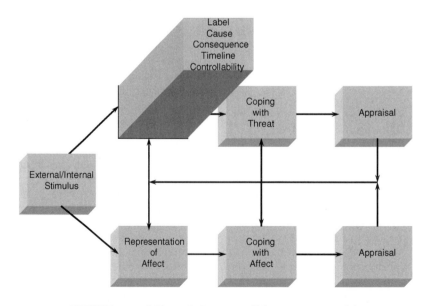

FIGURE 40.2. Self-regulation or parllel processing model.

many important judgments, including probability judgments (Slovic, Finucane, Peters, &
MacGregor, 2002). Zajonc (1980) proposed
that emotional reactions to stimuli are often
the earliest reactions. Under the affect heuristic
model, affect can be experienced first upon
consideration of a familiar technology, or it can
be the result of further information processing
(LeDoux, 1996; Peters, Västfjäll, Gärling, &
Slovic, 2006). In either event, affect then acts as
information, guiding decisions and judgments
such as risk and benefit perceptions. The affect
heuristic is substantially similar to models of
"risk as feelings" and "mood as information"
(Loewenstein et al., 2001; Schwarz & Clore,
2003), and it has much in common with dual
process theories discussed earlier (see, e.g.,
Cameron & Leventhal, 2003; Leventhal, 1970;
Leventhal, Diefenbach, & Leventhal, 1992;
Epstein, 1994).

Whereas some theories focus exclusively on
the use of mood states in judgments (e.g.,
Forgas, 1995; Schwarz & Clore, 2003), use of
the affect heuristic is characterized by reliance
on feelings attributed to an option or stimulus
and experienced while considering it in judgments and decisions. Alhakami and Slovic
(1994) proposed that the strength of positive or
negative affect associated with an activity (and
experienced while considering that activity)
guides perceptions of its risks and benefits.
Thus judgments about a technology such as a
new medical treatment may be based not only
on what people think about the treatment, but
also on how they feel about it. If feelings related to a technology are more positive, decision makers tend to judge its risks as low and
its benefits as high; if their feelings are more
negative, they tend to judge the opposite—risks
as high and benefits as low. For example, virtual colonoscopy is currently under much scrutiny for the detection of colon cancer. Individuals with positive affect toward this technology
(e.g., because they have learned that it is not invasive or that it is less embarrassing than actual
colonoscopy) may interpret new information
about risks and benefits in ways that are consistent with their affect (i.e., they may perceive
it as having low risk and high benefit).

Considerably less work has been done on the
other three proposed functions of affect. Affect
also can act as a "spotlight," focusing people's
attention on different information (e.g., numer-
ical cues, risks vs. benefits), depending on the
extent of their affect. First, the extent or type of

affective feelings (e.g., weak vs. strong affect,
or anger vs. fear) focuses the decision maker on
new information. Second, the new information
(rather than the initial feelings themselves) is
used to guide the judgment or decision. Affect
can also serve as a "motivator" for action or
the processing of information. For example, it
may provide an action tendency toward getting
a mammogram. Alternatively, it could change
the extent of deliberative effort the decision
maker puts forth. Finally, affect may serve as a
"common currency" in judgments and decisions allowing people to compare more effectively the values of very different decision options or information—in effect, to compare
apples to oranges (Cabanac, 1992). Montague
and Berns (2002) link this notion to "neural responses in the orbitofrontal–striatal circuit
which may support the conversion of disparate
types of future rewards into a kind of internal
currency, that is, a common scale used to compare the valuation of future behavioral acts or
stimuli" (p. 265). By translating more complex
thoughts into simpler emotional evaluations,
decision makers can compare and integrate
good and bad feelings, rather than attempt to
make sense out of a multitude of conflicting
logical reasons. This function is thus an extension of the affect-as-information function into
more complex decisions that require integration of information. It predicts that emotional
information can often be more easily and effectively integrated into complex judgments than
cognitive information can be.

INTEGRATING THE FUNCTIONS
OF AFFECT INTO
A SELF-REGULATION FRAMEWORK

We argue that the functions of affect should not
be examined as constructs by themselves, but
should be integrated into the larger body of
work that supports the self-regulation framework. There is considerable overlap between
the roles assigned to emotion in the parallel-
processing model and C-SHIP on the one hand,
and the functions of affect on the other. Thus,
from a theoretical point of view, a combination
of the two approaches seems readily achievable. Theoretical models need experimental
confirmation, and a greater effort must be
made to examine the role and functions of
emotion in both laboratory and field studies.
Examining the functions of emotion in medical

decision making would be a particularly fruitful approach. Medical decision making under uncertainty, such as the decision of whether to undergo mammography or genetic testing for susceptibility to breast cancer, is fraught with emotions. Yet few investigations have examined the role of emotions in such situations.

THE RELATIONSHIP BETWEEN FEAR AND BREAST CANCER SCREENING REVISITED

In our review of the literature on the role of emotions in breast cancer screening behavior, we have found provisional support for a positive relationship between negative emotions and such behavior. Some of the diverging results might be explained by differences in populations and measures of emotion, but none of these factors appears to consistently influence the direction of the effect. Some researchers (Bowen et al., 2004; Lerman et al., 1993; Schwartz et al., 2003) suggest that the effect of worry may best be characterized by an inverted-U curve: Very low and very high levels of worry may be associated with lower levels of screening behavior—the former because low levels emotion lack motivational force, and the latter because levels that are too high act as a barrier. Although intuitively attractive, this interpretation of the data is less plausible in the context of the literature on fear studies and its resulting theoretical developments.

The driving force behind a screening decision is likely to be a combination of factors. As suggested by the self-regulation approach, these factors consist of individual threat, vulnerability, and coping representations; emotional reactions; and societal and cultural determinants. In addition, research on heuristics and biases point to processing pitfalls that could potentially influence the information-processing sequence. Research on heuristics and biases within the health or cancer context is sparse; most of it has been conducted in the laboratory with non-health-related or non-cancer-related scenarios, and thus the influence of these variables in health-related decision situations is as yet unknown.

Many of the same points made about research focusing on cognitive variables and decision making can also be made with regard to research on emotion variables and decision making. Much of it lacks a health focus and is

therefore not readily transferable to decision making in the health or cancer context. Furthermore, researchers focusing on emotion variables often do so to the exclusion of cognitive variables, making it impossible to compare the individual contributions of each group of variables to the decision process.

As we have demonstrated, negative emotions can motivate, or in some cases can interfere with, cancer screening behavior. However, we do not currently understand the potential role that positive emotions—or the absence of negative emotions—may play. For example, are there some circumstances when a feeling of tranquility coupled with an objective assessment of costs and benefits may increase screening behavior? Or to what extent may screening behavior be prompted by the anticipation of relief from a current unpleasant anxiety state upon receiving good news? Anticipating one's affect in a particular situation is akin to role playing or the pre-living of a screening result. The role-playing/pre-living technique has recently been applied to facilitate decision making for genetic testing: At-risk individuals are asked to pre-live the emotional and cognitive consequences of both positive and negative genetic testing results (Diefenbach & Hamrick, 2003; Miller et al., 2001). However, it is necessary to examine the information-processing flow within that context more carefully, particularly the use and influence of heuristics and biases during the pre-living sequences. It is also critical to continue examining the degree to which individuals using the role-playing/pre-living technique can accurately predict their response to situations that may arise in real life.

Researchers interested in the diverse pathways between emotions and health should strive to incorporate the complex findings regarding emotions and health behavior that have been derived from diverse research areas into more comprehensive and integrative theoretical frameworks. With the notable exception of the C-SHIP framework and the parallel-processing model, efforts in model building have been sparse. However, model building should not consist of including an increasing number of variables in ever more complex models. In contrast, we suggest that researchers rigorously evaluate variables and their hypothesized relationships to other factors in a given model. These tests should be conducted both experimentally in laboratory settings that simulate the appropriate health contexts, as well as naturalistically in the field, employing both quantitative and qualitative methods. Only then can we be confident that our theoretical models are valid for predicting health-related behavior.

The role of emotions in cancer screening research needs further exploration. We hope that this chapter has sensitized researchers as well as clinicians to the necessity of examining and incorporating emotion variables in their research programs. Furthermore, we hope that cognitive researchers from areas that traditionally do not have a health focus will be persuaded to adopt such an outlook in their future research.

ACKNOWLEDGMENTS

This chapter was supported in part by grants from the National Institutes of Health (No. R01 CA104979, and No. P30 CA06927 to the Fox Chase Cancer Center Behavioral Research Core Facility), the Department of Defense (Nos. DAMD 17-01-01-1-0238 and DAMD 17-02-1-0382), and the American Cancer Society (No. TURSG 02-227-01). We are indebted to Joanne Buzaglo and Linda Fleisher for their valuable feedback, and to John Scarpato and Mary Anne Ryan for their technical assistance.

NOTE

1. Though the distinction between "affect" and "emotion" is clouded by the imprecision of language, affect is here understood to be a "basic invariant building block of emotional life derived from the human mind's capacity to engage in processes of valuation" (i.e., judging whether something is helpful or harmful; see also Russell & Barrett, 1999). It follows that affect is tantamount to a felt experience of valence—the specific quality of goodness or badness that both is experienced as a feeling state (with or without conscious awareness) and demarcates a positive or negative quality of a stimulus. Such feelings can be used as information for judgment and decision making (Schwarz & Clore, 1988), and this usage can be termed "the affect heuristic" (Slovic, Finucane, Peters, & MacGregor, 2002). By contrast, emotions, such as cancer-related worry, are in this context taken to be akin to what William James (1884) called "the more complicated cases in which a wave of bodily disturbance of some kind accompanies the perception of the interesting sights or sounds, or the passage of the exciting train of ideas" (p. 188). Both strong, visceral emotions such as fear and anger, and much subtler feelings—the "faint whisper[s] of emotion"

we call affects—can play a role in risk perceptions and behavior (e.g., Lerner & Keltner, 2000; Slovic & Peters, 2006).

REFERENCES

Ajzen, I. (1985). From intentions to actions: A theory of planned behavior. In J. Kuhl & J. Beckman (Eds.), *Action control: From cognition to behavior* (pp. 11–39). Berlin: Springer-Verlag.

Alhakami, A. S., & Slovic, P. (1994). A psychological study of the inverse relationship between perceived risk and perceived benefit. *Risk Analysis, 14,* 1085–1096.

Andersen, M. R., Smith, R., Meischke, H., Bowen, D., & Urban, N. (2003). Breast cancer worry and mammography use by women with and without a family history in a population-based sample. *Cancer Epidemiology, Biomarkers and Prevention, 12*(4), 314–320.

Aro, A. R., de Koning, H. J., Absetz, P., & Schreck, M. (1999). Psychosocial predictors of first attendance for organised mammography screening. *Journal of Medical Screening, 6*(2), 82–88.

Bandura, A. (1977). *Self-efficacy: The exercise of control.* New York: Freeman.

Bandura, A. (1986). *Social foundations of thought and action: A social cognitive theory.* Englewood Cliffs, NJ: Prentice Hall.

Bowen, D. J., Alfano, C. M., McGregor, B. A., & Andersen, M. R. (2004). The relationship between perceived risk, affect, and health behaviors. *Cancer Detection and Prevention, 28*(6), 409–417.

Burnett, C. B., Steakley, C. S., Slack, R., Roth, J., & Lerman, C. (1999). Patterns of breast cancer screening among lesbians at increased risk for breast cancer. *Women and Health, 29*(4), 35–55.

Cabanac, M. (1992). Pleasure: The common currency. *Journal of Theoretical Biology, 155,* 173–200.

Cameron, L. D., Leventhal, E. A., & Leventhal, H. (1995). Seeking medical care in response to symptoms and life stress. *Psychosomatic Medicine, 57,* 37–47.

Cameron, L. D., & Leventhal, H. (2003). Self-regulation, health, and illness: An overview. In L. D. Cameron & H. Leventhal (Eds.), *The self-regulation of health and illness behaviour* (pp. 1–14). London: Routledge.

Carver, C. S., Scheier, M. F., & Weintraub, J. K. (1989). Assessing coping strategies: A theoretically based approach. *Journal of Personality and Social Psychology, 56*(2), 267–283.

Champion, V. (1985). Use of the health belief model in determining frequency of breast self exam. *Research in Nursing and Health, 8,* 373–379.

Champion, V. (1987). The relationship of breast self-examination to health belief model variables. *Research in Nursing and Health, 10,* 375–382.

Champion, V. (1988). Attitudinal variables related to intention, frequency and proficiency of breast self-examination in women 35 and over. *Research in Nursing and Health, 11,* 283–291.

Cohen, S., & Wills, T. A. (1985). Stress, social support, and the buffering hypothesis. *Psychological Bulletin, 98,* 310–357.

Consedine, N. S., Magai, C., & Neugut, A. I. (2004). The contribution of emotional characteristics to breast cancer screening among women from six ethnic groups. *Preventive Medicine, 38*(1), 64–77.

Dabbs, J. M., Jr., & Leventhal, H. (1966). Effects of varying the recommendations in a fear-arousing communication. *Journal of Personality and Social Psychology, 4,* 525–531.

Damasio, A. R. (1994). *Descartes' error: Emotions, reason and the human mind.* New York: Avon.

Diefenbach, M. A., & Hamrick, N. (2003). Self-regulation and genetic testing. In L. D. Cameron & H. Leventhal (Eds.), *The self-regulation of health and illness behaviour* (pp. 314–331). London: Routledge.

Diefenbach, M. A., Miller, S. M., & Daly, M. B. (1999). Specific worry about breast cancer predicts mammography use in women at risk for breast and ovarian cancer. *Health Psychology, 18*(5), 532–536.

Ditto, P. H., & Hawkins, N. A. (2005). Advance directives and cancer decision making near the end of life. *Health Psychology, 24*(4, Suppl.), S63–S70.

Dollard, J., & Miller, N. (1950). *Personality and psychotherapy: An analysis in terms of learning, thinking and culture.* New York: McGraw-Hill.

Drossaert, C. C., Boer, H., & Seydel, E. R. (1996). Perceived risk, anxiety, mammogram uptake, and breast self-examination of women with a family history of breast cancer: The role of knowing to be at increased risk. *Cancer Detection and Prevention, 20*(1), 76–85.

Epstein, S. (1994). Integration of the cognitive and the psychodynamic unconscious. *American Psychologist, 49*(8), 709–724.

Epstein, S. A., Lin, T. H., Audrain, J., Stefanek, M., Rimer, B., & Lerman, C. (1997). Excessive breast self-examination among first-degree relatives of newly diagnosed breast cancer patients. *Psychosomatics, 38*(3), 253–261.

Finucane, M. L., Alhakami, A., Slovic, P., & Johnson, S. M. (2000). The affect heuristic in judgments of risks and benefits. *Journal of Behavioral Decision Making, 13,* 1–17.

Forgas, J. P. (1995). Mood and judgment: The affect infusion model (AIM). *Psychological Bulletin, 11,* 39–66.

Gram, I. T., & Slenker, S. E. (1992). Cancer anxiety and attitudes toward mammography among screening attenders, nonattenders, and women never invited. *American Journal of Public Health, 82*(2), 249–251.

Horowitz, M. J. (1991). *Person schemas and maladaptive interpersonal patterns.* Chicago: University of Chicago Press.

James, W. (1884). What is an emotion? *Mind, 9,* 188–205.

Janis, I. L. (1967). Effects of fear arousal on attitude change: Recent developments in theory and research. In L. Berkowitz (Ed.), *Advances in experimental social psychology* (Vol. 3, pp. 166–224). New York: Academic Press.

Janis, I. L., & Feshbach, S. (1953). Effect of fear-arousing communications. *Journal of Abnormal Psychology, 48*(1), 78–92.

Kahneman, D., & Tversky, A. (1982). The simulation heuristic. In D. Kahneman, P. Slovic, & A. Tversky (Eds.), *Judgement under uncertainty: Heuristics and biases* (pp. 201–208). New York: Cambridge University Press.

Kash, K. M., Holland, J. C., Halper, M. S., & Miller, D. G. (1992). Psychological distress and surveillance behaviors of women with a family history of breast cancer. *Journal of the National Cancer Institute, 84*(1), 24–30.

Lau, R. R., & Hartman, K. A. (1983). Common sense representations of common illnesses. *Health Psychology, 2,* 167–185.

Lauver, D. R., Kane, J., Bodden, J., McNeel, J., & Smith, L. (1999). Engagement in breast cancer screening behaviors. *Oncology Nursing Forum, 26*(3), 545–554.

Lazarus, R. S., & Folkman, S. (1984). *Stress, appraisal, and coping.* New York: Springer.

LeDoux, J. E. (1996). *The emotional brain.* New York: Simon & Schuster.

Lerman, C., Daly, M., Sands, C., Balshem, A., Lustbader, E., Heggan, T., et al. (1993). Mammography adherence and psychological distress among women at risk for breast cancer. *Journal of the National Cancer Institute, 85*(13), 1074–1080.

Lerman, C., Kash, K., & Stefanek, M. (1994). Younger women at increased risk for breast cancer: Perceived risk, psychological well-being, and surveillance behavior. *Journal of the National Cancer Institute Monographs, 16*(16), 171–176.

Lerman, C., Trock, B., Rimer, B. K., Boyce, A., Jepson, C., & Engstrom, P. F. (1991). Psychological and behavioral implications of abnormal mammograms. *Annals of Internal Medicine, 114*(8), 657–661.

Lerman, C., Trock, B., Rimer, B. K., Jepson, C., Brody, D., & Boyce, A. (1991). Psychological side effects of breast cancer screening. *Health Psychology, 10*(4), 259–267.

Lerner, J. S., & Keltner, D. (2000). Beyond valence: Toward a model of emotion-specific influences on judgment and choice. *Cognition and Emotion, 14*(4), 473–493.

Leventhal, H. (1970). Findings and theory in the study of fear communications. In L. Berkowitz (Ed.), *Advances in experimental social psychology* (Vol. 5, pp. 119–186). New York: Academic Press.

Leventhal, H. (1983). Behavioral medicine: Psychology in health care. In D. Mechanic (Ed.), *Handbook of health, health care, and the health professions* (pp. 709–743). New York: Free Press.

Leventhal, H. (1990). Emotional and behavioural processes. In M. Johnston & L. Wallace (Eds.), *Stress and medical procedures* (pp. 3–35). Oxford: Oxford University Press.

Leventhal, H., & Diefenbach, M. A. (1991). The active side of illness cognition. In J. A. Skelton & R. T. Croyle (Eds.), *Mental representation in health and illness* (pp. 247–272). New York: Springer-Verlag.

Leventhal, H., Diefenbach, M. A., & Leventhal, E. A. (1992). Illness cognition: Using common sense to understand treatment adherence and affect cognition interactions. *Cognitive Therapy and Research, 16,* 143–163.

Leventhal, H., & Niles, P. (1965). Persistence of influence for varying durations of exposure to threat stimuli. *Psychological Reports, 16,* 223–233.

Leventhal, H., & Patrick-Miller, L. (2000). Emotions and physical illness: Causes and indicators of vulnerability. In M. Lewis & J. H. Haviland-Jones (Eds.), *Handbook of emotions* (2nd ed., pp. 523–537). New York: Guilford Press.

Leventhal, H., & Singer, R. P. (1966). Affect arousal and positioning of recommendations in persuasive communications. *Journal of Personality and Social Psychology, 4,* 137–146.

Leventhal, H., Singer, R. P., & Jones, S. (1965). Effects of fear and specificity of recommendations upon attitudes and behavior. *Journal of Personality and Social Psychology, 2,* 20–29.

Leventhal, H., & Trembly, G. (1968). Negative emotions and persuasion. *Journal of Personality, 36,* 154–168.

Leventhal, H., & Watts, J. C. (1966). Sources of resistance to fear-arousing communications on smoking and lung cancer. *Journal of Personality, 34,* 155–175.

Leventhal, H., Watts, J. C., & Pagano, F. (1967). Effects of fear and instructions on how to cope with danger. *Journal of Personality and Social Psychology, 6,* 313–321.

Lindberg, N. M., & Wellisch, D. (2001). Anxiety and compliance among women at high risk for breast cancer. *Annals of Behavioral Medicine, 23*(4), 298–303.

Loewenstein, G. F., & Schkade, D. (1999). Wouldn't it be nice?: Predicting future feelings. In D. Kahneman, E. Diener, & N. Schwarz (Eds.), *Well-being: The foundations of hedonic psychology* (pp. 85–105). New York: Russell Sage Foundation.

Loewenstein, G. F., Weber, E. U., Hsee, C. K., & Welch, N. (2001). Risk as feelings. *Psychological Bulletin, 127*(2), 267–286.

McCaul, K. D., Branstetter, A. D., O'Donnell, S. M., Jacobson, K., & Quinlan, K. B. (1998). A descriptive study of breast cancer worry. *Journal of Behavioral Medicine, 21*(6), 565–579.

McCaul, K. D., Schroeder, D. M., & Reid, P. A. (1996). Breast cancer worry and screening: Some prospective data. *Health Psychology, 15*(6), 430–433.

Mellers, B. A., & McGraw, A. P. (2001). Anticipated emotions as guides to choice. *Current Directions in Psychological Science, 10,* 210–214.

Meyer, D., Leventhal, H., & Gutmann, M. (1985). Common-sense models of illness: The example of hypertension. *Health Psychology, 4,* 115–135.

Miller, S., Diefenbach, M., Krantz, D. S., Baum, A., & Academy of Behavioral Medicine Research. (1998). The cognitive–social health information-processing (C-SHIP) model: A theoretical framework for research in behavioral oncology. In D. S. Krantz & A. Baum (Eds.), *Technology and methods in behavioral medicine* (pp. 219–244). Mahwah, NJ: Erlbaum.

Miller, S. M., Diefenbach, M. A., Kruus, L., Ohls, L., Hanks, G., Bruner, D., et al. (2001). Psychological and screening profiles of first degree relatives of prostate cancer patients. *Journal of Behavioral Medicine, 24,* 247–258.

Miller, S. M., Shoda, Y., & Hurley, K. (1996). Applying cognitive–social theory to health-protective behavior: Breast self-examination in cancer screening. *Psychological Bulletin, 119*(1), 70–94.

Montague, R. P., & Berns, G. S. (2002). Neural economics and the biological substrates of valuation. *Neuron, 36,* 265–284.

Peters, E., Lipkus, I., & Diefenbach, M. (2006). The functions of affect in health communication and in the construction of health preferences. *Journal of Communication, 56,* S140–S162.

Peters, E., Västfjäll, D., Gärling, T., & Slovic, P. (2006). Affect and decision making: A "hot" topic. *Journal of Behavioral Decision Making, 19*(2), 79–85.

Prochaska, T. R., Keller, M. L., Leventhal, E. A., & Leventhal, H. (1987). Impact of symptoms and aging attribution on emotions and coping. *Health Psychology, 6,* 495–514.

Rogers, R. W., & Deckner, W. C. (1975). Effects of fear appeals and physiological arousal upon emotion, attitudes, and cigarette smoking. *Journal of Personality and Social Psychology, 32,* 222–230.

Rogers, R. W. & Thistlethwaite, D. L. (1970). Effects of fear arousal and reassurance on attitude change. *Journal of Personality and Social Psychology, 15,* 227–233.

Russell, J. A., & Barett, L. F. (1999). Core affect, prototypical emotional episodes, and other things called emotion: Dissecting the elephant. *Journal of Personality and Social Psychology, 76*(5), 805–819.

Salovey, P., & Birnbaum, D. (1989). Influence of mood on health-relevant cognitions. *Journal of Personality and Social Psychology, 57,* 539–551.

Scheier, M. F., & Carver, C. S. (1985). Optimism, coping, and health: Assessment and implications of generalized outcome expectancies. *Health Psychology, 4,* 219–247.

Schwarz, N. (1990). Feelings as information: Informational and motivational functions of affective states. In E. T. Higgins & R. M. Sorrentino (Eds.), *Handbook of motivation and cognition: Foundations of social behavior* (Vol. 2, pp. 527–561). New York: Guilford Press.

Schwarz, N., & Clore, G. L. (1988). How do I feel about it?: The informative function of affective states. In K. Fielder & J. Forgas (Eds.), *Affect, cognition and social behavior: New evidence and integrative attempts* (pp. 44–62). Toronto, ON: C. J. Hogrefe.

Schwarz, N., & Clore, G. L. (2003). Mood as information: 20 years later. *Psychological Inquiry, 14,* 296–303.

Schwartz, M. D., Taylor, K. L., & Willard, K. S. (2003). Prospective association between distress and mammography utilization among women with a family history of breast cancer. *Journal of Behavioral Medicine, 26*(2), 105–117.

Selye, H. (1951). *The physiology and pathology of exposure to stress.* Oxford: Acta.

Simon, H. (1967). Motivational and emotional controls of cognition. *Psychological Review, 74*(1), 29–39.

Slovic, P., Finucane, M. L., Peters, E., & MacGregor, D. G. (2002). The affect heuristic. In T. Gilovich, D. Griffin, & D. Kahneman (Eds.), *Heuristics and biases: The psychology of intuitive judgement* (pp. 397–420). Cambridge, UK: Cambridge University Press.

Slovic, P., & Peters, E. (2006). Risk Perception and Affect. *Current Directions in Psychological Science, 15*(6), 322–325.

Slovic, P., Peters, E., Finucane, M. L., & Macgregor, D. G. (2005). Affect, risk, and decision making. *Health Psychology, 24*(4, Suppl.), S35–S40.

Stefanek, M. E., & Wilcox, P. (1991). First degree relatives of breast cancer patients: Screening practices and provision of risk information. *Cancer Detection and Prevention, 15*(5), 379–384.

Stoller, E. P. (1984). Self-assessments of health by the elderly: The impact of informal assistance. *Journal of Health and Social Behavior, 25,* 260–270.

Sutton, S., Saidi, G., Bickler, G., & Hunter, J. (1995). Does routine screening for breast cancer raise anxiety?: Results from a three wave prospective study in England. *Journal of Epidemiology and Community Health, 49*(4), 413–418.

Tinley, S. T., Houfek, J., Watson, P., Wenzel, L., Clark, M. B., Coughlin, S., et al. (2004). Screening adherence in BRCA1/2 families is associated with primary physicians' behavior. *American Journal of Medical Genetics A, 125*(1), 5–11.

Tversky, A., & Kahneman, D. (1981). The framing of decisions and the psychology of choice. *Science, 211*(4481), 453–458.

Ubel, P. A., Loewenstein, G. F., Schwarz, N., & Smith, D. (2005). Misimagining the unimaginable: The disability paradox and healthcare decision making. *Health Psychology.*

U.S. Department of Health and Human Services. (2000). *Heathy people 2010.* Washington, DC: U.S. Government Printing Office.

Young, R. F., & Severson, R. K. (2005). Breast cancer screening barriers and mammography completion in older minority women. *Breast Cancer Research and Treatment, 89*(2), 111–118.

Zajonc, R. B. (1980). Feeling and thinking. Preferences need no inferences. *American Psychologist, 35,* 151–175.

Zajonc, R. B. (1984). On the primacy of affect. *American Psychologist, 39*(2), 117–123.

CHAPTER 41

Emotions, the Neuroendocrine and Immune Systems, and Health

MARGARET E. KEMENY and AVGUSTA SHESTYUK

Although emotions and other affective experiences have been linked to specific neural structures and circuits, much less is known about the relationships between emotions and the peripheral neuroendocrine and neuroimmune systems that contribute to physical health and disease. Most research on the linkages between psychological processes and these peripheral systems has focused on exposure to stressors and the experience of diffuse cognitive–affective states of mind, such as "stress" or "distress" (see Kemeny & Schedlowski, 2007). Alternatively, researchers have examined the peripheral physiological patterns associated with psychiatric disorders, including mood disorders (e.g., major depression). Despite the fact that emotional states are often considered central and most proximal mediators of the effects of environmental perturbation on peripheral physiology (Lazarus & Folkman, 1984), insufficient attention has been paid to the relations between specific emotions and these critically important regulatory systems.

An overarching assumption underlying much of the research in this area is that the physiological response to difficult, stressful, or threatening environmental perturbations is a generalized one. Hans Selye shaped the thinking on this topic for generations of researchers with his generality model, which proposes a core set of physiological responses that are common to all stressors—including activation of the hypothalamic–pituitary–adrenocortical (HPA) axis and impairment of immune function (Selye, 1956). Modern versions of Selye's generality model include many more psychological constructs than he envisioned. However, these modern adaptations remain essentially generality models, because "all roads" lead to a general state of distress. In other words, although individuals may respond to a particular event with different forms of affective, cognitive and behavioral response, it is the extent of resulting distress that is assumed to determine the physiological response. And distress is assumed to have a uniform relationship to these major physiological systems (Kemeny, 2003a).

The notion of an adaptive specificity has begun to be entertained in the fields of psychoneuroendocrinology and psychoneuroimmun-ology, however. For example, Herbert Weiner (1992) argued that "organisms meet . . . challenges and dangers by integrated behavioral, physiological patterns of response that are appropriate to the task" (p. 33). Specific conditions or environmental signals, then, elicit an integrated psychobiological response that includes a patterned array of neural and peripheral changes capable of preparing the organism to deal with the specific situation. For example, fleeing from a predator, grieving over a loss, and demonstrating one's social status require different kinds of psychological, physiological, and behavioral changes to respond adaptively to these situations (Weiner, 1992). Thus happiness is associated with approach behaviors, whereas fear in response to a threat to survival is associated with specific behavioral and physiological changes that facilitate flight, which in turn is different from physiological and behavioral manifestations of depressive affect (e.g., disengagement; Ekman, 1999; Levenson, 1994). This specificity is proposed to include the response of the HPA axis as well as the immune system. In addition, the specific nature of the physiological response depends not only on the characteristics of the environmental circumstance, but also on the cognitive appraisal of that circumstance and the specific emotional reaction (Kemeny, 2003). Increasing evidence supports specificity in the relationship among stressors, cognitive and affective responses, and peripheral physiology. For example, a recent meta-analysis found that all acute laboratory stressors did not activate the HPA axis. Instead, specific environmental characteristics were required to induce an increase in cortisol, as described in more detail below (Dickerson & Kemeny, 2004).

This chapter considers how specific neuroendocrine and immune changes may support adaptive behavioral responses to specific elicitors. The role of emotion in these integrated psychobiological responses to environmental perturbations is discussed. The chapter emphasizes the evidence linking affective experience with the neuroendocrine system (specifically, the HPA axis), as well as with critical functions of the immune system. In addition, we attempt to provide an initial overview of the relations between affective experience and central circuitry as a way of considering how these circuits mediate the relationship between affect and peripheral responses. The brain plays a key

role as a transducer of the effects of the environment on peripheral physiological responses. Neural mechanisms interpret elements of social environment; instantiate individuals' beliefs, expectations, and appraisals; and regulate (i.e., activate and inhibit) peripheral systems, including the HPA and immune systems.

In this chapter, we define "emotions" as short-duration, intensely felt states associated with distinctive behavioral predispositions and facial expressions that have evolved to coordinate responses to specific eliciting conditions (Ekman, 1994; Levenson, 1992). "Moods" are longer-term affective states that do not have unique facial signatures or eliciting conditions (Ekman, 1994) and often contain persistent cognitions (such as negative thoughts about the self with depressed mood). "Affective traits" are predispositions to experience specifics affects over time and across situations. "Mood disorders" are pathological variants of mood states that interfere with daily living and may require intervention.

Below we review several adaptive affective–motivational response patterns that involve the HPA and immune systems: the fight–flight response; the recuperative response and behavioral disengagement; and the positive approach response. The "fight–flight response" involves recognition of a threat that requires physical action and the mobilization of adequate physiological resources to fight or flee the threat. These responses are associated with emotions of fear (and, if persistent, anxiety) for the flight mode, and anger (and hostility) for the fight mode. The "recuperative response" and "behavioral disengagement" reflect physiological resource conservation processes that facilitate healing and disengagement from a threat. These responses are associated with negative affect and depression, as well as with shame and submissiveness. Finally, "positive approach responses" promote motivation and physiological homeostasis; depending on behavioral goals, they rely on resource building, mobilization, and conservation. These responses are associated with happiness, contentment, and excitement.

PSYCHOBIOLOGY OF FIGHT–FLIGHT RESPONSES

There is a long-standing recognition that organisms, even quite primitive ones, contain physiological systems adapted to respond effectively to danger and threat. The fight–fight system becomes activated in response to a threat to the central goal of preserving the physical self. This system mobilizes bodily processes that are required for threat-relevant physical actions (such as fighting and fleeing), and down-regulates restorative systems that are not critical to addressing a threat (such as reproduction, repair, and growth) (Sapolsky, 1993). Sapolsky argues that organisms engage in "resource building" at a physiological level until confronted with an emergency situation, at which time there is a shift to "resource utilization." For example, fighting requires energy, and activation of the HPA axis results in the release of cortisol, which mobilizes energy resources by stimulating the conversion of other substrates into glucose, a metabolic fuel. Cortisol also exerts a permissive effect on the sympathetic nervous system (SNS), allowing SNS products to activate the cardiovascular system (e.g., increasing heart rate) in preparation for physical exertion. A number of studies in animals and humans have demonstrated that exposure to physical and psychological threats can activate the HPA axis (Dickerson & Kemeny, 2004).

There is a growing literature documenting the effects of exposure to stressors and threats on the immune system, resulting in decrements in the functioning of various cell types. Some of the immune system changes observed during a threat, however, have been argued to be central components of the adaptive physiological response to the threat, rather than nonfunctional side effects of a more general stress response. In animal studies, Dhabhar and colleagues have demonstrated that acute exposure to a stressor or threat shunts white blood cells to the site of tissue damage or exposure to a pathogen, resulting in an enhancement of the local immune response (Dhabhar & McEwen, 1999; Viswanathan & Dhabhar, 2005). Dhabhar (2003) argues that these stress-induced immunological changes may be an adaptive preparation for the challenge of wounding or infection, which may occur during circumstances that involve fighting or fleeing. Just as soldiers about to fight an enemy leave the barracks and assume positions at battle stations, environmental dangers and threats cause immune cells to travel from the immune organs through the bloodstream to "battle stations" in the skin, in order to fight against infectious agents that may result from fight- or flight-induced

wounding. These effects are probably mediated via the activation of the SNS, a key system underlying other peripheral responses to fight–flight circumstances, since the SNS neurotransmitters influence trafficking of white blood cells and the expression of molecules that regulate immune cell trafficking (Ottaway & Husband, 1992).

At the same time, an increase in a subset of white blood cells, called "natural killer" (NK) cells, would be particularly effective at rapid and nonspecific killing of pathogens that enter the system in the context of fight- or flight-induced tissue injury (Kemeny & Gruenewald, 2000). NK cells can kill virally infected cells nonspecifically without prior exposure to the organism. Increases in the number and activity of NK cells immediately following exposure to an acute threat have been demonstrated (Segerstrom & Miller, 2004), while other types of white blood cells do not show this enhancement in most cases.

Fear and Anxiety

Real or perceived threat and its anticipation have been associated with a host of emotional responses, including fear, worry, and anxiety. Imminent threat (such as facing a predator) is likely to evoke fear, whereas an anticipation of a threatening or negative event (such as waiting to receive a punishment) is likely to evoke anxiety and apprehension. Physiological profiles (i.e., neural responses and peripheral activations) associated with these affective responses can be conceptualized in the framework of preparatory mobilization for active avoidance and escape from the threat (i.e., the "flight" responses). Thus fear and anxiety share similar patterns of central and peripheral activation, but can be differentiated based on whether the threatening stimulus is certain and imminent (i.e., requires immediate action) or is uncertain and anticipated (i.e., requires preparation for action) (Cox & Taylor, 1999).

Peripheral autonomic nervous system (ANS) responses associated with fear and anxiety, such as increased heart rate and respiration, are linked to noradrenergic activity, originating in the locus coeruleus (Charney, 2004). There is evidence that repeated noradrenergic activation may be linked to a greater risk of cardiovascular disease, especially in individuals with anxiety disorders (Kubzansky, Kawachi, Weiss, & Sparrow, 1998). Brain areas involved in orchestrating these ANS responses include the periaqueductal gray (PAG) and the brainstem autonomic nuclei (Price, 2005); these areas in turn are triggered by amygdala activation, which is hypothesized to play an assessment role in determining the salience and significance of external stimuli (Phelps & LeDoux, 2005). These norepinephrine-mediated responses are modulated by glutamate-dependent neuronal activity within the prefrontal regions and hippocampus (Cortese & Phan, 2005), which provide inhibitory regulation of the amygdala, PAG, and brainstem nuclei. Insufficient activity within the prefrontal network has been linked to the etiology and manifestation of anxiety disorders, which are marked by increased central and peripheral activation in response to an imagined, unrealistic, or unsubstantiated threat.

Physical and psychosocial threats known to elicit fear and anxiety can also activate the HPA axis and trigger cortisol release (Erickson, Drevets, & Schulkin, 2003; Sapolsky, 2005). HPA activation in these situations has been linked to enhanced memory for threatening events and may play a role in the development and manifestation of symptoms of posttraumatic stress disorder (PTSD; McNally, 1999). In fact, HPA dysregulation is one of the most prominent physiological features of PTSD. Individuals with this disorder demonstrate abnormally low baseline levels of cortisol secretion, but exaggerated reactivity of the HPA axis in response to external threats or internal glucocorticoid release (e.g., on the dexamethasone suppression test; Yehuda, 2000; Yehuda, Boisoneau, Mason, & Giller, 1993). Other anxiety disorders have a less clear pattern of HPA engagement. For example, panic attacks by themselves have been found insufficient in triggering HPA activation, but anticipatory anxiety seems to be more effective in eliciting cortisol release (Fraeff, Garcia-Leal, Del-Ben, & Guimaraes, 2005), and HPA activation has been found to precipitate panic attacks (Strohle & Holsboer, 2003).

In contrast to the ANS and HPA responses, there is less known about the relationship between immune system alterations with fear and anxiety. Naturalistic studies of self-relevant situations that produce genuine feelings of anxiety are more successful in eliciting immune effects than laboratory studies. For example, patients reporting higher levels of anxiety about cancer at their first outpatient visit had significantly lower levels of NK cell activity (which tests the ability of NK cells to kill tumor cells), suggesting that feelings of anxiety may have immunological correlates (Koga et al., 2001). In addition, intervention studies demonstrate an increase in immune functioning associated with a decrease in anxiety symptoms (Anderson et al., 2004). Furthermore, individuals with trait worry demonstrate distinct immune changes (e.g., fewer NK cells) in response to naturalistic stressors, such as the aftermath of an earthquake (Segerstrom, Solomon, Kemeny, & Fahey, 1998), or acute laboratory-induced stressors (Segerstrom, Glover, Craske, & Fahey, 1999).

Anxiety disorders have also been linked to compromised immune functioning. Specifically, changes in anxiety levels from pre- to posttreatment in patients with panic disorder have been associated with changes in proliferative responses to an *in vitro* stimulus and interleukin-2 (IL-2) cytokine production—two important aspects of immune cell function (Koh & Lee, 2004). However, such findings of abnormal immune functioning in anxiety disorders are not ubiquitous, as some studies report no association between anxiety disorders and proliferative capacity, NK cell activity, or the numbers of lymphocyte subsets (Schleifer, Keller, & Bartlett, 2002).

Anger and Hostility

Anger-related affective experiences, including hostility and aggression, have been linked to peripheral systems and health outcomes. "Anger" is "an unpleasant emotion ranging in intensity from irritation or annoyance to fury or rage" (Smith, 1994, p. 25), which often results from exposure to situations that involve the relational theme of unfair interference or harm (Lazarus, 1991). Anger involves the action tendency of inflicting harm through "aggression," which is defined as attacking, destructive, or hurtful behavior (Smith, 1994). "Hostility" has been defined as both an affective trait and a mood state; definitions usually include a cognitive propensity toward cynicism. Smith (1994) defines hostility as a negative attitude toward others that involves "a devaluation of the worth and motives of others, an expectation that others are likely sources of wrong-doing, a relational view of being in opposition toward others, and a desire to inflict harm or see others harmed" (p. 26).

Anger, hostility, and aggressiveness (collectively termed AHA) have been thought to contribute to cardiovascular disease since at least the 19th century. These anger-related responses are one of the most widely studied psychosocial risk factors for cardiovascular disease and mortality. Most studies support this link (e.g., Rozanski, Blumenthal, & Kaplan, 1999; Smith & Ruiz, 2002), including several recent prospective studies of initially healthy samples that have been controlled for confounding factors (Smith, Glazer, Ruiz, & Gallo, 2004). For example, hostility is strongly and independently associated with the development and progression of coronary artery disease (Boyle et al., 2004; Miller, Smith, Turner, Guijarro, & Hallet, 1996). Other cardiovascular outcomes predicted by hostility include high blood pressure, atherosclerosis, coronary artery calcification, and mortality (Suinn, 2001). Effect sizes can be as large as those associated with traditional risk factors, such as smoking and diet.

The psychophysiological reactivity model suggests that cardiovascular risk associated with hostility is due to exaggerated cardiovascular and neuroendocrine responses to stressors (including blood pressure, heart rate, epinephrine, and cortisol; Williams, Barefoot, & Shekelle, 1985). ANS and HPA concomitants of anger and hostility are thought to be linked to increased activity within the PAG and hypothalamus, and to inadequate inhibitory control from areas of the prefrontal cortex due to insufficient availability of serotonin (Gregg & Siegel, 2001; Davidson, Putnam, & Larson, 2000). Increasing evidence supports a relationship between cardiovascular and neuroendocrine reactivity to stressors, and the initiation and the progression of coronary artery disease (Rozanski et al., 1999; Smith & Ruiz, 2002). Other important physiological processes are also enhanced in stressful situations among hostile individuals, including cholesterol levels and protein mediators of inflammatory processes (see Smith et al., 2004). Interestingly, research supports the hypothesis that hostility predicts an exaggerated physiological response to stressors, particularly when the stressors are social (e.g., Smith & Gallo, 2001). For example, hostile individuals demonstrated great physiological reactivity to one task only when it included harassment. Conceptualizing this risk factor as a social process rather than as a function of personality alone is likely to lead to

important and interesting new directions for research in this area.

More recently, AHA constructs have been found to be associated with increased evidence of peripheral inflammation, which is known to predict increased mortality and morbidity—in particular, atherosclerosis and myocardial infarction (Ridker, Hennekens, Buring, & Rifai, 2000). For example, trait hostility, more so than self-reported anger and verbal aggression, has been associated with increased production of a proinflammatory cytokine (PIC) called tumor necrosis factor-α (TNF-α) (Suarez, Lewis, & Kuhn, 2002). TNF-α and other PICs play a critical role in orchestrating the inflammatory response. Overall, the association with inflammatory processes appears to depend on long term constructs such as hostility rather than short-term experiences of anger. In addition, AHA-related constructs have predicted decrements in cellular immunity. For example, higher levels of hostility coded from verbal and nonverbal behavior during a marital conflict task predicted decreases in immune function over the following 24-hour period. Specifically, individuals who behaved in a hostile way toward their spouses showed decreased ability of immune cells to proliferate in response to a stimulus, as well as decreased ability of NK cells to kill tumor targets (Kiecolt-Glaser et al., 1993).

Although the majority of studies in this area rely on self-report measures of AHA, more recent studies have included observer ratings of hostile behavior in social situations. Hostility defined on this basis in these behavioral assessment strategies is associated with increased facial expressions of anger and disgust (Brummett et al., 1998), reduced expressions of friendly appeasement (Prkachin & Silverman, 2002), and increased negative cardiovascular outcomes.

Unfortunately, few studies have directly compared other affective constructs, such as anxiety or depression, to anger and hostility as predictors of cardiovascular disease outcomes in the same studies. However, there is clearly less evidence for the role of these affects in this literature. Whether this is due to the popularity of hostility as a construct in this research area, or to a psychobiological specificity that suggests something unique and physiologically important about the neurobiology of anger and hostility, is an important issue and deserves scientific attention.

PSYCHOBIOLOGY OF DISENGAGEMENT

Whereas fear and anger reflect adaptive physiological responses to an imminent or anticipated threat and result in either fight or flight behaviors, exposure to an uncontrollable physical or psychosocial threat often activates emotional and physiological systems associated with behavioral disengagement and withdrawal. Behavioral disengagement is represented in a number of emotional responses, ranging from negative affect and depression (as responses to a personal loss or uncontrollable physical and psychosocial threat) to shame and embarrassment (as responses to a loss of social status or exposure to a social threat). These emotions and withdrawal behaviors are associated with a distinct pattern of central and peripheral activation, including diminished serotonergic and dopaminergic neuronal activity, abnormal prefrontal functioning, HPA dysregulation, and compromised immune functioning.

In particular, a number of physiological changes, such as increases in HPA activation, opioid-mediated analgesia, and lowered cellular immune function, are associated with goal disengagement in animals (Fleshner, Landenslager, Simons, & Maher, 1989; Miczek, Thompson, & Shuster, 1982; Stefanski & Ben-Eliyahu, 1996). Moreover, the role of the immune system in withdrawal behavior can be traced to a similar adaptive behavioral response called "behavioral recuperation." Following infection or injury, PICs are released by immunological cells to facilitate the immune response against the organism, for example. More recently, it has become clear that PICs play another critical role in response to infectious agents. These proteins act on the brain, causing what is known as "sickness behavior"—that is, inducing increases in sleep and decreases in social, sexual, aggressive, exploratory, and other behaviors. Careful animal work has shown that these behavioral changes are not functions of weakness or incapacitation, but represent a motivational shift (e.g., away from fight and flight) toward behavior that would support recuperation. This behavioral disengagement appears to be an adaptive response that allows the organism to conserve energy and thus to maximize recuperative physiological

processes, such as the maintenance of fever (Maier & Watkins, 1998).

PICs may play a significant role in other forms of adaptive "behavioral disengagement"—in particular, in uncontrollable contexts where disengagement may be the most adaptive response. Evidence suggests that animals are more likely to demonstrate an increase in the production of PICs in response to an uncontrollable stressor. For example, subordinate animals confronted with an attack from a dominant animal have been found to exhibit behavioral disengagement behaviors in conjunction with PIC release (Kinsey, Bailey, Sheridan, Padgett, & Avitsur, 2007). In such case, behavioral disengagement is more adaptive, as it minimizes the chance of an attack from the dominant animal (Kemeny, 2006a). Similarly, animals injected with PICs cease to display offensive behaviors in an aggressive encounter (Cirulli, De Acetis, & Alleva, 1998). Finally, uncontrollable acute social threats in humans have also been shown to increase levels of PICs, as discussed below (Ackerman, Martino, Heyman, Moyna, & Rabin, 1998; Dickerson, et al., 2007).

Negative Affect and Depression

Negative affect and depression have been linked to insufficient availability of serotonin and dopamine and to abnormal activation, especially within structures of the prefrontal cortex such as dorsolateral prefrontal cortex (DLPFC), ventromedial prefrontal cortex (VMPFC), and orbito-frontal cortex (OFC; Phan, Wager, Taylor, & Liberzon, 2004; Drevets, 1999). In particular, low concentrations of prefrontal dopamine and diminished activity in these regions have been linked to a loss of motivation, lack of goal-oriented behavior, and behavioral withdrawal in depression—symptoms commonly seen in individuals with organic prefrontal brain damage or frontal dementia (Rogers, Bradshaw, Pantelis, & Phillips, 1998). Moreover, abnormal patterns of prefrontal alpha electroencephalographic (EEG) asymmetry (i.e., relative increase in right-hemisphere activity relative to a decrease in left-hemisphere activity) have been observed during negative affect, in individuals at risk for depression, in individuals with current or remitted depression, or in those high in neuroticism (Davidson, 1992).

Abnormal activity in the prefrontal brain regions, and thus insufficient regulatory control exhibited during negative affect or depression, may account for the peripheral changes and dysregulation that accompany these emotions and may prompt behavioral withdrawal and disengagement. In humans, there is some empirical evidence that negative affect may lead to HPA activation and cortisol release; however, such evidence is limited, and observed effect sizes associated with the increases in cortisol are small compared to those elicited by physical or social threats (Dickerson, Gruenewald, & Kemeny, 2004). Findings of HPA dysregulation in clinical depression are more compelling, although the pattern of HPA dysregulation varies depending on depression subtype. Specifically, melancholic, but not atypical, depression has been linked to increased baseline cortisol secretion, abnormal slope of diurnal cortisol release, and limited HPA reactivity in response to acute laboratory stressors (Howland & Thase, 1999). Abnormal HPA activity in depression and negative affect may contribute to the deleterious effects on the immune system often observed during negative affect or depression, as described below. Moreover, patterns of prefrontal EEG asymmetry consistent with negative affect have been linked with lower antibody titers after vaccination for influenza (Davidson et al., 2003) and with lower NK cell activity (Davidson, Coe, Dolski, & Donzella, 1999; Kang et al., 1991).

The link between compromised immune functioning and depression has received much attention in recent years. In particular, studies have examined relations between major depressive episodes and immune status. Major depression has been associated with a variety of functional and phenotypic changes in the immune system, similar to those often observed in response to major life events and stressors (Irwin, Daniels, Bloom, & Weiner., 1986; Schleifer et al., 1984). Depression has been reliably associated with increases in neutrophils and decreases in B and T cells, as well as with deficiencies in the proliferative response and NK cell activity (Herbert & Cohen, 1993). These immune effects may be specific to an active state of depression, as they have been shown to be ameliorated with treatment (Irwin, Lacher, & Caldwell, 1992). Immune impairment is most likely to be observed in those individuals with major depression who are older, have melancholic depression, or have a sleep disorder—conditions commonly associated with abnormal HPA functioning (Irwin, 2001).

Furthermore, there is increasing evidence that clinical depression is associated with elevated levels and/or production of PICs, even when samples are controlled for medical conditions, medications, and health behaviors (Maes et al., 1994; Miller, Stetler, Carney, Freedland, & Banks, 2002). It has been proposed that that PICs may not only be consequences of major depression, but may also contribute to its etiology (Dantzer et al., 2001; Yirmiya, 1996; Yirmiya et al., 1999). In addition to the findings above, demonstrating in a number of studies that patients with major depression show evidence of increases in PICs, patients with inflammatory diseases (e.g., rheumatoid arthritis) often experience depression symptoms in excess of what is observed in individuals with diseases that are not directly linked to inflammation. Also, administration of cytokines such as interferon to boost the immune system during cancer or AIDS treatment often induces symptoms of clinical depression, such as dysphoria, anhedonia, fatigue, and apathy, within days of the first administration. These symptoms tend to remit when the cytokine treatment is discontinued. Finally, animals injected with PICs demonstrate the behavioral changes called sickness behavior—including motor retardation; lack of appetite, weight loss, and sleep disturbances; decreased sexual, social, and aggressive behavior; and anhedonia. These behavioral changes bear a striking resemblance to the vegetative symptoms of some forms of depression. Thus increases in these inflammatory molecules may play a causal role in the initiation or maintenance of depressive symptoms.

Shame and Submissiveness

In addition to the motive to protect the "physical self," humans and other animals are motivated to protect the "social self." Maintaining a sense of belonging and social connection appears to be a fundamental motive that is expressed across cultures. Threats to social connection can have a variety of adverse effects (Baumeister & Leary, 1995; Cacioppo et al., in press). In particular, contexts that include rejection, stigmatization, or discrimination are experienced as aversive, because they reflect a lack of social value or status and can result in drops in self-esteem (Baumeister & Leary, 1995). Social self-preservation theory argues that maintaining social status and value (i.e., social self-preservation) is a central motive in humans and other animals, akin to physical self-preservation (Dickerson, Gruenewald, & Kemeny, 2004). Threats to one's status or value, as in negative social evaluation, rejection, or stigmatization, can have a variety of psychological and physiological effects. If an individual is repeatedly exposed to evaluative and rejecting circumstances, such as those experienced in the context of low social status, persistent activation of these physiological systems may result in health risks.

Threats to the social self often involve conditions in which one may be negatively judged by others (i.e., social evaluative threat, or SET; Dickerson, Gruenewald, & Kemeny, 2004). SET can occur in performance contexts where important attributes are displayed in front of others, in a context where group membership is at risk or where an uncontrollable aspect of one's identity is made salient to others. Self-conscious emotions are frequent consequences of such contexts—notably shame, since this emotion is experienced when a core aspect of the self is judged to be defective or inferior by others (Gilbert, 1997; Tangney, 1995). The social nature of shame is fundamental to most historical and modern accounts of the emotion (e.g., Cooley, 1902; Benedict, 1946). For example, Darwin (1871/1899) argued that shame "relates almost exclusively to the judgment of others" (p. 114).

The motivational context, displays, and behaviors associated with shame suggest a link between this emotion and submissive behavior and withdrawal. For example, shame is elicited under social self-threat conditions and is associated with the motivation to disengage or withdraw (e.g., wanting to "shrink," "disappear," or avoid interpersonal interaction; Tangney, 1995). Submissive behavior in animals is elicited when social status is threatened; the behavior is consistent with the motive to disengage and withdraw. Characteristic displays of shame in humans are quite similar to displays of submission and appeasement in primates (e.g., gaze avoidance, head down, slumped posture, attempts to appear small; Gilbert, 1997; Keltner & Buswell, 1996).

Social self-preservation theory proposes that threats to the social self—such as threats to self-esteem, status, or acceptance—elicit an integrated psychobiological response that supports adaptive behavior in that context. Specifically, social self-threats provide a set of eliciting conditions for specific psychobiological changes that would support appeasement and behavioral disengagement. Recent research suggests that three components of this coordinated response may be central nervous system (CNS)-coordinated activation of the HPA, induced insensitivity of certain immune cells to the suppressive effects of cortisol, and increased production of PICs.

Although a variety of stressful circumstances can activate the HPA system, acute social threats are reliable and powerful elicitors of such activation. In a meta-analytic review of 208 acute laboratory stress studies, exposure to performance tasks in the presence of evaluative others, particularly in an uncontrollable context, was associated with substantially greater cortisol and adrenocorticotropic hormone responses than was exposure to other stressful tasks without social evaluation (Dickerson & Kemeny, 2004). Exposure to uncontrollable SET was also associated with slower recovery of cortisol to baseline levels.

An experimental test of the link between SET and cortisol increase demonstrated that performance tasks that had some degree of uncontrollability as well as an SET component (performance in front of an evaluative audience) induced a cortisol response, whereas the same uncontrollable task without SET did not (Gruenewald, Kemeny, Aziz, & Fahey, 2004). Although both conditions elicited a variety of emotions, the strongest effects were for shame and self-conscious emotions. The greater the shame reported, the greater the increase in cortisol in response to the SET. Other studies have also shown correlations between self-conscious emotions and cortisol (e.g., Lewis & Ramsay, 2002). Supporting the link between social evaluative processes and cortisol, fear of negative evaluation is a significant predictor of cortisol response to a laboratory-induced SET, with those reporting higher levels of such fear showing a greater cortisol response to the SET condition (Gruenewald et al., 2004).

At the same time, studies of primates demonstrate higher levels of cortisol associated with subordinate rank and submissive displays, suggesting that processes related to social status and submissive behavior in other animals may have been maintained and elaborated in humans as responses to social self-threats (Gilbert, 1997; Price, Sloman, Gardner, Gilbert, & Rohde, 1994). This HPA reactivity translates into greater basal cortisol levels, a slower response to challenge, and impaired sensitivity of the HPA axis to negative feedback regulation (Sapolsky, 2005). These effects have been argued to reflect the persistent exposure to social stressors and limited coping resources (Abbott et al., 2003).

HPA activation in response to SET is controlled by a specific neural network, consisting of cortical and subcortical structures. Animal research has shown that cortisol release in response to an acute physical or psychosocial threat is triggered by activity of the paraventricular nucleus (PVN) of the hypothalamus. In turn, activity of the PVN is regulated by limbic and higher cortical areas directly implicated in social cognition: the amygdala, hippocampus, anterior cingulate cortex, OFC, VMPFC, and DLPFC (Herman, Ostrander, Mueller, & Figueiredo, 2005; Floyd, Price, Ferry, Keay, & Bandler, 2001). These brain areas demonstrate greater activation in response to social stimuli and have been implicated in individuals' emotional, cognitive, and behavioral responses in the social context (Ochsner, 2004). For example, the OFC plays a crucial role in the appraisal of complex social situations and self-appraisal of social emotions, such that lesions in this area in humans result in failures to recognize or experience such emotions as shame and to monitor social behavior online (Beer, Heerey, Keltner, Scabini, & Knight, 2003; Beers, John, Scabini, & Knight, 2006). Given these patterns of brain activation in response to social cues and self-appraisal, it is likely that these brain areas feature prominently in the translation of social appraisals into peripheral physiological responses.

A second physiological response that would be adaptive in the context of social self-threat would be production of PICs. Social status disruption, which induces social submission and defeat, has been shown to increase production of PICs and to decrease sensitivity of immunological cells to down-regulation by glucocorticoids (i.e., glucocorticoid resistance, or GCR) in animals. The primary model of social threat utilized in this literature is a mouse model of social status disruption, in which an aggressive intruder is placed in the home cages of other animals, resulting in social defeat and subordination in the home-caged animals. Mice that are socially defeated show greater PIC production and greater GCR than do control animals that were not socially defeated (Avitsur, Stark, & Sheridan, 2001; Stark, Avitsur, Padgett, & Sheridan, 2001; Quan et al., 2001). The degree of submissive behavior is associated with the level of PIC production. By rendering immune cells insensitive to the suppressive effects of glucocorticoids, GCR causes increases in the production of PICs. Thus specific forms of social threat (i.e., social subordination and defeat) may cause increases in inflammatory processes in animals via GCR.

There is much less known about the impact of social status disruption on inflammatory processes in humans. Some studies indicate that acute social threat in humans increases PIC production. Recent findings suggest greater TNF-α production by peripheral blood mononuclear cells in an experimental context that involved performing stressful tasks with an evaluative audience, compared to performing these tasks without the evaluative audience (Dickerson et al., 2007). The increase in TNF-α production was correlated with the extent to which subjects described themselves as feeling more evaluated during the task, suggesting that cognitive appraisals of social threat may be a key mediator of these effects. In addition, induction of shame has been associated with increases in PICs. In one study, participants were either asked to write about a situation in which they blamed themselves or a neutral topic on three different days during one week. Those assigned to the self-blame condition showed increased levels of TNF-α receptor in oral mucosal transudate on each study day. Increases were correlated with self-reported increases in shame, but not with guilt or other emotions (Dickerson, Kemeny, Aziz, Kim, & Fahey, 2004).

Increases in cortisol, GCR, and PICs can be considered adaptive responses to relatively uncontrollable social status threats. As described earlier, increased levels of PICs would support the behavioral disengagement that would be adaptive in subordinate-ranked animals and would support submissive appeasement-related behavior, thus reducing the likelihood that the subordinate animal would provoke an attack.

GCR would prevent the increased cortisol levels induced by these social stressors from inhibiting the production of PICs.

PSYCHOBIOLOGY OF POSITIVE APPROACH

Whereas negative emotions, for the most part, are associated with withdrawal behaviors, positive emotions have been linked to approach behaviors and are thought to facilitate exploration, pleasure and comfort seeking, and affiliation. As such, positive emotions are likely to provide a psychological and physiological foundation for motivation and proactive behaviors. In fact, it is likely that positive affective states represent an affective baseline for healthy individuals (Seligman, 2002). Research suggests that psychologically healthy participants anticipate more positive than negative events, have a predominantly positive view of the self, and exhibit preferential processing of and brain activation in response to positive relative to negative or neutral stimuli (Taylor & Armor, 1996; Shestyuk, Deldin, Brand, & Deveney, 2005). Moreover, positive affective states have been linked, for the most part, to enhanced immune functioning and better overall health outcomes (Barak, 2006). However, it appears that the peripheral effects of positive emotions may be moderated by the level of physiological arousal—such that intense excitement would induce significant ANS, HPA, and immune changes, whereas calm contentment would not.

Positive emotions, such as happiness and pleasure, are associated with greater frontal left-hemisphere asymmetry (Davidson, 1992) and greater activation of the medial prefrontal regions and the basal ganglia (Parkinson, Cardinal, & Everitt, 2000). These processes are supported by monoamine neurotransmitter systems, with greater levels of serotonin associated with low-arousal contentment and pleasure, and greater levels of dopamine and norepinephrine associated with high-arousal excitement (Charney, 2004). Arousal can also moderate HPA activation. Specifically, some studies demonstrate a decrease in cortisol levels following positive mood induction or in correlation with trait positive affect (Berk et al., 1989; Buchanan, al'Absi, & Lovallo, 1999; Zachariae et al., 1991). In contrast, HPA activation has also been shown during induction of positive affect, which may result from experienced arousal (Pressman & Cohen, 2005), although there are few studies in this area. Similarly, induction of positive affect in studies that require active participation from participants has been shown to increase dopaminergic and noradrenergic neuronal activity, leading to elevations in heart rate and blood pressure (Ekman, Levenson, & Friesen, 1983; Futterman, Kemeny, Shapiro, & Fahey, 1994; Schwartz, Weinberger, & Singer, 1981).

Positive affect is also associated with changes in the immune system (Pressman & Cohen, 2005). For example, positive affect is positively correlated with secretory immunoglobulin A, an antibody found in the mucosal immune system (e.g., in saliva; Hucklebridge et al., 2000; Lambert & Lambert, 1995; McClelland & Cheriff, 1997). Moreover, daily positive affect has been linked with elevated levels of this antibody in response to a specific antigen measured on a daily basis (Stone, Cox, Valdimarsdottir, Jandorf, & Neale, 1987; Stone et al., 1994; but not Evans et al., 1993). Similarly, positive affect has been associated with increases in the number of certain subsets of white blood cells—a result similar to the one observed in response to acute stressors, suggesting a potential moderating role of arousal (Segerstrom & Miller, 2004).

Furthermore, laboratory induction of positive affect has been shown to lead to an increase in lymphocyte proliferative response to mitogenic stimulation (Futterman, Kemeny, Shapiro, Polonsky, & Fahey, 1992). These effects were not mediated by changes in cortisol in response to the manipulation. Positive mood induction may also result in increased levels of certain cytokines (IL-2, IL-3), while resulting in decreases in others (i.e., interferon-α and TNF-α; Mittwoch-Jaffe, Shalit, Srendi, & Yehuda, 1995). Moreover, Type I hypersensitivity to an allergen has been associated with positive affect in some studies (Kimata, 2001; Laidlaw, Booth, & Large, 1996), but not in others (Zachariae, Jorgensen, Egekvist, & Bjerring, 2001). Finally, induction of positive affect can lead to an increase in NK cell numbers, which is similar to the changes in response to negative affect and threatening stimuli (Futterman et al., 1994; Segerstrom & Miller, 2004). This effect is probably mediated by SNS arousal. Thus peripheral responses associated with positive emotions are both distinct from and similar to those elicited by negative emotions, depending on the level of arousal and behavioral engagement.

SUMMARY

There is increasing evidence that affective experiences are associated with important changes in peripheral regulatory systems intimately tied to health and disease. Further research in this area will be greatly benefited by, and may actually require, an integration of the frameworks and tools utilized in affective neuroscience with those of health psychology and psychoneuroimmunology. Although there are data on the neural substrates of specific emotions, as well as data on the link between these emotions and peripheral physiology, very few studies have attempted to define the pathway from the neural substrates of these affective experiences to peripheral physiological systems and then on to physical health indices (Kemeny, 2003b). No comprehensive mechanistic map of these relationships exists to form the basis for these studies. In the investigation of the role of affective experience in physical disease, it is critical that the CNS be investigated, since the brain is the most proximal physiological substrate through which psychological factors act on peripheral neural systems that affect pathophysiological mechanisms. Unfortunately, since the brain is rarely studied in this area of research, a critical step in the pathway remains unknown. An integration of the approaches in affective neuroscience with those utilized in health psychology and psychoneuroimmunology would form a strong basis for determining the complete pathway from emotional experience to peripheral response, including the neural circuitry involved in translating individual differences in affective response into important changes in the neuroendocrine and neuroimmune systems. These findings may then have tremendous value for understanding neural regulation of biological systems that play a significant role in health and disease.

REFERENCES

Abbott, D. H., Keverne, E. B., Bercovitch, F. B., Shively, C. A., Mendoza, S. P., Saltzman, C. T., et al. (2003). Are subordinates always stressed?: A comparative analysis of rank differences in cortisol levels among primates. *Hormones and Behavior, 43,* 67–82.
Anderson, N. B., Kaplan, R. M., Kumanyika, S.,

Salovey, P., Kawachi, I., Dunbar-Jacob, J., et al. (2004). *Encyclopedia of health and behavior.* Thousand Oaks, CA: Sage.
Avitsur, R., Stark, J. L., & Sheridan, J. F. (2001). Social stress induces glucocorticoid resistance in subordinate animals. *Hormones and Behavior, 39,* 247–257.
Barak, Y. (2006). The immune system and happiness. *Autoimmunity Reviews, 5,* 523–527.
Baumeister, R. F., & Leary, M. R. (1995). The need to belong: Desire for interpersonal attachment as a fundamental human motivation. *Psychological Bulletin, 117,* 497–529.
Beer, J. S., Heerey, E. A., Keltner, D., Scabini, D., & Knight, R. T. (2003). The regulatory function of self-conscious emotion: Insights from patients with orbitofrontal damage. *Journal of Personality and Social Psychology, 85,* 594–604.
Beer, J. S., John, O. P., Scabini, D., & Knight, R. T. (2006). Orbitofrontal cortex and social behavior: Integrating self-monitoring and emotion–cognition interactions. *Journal of Cognitive Neuroscience, 18,* 871–879.
Benedict, R. (1946). *The chrysanthemum and the sword.* Boston: Houghton Mifflin.
Berk, L. S., Tan, S. A., Fry, W. F., Napier, B. J., Lee, J. W., Hubbard, R. W., et al. (1989). Neuroendocrine and stress hormone changes during mirthful laughter. *American Journal of the Medical Sciences, 298,* 390–396.
Boyle, S. H., Williams, R. B., Mark, D. B., Brummett, B. H., Siegler, I. C., Helms, M. J., et al. (2004). Hostility as a predictor of survival in patients with coronary artery disease. *Psychosomatic Medicine, 66,* 629–632.
Brummett, B. H., Maynard, K. E., Babyak, M. A., Haney, T. L., Siegler, I. C., Helms, M. J., et al. (1998). Measures of hostility as predictors of facial affect during social interaction: Evidence for construct validity. *Annals of Behavioral Medicine, 20,* 168–173.
Buchanan, T. W., al'Absi, M., & Lovallo, W. R. (1999). Cortisol fluctuates with increases and decreases in negative affect. *Psychoneuroendocrinology, 24,* 227–241.
Cacioppo, J. T., Hawkley, L. C., Ernst, J. M., Burleson, M., Berntson, G. G., Nouriani, B., et al. (2006). Loneliness within a nomological net: An evolutionary perspective. *Journal of Research in Personality, 40,* 1054–1085.
Charney, D. S. (2004). Psychobiological mechanisms of resilience and vulnerability: Implications for successful adaptation to extreme stress. *American Journal of Psychiatry, 161,* 195–216.
Cirulli, F., De Acetis, L., & Alleva, E. (1998). Behavioral effects of peripheral interleukin-1 administration in adult CD-1 mice: Specific inhibition of the offensive components of intermale agonistic behavior. *Brain Research, 791,* 308–312.
Cooley, C. N. (1902). *Human nature and the social order.* New York: Scribner.

Cortese, B. M., & Phan, K. L. (2005). The role of glutamate in anxiety and related disorders. *CNS Spectrums, 10*, 820–830.

Cox, B. J., & Taylor, S. (1999). Anxiety disorders: Panic and phobias. In T. Millon, P. H. Blaney, & R. D. Davis (Eds.), *Oxford textbook of psychopathology* (pp. 81–113). New York: Oxford University Press.

Dantzer, R., Bluthe, R., Castanon, N., Cauvet, N., Capuron, L., Goodall, G., et al. (2001). Cytokine effects on behavior. In R. Ader, D. L. Felten, & N. Cohen (Eds.), *Psychoneuroimmunology* (3rd ed., Vol. 1, pp. 703–727). San Diego: Academic Press.

Darwin, C. (1899). *The descent of man* (2nd ed.). London: Murray. (Original work published 1871)

Davidson, R. J. (1992). Emotion and affective style: Hemispheric substrates. *Psychological Science, 3,* 39–43.

Davidson, R. J., Coe, C. C., Dolski, I., & Donzella, B. (1999). Individual differences in prefrontal activation asymmetry predict natural killer cell activity at rest and in response to challenge. *Brain, Behavior, and Immunity, 13,* 93–108.

Davidson, R. J., Kabat-Zinn, J., Schumacher, J., Rosenkranz, M., Muller, D., Santorelli, S. F., et al. (2003). Alterations in brain and immune function produced by mindfulness meditation. *Psychosomatic Medicine, 65,* 564–570.

Davidson, R. J., Putnam, K. M., & Larson, C. L. (2000). Dysfunction in the neural circuitry of emotion regulation: A possible prelude to violence. *Science, 290,* 1093–1095.

Dhabhar, F. S. (2003). Stress, leukocyte trafficking, and the augmentation of skin immune function. *Annals of the New York Academy of Sciences, 992,* 205–217.

Dhabhar, F. S., & McEwen, B. S. (1999). Enhancing versus suppressive effects of stress hormones on skin immune function. *Proceedings of the National Academy of Sciences of the USA, 96,* 1059–1064.

Dickerson, S. S., Gruenewald, T. L., & Kemeny, M. E. (2004). When the social self is threatened: Shame, physiology, and health. *Journal of Personality, 72,* 1191–1216.

Dickerson, S. S., & Kemeny, M. E. (2004). Acute stressors and cortisol responses: A theoretical integration and synthesis of laboratory research. *Psychological Bulletin, 130,* 355–391.

Dickerson, S. S., Kemeny, M. E., Aziz, N., Kim, K. H., & Fahey, J. L. (2004). Immunological effects of induced shame and guilt. *Psychosomatic Medicine, 66,* 124–131.

Dickerson, S. S., Gables, S., Kemeny, M. E., Aziz, N., Irwin, M., & Fahey, J. L. (2007). *Social evaluative threat induces increased production of TNF-α.* Manuscript in preparation.

Drevets, W. C. (1999). Prefrontal cortical–amygdalar metabolism in major depression. *Annals of the New York Academy of Sciences, 29,* 614–637.

Ekman, P. (1994). Moods, emotions, and traits. In P.

Ekman & R. J. Davidson (Eds.), *The nature of emotion: Fundamental questions* (pp. 56–58). New York: Oxford University Press.

Ekman, P. (1999). Basic emotions. In T. Dalgleish & M. Powers (Eds.), *Handbook of cognition and emotion.* Chichester, UK: Wiley.

Ekman, P., Levenson, R. W., & Friesen, W. V. (1983). Autonomic nervous system activity distinguishes among emotions. *Science, 221,* 1208–1210.

Erickson, K., Drevets, W., & Schulkin, J. (2003). Glucocorticoid regulation of diverse cognitive functions in normal and pathological emotional states. *Neuroscience and Biobehavioral Reviews, 27,* 233–246.

Evans, P., Bristow, M., Hucklebridge, F., Clow, A., & Walters, N. (1993). The relationship between secretory immunity, mood and life-events. *British Journal of Psychology, 32,* 227–236.

Fleshner, M., Laudenslager, M. L., Simons, L., & Maier, S. F. (1989). Reduced serum antibodies associated with social defeat in rats. *Physiology and Behavior, 45,* 1183–1187.

Floyd, N. S., Price, J. L., Ferry, A. T., Keay, K. A., & Bandler, R. (2001). Orbitomedial prefrontal cortical projections to hypothalamus in the rat. *Journal of Comparative Neurology, 432,* 307–328.

Fraeff, F. G., Garcia-Leal, C., Del-Ben, C. M., & Guimaraes, F. S. (2005). Does the panic attack activate the hypothalamic–pituitary–adrenal axis? *Anais da Academia Brasileira de Ciencias, 77,* 477–491.

Futterman, A. D., Kemeny, M. E., Shapiro, D., & Fahey, J. L. (1994). Immunological and physiological changes associated with induced positive and negative mood. *Psychosomatic Medicine, 56,* 499–511.

Futterman, A. D., Kemeny, M. E., Shapiro, D., Polonsky, W., & Fahey, J. L. (1992). Immunological variability associated with experimentally-induced positive and negative affective states. *Psychological Medicine, 22,* 231–238.

Gilbert, P. (1997). The evolution of social attractiveness and its role in shame, humiliation, guilt and therapy. *British Journal of Medical Psychology, 70,* 113–147.

Gregg, T. R., & Siegel, A. (2000). Brain structures and neurotransmitters regulating aggression in cats: Implications for human aggression. *Science, 289,* 591–594.

Gruenewald, T. L., Kemeny, M. E., Aziz, N., & Fahey, J. L. (2004). Acute threat to the social self: Shame, social self-esteem and cortisol activity. *Psychosomatic Medicine, 66,* 915–924.

Herbert, T. B., & Cohen, S. (1993). Depression and immunity: A meta-analytic review. *Psychological Bulletin, 113,* 472–486.

Herman, J. P., Ostrander, M. M., Mueller, N. K., & Figueiredo, H. (2005). Limbic system mechanisms of stress regulation: Hypothalamo–pituitary–adrenocortical axis. *Progress in Neuro-Psychopharmacology and Biological Psychiatry, 29,* 1201–1213.

Howland, R. H., & Thase, M. E. (1999). Affective disorders: Biological aspects. In T. Millon, P. H. Blaney, & R. D. Davis (Eds.), *Oxford textbook of psychopathology* (pp. 166–202). New York: Oxford University Press.

Hucklebridge, F., Lambert, S., Clow, A., Warburton, D. M., Evans, P. D., & Sherwood, N. (2000). Modulation of secretory immunoglobulin a in saliva; response to manipulation of mood. *Biological Psychology, 53*, 25–35.

Irwin, M. (2001). Depression and immunity. In R. Ader, D. L. Felten, & N. Cohen (Eds.), *Psychoneuroimmunology* (3rd ed., Vol. 2, pp. 383–398). San Diego: Academic Press.

Irwin, M., Daniels, M., Bloom, E. T., & Weiner, H. (1986). Life events, depression, and natural killer cell activity. *Psychopharmacology Bulletin, 22*, 1093–1096.

Irwin, M., Lacher, U., & Caldwell, C. (1992). Depression and reduced natural killer cytotoxicity: A longitudinal study of depressed patients and control subjects. *Psychological Medicine, 22*, 1045–1050.

Kang, D. H., Davidson, R. I., Coe, C. L., Wheeler, R. W., Tomarken, A. J., & Ershler, W. B. (1991). Frontal brain asymmetry and immune function. *Behavioral Neuroscience, 105*, 860–869.

Keltner, D., & Buswell, B. N. (1996). Evidence for the distinctness of embarrassment, shame, and guilt: A study of recalled antecedents and facial expressions of emotion. *Cognition and Emotion, 10*, 155–171.

Kemeny, M. E. (2003a). The psychobiology of stress. *Current Directions in Psychological Science, 12*, 124–128.

Kemeny, M. E. (2003b). An interdisciplinary research model to investigate psychosocial cofactors in disease: Application to HIV-1 pathogenesis. *Brain Behavior and Immunity, 17*, 62–72.

Kemeny, M. E. (2006a). Psychoneuroimmunology. In H. Friedman & R. Silver (Eds.), *Foundations of health psychology* (pp. 92–116). New York: Oxford University Press.

Kemeny, M. E., & Gruenewald, T. L. (2000). Affect, cognition, the immune system and health. *Progress in Brain Research, 122*, 291–308.

Kemeny, M. E., & Schedlowski, M. (2007). Understanding the interaction between psychosocial stress and immune-related disease: A stepwise progression. *Brain, Behavior and Immunity, 21*, 1009–1018.

Kiecolt-Glaser, J. K., Malarkey, W. B., Chee, M., Newton, T., Cacioppo, J. T., Mao, H. Y., et al. (1993). Negative behavior during marital conflict is associated with immunological down-regulation. *Psychosomatic Medicine, 55*, 410–412.

Kimata, H. (2001). Effect of humor on allergen-induced wheal reactions. *Journal of the American Medical Association, 285*, 738.

Kinsey, S. G., Bailey, M. T., Sheridan, J. F., Padgett, D. A., & Avitsur, R. (2007). Prepeated social defeat causes increased anxiety-like behavior and alters

splenocyte function in C57BL/6 and CD-1 mice. *Brain, Behavior, and Immunity, 21*, 458–466.

Koga, C., Itoh, K., Aoki, M., Suefuji, Y., Yoshida, M., Asosina, S., et al. (2001). Anxiety and pain suppress the natural killer cell activity in oral surgery outpatients. *Oral Surgery, Oral Medicine, Oral Pathology, Oral Radiology, and Endodontics, 91*, 654–658.

Koh, K. B., & Lee, Y. (2004). Reduced anxiety level by therapeutic interventions and cell-mediated immunity in panic disorder patients. *Psychotherapy and Psychosomatics, 73*, 286–292.

Kubzansky, L. D., Kawachi, I., Weiss, S. T., & Sparrow, D. (1998). Anxiety and coronary heart disease: A synthesis of epidemiological, psychological, and experimental evidence. *Annals of Behavioral Medicine, 20*, 47–58.

Laidlaw, T. M., Booth, R. J., & Large, R. G. (1996). Reduction in skin reactions to histamine after a hypnotic procedure. *Psychosomatic Medicine, 58*, 242–248.

Lambert, R. B., & Lambert, N. K. (1995). The effects of humor on secretory immunoglobulin A levels in school-aged children. *Pediatric Nursing, 21*, 16–19.

Lazarus, R. S. (1991). *Emotion and adaptation.* London: Oxford University Press.

Lazarus, R. S., & Folkman, S. (1984). *Stress, appraisal, and coping.* New York: Springer.

Levenson, R. W. (1992). Autonomic nervous system differences among emotions. *Psychological Science, 3*, 23–27.

Levenson, R. W. (1994). The search for autonomic specificity. In P. Ekman & R. J. Davidson (Eds.), *The nature of emotion: Fundamental questions* (pp. 252–257). New York: Oxford University Press.

Lewis, M., & Ramsay, D. (2002). Cortisol response to embarrassment and shame. *Child Development, 73*, 1034–1045.

Maes, M., Scharpe, S., Meltzer, H. Y., Okayli, G., Bosmans, E., D'Hondt, P., et al. (1994). Increased neopterin and interferon-gamma secretion and lower availability of L-tryptophan in major depression: Further evidence for an immune response. *Psychiatry Research, 54*, 143–160.

Maier, S. F., & Watkins, L. R. (1998). Cytokines for psychologists: Implications of bidirectional immune-to-brain communication for understanding behavior, mood, and cognition. *Psychological Review, 105*, 83–107.

McClelland, D. C., & Cheriff, A. D. (1997). The immunoenhancing effects of humor on secretory IgA and resistance to respiratory infections. *Psychology and Health, 12*, 329–344.

McNally, R. J. (1999). Posttraumatic stress disorder. In T. Millon, P. H. Blaney, & R. D. Davis (Eds.), *Oxford textbook of psychopathology* (pp. 144–165). New York: Oxford University Press.

Miczek, K. A., Thompson, M. L., & Shuster, L. (1982). Opioid-like analgesia in defeated mice. *Science, 215*, 1520–1522.

Miller, G. E., Stetler, C. A., Carney, R. M., Freedland, K. E., & Banks, W. A. (2002). Clinical depression and inflammatory risk markers for coronary heart disease. *American Journal of Cardiology, 90,* 1279–1283.

Miller, T. Q., Smith, T. W., Turner, C. W., Guijarro, M. L., & Hallet, A. J. (1996). A meta-analytic review of research on hostility and physical health. *Psychological Bulletin, 119,* 322–348.

Mittwoch-Jaffe, T., Shalit, F., Srendi, B., & Yehuda, S. (1995). Modification of cytokine secretion following mild emotional stimuli. *NeuroReport, 6,* 789–792.

Ochsner, K. N. (2004). Current directions in social cognitive neuroscience. *Current Opinion in Neurobiology, 14,* 254–258.

Ottaway, C. A., & Husband, A. J. (1992). Central nervous system influences on lymphocyte migration. *Brain, Behavior, and Immunity, 6,* 97–116.

Parkinson, J. A., Cardinal, R. N., & Everitt, B. J. (2000). Limbic cortical–ventral striatal systems underlying appetitive conditions. *Progress in Brain Research, 126,* 263–285.

Phan, K. L., Wager, T. D., Taylor, S. F., & Liberzon, I. (2004). Functional neuroimaging studies of human emotions. *CNS Spectrums, 9,* 258–266.

Phelps, E. A., & LeDoux, J. E. (2005). Contributions of the amygdala to emotion processing: From animal models to human behavior. *Neuron, 48,* 175–187.

Pressman, S., & Cohen, S. (2005). Does positive affect influence health? *Psychological Bulletin, 131,* 925–971.

Price, J., Sloman, L., Gardner, R., Jr., Gilbert, P., & Rohde, P. (1994). The social competition hypothesis of depression. *British Journal of Psychiatry, 164,* 309–315.

Price, J. L. (2005). Free will versus survival: Brain systems that underlie intrinsic constraints on behavior. *Journal of Comparative Neurology, 493,* 132–139.

Prkachin, K. M., & Silverman, B. E. (2002). Hostility and facial expression in young men and women: Is social regulation more important than negative affect? *Health Psychology, 21,* 33–39.

Quan, N., Avitsur, R., Stark, J., He, L., Shah, M., Caliguiri, M., et al. (2001). Social stress increases susceptibility to endotoxic shock. *Journal of Neuroimmunology, 115,* 36–45.

Ridker, P. M., Hennekens, C. H., Buring, J. E., & Rifai, N. (2000). C-reactive protein and other markers of inflammation in the prediction of cardiovascular disease in women. *New England Journal of Medicine, 342,* 836–843.

Rogers, M. A., Bradshaw, J. L., Pantelis, C., & Phillips, J. G. (1998). Frontostriatal deficits in unipolar major depression. *Brain Research Bulletin, 47,* 297–310.

Rozanski, A., Blumenthal, J. A., & Kaplan, J. (1999). Impact of psychological factors on the pathogenesis of cardiovascular disease and implications for therapy. *Circulation, 99,* 2192–2217.

Sapolsky, R. M. (1993). Endocrinology alfresco: Psychoendocrine studies of wild baboons. *Recent Progress in Hormone Research, 48,* 437–468.

Sapolsky, R. M. (2005). The influence of social hierarchy on primate health. *Science, 308,* 648–652.

Schleifer, S. J., Keller, S. E., & Bartlett, J. A. (2002). Panic disorder and immunity: Few effects on circulating lymphocytes, mitogen response, and NK cell activity. *Brain, Behavior, and Immunity, 16,* 698–705.

Schleifer, S. J., Keller, S. E., Meyerson, A. T., Raskin, M. J., Davis, K. L., & Stein, M. (1984). Lymphocyte function in major depressive disorder. *Archives of General Psychiatry, 41,* 484–486.

Schwartz, G. E., Weinberger, D. A., & Singer, J. A. (1981). Cardiovascular differentiation of happiness, sadness, anger, and fear following imagery and exercise. *Psychosomatic Medicine, 43,* 343–364.

Segerstrom, S. C., Glover, D. A., Craske, M. G., & Fahey, J. L. (1999). Worry affects the immune response to phobic fear. *Brain, Behavior, and Immunity, 13,* 80–92.

Segerstrom, S. C., & Miller, G. E. (2004). Psychological stress and the human immune system: A meta-analytic study of 30 years of inquiry. *Psychological Bulletin, 130,* 601–630.

Segerstrom, S. C., Solomon, G. F., Kemeny, M. E., & Fahey, J. L. (1998). Relationship of worry to immune sequelae of the Northridge earthquake. *Journal of Behavioral Medicine, 21,* 433–450.

Seligman, M. E. P. (2002). Positive psychology, positive prevention, and positive therapy. In C. R. Snyder & S. J. Lopez (Eds.), *Handbook of positive psychology* (pp. 3–9). New York: Oxford University Press.

Selye, H. (1956). *The stress of life.* New York: McGraw-Hill.

Shestyuk, A. Y., Deldin, P. J., Brand, J. E., & Deveney, C. M. (2005). Reduced sustained brain activity during processing of positive emotional stimuli in major depression. *Biological Psychiatry, 57,* 1089–1096.

Smith, T. W. (1994). Concepts and methods in the study of anger, hostility, and health. In A. W. Siegman & T. W. Smith (Eds.), *Anger, hostility and the heart* (pp. 23–42). Hillsdale, NJ: Erlbaum.

Smith, T. W., & Gallo, L. C. (2001). Personality traits as risk factors for physical illness. In A. Baum, T. Revenson, & J. Singer (Eds.), *Handbook of health psychology* (pp. 139–172). Mahwah, NJ: Erlbaum.

Smith, T. W., Glazer, K., Ruiz, J. M., & Gallo, L. C. (2004). Hostility, anger, aggressiveness, and coronary heart disease: An interpersonal perspective on personality, emotion, and health. *Journal of Personality, 72,* 1217–1270.

Smith, T. W., & Ruiz, J. M. (2002). Psychosocial influences on the development and course of coronary heart disease: Current status and implications for research and practice. *Journal of Consulting and Clinical Psychology, 7,* 548–568.

Stark, J., Avitsur, R., Padgett, D. A., & Sheridan, J. F. (2001). Social stress induces glucocorticoid resistance in macrophages. *American Journal of Physiology:*

Regulatory, Integrative and Comparative Physiology, 280, 1799–1805.

Stefanski, V., & Ben-Eliyahu, S. (1996). Social confrontation and tumor metastasis in rats: Defeat and beta-adrenergic mechanisms. *Physiology and Behavior, 60,* 277–282.

Stone, A. A., Cox, D. S., Valdimarsdottir, H., Jandorf, L., & Neale, J. M. (1987). Evidence that secretory IgA antibody is associated with daily mood. *Journal of Personality and Social Psychology, 52,* 988–993.

Stone, A. A., Neale, J. M., Cox, D. S., Napoli, A., Valdimarsdottir, H., & Kennedy-Moore, E. (1994). Daily events are associated with a secretory immune response to an oral antigen in men. *Health Psychology, 13,* 440–446.

Strohle, A., & Holsboer, F. (2003). Stress responsive neurohormones in depression and anxiety. *Pharmacopsychiatry, 36,* S207–S214.

Suarez, E. C., Lewis, J. G., & Kuhn, C. (2002). The relation of aggression, hostility, and anger to lipopolysaccharide-stimulated tumor necrosis factor (TNF)-alpha by blood monocytes from normal men. *Brain, Behavior and Immunity, 16,* 675–684.

Suinn, R. M. (2001). The terrible twos—anger and anxiety: Hazardous to your health. *American Psychologist, 56,* 27–36.

Tangney, J. (1995). Recent advances in the empirical study of shame and guilt. *American Behavioral Scientist, 38,* 1132–1145.

Taylor, S. E., & Armor, D. A. (1996). Positive illusions and coping with adversity. *Journal of Personality, 64,* 873–898.

Viswanathan, K., & Dhabhar, F. S. (2005). Stress-induced enhancement of leukocyte trafficking into sites of surgery or immune activation. *Proceedings of the National Academy of Sciences of the USA, 102,* 5808–5813.

Weiner, H. (1992). *Perturbing the organism: The biology of stressful experiences.* Chicago: University of Chicago Press.

Williams, R. B., Jr., Barefoot, J. C., & Shekelle, R. (1985). The health consequences of hostility. In M. A. Chesney & R. H. Rosenman (Eds.), *Anger and hostility in cardiovascular and behavioral disorders* (pp. 173–185). New York: Hemisphere.

Yehuda, R. (2000). Biology of posttraumatic stress disorder. *Journal of Clinical Psychiatry, 61,* S14–S21.

Yehuda, R., Boisoneau, D., Mason, J. W., & Giller, E. L. (1993). Glucocorticoid receptor number and cortisol excretion in mood, anxiety, and psychotic disorders. *Biological Psychiatry, 34,* 18–25.

Yirmiya, R. (1996). Endotoxin produces a depressive-like episode in rats. *Brain Research, 711,* 163–174.

Yirmiya, R., Weidenfeld, J., Pollak, U., Morag, M., Morag, A., Avitsur, R., et al. (1999). Cytokines, "depression due to a general medical condition," and antidepressant drugs. In R. Dantzer, E. Wollman, & R. Yirmiya, (Eds.), *Cytokines, stress and depression* (pp. 283–316). New York: Kluwer Academic.

Zachariae, R., Bjerring, P., Zachariae, C., Arendt-Nielsen, L., Nielsen, T., Eldrup, E., et al. (1991). Monocyte chemotactic activity in sera after hypnotically induced emotional states. *Scandinavian Journal of Immunology, 34,* 71–79.

Zachariae, R., Jorgensen, M. M., Egekvist, H., & Bjerring, P. (2001). Skin reactions to histamine of healthy subjects after hypnotically induced emotions of sadness, anger, and happiness. *Allergy, 56,* 734–740.

CHAPTER 42

Health-Promoting and Health-Damaging Effects of Emotions

The View from Developmental Functionalism

NATHAN S. CONSEDINE

Nothing vivifies, and nothing kills, like the emotions.
—JOSEPH ROUX

It may have taken the social sciences the best part of 200 years to subject Roux's observation to systematic scrutiny, but the field of emotions and health has gained increasing coherence and momentum across the last few decades. Monographs (Zautra, 2003), book chapters (Leventhal & Patrick-Miller, 2000; Mayne, 2001), papers in special journal issues (Andersen, 2002; Hamilton & Malcarne, 2004; Stefanek & McDonald, 2003; Zautra, Davis, & Smith, 2004), and review articles (Consedine, Magai, Krivoshekova, Ryzewicz, & Neugut, 2004; Mayne, 1999; Smith, Glazer, Ruiz, & Gallo, 2004) are appearing with increasing regularity. Admittedly, the field (and the current chapter) might currently be better termed the study of emotions and *disease*, with one review suggesting that studies of negative emotions outnumber those on positive emotions by 11:1 (Mayne, 1999). Nonetheless, and despite differences in emphasis, numerous psychological, physiological, immunological, epi-demiological, prevention, and intervention researchers have begun to document the pervasiveness with which emotions relate to health outcomes.

REVIEW OF THE LITERATURE

There are several ways in which one could review and arrange this blossoming literature— by disease outcome, by emotion, or by mechanism/pathway. In the interests of space, however, and with an eye toward demonstrating the pervasiveness of emotion's relations with health outcomes, I have chosen to arrange studies and theory relating emotions to health outcomes within a framework emphasizing five points along a disease progression spectrum (see Figure 42.1): primary causation and prevention, secondary causation and prevention, symptom sensitivity, detection/screening, and treatment choice/adherence. The current chap-

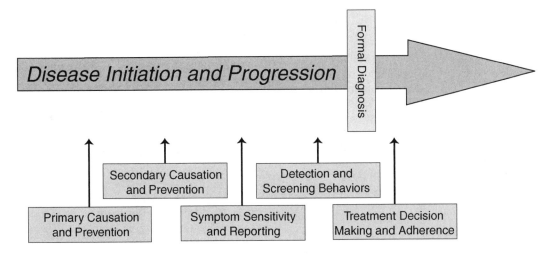

FIGURE 42.1. Organizational model describing five points at which emotions can relate to health.

ter emphasizes these five more "psychological" aspects of emotions and health, and readers are referred to other sources for more comprehensive discussions of the physiological, neurohormonal, and immunological effects of emotions (see, e.g., Kemeny & Shestyuk, Chapter 41, this volume). Following a brief overview of how emotions relate to health at each point, a brief critique of the field as a whole is given, and areas for future research are suggested.

Primary Causative/Preventive Aspects

Greater levels of negative affect (NA) have been implicated in a full panorama of diseases, ranging from heart disease (Donker, 2000) and cancer (Reiche, Morimoto, & Nunes, 2006) to arthritis (Kiecolt-Glaser, McGuire, Robles, & Glaser, 2002), diabetes (Carnethon, Kinder, Fair, Stafford, & Fortmann, 2003), AIDS (Moscowitz, 2003), and the common cold (Cohen et al., 1998). Most extensively researched in the context of cardiovascular disease, such types of NA as anger, anxiety, and depression have been implicated in basic disease processes (Krantz & McCeney, 2002; Sirois & Burg, 2003), immunological functioning (Baum & Pozluszny, 1999), incidence (Rugulies, 2002), and early mortality (Harburg, Julius, Kaciroti, Gleiberman, & Schork, 2003). In a large number of cases, the health-deleterious impact of greater negative emotion is found longitudinally (Kubzansky, Cole, Kawachi, Vokonas, & Sparrow, 2006), and even when health behaviors are controlled for (Consedine, Magai, Cohen, & Gillespie, 2002). At this level, excessive NA appears to promote disease and ill health.

Although positive affect (PA) is proportionally underrepresented in the literature, more recent data indicate that forms of PA may also be associated with health outcomes, including mortality (see reviews in Chesney et al., 2005; Pressman & Cohen, 2005; Richman et al., 2005). PA predicted superior health across both 5 weeks (Pettit, Kline, Gencoz, Gencoz, & Joiner, 2001) and 2 years (Ostir, Markides, Black, & Goodwin, 2000), even when baseline health, NA, health behaviors, and (in one study) self-report biases were controlled (Pettit et al., 2001). Global measures of PA have been shown to predict lower readmission among hospitalized older adults (Middleton & Byrd, 1996) and lower mortality among patients with HIV (Moskowitz, 2003), while the related construct of optimism may protect against pulmonary decline (Kubzansky et al., 2002). Hope has been linked to increased survival time in patients with cancer (Gottschalk, 1985), while curiosity has been linked to lower hypertension and diabetes (Richman et al., 2005) and to lower mortality (Silvia, 2001; Swan & Carmelli, 1996). Recent work suggests that PA may have health-promoting benefits for physiology in general (Fredrickson & Levenson, 1998) and for hormone production and immune parameters in particular (Cohen, Doyle, Turner, Alper, & Skoner, 2003), or that positive emotions may facilitate health-promoting cognitive styles (Tugade, Fredrickson, & Barrett, 2004).

Secondary Causative/Preventive Aspects of Behavior

A second point at which emotions influence health and disease processes lies in their relations with behaviors that are often "aimed" at the regulation of emotional states, but that also promote either health or disease (Brigham, Henningfield, & Stitzer, 1991). Although the role of NA in the *initiation* of unhealthy behavior profiles is less well established than its roles in *maintenance* and *relapse* (see Kassel, Stroud, & Paronis, 2003, on this issue), a voluminous literature implicates greater NA in several key health behaviors—notably the use of cigarettes (Kassel et al., 2003), the consumption of high-fat/sugar "comfort" foods (Dube, LeBel, & Lu, 2005), overeating (Arnow, Kenardy, & Agras, 1995), drug/alcohol use (Wills, Sandy, Shinar, & Yaeger, 1999; Witkiewitz & Marlatt, 2004), and reduced exercise (Kawachi, Sparrow, Spiro, Vokonas, & Weiss, 1996).

As in other areas of emotions–health research, more work has been done regarding the role of NA than on that of PA. There are, however, a growing number of exceptions (see Pressman & Cohen, 2005). In one recent study of 1,093 women participating in a worksite health promotion intervention, PA and coping both predicted self-reported health and exercise (Kelsey, DeVellis, Begum, Belton, & Hooten, 2006). Other work has linked greater PA to greater levels of exercise and better nutrition (Griffin, Friend, Eitel, & Lobel, 1993), although the motivation to up-regulate PA has been linked to several risky behaviors, including unprotected sex (Kalichman et al., 1994) and preferences for stimulant use (Adams et al., 2003).

Symptom Perception and Sensitivity

Third, aspects of emotions appear related to *reports* of health symptoms and to symptom sensitivity. One line of research suggests that at least a part of the general relation between forms of NA and poorer health reflects differences in the tendency to attend to (or complain about) somatic symptoms—a methodological nuisance factor (see reviews in Van Diest et al., 2005; Watson & Pennebaker, 1989). Consistent with this view, several longitudinal studies have shown state NA, to be a better predictor of self-reported health symptoms than trait NA (Brown & Moskowitz, 1997; Charles & Almeida, 2006; Leventhal, Hansell, Diefenbach, Leventhal, & Glass, 1996).

Others have, however, argued that trait NA is not necessarily most usefully viewed as a *biasing* factor in reports of illness or health care (Mora, Robitaille, Leventhal, Swigar, & Leventhal, 2002). According to these authors, older adults with high trait NA—particularly anxiety—will be cognitively more attentive to their somatic state and have greater expertise in differentiating current symptoms from their baseline somatic background (Mora et al., 2002). Such a claim is consistent with other work suggesting that nondepressed people generally tend to underreport disease symptomatology, while depressed persons report symptoms more accurately (see Mayne, 2001). The effect of NA on reporting may also vary with the specificity of the symptoms being assessed; "vague," systemic symptoms appear to be more strongly related than local, specific symptoms to NA (Van Diest et al., 2005). Positive emotions have scarcely been researched at this interface. Although PA is thought to promote a number of advantageous perceptual and coping changes (see, e.g., Folkman & Moskowitz, 2004; Fredrickson & Losada, 2005), how (if at all) such advantages might be evident in the context of symptom perception and sensitivity is presently unclear.

Detection and Screening Behaviors

One of the most active areas of behavioral emotions–health research focuses on how emotions—particularly fear/anxiety, depression, and embarrassment—relate to the frequency of medical contacts, as well as to detection and screening behaviors. Clinically significant levels of NA generally predict more frequent contact with physicians, even when health status is controlled for; this finding is best documented in the case of depression and anxiety (Tweed, Goering, Lin, & Williams, 1998). Distress and/or depression have been linked to more frequent physician visits (Callahan, Hui, Nienaber, Musick, & Tierney, 1994; Karlsson, Lehtinen, & Joukamaa, 1995), perhaps more strongly among women (Larsen, Schroll, & Avlund, 2006). Discrete emotions have also begun to be studied in this context. A recent study of 345 older adults found that anger, but not fear, predicted increases in the number of physicians' visits but not admissions; sadness interacted with gender such that it related to more admissions for men, but fewer for women (McKeen, Chipperfield, & Campbell, 2004).

A large literature has examined how fear-related constructs relate to cancer screening (Dale, Bilir, Han, & Meltzer, 2005; Hay, Buckley, & Ostroff, 2005). In general, greater anxiety or worry appears to facilitate screening among women, at least when operationalized in terms of trait anxiety or fear of cancer (Consedine, Magai, Krivoshekova, et al., 2004), and trait anxiety appears to predict more frequent prostate screening among men (Dale et al., 2005). It is worth noting, however, that research in both men's (Consedine, Morgenstern, Kudadjie-Gyamfi, Magai, & Neugut, 2006) and women's (Andersen, Smith, Meischke, Bowen, & Urban, 2003; Diefenbach, Miller, & Daly, 1999) screening has found evidence of nonlinearities in the relation between anxiety and screening (Miller & Diefenbach, 1998). Such findings suggest that there may be "threshold" rather than "dose" effects for anxiety's relation to screening.

Whereas anxiety generally appears to enhance the frequency of health-promoting medical contacts, other types of NA appear to have more complex (and potentially less salutary) relations with health. Although depression appears to predict more frequent medical contact in general, it has also been associated with less frequent mammography (Husaini et al., 2001), and a greater likelihood of late-stage breast cancer diagnosis (Desai, Bruce, & Kasl, 1999), although at least one study found no relation with Pap smear frequency (Pirraglia, Sanyal, Singer, & Ferris, 2004). Greater embarrassment has been found to relate negatively to general medical visits (Consedine, Krivoshekova, & Harris, 2007), dental visit frequency (Moore, Brodsgaard, & Rosenberg, 2004), and help seeking for incontinence (Hagglund, Walker-Engstrom, Larsson, & Leppert, 2003), as well as to be associated with less frequent breast (Consedine, Magai, & Neugut, 2004), testicular (Gascoigne, Mason, & Roberts, 1999), cervical (Taylor et al., 2002), and colon (Farraye et al., 2004) cancer screenings.

Treatment Decision Making and Adherence

Persons diagnosed with a serious health threat or disease are confronted with a bewildering array of information, advice, demands, and treatment options (Lam, Fielding, Chan, Chow, & Or, 2005). Having eventually embarked on a treatment course and experienced any possible benefits and side effects, such persons must then decide whether to persist with the adopted treatment/adhere to physician recommendations. Both initial treatment decision making (TDM) and adherence are inevitably complex and highly demanding processes that naturally lend themselves to emotions-based analyses.

Despite the presence of multiple, unclear, and/or competing goals in TDM contexts (Broadstock & Michie, 2000), most studies of TDM assume a high degree of rationality (Lam et al., 2005). The consequence of this orientation is that despite the importance of *anticipated* benefits and costs of treatment options (Lam et al., 2005), including emotional costs and benefits, there are few studies of emotions in TDM. Moreover, such research has tended to conceptualize affect as an outcome factor that must be weighed against treatment efficacy.

In some of the few studies to date of TDM and emotions, women reporting greater intrusive thinking and cancer worry are more likely to choose tamoxifen treatment for breast cancer risk (Bober, Hoke, Duda, Regan, & Tung, 2004), and health-related quality of life has been related to the decision to modify chemotherapy treatment (Detmar, Muller, Schnornagel, Wever, & Aaronson, 2002). Other work suggests that anticipated consequences of treatment decisions with a high affective content (e.g., losing hair, weight gain) are influential in determining adjuvant breast cancer treatment decisions (Lam et al., 2005), and it has been argued that anxiety and depression interfere with TDM (Petersen et al., 2003).

One interesting question that emerges in this research lies in examining exactly what comprises a "good decision." Research conducted within the "affective heuristic" (Slovic, Peters, Finucane, & MacGregor, 2005) or "risk-as-feelings" (Loewenstein, Weber, Hsee, & Welch, 2001) models discriminates between fast, instinctive, and intuitive reactions to threat (risk as feelings) and more effortful, logical, and reasoned efforts to manage risk (risk as analysis). Importantly for TDM researchers, factors such as age, cognitive load, stress, and ill health may increase the reliance on less analytic and more affectively driven styles (Slovic et al., 2005). In the context of cancer TDM, this might produce situations in which high levels of cancer-related anxiety and restrictive regulatory styles— evident in several minority groups—promote rapid (or even preemptive) TDM as the process becomes more heavily influenced by affective considerations.

While treatment adherence is inherently a behavioral and motivational issue, there has been comparatively little research on the role of emotions in adherence. Depression has been related to poorer adherence to medications for hypertension (Carney et al., 1998; Kaplan, Bhalodkar, Brown, Wflite, & Brown, 2004; Wang et al., 2002) and HIV (Van Servellen, Chang, Garcia, & Lombardi, 2002), as well as to dialysis (Brownbridge & Fielding, 1994), and oral hypoglycemic treatments for diabetes (Kalsekar et al., 2006); it has also been linked to withdrawal from dialysis (McDade-Montez, Christensen, Cvengros, & Lawton, 2006). It remains unclear whether such effects are caused by greater sensitivity to side effects or are a consequence of intense emotions' dominating coping efforts at the expense of problem-focused efforts (see Cameron, Petrie, Ellis, Buick, & Weinman, 2005).

The relations between anxiety and adherence appear complex. Perhaps surprisingly, anxiety has been shown to predict lower adherence to HIV medication (Van Servellen et al., 2002) and dialysis (Brownbridge & Fielding, 1994) regimens, although few studies controlling for the large number of confounds in adherence have been conducted. A meta-analysis of these two affects (DiMatteo, Lepper, & Croghan, 2000) found that the association between anxiety and nonadherence was variable, but reported a strong negative relation between depression and nonadherence (odds ratio [OR] = 3.03).

Again, PA remains understudied. One study reported that positive states of mind predicted adherence to HIV treatment and partially mediated the relation between social support and adherence (Gonzalez et al., 2004), although other work has suggested that the optimism– adherence link may be nonlinear for antiretroviral therapy adherence (Milam, Richardson, Marks, Kemper, & McCutchan, 2004). Another study suggested that lower quality of life marginally predicted (OR = 1.3) tamoxifen (a breast cancer treatment) discontinuance over a 2-year period (Fink, Gurwitz, Rakowski, Guadagnoli, & Silliman, 2004).

A CRITIQUE ON THE STATE OF THE ART

Although emotions–health research has made considerable progress in recent years, a number of key issues remain unclear. Although some of these issues are empirical and are likely to be clarified by ongoing research, several pressing concerns are theoretical and stem from the field's historical origins (Donker, 2000; Friedman & Booth-Kewley, 1987; Smith, 1992) and ongoing applied focus. It has been noted that many datasets used to examine emotion–health relations were "pressed into service" after the fact, with the consequences that basic psychometric issues are frequently ignored (Smith, 1992) and observations are infrequently placed within broader theoretical contexts (Friedman & Booth-Kewley, 1987; Miller et al., 2004). Below, a selection of the global issues confronting emotions and health research are described, and some suggestions regarding the field's development are given.

Function

The emotions are thought to represent adaptations that evolved over time to deal with recurrent adaptive challenges or opportunities, and thus they are viewed as serving key social, physiological, cognitive, and motivational functions (Consedine & Magai, 2006; Frijda, 1994; Keltner & Gross, 1999). Whether health may represent one of these challenges is unclear, as is the question of whether the emotions have functions that are specifically related to health or whether the relations between emotions and health arise epiphenomenally with respect to non-health-related functions (e.g., Mayne, 2001). There is a marked difference between an emotion's having consequences for health and the emotion's having evolved *because* of these consequences (Consedine, Magai, & Bonanno, 2002).

Few of the discrete emotions thus far considered by health researchers have any obvious health-related functions. Nonetheless, understanding what emotions are designed or "meant" for is critical to the advancement of the field, because it provides guidance in the search for mechanisms. Because each emotion has evolved to solve specific adaptive challenges, each involves a coordinated response among physiological (Larsen, Berntson, Poehlmann, Ito, & Caccioppo, Chapter 11, this volume), cognitive (Stein, Hernandez, & Trabasso, Chapter 35, this volume), and motivational (Consedine, Magai, Krivoshekova, et al., 2004), systems that, in total, is aimed towards addressing that challenge. Understanding the purpose of emotional response sets allows researchers to "fill" the explanatory gap between emotions and health outcomes in a systematic and theoretically driven way.

Mechanisms

Perhaps because emotions are so central to human functioning, they appear to affect health processes at a large number of points across the health–disease spectrum; the mechanisms linking them are multiple and complex. Below, three major classes of mechanisms are briefly reviewed, with an eye toward considering how descriptions of the functions of emotions in regard to three different components (physiological, experiential/motivational, and cognitive) may supplement existing accounts.

Historically, the mechanisms thought to explain the link between emotions and health have been classed as either "direct" or "indirect," depending on whether a particular model suggests that emotions have a direct impact on health via their role in generating autonomic and immunological changes, or whether they are linked through mediated (indirect) pathways. One grouping of direct-pathway explanations—the arousal, accumulation, or "wear-and-tear" models—suggests that the autonomic and immunological changes associated with emotions such as anxiety and anger are what create health risk; such a view (albeit in reverse) is also evident in recent models examining positive emotions (Fredrickson & Losada, 2005; Moskowitz, 2003; Tugade et al., 2004). Although this approach may have more difficulty in accounting for direct links between depressed (nonarousing) affects and health, the general notion that the activation of the negative emotions was historically adaptive (Levenson, 1994), but has become vestigial and now damages and/or impairs autonomic and immune systems when repeated or chronic, has garnered an impressive body of support (Mayne, 2001).

A second grouping of models conceptualizes the emotion–health relation as indirect, arising predominantly as a result of emotion's strong motivational functions. Models examining the effects of emotions on health via health behav-

iors, screening, and adherence have tended to be motivationally hedonic (e.g., Chapman & Coups, 2006; Consedine, Magai, Krivoshekova, et al., 2004); health-relevant behaviors are argued to occur *in order to regulate either experienced or anticipated affect*. For example, many behaviors with implications for poorer health (e.g., poor dietary preferences; cigarette, alcohol, and drug use) are enacted because they help people minimize the experience of negative emotions and maximize the experience of positive emotions.

However, in the context of detection, screening, and adherence behaviors, experienced negative emotion appears to have diverse effects on health behavior, *depending on the affect in question*. It is at this point that the functionalist approach to discrete emotions becomes most useful. Moderate levels of fear/anxiety, be they general or specific to a condition, generally appear to promote health-enhancing behavior profiles. Functionally, when people are anxious, their cognitive processes and motivational priorities shift. They begin to evaluate the environment for the source of the threat and to engage in information- and support-seeking behaviors, as well as in behaviors that consciously or unconsciously serve to ameliorate the unpleasant experience of anxiety (Consedine, Magai, Krivoshekova, et al., 2004). Thus, despite the fact that fear did not evolve in order to increase medical care seeking or screening, fear of a disease outcome appears to motivate behaviors that reduce risk so long as efficacy requirements are met (Mayne, 2001).

Conversely, emotional syndromes such as depression have been generally linked to health-deleterious behaviors, poorer cancer screening, and poorer adherence. Given that depressed affects such as sadness induce passivity rather than overt activity (Brehm, 1999), and are thought to function by motivating an individual to *cease* directing effort toward a lost goal (Campos & Barrett, 1984)—thus conserving systemic resources (Clark & Watson, 1994)—these relationships are perhaps not surprising. Given that depressed affect naturally lends itself to behavioral passivity, future research might benefit from considering the nature of these "lost" goals, examining whether they relate to health states, and considering how best to activate competing goal and affective states that facilitate less unhealthy behavioral profiles.

A final pathway that has received increasing attention in recent times has involved the consideration of how emotions compete with, relate to, and are manifest in health-relevant cognitive processes. For health researchers interested in emotions, engaging at this interface has been a necessary step, as most psychological models of health behavior remain heavily cognitive in orientation (Jessop, Rutter, Sharma, & Albery, 2004; Ogden, 2003; Zautra et al., 2004)—stressing characteristics such as perceptions of threat and risk, illness representations, beliefs, knowledge, self- and treatment efficacy, and outcome expectancies. Some theories view emotions as affecting health only through cognitive pathways (e.g., Witte, 1998); others view cognitive factors as operating via affective channels (Cameron & Diefenbach, 2001; Chapman & Coups, 2006; Loewenstein et al., 2001; Mellers & McGraw, 2001); and still others incorporate both emotional and cognitive elements (Cameron & Leventhal, 1995; Leventhal, Diefenbach, & Leventhal, 1992; Miller & Diefenbach, 1998). Clearly, there exists a recurrent, if unilluminating, tension between cognitive and affective approaches to human behavior.

In many ways, however, such competition is unnecessary for emotion researchers. It is well established within emotion theory that many functions are enacted through cognitive channels (Keltner, Ellsworth, & Edwards, 1993); thus emotions are likely to affect health behaviors via cognitive pathways. Take an emotion such as sadness. In addition to motivationally preventing continued investment in a "lost cause," sadness produces "dwelling" on the lost object—a cognitive process that allows the organism time for introspection, rearrangement of compromised goal commitments, and construction of contingency-based plans to deal with the loss (Consedine & Magai, 2006).

In regard to forms of NA, it has been noted above that the relation between symptom reporting and greater NA—perhaps particularly depression—may arise because depressed affect either promotes introspection and greater attention to symptoms (Mora et al., 2002) or eliminates positivistic biases (Mayne, 2001), perhaps leading to a greater likelihood of interpreting symptoms as threatening and responding with care-seeking behavior. Conversely, however, depressed affect is known to be associated with hopeless/helplessness, which may equate with low self- and treatment efficacy.

This relation may help explain the links between depression on the one hand and low screening (Husaini et al., 2001) and poor adherence (DiMatteo et al., 2000) on the other.

It has been suggested that in contrast to negative emotions, which tend to narrow attentional focus, PA may have health benefits in broadening the scope of attention (Fredrickson & Losada, 2005), producing thorough yet flexible information-processing strategies (Isen, 1999), improving outcome expectancies (Erez & Isen, 2002), and improving medical diagnostic reasoning (Isen, Chapter 34, this volume). Although it has been suggested that cognitive interventions have proven comparatively ineffective in areas such as adherence (Beswick et al., 2005), the role of cognitive processes in health behavior is a key one, and continued work examining how emotions influence or are manifest in health-promoting or health-deleterious cognitive processing is clearly needed.

Specificity: I. Discrete Emotions

Examining studies of the emotions–health interface while recalling their evolutionary design tends to suggest that research on more specific classes of affect—discrete emotions—will prove critical in disentangling the complex links between emotions and health. Although most research has concentrated on broad affective constructs—anxiety, depression, and anger/hostility (Dickerson, Gruenewald, & Kemeny, 2004)—theory regarding the functions of discrete emotions provides guidance for understanding their likely physiological, motivational, and cognitive correlates, and thus their impact on health outcomes. Table 42.1 summarizes the current literature regarding 10 discrete emotions taken from Izard (1991), as well as embarrassment and global PA and NA.

As can be seen in this summary, global PA and NA as well as fear/anxiety and sadness/depression have been the most systematically examined affects across the disease spectrum. Joy, interest, shame, and particularly anger/hostility have received some attention, although only in primary and secondary causative arenas. The research on other discrete emotions—contempt, disgust, embarrassment, guilt, and surprise—either remains isolated in only considering a specific intersection or does not exist at this point. Although relations between con-

TABLE 42.1. Summary of What Current Data Suggest Regarding How Two Global Affects and 11 Discrete Emotions Relate to Health at Five Points of Health Interface

Affective construct	Point of interface				
	Primary causative	Secondary causative	Symptom sensitivity	Detection and screening	Decisions and adherence
Global NA	– –	– –	+	+ / –	+ / –
Global PA	+ +	+ / –	?	?	+
Fear/anxiety	–	+ / –	+ / –	+ / –	+ / –
Anger/hostility	– –	– –	?	?	?
Contempt	?	?	?	?	?
Disgust	?	?	?	?	?
Sadness/depression	– –	– –	+	– –	– –
Shame	– –	–	?	?	?
Embarrassment	?	?	?	+ / –	?
Guilt	?	+ / –	?	?	?
Joy	+ +	+	?	?	?
Interest	+ / –	+ / –	?	?	?
Surprise	?	?	?	?	?

Note. ++, clear suggestion of health-promoting effects; – –, clear suggestion of health-deleterious effects; +, preliminary data suggesting some health-promoting impact; –, preliminary data suggesting some health-deleterious impact; +/–, mixed effects.

tempt and surprise appear unlikely from a theoretical point of view, there are good reasons to suspect that disgust, embarrassment, and guilt should relate to health outcomes. These three emotions are discussed briefly below.

Disgust

Despite the fact that disgust is the only discrete emotion with clear health-related functions, it has received almost no empirical attention. Fundamentally, disgust functions to obviate threats to physical health by encouraging spitting or the ejection of a noxious substance (Rozin & Fallon, 1987; Rozin, Lowery, Imada, & Haidt, 1997), and it is associated with a desire to avoid contamination (Davey & Bond, 2006). Disgust may influence dietary choices (Hamilton, 2006), obsessional behavior (Rachman, 2004), and sexual symptom reporting (Berman et al., 2003).

Guilt

A second emotion that theory implies should have relevance for the cessation of unhealthy behaviors and the motivation of healthy behaviors is guilt (Lindsey, 2005). Experiences of guilt serve a key function in moving an individual toward positive reparation and change (Dearing, Stuewig, & Tangney, 2005). A few studies have linked guilt to exercise motivation (Eyler & Vest, 2002), to attempts to make subsequent dietary or exercise-related improvements (Sukhdial & Boush, 2004), and to reduced odds of substance abuse problems (Dearing et al., 2005).

Embarrassment

Finally, because embarrassment is thought to have evolved to prevent social ostracism arising from norm violations, awkward interactions, and negative evaluations, the experience of embarrassment appears to motivate avoidance of potential eliciting situations (Consedine et al., 2007). Failures in privacy regulation constitute a key source of embarrassment (Keltner & Anderson, 2000); thus many medical contexts (particularly cancer screenings, which often involve intimate examinations) are avoided. However, because embarrassment also arises due to physical inadequacies (Keltner & Buswell, 1996), such as bad breath or being obese, anticipated embarrassment may potentially lead individuals to engage in health-promoting behaviors that prevent embarrassment.

Specificity: II. Discrete Elicitors

Understanding the role of emotions in health behavior is predicated on a clear understanding of the emotions' elicitors. Specifically, because of the likely motivational and cognitive pathways linking several discrete emotions to behavioral outcomes, knowing *exactly* what it is that (for example) frightens or embarrasses a person is probably critical in understanding when emotions will and will not promote health (Consedine et al., 2007). In the context of breast cancer screening, for example, it has been argued that fears pertaining to the screening context (e.g., fear of pain or of the medical establishment) will produce avoidance of the fear-inducing situation, and screening will therefore be infrequent. Conversely, where fears relate to the disease and expectancies are that screening will reduce anxiety, greater fear generally facilitates screening (Consedine, Magai, Krivoshekova, et al., 2004). Similarly, although experienced or anticipated embarrassment is typically a barrier to medical contacts (see above), it has been argued that understanding exactly what embarrasses people (and thus deters them from medical contacts) is a necessary precursor to developing interventions designed to reduce the impact of this barrier (Consedine et al., 2007). In differentiating among elicitors, this study also demonstrated that some elements of embarrassment *facilitated* certain classes of medical contact (Consedine et al., 2007). Future research that further discriminates among the elicitors of emotions as they relate to health is likely to prove of equal benefit.

Anticipated versus Actual Emotions

The functionalist view of emotions reminds us that emotions can be motivational in terms of both experience and anticipation. Some infrequently studied discrete emotions (such as shame, guilt, and embarrassment) are thought to motivate prosocial choices *predominantly* in anticipation—through prompting behaviors that prevent the occurrence of these emotions (Frijda, 1994), and by motivating the acquisition of experiences, skills, or attributes that foreclose on potentially unpleasant experiences (Izard, 1991). This perspective on emotion coheres nicely with the growing field of "affective forecasting," which suggests that despite the ultimate inaccuracy of such "forecasts" (Connolly & Reb, 2005), people nonetheless pay considerable attention to the anticipated affective consequences when making choices (Chapman & Coups, 2006), and to the inherent tradeoffs between short- and long-term benefits (as in the case of diet or exercise; Chapman et al., 2001). In one recent study of worry, regret, and influenza vaccination decisions, for example, it was found that persons who did not obtain vaccinations in Year 1 were more likely to get vaccinated in a subsequent year *if* they anticipated and experienced high levels of worry and regret (Chapman & Coups, 2006). Differentiating the relative contribution of experienced and anticipated affect to health behaviors, screening, and TDM, as well as examining how the predicted relations evolve with the experience of estimation–outcome contingencies, will be exciting areas for future research.

Model Generalizability

Finally, it is worth noting that few studies examining emotion–health links have specifically considered whether the relations between emotions and health outcomes are the same across groups (Consedine, Magai, & Bonanno, 2002). There are questions regarding model generalizability across genders (Van Diest et al., 2005) and ethnicities (Fredrickson et al., 2000). In my own opinion, sufficient data have been provided to make it seem likely that cultural variables moderate many vectors linking emotions and health. In one study, while NA predicted sleep disturbance in all groups, the effect was reduced among black English-speaking Caribbeans (Consedine, Magai, Cohen, et al., 2002). Other work found that although greater anger predicted reports of worse health in general, anger was related to *better* health in several groups of minority women (Consedine, Magai, & Horton, 2005). Conversely, while trait sadness was positively associated with somatic symptoms among U.S.-born white men and Dominican men, they were negatively associated with symptoms among black English-speaking Caribbean men, and the relation for anger also differed marginally across groups (Consedine, Magai, et al., 2006).

In addition, there may well be gender differences in the relations between negative emotions and disease or symptom clusters. One study of 1,017 university students found that different symptom characteristics—severity, and somatic versus psychic nature—were differentially related to NA in men and women (Van Diest et al., 2005). Specifically, high-NA women tended to report more severe symptoms, while high-NA men tended to report more common, nonspecific symptoms. Other research based in emotion theory suggests that the emotion/personality variables that best explained variance in cardiovascular disease scores differed between men and women; anxiety predicted disease for women, and hostility predicted disease for men (Consedine, Magai, & Chin, 2004).

In part because the mechanisms linking emotions and health outcomes are so complex, there is little theory to explain why global NA and some discrete emotions appear to pose different risks to persons from different ethnic and gender groups. We have argued that reconciling these complex data is likely to require considering whether the presence or absence of an emotion is telling us the same thing about persons from different ethnic groups (Consedine, Magai, et al., 2006). Cultural psychology suggests that the experiences of emotions such as anger in persons among different cultures and contexts (gender, nationality, developmental, religious, socioeconomic) may be quite different (Mesquita & Leu, 2007). For example, the discrepancy between ideals and actual emotion may be as informative in terms of health as the emotions themselves (see Tsai, Knutson, & Fung, 2006). The extent to which emotions "fit" their sociocultural contexts may be an important determinant of their impact on health—or, conversely, reports of emotions that are infrequent within such contexts (e.g., sadness for men, anger for women) may be indexing a more balanced emotional repertoire that predicts superior health outcomes (Consedine, Magai, et al., 2006). Although such competing explanatory possibilities have yet to be examined, the fact that models relating emotions and health do not appear to generalize easily across groups illuminates inadequacies in existing theory and suggests that our understanding of mechanisms is probably incomplete. Given the disparities that exist in most domains of health, research that systematically tests models across age, gender, ethnic, cultural, national, and socioeconomic groups is clearly needed.

CONCLUDING REMARKS

Human lives are born, lived, and ended in the presence of emotions. Emotions act as a major interface among the intrapersonal, sociocultural, and biological spheres of human functioning, providing a near-seamless bridge between person and environment. As such, the fact that they relate to a large number of health behaviors and health outcomes is not surprising. What have perhaps been less readily foreseen in the relations between emotions and health are the sheer pervasiveness of the links, the manifold pathways, and the litany of likely mechanisms and moderators. Although negative emotions are broadly thought to cause worse health (and positive emotions better health), the review provided above suggests that matters are vastly more complex—with variations arising depending on whether one considers direct physiological pathways, health behaviors, symptom sensitivity, screening and detection, or TDM and adherence phases of health and disease processes.

Comprehending the mechanisms underlying these links is a process that emotion researchers have only just begun, and a number of areas would benefit from further research. Some of these have been described above. Nonetheless, there exist considerable grounds for encouragement. Emotion–health researchers have access to a strongly theoretical tradition that describes the impact of emotions on physiological, motivational, cognitive, and behavioral systems, and that can thus inform their search for mechanisms.

ACKNOWLEDGMENTS

I would like to thank Carol Magai, Ratja Mesquita, and Judith Moskowitz for their helpful comments on earlier versions of this chapter.

REFERENCES

Adams, J. B., Heath, A. J., Young, S. E., Hewitt, J. K., Corley, R. P., & Stallings, M. C. (2003). Relationships between personality and preferred substance and motivations for use among adolescent substance abusers. *American Journal of Drug and Alcohol Abuse, 29,* 691–712.

Andersen, B. L. (2002). Biobehavioral outcomes following psychological interventions for cancer patients.

Journal of Consulting and Clinical Psychology, 70, 590–610.

Andersen, M. R., Smith, R., Meischke, H., Bowen, D., & Urban, N. (2003). Breast cancer worry and mammography use by women with and without a family history in a population-based sample. *Cancer Epidemiology, Biomarkers, and Prevention, 12,* 314–320.

Arnow, B., Kenardy, J., & Agras, W. S. (1995). The Emotional Eating Scale: The development of a measure to assess coping with negative affect by eating. *International Journal of Eating Disorders, 18,* 79–90.

Baum, A., & Pozluszny, D. M. (1999). Health psychology: Mapping biobehavioral contributions to health and illness. *Annual Review of Psychology, 50,* 137–163.

Berman, L., Berman, J., Felder, S., Pollets, D., Chhabra, S., Miles, M., et al. (2003). Seeking help for sexual function complaints: What gynecologists need to know about the female patient's experience. *Fertility and Sterility, 79,* 572–576.

Beswick, A. D., Rees, K., West, R. R., Taylor, F. C., Burke, M., Griebsch, I., et al. (2005). Improving uptake and adherence in cardiac rehabilitation: Literature review. *Journal of Advanced Nursing, 49,* 538–555.

Bober, S. L., Hoke, L. A., Duda, R. B., Regan, M. M., & Tung, N. M. (2004). Decision-making about tamoxifen in women at high risk for breast cancer: Clinical and psychological factors. *Journal of Clinical Oncology, 22,* 4951–4957.

Brehm, J. W. (1999). The intensity of emotion. *Personality and Social Psychology Review, 3,* 2–22.

Brigham, J., Henningfield, J. E., & Stitzer, M. L. (1991). Smoking relapse: A review. *International Journal of the Addictions, 25,* 1239–1255.

Broadstock, M., & Michie, S. (2000). Processes of patient decision making: Theoretical and methodological issues. *Psychology and Health, 15,* 191–204.

Brown, K. W., & Moskowitz, D. S. (1997). Does unhappiness make you sick?: The role of affect and neuroticism in the experience of common physical symptoms. *Journal of Personality and Social Psychology, 72,* 907–917.

Brownbridge, G., & Fielding, D. M. (1994). Psychosocial adjustment and adherence to dialysis treatment regimes. *Pediatric Nephrology, 8,* 744–749.

Callahan, C. M., Hui, S. L., Nienaber, N. A., Musick, B. S., & Tierney, W. M. (1994). Longitudinal study of depression and health-services use among elderly primary-care patients. *Journal of the American Geriatrics Society, 42,* 833–838.

Cameron, L. D., & Diefenbach, M. A. (2001). Responses to information about psychosocial consequences of genetic testing for breast cancer susceptibility: Influences of cancer worry and risk perceptions. *Journal of Health Psychology, 6,* 47–59.

Cameron, L. D., & Leventhal, H. (1995). Vulnerability beliefs, symptom experiences and the processing of health threat information: A self-regulatory perspective. *Journal of Applied Social Psychology, 25,* 1859–1883.

Cameron, L. D., Petrie, K. J., Ellis, C. J., Buick, D., & Weinman, J. A. (2005). Trait negative affectivity and responses to a health education intervention for myocardial infarction patients. *Psychology and Health, 20,* 1–18.

Campos, J. J., & Barrett, K. C. (1984). Toward a new understanding of emotions and their development. In C. E. Izard, J. Kagan & R. B. Zajonc (Eds.), *Emotions, cognition, and behavior* (pp. 229–263). Cambridge, UK: Cambridge University Press.

Carnethon, M. R., Kinder, L. S., Fair, J. M., Stafford, R. S., & Fortmann, S. P. (2003). Symptoms of depression as a risk factor for incident diabetes: Findings from the National Health and Nutrition Examination Epidemiologic Follow-Up study, 1971–1992. *American Journal of Epidemiology, 158,* 416–423.

Carney, R. M., Freedland, K. E., Eisen, S. A., Rich, M. W., Skala, J. A., & Jaffe, A. S. (1998). Adherence to a prophylactic medication regimen in patients with symptomatic versus asymptomatic ischemic heart disease. *Behavioral Medicine, 24,* 35–39.

Chapman, G. B., Brewer, N. T., Coups, E. J., Brownlee, S., Leventhal, H., & Leventhal, E. A. (2001). Value for the future and preventive health behavior. *Journal of Experimental Psychology: Applied, 7,* 235–250.

Chapman, G. B., & Coups, E. J. (2006). Emotions and preventive health behavior: Worry, regret, and influenza vaccination. *Health Psychology, 25,* 82–90.

Charles, S. T., & Almeida, D. M. (2006). Daily reports of symptoms and negative affect: Not all symptoms are the same. *Psychology and Health, 21,* 1–17.

Chesney, M. A., Darbes, L. A., Hoerster, K., Taylor, J. M., Chambers, D. B., & Anderson, D. E. (2005). Positive emotions: Exploring the other hemisphere in behavioral medicine. *International Journal of Behavioral Medicine, 12,* 50–58.

Clark, L. A., & Watson, D. (1994). Distinguishing functional from dysfunctional affective bursts. In P. Ekman & R. J. Davidson (Eds.), *The nature of emotion: Fundamental questions* (pp. 131–136). New York: Oxford University Press.

Cohen, S., Doyle, W. J., Turner, R. B., Alper, C. M., & Skoner, D. P. (2003). Emotional style and susceptibility to the common cold. *Psychosomatic Medicine, 65,* 652–657.

Cohen, S., Frank, E., Doyle, W. J., Skoner, D. P., Rabin, B. S., & Gwaltney, J. M. (1998). Types of stressors that increase susceptibility to the common cold in health adults. *Health Psychology, 17,* 214–223.

Connolly, T., & Reb, J. (2005). Regret in cancer-related decisions. *Health Psychology, 24,* S29–S34.

Consedine, N. S., Krivoshekova, Y. S., & Harris, C. R. (2007). Bodily embarrassment and judgment concern as separable factors in the measurement of medical embarrassment: Psychometric development and links to treatment-seeking outcomes. *British Journal of Health Psychology, 12,* 439–462.

Consedine, N. S., & Magai, C. (2006). Emotion development in adulthood: A developmental functionalist review and critique. In C. Hoare (Ed.), *The Oxford handbook of adult development and learning* (pp. 209–244). New York: Oxford University Press.

Consedine, N. S., Magai, C., & Bonanno, G. A. (2002). Moderators of the emotion inhibition–health relationship: A review and research agenda. *Review of General Psychology, 6,* 204–228.

Consedine, N. S., Magai, C., & Chin, S. (2004). Hostility and anxiety fear differentially predict coronary heart disease in men and women. *Sex Roles, 50,* 63–75.

Consedine, N. S., Magai, C., Cohen, C. I., & Gillespie, M. (2002). Ethnic variation in the impact of negative affect and emotion inhibition on the health of older adults. *Journal of Gerontology: Series B: Psychological Sciences, 57B,* 396–408.

Consedine, N. S., Magai, C., & Horton, D. (2005). Ethnic variation in the impact of emotion and emotion regulation on health: A replication and extension. *Journals of Gerontology: Psychological Sciences, 60B,* P165–P173.

Consedine, N. S., Magai, C., Krivoshekova, Y. S., Ryzewicz, L., & Neugut, A. I. (2004). Fear, anxiety, worry, and breast cancer screening behavior: A critical review. *Cancer Epidemiology, Biomarkers, and Prevention, 13,* 501–510.

Consedine, N. S., Magai, C., Kudadjie-Gyamfi, E. K., Kaluk Longfellow, J., Ungar, T. M., & King, A. R. (2006). Stress versus discrete negative emotion in the prediction of physical complaints: Does predictive utility vary across groups? *Cultural Diversity and Ethnic Minority Psychology, 12,* 541–557.

Consedine, N. S., Magai, C., & Neugut, A. I. (2004). The contribution of emotional characteristics to breast cancer screening among women from six ethnic groups. *Preventive Medicine, 38,* 64–77.

Consedine, N. S., Morgenstern, A. H., Kudadjie-Gyamfi, E., Magai, C., & Neugut, A. I. (2006). Prostate cancer screening behavior in men from seven ethnic groups: The fear factor. *Cancer Epidemiology, Biomarkers, and Prevention, 15,* 228–237.

Dale, W., Bilir, P., Han, M., & Meltzer, D. (2005). The role of anxiety in prostate carcinoma. *Cancer, 104,* 467–478.

Davey, G. C. L., & Bond, N. (2006). Using controlled comparisons in disgust psychopathology research: The case of disgust, hypochondriasis and health anxiety. *Journal of Behavior Therapy and Experimental Psychiatry, 37,* 4–15.

Dearing, R. L., Stuewig, J., & Tangney, J. P. (2005). On the importance of distinguishing shame from guilt: Relations to problematic alcohol and drug use. *Addictive Behaviors, 30,* 1392–1404.

Desai, M. M., Bruce, M. L., & Kasl, S. V. (1999). The effects of major depression and phobia on stage at diagnosis of breast cancer. *International Journal of Psychiatry in Medicine, 29,* 29–45.

Detmar, S. B., Muller, M. J., Schnornagel, J. H., Wever, L. D. V., & Aaronson, N. K. (2002). Role of health-related quality of life in palliative chemotherapy treatment decisions. *Journal of Clinical Oncology, 20,* 1056–1062.

Dickerson, S. S., Gruenewald, T. L., & Kemeny, M. E. (2004). When the social self is threatened: Shame, physiology, and health. *Journal of Personality, 72,* 1191–1216.

Diefenbach, M. A., Miller, S. M., & Daly, M. B. (1999). Specific worry about breast cancer predicts mammography use in women at risk for breast and ovarian cancer. *Health Psychology, 18,* 532–536.

DiMatteo, M. R., Lepper, H. S., & Croghan, T. W. (2000). Depression is a risk factor for noncompliance with medical treatment: Meta-analysis of the effects of anxiety and depression on patient adherence. *Archives of Internal Medicine, 160,* 2101–2107.

Donker, F. J. S. (2000). Cardiac rehabilitation: A review of current developments. *Clinical Psychology Review, 20,* 923–943.

Dube, L., LeBel, J. L., & Lu, J. (2005). Affect asymmetry and comfort food consumption. *Physiology and Behavior, 86,* 559–567.

Erez, A., & Isen, A. M. (2002). The influence of positive affect on the components of expectancy motivation. *Journal of Applied Psychology, 87,* 1055–1067.

Eyler, A. A., & Vest, J. R. (2002). Environmental and policy factors related to physical activity in rural white women. *Women and Health, 36,* 111–121.

Farraye, F. A., Wong, M., Hurwitz, S., Puleo, E., Emmons, K., Wallace, M. B., et al. (2004). Barriers to endscopic colorectal cancer screening: Are women different from men? *American Journal of Gastroenterology, 99,* 341–349.

Fink, A. K., Gurwitz, J., Rakowski, W., Guadagnoli, E., & Silliman, R. A. (2004). Patient beliefs and tamoxifen discontinuance in older women with estrogen receptor-positive breast cancer. *Journal of Clinical Oncology, 22,* 3309–3315.

Folkman, S., & Moskowitz, J. T. (2004). Coping: Pitfalls and promise. *Annual Review of Psychology, 55,* 745–774.

Fredrickson, B. L., & Levenson, R. W. (1998). Positive emotions speed recovery from the cardiovascular sequelae of negative emotions. *Cognition and Emotion, 12,* 191–220.

Fredrickson, B. L., & Losada, M. F. (2005). Positive affect and the complex dynamics of human flourishing. *American Psychologist, 60,* 678–686.

Fredrickson, B. L., Maynard, K. E., Helms, M. J., Haney, T. L., Siegler, I. C., & Barefoot, J. C. (2000). Hostility predicts magnitude and duration of blood pressure responses to anger. *Journal of Behavioral Medicine, 23,* 229–243.

Friedman, H. S., & Booth-Kewley, S. (1987). The "disease-prone personality": A meta-analytic view of the construct. *American Psychologist, 42,* 539–555.

Frijda, N. H. (1994). Emotions are functional, most of the time. In P. Ekman & R. J. Davidson (Eds.), *The nature of emotion: Fundamental questions* (pp. 112–122). New York: Oxford University Press.

Gascoigne, P., Mason, M. D., & Roberts, E. (1999). Factors affecting presentation and delay in patients with testicular cancer: Results of a qualitative study. *Psycho-Oncology, 8,* 144–154.

Gonzalez, J. S., Penedo, F. J., Antoni, M. H., Durdan, R. E., Fernandez, M. I., McPherson-Baker, S., et al. (2004). Social support, positive states of mind, and HIV treatment adherence in men and women living with HIV/AIDS. *Health Psychology, 23,* 413–418.

Gottschalk, L. A. (1985). Hope and other deterrents to illness. *American Journal of Psychotherapy, 39,* 515–524.

Griffin, K. W., Friend, R., Eitel, P., & Lobel, M. (1993). Effects of environmental demands, stress, and mood on health practices. *Journal of Behavioral Medicine, 16,* 643–661.

Hagglund, D., Walker-Engstrom, M. L., Larsson, G., & Leppert, J. (2003). Reasons why women with long-term urinary incontinence do not seek professional help: A cross-sectional population-based cohort study. *International Urogynecology Journal and Pelvic Floor Dysfunction, 14,* 296–304.

Hamilton, M. (2006). Disgust reactions to meat among ethically and health motivated vegetarians. *Ecology of Food and Nutrition, 45,* 125–158.

Hamilton, N. A., & Malcarne, V. L. (2004). Cognition, emotion, and chronic illness. *Cognitive Therapy and Research, 28,* 555–557.

Harburg, E., Julius, M., Kaciroti, N., Gleiberman, L., & Schork, M. A. (2003). Expressive/suppressive anger-coping responses, gender, and types of mortality: A 17-year follow-up (Tecumseh, Michigan, 1971–1988). *Psychosomatic Medicine, 65,* 588–597.

Hay, J. L., Buckley, T. R., & Ostroff, J. S. (2005). The role of cancer worry in cancer screening: A theoretical and empirical review of the literature. *Psycho-Oncology, 14,* 517–534.

Husaini, B. A., Sherkat, D. E., Bragg, R., Levine, R., Emerson, J. S., Mentes, C. M., et al. (2001). Predictors of breast cancer screening in a panel study of African American women. *Women and Health, 34,* 35–51.

Isen, A. M. (1999). Positive affect. In T. Dalgleish & M. Power (Eds.), *Handbook of cognition and emotion* (pp. 521–539). New York: Wiley.

Izard, C. E. (1991). *The psychology of emotions.* New York: Plenum Press.

Jessop, D. C., Rutter, D. R., Sharma, D., & Albery, I. P. (2004). Emotion and adherence to treatment in people with asthma: An application of the emotional Stroop paradigm. *British Journal of Psychology, 95,* 127–147.

Kalichman, S. C., Johnson, J. R., Adair, V., Rompa, D., Multhauf, K., & Kelly, J. A. (1994). Sexual Sensation Seeking: Scale development and predicting AIDS-risk behavior among homosexually active men. *Journal of Personality Assessment, 62,* 385–397.

Kalsekar, I. D., Madhavan, S. S., Amonkar, M. M., Makela, E. H., Scott, V. G., Douglas, S. M., et al. (2006). Depression in patients with Type 2 diabetes: Impact on adherence to oral hypoglycemic agents. *Annals of Pharmacotherapy, 40,* 605–611.

Kaplan, R. C., Bhalodkar, N. C., Brown, E. J., Wflite, J., & Brown, D. L. (2004). Race, ethnicity, and sociocultural characteristics predict noncompliance with lipid-lowering medications. *Preventive Medicine, 39,* 1249–1255.

Karlsson, H., Lehtinen, V., & Joukamaa, M. (1995). Are frequent attenders of primary health-care distressed? *Scandinavian Journal of Primary Health Care, 13,* 32–38.

Kassel, J. D., Stroud, L. R., & Paronis, C. A. (2003). Smoking, stress, and negative affect: Correlation, causation, and context across stages of smoking. *Psychological Bulletin, 129,* 270–304.

Kawachi, I., Sparrow, D., Spiro, A., Vokonas, P., & Weiss, S. T. (1996). A prospective study of anger and coronary heart disease: The Normative Aging Study. *Circulation, 94,* 2090–2095.

Kelsey, K. S., DeVellis, B. M., Begum, M., Belton, L., & Hooten, E. G. (2006). Positive affect, exercise and self-reported health in blue-collar women. *American Journal of Health Behavior, 30,* 199–207.

Keltner, D., & Anderson, C. (2000). Saving face for Darwin: The functions and uses of embarrassment. *Current Directions in Psychological Science, 9,* 187–192.

Keltner, D., & Buswell, B. N. (1996). Evidence for the distinctiveness of embarrassment, shame, and guilt: A study of recalled antecedents and facial expressions of emotion. *Cognition and Emotion, 10,* 155–171.

Keltner, D., Ellsworth, P. C. E., & Edwards, K. (1993). Beyond simple pessimism: Effects of sadness and anger on social perception. *Journal of Personality and Social Psychology, 64,* 740–752.

Keltner, D., & Gross, J. J. (1999). Functional accounts of emotions. *Cognition and Emotion, 13,* 467–480.

Kiecolt-Glaser, J. K., McGuire, L., Robles, T. F., & Glaser, R. (2002). Emotions, morbidity, and mortality: New perspectives from psychoneuroimmunology. *Annual Review of Psychology, 53,* 83–107.

Krantz, D. S., & McCeney, M. K. (2002). Effects of psychological and social factors on organic disease: A critical assessment of research on coronary heart disease. *Annual Review of Psychology, 53,* 341–369.

Kubzansky, L. D., Cole, S. R., Kawachi, I., Vokonas, P., & Sparrow, D. (2006). Shared and unique contributions of anger, anxiety, and depression to coronary heart disease: A prospective study in the Normative Aging Study. *Annals of Behavioral Medicine, 31,* 21–29.

Kubzansky, L. D., Wright, R. J., Cohen, S., Weiss, S., Rosner, B., & Sparrow, D. (2002). Breathing easy: A prospective study of optimism and pulmonary function in the normative aging study. *Annals of Behavioral Medicine, 24,* 345–353.

Lam, W. W. T., Fielding, R., Chan, M., Chow, L., & Or, A. (2005). Gambling with your life: The process of breast cancer treatment decision making in Chinese women. *Psycho-Oncology, 14,* 1–15.

Larsen, K., Schroll, M., & Avlund, K. (2006). Depressive symptomatology at age 75 and subsequent use of health and social services. *Archives of Gerontology and Geriatrics, 42*, 125–139.

Levenson, R. W. (1994). Human emotion: A functional view. In P. Ekman & R. J. Davidson (Eds.), *The nature of emotion: Fundamental questions* (pp. 123–126). New York: Oxford University Press.

Leventhal, E. A., Hansell, S., Diefenbach, M., Leventhal, H., & Glass, D. C. (1996). Negative affect and self-report of physical symptoms: Two longitudinal studies of older adults. *Health Psychology, 15*, 193–199.

Leventhal, H., Diefenbach, M., & Leventhal, E. A. (1992). Illness cognition: Using common sense to understand treatment adherence and affect cognition interactions. *Cognitive Therapy and Research, 16*, 143–163.

Leventhal, H., & Patrick-Miller, L. (2000). Emotions and physical illness: Causes and indicators of vulnerability. In M. Lewis & J. M. Haviland-Jones (Eds.), *Handbook of emotions* (2nd ed., pp. 523–537). New York: Guilford Press.

Lindsey, L. L. M. (2005). Anticipated guilt as behavioral motivation: An examination of appeals to help unknown others through bone marrow donation. *Human Communication Research, 31*, 453–481.

Loewenstein, G. F., Weber, E. U., Hsee, C. K., & Welch, N. (2001). Risk as feelings. *Psychological Bulletin, 127*, 267–286.

Mayne, T. J. (1999). Negative affect and health: The importance of being earnest. *Cognition and Emotion, 13*, 601–635.

Mayne, T. J. (2001). Emotions and health. In T. J. Mayne & G. A. Bonanno (Eds.), *Emotions: Current issues and future directions* (pp. 361–397). New York: Guilford Press.

McDade-Montez, E. A., Christensen, A. J., Cvengros, J. A., & Lawton, W. J. (2006). The role of depression symptoms in dialysis withdrawal. *Health Psychology, 25*, 198–204.

McKeen, N. A., Chipperfield, J. G., & Campbell, D. W. (2004). A longitudinal analysis of discrete negative emotions and health-services use in elderly individuals. *Journal of Aging and Health, 16*, 204–227.

Mellers, B. A., & McGraw, A. P. (2001). Anticipated emotions as guides to choice. *Current Directions in Psychological Science, 10*, 210–214.

Mesquita, B., & Leu, J. (2007). The cultural psychology of emotion. In S. Kitayama & D. Cohen (Eds.), *Handbook of cultural psychology* (pp. 734–759). New York: Guilford Press.

Middleton, R. A., & Byrd, E. K. (1996). Psychosocial factors and hospital readmission status of older persons with cardiovascular disease. *Journal of Applied Rehabilitation Counseling, 27*, 3–10.

Milam, J. E., Richardson, J. L., Marks, G., Kemper, C. A., & McCutchan, A. J. (2004). The roles of dispositional optimism and pessimism in HIV disease progression. *Psychology and Health, 19*, 167–181.

Miller, S. M., Bowen, D. J., Campbell, M. K., Diefenbach, M. A., Gritz, E. R., Jacobsen, P. B., et al. (2004). Current research promises and challenges in behavioral oncology: Report from the American Society of Preventive Oncology Annual Meeting, 2002. *Cancer Epidemiology, Biomarkers, and Prevention, 13*, 171–180.

Miller, S. M., & Diefenbach, M. A. (1998). The cognitive–social health information processing (C-SHIP) model: A theoretical framework for research in behavioral oncology. In D. Krantz & A. Baum (Eds.), *Technology and methods in behavioral medicine* (pp. 219–243). Mahwah, NJ: Erlbaum.

Moore, R., Brodsgaard, I., & Rosenberg, N. (2004). The contributions of embarrassment to phobic dental anxiety: A qualitative research study. *BMC Psychiatry, 4*(10). Available online at *www.biomedcentral. com/content/pdf/1471-244X-4-10.pdf*

Mora, P. A., Robitaille, C., Leventhal, H., Swigar, M., & Leventhal, E. A. (2002). Trait negative affect relates to prior-week symptoms, but not to reports of illness episodes, illness symptoms, and care seeking among older persons. *Psychosomatic Medicine, 64*, 436–449.

Moskowitz, J. T. (2003). Positive affect predicts lower risk of AIDS mortality. *Psychosomatic Medicine, 65*, 620–626.

Ogden, J. (2003). Some problems with social cognition models: A pragmatic and conceptual analysis. *Health Psychology, 22*, 424–428.

Ostir, G. V., Markides, K. S., Black, S. A., & Goodwin, J. S. (2000). Emotional well-being predicts subsequent functional independence and survival. *Journal of the American Geriatrics Society, 48*, 473–478.

Petersen, S., Schwartz, R. C., Sherman-Slate, E., Frost, H., Straub, J. L., & Damjanov, N. (2003). Relationship of depression and anxiety to cancer patients' medical decision making. *Psychological Reports, 93*, 323–334.

Pettit, J. W., Kline, J. P., Gencoz, T., Gencoz, F., & Joiner, T. E. (2001). Are happy people healthier?: The specific role of positive affect in predicting self-reported health symptoms. *Journal of Research in Personality, 35*, 521–536.

Pirraglia, P. A., Sanyal, P., Singer, D. E., & Ferris, T. G. (2004). Depressive symptom burden as a barrier to screening for breast and cervical cancers. *Journal of Women's Health, 13*, 731–738.

Pressman, S. D., & Cohen, S. (2005). Does positive affect influence health? *Psychological Bulletin, 131*, 925–971.

Rachman, S. (2004). Fear of contamination. *Behaviour Research and Therapy, 42*, 1227–1255.

Reiche, E. M. V., Morimoto, H. K., & Nunes, S. O. V. (2006). Stress and depression-induced immune dysfunction: Implications for the development and progression of cancer. *International Review of Psychiatry, 17*, 515–527.

Richman, L. S., Kubzansky, L., Maselko, J., Kawachi, I., Choo, P., & Bauer, M. (2005). Positive emotion and health: Going beyond the negative. *Health Psychology, 24,* 422–429.

Rozin, P., & Fallon, A. E. (1987). A perspective on disgust. *Psychological Review, 94,* 23–41.

Rozin, P., Lowery, L., Imada, S., & Haidt, J. (1997). The CAD triad hypothesis: A mapping between three moral emotions (contempt, anger, disgust) and three moral codes (community, autonomy, divinity). *Journal of Personality and Social Psychology, 76,* 574–586.

Rugulies, R. (2002). Depression as a predictor for coronary heart disease: A review and meta-analysis. *American Journal of Preventive Medicine, 23,* 51–61.

Silvia, P. (2001). Interest and interests: The psychology of constructive capriciousness. *Review of General Psychology, 5,* 279–290.

Sirois, B. C., & Burg, M. M. (2003). Negative emotion and coronary heart disease. *Behavioral Modification, 27,* 83–102.

Slovic, P., Peters, E., Finucane, M. L., & MacGregor, D. G. (2005). Affect, risk, and decision making. *Health Psychology, 24,* S35–S40.

Smith, T. W. (1992). Hostility and health: Current status of a psychosomatic hypothesis. *Health Psychology, 11,* 139–150.

Smith, T. W., Glazer, K., Ruiz, J. M., & Gallo, L. C. (2004). Hostility, anger, aggressiveness, and coronary heart disease: An interpersonal perspective on personality, emotion, and health. *Journal of Personality, 72,* 1217–1270.

Stefanek, M., & McDonald, P. G. (2003). Editorial: Biological mechanisms of psychosocial effects on disease: Implications for cancer control. Introduction to the special issue. *Brain, Behavior, and Immunity, 17,* S1–S4.

Sukhdial, A., & Boush, D. M. (2004). Eating guilt: Measurement and relevance to consumer behavior. *Advances in Consumer Research, 31,* 575–576.

Swan, G. E., & Carmelli, D. (1996). Curiosity and mortality in aging adults: A 5-year follow-up of the Western Collaborative Group Study. *Psychology and Aging, 11,* 449–453.

Taylor, V. M., Jackson, J. C., Tu, S.-P., Yasui, Y., Schwartz, S. M., Kuniyuki, A., et al. (2002). Cervical cancer screening among Chinese Americans. *Cancer Detection and Prevention, 26,* 139–145.

Tsai, J. L., Knutson, B., & Fung, H. H. (2006). Cultural variation in affect valuation. *Journal of Personality and Social Psychology, 90,* 288–307.

Tugade, M. M., Fredrickson, B. L., & Barrett, L. F. (2004). Psychological resilience and positive emotional granularity: Examining the benefits of positive emotions on coping and health. *Journal of Personality, 72,* 1161–1190.

Tweed, D. L., Goering, P., Lin, E., & Williams, J. I. (1998). Psychiatric morbidity and physician visits: Lessons from Ontario. *Medical Care, 36,* 573–585.

Van Diest, I., De Peuter, S., Eertmans, A., Bogaerts, K., Victoir, A., & Van den Bergh, O. (2005). Negative affectivity and enhanced symptom reports: Differentiating between symptoms in men and women. *Social Science and Medicine, 61,* 1835–1845.

Van Servellen, G., Chang, B., Garcia, L., & Lombardi, E. (2002). Individual and system level factors associated with treatment nonadherence in human immunodeficiency virus-infected men and women. *AIDS Patient Care and Studies, 16,* 269–281.

Wang, P. S., Bohn, R. L., Knight, E., Glynn, R. J., Mogun, H., & Avorn, J. (2002). Noncompliance with antihypertensive medications: The impact of depressive symptoms and psychosocial factors. *Journal of General Internal Medicine, 17,* 504–511.

Watson, D., & Pennebaker, J. W. (1989). Health complaints, stress, and distress: Exploring the central role of negative affectivity. *Psychological Review, 96,* 234–254.

Wills, T. A., Sandy, J. M., Shinar, O., & Yaeger, A. (1999). Contributions of positive and negative affect to adolescent substance use: Test of a bidirectional model in a longitudinal study. *Psychology of Addictive Behaviors, 13,* 327–338.

Witkiewitz, K., & Marlatt, G. A. (2004). Relapse prevention for alcohol and drug problems: That was Zen, this is Tao. *American Psychologist, 59,* 224–235.

Witte, K. (1998). Fear as motivator, fear as inhibitor: Using the extended parallel process model to explain fear appeal successes and failures. In P. A. Andersen & L. K. Guerrero (Eds.), *Handbook of communication and emotion: Research, theory, application, and contexts* (pp. 423–450). San Diego, CA: Academic Press.

Zautra, A. J. (2003). *Emotions, stress, and health.* New York: Oxford University Press.

Zautra, A. J., Davis, M. C., & Smith, B. W. (2004). Emotions, personality, and health: Introduction to the special issue. *Journal of Personality, 72,* 1097–1104.

CHAPTER 43

Emotion Disturbances as Transdiagnostic Processes in Psychopathology

ANN M. KRING

Emotion disturbances are ubiquitous in psychopathology. Even a cursory glance at the current version of the American diagnostic system—the *Diagnostic and Statistical Manual of Mental Disorders*, fourth edition, text revision (DSM-IV-TR; American Psychiatric Association, 2000)—reveals that nearly all the diagnostic categories include symptoms that tap one type of emotion disturbance or another (see Table 43.1). These disturbances span both positive and negative emotions, and they include excesses of emotion (as in the case of specific and social phobias, with marked and persistent fear); deficits in emotion (as in the case of narcissistic personality disorder, with a lack of empathy); social emotional problems (as in autistic disorder, with a lack of emotional reciprocity); and regulation problems (as in borderline personality disorder, with difficulties in controlling anger). The pervasiveness of emotion disturbances in psychopathology suggests the potential for commonalities across disorders. Indeed, there may be emotional distur-

bances that are central to a number of different disorders; yet the manifestation of these disturbances may differ from disorder to disorder, thus helping to account for the different symptom constellations across disorders. In this chapter, I consider the utility of adopting a transdiagnostic approach to understanding emotion disturbances in psychopathology across several levels, including descriptive phenomenology, etiology, and treatment.

CONSTRAINING EMOTION AND AFFECT

Emotions have developed through the course of human evolutionary history to prepare organisms to act in response to a number of environmental stimuli and challenges. This account suggests that emotions, under most circumstances, serve a number of important intra- and interpersonal functions (e.g., Frijda, 1986; Keltner & Kring, 1998; Lang, Bradley, &

TABLE 43.1. Emotion-Based Symptoms in DSM-IV-TR Disorders

Disorders	Symptoms
Schizophrenia and other psychotic disorders	
Schizophrenia	
Schizoaffective disorder	
Schizophreniform disorder	Affective flattening, anhedonia
Mood disorders	
Major depressive episode	Depressed mood, anhedonia
Dysthymia	Depressed mood
Manic or hypomanic episode	Elevated, expansive, or irritable mood
Anxiety disorders	
Panic disorder	Intense fear or discomfort
Agoraphobia	Anxiety
Specific and social phobias	Marked and persistent fear, anxious anticipation
Obsessive–compulsive disorder	Marked anxiety or distress
Posttraumatic stress disorder	Irritability, anger, distress, anhedonia, restricted range of affect
Acute stress disorder	Anxiety or increased arousal
Generalized anxiety disorder	Excessive anxiety and worry, irritability
Somatoform disorders	
Hypochondriasis	Preoccupation with fears of having disease
Eating disorders	
Anorexia nervosa	Fear of gaining weight
Sleep disorders	
Sleep terror disorder	Intense fear and signs of autonomic arousal
Circadian rhythm sleep disorder, nightmare disorder	Clinically significant distress
Impulse control disorders	
Pathological gambling	Irritability, dysphoric mood
Trichotillomania	Tension; pleasure or relief after hair pulling
Intermittent explosive disorder	Rage, anger
Pyromania, kleptomania	Tension or excited mood
Adjustment disorders	Marked distress
Personality disorders	
Paranoid personality disorder	Quickness to react angrily
Schizoid personality disorder	Emotional coldness, detachment, flattened affect
Schizotypal personality disorder	Inappropriate or constricted affect, excessive social anxiety
Antisocial personality disorder	Lack of remorse, irritability
Borderline personality disorder	Affective instability due to marked reactivity of mood, inappropriate intense anger, or difficulty controlling anger
Histrionic personality disorder	Rapidly shifting and shallow expressions of emotion
Narcissistic personality disorder	Lack of empathy
Avoidant personality disorder	Fear of criticism, disapproval, or rejection
Dependent personality disorder	Fear of being unable to care for self, being left alone
Substance-related disorders	
Alcohol intoxication	Mood lability
Alcohol withdrawal	Anxiety
Amphetamine and cocaine intoxication	Euphoria or affective blunting; anxiety, tension, anger
Amphetamine and cocaine withdrawal	Dysphoric mood

(continued)

TABLE 43.1. *(continued)*

Disorders	Symptoms
Substance-related disorders (cont.)	
Caffeine intoxication	Nervousness, excitement
Cannabis intoxication	Euphoria, anxiety
Dementias	
Dementia due to Pick's disease	Emotional blunting
Dementia due to Huntington's disease	Depression, irritability, anxiety
Childhood disorders	
Autistic disorder, Asperger's disorder nonverbal behaviors, such as facial expression	Lack of emotional reciprocity; marked impairment in
Separation anxiety disorder	Distress, worry, fearfulness
Oppositional defiant disorder	Quickness to lose temper, get angry, be annoyed by others
Childhood disintegrative disorder	Impairment in nonverbal behaviors; lack of social or emotional reciprocity
Other conditions	
Bereavement	Guilt

Cuthbert, 1990; Levenson, 1994). As I have argued elsewhere, the functions of emotion in persons with psychopathology are comparable to those for persons without psychopathology (Keltner & Kring, 1998; Kring & Bachorowski, 1999). However, emotion disturbances in psychopathology interfere with the achievement of emotion-related functions. For example, the absence of facial expressions in a patient with schizophrenia may evoke negative responses from others (Krause, Steimer-Krause, & Hufnagel, 1992), thus negatively affecting his or her social relationships and interactions (e.g., Hooley, Richters, Weintraub, & Neale, 1987).

Emotions are typically considered to have multiple components, including expression, experience, and physiology. The extent to which these emotion components correspond with one another or cohere remains a topic of debate (e.g., Barrett, 2006a; Bradley & Lang, 2000; Mauss, Levenson, McCarter, Wilhelm, & Gross, 2005). Functionalist accounts of emotion suggest that coherence among components is adaptive (e.g., Levenson, 1994), but the empirical data supporting coherence are mixed (Barrett, 2006a). There are a number of reasons why particular emotion components may not cohere in any given study—including sample characteristics, emotion elicitation methods, emotion component measurements,

and data-analytic techniques, as well as whether even under ideal circumstances, emotion coherence is the exception rather than the norm. Nevertheless, the lack of coherence across multiple emotions, situations, and contexts has been observed in different psychological disorders (e.g., schizophrenia, psychopathy) and has been considered an emotional disturbance (e.g., Kring, 2001).

Although the terms "affect" and "emotion" are used interchangeably in the psychopathology literature, there are important conceptual and empirical distinctions between the terms. Generally speaking, "affect" is most often used in reference to feeling states, whereas "emotion" is used in reference to multiple components (only one of which is a feeling state). Barrett and colleagues have distinguished "core affect" from the more generic term "affect." Core affect reflects neurophysiological states that are an omnipresent indicator of a person(s relationship to his or her environment at any given time (Barrett, 2006a; Barrett, Mesquita, Ochsner, & Gross, 2007; Russell, 2003; Barrett & Russell, 1999). Core affect is experienced as feelings of pleasure or displeasure, and to a lesser extent arousal or activation (Barrett, 2006a; Barrett et al., 2007). Although core affect is observed across cultures, there are nevertheless important individual and cultural differences (Barrett, 2006b; Mesquita &

Karasawa, 2002) that may be important for understanding disturbances in core affect in psychopathology.

THE TRANSDIAGNOSTIC APPROACH

In a recent and influential book, Harvey, Watkins, Mansell, and Shafran (2004) have reviewed the literature on cognitive and behavioral maintaining processes in psychopathology. Rather than organizing their book by disorder, they have instead adopted a transdiagnostic perspective, reviewing the evidence for common processes across different disorders. Their analysis points to an accumulating body of evidence of disruptions in a number of processes, such as attention, memory, reasoning, and avoidance, that are common across more than one adult disorder and that serve to maintain or exacerbate the symptoms of these disorders. Similar conclusions have been reached regarding common cognitive maintaining processes across the eating disorders (Fairburn, Cooper, & Shafran, 2003), and treatment approaches that target transdiagnostic processes across disorders have recently been developed for depression, anxiety, and eating disorders (e.g., Barlow, Allen, & Choate, 2004; Fairburn et al., 2003; Norton, Hayes, & Hope, 2004).

Harvey et al. (2004) have argued that there are a number of key advantages to adopting a transdiagnostic perspective in psychopathology. First, the transdiagnostic perspective may help to account for the high rates of comorbidity among the current DSM disorders. Indeed, comorbidity is the norm rather than the exception. In the National Comorbidity Survey (NCS), Kessler et al. (1994) found that nearly 80% of individuals with a lifetime diagnosis of one disorder had received at least one other lifetime diagnosis. In the NCS replication study, 45% of people who met criteria for one diagnosis in the prior 12 months met criteria for at least one more diagnosis (Kessler, Chiu, Demler, & Walters, 2005). Other studies have found similarly high rates of comorbidity. For example, nearly two-thirds of individuals with depression meet diagnostic criteria for an anxiety disorder (e.g., Mineka, Watson, & Clark, 1998), and as many as 50% of individuals who meet criteria for an anxiety disorder are depressed (e.g., Brown et al., 2001). The high level of comorbidity may well reflect problems

in the current diagnostic system (e.g., poor discriminant validity). However, the rampant comorbidity also suggests that there may be common symptoms or processes across disorders, including emotional processes.

Second, a transdiagnostic approach may be useful for developing and evaluating treatments. For example, recent theory and empirical data point to the notion that currently available treatments for anxiety and depression are changing common aspects of these disorders, rather than disorder-specific aspects (e.g., Barlow et al., 2004; Hayes, Strosahl, & Wilson, 1999; Persons, Roberts, & Zalecki, 2003). In addition, evidence from treatment outcome studies suggests that interventions for one disorder (e.g., depression) are also effective in treating other disorders (e.g., generalized anxiety disorder) (e.g., Brown & Barlow, 1992; Tsao, Mystkowski, Zucker, & Craske, 2002). A transdiagnostic perspective may illuminate the common mechanisms or processes across disorders, which may then be more directly targeted in treatment.

A transdiagnostic approach to emotion disturbances in psychopathology has been suggested, sometimes implicitly, by other theorists, researchers, and clinicians (e.g., Barlow et al., 2004; Patrick & Bernat, 2006; Thayer & Brosschot, 2005). However, the reach of such an approach has been fairly limited thus far, for at least two reasons. First, some disorders lend themselves more clearly to such an approach than others, given their comorbidities, comparable treatments, and treatment responses. For example, mood and anxiety disorders—two broad categories that are collectively referred to as the "emotional disorders" (e.g., Barlow, 2004; Watson, 2005)—have been discussed in transdiagnostic terms across many levels. Other disorders that may well benefit from a transdiagnostic approach (e.g., personality disorders) have not yet stimulated much transdiagnostic theory and research. Many of the examples of the transdiagnostic approach to emotion disturbances in psychopathology illustrated throughout the chapter will involve the mood and anxiety disorders.

A second reason why the transdiagnostic approach to emotion disturbances has been fairly limited is probably the fact that the prevailing paradigm in psychopathology research over the past several decades has been "disorder-centric." That is, most investigations are designed to answer questions about the symptoms, causes, and treatments of individual disorders. In the realm of emotion and psychopathology, studies are typically designed to study a particular emotion disturbance in a particular disorder. For example, the literature is packed with studies of particular emotion disturbances (e.g., facial emotion perception deficits) in putatively distinct disorders (e.g., depression, borderline personality disorder, schizophrenia), with little consideration of the possibility that the emotion disturbance may cut across these disorders. Such disorder-centric research is perpetuated by the field's relatively greater emphasis on internal validity (e.g., tightly controlled study of one disorder) over external validity (e.g., naturalistic study of comorbid disorders), as reflected in editorial practices at top-flight journals and funding priorities at granting agencies. As such, the entry point for a majority of psychopathology studies is typically a single disorder rather than multiple disorders, with relatively less emphasis on mechanisms or processes (such as emotion disturbances) that may cut across traditional diagnostic boundaries. Unfortunately, this disorder-centric focus overlooks the fact that most disorders do not occur in "pure" form, and thus conclusions regarding specificity of emotion disturbances in X disorder may not be particularly informative with respect to understanding X disorder as it more commonly occurs in combination with Y disorder.

Despite these challenges, the promise of a transdiagnostic approach to emotion disturbances in psychopathology is evident at many levels. First, a transdiagnostic approach can inform the ways in which different disorders are classified. In other words, examining emotion-related commonalities at the symptom level may help to account for the high levels of comorbidity in the current diagnostic system, and in turn may provide guidance on refining diagnostic categories. Second, a transdiagnostic approach can be informative with respect to identifying common emotion-related causal and/or maintaining processes across disorders. Third, a transdiagnostic approach can be useful for treatment development, with an emphasis on changing emotion processes. In the remaining sections of this chapter, I consider the relative merits of adopting a transdiagnostic approach to emotion disturbances in psychopathology across these three levels: descriptive phenomenology, etiology, and treatment.

DESCRIPTIVE PSYCHOPATHOLOGY AND DIAGNOSIS

In an effort to spur the field toward greater attention to emotion and psychopathology, Berenbaum, Raghavan, Le, Vernon, and Gomez (2003) have proposed a separate taxonomy of emotional disturbances as a companion to the current diagnostic system. Their taxonomy parses specific emotion (e.g., shame, guilt, happiness, fear) disturbances into three broad areas of disruption: "valence," "intensity/regulation," and "disconnections." Each of the broad categories is further subdivided to achieve greater specificity of particular emotion disturbances. Emotional valence disturbances can involve pleasant or unpleasant emotions, as well as too much or too little of these emotions. For example, the limited experience of pleasure (i.e., anhedonia) that characterizes depression and schizophrenia, as well as the excess of fear in panic disorder, would constitute valence disturbances. Emotional intensity/regulation disturbances are defined as over- or underregulation of both pleasant and unpleasant emotions. For example, mania, which is characterized by excesses in both pleasant (joy, euphoria) and unpleasant (irritability) emotions, would be construed as an emotional intensity/regulation disturbance. Disconnection disturbances reflect disconnections between the expressive component of emotion and other components, as in schizophrenia, where patients experience strong feelings yet do not express them outwardly (e.g., Berenbaum & Oltmanns, 1992; Kring & Neale, 1996; Kring & Earnst, 1999). Disconnection disturbances also reflect a lack of conscious awareness of one's own emotional responses. Berenbaum et al. (2003) conclude their paper with nine recommendations for future research, but these do not explicitly include the possibility of examining these disturbances across disorders. Instead, the recommendations are geared toward amplifying our understanding of specific disorders; examining emotion disturbances independently from diagnosed disorders; modifying treatments for specific disorders by targeting emotion disturbances; and examining similarities and differences in the disturbances across gender, culture, and the lifespan. Although these are certainly important goals for future research, the transdiagnostic implications of this taxonomy are also ripe for further investigation.

In a commentary on Berenbaum et al.'s article, Watson (2003) has argued that including the taxonomy as a companion to the current diagnostic system would add unnecessary complexity and serve to further reify already problematic diagnostic categories. Although he does not suggest a transdiagnostic approach, Watson has nonetheless argued for "scrapping these heterogeneous diagnostic categories and focusing instead on homogeneous symptom clusters" (p. 237). In this view, focusing on the current DSM symptoms, many of which reflect emotion disturbances, may be a more fruitful way of classifying psychopathology.

More recently, Watson (2005) has expanded upon this idea, arguing that the current configuration of mood disorders and anxiety disorders ought to be replaced with a different configuration. Specifically, he proposes a quantitative hierarchical model to account for the high levels of comorbidity between mood and anxiety disorders, drawing upon structural analyses of the diagnostic symptoms at both the phenotypic and genotypic levels. His model includes an overarching domain referred to as "emotional disorders." This would consist of three subdomains, including what Watson calls "distress disorders" (generalized anxiety disorder, posttraumatic stress disorder, major depressive disorder, dysthymia), "bipolar disorders" (bipolar I and II disorders, cyclothymia), and "fear disorders" (specific and social phobias, panic disorder, agoraphobia). Watson's proposal is more than a simple reshuffling of diagnostic categories, and this approach is certainly a more rational and empirically supported approach to situating the mood and anxiety disorders in the diagnostic system than is the current, purely phenomenological approach. The model also points to the promise of a transdiagnostic approach to the descriptive phenomenology of mental disorders.

Indeed, part of the impetus for Watson's (2005) proposed model has come from the influential theory and research on common and distinct emotion disturbances in the mood and anxiety disorders. Clark and Watson (1991) originally proposed the tripartite model to account for the relationship between anxiety and depression (see also Watson, Clark, et al., 1995; Watson, Weber, et al., 1995; Watson, Weise, Vaidya, & Tellegen, 1999). In this model, a general distress factor characterized by high levels of negative activation (NA) is common to both anxiety and depression; a sec-

ond factor, characterized by low levels of positive activation (PA) or pleasurable engagement with the environment, is specific to depression; and a third factor, variously referred to as "anxious arousal" (AA) or "somatic arousal," is specific to anxiety. A revision to the model was later proposed, to account better for the heterogeneity among the anxiety disorders (Mineka et al., 1998). The revised model, termed the integrative hierarchical model, followed from additional data suggesting that high levels of AA are more characteristic of panic disorder in particular than of the anxiety disorders in general (Brown, Chorpita, & Barlow, 1998; Zinbarg & Barlow, 1996).

Watson (2005) has argued that data generated from the integrative hierarchical model thus far are not sufficient to account fully for the comorbidity among the mood and anxiety disorders. Thus he has proposed the new quantitative model to account better for the extensive comorbidities, while at the same time retaining the current diagnostic categories (i.e., a disorder-centric approach). An alternative to Watson's model is the dissection of mood and anxiety disorders into categories based on emotion-related difficulties. Thus, instead of separate categories for the different mood and anxiety disorders, there might be an overarching category of general distress disorders with subdomains of low-PA disorders and high-AA disorders. Brown et al. (1998) proposed such a structural model, showing that many of the anxiety disorders and depression were better accounted for by the emotion-based factors of NA, PA, and AA, though they did not explicitly call for the scrapping of the specific mood and anxiety disorder categories. More recently, Barlow and colleagues have pushed this idea further, noting that "*DSM-IV* emotional disorder categories do not qualify in any sense as real entities . . . but do seem to be useful concepts or constructs that emerge as "blips" on a general background of NAS [negative affect syndrome]" (Barlow et al., 2004, p. 212), and suggesting that future revisions of the DSM may do well to eliminate many of the current categories of disorders (Moses & Barlow, 2006). This is a fairly radical proposal, but perhaps one whose time has (nearly) come.

It is true that the field's disorder-centric approach, which has been central at least since the development of DSM-III (Wilson, 1993), has proven to be advantageous in the diagnosis, assessment, and treatment of various disorders. Furthermore, reconfiguring the current diagnostic categories based only on emotion-related disturbances might leave out much clinically relevant information. However, a transdiagnostic approach would not necessarily have to supplant the current diagnostic categories for it to inform our understanding of the symptoms of various disorders. Indeed, mental disorders do not just consist of emotion-related symptoms. Different symptoms reflect other processes, including cognitive (e.g., inattention, thought disorder), behavioral (e.g., avoidance), and interpersonal (e.g., no close friends or confidants) processes. However, understanding the emotion-related symptoms that cut across disorders may help to refine the current diagnostic categories without necessarily reconfiguring them, as Watson (2005) has suggested. For example, knowing that individuals with depression and panic disorder share the heightened experience of NA, even though panic is also characterized by AA and depression is characterized by low PA, provides key information about similarities and differences between these two disorders that is not readily acknowledged in the current diagnostic system.

CAUSAL AND MAINTAINING PROCESSES

There have been several recent reviews of emotion disturbances in psychopathology (e.g., Kring & Werner, 2004; Rottenberg & Johnson, 2007). Instead of duplicating these efforts, I focus here on candidate transdiagnostic emotion disturbances that may reflect causal or maintaining processes. There are many points along the temporal course of disorders at which a transdiagnostic perspective may be informative (Barnett & Gotlib, 1988; Harvey et al., 2004). Specifically, transdiagnostic emotion disturbances may be antecedents (i.e., predisposing or vulnerability factors), concomitants, or consequences (i.e., perpetuating or maintaining factors). For an emotion disturbance to be considered an antecedent transdiagnostic process, it must be shown to precede the onset of a disorder. Disturbances that are observed during active episodes of disorders may be more accurately construed as concomitant transdiagnostic processes, and disturbances that persist after active episodes have abated might be considered consequences or maintaining processes. Much of the evidence to date regarding specific

emotion disturbances in particular disorders is most readily interpreted as evidence for maintaining processes. There has been less theoretical, conceptual, and empirical work on possible transdiagnostic causal or maintaining emotion processes than in the domains of phenomenology and treatment. Indeed, the disorder-centric focus of research has been particularly dominant in studies of possible etiological emotion disturbances, making integration across disorders more of a challenge. Although space constraints preclude me from considering all possible transdiagnostic emotion disturbances, I briefly consider four promising candidates here: core affect, emotion awareness, emotion regulation, and emotion disconnections.

Core Affect

As discussed earlier, Barrett and colleagues define "core affect" as neurophysiological states that are experienced as pleasant or unpleasant and are ever-present indicators of a person's relationship to his or her environment (Barrett, 2006a; Barrett et al., 2007; Russell, 2003; Barrett & Russell, 1999). Findings from several studies that have measured reports of feeling states have indicated that the experience of excessive unpleasant affect (although it is not necessarily conceived of as "core affect") is common across many different disorders, including depression (for a review, see Mineka et al., 1998), the anxiety disorders (Mineka et al., 1998), eating disorders (e.g., Stice, 2001), schizophrenia (for a review, see Kring, 2001), substance-related disorders (e.g., Kassel, Stroud, & Paronis, 2003), and a number of personality disorders (e.g., Berenbaum et al., 2006; Huperich, 2005; Putnam & Silk, 2005). Integrating findings across behavioral and brain imaging studies, Barrett et al. (2007) have suggested that disturbances in core affect may reflect an important emotion-related transdiagnostic process in psychopathology. Indeed, the conceptual, theoretical, and empirical advances regarding core affect among healthy individuals are ripe for translation into the realm of psychopathology.

Emotion Awareness

Barrett and Gross (2001) have argued that knowledge and awareness of one's emotions are necessary prerequisites to effective emotion regulation. However, simply having knowledge about emotion is not sufficient; rather, greater accessibility of that emotion knowledge is believed to promote effective emotion regulation. Individuals who describe their feelings in a more differentiated manner (e.g., "sad," "confused," "elated") rather than more globally (e.g., "good," "bad") have greater accessibility to and awareness of emotion knowledge and use this knowledge when the regulation of emotion may be necessary (Barrett, Gross, Christensen, & Benvenuto, 2001).

What is the evidence for emotion awareness difficulties in psychopathology? Although being aware of how one feels is at the heart of most types of psychotherapy, surprisingly little research has explicitly examined emotion awareness in psychopathology and how it may wax or wane with the exacerbation and remission of symptoms. There is some evidence suggesting that patients with schizophrenia do not differ from individuals without schizophrenia in terms of their emotion knowledge. However, patients with schizophrenia differentiate less among emotional states, and thus may be less effective at emotion regulation (Kring, Barrett, & Gard, 2003). Clinical conceptualizations of borderline personality disorder include the notion that patients have difficulty distinguishing among different emotional states (e.g., Westen, 1991), but the empirical confirmation of this notion is needed. A recent investigation of schizotypal personality disorder symptoms found that such symptoms were associated with poor emotion clarity, but more attention to emotions (Berenbaum et al., 2006).

Related to emotion awareness, the construct of "alexithymia" refers to difficulties in verbalizing feelings. The most widely used measure of this construct, the Toronto Alexithymia Scale (Bagby, Parker, & Taylor, 1994), includes two subscales that appear important to emotion awareness: difficulty in identifying feelings and difficulty in describing feelings. This measure has been widely used in correlational studies of psychiatric symptoms (e.g., Grabe, Spitzer, & Freyberger, 2004; Parker, Bagby, & Taylor, 1991), anxiety disorders (e.g., Frewin, Pain, Dozois, & Lanius, 2006; Parker, Taylor, Bagby, & Acklin, 1993; Turk, Heimberg, Luterek, Mennin, & Fresco, 2005), eating disorders (e.g., Cochrane et al., 1993), personality disorders (e.g., Berenbaum, 1996), substance-related disorders (e.g., Speranza et al., 2004), and insomnia (e.g., Lundh & Broman, 2006).

However, the linkages between this construct and the various disorders are not always replicated across studies. Additional work is thus needed to clarify alexithymia as a transdiagnostic process, beyond correlations between the one measure and symptoms within disorders.

Emotion Regulation

Emotion regulation problems have been at the forefront of discussions about emotion disturbances in psychopathology for at least the last 10 years (e.g., Barlow et al., 2004; Gross & Muñoz, 1995; Kring & Werner, 2004; Linehan, 1993). Broadly, emotion regulation refers to processes that serve to modify what we feel, when we feel it, and how we use that feeling to guide behavior (e.g., Gross, 1998). Many current diagnostic criteria explicitly refer to emotion regulation difficulties. For example, the criteria "difficulty controlling anger" in borderline personality disorder; "efforts to avoid feelings" in posttraumatic stress disorder (PTSD); "difficulty controlling worry" in generalized anxiety disorder; and "rapidly shifting expressions of emotion" in histrionic personality disorder all point to difficulties in regulating emotions.

Despite the perceived importance of emotion regulation deficits in psychopathology, it is difficult to integrate the literatures across disorders, because of the myriad approaches to constraining the concept of emotion regulation across studies. For example, some researchers do not distinguish emotional responding from regulation, following from theory that suggests the processes are indistinguishable (e.g., Campos, Frankel, & Camras, 2004; Davidson, 2000). Other studies examine emotion regulation within the individual, whereas still other studies examine emotion regulation from the outside (e.g., having others provide soothing to down-regulate negative emotion). Disentangling emotion from emotion regulation remains a critical challenge for the field (Rottenberg & Gross, 2003). Greater conceptual clarity will advance our understanding of how emotion regulation difficulties may be linked across different disorders.

A close cousin to emotion regulation is the time course, or chronometry, of emotional responses (e.g., Davidson, 1998). Emotional responses are not wholly temporally constrained by the presence of an eliciting stimulus, but instead vary in their peak and duration in ways that may hold important information about the nature of emotion disturbances in psychopathology. Two elements of the time course of an emotional response that have been studied in healthy populations are (1) the time from the onset to the peak intensity of the response, and (2) the recovery time, or the time it takes for the emotional response to resolve. This latter process, recovery time, is a probable transdiagnostic emotion disturbance that remains a topic for future research. For example, the prolonged experience of NA associated with depression, generalized anxiety disorder, and eating disorders, or the prolonged experience of PA associated with bipolar disorder, may reflect a difficulty in the recovery time of emotional responding (e.g., Tomarken & Keener, 1998).

Emotion Disconnections

A good deal of evidence indicates that patients with schizophrenia report experiencing strong emotions in response to a variety of emotionally evocative stimuli (films, pictures, social interactions); yet they do not often display these feelings outwardly (for reviews, see Kring, 2001; Kring & Werner, 2004). In other words, these patients' outward displays of emotion are not often accurate reflections of their experienced emotion, indicating a disconnection between emotion response components. There is some evidence to suggest that this disconnection may be present prior to the onset of the illness. Walker, Grimes, Davis, and Smith (1993) analyzed home movies of adults with schizophrenia that were made before the adults developed schizophrenia. They found that girls displayed fewer joy expressions, and that both boys and girls displayed more negative facial expressions, compared to their healthy siblings.

Studies using the emotion-modulated startle paradigm (Lang et al., 1990) have observed a different disconnection among individuals with psychopathy. Compared to healthy controls, these individuals showed comparable startle inhibition during exposure to pleasant stimuli, but they did not show startle potentiation during exposure to aversive stimuli (e.g., Patrick, 1994; Patrick, Bradley, & Lang, 1993). However, the individuals with psychopathy did not differ from controls in their reported emotional experience to the aversive stimuli. Additional evidence for this disconnection has been found

in imagery studies (Patrick, Cuthbert, & Lang, 1994) and incidental memory paradigms (Christianson et al., 1996).

In both of the examples above, patients' reports of emotional experience were indistinguishable from healthy controls, but their behavioral or psychophysiological responses differed. It may well be that such emotion disturbances are better construed as reflecting a relatively intact core affect system with corresponding behavioral system disturbances.

TREATMENT DEVELOPMENT AND EVALUATION

Although medication is a common form of treatment for many different disorders, very few investigations have explicitly adopted a transdiagnostic approach to evaluating pharmacological treatment. Nevertheless, the evidence that particular medications may be effective for multiple disorders is hiding in plain sight. For example, studies have found that antidepressant medications are effective at reducing the symptoms of several other disorders, including specific and social phobias (e.g., Stein et al., 1998; Van Ameringen et al., 2001), panic disorder (White & Barlow, 2002), generalized anxiety disorder (Lydiard & Monnier, 2004), obsessive–compulsive disorder (Steketee & Barlow, 2002), posttraumatic stress disorder (Brady et al., 2000), some of the personality disorders (e.g., Rinne, van den Brink, Wouters, & van Dyck, 2002), and eating disorders (e.g., Walsh et al., 2000). Following from such evidence, medications that were originally approved by the U.S. Food and Drug Administration (FDA) for the treatment of depression have since received approval (or an "indication," in FDA terminology) for the treatment of other disorders. For example, paroxetine (Paxil) was later approved for the treatment of obsessive–compulsive disorder, panic disorder, generalized anxiety disorder, and social anxiety; fluoxetine (Prozac) was later approved for the treatment of obsessive–compulsive disorder and bulimia nervosa; sertraline (Zoloft) was later approved for the treatment of obsessive–compulsive disorder, panic disorder, social anxiety, and PTSD.

Although it may be the case that antidepressant medications are rather blunt instruments for targeting the general distress that is common across disorders, little research has directly examined the emotion-related mechanisms by which the medications might exert their transdiagnostic effects. However, we know that the selective serotonin reuptake inhibitors work on the neurotransmitter serotonin (as well as others, including dopamine; e.g., Svenningsson et al., 2002), functionally leaving more serotonin in the synapse, and that disruptions in serotonin have been implicated in depression (e.g., Thase, Jindal, & Howland, 2002), anxiety disorders (e.g., Stein, 1998), and eating disorders (e.g., Carrasco, Dyaz-Marsa, Hollander, Cesar, & Saiz-Ruiz, 2000; Kaye et al., 1998). We also know a good deal about how serotonin works throughout the brain, and perhaps not surprisingly, this neurotransmitter is heavily concentrated in areas of the brain linked with emotion (e.g., Barrett et al., 2007; Wrase et al., 2006). Finally, research has indicated that serotonin levels are associated with PA among healthy individuals (e.g., Duffy et al., 2006; Zald & Depue, 2001). The building blocks are thus available for constructing a transdiagnostic approach to medication treatment that explicitly links pharmacology, neuroscience, and emotion. Much of this integrative work remains to be done, but it is certainly a fruitful avenue for future research.

Historically, different forms of psychotherapy were conceived of as treatments that could be applied across disorders or clinical problems (e.g., psychoanalysis). Furthermore, despite the distinctly different theoretical traditions underpinning various types of psychotherapy (e.g., psychodynamic, interpersonal, gestalt, client-centered, behavioral), each of these traditions has included some consideration of emotion (for reviews, see Greenberg, 2002b; Greenberg & Safran, 1987). One form of psychotherapy that is relevant to the focus of this chapter is emotion-focused therapy (EFT), which was developed by Leslie Greenberg (e.g., Greenberg, 2002a). Boiled down to its essence, EFT is based on the idea that some emotions are adaptive, whereas others are maladaptive. Maladaptive emotions are based on an underlying loneliness, abandonment, worthlessness, anger, or inadequacy, and they can interfere with a person's relationships and overall functioning. The primary therapeutic goal is for a client to become more aware of these maladaptive emotions, to understand the source of these feelings, and to learn emotion regulation skills. According to Greenberg (2002a), EFT is better

suited to particular types of clinical conditions (including depression and generalized anxiety disorder) and less well suited to others (such as panic disorder). Unfortunately, data regarding the efficacy of this treatment are limited. No randomized controlled clinical trials have been conducted, although smaller studies examining the process of change within EFT indicate that the treatment is effective for some clinical problems (Greenberg, 2002a). The theoretical foundations of this treatment continue to be enhanced by research in emotion, emotion and psychopathology, and affective neuroscience (e.g., Greenberg, 2002b, 2004, and Chapter 6 of this volume); a worthwhile endeavor for future research would be to examine whether this treatment is effective in targeting transdiagnostic emotion-related disturbances.

The shift to more disorder-specific psychotherapeutic approaches perhaps began in the late 1950s, with the pioneering work of Joseph Wolpe (1958), who developed systematic desensitization for the treatment of specific phobias. Additional disorder-specific psychotherapies were developed in the 1960s, as cognitive-behavioral therapies became more prominent. A number of other influences in the field since the 1970s have converged to solidify a disorder-specific approach to treatment development. These have included the greater demand to show that psychotherapy is effective; the development of the DSM-III, which was heavily influenced by the medical model (Wilson, 1993); the sophistication of research methods to evaluate treatment outcomes (e.g., Barlow, 2004; Westen, Novotny, & Thompson-Brenner, 2004); the emphasis on evidence-based practice (e.g., Barlow, 1996; Chambless & Hollon, 1998; Kendall, 1998); the efforts to position psychology as a health care profession and thus in the larger health care context (e.g., Johnson, 2001); and the observation that psychological treatments tailored to specific disorders are as effective as, or more effective than, other types of interventions. Indeed, as Barlow (2004) has noted, "few would argue that diversity in procedures to address specific aspects of pathology is not necessary" (p. 873).

The disorder-specific approach to treatment development, particularly in the context of empirically supported treatments (Chambless & Hollon, 1998), has spawned a large number of individual treatment protocols and manuals. This proliferation of different treatment protocols has undoubtedly benefited countless individuals who have received these treatments, as they have been shown to be effective (Nathan & Gorman, 2002). However, the sheer magnitude of treatment protocols has become a bit overwhelming to treatment professionals, with respect to both learning the varied protocols and disseminating them to a broader range of treatment providers (Barlow et al., 2004; Persons, 2005). Furthermore, the reality in clinical practice is that providers often select bits and pieces from a number of different protocols, in order to provide the best possible treatment for a given individual patient (Persons, 2005). Partly in reaction to this overwhelming number of treatment protocols, there has recently been a call for more unified treatments across disorders. This conversation has been situated primarily within the mood and anxiety disorders, and it has been informed by research on emotion-related disturbances that are common across these disorders.

Following from research on the structural configuration of descriptive phenomenology and shared etiologies across mood and anxiety disorders, Barlow and colleagues have proposed a unified treatment for these disorders (Barlow et al., 2004; Moses & Barlow, 2006). The focus of this intervention is on putative emotion-related mechanisms that may be driving the emotion disturbances that cut across mood and anxiety disorders. The treatment has three main components: (1) altering cognitive reappraisals, a key component in emotion regulation processes; (2) preventing emotional avoidance; and (3) changing emotion action tendencies, or replacing emotion behaviors associated with fear and anxiety with behaviors related to positive emotions. These key components of the intervention have their origin in basic science in emotion, in both healthy and disordered individuals. Time will tell whether the intervention is as effective as other available treatments. Because the intervention is designed to target emotion-related mechanisms that cut across disorders, it is transdiagnostic at heart, and it seems likely that it will pay off. Indeed, there has been a call for more treatments to target mechanisms rather than disorders per se. For example, Rosen and Davison (2003) have argued that we should be defining empirically supported principles of change rather than empirically supported treatments.

Other recent treatments have been designed to target emotional disturbances, such as Mennin and colleagues' emotion regulation treatment for generalized anxiety disorder (e.g., Mennin, 2004). Though this intervention was designed around the emotion regulation problems associated with generalized anxiety disorder, it seems probable that it would be useful for a number of disorders with similar difficulties in emotion regulation, such as an inability to down-regulate intense negative emotions and a lack of awareness of negative emotions.

SUMMARY AND CONCLUSIONS

Advances in affective neuroscience and basic behavioral research in emotion have greatly contributed to our understanding of emotion disturbances in psychopathology. Indeed, methods, theories, and measures developed in these domains have allowed us to achieve greater clarity regarding the reach of emotion disturbances across many different disorders. With this clarity has come the realization that many of the observed emotion disturbances may be common across disorders. Progress in understanding the reach of transdiagnostic emotion disturbances has begun to be achieved at the levels of descriptive phenomenology and treatment. Although transdiagnostic treatment approaches targeting emotion disturbances are grounded in theory regarding emotion-based mechanisms, more work is needed to unpack the nature of transdiagnostic etiological processes that are emotion-based.

REFERENCES

American Psychiatric Association. (2000). *Diagnostic and statistical manual of mental disorders* (4th ed., text rev.). Washington, DC: Author.

Bagby, M. R., Parker, J. D. A., & Taylor, G. J. (1994). The twenty-item Toronto Alexithymia Scale: I. Item selection and cross validation of the factor structure. *Journal of Psychosomatic Research, 38,* 23–32.

Barlow, D. H. (1996). The effectiveness of psychotherapy: Science and policy. *Clinical Psychology: Science and Practice, 1,* 109–122.

Barlow, D. H. (2004). Psychological treatments. *American Psychologist, 59,* 869–878.

Barlow, D. H., Allen, L. B., & Choate, M. L. (2004). Toward a unified treatment for emotional disorders. *Behavior Therapy, 35,* 205–230.

Barnett, P. A., & Gotlib, I. H. (1988). Psychosocial functioning and depression: Distinguishing among antecedents, concomitants, and consequences. *Psychological Bulletin, 104*, 97–126.

Barrett, L. F. (2006a). Solving the emotion paradox: Categorization and the experience of emotion. *Personality and Social Psychology Review, 10*, 20–46.

Barrett, L. F. (2006b). Valence is a basic building block of emotional life. *Journal of Research in Personality, 40*, 35–55.

Barrett, L. F., & Gross, J. J. (2001). Emotional intelligence: A process model of emotion representation and regulation. In T. J. Mayne & G. A. Bonanno (Eds.), *Emotions: Current issues and future directions* (pp. 286–310). New York: Guilford Press.

Barrett, L. F., Gross, J. J., Christensen, T. C., & Benvenuto, M. (2001). Knowing what you're feeling and knowing what to do about it: Mapping the relation between emotion differentiation and emotion regulation. *Cognition and Emotion, 15*, 713–724.

Barrett, L. F., Mesquita, B., Ochsner, K., & Gross, J. J. (2007). The experience of emotion. *Annual Review of Psychology, 58*, 373–403.

Barrett, L. F., & Russell, J. A. (1999). The structure of current affect: Controversies and emerging consensus. *Current Directions in Psychological Science, 8*, 10–14.

Berenbaum, H. (1996). Childhood abuse, alexithymia, and personality disorder. *Journal of Psychosomatic Research, 41*, 585–595.

Berenbaum, H., Boden, M. T., Baker, J. P., Dizen, M., Thompson, R. J., & Abramowitz, A. (2006). Emotional correlates of the different dimensions of schizotypal personality disorder. *Journal of Abnormal Psychology, 115*, 359–368.

Berenbaum, H., & Oltmanns, T. F. (1992). Emotional experience and expression in schizophrenia and depression. *Journal of Abnormal Psychology, 101*, 37–44.

Berenbaum, H., Raghavan, G., Le, H.-N., Vernon, L. L., & Gomez, J. J. (2003). A taxonomy of emotional disturbances. *Clinical Psychology: Science and Practice, 10*, 206–226.

Bradley, M. M., & Lang, P. J. (2000). Measuring emotion: Behavior, feeling, and physiology. In R. D. Lane & L. Nadel (Eds.), *Cognitive neuroscience of emotion* (pp. 242–276). New York: Oxford University Press.

Brady, K., Pearlstein, T., Asnis, G. M., Baker, D., Rothbaum, B., Sikes, R., & Farfel, G. U. (2000). Efficacy and safety of sertraline treatment of posttraumatic stress disorder. *Journal of the American Medical Association, 283*, 1837–1844.

Brown, T. A., & Barlow, D. H. (1992). Comorbidity among anxiety disorders: Implications for treatment and DSM-IV. *Journal of Consulting and Clinical Psychology, 60*, 835–44.

Brown, T. A., Campbell, L. A., Lehman, C. L., et al. (2001). Current and lifetime comorbidity of the DSM-IV anxiety and mood disorders in a large clinical sample. *Journal of Abnormal Psychology, 110*, 585–599.

Brown, T. A., Chorpita, B., & Barlow, D. H. (1998). Structural relationships among dimensions of the *DSM-IV* anxiety and mood disorders and dimensions of negative affect, positive affect, and autonomic arousal. *Journal of Abnormal Psychology, 107*, 179–192.

Campos, J. J., Frankel, C. B., & Camras, L. (2004). On the nature of emotion regulation. *Child Development, 75*, 377–394.

Carrasco, J. L., Dyaz-Marsa, M., Hollander, E., Cesar, J., & Saiz-Ruiz, J. (2000). Decreased monoamine oxidase activity in female bulimia. *European Neuropsychopharmacology, 10*, 113–117.

Chambless, D., & Hollon, S. (1998). Defining empirically supported therapies. *Journal of Consulting and Clinical Psychology, 66*, 7–18.

Christianson, S. A., Forth, A. E., Hare, R. D., Strachan, C., Lidberg, L., & Thorell, L. H. (1996). Remembering details of emotional events: A comparison between psychopathic and nonpsychopathic offenders. *Personality and Individual Differences, 20*, 437–443.

Clark, L. A., & Watson, D. (1991). Tripartite model of anxiety and depression: Psychometric evidence and psychometric implications. *Journal of Abnormal Psychology, 100*, 316–336.

Cochrane, C. E., Brewerton, T. D., Wilson, D. B., & Hodges, E. L. (1993). Alexithymia in the eating disorders. *International Journal of Eating Disorders, 14*, 219–228.

Davidson, R. J. (1998). Affective style and affective disorders: Perspectives from affective neuroscience. *Cognition and Emotion, 12*, 307–330.

Davidson, R. J. (2000). The functional neuroanatomy of affective style. In R. D. Lane & L. Nadel (Eds.), *Cognitive neuroscience of emotion* (pp. 371–388). New York: Oxford University Press.

Duffy, M. E., Stewart-Knox, B. J., McConville, C., Bradbury, I., O'Connor, J., Helander, A., et al. (2006). The relationship between whole blood serotonin and subjective mood in apparently healthy postmenopausal women. *Biological Psychiatry, 73*, 165–168.

Fairburn, C. G., Cooper, Z., & Shafran, R. (2003). Cognitive behavioural treatment for eating disorders: A transdiagnostic theory and treatment. *Behaviour Research and Therapy, 41*, 509–528.

Frewin, P. A., Pain, C., Dozois, D. J. A., & Lanius, R. A. (2006). Alexithymia in PTSD: fMRI and psychometric studies. *Annals of the New York Academy of Sciences, 1071*, 397–400.

Frijda, N. (1986). *The emotions.* Cambridge, UK: Cambridge University Press.

Grabe, H. J., Spitzer, C., & Freyberger, H. J. (2004). Alexithymia and personality in relation to dimensions of psychopathology. *American Journal of Psychiatry, 161*, 1299–1301.

Greenberg, L. S. (2002a). *Emotion-focused therapy: Coaching clients to work through their feelings.* Washington, DC: American Psychological Association.

Greenberg, L. S. (2002b). Integrating and emotion-focused approach to treatment into psychotherapy integration. *Journal of Psychotherapy Integration*, 12, 154–189.

Greenberg, L. S. (2004). Emotion-focused therapy. *Clinical Psychology and Psychotherapy*, 11, 3–16.

Greenberg, L. S., & Safran, J. D. (1987). *Emotion in psychotherapy*. New York: Guilford Press.

Gross, J. J. (1998). The emerging field of emotion regulation: An integrative review. *Review of General Psychology*, 2, 271–299.

Gross, J. J., & Muñoz, R. F. (1995). Emotion regulation and mental health. *Clinical Psychology: Science and Practice*, 2, 151–164.

Harvey, A., Watkins, E., Mansell, W., & Shafran, R. (2004). *Cognitive behavioural processes across psychological disorders: A transdiagnostic approach to research and treatment*. New York: Oxford University Press.

Hayes, S. C., Strosahl, K. D., & Wilson, K. G. (1999). *Acceptance and commitment therapy: An experiential approach to behavior change*. New York: Guilford Press.

Hooley, J. M., Richters, J. E., Weintraub, S., & Neale, J. M. (1987). Psychopathology and marital distress: The positive side of positive symptoms. *Journal of Abnormal Psychology*, 96, 27–33.

Huperich, S. K. (2005). Differentiating avoidant and depressive personality disorders. *Journal of Personality Disorders*, 19, 659–673.

Johnson, N. G. (2001, April). President's column: Psychology's mission includes health: An opportunity. *Monitor on Psychology*, 32(4). Retrieved from *www.apa.org/monitor/apr01/pc.html*

Linehan, M. M. (1993). *Cognitive-behavioral treatment of borderline personality disorder*. New York: Guilford Press.

Kassel, J. D., Stroud, L. R., & Paronis, C. A. (2003). Smoking, stress, and negative affect: Correlation, causation, and context across stages of smoking. *Psychological Bulletin*, 129, 270–304.

Kaye, W. H., Greeno, C. G., Moss, H., Fernstrom, J., Lilenfeld, L. R., Wahlund, B., et al. (1998). Alterations in serotonin activity and platelet monoamine oxidase and psychiatric symptoms after recovery from bulimia nervosa. *Archives of General Psychiatry*, 55, 927–935.

Keltner, D., & Kring, A. M. (1998). Emotion, social function, and psychopathology. *Review of General Psychology*, 2, 320–342.

Kendall, P. C. (1998). Empirically supported psychological therapies. *Journal of Consulting and Clinical Psychology*, 66, 3–6.

Kessler, R. C., Chiu, W. T., Demler, O., & Walters, E. (2005). Prevalence, severity, and comorbidity of 12 month DSM-IV disorders in the National Comorbidity Survey replication. *Archives of General Psychiatry*, 62, 617–627.

Kessler, R. C., McGonagle, K. A., Zhao, S., Nelson, C. B., Hughes, M., Eshleman, S., et al. (1994). Lifetime and 12-month prevalence of *DSM-III-R* psychiatric disorders in the United States: Results from the National Comorbidity Survey. *Archives of General Psychiatry*, 51, 8–19.

Krause, R., Steimer-Krause, E., & Hufnagel, H. (1992). Expression and experience of affects in paranoid schizophrenia. *Revue Européenne de Psychologie Appliquée*, 42, 131–138.

Kring, A. M. (2001). Emotion and psychopathology. In T. J. Mayne & G. Bonanno (Eds.), *Emotion: Current issues and future directions* (pp. 337–360). New York: Guilford Press.

Kring, A. M., & Bachorowski, J.-.A. (1999). Emotion and psychopathology. *Cognition and Emotion*, 13, 575–599.

Kring, A. M., Barrett, L. F., & Gard, D. E. (2003). On the broad applicability of the circumplex: Representations of affective knowledge in schizophrenia. *Psychological Science*, 14, 207–214.

Kring, A. M., & Earnst, K. S. (1999). Stability of emotional responding in schizophrenia. *Behavior Therapy*, 30, 373–388.

Kring, A. M., & Neale, J. M. (1996). Do schizophrenic patients show a disjunctive relationship among expressive, experiential, and psychophysiological components of emotion? *Journal of Abnormal Psychology*, 105, 249–257.

Kring, A. M., & Werner, K. H. (2004). Emotion regulation in psychopathology. In P. Philippot & R. S. Feldman (Eds.), *The regulation of emotion* (pp. 359–385). Mahwah, NJ: Erlbaum.

Lang, P. J., Bradley, M. M., & Cuthbert, B. N. (1990). Emotion, attention, and the startle reflex. *Psychological Review*, 97, 377–395.

Levenson, R. W. (1994). Human emotion: A functional view. In P. Ekman & R. J. Davidson (Eds.), *The nature of emotion* (pp. 123–126). New York: Oxford University Press.

Lundh, L.-G., & Broman, E.-L. (2006). Alexithymia and insomnia. *Personality and Individual Differences*, 40, 1615–1624.

Lydiard, R. B., & Monnier, J. (2004). Pharmacological treatment. In R. G. Heimberg, C. L. Turk, & D. S. Mennin (Eds.), *Generalized anxiety disorder* (pp. 351–381). New York: Guilford Press.

Mauss, I., Levenson, R. W., McCarter, L., Wilhelm, F., & Gross, J. J. (2005). The tie that binds?: Coherence among emotion experience, behavior, and physiology. *Emotion*, 5, 175–190.

Mennin, D. (2004). Emotion regulation therapy for generalized anxiety disorder. *Clinical Psychology and Psychotherapy*, 11, 17–29.

Mesquita, B., & Karasawa, M. (2002). Different emotional lives. *Cognition and Emotion*, 16, 127–141.

Mineka, S., Watson, D., & Clark, L. A. (1998). Comorbidity of anxiety and unipolar mood disorders. *Annual Review of Psychology*, 49, 377–412.

Moses, E. B., & Barlow, D. H. (2006). A new unified treatment approach for emotional disorders based on emotion science. *Current Directions in Psychological Science, 15*, 146–150.

Nathan, P. E., & Gorman, J. M. (Eds.). (2002). *A guide to treatments that work*. London: Oxford University Press.

Norton, P. J., Hayes, S. A., & Hope, D. A. (2004). Effects of a transdiagnostic group treatment for anxiety disorders on secondary depression. *Depression and Anxiety, 20*, 198–202.

Parker, J. D. A., Bagby, M., & Taylor, G. J. (1991). Alexithymia and depression: Distinct or overlapping constructs? *Comprehensive Psychiatry, 32*, 387–394.

Parker, J. D. A., Taylor, G. J., Bagby, R. M., & Acklin, M. W. (1993). Alexithymia in panic disorder and simple phobia: A comparative study. *American Journal of Psychiatry, 150*, 1105–1107.

Patrick, C. J. (1994). Emotion and psychopathy: Startling new insights. *Psychophysiology, 31*, 319–330.

Patrick, C. J., & Bernat, E. M. (2006). The construct of emotion as a bridge between personality and psychopathology. In R. F. Krueger & J. L. Tackett (Eds.), *Personality and psychopathology* (pp. 174–209). New York: Guilford Press.

Patrick, C. J., Bradley, M. M., & Lang, P. J. (1993). Emotion in the criminal psychopath: Startle reflex modulation. *Journal of Abnormal Psychology, 102*, 82–92.

Patrick, C. J., Cuthbert, B. N., & Lang, P. J. (1994). Emotion in the criminal psychopath: Fear image processing. *Journal of Abnormal Psychology, 103*, 523–534.

Persons, J. B. (2005). Empiricism, mechanism, and the practice of cognitive-behavior therapy. *Behavior Therapy, 36*, 107–118.

Persons, J. B., Roberts, N. A., & Zalecki, C. (2003). Anxiety and depression change together during treatment. *Behavior Therapy, 34*, 149–163.

Putnam, K. M., & Silk, K. R. (2005). Emotion dysregulation and the development of borderline personality disorder. *Development and Psychopathology, 17*, 899–925.

Rinne, T., van den Brink, W., Wouters, L., & van Dyck, R. (2002). SSRI treatment of borderline personality disorder: A randomized, placebo-controlled clinical trial for female patients with borderline personality disorder. *American Journal of Psychiatry, 159*, 2048–2054.

Rosen, G. M., & Davison, G. C. (2003). Psychology should list empirically supported principles of change (ESPs) and not credential trademarked therapies or other treatment packages. *Behavior Modification, 27*, 300–312.

Rottenberg, J., & Gross, J. J. (2003). When emotion goes wrong: Realizing the promise of affective science. *Clinical Psychology: Science and Practice, 10*, 227–232.

Rottenberg, J., & Johnson, S. L. (Eds.). (2007). *Emotion and psychopathology: Bridging affective and clinical science*. Washington, DC: American Psychological Association.

Russell, J. A. (2003). Core affect and the psychological construction of emotion. *Psychological Review, 110*, 145–172.

Speranza, M., Corcos, M., Stéphan, P., Loas, G., Pérez-Diaz, F., Lang, F., et al. (2004). Alexithymia, depressive experiences, and dependency in addictive disorders. *Substance Use and Misuse, 39*, 567–595.

Stein, M. B. (1998). Neurobiological perspectives on social phobia: From affiliation to zoology. *Biological Psychiatry, 44*, 1277–1285.

Stein, M. B., Liebowitz, M. R., Lydiard, R. B., Pitts, C. D., Bushnell, W., & Gergel, I. (1998). Paroxetine treatment of generalized social phobia (social anxiety disorder): A randomized clinical trial. *Journal of the American Medical Association, 280*, 708–713.

Steketee, G., & Barlow, D. H. (2002). Obsessive–compulsive disorder. In D. H. Barlow, *Anxiety and its disorders: The nature and treatment of anxiety and panic* (pp. 516–550). New York: Guilford Press.

Stice, E. (2001). A prospective test of the dual-pathway model of bulimic pathology: Mediating effects of dieting and negative affect. *Journal of Abnormal Psychology, 110*, 124–135.

Svenningsson, P., Tzavara, E. T., Witkin, J. M., Fienberg, A. A., Nomikos, G. G., & Greengard, P. (2002). Involvement of striatal and extrastriatal DARPP-32 in biochemical and behavioral effects of fluoxetine (Prozac). *Proceedings of the National Academy of Sciences of the USA, 99*, 3182–3187.

Thase, M. E., Jindal, R., & Howland, R. H. (2002). Biological aspects of depression. In C. L. Hammen & I. H. Gotlib (Eds.), *Handbook of depression* (pp. 192–218). New York: Guilford Press.

Thayer, J. F., & Brosschot, J. F. (2005). Psychomatics and psychopathology: Looking up and down from the brain. *Psychoneuroendocrinology, 30*, 1050–1058.

Tomarken, A. J., & Keener, A. D. (1998). Frontal brain asymmetry and depression: A self-regulatory perspective. *Cognition and Emotion, 12*. 387–420.

Tsao, J. C. I., Mystkowski, J. L., Zucker, B. G., & Craske, M. G. (2002). Effects of cognitive behavioral therapy for panic disorder on comorbid conditions: Replication and extension. *Behaviour Therapy, 33*, 493–509.

Turk, C. L., Heimberg, R. G., Luterek, J. A., Mennin, D. S., & Fresco, D. M. (2005). Emotion dysregulation in generalized anxiety disorder: A comparison with social anxiety disorder. *Cognitive Therapy and Research, 29*, 89–106.

Van Ameringen, M. A., Lane, R. M., Walker, J. R., Bowen, R. C., Chokka, P. R., Goldner, E. M., et al. (2001). Sertraline treatment of generalized social phobia: A 20-week, double-blind, placebo-controlled study. *American Journal of Psychiatry, 158*, 275–281.

Walker, E. F., Grimes, K. E., Davis, D. M., & Smith, A. J. (1993). Childhood precursors of schizophrenia:

Facial expressions of emotion. *American Journal of Psychiatry, 150,* 1654–1660.

Walsh, B. T., Agras, S. W., Devlin, M. J., Fairburn, C. G., Wilson, G. T., Kahn, C., & Chally, M. K. (2000). Fluoxetine for bulimia nervosa following poor response to psychotherapy. *American Journal of Psychiatry, 157,* 1332–1334.

Watson, D. (2003). Subtypes, specifiers, epicycles, and eccentrics: Toward a more parsimonious taxonomy of psychopathology. *Clinical Psychology: Science and Practice, 10,* 233–238.

Watson, D. (2005). Rethinking the mood and anxiety disorders: A quantitative hierarchical model for *DSM-V. Journal of Abnormal Psychology, 114,* 522–536.

Watson, D., Clark, L. A., Weber, K., Assenheimer, J. S., Strauss, M. E., & McCormick, R. A. (1995). Testing a tripartite model II: Exploring the symptom structure of anxiety and depression in student, adult, and patient samples. *Journal of Abnormal Psychology, 104,* 15–25.

Watson, D., Weber, K., Assenheimer, J. S., Clark, L. A., Strauss, M. E., & McCormick, R. A. (1995). Testing a tripartite model I: Evaluating the convergent and discriminant validity of anxiety and depression scales. *Journal of Abnormal Psychology, 104,* 3–14.

Watson, D., Weise, D., Vaidya, J., & Tellegen, A. (1999). The two general activation systems of affect: Structural findings, evolutionary considerations, and psychobiological evidence. *Journal of Personality and Social Psychology, 76,* 820–838.

Westen, D. (1991). Cognitive-behavioral interventions in the psychoanalytic psychotherapy of borderline personality disorders. *Clinical Psychology Review, 11,* 211–230.

Westen, D., Novotny, C. M., & Thompson-Brenner, H. (2004). The empirical status of empirically supported psychotherapies: Assumptions, findings, and reporting in controlled clinical trials. *Psychological Bulletin, 130,* 631–663.

White, K. S., & Barlow, D. H. (2002). Panic disorder and agoraphobia. In D. H. Barlow, *Anxiety and its disorders: The nature and treatment of anxiety and panic* (pp. 328–379). New York: Guilford Press.

Wilson, M. (1993). DSM-III and the transformation of American psychiatry: A history. *American Journal of Psychiatry, 150,* 399–410.

Wolpe, J. (1958). *Psychotherapy by reciprocal inhibition.* Stanford, CA: Stanford University Press.

Wrase, J., Reimold, M., Puls, I., Kienast, T., & Heinz, A. (2006). Serotonergic dysfunction: Brain imaging and behavioral correlates. *Cognitive, Affective, and Behavioral Neuroscience, 6,* 53–61.

Zald, D. H., & Depue, R. A. (2001). Serotonergic functioning correlates with positive and negative affect in psychiatrically healthy males. *Personality and Individual Differences, 30,* 71–86.

Zinbarg, R. E., & Barlow, D. H. (1996). Structure of anxiety and the anxiety disorders: A hierarchical model. *Journal of Abnormal Psychology, 105,* 181–193.

PART VIII

SELECT EMOTIONS

CHAPTER 44

Fear and Anxiety
Overlaps and Dissociations

ARNE ÖHMAN

Fear is a ubiquitous experience among humankind that can be traced back to a distant mammalian heritage. Recent world events, with terrorist attacks randomly striking innocent bystanders at many places, highlight the long-standing insight that fear is an inevitable part of human existence. Throughout human history, fear and its close ally, anxiety, provide recurrent themes for people pondering their existential predicament and have inspired frequent artistic representations. In a clinical context, the vicissitudes of fear and anxiety have been understood as keys to the dynamics of psychopathology—whether these are conceptualized in terms of a learnable drive supporting escape and avoidance, or as the targets of psychologically distorting defense mechanisms. The ubiquity and controversial status of fear and anxiety have made them central topics for research and reflection; they have generated a voluminous literature (see, e.g., Barlow, 2002;

Bourke, 2006; Tuma & Maser, 1985), only a tiny fraction of which can be represented in this chapter.

The point of departure for this chapter is that fear and anxiety are closely related emotional phenomena originating in evolved mammalian defense systems. Nonetheless, in spite of their overlap, research during the last decade has started to unravel important differences between them. The chapter starts with a brief conceptual overview and proceeds to consider the situational contexts of fear in an evolutionary perspective. A model of fast, unconscious mechanisms in the generation of fear is presented and discussed in relation to behavioral data from backward-masking and attentional paradigms. Then follows a section devoted to the biology of fear and anxiety, reviewing neuroanatomical, genetic, and psychophysiological data that collectively provide a distinction between them. The chapter concludes with a discussion of the implications of the knowledge presented in prior sections for the clinical understanding of fear and anxiety.

THE PHENOMENA OF FEAR AND ANXIETY

Fear and anxiety are obviously overlapping, aversive, activated states centered on threat. They both involve intense negative feelings and strong bodily manifestations. Subjectively, however, they take somewhat different forms. Fear denotes dread of impending disaster and an intense urge to defend oneself, primarily by getting out of the situation. Clinical anxiety, on the other hand, has been described as an ineffable and unpleasant feeling of foreboding (Lader & Marks, 1973). Accordingly, the glossary of the *Diagnostic and Statistical Manual of Mental Disorders*, fourth edition, text revision (DSM-IV-TR; American Psychiatric Association [APA], 2000), uses the term "anxiety" to denote "apprehensive anticipation of future danger or misfortune accompanied by a feeling of dysphoria or somatic symptoms of tension" (p. 820). "Fear" is said to differ from anxiety primarily in having an identifiable eliciting stimulus. In a sense, therefore, anxiety is often "prestimulus" (i.e., anticipatory to [more or less real] threatening stimuli), whereas fear is "poststimulus" (i.e., elicited by a defined fear stimulus).

As eloquently argued by Epstein (1972), external stimuli are insufficient to distinguish fear and anxiety. He concluded that fear is related to coping behavior, particularly escape and avoidance. However, when coping attempts fail (e.g., because the situation is uncontrollable), fear is turned into anxiety. In Epstein's view, then, "*fear* is an avoidance motive. If there were no restraints, internal or external, fear would support the action of flight. *Anxiety* can be defined as unresolved fear, or, alternatively, as a state of undirected arousal following the perception of threat" (1972, p. 311). In fear, therefore, it is an obvious (albeit not necessarily clearly perceived) danger located in space and time that must be dealt with; in anxiety, on the other hand, the nature and location of the threat remain more obscure and thus are difficult to cope with by active defensive maneuvers.

Fear may be focused on external sources, as in *phobias*. Or anxiety may be situationally unfocused, as in free-floating or *generalized anxiety*. The latter may come in the form of *episodic panic attacks* (i.e., as sudden emotional surges dominated by physical symptoms, sometimes with and sometimes without clear precipitants), which form the backbone of *panic disorder* (PD). Or it may be a relatively constant mental preoccupation with more or less reasonable threats and dangers—associated with somatic symptoms—as in *generalized anxiety disorder* (GAD).

As these descriptions imply, fear and anxiety can be regarded both as *emotional states*, evoked in a particular context and having a limited duration, and as *personality traits*, characterizing individuals across time and situations (e.g., Spielberger, 1972; Rapee, 1991). The differences between clinical and normal fear/anxiety include that the former is more recurrent and persistent; that its intensity is unreasonable, given the objective danger or threat; that it tends to paralyze individuals, making them helpless and unable to cope; and that it results in impeded psychosocial or physiological functioning (e.g., Lader & Marks, 1973).

THE SITUATIONAL CONTEXT OF FEAR AND ANXIETY

Basically, fear is a functional emotion with a deep evolutionary origin, reflecting the fact that earth has always been a hazardous environment to inhabit. Staying alive is a prerequisite for the basic goal of biological evolution—sending genes on to subsequent generations. Hence even the most primitive of organisms have developed defense responses to deal with life threats in their environment, whether these are unhealthy chemicals in the surroundings, circumstances suggesting a hunting predator, or aggressive conspecifics. Viewed from the evolutionary perspective, fear is central to mammalian evolution. As a product of natural selection, it is shaped and constrained by evolutionary contingencies. Our evolutionary history is obvious in the fears and phobias that we humans exhibit and readily learn. We are more likely to fear events and situations that provided threats to the survival of our ancestors, such as potentially deadly predators, heights, and wide-open spaces, than to fear the most frequently encountered potentially deadly objects in our contemporary environment, such as handguns or motorcycles (Öhman & Mineka, 2001; Seligman, 1971).

Traumatic Situations

Extreme danger jeopardizing one's life (or the lives of close kin) elicits intense fright and may have long-lasting consequences in the form of posttraumatic stress disorder (PTSD). Trauma may involve natural catastrophes, such as floods or hurricanes destroying homes or communities; or it may involve seeing others being seriously injured or killed as a result of an accident or physical violence. If the trauma results in PTSD, the traumatic event is persistently reexperienced (e.g., in the form of "flashbacks"); stimuli or events associated with the trauma are avoided; and the person feels generally numbed with regard to emotions. Common anxiety symptoms experienced by persons suffering from PTSD include sleep and concentration difficulties, irritability or anger outbursts, hypervigilance, and exaggerated startle. Some events, such as torture, frequently result in PTSD, whereas others, such as natural disasters or car accidents, only occasionally result in the disorder (APA, 2000).

Commonly Feared and Potentially Phobic Situations

Survival considerations, either contemporary or in an evolutionary perspective, are relevant for most situational dimensions of human fears. Arrindell, Pickersgill, Merckelbach, Ardon, and Cornet (1991) reviewed studies factor-analyzing questionnaire data on self-reported fear, arguing that the results from nearly 200 studies fit a simple structure involving four factors. The first factor was "fears about interpersonal events or situations." It included fears of criticism and social interaction, rejection, conflicts, and evaluation, but also interpersonal aggression and display of sexual and aggressive scenes. The second factor was "fears related to death, injuries, illness, blood, and surgical procedures." This factor had a quite heterogeneous content, with fear of bodily ailments, illness, and death as the common theme. The third factor, "fear of animals," included common domestic animals; other small, often harmless animals; and creeping and crawling animals such as insects and reptiles. Finally, "agoraphobic fears" was the fourth factor. It involved fear of entering public places (such as stores or shopping malls) and crowds, but also fear of closed spaces (such as elevators, theaters, or churches) or places lacking an escape route to a safe haven (such as bridges and tunnels, and traveling alone in trains, buses, or airplanes).

All these four factors represent situations of relevance for human evolution. Human history is replete with examples of how social conflicts that have escalated out of control can create potentially deadly dangers, not to speak of the social threat in terms of the defeat and humiliation they may involve (Öhman, 1986). Thus it comes as no surprise that social interactions are sometimes feared. For fear of death and illness, and associated bodily conditions, there is no need to elaborate the potential survival threat. Although many animals are friendly and sought as companions, there is no question that animals as predators have posed recurrent threats that have been an important force in shaping the evolution of humankind. Indeed, it is reasonable to give reptiles a privileged position as the prototypical predators (Isbell, 2006; Öhman, 1986; Öhman, Dimberg, & Öst, 1985; Öhman & Mineka, 2001, 2003). Finally, agoraphobic fears center on the lack of security inherent in separation from safe bases and kin, and the avoidance of places associated with panic and feelings of discomfort.

These factors correspond to four prominent types of *phobias* (intense fright and avoidance of specific situations or events): social phobia, blood phobia, animal phobia, and agoraphobia. Furthermore, the second factor incorporates fears often encountered in PD, such as fears or syncope, and in obsessive–compulsive disorder (OCD), such as contamination. Departing from a preparedness perspective on phobias (Seligman, 1971), my colleagues and I (Öhman et al., 1985; Öhman & Mineka, 2001) have argued that these fears reflect basic, evolutionarily shaped behavioral systems. Specifically, we have suggested that social fears originated in a dominance–submissiveness system, the adaptive function of which was to promote social order by facilitating the establishment of dominance hierarchies. Animal fears, on the other hand, are attributed to a predatory defense system, originating in the fear of the exclusive predators of early mammals—snakes and reptiles—and later in fear of venomous snakes among monkeys and apes (Isbell, 2006).

These evolved systems involve stimuli for which organisms were adaptively shaped by evolution to associate easily with fear and defense. By co-occurring with actual danger, they may through Pavlovian fear conditioning be compromised into producing social and animal phobias when the fear responses they engender become conditioned to stimuli that actually are harmless in the ecology of modern humans (Öhman & Mineka, 2001). The basic argument is that evolution has equipped humans with a propensity to associate fear with situations that threatened the survival of their ancestors (Seligman, 1971). Hence, although humans in general are prepared to acquire some fears (e.g., snake fears) easily, some individuals are more prepared than others to develop fears of particular situations. Thus the development of phobias is jointly determined by genetic predispositions and specific environmental exposures. We have tested these ideas (see reviews by Dimberg & Öhman, 1996; McNally, 1987; Öhman, 1993; Öhman & Mineka, 2001) in autonomic conditioning experiments primarily comparing acquisition and resistance to extinction of skin conductance conditioning to potentially phobic (e.g., snakes, spiders, angry faces) and neutral (e.g., flowers, mushrooms, neutral faces, or friendly faces) stimuli. The general finding has been that responses conditioned to potentially phobic stimuli show enhanced resistance to extinction, compared to responses conditioned to neutral stimuli (Öhman & Mineka, 2001; Dimberg & Öhman, 1996). Examples of data on skin conductance responses from a single cue conditioning paradigm are given in Figure 44.1.

THE ROLE OF UNCONSCIOUS PROCESSES IN ANXIETY AND FEAR

This section of the chapter focuses on the psychological mechanisms underlying the adaptive input–output relationships for fear and anxiety that have been discussed in previous sections. A model is presented that emphasizes the role of automatic, unconscious processes in the generation of fear and anxiety.

A Functional Perspective on Fear and Anxiety

As I have pointed out earlier (Öhman, 1993) defense responses are of little use unless they are appropriately elicited. Thus they require perceptual systems that can effectively locate

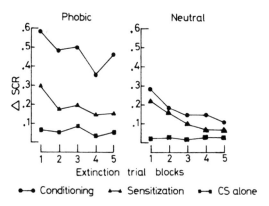

FIGURE 44.1. Extinction of skin conductance responses (SCRs) in subjects who were conditioned to potentially phobic stimuli (pictures of snakes; left panel) or neutral stimuli (pictures of houses; right panel) by receiving them paired with electric shock (unconditioned stimulus). Control subjects had the pictures and the shocks unpaired ("Sensitization") or were only exposed to pictures ("CS alone"). It is obvious that potentially phobic conditioned stimuli resulted in much larger resistance to extinction than did neutral conditioned stimuli. Data from Öhman, Eriksson, and Olofsson (1975).

threat. Clearly, false negatives (i.e., failing to elicit defense to a potentially hazardous stimulus) are more evolutionarily costly than false positives (i.e., eliciting the response to a stimulus that in effect is harmless). In an evolutionary perspective, therefore, it is likely that perceptual systems are biased toward discovering threat. Indeed, this provides an evolutionary reason for why there are anxiety disorders. To guarantee effective defense when life is at stake, the system is biased to "play it safe" by sometimes activating defense to what on closer examination turn out to be nondangerous contexts. Responses of the latter type may seem unnecessary and unreasonable, and may be understood as "irrational anxiety" by both observers and the responder.

Effective defense must be quickly activated. Consequently, there is a premium for early detection of threat. Furthermore, threat stimuli must be detected wherever they occur in the perceptual field, independently of the current direction of attention. Coupled with the bias toward false positives, these factors imply that discovery of threat is better based on a quick, superficial analysis of potentially dangerous stimuli (wherever they are) than on an effortful, detailed, and complete extraction of the meaning of one particular stimulus (LeDoux, 1996; Öhman, 1986). Therefore, the functional, evolutionary perspective suggests that the burden of threat discovery should be placed on early, parallel-processing perceptual mechanisms, which define threat on the basis of relatively simple stimulus features.

Automatic Information-Processing Routines to Discover Threat

My colleagues and I (Öhman, 1986, 1993; Öhman et al., 1985; Öhman, Flykt, & Lundqvist, 2000; Öhman & Wiens, 2004) have developed a theoretical perspective on the generation of emotion that is consistent with the functional scenario discussed above. Originating in a model of orienting response activation (Öhman, 1979), the perspective rests on a distinction between "automatic" and "controlled" or "strategic" information processing (e.g., Posner, 1978; Schneider, Dumais, & Shiffrin, 1984) to argue that many perceptual channels can be automatically and simultaneously monitored for potential threat. When stimulus events implying threat are located by the automatic system, attention is drawn to the stimulus, as the control for its further analysis is transferred to the strategic level of information processing.

The switch of control from automatic to strategic information processing is associated with activation of physiological responses—particularly the orienting response as indexed by, for example, skin conductance responses and heart rate deceleration (Öhman, 1979; Öhman, Hamm, & Hugdahl, 2000). The automatic system is involuntary, in the sense that it is hard to suppress consciously once it is initiated; it does not interfere with focal attention; it is not easily distracted by attended activities; and it is typically not available for conscious introspection (Schneider et al., 1984). Controlled or strategic information processing, on the other hand, is governed by intentions. It is resource- or capacity-limited, in the sense that interference is marked between strategically controlled tasks; it works sequentially rather than in parallel; it requires effort; and it is more readily available to consciousness (Schneider et al., 1984).

This conceptualization suggests that the automatic sensory monitoring processes have a capacity for sensory events exceeding that of the controlled or strategic processes. Thus they can keep track of many channels, only one of which can be selected for strategic processing. Sensory messages have to compete for access to the strategic processing channel for complete sensory analysis. Given the survival contingencies implied by potential threats in the external and internal environment, it is a natural assumption that events implying some degree of threat should have selection priority for strategic processing. This theoretical analysis suggests that anxiety and fear are activated as correlates to recruitment of defense responses after quick, unconscious analyses of stimuli. As a result of these analyses, threatening stimuli are selected for further conscious, controlled processing. Because they are located by automatic perceptual mechanisms, the person is not necessarily aware of the eliciting stimuli, which may result in episodes of anxiety. Indeed, what appear from the inside to be "spontaneous" episodes of anxiety may in fact be the results of unconscious stimulation. These theoretical principles are illustrated in the schematic model shown in Figure 44.2.

Experimental Test of the Model: Unconscious Activation of Phobias

Backward Masking

The central theoretical tenet of this model is that responses of anxiety or fear can be elicited after only a preliminary, unconscious analysis of the stimulus. Its empirical examination, therefore, requires a means of presenting fear stimuli outside of the subject's awareness. Such a means is provided by backward masking, which has been held to be the potentially most fruitful avenue to unconscious perception (Holender, 1986; Öhman, 1999). Thus if backwardly masked fear stimuli were presented to fearful subjects, and these stimuli still elicited physiological responses suggesting activation of fear/anxiety even though conscious recognition could be ruled out, the theoretical notions advanced here would receive experimental support.

Unconscious Phobic Responses

We (Öhman & Soares, 1994) selected research participants who feared snakes but not spiders, or vice versa. Participants in the control group feared neither stimulus. In the experiment, participants were exposed to series of pictures of

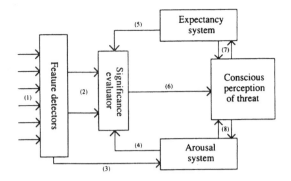

FIGURE 44.2. A schematic version of the model of emotion activation presented in the text. External stimuli (1) make contact with "feature detectors," detecting potentially significant stimuli on the basis of signal features. If such features are present, information is passed on (2) to the "significance evaluator" and (3) to the "arousal system," which initiates a surge of autonomic activity to prepare action. Feedback is then provided (4) to tune the significance evaluator for threat evaluation, which is also biased (5) by an "expectancy system," which relies on the organization of emotion in memory. These inputs are evaluated (still unconsciously) by the significance evaluator, which then can call on (6) a system for "conscious perception of threat" for an elaborated analysis of the stimulus in interaction with the expectancy system (7) and the arousal system (8). See Öhman (2000) for a more detailed presentation of the model.

snakes and spiders, with pictures of flowers and mushrooms serving as controls, while skin conductance responses were measured. In the first series, presentations were effectively masked by similar pictures that were grossly similar to the target stimuli in colors and texture, but lacked any recognizable central object. A pilot experiment using a forced-choice recognition procedure ascertained that both fearful and nonfearful participants consistently failed to identify the target with the masking parameters used. The masks interrupted presentation of the target stimuli after 30 milliseconds of exposure and remained on for 100 milliseconds during the masked presentation series. In the following series of presentations, the stimuli were presented unmasked. After these series, the participants rated the stimuli for arousal, valence, and control/dominance during separately presented masked and nonmasked rating series. Figure 44.3 shows skin conductance responses to masked (a) and nonmasked (b) presentations of the stimuli. It is evident that the fearful participants responded specifically to their feared stimulus, but did not differ from controls for the other stimulus categories, independently of masking. This enhanced responding to the feared stimulus cannot be attributed to conscious perception. Nevertheless, parallel data were obtained for all three rating dimensions, which suggests

that some aspect of the masked stimulation became indirectly available to the conscious system (maybe through bodily feedback). Thus the fearful participants rated themselves as more disliking, more aroused, and less in control when exposed to masked presentations of their feared stimulus.

Conditioning of Unconscious Effects

The data presented in Figure 44.3 support the notion of fear as elicitable after only preliminary, preattentive, automatic, and unconscious analyses of the stimulus. Consistent with a prepared Pavlovian conditioning perspective on phobias, we (Öhman & Soares, 1993; Soares & Öhman, 1993a, 1993b) demonstrated that Pavlovian conditioning to unmasked presentations of fear-relevant stimuli (snakes and spiders) in nonfearful individuals resulted in conditioned skin conductance responses that survived backward masking. Conditioning to fear-irrelevant stimuli (flowers and mushrooms), on the other hand, resulted in more elusive responses that were abolished by masking.

Similar data were obtained for another class of fear-relevant stimuli, angry faces, which were masked by neutral faces (Esteves, Dimberg, & Öhman, 1994; Parra, Esteves, Flykt, & Öhman, 1997). Furthermore, we

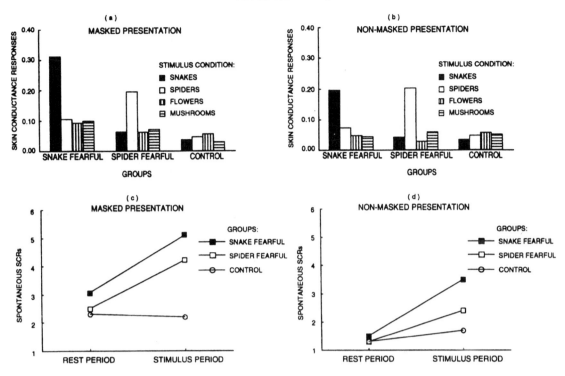

FIGURE 44.3. Upper panels (a and b) show skin conductance responses from snake-fearful, spider-fearful, and nonfearful control participants to effectively masked (a) and nonmasked (b) presentations of pictures of snakes, spiders, flowers, and mushrooms. Fearful subjects showed elevated responding to their feared stimulus even if it was prevented from entering conscious perception by backward masking (a). Lower panels (c and d) show spontaneous skin conductance responses (SCRs) in the intervals between stimulation. Whereas controls did not change from rest during stimulation, the fearful subjects showed enhanced spontaneous responding, suggesting that they became anxious after both masked (c) and nonmasked (d) presentations of feared stimuli. Data from Öhman and Soares (1994).

(Esteves, Dimberg, Parra, & Öhman, 1994) reported that skin conductance responses could be conditioned to masked fear-relevant, but not to masked fear-irrelevant, stimuli. That is, after conditioning to masked angry or happy faces, subjects showed enhanced responding to subsequent nonmasked presentations of angry but not happy faces. Similarly, we (Öhman & Soares, 1998) demonstrated unconscious conditioning to masked snakes or spiders, but not to masked flowers or mushrooms. Thus not only could emotional responses be elicited to masked stimuli, but they could also be learned to such stimuli, provided that they were evolutionarily fear-relevant. We (Öhman & Mineka, 2001) concluded that these types of preattentive effects are best interpreted in terms of the ability of biologically fear-relevant stimuli to access directly a basic, noncognitive level of conditioning.

Fear-Relevant Stimuli as Guides to Attention

The model suggests that fear-relevant stimuli recruit attention by providing a switch from automatic to controlled processing of the stimulus. Thus automatic perceptual processes may locate emotionally relevant stimuli at a preattentive level, and then call on controlled processing resources in order to deal with the situation. Examining this hypothesis, we (Öhman, Flykt, & Esteves, 2001) demonstrated fast detection of evolutionarily fear-relevant stimuli (pictures of snakes and spiders) in a complex array of stimuli (pictures of flowers and mushrooms) by research participants selected to be nonfearful or specifically fearful of snakes or spiders. The research used a visual search paradigm, in which the participants were instructed to detect a discrepant target stimulus among different exemplars of a background category of stimuli. For example, the target could be a snake picture presented among distractor pictures of flowers. All participants were faster to locate snakes and spiders among flowers and mushrooms than vice versa; this advantage for fear-relevant targets, in contrast to the detection of neutral targets, was independent of the number of distractors in the display, which suggests that the detection of snakes and spiders had a preattentive origin (see, e.g., Eastwood et al., 2005). The basic finding that threatening animals are more quickly detected than plants in complex displays has been replicated in several laboratories (even though the interpretations of these effects may differ; see Brosch & Sharma, 2005; Flykt, 2004; Lipp, 2006; Lipp et al., 2004; Lipp, Derakshan, Waters, & Logies, 2004). Similarly, visual search studies that have examined detection of schematic facial target stimuli showing different emotions among distractor faces consistently report faster detection of threatening (angry) than friendly (happy) targets (Eastwood, Smilek, & Merikle, 2001; Fox et al., 2000; Mather & Knight, 2006; Öhman, Lundqvist, & Esteves, 2001; Tipples, Atkinson, & Young, 2002). This effect is obvious with both neutral and emotional distractors, and it is specific for threatening rather than negative faces (Öhman, Lundqvist, & Esteves, 2001). Furthermore, it is closely related to emotional ratings of the stimuli, and the threat advantage is primarily conveyed by the upper part of the face (Lundqvist & Öhman, 2005; Tipples et al., 2002).

Snake-fearful participants were as quick as the controls in detecting spiders, but they were still faster in detecting snakes, and vice versa for spider-fearful participants (Öhman, Flykt, & Esteves, 2001). Thus people in general appear to be sensitive to evolutionarily relevant fear stimuli, and this sensitivity seems to be further enhanced in individuals for whom the stimuli actually elicit fear.

Rinck, Reinecke, Ellwart, Heuer, and Becker (2005) confirmed that spider-phobic participants were quicker to detect spiders than neutral stimuli (beetles and butterflies) among neutral distractors (dragonflies), whereas nonanxious controls were slower than the phobic individuals for spiders but not for beetles and butterflies. In addition, the phobic participants were slower to detect dragonflies among spiders than among beetles and butterflies, which suggests that phobic stimuli in fact were more difficult to ignore as distractors than were neutral pictures when the primary task was to find neutral targets. Similarly, examining participants that were high and low in social anxiety, we (Juth, Lundqvist, Karlsson, & Öhman, 2005) found that those high in social anxiety detected schematic threatening targets more accurately than friendly targets, particularly when social anxiety was elevated by a critical observer in the room, and when the distractors were emotional (i.e., happy for angry targets, and angry for happy targets).

Miltner, Kriechel, Hecht, Trippe, and Weiss (2004) instructed spider-fearful and nonfearful participants to search for a neutral (mushroom) target among neutral distractors (flowers). On occasional trials, however, a spider was presented among the flower distractors. Even though the voluntarily controlled attention was occupied in searching for the designated mushroom targets, the occasional spider among the distractor captured the attention of the spider-fearful but not the control participants, which resulted in prolonged search times for the target mushroom. Taken together, these studies show that fear stimuli can be automatically detected and guide attention, both under conditions of top-down attentional control (Öhman, Flykt, & Esteves, 2001; Rinck et al., 2005), and in a stimulus-driven mode when they are unexpectedly presented outside the attentional focus (Miltner et al., 2004). In addition, if stimuli are actively feared (e.g., spiders in spider phobia), they also interfere with the detection of neutral targets when serving as a class of distractors to be ignored in a top-down mode (Rinck et al., 2005). Whereas the former two effects suggest that feared stimuli are effective in *shifting* and *engaging* attention, the latter effect suggests, in addition, that it is more difficult to *disengage* attention from an actively feared stimulus (see Posner & Peterson, 1990).

Processing Biases in Anxiety

There is a large literature (see reviews by Mathews & MacLeod, 1994; Mineka, Rafaeli, & Yovel, 2003; Mogg & Bradley, 1998) on cognitive functions in anxiety, which documents that trait anxiety is associated with an attentional bias to focus on threatening information in the surroundings. As Mathews (1990) put it, "anxiety and worry are associated with an automatic processing bias, initiated prior to awareness, but serving to attract attention to environmental threat cues, and thus facilitating the acquisition of threatening information" (p. 462). This view is consistent with the functional perspective on fear and anxiety presented above. Accordingly, participants selected for high trait anxiety or for fulfilling diagnostic criteria for an anxiety disorder (particularly GAD) preferentially direct their attention toward threatening stimuli in different experimental tasks (for reviews, see Mathews & MacLeod, 1994; Mogg & Bradley, 1998).

MacLeod, Mathews, and Tata (1986) developed a dot probe detection procedure in which participants were presented with two briefly displayed words, one shown above and the other below a fixation cross that forewarned the words. When the words disappeared, a dot appeared at the previous location of one of the words. On some critical trials one of the words was threat-related and the other neutral. MacLeod et al. (1986) reported that patients with GAD were faster to respond to dots appearing at the location previously occupied by a threat word than at the location occupied by a neutral word, which implied that the patients' attention was preferentially directed toward the threatening words.

The dot probe paradigm can be modified for use with pictorial threatening and neutral stimuli. Following presentation of a central fixation cross, Bradley et al. (1997) briefly presented two pictures of faces, one showing an emotional and the other a neutral expression, side by side, one at each side of the cross. When the faces disappeared, a dot probe appeared at one of the locations of the previously presented faces, and the participants were instructed to indicate its position (left or right) on the screen. As assessed by response latencies to the probes, the results showed a bias away from angry (compared to happy and neutral) faces in nonanxious participants, and a bias for looking at the angry faces among participants selected for high trait anxiety (Bradley, Mogg, Falla, & Hamilton, 1998). Furthermore, recordings of eye movements showed that individuals with GAD more frequently and rapidly looked first at threatening rather than neutral faces (Mogg, Millar, & Bradley, 2000).

The dot probe paradigm (with words—e.g., Mogg, Bradley, & Williams, 1995; or with threatening and neutral faces—Mogg & Bradley, 1999) can be used with masked stimuli. Using a dot probe procedure with pictures, Mogg and Bradley (2002) presented briefly (for 17 milliseconds) pairs of pictures of the same

actor displaying an emotional (threatening or happy) and a neutral facial expression, and then this stimulus pair was immediately masked by another pair of pictures of scrambled faces (for 68 milliseconds). The results showed that anxious individuals (particularly those with social anxiety) preferentially oriented their attention to the location of the masked threatening faces, thus supporting a preattentive origin for the threat bias.

Anxiety and Difficulties in Disengaging Attention from Threat

Taken together, the data reviewed in this section are quite consistent in showing not only that fear-relevant stimuli often guide attention among nonselected participants, but also that this effect is potentiated by high anxiety. Furthermore, these biases for threat are likely to have preattentive origins. However, there are alternative interpretations of the nature of the reported attentional bias in the dot probe paradigm. If we assume (for the sake of the argument) that there is no bias of shifting attention to the threatening stimulus in the dot probe paradigm, participants are initially as likely to focus on the threatening as on the neutral stimulus. However, when they happen to focus on the threatening stimulus, they may have difficulties in disengaging attention, which will slow their detection latency when they have to shift attention to a dot appearing at the location of the neutral stimulus. Because they do not get stuck in this way on neutral stimuli, there is no interference with moving the attention to dots appearing behind the threatening stimuli. Thus one would generally expect slower response latencies to neutral than to threatening stimuli—not because of fast detection of the latter, but because of slow detection of neutral stimuli due to slow disengagement from threatening stimuli.

These interpretational hazards led Fox, Russo, Bowles, and Dutton (2001) to develop paradigms for stringent testing of the hypothesis that the effect of anxiety on threat detection is primarily due to slow disengagement of attention from threatening stimuli. They used a paradigm adopted from Posner, Inhoff, Friedrich, and Cohen (1987). A trial was initiated by the appearance of a fixation cross in the center of a screen between two laterally placed boxes. With the cross still on, a neutral or threatening cue (a word or a face, depending on the experiment) was briefly (for 100 milliseconds) presented in one of two boxes. The cue disappeared and was followed by a dot probe in the same box in the majority of (e.g., 75%) the trials (valid cueing) or a dot in the other box on the remaining trials (invalid cueing). Invalid cueing carries a cost in terms of slowed reaction time, because attention has to be disengaged from the validly cued location before it can be moved to the other location (Posner et al., 1987). Across four experiments, Fox et al. (2001) reported consistently longer reaction times to invalidly than validly cued dots. This effect was enhanced if the cue was a threatening word or face (compared to positive words or happy faces)—*but only for highly anxious participants.* These findings suggest that high-anxiety individuals were slow to shift the attention to a new location once they had engaged their attention in a threatening stimulus. Thus the attention of people with high anxiety may get stuck on threatening events around them, which may interfere with flexible deployments of attention according to current performance demands. Subsequent research from Fox's group has confirmed this effect (Fox, Russo, & Dutton, 2002) and demonstrated that it is specific to threatening (angry, fearful) rather than to negative (sad) faces (Georgiou et al., 2005).

For people preferentially attending to threatening events and objects in the environment, the world will appear a dangerous and risky place, which is likely to influence their mood state negatively. An attentional bias for threat, therefore, may be an important factor maintaining anxiety over time in a vicious circle (where anxiety promotes a bias for threat, the result of which is more anxiety promoting further threat bias, etc.). Furthermore, people who have difficulties disengaging attention from threatening information will be preoccupied by threat. If the threatening event that holds attention in this way is mental (a memory, thought, or image), this is tantamount to getting stuck on ruminative worry. Thus the central symptom of GAD may result from problems with the control of attention.

TOWARD A NEUROBIOLOGY OF FEAR AND ANXIETY

The Amygdala and Fear

LeDoux (1996) has described the neuroarchitecture of a system that accounts for many of the behavioral findings reviewed above. He and his coworkers have demonstrated a direct neural link from auditory nuclei (medial geniculate body) in the thalamus to the "significance evaluator" and "fear effector system" in the lateral and central amygdala, respectively. This monosynaptic link provides immediate information to the amygdala of gross features of emotionally relevant auditory stimuli. It bypasses the traditionally emphasized thalamocortical sensory pathway, which gives full meaning to the stimulus, and the cortico-amygdala link, which is presumed to activate emotion. It is described as a "quick and dirty" transmission route: It "probably does not tell the amygdala much about the stimulus, certainly not much about Gestalt or object properties of the stimulus, but it at least informs the amygdala that the sensory receptors of a given modality have been activated and that a significant stimulus may be present" (LeDoux, 1990, p. 172), so that the amygdala can start early activation of defense responses. This system is explicitly postulated to be adaptively biased toward false positives rather than false negatives. This is because it is less costly to abort falsely initialized defense responses than to fail to elicit defense when the threat is real.

Tests of the Amygdala Model in Humans

LeDoux's model is primarily based on data resulting from experiments manipulating the rodent brain. However, in recent years, data on brain imaging in humans supporting the model have started to appear.

Activation of the Human Amygdala by Fear Stimuli

The most basic implication of LeDoux's model, of course, is that fear stimuli of the type that I have been discussing actually engage the amygdala. This assertion is supported by a range of studies (see, e.g., Phelps, 2006). For example, my colleagues and I (Carlsson et al., 2004) reported positron emission tomography data from participants who, like those in an earlier study (Öhman & Soares, 1994; see Figure 44.3), were selected to be afraid of spiders but not snakes, and vice versa. They showed bilateral activation of the amygdala to phobic pictures (e.g., snakes for snake-phobic participants) as compared to fear-relevant but nonfeared pictures (e.g., spiders), as well as reliable activations of the midbrain periaqueductal gray, the insula, and the anterior cingulate cortex. Very similar data were reported by Straube, Mentzel, and Miltner (2006) and Sabatinelli, Bradley, Fitzsimmons, and Lang (2005), using functional magnetic resonance imaging and spider-phobic participants. Amygdala activations, however, were conspicuously absent in earlier brain imaging studies of individuals with specific phobias challenged by their phobic objects in video clips or *in vivo* (e.g., Fredrikson et al., 1993; Fredrikson, Wik, Annas, Ericson, & Stone-Elander, 1995; Rauch et al., 1995). These failures can probably be attributed to the use of lengthy stimulus presentations rather than repeated short stimulations, because the amygdala is likely to respond best to the onset of an effective fear stimulus (e.g., Carlsson et al., 2004). In addition, many studies have reported larger responses to emotional (e.g., fearful) than to neutral faces (e.g., Anderson, Christoff, Panitz, De Rosa, & Gabrieli, 2003).

Amygdala Activation by Unconsciously Presented Stimuli

Because of its emphasis on the subcortical input to the amygdala, the LeDoux model implies that it should be possible to activate the amygdala by stimuli that are not consciously perceived. This prediction was supported in the Carlsson et al. (2004) study, which reported reliable amygdala activation (compared to neutral pictures) both for masked phobic pictures (e.g., snakes for snake phobics) and for masked fear-relevant but nonphobic (e.g., spiders) pictures. Furthermore, we (Morris, Öhman, & Dolan, 1998) demonstrated specific activation of the amygdala by masked conditioned angry faces in human subjects, and Whalen et al. (1998) demonstrated significant amygdala activation to masked fearful faces.

Binocular rivalry is an alternative method to backward masking for presenting stimuli outside of awareness. If two different stimuli are separately projected on corresponding retinal locations in the two eyes, rather than appearing as a mixture, they will compete to determine the percept. Given that the two stimuli are roughly matched in salience, the percept will spontaneously shift between them. However, if one stimulus is in some sense more salient than the other, the latter will be suppressed, which implies that it is presented outside of the participant's awareness. Two studies have reported reliable amygdala activation to suppressed pictures of fearful faces in a binocular rivalry paradigm (Pasley, Mayes, & Schultz, 2004;

Williams, Morris, McGlone, Abbott, & Mattingley, 2004), thus providing converging evidence to the effect that the amygdala can be activated by nonconsciously perceived threat stimuli.

Amygdala Activation by Nonattended Fear Stimuli

The notion of a direct subcortical link to the amygdala implies that it should be possible to activate the amygdala by nonattended stimuli. Vuilleumier, Armony, Driver, and Dolan (2001) examined this notion by exposing their participants to pairs of pictures of faces and houses that were either horizontally or vertically arranged around a fixation cross. Attention was manipulated by requiring the participants to judge whether the pairs of faces or houses showed identical pictures on different trials. In contrast to the fusiform facial area, whose response to fearful faces was enhanced when faces were attended to, amygdala activation was larger to fearful than to neutral faces regardless of whether faces or houses were attended to. Thus these data support the hypothesis that the amygdala can be activated by nonattended stimuli.

This conclusion was further supported by Anderson et al. (2003) in a similar paradigm, in which participants attended to either faces (showing fear, disgust, or a neutral expression) or houses in different colors that were superimposed on each other. In support of the hypothesis that the amygdala activation is independent of attention to the eliciting stimulus, these authors reported that the amygdala response to fearful faces did not differ as a function of whether the faces were attended or not.

Finally, Straube et al. (2006) required their spider-phobic participants either to identify whether pictures showed a spider or a mushroom, or to perform a perceptual judgment task on a circle superimposed on spiders or mushrooms. Amygdala responses to spiders (relative to mushrooms) were larger in phobic than in nonphobic participants. Furthermore, in contrast to the responses in other structures (e.g., insula, anterior cingulate, dorsomedial prefrontal cortex), in which the responses to spiders were smaller during the perceptual task, the amygdala responses were as large during this task as when participants focused on spiders and mushroom pictures in the picture identification task. These results again support independence of the amygdala to attentional conditions.

Amygdala Facilitation of Visual Perception

The amygdala is richly connected with the neocortex. However, these connections are biased, in the sense that the amygdala projects to many more cortical areas than it receives input from (Emery & Amaral, 2000; LeDoux, 1996). With regard to the visual system, it receives input from the primary visual cortex (V1) and the inferotemporal cortex (IT); however, it has efferent pathways to all the major way stations in the ventral visual processing stream, as well as the lateral and medial orbito-frontal cortices (Emery & Amaral, 2000). This anatomical organization might suggest that the amygdala tunes perceptual processing in order to facilitate perception of potentially threatening events.

To test this idea, Phelps, Ling, and Carrasco (2006) performed an experiment in which they briefly cued a perceptual task (judging line orientations as a function of contrast between lines and background) by fearful or neutral faces. Confirming that emotion facilitates perception of low-level visual features, their data showed improved contrast sensitivity (i.e., more accurate judgment of line orientation at lower spatial contrasts between line and background) after fearful as opposed to neutral faces. This effect, however, was not obtained with inverted faces, which provides support for the emotional (amygdala?) origin of the effect. Furthermore, in a second experiment, Phelps et al. (2006) showed that this enhanced contrast sensitivity was stronger for emotional than for neutral upright (but not inverted) faces in both focused- and divided-attention conditions, suggesting that it did not depend on attention. However, the emotion effect was larger with focused than with divided attention, which implies that the effect of emotion was potentiated by attention.

Vuilleumier, Richardson, Armony, Driver, and Dolan (2004), in a study of patients with focal amygdala and hippocampal lesions, provided data indicating that these types of perceptual effects may be mediated by the amygdala. They replicated previously demonstrated emotional enhancement of an early cortical area involved in vision, the fusiform cortex, to fearful faces (e.g., Vuilleumier et al., 2001) in normal controls and patients with focal hippocampal lesions. However, such emotional enhancement was not observed in the patients with focused amygdala lesions (with or without hippocampal lesions). Thus these findings imply that the amygdala is rapidly activated in order to prime early visual processing of emotional stimuli, as suggested by LeDoux (1996) and as behaviorally demonstrated by Phelps et al. (2006).

Amygdala Activation in the Absence of Relevant Sensory Cortex

The notion of a direct route from sensory organs to the amygdala implies that it should be possible to activate the amygdala even if cortical processing of the fear stimulus is impossible because of lesions in the relevant sensory cortices. To examine this prediction, Morris, deGelder, Weiskrantz, and Dolan (2001) examined a patient with lesions in V1, resulting in "blindsight"—a condition in which a person denies any visual experience from stimulations in the blind spot, yet is able to locate and sometimes to discriminate stimuli in the blind field. When the patient with blindsight examined by Morris et al. (2001) was exposed to faces in the blind field, he showed reliable activation of the right amygdala to fearful as compared to neutral faces. Furthermore, similar results were obtained in a patient whose extensive occipital lesion was associated with total blindness without any signs of residual vision (Pegna, Khateb, Lazeyras, & Seqhier, 2005).

Is There a Subcortical Pathway to the Amygdala?

To examine the route to nonconscious amygdala activation, we (Morris, Öhman, & Dolan, 1999) used our earlier data (Morris et al., 1998) to examine the neural connectivity between the amygdala and other brain regions when the amygdala was activated by masked stimuli. In support of the hypothesis (LeDoux, 1996), we reported that activation of the right amygdala by masked stimuli could be reliably predicted from activation of subcortical way stations in the visual systems (such as the superior colliculus and the right pulvinar nucleus of the thalamus), but not from any cortical regions.

Liddell et al. (2005) examined the effect of masked fearful versus masked neutral faces on anatomically defined regions of interest. Confirming our connectivity data (Morris et al., 1999) they found reliable activation to masked fearful faces in the left superior colliculi, the left pulvinar, and bilateral amygdalae. In addition, they found activation in the locus coeruleus and the anterior cingulate.

In an ingenious elaboration of the low-road concept, Vuilleumier, Armony, Driver, and Dolan (2003) suggested that the amygdala operates primarily on gross, low-frequency information, because it is served by large, rapidly conducting neurons. Accordingly, they filtered the spatial frequency of pictures of faces to produce facial stimuli that retained only high- or low-frequency spatial information. Their results showed that amygdala responses were larger for low-frequency faces, provided that they showed expressions of fear. Moreover, they demonstrated activation of the pulvinar and superior colliculus by low-frequency but not high-frequency fearful faces. Thus these results suggest that there is a distinct superior colliculus–pulvinar pathway to the amygdala that operates primarily on low-frequency information.

Finally, in a powerful new hypothesis of the evolutionary origin of the visualization of the primate brain, Isbell (2006) argued that the koniocellular pathways that connect the superior colliculi and the pulvinar with the lateral geniculate and the visual cortex (V2 area) was driven by the evolutionary functionality of these pathways in detecting venomous, potentially deadly snakes hidden on the ground and in foliage.

The low-road hypothesis has been controversial, and it has influential challengers (e.g., Pessoa, 2005; Pessoa, McKenna, Gutierrez, & Ungerleider, 2002; Rolls, 1999). A recurrent theme has been that input from IT is necessary for the evidence suggesting discriminatory behavior by the amygdala to facial emotion. However, Pasley et al. (2004), who reported amygdala activation to fearful faces suppressed from awareness by binocular rivalry, demonstrated that areas of the IT that responded to faces under normal viewing did not discriminate faces from objects under conditions of binocular rivalry. If we assume that the binocular rivalry suppressed the V1, these data strongly suggest a subcortical origin of the visual input that allowed the amygdala to discriminate suppressed fearful from suppressed neutral faces.

In summary, the data reviewed here provide substantial support for LeDoux's (1996) conception of dual input to the amygdala, thus supporting a neural underpinning for the behavioral data from masking and attention paradigms.

Toward a Psychobiological Distinction between Fear and Anxiety

A distinction between fear and anxiety that is broadly consistent with Epstein's (1972) ideas, but couched in terms of neuroanatomical structure, has recently been proposed.

The Neuroanatomy of Fear and Anxiety: Related but Distinct

Davis and his colleagues (Davis, 1998; Davis & Shi, 1999; Walker, Toufexis, & Davis, 2003) propose that both fear and anxiety are related to the extended amygdala complex, which reaches from the medial temporal lobe to the ventral striatum. The central nucleus of the amygdala mediates acute fear responses to specific stimuli, whereas the anatomically closely related bed nucleus of the stria terminalis mediates anxiety (i.e., more long-lasting, tonic responses to aversive contexts without a necessary, discrete eliciting stimulus). Both these structures receive input from the basolateral amygdala complex. Because they both have efferent connections to the same set of anatomical targets in the hypothalamus and brainstem that control and coordinate behavioral signs of fear and anxiety (autonomic responses, defensive reflexes, etc.), this distinction retains the largely overlapping response output of fear and anxiety. Nonetheless, Davis's group has shown that the involved structures can also be dissociated.

At the behavioral level, Davis and colleagues (see, e.g., Davis, 2000, for references) use the startle reflex as the measure of fear. "Startle" is a defensive reflex elicited by any abrupt, unexpected, and relatively intense stimulus that "makes us jump." In its complete form it involves the whole body, with a defensive forward thrust of the head and trunk, and with a spreading wave of flexor movements along the neural axis. In rats it is measured as whole-body startle, and in humans it is commonly measured by one of its components, the eye-blinking response. Movie directors demonstrate their insight into startle reflex dynamics by making the audience jump to an abrupt cut (often coinciding with a sudden noise) that culminates a fright-inducing sequence. This is an example of "fear-potentiated startle." In the psychological laboratory, fear-potentiated startle denotes evidence of an enhanced startle reflex to auditory probe stimuli presented against a fear-inducing as compared to a neutral background stimulus (Lang, Bradley, & Cuthbert, 1990). This effect is mediated by the central nucleus of the amygdala (Davis, 2000; Lang, Davis, & Öhman, 2000).

The secretion of corticotropin-releasing hormone (CRH), which triggers the various bodily changes (via the pituitary) that are commonly used as indices of stress and anxiety, is activated by cells in the hypothalamus, but it also acts as a neurotransmitter in the brain. Infusion of CRH in the brains of rats results in strong and relatively long-lasting startle potentiation, which is mediated not by the amygdala but by dense CRH receptors in the bed nucleus of the stria terminalis (Davis & Shi, 1999; Walker et al., 2003). Thus there is a double-dissociation effect: Lesion of the central nucleus of the amygdala blocks fear-potentiated startle by conditioned fear stimuli, but has no effect on the CRH-enhanced startle; lesion of the bed nucleus of the stria terminalis, on the other hand, blocks CRH-enhanced startle but has no effect on conditioned startle potentiation. Furthermore, the acute fear response ("freezing") in rats to uncontrollable foot shock is abolished by amygdala lesion, but the more long-term escape deficit to aversive stimuli that results from uncontrollable shock ("learned helplessness") is dependent on an intact bed nucleus of the stria terminalis (see review by Walker et al., 2003).

To conclude, therefore, even though fear and anxiety are overlapping responses, they can be distinguished in terms of stimuli (presence vs. absence of a discrete eliciting stimulus), behavior (coping vs. noncoping), and neuroanatomy (central nucleus of the amygdala vs. bed nucleus of the stria terminalis).

The Behavioral Genetics of Fear- and Anxiety-Related Disorders

A distinction between primarily fear-related disorders such as the specific phobias on the one hand, and primarily anxiety-related disorders (PD, GAD, PTSD) and depression on the other, is emerging in the behavioral genetics literature. These investigations use data on the comorbidity of DSM anxiety disorders in large samples of mono- and dizygotic twins to model variance in these disorders that can be attributed to genes versus shared and unique environmental influences. The results suggest that a model incorporating two additive genetic factors (as well as shared and unique environmental factors) provides a good fit to data on six DSM anxiety disorders in large samples of male and female twins (Hettema, Prescott, Myers, Neale, & Kendler, 2005). One genetic factor showed substantial loadings for the studied specific phobias (animal, situational), but low loadings for social phobia, GAD, PD, and agoraphobia.

The other genetic factor had high loadings for GAD, PD, and agoraphobia; some loading for social phobia; and virtually zero loadings for the two diagnoses of specific phobias. Furthermore, a twin study on Vietnam veterans demonstrated considerable genetic overlap among PTSD, GAD, and PD (Chantarujikapong et al., 2001). Indeed, the behavioral genetics literature is consistent in attributing specific phobias on the one hand, and GAD, PD, and sometimes depression on the other, to distinctly different genetic factors (Kendler, Prescott, Myers, & Neale, 2003). Our analysis would then imply that this second factor is an anxiety factor, which potentially is related to the bed nucleus of the stria terminalis. These conclusions are schematically illustrated in Figure 44.4.

Psychophysiological Data from Patients with DSM Anxiety Disorders

The distinction between specific phobias on the one hand, and PD, GAD, and PTSD on the other, is vindicated by psychophysiological data. Individuals diagnosed with specific phobias, and particularly animal phobias, show a distinct psychophysiological response when exposed to their feared stimuli. For example, we (Globisch, Hamm, Esteves, & Öhman, 1999) exposed student volunteer participants who were specifically fearful (if not phobic) of snakes or spiders to pictures of snakes or spiders, household objects (neutral), and erotica and cute animals (positive). The fearful participants rated snake/spider pictures as much more unpleasant and arousing than neutral and positive pictures, compared to controls. Furthermore, they showed clearly larger skin conductance responses to pictures of their feared animals than controls did, and their responses to these animals were larger than their responses to neutral or positive pictures. As expected from previous data (e.g., Hamm, Cuthbert, Globisch, & Vaitl, 1997; Hare & Blevings, 1975), fearful participants showed a

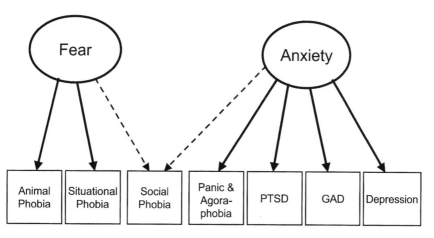

FIGURE 44.4. The genetic structure of fear-related and anxiety-related disorders (based on behavioral genetics data reported by Hettema et al., 2005, and Chantarujikapong et al., 2001). There is one set of genes ("Fear") influencing specific phobias (animal and situational phobias), and another ("Anxiety") influencing panic disorder and agoraphobia, posttraumatic stress disorder (PTSD), generalized anxiety disorder (GAD), and depression. Social phobia shows relations to both clusters. These clusters may be related to different neural structures (central nucleus of the amygdala vs. bed nucleus of the stria terminalis), differences in psychophysiological reactivity (enhanced responses to fear stimuli vs. elevated resting levels and blunted stress responses), and different attention biases (shift of attention to threat vs. failure to disengage from threat).

strong heart rate acceleration to snake/spider pictures, which was in marked contrast to the deceleration shown by controls to these animals, and to the small and indistinguishable response shown by both groups to neutral stimuli. The startle data showed a rapid relative startle potentiation to feared compared to neutral stimuli, which was obvious to probes presented as early as 300 milliseconds after picture onset, and then remained (and even increased) for at least 4 seconds of picture viewing. Controls, on the other hand, showed a rapid relative startle inhibition to animal stimuli that lasted for more than a second. In concert, these data show that enhanced (phobic) fear to animal stimuli is associated with a distinct psychophysiological response suggesting activation of fight–flight behavior, which clearly differs from the pattern elicited by these stimuli in nonfearful participants. This distinct stimulus-elicited fear response in specific phobias contrasts with the psychophysiological response to stress seen in PD and GAD. In spite of the clinical description (confirmed by self-report data) of panic as involving a surge of sympathetic activation much like that in fear responses (Öhman, 1993), research shows that PD and GAD are associated primarily with high resting autonomic activity, and, if any-

thing, less acute reactivity to common stress tasks (Hoehn-Saric & MacLeod, 2000).

Cuthbert et al. (2003) examined psychophysiological responses across the whole spectrum of DSM anxiety disorders in patients engaged in imagery of different fear scenes (Lang, 1979). When cued, the patients were instructed to imagine fear scenes based on previously learned sentences briefly describing personal fear experiences (referring to "the worst fear you ever experienced"), standard danger scenes ("Taking a shower, alone in the house, I hear the sound of someone forcing the door, and I panic"), social fear scenes ("My heart pounds in the suddenly silent room; everyone is watching me . . . ") or neutral control scenes ("Soft music is playing on the stereo as I snooze lazily on my favorite chair").

In spite of small differences between patient groups in ratings of fear and vividness of imagery, heart rate increases when imagining the fear scenes were larger in the participants with specific or social phobia than in the participants with PTSD, PD, or no disorder, who did not differ among each other. The group with specific phobia showed considerably more startle potentiation than the other diagnostic groups when imagining not only their own personal fear scene, but also the other fear scenes.

These results are consistent with previous data showing larger heart rate responses during fear imagery for individuals with specific phobias than for those with social phobia (Cook, Melamed, Cuthbert, McNeil, & Lang, 1988; McNeil, Vrana, Melamed, Cuthbert, & Lang, 1993), who both showed larger responses than those with agoraphobia (Cook et al., 1988). Similarly, Lang, McTeague, and Cuthbert (2005) observed larger fear-potentiated startle to fear imagery in patients with specific or social phobia than in patients with PD or GAD.

Keane et al. (1998) examined psychophysiological responses to a standard stress task (mental arithmetic), a standardized series of combat pictures and sounds, and personalized mental imagery scripts of experienced traumas (using the Lang [1979] methodology) in more than 1,200 Vietnam veterans (see also the review by Orr & Roth, 2000). Veterans with a current PTSD diagnosis showed larger heart rate, skin conductance, and systolic and diastolic blood pressure responses to both standard combat and imagined personal trauma scenes than veterans never diagnosed with PTSD. Veterans with a lifetime but not a current PTSD diagnosis in general were intermediate to the other two groups. In addition, the group with a current diagnosis showed higher resting heart rate and skin conductance, but lower heart rate and diastolic blood pressure responses to standard stress, than the other two groups.

Like the patients with PTSD examined by Keane et al. (1998), the patients with PD examined by Cuthbert et al. (2003) showed elevated heart rate between imagery trials. These data conform to those reported by Hoehn-Saric and MacLeod (2000) showing elevated base levels of heart rate and skin conductance, but, if anything, less reactivity to common stress tasks, in patients with PD and GAD.

There are also interesting differences between patients with specific phobias on the one hand, and those with PD, GAD, or PTSD on the other, in self-reported anxiety and comorbidity for other DSM anxiety disorders and depression. Whereas those with specific phobias did not differ from controls in self-reported anxiety, patients diagnosed with social phobia, PTSD, PD, or GAD showed elevated levels of self-reported anxiety and depression (Cuthbert et al., 2003; Lang et al., 2005). Likewise, in agreement with other data (Brown, Campbell, Lehman, Grisham, & Mancill, 2001), a majority of patients diagnosed with PTSD, PD, or GAD had comorbidity for an additional DSM anxiety or mood disorder, whereas this was less frequent among patients with social phobia and particularly infrequent among patients diagnosed with specific phobias (Cuthbert et al., 2003; Lang et al., 2005).

Overall, the data reviewed in this section show that specific phobia is associated with a distinct fear response, as indexed by startle potentiation and strong heart rate acceleration when patients are exposed to their feared objects. In addition, they show little evidence of elevated general anxiety levels, and only modest comorbidity with other DSM anxiety and mood disorders. Patients with social phobia likewise show enhanced startle potentiation and accelerative heart rate responses when imagining fear scenes, but they also show some elevation in anxiety scores (Cuthbert et al., 2003; Lang et al., 2005), compared to controls and patients with specific phobias. Patients with PTSD appear to show both patterns, with enhanced psychophysiological responses to trauma-related scenes and elevated resting heart rate and skin conductance levels (Orr & Roth, 2000); they also exhibit enhanced self-reported anxiety and depression, and considerable comorbidity for DSM anxiety and depressive disorders. These data converge nicely with the previously reviewed neuroanatomical and behavioral genetics results, suggesting that similar distinctions between fear and anxiety are emerging in all three of these research fields.

CONCLUDING DISCUSSION

To recapitulate, I have started with the obvious communality between fear and anxiety, and then launched a discussion of differences with respect to coping with an implied threat (Epstein, 1972). In fear, organisms try to cope with the danger, but in anxiety, the situation does not allow effective means of coping. The theoretical perspective I have presented stresses the role of rapid early information-processing mechanisms in fear activation. Here, both fear and anxiety have a joint origin in an unconscious mobilization to an as yet poorly defined threat. With more time to appraise the situation, the emotion can be resolved into fear when reflexive (or highly preferred) coping options are available, or can turn into anxiety when they are not.

A cognitive-psychobiological model has been presented, which is broadly consistent with behavioral data on the effect of masking on responses to fear stimuli and on the power of fear or anxiety stimuli to guide attention. This model has an empirically well-founded neural underpinning. However, in contrast to my previous position (Öhman, 1993) converging data now appear to support a model with fundamental differences between fear and anxiety in terms of genetics, neuroanatomy, and psychophysiological reactivity.

Behavioral genetic studies suggest that specific phobias on the one hand, and GAD, PD, and PTSD on the other, are related to different genetic factors (Hettema et al., 2005). This information converges with the neuroanatomical distinction between the central nucleus of the amygdala as related to fear and the bed nucleus of the stria terminalis as related to anxiety (Walker et al., 2003). Furthermore, there are distinct psychophysiological responses for specific phobias (Cuthbert et al., 2003). There is a suggestion in the data on attention, fear, phobias, and anxiety that fear stimuli promote reflexive shifts in focal attention. The attentional bias of anxious individuals (and particularly patients diagnosed with GAD), on the other hand, primarily concerns difficulties of disengaging attention from threatening stimuli once they have become the focus of attention (Fox et al., 2001). Social phobia appears intermediate to the two genetic factors (Hettema et al., 2005), as well as to the two patterns of psychophysiological reactivity (Lang et al., 2005). Finally, PTSD belongs genetically to the anxiety factor, but psychophysiologically it involves both enhanced reactivity to feared stimuli and elevated basal levels of psychophysiological activity (Keane et al., 1998).

Thus it is reasonable to talk about specific phobias as exclusively fear-related disorders, PD and perhaps particularly GAD as primary anxiety-related disorders, and social phobia and PTSD as mixed fear- and anxiety-related disorders. This conclusion is further supported by data on comorbidity, which show only modest comorbidity with other DSM anxiety disorders and depression for specific phobias; some such comorbidity for social phobia; and considerable such comorbidity for PTSD, PD, and GAD (Brown et al., 2001).

As a final note, it is important to remember that the modeled genetic factors are independent and additive. This means that principles of fear may be operating in other DSM anxiety disorders besides phobias. For example, fear conditioning is an important factor producing many of the symptoms of PTSD (e.g., Öhman & Mineka, 2001), but factors shared with PD and GAD are also important for understanding other PTSD symptoms, such as the elevated physiological levels suggesting a generalized stress impact. Similarly, the neuroendocrine response patterns that may predispose for PD, GAD, and PTSD also seems to facilitate fear conditioning (LeDoux, 1996). What makes specific phobias unique is that they tend to have one central problem, which is best conceptualized in terms of fear. For the other DSM anxiety disorders, fear may be one of the components; however, it is then embedded in a much wider context of emotional agitation, which is best conceptualized in terms of anxiety.

REFERENCES

American Psychiatric Association (APA). (2000). *Diagnostic and statistical manual of mental disorders* (4th ed., text rev.). Washington, DC: Author.

Anderson, A. K., Christoff, K., Panitz, D., De Rosa, E., & Gabrieli, J. D. E. (2003). Neural correlates of the automatic processing of threat facial signals. *Journal of Neuroscience, 23,* 5627–5633.

Arrindell, W. A., Pickersgill, M. J., Merckelbach, H., Ardon, M. A., & Cornet, F. C. (1991). Phobic dimensions: III. Factor analytic approaches to the study of common phobic fears: An updated review of findings obtained with adult subjects. *Advances in Behaviour Research and Therapy, 13,* 73–130.

Barlow, D. H. (2002). *Anxiety and its disorders: The nature and treatment of anxiety and panic* (2nd ed.). New York: Guilford Press.

Bourke, J. (2006). *Fear: A cultural history.* Emeryville, CA: Shoemaker & Hoard.

Bradley, B. P., Mogg, K., Falla, S. J., & Hamilton, L. R. (1998). Attentional bias for threatening facial expressions in anxiety: Effect of stimulus duration. *Cognition and Emotion, 12,* 737–753.

Bradley, B. P., Mogg, K., Millar, N., Bonham-Carter, C., Fergusson, E., Jenkins, J., et al. (1997). Attentional biases for emotional faces. *Cognition and Emotion, 11,* 25–42.

Brosch, T., & Sharma, D. (2005). The role of fear-relevant stimuli in visual search: A comparison of phylogenetic and ontogenetic stimuli. *Emotion, 5,* 360–364.

Brown, T. A., Campbell, L. A., Lehman, C. L., Grisham, J. R., & Mancill, R. B. (2001). Current and lifetime comorbidity of the DSM-IV anxiety and mood disorders in a large clinical sample. *Journal of Abnormal Psychology, 110,* 585–599.

Carlsson, K., Petersson, K. M., Lundqvist, D., Karlsson, A., Ingvar, M., & Öhman, A. (2004). Fear and the amygdala: Manipulation of awareness generates differential cerebral responses to phobic and fear-relevant (but non-feared) stimuli. *Emotion, 4,* 340–353.

Chantarujikapong, S. I., Scherrer, J. F., Xian, H., Eisen, S. A., Lyons, M. J., Goldberg, J., et al. (2001). A twin study of generalized anxiety disorder symptoms, panic disorder symptoms, and post-traumatic stress disorder in men. *Psychiatry Research, 103,* 133–145.

Cook, E. W., III, Melamed, B. G., Cuthbert, B. N., McNeil, D. W., & Lang, P. J. (1988). Emotional imagery and the differential diagnosis of anxiety. *Journal of Consulting and Clinical Psychology, 56,* 734–740.

Cuthbert, B. N., Lang, P. J., Strauss, C., Drobes, D., Patrick, C. J., & Bradley, M. M. (2003). The psychophysiology of anxiety disorder: Fear memory imagery. *Psychophysiology, 40,* 407–422.

Davis, M. (1998). Are different parts of the extended amygdala involved in fear versus anxiety? *Biological Psychiatry, 44,* 1239–1247.

Davis, M. (2000). The role of the amygdala in conditioned and unconditioned fear and anxiety. In J. P. Aggleton (Ed.), *The amygdala* (2nd ed., pp. 213–288). New York: Oxford University Press.

Davis, M., & Shi, C. (1999). The extended amygdala: Are the central nucleus of the amygdala and the bed nucleus of the stria terminalis differentially involved in fear versus anxiety? *Annals of the New York Academy of Sciences, 877,* 281–291.

Dimberg, U., & Öhman, A. (1996). Behold the wrath: Psychophysiological responses to facial stimuli. *Motivation and Emotion, 20,* 149–182.

Eastwood, J. D., Smilek, D., & Merikle, P. M. (2001). Differential attentional guidance by unattended faces expressing positive and negative emotion. *Perception and Psychophysics, 63,* 1004–1013.

Eastwood, J. D., Smilek, D., Oakman, J. M., Farvolden, P., van Ameringen, M., Mancini, C., et al. (2005). Individuals with social phobia are biased to become aware of negative faces. *Visual Cognition, 12,* 159–179.

Emery, N. J., & Amaral, D. G. (2000). The role of the amygdala in primate social cognition. In R. D. Lane & L. Nadel (Eds.), *Cognitive neuroscience of emotion* (pp. 156–191). New York Oxford University Press.

Epstein, S. (1972). The nature of anxiety with emphasis upon its relationship to expectancy. In C. D. Spielberger (Ed.), *Anxiety: Current trends in theory and research* (Vol. 2, pp. 291–337). New York: Academic Press.

Esteves, F., Dimberg, U., & Öhman, A. (1994). Automatically elicited fear: Conditioned skin conductance responses to masked facial expressions. *Cognition and Emotion, 8,* 393–413.

Esteves, F., Dimberg, U., Parra, C., & Öhman, A. (1994). Nonconscious associative learning: Pavlov-ian conditioning of skin conductance responses to masked fear-relevant facial stimuli. *Psychophysiology, 31,* 375–385.

Flykt, A. (2004). Visual search with biological threat stimuli: Accuracy, reaction times, and heart rate changes. *Emotion, 5,* 349–353.

Foa, E. B., & McNally, R. J. (1986). Sensitivity to feared stimuli in obsessive–compulsives: A dichotic listening analysis. *Cognitive Therapy and Research, 10,* 477–486.

Fox, E., Lester, V., Russo, R., Bowles, R. J., Pichler, A., & Dutton, K. (2000). Facial expressions of emotion: Are angry faces detected more efficiently? *Cognition and Emotion, 14,* 61–92.

Fox, E., Russo, R., Bowles, R., & Dutton, K. (2001). Do threatening stimuli draw or hold visual attention in subclinical anxiety? *Journal of Experimental Psychology: General, 130,* 681–700.

Fox, E., Russo, R., & Dutton, K. (2002). Attentional bias for threat: Evidence for delayed disengagement form emotional faces. *Cognition and Emotion, 16,* 355–379.

Fredrikson, M., Wik, G., Annas, P., Ericson, K., & Stone-Elander, S. (1995). Functional neuroanatomy of visually elicited simple phobic fear: Additional data and theoretical analysis. *Psychophysiology, 32,* 43–48.

Fredrikson, M., Wik, G., Greitz, T., Eriksson, L., Stone-Elander, S., Ericson, K., & Sedvall, G. (1993). Regional cerebral blood flow during experimental fear. *Psychophysiology, 30,* 126–130.

Georgiou, G. A., Bleakley, C., Hayward, J., Russo, R., Dutton, K., Eltiti, S., et al. (2005). Focusing on fear: Attentional disengagement from emotional faces. *Visual Cognition, 12,* 145–158.

Globisch, J., Hamm, A. O., Esteves, F., & Öhman, A. (1999). Fear appears fast: Temporal course of startle reflex potentiation in animal fearful subjects. *Psychophysiology, 36,* 66–75.

Hamm, A. O., Cuthbert, B. N., Globisch, J., & Vaitl, D. (1997). Fear and the startle reflex: Blink modulation and autonomic response patterns in animal and mutilation fearful subjects. *Psychophysiology, 34,* 97–107.

Hare, R. D., & Blevings, G. (1975). Defensive responses to phobic stimuli. *Biological Psychology, 3,* 1–13.

Hettema, J. M., Prescott, C. A., Myers, J. M., Neale, M. C., & Kendler, K. S. (2005). The structure of genetic and environmental risk factors for anxiety disorders in men and women. *Archives of General Psychiatry, 62,* 182–189.

Hoehn-Saric, R., & McLeod, D. R. (2000). Anxiety and arousal: Physiological changes and their perception. *Journal of Affective Disorders, 61,* 217–224.

Holender, D. (1986). Semantic activation without conscious identification in dichotic listening, parafoveal vision, and visual masking: A survey and appraisal. *Behavioral and Brain Sciences, 9,* 1–66.

Isbell, L. A. (2006). Snakes as agents of evolutionary

change in primate brains. *Journal of Human Evolution*, *51*, 1–35.

Juth, P., Lundqvist, D., Karlsson, A., & Öhman, A. (2005). Looking for foes and friends: Perceptual and emotional factors when finding a face in the crowd. *Emotion*, *5*, 379–395.

Keane, T. M., Kolb, L. C., Kaloupek, D. G., Orr, S. P., Blanchard, E. B., Thomas, R. G., et al. (1998). Utility of psychophysiological measurement in the diagnosis of posttraumatic stress disorder: Results from the Department of Veterans Affairs Cooperative Study. *Journal of Consulting and Clinical Psychology*, *66*, 914–923.

Kendler, K. S., Prescott, C. A., Myers, J., & Neale, M. C. (2003). The structure of genetic and environmental risk factors for common psychiatric and substance use disorders in men and women. *Archives of General Psychiatry*, *60*, 929–937.

Lader, M., & Marks, I. (1973). *Clinical anxiety*. London: Heinemann.

Lang, P. J. (1979). A bio-informational theory of emotional imagery. *Psychophysiology*, *16*, 495–512

Lang, P. J., Bradley, M. M., & Cuthbert, B. N. (1990). Emotion, attention, and the startle reflex. *Psychological Review*, *97*, 377–395.

Lang, P. J., Davis, M., & Öhman, A. (2000). Fear and anxiety: Animal models and human cognitive psychophysiology. *Journal of Affective Disorders*, *61*, 137–159.

Lang, P. J., McTeague, L. M., & Cuthbert, B. N. (2005). Fear startle, and the anxiety disorder spectrum. In B. Rothbaum (Ed.) *Pathological anxiety: Emotional processing in etiology and treatment* (pp. 56–77). New York: Guilford Press.

LeDoux, J. E. (1990). Fear pathways in the brain: Implications for a theory of the emotional brain. In P. F. Brain, S. Parmigiani, R. J. Blanchard, & D. Mainardi (Eds.), *Fear and defence* (pp. 163–177). London: Harwood.

LeDoux, J. E. (1996). *The emotional brain*. New York: Simon & Schuster.

Liddell, B. J., Brown, K. J., Kemp, A. H., Barton, M. J., Das, P., Peduto, A., et al. (2005). A direct brainstem–amygdala–cortical "alarm" system for subliminal signals of fear. *NeuroImage*, *24*, 235–243.

Lipp, O. V. (2006). Of snakes and flowers: Does preferential detection of pictures of fear-relevant animals in visual search reflect on fear-relevance? *Emotion*, *6*, 296–308.

Lipp, O. V., Derakshan, N., Waters, A., & Logies, S. (2004). Snakes and cats in the flower bed: Fast detection is not specific to pictures of fear-relevant stimuli. *Emotion*, *4*, 233–250.

Lundqvist, D., & Öhman, A. (2005). Emotion regulates attention: The relation between facial configuration, facial emotion, and visual attention. *Visual Cognition*, *12*, 51–84.

MacLeod, C., Mathews, A., & Tata, P. (1986). Attentional bias in emotional disorders. *Journal of Abnormal Psychology*, *95*, 15–20.

MacLeod, C., & Rutherford, E. M. (1992). Anxiety and the selective processing of emotional information: Mediating roles of awareness, trait and state variables, and personal relevance of stimulus materials. *Behaviour Research and Therapy*, *30*, 479–491.

Mather, M., & Knight, M. R. (2006). Angry faces get noticed quickly: Threat detection is not impaired among older adults. *Journal of Gerontology: B. Psychological Science*, *61*, 54–57.

Mathews, A. (1990). Why worry?: The cognitive function of anxiety. *Behaviour Research and Therapy*, *28*, 455–468.

Mathews, A., & MacLeod, C. (1994). Cognitive approaches to emotion and emotional disorders. *Annual Review of Psychology*, *45*, 25–50.

McNally, R. J. (1987). Preparedness and phobias: A review. *Psychological Bulletin*, *101*, 283–303.

McNeil, D. W., Vrana, S. R., Melamed, B. G., Cuthbert, B. N., & Lang, P. J. (1993). Emotional imagery in simple and social phobia: Fear versus anxiety. *Journal of Abnormal Psychology*, *102*, 212–225.

Miltner, W. H. R., Kriechel, S., Hecht, H., Trippe, R., & Weiss, T. (2004). Eye movements and behavioral responses to threatening and nonthreatening stimuli during visual search in phobic and nonphobic subjects. *Emotion*, *4*, 323–339.

Mineka, S., Rafaeli, E., & Yovel, I. (2003). Cognitive biases in emotional disorders: Information processing and social-cognitive perspectives. In R. J. Davidson, K. R. Scherer, & H. H. Goldsmith (Eds.). *Handbook of affective sciences* (pp. 976–1009). New York: Oxford University Press.

Mogg, K., & Bradley, B. P. (1998). A cognitive–motivational analysis of anxiety. *Behaviour Research and Therapy*, *36*, 809–848.

Mogg, K., & Bradley, B. P. (1999). Orienting attention to threatening facial expressions presented under conditions of restricted awareness. *Cognition and Emotion*, *13*, 713–740.

Mogg, K., & Bradley, B. P. (2002). Selective orienting of attention to masked threat faces in social anxiety. *Behaviour Research and Therapy*, *40*, 1403–1414.

Mogg, K., Bradley, B. P., & Williams, R. (1995). Attentional bias in anxiety and depression: The role of awareness. *British Journal of Clinical Psychology*, *34*, 17–36.

Mogg, K., Millar, N., & Bradley, B. P. (2000). Biases in eye movement to threatening facial expression in generalized anxiety disorder and depressive disorder. *Journal of Abnormal Psychology*, *109*, 695–704.

Morris, J. S., deGelder, B., Weiskrantz, L., & Dolan, R. J. (2001). Differential extrageniculostriate and amygdala responses to presentation of emotional faces in a cortically blind field. *Brain*, *124*, 1241–1252.

Morris, J. S., Öhman, A., & Dolan, R. J. (1998). Conscious and unconscious emotional learning in the human amygdala. *Nature*, *393*, 467–470.

Morris, J. S., Öhman, A., & Dolan, R. J. (1999). A

subcortical pathway to the right amygdala mediating "unseen" fear. *Proceedings of the National Academy of Sciences USA, 96,* 1680–1685.

Öhman, A. (1979). The orienting response, attention, and learning: An information processing perspective. In H. D. Kimmel, E. H. van Olst, & J. F. Orlebeke (Eds.), *The orienting reflex in humans* (pp. 443–472). Hillsdale, NJ: Erlbaum.

Öhman, A. (1986). Face the beast and fear the face: Animal and social fears as prototypes for evolutionary analyses of emotion. *Psychophysiology, 23,* 123–145.

Öhman, A. (1993). Fear and anxiety as emotional phenomena: Clinical phenomenology, evolutionary perspectives, and information processing mechanisms. In M. Lewis & J. M. Haviland (Eds.) *Handbook of emotions* (pp. 511–536). New York: Guilford Press.

Öhman, A. (1999). Distinguishing unconscious from conscious emotional processes: Methodological considerations and theoretical implications. In T. Dalgleish & M. Power (Eds.), *Handbook of cognition and emotion* (pp. 321–352). Chichester, UK: Wiley.

Öhman, A. (2000). Fear and anxiety: Evolutionary, cognitive, and clinical perspectives. In M. Lewis & J. M. Haviland-Jones (Eds.), *Handbook of emotions* (2nd ed., pp. 573–593). New York: Guilford Press.

Öhman, A., Dimberg, U., & Öst, L.-G. (1985). Animal and social phobias: Biological constraints on learned fear responses. In S. Reiss & R. R. Bootzin (Eds.), *Theoretical issues in behavior therapy* (pp. 123–175). New York: Academic Press.

Öhman, A., Eriksson, A., & Olofsson, C. (1975). One trial learning and superior resistance to extinction of autonomic responses conditioned to potentially phobic stimuli. *Journal of Comparative and Physiological Psychology, 88,* 619–627.

Öhman, A., Flykt, A., & Esteves, F. (2001). Emotion drives attention: Detecting the snake in the grass. *Journal of Experimental Psychology: General, 130,* 466–478.

Öhman, A., Flykt, A., & Lundqvist, D. (2000). Unconscious emotion: Evolutionary perspectives, psychophysiological data, and neuropsychological mechanisms. In R. Lane & L. Nadel (Eds.), *The cognitive neuroscience of emotion* (pp. 296–327). New York: Oxford University Press.

Öhman, A., Hamm, A. O., & Hugdahl, K. (2000). Cognition and the autonomic nervous system: Orienting, anticipation, and conditioning. In J. T. Cacioppo, L. G. Tassinary, & G. G. Berntson (Eds.), *Handbook of psychophysiology* (pp. 533–575). New York: Cambridge University Press.

Öhman, A., Lundqvist, D., & Esteves, F. (2001). The face in the crowd revisited: An anger superiority effect with schematic stimuli. *Journal of Personality and Social Psychology, 80,* 381–396.

Öhman, A., & Mineka, S. (2001). Fears, phobias, and preparedness: Toward an evolved module of fear and fear learning. *Psychological Review, 108,* 483–522.

Öhman, A., & Mineka, S. (2003). The malicious serpent: Snakes as a prototypical stimulus for an evolved module of fear. *Current Directions in Psychological Science, 12,* 2–9.

Öhman, A., & Soares, J. J. F. (1993). On the automaticity of phobic fear: Conditioned skin conductance responses to masked fear-relevant stimuli. *Journal of Abnormal Psychology, 102,* 121–132.

Öhman, A., & Soares, J. J. F. (1994). "Unconscious anxiety": Phobic responses to masked stimuli. *Journal of Abnormal Psychology, 103,* 231–240.

Öhman, A., & Soares, J. J. F. (1998). Emotional conditioning to masked stimuli: Expectancies for aversive outcomes following nonrecognized fear-relevant stimuli. *Journal of Experimental Psychology: General, 127,* 69–82.

Öhman, A., & Wiens, S. (2004). The concept of an evolved fear module and cognitive theories of anxiety. In A. S. R. Manstead, N. Frijda, & A. Fischer (Eds.), *Feelings and emotions: The Amsterdam Symposium* (pp. 58–80). Cambridge, UK: Cambridge University Press.

Orr, S. P., & Roth, W. T. (2000). Psychophysiological assessment: Clinical applications for PTSD. *Journal of Affective Disorders, 61,* 225–240.

Parra, C., Esteves, F., Flykt, A., & Öhman, A. (1997). Pavlovian conditioning to social stimuli: Backward masking and the dissociation of implicit and explicit cognitive processes. *European Psychologist, 2,* 106–117.

Pasley, B. N., Mayes, L. C., & Schultz, R. T. (2004). Subcortical discrimination of unperceived objects during binocular rivalry. *Neuron, 42,* 163–172.

Pegna, A., Khateb, A., Lazeyras, F., & Seqhier, M. (2005). Discriminating emotional faces without primary visual cortices involves the right amygdala, *Nature Neuroscience, 8,* 24–25.

Pessoa, L. (2005). To what extent are emotional visual stimuli processed without attention and awareness? *Current Opinion in Neurobiology, 15,* 188–196.

Pessoa, L., McKenna, M., Gutierrez, E., & Ungerleider, L. G. (2002). Neural processing of emotional faces requires attention. *Proceedings of the National Academy of Sciences of the USA, 99,* 11458–11463.

Phelps, E. A. (2006). Emotion and cognition: Insights from studies of the human amygdala. *Annual Review of Psychology, 57,* 27–53.

Phelps, E. A., Ling, S., & Carasco, M. (2006). Emotion facilitates perception and potentiates the perceptual benefits of attention. *Psychological Science, 17,* 292–299.

Posner, M. I. (1978). *Chronometric explorations of mind.* Hillsdale, NJ: Erlbaum.

Posner, M. I., Inhoff, A. W., Friedrich, F. J., & Cohen, A. (1987). Isolating attentional systems: A cognitive-anatomical analysis. *Psychobiology, 15,* 107–121.

Posner, M. I., & Peterson, S. E. (1990). The attention system of the human brain. *Annual Review of Neuroscience, 13,* 25–42.

Rapee, R. M. (1991). Generalized anxiety disorder: A review of clinical features and theoretical concepts. *Clinical Psychology Review, 11*, 419–440.

Rauch, S. L., Savage, C. R., Nathaniel, M. A., Miguel, E., Baer, L., Breiter, H. C., et al. (1995). A positron emission tomographic study of simple phobic symptom provocation. *Archives of General Psychiatry, 52*, 20–28.

Rinck, M., Reinecke, A., Ellwart, T., Heuer, K., & Becker, E. S. (2005). Speeded detection and increased distraction in fear of spiders: Evidence from eye movements. *Journal of Abnormal Psychology, 114*, 235–248.

Rolls, E. T. (1999). *The brain and emotion.* Oxford, UK: Oxford University Press.

Sabatinelli, D., Bradley, M. M. M., Fitzsimmons, J. R., & Lang, P. J. (2005). Parallel amygdala and inferotemporal activation reflect emotional intensity and fear relevance. *NeuroImage, 24*, 1265–1270.

Schneider, W., Dumais, S. T., & Shiffrin, R. M. (1984). Automatic and control processing and attention. In R. Parasuraman & D. R. Davies (Eds.), *Varieties of attention* (pp. 1–27). Orlando, FL: Academic Press.

Seligman, M. E. P. (1971). Phobias and preparedness. *Behavior Therapy, 2*, 307–320.

Soares, J. J. F., & Öhman, A. (1993a). Backward masking and skin conductance responses after conditioning to non-feared but fear-relevant stimuli in fearful subjects. *Psychophysiology, 30*, 460–466.

Soares, J. J. F., & Öhman, A. (1993b). Preattentive processing, preparedness, and phobias: Effects of instruction on conditioned electrodermal responses to masked and non-masked fear-relevant stimuli. *Behaviour Research and Therapy, 31*, 87–95.

Spielberger, C. D. (1972). Anxiety as an emotional state. In C. D. Spielberger (Ed.), *Anxiety: Current trends in theory and research* (Vol. 1, pp. 23–49). New York: Academic Press.

Straube, T., Mentzel, H.-J., & Miltner, W. H. R. (2006). Neural mechanisms of automatic and direct processing of phobigenic stimuli in specific phobia. *Biological Psychiatry, 59*, 162–170.

Tipples, J., Atkinson, A. P., & Young, A. W. (2002). The eyebrow frown: A salient social signal. *Emotion, 2*, 288–296.

Tuma, A. H., & Maser, J. D. (Eds.). (1985). *Anxiety and the anxiety disorders.* Hillsdale, NJ: Erlbaum.

Vuilleumier, P., Armony, J. L., Driver, J., & Dolan, R. J. (2001). Effects of attention and emotion on faces processing in the human brain: An event-related fMRI study. *Neuron, 30*, 829–841.

Vuilleumier, P., Armony, J. L., Driver, J., & Dolan, R. J. (2003). Distinct spatial frequency sensitivities for processing faces and emotional expressions. *Nature Neuroscience, 6*, 624–631.

Vuilleumier, P., Richardson, M. P., Armony, J. L., Driver, J., & Dolan, R. (2004). Distant influences of amygdala lesion on visual cortical activation during emotional face processing. *Nature Neuroscience, 7*, 1271–1278.

Walker, D. L., Toufexis, D. J., & Davis, M. (2003). Role of the bed nucleus of the stria terminalis versus the amygdala in fear, stress, and anxiety. *European Journal of Pharmacology, 463*, 199–216.

Whalen, P. J., Rauch, S. L., Etcoff, N. L., McInerney, S. C., Lee, M. B., & Jenike, M. A. (1998). Masked presentations of emotional facial expressions modulate amygdala activity without explicit knowledge. *Journal of Neuroscience, 18*, 411–418.

Wilson, E. J., MacLeod, C., Mathews, A., & Rutherford, E. M. (2006). The causal role of interpretive bias in anxiety reactivity. *Journal of Abnormal Psychology, 115*, 103–111.

CHAPTER 45

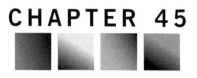

The Development of Anger and Hostile Interactions

ELIZABETH A. LEMERISE and KENNETH A. DODGE

Since the publication of the first and second editions of this volume (Lewis & Haviland, 1993; Lewis & Haviland-Jones, 2000), research on emotions has grown to the point where emotion is a major focus in the sixth edition of the *Handbook of Child Psychology* (Eisenberg, 2006). Here we trace the normative development of anger in infants and children, with the thesis that anger develops and comes to be regulated in the context of transactions with the social environment (Parke, 1994). Also, individual differences in abilities/capacities and developmental changes contribute to this transaction and shed light on important processes (Bugenthal & Grusec, 2006). The literature reviewed here includes studies on infants' and children's expression of anger; their reactions to and appraisal of anger; their regulation of and/or coping with anger in themselves and others; and their understanding of anger, including display rules. We also consider socialization processes relevant to anger, and both adaptive and maladaptive aspects of anger and angry interactions.

THE FUNCTIONAL SIGNIFICANCE OF ANGER

Although emotion theorists do not agree on whether anger is a primary human emotion (Izard, 1991) or is differentiated from a generalized distress state (Camras, 1992), they do agree that anger serves a variety of adaptive functions. Anger organizes and regulates physiological and psychological processes related to self-defense and mastery and regulates social and interpersonal behaviors (Izard & Kobak, 1991; Lewis, Sullivan, Ramsay, & Alessandri, 1992; Saarni, Campos, Camras, & Witherington, 2006). From a functionalist perspective on emotion, when there is an obstacle to goal attainment, anger's function is to overcome obstacles in order to achieve goals (Saarni et al., 2006). Despite its adaptive significance, anger poses difficulties for social organisms in that it repels others (Marsh, Ambady, & Kleck, 2005), incurring long-term costs. Thus the regulation and appropriate expression of anger are key developmental tasks. Individuals must learn their culture's "display rules," which concern when, to whom, and how to express emotions in culturally acceptable ways. Indirect socialization of display rules can be observed quite early in infancy (Malatesta & Haviland, 1982). Anger regulates interpersonal behavior and comes to be regulated in an interpersonal context via socialization by caregivers, peers, and the larger social context (Oatley & Jenkins, 1996). Problems in regulating and appropriately expressing anger appropriately have implications for social functioning (Eisenberg, Fabes, Nyman, Bernzweig, & Pineulas, 1994; Murphy, Shepard, Eisenberg, & Fabes, 2004), as well as for the development of psychopathology and disease (Barefoot, Dodge, Peterson, Dahlstrom, & Williams, 1989; Casey & Schlosser, 1994; Cole, Teti, & Zahn-Waxler, 2003; Suinn, 2001).

THE DEVELOPMENTAL COURSE OF ANGER AND ITS REGULATION

Anger in Infants and Toddlers

Validity of Infant Anger

The question of whether young infants display discrete negative emotions (including anger), or a more generalized distress reaction, is the topic of an ongoing debate (Bennett, Bendersky, & Lewis, 2002, 2004; Camras, 2004; Camras, Sullivan, & Michel, 1993; Izard, 2004; Izard et al., 1995; Oster, Hegley, & Nagel, 1992). In part, this debate reflects the inherent difficulties in studying infants. Although objective methods for coding infants' facial expressions of emotion are available (MAX and AFFEX; Izard, 1983; Izard, Dougherty, & Hembree, 1983), some researchers have questioned whether infant facial expressions reflect internal states (Saarni et al., 2006). Another source of difficulty lies in finding situations that reliably elicit particular emotions (Bennett et al., 2002, 2004; Camras, 2004; Izard, 2004). Similar problems arise when considering data that young infants respond differentially to naturally presented, multimodal emotion displays, especially in their mothers (e.g., Kahana-Kalman & Walker-Andrews, 2001; Montague & Walker-Andrews, 2001), because it is not clear what cues are driving the responses or what the responses mean regarding infants' understanding of expressions (see Saarni et al., 2006). Unfortunately, this debate has had an inhibiting ef-

fect on research on infant anger. In the remainder of this section, we summarize studies that examine anger in the first year. As a group, these studies used MAX/AFFEX—coding schemes that yield discrete codes for negative emotions.

Early Development of Anger

In previous editions of this chapter (Lemerise & Dodge, 1993, 2000), we reviewed work by Stenberg and Campos (1990) and Izard, Hembree, and Hueber (1987) suggesting that the first clear expressions of anger emerge at about 4 months of age, and that anger expressions are targeted to a social figure by 7 months. These expressions have been observed in response to arm restraint (Stenberg & Campos, 1990) and inoculations (Izard et al., 1987). Field and colleagues (e.g., Field et al., 2005; Pickens & Field, 1993; see also Reissland, Shepherd, & Herrera, 2005) have observed anger expressions in infants as young as 3 months during face-to-face interactions with mothers, particularly in infants of depressed mothers. Anger expressions have been observed in infants as young as 2 months in the context of a contingency-learning paradigm (Lewis, Alessandri, & Sullivan, 1990). In this paradigm, infants learn that an arm-pulling response produces an interesting display. Goal blockage is introduced by removing the contingency between arm pulling and the display, thus fulfilling the functionalist definition of an anger-eliciting situation wherein the infant's goal can be specified with greater certainty than in arm restraint, for example. At extinction, anger (but not sadness) is associated with arm pulling, and the highest levels of joy, interest, and arm pulling occur when the contingency is reinstated (Lewis et al., 1990, 1992; Sullivan & Lewis, 2003; Sullivan, Lewis, & Alessandri, 1992). Lewis and Ramsay (2005) replicated these results in 4- to 6-month-olds with contingency learning and a still-face procedure; sadness, but not anger, was found to relate to cortisol responses, supporting the hypothesis that sadness and anger are distinct in young infants.

A study by Buss and Goldsmith (1998) also underscores the adaptive significance of anger. In separate sessions, 6-, 12-, and 18-month-old infants were exposed to two anger-eliciting stimuli (a barrier problem and arm restraint) and two fear-eliciting stimuli, which elicited the predicted emotions. Anger and fear were distinct and not significantly related to one another, as might be expected if they were really "distress." Infants used different regulatory strategies for anger and fear; these regulatory behaviors reduced their anger, but not their fear, expressions. Buss and Goldsmith concluded that the emotion regulation literature's almost exclusive focus on negative emotion as a global construct has obscured important between-emotion differences in infants' regulatory strategies.

Factors Affecting the Development of Anger

The body of work reviewed suggests that anger is associated with infants' attempts to master the physical environment, and that anger elicits behavioral strategies from infants that serve regulatory functions and contribute to problem solving. An infant's anger can also be a social signal, mobilizing a reaction from the caregiver that assists the infant in modulating distress. At the same time, however, caregivers' socialization goals are to encourage positive and neutral emotions and to minimize negative emotions. Differential responding to positive and negative emotions by caregivers is related to the increasing frequency of positive and neutral expressions over time; also, mothers are more likely to reinforce sadness than anger (Malatesta, Culver, Tesman, & Shepard, 1989; Malatesta & Haviland, 1982). Children as young as 24 months appear to be responsive to these differential responses to negative emotions. In laboratory situations designed to elicit fear and anger, children did exhibit the targeted emotions, *except* when they looked at their mothers; during these looks, sad expressions were more likely (Buss & Kiel, 2004).

Campos and colleagues have suggested that infants' evolving abilities alter transactions with their environments (Campos et al., 2000; Campos, Kermoian, & Zumbahlen, 1992). For example, Campos et al. (1992) reported that the onset of locomotion is associated with parent report of anger in both infants and parents, as well as with the perception that the infants are more autonomous and responsible.

Campos et al.'s (1992) work also suggests that seeing an infant as autonomous is linked to a parent's using direct socialization strategies and being less permissive. The child's increasing autonomy makes it more likely that the parent and child will find themselves at cross-purposes. In Goodenough's (1931) classic

monograph, as children moved from infancy to toddlerhood, parents became less permissive of anger and used a variety of strategies, such as coaxing, diversion of attention, ignoring, and physical restraint, to discourage it. With increasing age, ignoring continued to be used for girls, whereas boys received more attention for anger in the form of power-assertive measures such as threats, spankings, and deprivation of privileges (Goodenough, 1931; see also Radke-Yarrow & Kochanska, 1990).

Although direct socialization methods are used more with older children, caregivers do not abandon indirect socialization methods. Denham (1993) found that mothers and their 2-year-olds responded contingently to each other's emotion displays, and that mothers seemed to have agendas similar to those reported by Malatesta and Haviland (1982; i.e., maximizing positive and neutral emotions, minimizing negative emotions). Mothers who responded to toddlers' anger with calm neutrality or cheerful displays had toddlers who showed interest in the environment, positive emotions, and positive responses to strangers in their mothers' absence. On the other hand, as Crockenberg (1985) demonstrated, angry maternal responding to toddlers' difficult behaviors is associated with toddlers' persisting in angry, noncompliant behavior and a lower likelihood of empathic responding to others. Thus socialization practices that act to modulate toddlers' negative arousal may make possible more competent and empathic behavior, whereas socialization practices that exacerbate system arousal may hinder social development.

Another mechanism of indirect socialization involves exposure to interadult anger. Infants as young as 3 months respond differentially to mothers' natural (multimodal) displays of emotion, including anger (e.g., Haviland & Lelwica, 1987), and 5-month-old infants respond differentially to positively and negatively toned infant-directed vocalizations in their own and unfamiliar languages (Fernald, 1993). According to maternal diaries of naturally occurring emotions, children as young as 12 months may stare or "freeze," look concerned or frown, or show distress by whimpering when witnessing others' angry interactions. Slightly older children engage in social referencing (Walden & Ogan, 1988) of their mothers (Radke-Yarrow & Kochanska, 1990), in order to learn how to interpret social stimuli.

Beginning at 16–18 months, toddlers use more direct strategies, such as covering their ears, leaving the room, intervening verbally and/or physically (Cummings, Zahn-Waxler, & Radke-Yarrow, 1981; Radke-Yarrow & Kochanska, 1990), or behaving aggressively. Data from a laboratory study suggest that exposure to emotionally arousing situations creates expectancies about adults' interactions (Jenkins, Franco, Dolins, & Sewell, 1995). Jenkins et al. argued that interadult anger influences children's models of relationships, which are used to interpret future interactions (see also Dodge, Bates, & Pettit, 1990; Schwartz, Dodge, Pettit, & Bates, 1997).

Complicating the picture of the normative development of anger, there are individual differences in infants' "anger-proneness," considered to be a component of temperament. Calkins, Dedman, Gill, Lomax, and Johnson (2002) compared 6-month-olds on "frustration reactivity, . . . a pattern of negative affect characterized by anger and low tolerance for frustration" (p. 176). Based on a composite measure derived from three laboratory frustration tasks and maternal reports of distress, infants were classified as easily frustrated versus not easily frustrated. The easily frustrated infants displayed greater physiological reactivity (which they were less able to regulate), poorer attention, and higher activity levels. Calkins and colleagues suggested that the implications of greater frustration reactivity may depend on the extent to which infants receive support in their environments for managing their affect. Support for this hypothesis is found in longitudinal work by Kochanska and colleagues. Kochanska, Aksan, and Carlson (2005) found that maternal responsiveness and security of attachment with fathers promoted later receptive cooperation with parents in anger-prone 7-month-olds. Kochanska (2001) also found that while securely attached children became less angry from 14 to 33 months, insecurely attached children increased in negative emotional expressivity; disorganized attachment was associated with large increases in anger and decreases in fear (see also Lyons-Ruth, Alpern, & Repacholi, 1993; Shaw, Owens, Vondra, Keenan, & Winslow, 1996).

In summary, the emergence of anger in infants remains a topic of theoretical and methodological debate. An answer to this question awaits the resolution of the thorny issue of how to measure infants' emotions reliably and validly. However, the perception of infants as autonomous and responsible, coincident with the emergence of locomotion, is associated with parental reports of infant anger. It may be that locomoting infants' goals are clearer to adult observers, and that the infants' response to goal blockage is thus easier to interpret as anger. Research from a variety of investigators suggests that anger is an important energizer of infants' adaptive behavior. However, the onset of locomotion often places infants' goals at odds with those of caregivers, increasing the incidence of anger between them. Parents become less permissive of angry outbursts, and socialization of anger becomes more direct. Toddlers' social-emotional competence has been linked to maternal socialization practices that modulate strong negative emotions and encourage positive and neutral ones.

Anger and Its Regulation in Preschool-Age Children

Preschoolers continue to learn to coordinate their goals with those of others and are thus expected to show increasing control of anger. Peers emerge as important new socializers of anger, and language affords children a new way to express emotions and gives parents a powerful tool in socializing emotion. However, preschoolers still have relatively poor control over their emotion displays. An important developmental task involves learning to manage arousal in service of goals for play and affiliation with peers (Parker & Gottman, 1989). Emotion socialization processes in the family contribute to social competence with peers and at preschool (e.g., Denham, 1998; Dunn & Brown, 1994; Gottman, Katz, & Hooven, 1997).

The Expression and Socialization of Anger in the Family Context

Parents can indirectly influence children's expressivity through contingent emotion displays during dyadic interaction. Also, with the advent of language, parents can teach or coach children about emotion. Finally, parents influence children's opportunities to learn about emotion by regulating their access to peers, stimulating games, and television programs, and by protecting versus exposing them to emotional displays and arguments (Eisenberg, Cumberland, & Spinrad, 1998; Parke, 1994).

Because preschoolers generally have poorer control of their emotion displays than do older children, observational methods in the home and laboratory are often used to study emotions at this age. Across home and laboratory settings, evidence indicates that negative affect (especially anger) in the context of parent–child interaction—particularly if it is intense, reciprocated, and/or more frequent than for most children and parents—is associated with poorer child outcomes (Carson & Parke, 1996; Cole et al., 2003; Denham, Mitchell-Copeland, Strandberg, Auerbach, & Blair, 1997; Hayden, Klein, & Durbin, 2005; Rubin, Burgess, Dwyer, & Hastings, 2003; Snyder, Stoolmiller, Wilson, & Yamamoto, 2003). In contrast, "emotion coaching" (combining low anger with verbal strategies) is positively correlated with social competence (Denham et al., 1997; Dunn & Brown, 1994; Garner & Spears, 2000; Gottman et al., 1997). Also, converging evidence demonstrates that parental sensitive responding, particularly as manifested in secure attachment, is protective for children who are anger-prone (e.g., Denham, Blair, Schmidt, & DeMulder, 2002; Kochanska, 2001).

Parents socialize children's anger by regulating their exposure to angry situations, either intentionally or unintentionally. Children of all ages find adults' anger stressful; exposure to interadult anger may sensitize children toward anger, making it more likely that they will be aggressive (Cummings, 1994; Schudlich, Shamir, & Cummings, 2004; Schwartz et al., 1997). Children's negative emotionality may exacerbate these effects (Davies & Cummings, 1995). Children older than 6 years show increasing sensitivity to whether conflicts are resolved and are less upset by resolved conflicts, but even 4- to 5-year-olds are somewhat sensitive to this information (El-Sheikh & Cummings, 1995; Shifflett-Simpson & Cummings, 1996).

The Expression and Socialization of Anger in the Peer Context

Preschoolers' emotion regulation skills equip them, for better or worse, for interactions with peers. Peer interactions provide a unique context for becoming more socially competent and learning to manage one's emotions, particularly when in conflict with peers (e.g., Putallaz & Sheppard, 1992). Children who are high in negative emotionality play less with peers over time (Fabes, Hanish, Martin, & Eisenberg, 2002), thus missing important socialization experiences. Poorly regulated anger is predictive of conduct problems (Cole et al., 2003; Rydell,

Berlin, & Bohlin, 2003) and lower levels of empathy (Strayer & Roberts, 2004), whereas preschoolers' emotion knowledge and emotion regulation skills predict social competence with peers both concurrently and longitudinally (Denham, et al., 2003; Denham, Caverly, et al., 2002; Eisenberg, et al., 1997).

Arsenio and colleagues have examined preschool children's affect both during and outside conflicts. Arsenio and Killen (1996) videotaped and coded with AFFEX triads of preschoolers during table play. Conflict initiators displayed more positive affect during conflicts, whereas recipients expressed more anger and sadness. Children who were "happy initiators" were more likely to be angry and surprised when they were targets of conflict. Recipients of conflict who exhibited higher levels of anger and sadness were more at risk for both initiating and being the targets of conflicts. Similar findings were reported for conflict and aggression observed during free play (Arsenio, Cooperman, & Lover, 2000; Arsenio & Lover, 1997). Also, anger expressed outside conflict situations predicted both initiation of aggression and anger during aggression.

Another approach to studying anger in preschoolers is to present hypothetical situations and to elicit verbal or behavioral responses. An advantage of this method is that anger-eliciting situations can be presented in a standardized manner. When researchers are studying naturally occurring conflicts/anger, not all children exhibit the behaviors of interest, and the circumstances surrounding conflict events vary widely and nonrandomly across participants (Murphy & Eisenberg, 1997). Denham, Bouril, and Belouad (1994) presented preschoolers with hypothetical provocation and peer entry situations, and asked them how they would feel and what they would do. Children who said that they would be angry were more likely to select aggression and less likely to pick prosocial behavior as responses. In the classroom, these children were less expressive; teachers were more likely to rate them as miserable/fearful. Eisenberg, Fabes, Minore, et al. (1994) used a puppet paradigm in which preschoolers acted out responses to hypothetical conflict situations. Children's puppet enactments related well to observed anger reactions at preschool and to reports from mothers and teachers about how the children handled conflict. High levels of emotionality were associated with high levels of aggression and less friendliness enacted with puppets. Murphy and

Eisenberg (1997) found that boys' friendly responses to hypothetical provocateurs were related to socializers' reports of high self-regulation and low emotional intensity. Across studies, negative emotionality, especially anger, is associated with aggression in preschoolers.

Preschoolers' Knowledge about Anger

Preschoolers exhibit increasing understanding of the situational determinants of emotion and rules guiding the display of emotions; this knowledge predicts social competence both concurrently and longitudinally (Denham, 1998; Denham et al., 2003). Using hypothetical-situation methodology, Zeman, Penza, Shipman, and Young (1997) investigated the effects of social partner (mother, father, friend) on 4-year-olds' use of display rules and expectancies about managing emotion. Children reported that they would feel angry most often and regulate emotion more with mothers and friends than with fathers. Children expected mothers and fathers to be more receptive than friends to displays of emotion; they were more likely to report that they would express negative emotions when they expected to receive support or assistance. Thus 4-year-olds demonstrated an awareness of display rules and a sensitivity to the role of context in their use.

In summary, during the preschool period demands are placed on children by family and peers to regulate and express emotions in socially constructive ways. Children make great strides in controlling emotion displays and understanding situational determinants of emotion and display rules. Some children, however, begin to show deficits in managing emotions, especially anger; these difficulties predict poorer social functioning and problem behaviors.

Anger and Its Regulation in School-Age Children

A number of factors converge to make the peer context salient for school-age children. With school entry, children spend more time with peers and are exposed to a greater number and variety of peers. School-age children acquire information about their own competencies by comparing themselves to peers; across the elementary school years, children increase in their use of social comparison (Stipek & MacIver, 1989). Children show increasing sensitivity to their position relative to peers; being accepted by peers and having friends assume great importance (Parker & Gottman, 1989), making peer group norms for emotion regulation especially significant. Parker and Gottman contend that children learn a great deal about display rules from the reactions of peers to their own and others' emotion displays. Moreover, the peer norm during middle childhood is to avoid emotionality and give the impression of "being 'cool'—calm, unruffled, and always under emotional control" (Parker & Gottman, 1989, p. 116).

Research on children's use and understanding of display rules supports Parker and Gottman's (1989) view. Children expect more negative reactions from peers than parents for expressing anger and sadness, and report using display rules more with friends than with parents (Zeman & Shipman, 1998). Children expect little support for expressing anger, particularly via sulking or aggression (Zeman & Shipman, 1996; Shipman, Zeman, Nesin, & Fitzgerald, 2003), and report more masking of anger than of other emotions (Underwood, 1997). Also, they see anger as hard to control, reporting lower self-efficacy for controlling anger than sadness (Zeman & Shipman, 1997). Underwood (1997) found no peer status differences in emotion display rule knowledge, indicating that these peer group norms are quite salient for all children.

Given the peer group norms for controlling one's emotions, it is not surprising that indices of peer group acceptance during middle childhood are related to children's skills at reading and managing emotions, including anger (Bryant, 1992; Cassidy, Parke, Butkovsky, & Braungart, 1992; Hubbard & Coie, 1994; Vosk, Forehand, & Figueroa, 1983). In contrast, poor regulation of negative emotions, especially anger, is associated with peer rejection (Eisenberg, Fabes, Guthrie, & Reiser, 2000) and victimization (Hanish et al., 2004).

Research and theory on social information processing (SIP) provide a mechanism for understanding how anger influences social behavior (Crick & Dodge, 1994; Lemerise & Arsenio, 2000). One important process in regulating anger responses is a child's skill in interpreting others' intentions in social situations. Children who are relatively poor at interpreting peers' intentions, especially prosocial and benign intentions, are unlikely to be socially popular with peers (Dodge, Murphy, &

Buchsbaum, 1984) and are likely to display aggressive behavior toward peers (Dodge, Pettit, McClaskey, & Brown, 1986). Biases in interpretations of peers' intentions are particularly relevant to anger and aggression responses. Children who are biased toward attributing hostile intent in peers are likely to display anger, behave aggressively, and grow in aggression across development (Dodge, 1980; Dodge & Pettit, 2003). Converging evidence shows that harsh parenting contributes to anger perception bias and to later aggression and conduct problems (Fine, Trentacosta, Izard, Mostow, & Campbell, 2004; Pollack, 2003; Schultz, Izard, & Bear, 2004; Schultz & Shaw, 2003). Also, aggressive individuals report experiencing more anger and being less in control of their anger than do nonaggressive children and adolescents (Camodeca & Goossens, 2005; DiLiberto, Katz, Beauchamp, & Howells, 2002; Graham, Hudley, & Williams, 1992; Orobio de Castro, Merk, Koops, Veerman, & Bosch, 2005). Other research has shown that aggressive children are more susceptible to anger expressed by others. In videotaped hypothetical situations, provocateurs' angry emotion displays have been found to facilitate hostile social goals and problem solving, whereas provocateurs' happy displays suppress hostile goals and are associated with friendlier problem-solving responses in aggressive children (Lemerise, Fredstrom, Kelley, Bowersox, & Waford, 2006; Lemerise, Gregory, & Fredstrom, 2005).

In other SIP research, arousal has been experimentally manipulated via staged situations. For example, when a "threat" was staged, rejected–aggressive boys made more SIP errors of presumed hostility and more hostile attributions than did adjusted–nonaggressive boys (Dodge & Somberg, 1987). Similar results were reported in a study using a manipulation that involved unjustly losing a computer game (Orobio de Castro, Slot, Bosch, Koops, & Veerman, 2003). These studies suggest that for aggressive children, feelings of anger may "short-circuit" evaluations of intent, leading to aggressive responding. This interpretation receives support in a study that examined second graders' nonverbal behavior and physiological reactivity in the context of a manipulation where children lost a board game to a confederate who obviously cheated. Reactive aggression (Dodge & Coie, 1987) was positively related to nonverbal expression of anger and physiological reactivity, both of which in-

creased throughout the course of the game for those high in reactive aggression. On the other hand, children low in reactive aggression displayed low and steady levels of nonverbal expressions of anger and physiological reactivity throughout the game (Hubbard et al., 2002; see also Hubbard, 2001; Underwood & Hurley, 1999; Waschbusch et al., 2002).

The research on school-age children suggests individual differences in the ability to deal with anger and provocative situations. Rejected and/or aggressive children have difficulty regulating their anger in provocative situations, and this contributes to goals and responses that are less socially competent and constructive. Converging research suggests that individual differences in negative emotionality and regulation contribute to peer status differences in emotion-related skills and social competence. Children who are high in regulatory skills and low in negative emotionality, general emotional intensity, and nonconstructive coping show high-quality social functioning, both concurrently and longitudinally (Eisenberg et al., 1997, 2005; Murphy & Eisenberg, 1996; Rydell et al., 2003). Moreover, interventions for children with conduct problems that include training in the recognition and management of anger have shown some degree of success (e.g., Greenberg & Kusche, 1993; Lochman & Wells, 2004; Weiss, Harris, Catron, & Han, 2003).

SUMMARY AND CONCLUSIONS

Examination of the developmental course of anger and its regulation reveals that the role and meaning of anger in a child's repertoire change developmentally. For infants, the expression of anger is often associated with being effective. When someone is restraining an infant's movement, or a barrier is placed between the infant and a desirable object, anger energizes and organizes behaviors (e.g., struggling, pushing away the barrier) that "work" in the sense that they reduce anger and obtain goals. Infants' angry signals are also effective in producing responses that reduce anger and increase the infants' sense of efficacy. However, the onset of locomotion changes parents' views of infants; they see infants as autonomous, responsible, and angry, and they are more likely to report getting angry with their infants. Thus the "rules" appear to change at this point, and parents begin to socialize the expression of anger more actively. Although children begin to learn that anger doesn't *always* work, they still find that it is effective in obtaining instrumental goals (Patterson, Littman, & Bricker, 1967).

The process of socializing anger and its regulation is complex. The role of children's temperament seems to be important, but we know less about how parents' temperament contributes to the process. Clearly, some children experience emotions more intensely and have more difficulty regulating their emotions, and these characteristics have long-term implications for their social functioning. In several studies, socialization techniques that combine minimization of negative emotions with emotion coaching have been found to facilitate empathy and prosocial responding, and thus to promote emotional and social competence. However, it is less clear whether these techniques work equally well with children who vary in emotional intensity and self-regulation skills.

As children move from infancy to early childhood, their social circle widens, and peers become important elicitors and socializers of anger. Children must learn to coordinate their goals with those of others who are much less indulgent than parents. Affiliative goals play a crucial role in motivating children to control arousal in order to sustain the exciting and enjoyable activity of play with peers and to maintain friendship. Children's temperamental profiles and/or their socialization experiences in the family may prepare them to function more or less effectively with peers. Difficulties with peers may further reduce children's opportunities and motivation to learn to manage anger in ways that preserve relationships.

By elementary school, children with deficits in anger regulation are at risk for problem behaviors, and children who have been diagnosed with externalizing disorders show deficits in the expression, appraisal, and regulation of emotions, particularly anger. These findings underscore the importance of continuing to study how anger and other emotions regulate and come to be regulated in the context of social interactions.

In conclusion, progress has been made in the study of anger and its development. The results reviewed here have considerable applied significance for those working with children who have difficulties with peers, as well as more serious problems. Continued progress depends on resolving methodological debates and developing new techniques to study anger.

REFERENCES

Arsenio, W., Cooperman, S., & Lover, A. (2000). Affective predictors of preschool children's aggression and peer acceptance: Direct and indirect effects. *Developmental Psychology, 36*, 438–448.

Arsenio, W., & Killen, M. (1996). Conflict-related emotions during peer disputes. *Early Education and Development, 7*, 43–57.

Arsenio, W., & Lover, A. (1997). Emotions, conflicts and aggression during preschoolers' free play. *British Journal of Developmental Psychology, 15*, 531–542.

Barefoot, J. C., Dodge, K. A., Peterson, B. L., Dahlstrom, W. G., & Williams, X. B. (1989). The Cook–Medley Hostility Scale: Item content and ability to predict survival. *Psychosomatic Medicine, 51*, 46–57.

Bennett, D. S., Bendersky, M., & Lewis, M. (2002). Facial expressivity at 4 months: A context by expression analysis. *Infancy, 3*(1), 97–113.

Bennett, D. S., Bendersky, M., & Lewis, M. (2004). On specifying specificity: Facial expressions at 4 months. *Infancy, 6*(3), 425–429.

Bryant, B. K. (1992). Conflict resolution strategies in relation to children's peer relations. *Journal of Applied Developmental Psychology, 13*, 35–50.

Bugenthal, D. B., & Grusec, J. E. (2006). Socialization processes. In W. Damon & R. M. Lerner (Series Eds.) & N. Eisenberg (Vol. Ed.), *Handbook of child psychology: Vol. 3. Social, emotional, and personality development* (6th ed., pp. 366–428). Hoboken, NJ: Wiley.

Buss, K. A., & Goldsmith, H. H. (1998). Fear and anger regulation in infancy: Effects on the temporal dynamics of affective expression. *Child Development, 69*, 359–374.

Buss, K. A., & Kiel, E. J. (2004). Comparison of sadness, anger, and fear facial expressions when toddlers look at their mothers. *Child Development, 75*, 1761–1773.

Calkins, S. D., Dedmon, S. E., Gill, K. L., Lomax, L. E., & Johnson, L. M. (2002). Frustration in infancy: Implications for emotion regulation, physiological processes, and temperament. *Infancy, 3*(2), 175–197.

Camodeca, M., & Goossens, F. A. (2005). Aggression, social cognitions, anger and sadness in bullies and victims. *Journal of Child Psychology and Psychiatry, 46*(2), 186–197.

Campos, J. J., Anderson, D., Barbu-Roth, M., Hubbard, E., Herenstein, M., & Witherington, D. (2000). Travel broadens the mind. *Infancy, 1*, 149–219.

Campos, J. J., Kermoian, R., & Zumbahlen, M. R. (1992). Socioemotional transformations in the family system following infant crawling onset. In N. Eisenberg & R. Fabes (Eds.), *New directions for child development: Vol. 55. Emotion and its regulation in early development* (pp. 25–40). San Francisco: Jossey-Bass.

Camras, L. A. (1992). Expressive development and basic emotions. *Cognition and Emotion, 6*, 269–283.

Camras, L. A. (2004). An event–emotion or event–expression hypothesis?: A comment on the commentaries on Bennett, Bendersky, and Lewis (2002). *Infancy*, 6(3), 431–433.

Camras, L. A., Sullivan, J., & Michel, G. (1993). Do infants express discrete emotions?: Adult judgments of facial, vocal, and body actions. *Journal of Nonverbal Behavior*, 17, 171–186.

Carson, J. L., & Parke, R. D. (1996). Reciprocal negative affect in parent–child interactions and children's peer competence. *Child Development*, 67, 2217–2226.

Casey, R. J., & Schlosser, S. (1994). Emotional responses to peer praise in children with and without a diagnosed externalizing disorder. *Merrill–Palmer Quarterly*, 40, 60–81.

Cassidy, J., Parke, R. D., Butkovsky, L., & Braungart, J. M. (1992). Family–peer connections: The roles of emotional expressiveness within the family and children's understanding of emotions. *Child Development*, 63, 603–618.

Cole, P. M., Teti, L. O., & Zahn-Waxler, C. (2003). Mutual emotion regulation and the stability of conduct problems between preschool and early school age. *Development and Psychopathology*, 15, 1–18.

Crick, N. R., & Dodge, K. A. (1994). A review and reformulation of social-information-processing mechanisms of children's social adjustment. *Psychological Bulletin*, 115, 74–101.

Crockenberg, S. (1985). Toddlers' reactions to maternal anger. *Merrill–Palmer Quarterly*, 31, 361–373.

Cummings, E. M. (1994). Marital conflict and children's functioning. *Social Development*, 3, 16–36.

Cummings, E. M., Zahn-Waxler, C., & Radke-Yarrow, M. (1981). Young children's responses to expressions of anger and affection by others in the family. *Child Development*, 52, 1274–1282.

Davies, P. T., & Cummings, E. M. (1995). Children's emotions as organizers of their reactions to interadult anger: A functionalist perspective. *Developmental Psychology*, 31, 677–684.

Denham, S. A. (1993). Maternal emotional responsiveness and toddlers' social-emotional competence. *Journal of Child Psychology and Psychiatry*, 34, 715–728.

Denham, S. A. (1998). *Emotional development in young children*. New York: Guilford Press.

Denham, S. A., Blair, K. A., DeMulder, E., Levitas, J., Sawyer, K., Auerbach-Major, S., et al. (2003). Preschool emotional competence: Pathway to social competence? *Child Development*, 74, 238–256.

Denham, S. A., Blair, K. A., Schmidt, M., & DeMulder, E. (2002). Compromised emotional competence: Seeds of violence sown early? *American Journal of Orthopsychiatry*, 72, 70–82.

Denham, S. A., Bouril, B., & Belouad, F. (1994). Preschoolers' affect and cognition about challenging peer situations. *Child Study Journal*, 24, 1–21.

Denham, S. A., Caverly, S., Schmidt, M., Blair, K. DeMulder, E., Caal, S., et al. (2002). Preschool understanding of emotions: Contributions to classroom anger and aggression. *Journal of Child Psychology and Psychiatry*, 43(7), 1–16.

Denham, S. A., Mitchell-Copeland, J., Strandberg, K., Auerbach, S., & Blair, K. (1997). Parental contributions to preschoolers' emotional competence: Direct and indirect effects. *Motivation and Emotion*, 27, 65–86.

DiLiberto, L., Katz, R. C., Beauchamp, K. L., & Howells, G. N. (2002). Using articulated thoughts in simulated situations to assess cognitive activity in aggressive and nonaggressive adolescents. *Journal of Child and Family Studies*, 11(2), 179–189.

Dodge, K. A. (1980). Social cognition and children's aggressive behavior. *Child Development*, 51, 162–170.

Dodge, K. A., Bates, J. E., & Pettit, G. S. (1990). Mechanisms in the cycle of violence. *Science*, 250, 1678–1683.

Dodge, K. A., & Coie, J. D. (1987). Social-information-processing factors in reactive and proactive aggression in children's peer groups. *Journal of Personality and Social Psychology*, 53, 1146–1158.

Dodge, K. A., Murphy, R. R., & Buchsbaum, K. (1984). The assessment of intention-cue detection skills in children: Implications for developmental psychopathology. *Child Development*, 55, 163–173.

Dodge, K. A., & Pettit, G. S. (2003). A biopsychosocial model of the development of chronic conduct problems in adolescence. *Developmental Psychology*, 39(2), 349–371.

Dodge, K. A., Pettit, G. S., McClaskey, C. L., & Brown, M. (1986). Social competence in children. *Monographs of the Society for Research in Child Development*, 51(2, Serial No. 213).

Dodge, K. A., & Somberg, D. R. (1987). Hostile attributional biases among aggressive boys are exacerbated under conditions of threat to the self. *Child Development*, 58, 213–224.

Dunn, J., & Brown, J. (1994). Affect expression in the family, children's understanding of emotion, and their interaction with others. *Merrill–Palmer Quarterly*, 40, 120–137.

Eisenberg, N. (2006). Introduction. In W. Damon & R. M. Lerner (Series Eds.) & N. Eisenberg (Vol. Ed.), *Handbook of child psychology: Vol. 3. Social, emotional, and personality development* (6th ed., pp. 1–23). Hoboken, NJ: Wiley.

Eisenberg, N., Cumberland, A., & Spinrad, T. L. (1998). Parental socialization of emotion. *Psychological Inquiry*, 9, 241–273.

Eisenberg, N., Fabes, R. A., Guthrie, I. K., & Reiser, M. (2000). Dispositional emotionality and regulation: Their role in predicting the quality of social functioning. *Journal of Personality and Social Psychology*, 78, 136–157.

Eisenberg, N., Fabes, R. A., Minore, D., Mathy, R., Hanish, L., & Brown, T. (1994). Children's enacted interpersonal strategies: Their relations to social behavior and negative emotionality. *Merrill–Palmer Quarterly*, 40, 212–232.

Eisenberg, N., Fabes, R. A., Nyman, M., Bernzweig, J., & Pinuelas, A. (1994). The relations of emotionality and regulation to children's anger-related reactions. *Child Development*, 65, 109–128.

Eisenberg, N., Fabes, R. A., Shepard, S. A., Murphy, B. C., Guthrie, I. K., Jones, S., et al. (1997). Contemporaneous and longitudinal prediction of children's social functioning from regulation and emotionality. *Child Development, 68,* 642–664.

Eisenberg, N., Sadovsky, A., Spinrad, T. L., Fabes, R. A., Losoya, S. H., Valiente, C., et al. (2005). The relations of problem behavior status to children's negative emotionality, effortful control, and impulsivity: Concurrent relations and prediction of change. *Developmental Psychology, 41,* 193–211.

El-Sheikh, M., & Cummings, E. M. (1995). Children's responses to angry adult behavior as a function of experimentally manipulated exposure to resolved and unresolved conflict. *Social Development, 4,* 75–91.

Fabes, R. A., Hanish, L. D., Martin, C. L., & Eisenberg, N. (2002). Young children's negative emotionality and social isolation: A latent growth curve analysis. *Merrill–Palmer Quarterly, 48,* 284–307.

Fernald, A. (1993). Approval and disapproval: Infant responsiveness to vocal affect in familiar and unfamiliar languages. *Child Development, 64,* 657–674.

Field, T., Hernandez-Reif, M., Vera, Y., Gil, K., Diego, M., Bendell, D., et al. (2005). Anxiety and anger effects on depressed mother–infant spontaneous and imitative interactions. *Infant Behavior and Development, 28*(1), 1–9.

Fine, S. E., Trentacosta, C. J., Izard, C. E., Mostow, A. J., & Campbell, J. L. (2004). Anger perception, caregivers' use of physical discipline, and aggression in children at risk. *Social Development, 13,* 213–228.

Garner, P. W., & Spears, F. M. (2000). Emotion regulation in low-income preschoolers. *Social Development, 9,* 226–245.

Goodenough, F. L. (1931). *Anger in young children.* Minneapolis: University of Minnesota Press.

Gottman, J. M., Katz, L. F., & Hooven, C. (1997). *Meta-emotion: How families communicate emotionally.* Mahwah, NJ: Erlbaum.

Graham, S., Hudley, C., & Williams, E. (1992). Attributional and emotional determinants of aggression among African-American and Latino young adolescents. *Developmental Psychology, 28,* 731–740.

Greenberg, M. T., & Kusche, C. A. (1993). *Promoting social and emotional development in deaf children: The PATHS Project.* Seattle: University of Washington Press.

Hanish, L. D., Eisenberg, N., Fabes, R. A., Spinrad, T. L., Ryan, P., & Schmidt, S. (2004). The expression and regulation of negative emotions: Risk factors for young children's peer victimization. *Development and Psychopathology, 16,* 335–353.

Haviland, J. M., & Lelwica, M. (1987). The induced affect response: 10-week-old infants' responses to three emotion expressions. *Developmental Psychology, 23,* 97–104.

Hayden, E. P., Klein, D. N., & Durbin, C. E. (2005). Parent reports and laboratory assessments of child temperament: A comparison of their associations with risk for depression and externalizing disorders.

Journal of Psychopathology and Behavioral Assessment, 27, 89–100.

Hubbard, J. A. (2001). Emotion expression processes in children's peer interaction: The role of peer rejection, aggression, and gender. *Child Development, 72,* 1426–1438.

Hubbard, J. A., & Coie, J. D. (1994). Emotional correlates of social competence in children's peer relationships. *Merrill–Palmer Quarterly, 40,* 1–20.

Hubbard, J. A., Smithmyer, C. M., Ramsden, S. R., Parker, E. H., Flanagan, K. D., Dearing, K. F., et al. (2002). Observational, physiological, and self report measures of children's anger: Relations to reactive versus proactive aggression. *Child Development, 73,* 1101–1118.

Izard, C. E. (1983). *The Maximally Discriminative Facial Movement Coding System (MAX)* (rev. ed.). Newark: Instructional Resources Center, University of Delaware.

Izard, C. E. (1991). *The psychology of emotions.* New York: Plenum Press.

Izard, C. E. (2004). The generality–specificity issue in infants' emotion responses: A comment on Bennett, Bendersky, and Lewis (2002). *Infancy, 6*(3), 417–423.

Izard, C. E., Dougherty, L., & Hembree, E. A. (1983). *A System for Identifying Affect Expressions by Holistic Judgments (AFFEX) (rev. ed.).* Newark: Computer Network Services and University Media Services, University of Delaware.

Izard, C. E., Fantauzzo, C. A., Castle, J. M., Haynes, O. M., Rayias, M. F., & Putnam, P. H. (1995). The ontogeny and significance of infants' facial expressions in the first nine months of life. *Developmental Psychology, 31,* 997–1013.

Izard, C. E., Hembree, E. A., & Huebner, R. R. (1987). Infants' emotion expressions to acute pain: Developmental change and stability of individual differences. *Developmental Psychology, 23,* 105–113.

Izard, C. E., & Kobak, R. R. (1991). Emotions system functioning and emotion regulation. In J. Garber & K. A. Dodge (Eds.), *The development of emotion regulation and dysregulation* (pp. 303–321). New York: Cambridge University Press.

Jenkins, J. M., Franco, F., Dolins, F., & Sewell, A. (1995). Toddlers' reactions to negative emotion displays: Forming models of relationships. *Infant Behavior and Development, 18,* 273–281.

Kahana-Kalman, R., & Walker-Andrews, A. S. (2001). The role of person familiarity in young infants' perception of emotional expressions. *Child Development, 72,* 352–369.

Kochanska, G. (2001). Emotional development in children with different attachment histories: The first three years. *Child Development, 72,* 474–490.

Kochanska, G., Aksan, N., & Carlson, J. J. (2005). Temperament, relationships, and young children's receptive cooperation with their parents. *Developmental Psychology, 41,* 648–660.

Lemerise, E. A., & Arsenio, W. F. (2000). An integrated model of emotion processes and cognition in social information processing. *Child Development*, *71*, 107–118.

Lemerise, E. A., & Dodge, K. A. (1993). The development of anger and hostile interactions. In M. Lewis & J. M. Haviland (Eds.), *Handbook of emotions* (pp. 537–546). New York: Guilford Press.

Lemerise, E. A., & Dodge, K. A. (2000). The development of anger and hostile interactions. In M. Lewis & J. M. Haviland-Jones (Eds.), *Handbook of emotions* (2nd ed., pp. 594–606). New York: Guilford Press.

Lemerise, E. A., Fredstrom, B. K., Kelley, B. M., Bowersox, A. L., & Waford, R. N. (2006). Do provocateurs' emotion displays influence children's social goals and problem solving? *Journal of Abnormal Child Psychology*, *34*, 559–571.

Lemerise, E. A., Gregory, D. S., & Fredstrom, B. K. (2005). The influence of provocateurs' emotion displays on the social information processing of children varying in social adjustment and age. *Journal of Experimental Child Psychology*, *90*, 344–366.

Lewis, M., Alessandri, S. M., & Sullivan, M. W. (1990). Violation of expectancy, loss of control, and anger expressions in young infants. *Developmental Psychology*, *26*, 745–751.

Lewis, M., & Haviland, J. M. (Eds.). (1993). *Handbook of emotions*. New York: Guilford Press.

Lewis, M., & Haviland-Jones, J. M. (Eds.). (2000). *Handbook of emotions* (2nd ed.). New York: Guilford Press.

Lewis, M., & Ramsay, D. (2005). Infant emotional and cortisol responses to goal blockage. *Child Development*, *76*, 518–530.

Lewis, M., Sullivan, M. W., Ramsay, D., & Alessandri, S. M. (1992). Individual differences in anger and sad expressions during extinction: Antecedents and consequences. *Infant Behavior and Development*, *15*, 443–452.

Lochman, J. E., & Wells, K. C. (2004). The coping power program for preadolescent boys and their parents: Outcome effects at the 1-year follow-up. *Journal of Consulting and Clinical Psychology*, *72*, 571–578.

Lyons-Ruth, K., Alpern, L., & Repacholi, B. (1993). Disorganized infant attachment classification and maternal psycho-social problems as predictors of hostile–aggressive behavior in the preschool classroom. *Child Development*, *64*, 572–585.

Malatesta, C. Z., Culver, C., Tesman, J. R., & Shepard, B. (1989). The development of emotion during the first two years of life. *Monographs of the Society for Research in Child Development*, *54*(1–2, Serial No. 219).

Malatesta, C. Z., & Haviland, J. M. (1982). Learning display rules: The socialization of emotion expression in infancy. *Child Development*, *53*, 991–1003.

Marsh, A. A., Ambady, N., & Kleck, R. E. (2005). The effects of fear and anger facial expressions on approach- and avoidance-related behaviors. *Emotion*, *5*, 119–124.

Montague, D. P. F., & Walker-Andrews, A. S. (2001). Peekaboo: A new look at infants' perception of emotion expressions. *Developmental Psychology*, *37*, 826–838.

Murphy, B. C., & Eisenberg, N. (1996). Provoked by a peer: Children's anger-related responses and their relations to social functioning. *Merrill–Palmer Quarterly*, *42*, 103–124.

Murphy, B. C., & Eisenberg, N. (1997). Young children's emotionality: Regulation and social functioning and their responses when they are targets of a peer's anger. *Social Development*, *6*, 18–36.

Murphy, B. C., Shepard, S. A., Eisenberg, N., & Fabes, R. A. (2004). Concurrent and across time prediction of young adolescents' social functioning: The role of emotionality and regulation. *Social Development*, *13*, 56–86.

Oatley, K., & Jenkins, J. M. (1996). *Understanding emotions*. Oxford: Blackwell.

Orobio de Castro, B., Merk, W., Koops, W., Veerman, J. W., & Bosch, J. D. (2005). Emotions in social information processing and their relations with reactive and proactive aggression in referred aggressive boys. *Journal of Clinical Child and Adolescent Psychology*, *34*, 105–116.

Orobio de Castro, B., Slot, N. W., Bosch, J. D., Koops, W., & Veerman, J. W. (2003). Negative affect exacerbates hostile attributions of intent in highly aggressive boys. *Journal of Clinical Child and Adolescent Psychology*, *32*, 57–66.

Oster, H., Hegley, D., & Nagel, L. (1992). Adult judgments and fine-grained analysis of infant facial expressions: Testing the validity of a priori coding formulas. *Developmental Psychology*, *28*, 1115–1131.

Parke, R. D. (1994). Progress, paradigms, and unresolved problems: A commentary on recent advances in our understanding of children's emotions. *Merrill–Palmer Quarterly*, *40*, 157–169.

Parker, J. G., & Gottman, J. M. (1989). Social and emotional development in a relational context: Friendship interaction from early childhood to adolescence. In T. J. Berndt & G. W. Ladd (Eds.), *Peer relationships in child development* (pp. 95–131). New York: Wiley.

Patterson, G. R., Littman, R. A., & Bricker, W. (1967). Assertive behavior in children: A step toward a theory of aggression. *Monographs of the Society for Research in Child Development*, *32*(5, Serial No. 113).

Pickens, J., & Field, T. (1993). Facial expressivity in infants of depressed mothers. *Developmental Psychology*, *29*, 986–988.

Pollack, S. D. (2003). Selective attention to facial emotion in physically abused children. *Journal of Abnormal Psychology*, *112*(3), 323–338.

Putallaz, M., & Sheppard, B. H. (1992). Conflict management and social competence. In C. U. Shantz & W. W. Hartup (Eds.), *Conflict in child and adolescent development* (pp. 330–355). New York: Cambridge University Press.

Radke-Yarrow, M., & Kochanska, G. (1990). Anger in

young children. In N. L. Stein, B. Leventhal, & T. Trabasso (Eds.), *Psychological and biological approaches to emotion* (pp. 297–310). Hillsdale, NJ: Erlbaum.

Reissland, N., Shepherd, J., & Herrera, E. (2005). Teasing play in infancy: Comparing mothers with and without self-reported depressed mood during play with their babies. *European Journal of Developmental Psychology*, 2(3), 271–283.

Rubin, K. H., Burgess, K. B., Dwyer, K. D., & Hastings, P. (2003). Predicting preschoolers' externalizing behaviors from toddler temperament, conflict, and maternal negativity. *Developmental Psychology*, 39, 164–176.

Rydell, A., Berlin, L., & Bohlin, G. (2003). Emotionality, emotion regulation, and adaptation in 5- to 8-year old children. *Emotion*, 3, 30–47.

Saarni, C., Campos, J. J., Camras, L. A., & Witherington, D. (2006). Emotional development: Action, communication, and understanding. In W. Damon & R. M. Lerner (Series Eds.) & N. Eisenberg (Vol. Ed.), *Handbook of child psychology: Vol. 3. Social, emotional, and personality development* (pp. 226–299). Hoboken, NJ: Wiley.

Schudlich, T. D. D. R., Shamir, H., & Cummings, E. M. (2004). Marital conflict, children's representations of family relationships, and children's dispositions towards peer conflict strategies. *Social Development*, 13, 171–192.

Schultz, D., Izard, C. E., & Bear, G. (2004). Children's emotion processing: Relations to emotionality and aggression. *Development and Psychopathology*, 16, 371–387.

Schultz, D., & Shaw, D. S. (2003). Boys' maladaptive social information processing, family emotional climate, and pathways to early conduct problems. *Social Development*, 12, 440–460.

Schwartz, D., Dodge, K. A., Pettit, G. S., & Bates, J. E. (1997). The early socialization of aggressive victims of bullying. *Child Development*, 68, 665–675.

Shaw, D. S., Owens, E. B., Vondra, J. I., Keenan, K., & Winslow, E. B. (1996). Early risk factors and pathways in the development of early disruptive behavior problems. *Development and Psychopathology*, 8, 679–699.

Shifflett-Simpson, K., & Cummings, E. M. (1996). Mixed message resolution and children's responses to interadult conflict. *Child Development*, 67, 437–448.

Shipman, K. L., Zeman, J., Nesin, A. E., & Fitzgerald, M. (2003). Children's strategies for displaying anger and sadness: What works with whom? *Merrill–Palmer Quarterly*, 49, 100–122.

Snyder, J., Stoolmiller, M., Wilson, M., & Yamamoto, M. (2003). Child anger regulation, parental responses to children's anger displays, and early child antisocial behavior. *Social Development*, 12, 335–360.

Stenberg, C. R., & Campos, J. J. (1990). The development of anger expressions in infancy. In N. L. Stein, B. Leventhal, & T. Trabasso (Eds.), *Psychological and biological approaches to emotion* (pp. 297–310). Hillsdale: NJ: Erlbaum.

Stipek, D., & MacIver, D. (1989). Developmental changes in children's assessment of intellectual competence. *Developmental Psychology*, 60, 521–538.

Strayer, J., & Roberts, W. (2004). Empathy and observed anger and aggression in five-year-olds. *Social Development*, 13, 1–13.

Suinn, R. M. (2001). The terrible twos—anger and anxiety: Hazardous to your health. *American Psychologist*, 56, 27–36.

Sullivan, M. W., & Lewis, M. (2003). Contextual determinants of anger and other negative expressions in young infants. *Developmental Psychology*, 39, 693–705.

Sullivan, M. W., Lewis, M., & Alessandri, S. M. (1992). Cross-age stability in emotional expressions during learning and extinction. *Developmental Psychology*, 28, 58–63.

Underwood, M. K. (1997). Peer social status and children's understanding of the expression and control of positive and negative emotions. *Merrill–Palmer Quarterly*, 43, 610–634.

Underwood, M. K., & Hurley, J. C. (1999). Emotion regulation in peer relationships during middle childhood. In L. Balter & C. Tamis-LeMonda (Eds.), *Child psychology: A handbook of contemporary issues* (pp. 58–87). Philadelphia: Psychology Press.

Vosk, B. N., Forehand, R., & Figueroa, R. (1983). Perceptions of emotions by accepted and rejected children. *Journal of Behavioral Assessment*, 5, 151–160.

Walden, T. A., & Ogan, T. A. (1988). The development of social referencing. *Child Development*, 59, 1230–1240.

Waschbusch, D. A., Pelham, W. E., Jennings, J. R., Greiner, A. R., Tarter, R. E., & Moss, H. B. (2002). Reactive aggression in boys with disruptive behavior disorders: Behavior, physiology and affect. *Journal of Abnormal Child Psychology*, 30, 641–656.

Weiss, B., Harris, V., Catron, T., & Han, S. H. (2003). Efficacy of the RECAP intervention program for children with concurrent internalizing and externalizing problems. *Journal of Consulting and Clinical Psychology*, 71, 364–374.

Zeman, J., Penza, S., Shipman, K., & Young, G. (1997). Preschoolers as functionalists: The impact of social context on emotion regulation. *Child Study Journal*, 27, 41–67.

Zeman, J., & Shipman, K. (1996). Children's expression of negative affect: Reasons and methods. *Developmental Psychology*, 32, 842–849.

Zeman, J., & Shipman, K. (1997). Social-contextual influences on expectancies for managing anger and sadness: The transition from middle childhood to adolescence. *Developmental Psychology*, 33, 917–924.

Zeman, J., & Shipman, K. (1998). Influence of social context on children's affect regulation: A functionalist perspective. *Journal of Nonverbal Behavior*, 22(3), 141–165.

CHAPTER 46

Self-Conscious Emotions
Embarrassment, Pride, Shame, and Guilt

MICHAEL LEWIS

In Chapter 18, I have suggested a model for the emergence of emotional life in the first 3 to 4 years of life. Here, I focus on a unique set of emotions that emerge late and that require certain cognitive abilities for their elicitation. Whereas the emotions that appear early, such as joy, sadness, fear, and anger, have received considerable attention, these later-appearing emotions have received relatively little attention. There are likely to be many reasons for this. One reason is that these self-conscious emotions cannot be described solely by examining a particular set of facial movement; they necessitate the observation of bodily action more than facial cues (Darwin, 1872/1965).

A second reason for their neglect is the realization that there are no clear, specific elicitors of these particular emotions, although some researchers have claimed otherwise (e.g., Izard, 1979). Whereas happiness can be elicited by seeing a significant other, and fear can be elicited by the approach of a stranger, there are few specific situations that will elicit shame, pride, guilt, or embarrassment. These self-conscious emotions are likely to require classes of events

that can only be identified by the individuals themselves. Consider pride. What kinds of elicitors are necessary for pride to take place? Pride requires a large number of factors, all having to do with cognitions related to the self (Lewis, 1992; Tracy & Robins, 2004). Pride occurs when one makes a comparison or evaluates one's behavior vis-à-vis some standard, rule, or goal (SRG) and finds that one has succeeded. Shame or guilt, on the other hand, occurs when such an evaluation leads to the conclusion that one has failed.

The elicitation of self-conscious emotions involves elaborate cognitive processes that have, at their heart, the notion of self. Although some theories—psychoanalysis, for example (see Freud, 1936/1963, and Erikson, 1950)—have argued for some universal elicitors of shame, such as failure at toilet training or exposure of the backside, the idea of an automatic, noncognitive elicitor of these emotions seems unlikely. Cognitive processes must be the elicitors of these complex emotions. It is the way we think or what we think about that becomes the elicitor of pride, shame, guilt, or embarrassment. There may be a one-to-one correspondence between thinking certain thoughts and the occurrence of a particular emotion; however, in the case of this class of emotions, the elicitor is likely to be some cognitive event. This does not mean that the earlier emotions, those called "primary" or "basic," are elicited by noncognitive events. Cognitive factors may play a role in the elicitation of any emotion; however, the nature of the cognitive events are much less articulated and differentiated in the earlier ones (Plutchik, 1980).

In order to explore these self-conscious emotions, we need first to articulate the role of self in their elicitation. Following this, an attempt at a working definition through a cognitive–attributional model is presented. The chapter focuses on shame, pride, guilt, and embarrassment, although other self-conscious emotions could be included—for example, jealousy, empathy, and envy.

THE ROLE OF SELF

Elsewhere, I have attempted to clarify those specific aspects of self that are involved in self-conscious emotions—in particular, the self-conscious evaluative emotions (Lewis, 2003). Self-conscious evaluative emotions first involve a set of standards, rules, or goals (SRGs). These SRGs are inventions of the culture that are transmitted to children and involve their learning of, and willingness to consider, these SRGs as their own. This process of incorporating the SRGs has been discussed by Stipek, Recchia, and McClintic (1992). What is apparent from the work of Stipek et al. is that the process of incorporation starts quite early in life. SRGs imply self-evaluation, for it would make little sense if we had SRGs but had no evaluation of our action in regard to them.

Having self-evaluative capacity allows for two distinct outcomes: We can evaluate our behavior and hold ourselves responsible for the action being evaluated, or we can hold ourselves not responsible. In the attribution literature, this distinction has been called an "internal" or an "external" attribution, respectively (Weiner, 1986).

If we conclude that we are not responsible, then evaluation of our behavior ceases. However, if we evaluate ourselves as responsible, then we can evaluate our behavior as successful or unsuccessful vis-à-vis the SRGs. The deter-mination of success and failure resides within an individual and is based on the nature of the standard that is set. For example, if a student believes that only receiving an A in an exam constitutes success, then receiving a B represents a failure for that student. On the other hand, a B may be considered a success by another.

Still another cognition related to the self has to do with the evaluation of the self in terms of specific or global attributions. "Global self-attributions" refer to the whole self, while "specific self-attributions" refer to specific features or actions of the self (see Beck, 1979; Elliot & Dweck, 2005). In almost every one of these processes, a concept of the self needs to be considered.

The need for cognitive elicitors having to do with the self was known to Darwin (1872/1965). Darwin not only described the basic, primary, or early emotions, but also dealt with the self-conscious emotions. Darwin saw these later emotions as involving the self, although he was not able to distinguish between the various types (see Tomkins, 1963, for a similar problem). For example, Darwin believed that blushing, which could be a sign of either shyness, embarrassment, shame, or guilt, was caused by how we appear to others; as he put it, "the thinking about others, thinking of us . . . excites a blush" (Darwin, 1872/1965, p. 325). His observation in regard to blushing indicates his concern with two issues: the issue of appearance and the issue of consciousness. He repeatedly made the point that these emotions depend on sensitivity to the opinion of others, whether good or bad. Thus the distinction between emotions that require opinion or thought of others and emotions that do not suggests that two different kinds of cognitive processes are involved.

The distinction between self-conscious emotions and primary or basic emotions remains of concern. The idea that there is a basic set of emotions grows out of the idea of human instincts or propensities. If they are basic, prewired, or genetically given, they are likely to be limited in number. Although we recognize an enormous variety of emotions, the existence of each one as a unique and discrete "wiring" is too burdensome a characterization of the nervous system. Instead of positing this complex set of emotions, many have argued that there are only a few select basic, primary, or pure emotions (see Oatley & Johnson-Laird, 1987, and Ortony, Clore, & Collins, 1988, for contrary views). In order to resolve this problem in regard to self-conscious emotions, we might instead make the distinction between emotions that involve few or simple cognitive processes and emotions that involve complex cognitive processes (Darwin, 1872/1965; Plutchik, 1980).

TOWARD A WORKING DEFINITION

Trying to distinguish among the different types of self-conscious emotions (e.g., embarrassment, shyness, shame, and guilt) is not easy. As Darwin's analysis makes clear, all of these emotions are likely to produce blushing. Since Darwin viewed blushing as a human species-specific behavior, he also viewed these emotions as unique to humans. However, blushing occurs with any one of these emotions (or, as in most cases, not at all), so it is clear that blushing cannot be used to distinguish between them.

One can turn to the psychoanalytic literature; however, its focus on guilt rather than shame (see Broucek, 1991, and Lansky & Morrison, 1997, for exceptions) makes this literature suspect. For example, Freud (1905/1953) discussed the function of guilt but said little about shame. For Freud, the superego—the mechanism by which the standards of the parents are incorporated into the self, specifically via the child's fear that the parents will respond to transgression by withdrawal of love or even by punishment—is the initial source of the feeling of guilt. Freud's discussion of guilt in relationship to the superego is similar to his discussion of guilt in relation to the instinctual drives and their expression. For Freud, anxiety or fear is translatable directly into guilt. The two stages in the development of the sense of guilt related to the superego are (1) the fear of authority and (2) the fear of the superego itself, once the authority standards are incorporated. In the well-developed superego, the sense of guilt arises not only when a violation is committed, but even when a violation is being anticipated.

The guilt that Freud focuses on is not a guilt related to the whole self, but rather a guilt related to one's action. For Freud, guilt is a specific and focused response to a transgression that can be rectified by abstinence and penance. Freud's focus on guilt, not shame, can also be found in his discussion of psychopathology. It is to be found in the overdeveloped sense of guilt resulting from an overdeveloped ego. Within normal functioning, the superego condemns the ego; this condemnation in turn gives rise to normal guilt. When Freud did mention shame, he usually did so in the context of drives and impulses that require restriction. So, for example, in discussing the impulses having to do with the erogenous zones, he stated that these impulses

> would seem in themselves to be perverse—that is, to arise from erogenic zones, and to derive their activity from instincts which, in view of the direction of the subjects' development, can arouse only unpleasant feelings. They [the impulses] consequently evoke opposing mental forces [reacting impulses] which, in order to suppress this displeasure affectively, build up the mental dams of . . . disgust, shame and morality. (Freud, 1905/1953, p. 178)

Erikson had no more success in distinguishing between shame and guilt than the earlier psychoanalysts had. Erikson turned more to the Darwinian view when he suggested that shame arises when "one is completely exposed and conscious of being looked at, in a word, self-conscious" (1950, pp. 223–224). Again, this self-consciousness is an undifferentiated state of being—that is, shame, shyness, embarrassment, and guilt. Erikson tried to differentiate these terms, but was not completely successful. For example, he discussed "visual shame" versus "auditory guilt," but did not develop this concept. I imagine that the reference to visual shame is based on Darwin's theory that shame derives from being looked at, and that in feeling shame, one wishes to hide one's face and to disappear. Although Erikson held to a more interactional view, one involving self and self-consciousness, he also indicated that the conditions necessary for feeling shame include being in an upright and exposed position. As he stated, "Clinical observation leads me to believe that shame has much to do with a consciousness of having a front and a back, especially a 'behind' " (Erikson, 1950, pp. 223–224). Erikson believed that shame is related to specific body acts, particularly toilet functions. Erikson's theory of ego challenges offers the clearest differentiation between shame and guilt, their place in human life, and events likely to elicit them. Erikson's second challenge is autonomy versus shame and doubt. Autonomy is the attempt of the child to achieve, to do for him- or herself—an attempt that is related to a developing sense of the self. Achieving muscular control, including control of the elimination of body waste, is the socialization and the developmental challenge at this life stage. Shame and doubt arise during this stage as the counterpoints to autonomy, the successful achievement. In other words, shame and doubt arise from the child's inability to control bodily functions fully. It is only after this basic ego task that the third ego task, initiative versus guilt, becomes significant. Here Erikson suggested that guilt has a reparative function. Erikson's developmental sequence indicates a recognition that shame and guilt are different emotions—that shame precedes guilt, and that they are associated in counterpoint with different ego tasks. It also leads to the commonly held psychoanalytic view that guilt is a more mature emotion than shame.

There is very little agreement as to the specific elicitors of shame, guilt, or embarrassment. Many events are capable of eliciting any one of them. No particular stimulus event has been identified as the trigger for shame and guilt. It would be easier to understand these self-conscious emotions if we could specify the class of external events likely to elicit them. If it were true that shame and guilt are similar to anxiety and that they reflect the subject's fear of uncontrollable impulses, then we could consider the causes of shame to be sexual or aggressive impulses. Alternatively, if we could prove that situations having to do with toilet or genital functions are likely to elicit shame, or if we could prove that the way we appear physically or how we behave in front of others may automatically elicit embarrassment, we could then specify situations that would help us to define these self-conscious emotions and increase our understanding of what causes them. There is no such clear cause-and-effect pattern—no event that can be used consistently as an elicitor of each of these self-conscious emotions.

Alternative theories having to do with self psychology are necessary. Success or failure vis-à-vis our SRGs is likely to produce a signal to the self that results in self-reflection (see Mandler, 1975, for a discussion of events likely to cause self-reflection). This cognitive reflective process gives rise to self-attribution and to the specific emotions that accompany the different types of self-attribution. The importance

of such a view resides in three important factors. First, the model does not attempt to specify what constitutes success or failure, or how the person goes about evaluating success or failure. Second, the model does not specify any particular SRG. In other words, it is not clear whether there are any specific stimuli that uniquely contribute to any of the self-conscious emotions. Third, the model assumes that self-attributions leading to specific emotions are internal events that reside in people themselves, although the SRGs are taught by others.

Although this model is based on a phenomenological and cognitive–attributional model, self-conscious emotions are not just epiphenomenological and therefore deserve "lower status" than the cognitive–attributional processes themselves. These self-conscious emotions may have discrete and specific locations, as well as specific processes that are themselves "bodily" in nature (see Lindquist & Barrett, Chapter 32, and Niedenthal, Chapter 36, this volume). For example, shame but not embarrassment leads to increases in cortisol responses (Lewis & Ramsay, 2002). The cognitions associated with these emotions may serve simply as elicitors of specific emotions in the same way as do other stimuli, such as the social behavior of others, loud noises, or sudden and uncontrolled events. Specific emotions can be elicited through a variety of attributions. The idea that cognitions can lead to emotions has been poorly received by some, who believe that this idea implies that cognitions have real status, while emotions are epiphenomenological and certainly not bodily (Schachter & Singer, 1962). We need to give emotions the same status as cognitions. Just as cognitions can lead to emotions, emotions can lead to cognitions. The theory implies no status difference.

A COGNITIVE–ATTRIBUTIONAL THEORY

Figure 46.1 presents a structural model for defining various self-conscious emotions. In the figure, A, B, and C represent cognitive processes that serve as stimuli for these emotions.

Standards, Rules, and Goals

The first feature of the model has to do with the SRGs that govern our behavior. All of us have beliefs about what is acceptable for others

A. STANDARDS AND RULES

B. EVALUATION

SUCCESS	FAILURE	C. ATTRIBUTION OF SELF
HUBRIS	SHAME	GLOBAL
PRIDE	GUILT/ REGRET	SPECIFIC

FIGURE 46.1. Structural model for the elicitation of self-conscious evaluative emotions. From Lewis (1992). Copyright 1992 by Michael Lewis. Reprinted by permission.

and for ourselves with regard to standards having to do with actions, thoughts, and feelings. This set of beliefs, or SRGs, constitutes the information one acquires through culturalization in a particular society. SRGs differ across different societies, across groups within societies, across different time epochs, and among individuals of different ages. The standards of our culture are varied and complex, yet each of us knows at least some of them. Moreover, each of us has a unique set. To become a member of any group requires that we learn them. I can think of no group that does not have SRGs, or in which violations of SRGs does not lead to negative sanctions. These SRGs are acquired through a variety of processes. They are always associated with human behavior, including thinking, action, and feeling. They are prescribed by the culture, including the culture at large, as well as by the influences of specific groups, such as clan, peers, and family.

It is safe to claim that by the age of 1 year, children are beginning to learn the appropriate action patterns reflecting the SRGs of the culture. By the second year of life, children show some understanding about appropriate and inappropriate behavior (Heckhausen, 1984). The acquisition of these SRGs continues across the lifespan; however, some emerge early.

Evaluation

The evaluation of one's actions, thoughts, and feelings in terms of SRGs is the second cognitive–evaluative process that serves as a stimulus for self-conscious emotions. Two major aspects of this process are considered; the first has to do with the internal and external aspects of evaluation. For the model to work in

describing the process of eliciting emotions, internal evaluation, as opposed to either no evaluation or external evaluation, is necessary. Individuals differ in their characteristic evaluative responses. Moreover, situations differ in the likelihood that they will cause a particular evaluative response. The second consideration has to do with how individuals make a determination about success or failure in regard to any specific standard. Research seems to indicate that by the beginning of the third year of life, children already have SRGs and seem to show distress when they violate them (Lewis, Alessandri, & Sullivan, 1992; Stipek, 1983).

Responsibility

Within the field of attributional studies, the problem of responsibility has received considerable attention (Weiner, 1986). Often when people violate SRGs, they do not attribute the failure to themselves; they may explain their failure in terms of chance or the actions of others (Seligman et al., 1984). Determining responsibility is a function both of situational factors and of individual characteristics. There are people who are likely to blame themselves no matter what happens. Dweck and associates, in studying causes of success and failure within academic fields, found that many children blamed their success or failure on external forces and not themselves, although there were as many who were likely to evaluate success and failure in terms of their own actions (see Dweck & Leggett, 1988, for one example). Interestingly, sex differences emerged: In academic achievement, boys were more apt to hold themselves responsible for their success and others for their failure, whereas girls were apt to blame others for their success and themselves for their failure.

Success or Failure

Another feature of the self-evaluation process has to do with the socialization of what constitutes success or failure. Once one has assumed responsibility (internal evaluation), exactly how one comes to evaluate an action, thought, or feeling as a success or a failure is not well understood. This aspect of self-evaluation is particularly important because, as we can see from Figure 46.1, the same SRGs can result in radically different feelings, depending upon whether success or failure is attributed to oneself.

Many factors are involved in producing inaccurate or unique evaluations of success or failure. These include early failures in the self-system leading to narcissistic disorders (see Morrison, 1989), harsh socialization experiences, and high levels of reward for success or punishment for failure (see Alessandri & Lewis, 1996). The evaluation of one's behavior in terms of success and failure is a very important aspect of the organization of plans and the determination of new goals and new plans.

Attribution about Self

As noted earlier, another attribution in regard to the self has to do with "global" or "specific" self-attribution (Beck, 1979). Global attribution refers to an individual's propensity to focus on the total self. Thus, for any particular behavior violation, some individuals, some of the time, are likely to focus on the totality of the self; they use such self-evaluative phrases as "Because I did this, I am bad [or good]." Janoff-Bulman's (1979) distinction between "characterological" and "behavioral" self-blame is particularly relevant here.

On such occasions the focus is upon the self, both as object and as subject. The self becomes embroiled in the self. It becomes embroiled because the evaluation of the self by the self is total. There is no way out. The focus is not on an individual's behavior, but on the total self. There is little wonder that in using such global attribution people can think of nothing else, and they become confused and speechless (H. B. Lewis, 1971). They tend to focus upon themselves, not upon their action. Because of this, they are unable to act and are driven

from the field of action into hiding or disappearing.

"Specific" attribution refers to individuals' propensity in some situations, some of the time, to focus on specific actions of the self. That is, their self-evaluation is not global, but specific. It is not the total self that has done something wrong or good; instead, particular specific behaviors are judged. At such times as these, individuals will use such evaluative phrases as "What I did was wrong. I mustn't do it again." Notice that for such occurrences, an individual's focus is not on the totality of the self, but on the specific behavior of the self in a specific situation. The focus here is on the behavior of the self in interaction with objects or persons. Here attention is on the actions of the self or the effect on other selves.

Global versus specific self-focus may be a personality style. Global attributions for negative events are generally uncorrelated with global attributions for positive events. It is only when positive or negative events are taken into account that relatively stable and consistent attributional patterns are observed. Some individuals are likely to be stable in their global and specific evaluations; under most conditions of success or failure, these subjects are likely to maintain a global or specific posture in regard to self-attribution. In the attribution literature, such dispositional factors have important consequences upon a variety of fixed "personality patterns." So, for example, depressed individuals are likely to make stable global attributions, whereas nondepressed individuals are less likely to be stable in their global attributions (Beck, 1979).

In addition to the dispositional factors relating to specific or global attributions (Kochanska, 1997), there are likely to be situational constraints as well. Some have called these "prototypic situations." That is, although there are dispositional factors, not all people all the time are involved in either global or specific attributions. Unfortunately, these situational factors have not been well studied. It seems reasonable that certain classes of situations should be more likely than others to elicit a particular focus, but exactly what classes of stimuli are likely to elicit global or specific attributions remain unknown. Another way to view this distinction has been made by Dweck (e.g., Dweck, Hong, & Chiu, 1993). In her work, Dweck has referred to two styles that are quite similar to specific and global. She has referred to them as "task focus" and "self/performance focus." In task focus, attention is paid to a specific action; in self/performance focus, attention is on the whole self.

MAKING SENSE OF THE MODEL

Given these three sets of activities—(1) the establishment of one's SRGs; (2) the evaluation of success or failure of one's action in regard to these; and (3) the attribution of the self, in terms of both responsibility (external vs. internal) and self-focus (global vs. specific)—it is now possible to see how these factors bear on self-conscious emotional states. This model is symmetrical in relation to positive and negative self-conscious emotions. It is the cognitive–evaluative process of the organism itself that elicits these states. The model distinguishes among four emotional states.

Shame

Shame is the product of a complex set of cognitive activities: individuals' evaluation of their actions in regard to their SRGs and their global evaluation of the self. The phenomenological experience of a person having shame is that of a wish to hide, disappear, or die (H. B. Lewis, 1971; Lewis, 1992). It is a highly negative and painful state that also results in the disruption of ongoing behavior, confusion in thought, and an inability to speak. The physical action accompanying shame is a shrinking of the body, as though to disappear from the eye of the self or the other. Because of the intensity of this emotional state, the global attack on the self-system, all that individuals can do when presented with such a state is to attempt to rid themselves of it. However, since it is a global attack on the self, people have great difficulty in dissipating this emotion. There are specific actions individuals employ when shamed in efforts to undo the shame state, such as reinterpretation, self-splitting (multiple personalities), or forgetting (repression); see Lewis (1992) for a fuller discussion.

Shame is not produced by any specific situation, but rather by the individual's interpretation of the event. Even more important is that shame is not related necessarily to the event's being public or private. Although many hold that shame is a public failure, this need not be so. Failure, attributed to the whole self, can be either public or private. Shame may be public, but it is as likely to be private. Each of us can think of private events when we say to ourselves, "I'm ashamed of having done that." Shame can center around moral action as well. Thus, when persons violate some moral SRG, they are ashamed.

Guilt

The emotional state of guilt or regret is produced when individuals evaluate their behavior as failure but focus on the specific features or actions of the self that led to the failure. Unlike the focus in shame on the global self, the focus in guilt is on the self's actions and behaviors that are likely to repair the failure. From a phenomenological point of view, individuals are pained by their failure, but this pained feeling is directed to the cause of the failure or the object of harm. Because the cognitive–attributional process focuses on the action of the self rather than on the totality of self, the feeling that is produced—guilt—is not as intensely negative as shame and does not lead to confusion and to the loss of action. In fact, the emotion of guilt always has associated with it a corrective action that an individual can take (but does not necessarily take) to repair the failure. Rectification of the failure and preventing it from occurring again are the two possible corrective paths. Whereas in shame we see the body hunched over itself in an attempt to hide and disappear, in guilt we see individuals moving in space as if trying to repair their action (see Barrett & Zahn-Waxler, 1987). The marked postural differences that accompany guilt and shame are helpful both in distinguishing these emotions and in measuring individual differences. We might point to blushing as a measure also distinguishing guilt from shame; however, because of the variability in the likelihood of individuals to blush, the use of blushing is not an accurate index.

Because in guilt the focus is on the specific, individuals are capable of ridding themselves of this emotional state through action. The corrective action can be directed toward the self as well as toward the other; thus, unlike shame, which is a melding of the self as subject and object, in guilt the self is differentiated from the object. As such, the emotion is less intense and more capable of dissipation. Moreover, it should be unrelated to maladaptive behavior. The problem is that guilt may merge into shame; thus two types of guilt might be considered, guilt and maladaptive guilt. The expectation would be that guilt would not be correlated with shame, while maladaptive guilt would be (Tangney & Dearing, 2002). Thus, should the corrective action not be forthcoming—in either thought, feeling, or deed—it is possible that a guilt experience can be converted into one of shame (H. B. Lewis, 1971). Here, then, is another difference between shame and guilt. We can be ashamed of our guilty action, but we cannot be guilty over being ashamed, suggesting a levels difference and a directional difference in the experiencing of these emotions. The emotion of guilt lacks the negative intensity of shame. It is not self-destroying, and as such can be viewed as a more useful emotion in motivating specific and corrective action. However, because it is less intense, it may not convey the motivation necessary for change or correction.

Hubris

Hubris is defined as exaggerated pride or self-confidence, often resulting in retribution. It is an example of pridefulness—something dislikable and to be avoided. Hubris is a consequence of an evaluation of success in regard to one's SRGs where the focus is on the global self. In this emotion, the individual focuses on the total self as successful. Hubris is associated with such descriptions as "puffed up." In extreme cases, it is associated with grandiosity or with narcissism (Morrison, 1989). Mueller and Dweck (1998) have shown that too much praise of children may result in negative achievement performance; the assumed mechanism may be that such high levels of praise may elicit a global self-focus rather than a specific focus—or, to use Dweck's terms, may lead to a self/performance focus rather than a task focus. The global self-focus can lead in time to shame over failure. Given this powerful negative state, the desire to avoid it can lead to not taking responsibility for the failure on the one hand, and to assuming success where others see failure on the other. These two features have been associated with narcissistic disorders (Lansky & Morrison, 1997). Hubris occurs because of the global or self/performance focus. Because of the global nature of the attributions of this emotion, it is likely to be transient, and in order to be able to maintain this state, one must either alter standards or reevaluate what consti-

tutes success. Unlike shame, it is highly positive and emotionally rewarding; that is, one feels good about oneself.

Hubris is, however, an emotion difficult to sustain, since there is no specific action that precipitates the feeling. Because such feelings are addictive, people prone to hubris derive little satisfaction from the emotion. Consequently, they seek out and invent situations likely to repeat this emotional state. They can do this either by altering their SRGs or by reevaluating what constitutes success in their actions, thoughts, or feelings.

From the outside, other people observe the individuals having hubris with some disdain. Hubristic people have difficulty in their interpersonal relations, since their own hubris is likely to interfere with the wishes, needs, and desires of others, in which case there is likely to be an interpersonal conflict. Moreover, given the contemptuousness associated with hubris, the other persons are likely to be shamed by the nature of the actions of the persons having this emotion. The three problems associated with hubris, therefore, are that (1) it is a transient but addictive emotion; (2) it is not related to a specific action, and thus requires altering patterns of goal setting or evaluation of what constitutes success; and (3) it interferes with interpersonal relationships because of its contemptuous and insolent nature. In its extreme form, it is quite similar to narcissism.

Pride

Pride, on the other hand, is the consequence of a successful evaluation of a specific action. The phenomenological experience is joy over an action, thought, or feeling well done. Here, the focus of pleasure is specific and related to a particular behavior. In pride, the self and object are separated, as in guilt (see Tracy & Robins, 2004). Unlike shame and hubris, where subject and object are fused, pride occurs when people focus on their actions; the persons are engrossed in the specific actions that give them pride. Stipek et al. (1992) have likened this state to achievement motivation. Because this positive state is associated with a particular action, individuals have available to themselves the means by which they can reproduce the state. Notice that, unlike hubris, pride's specific focus allows for action. Because of the general use of the term "pride" to refer to "hubris," "efficacy," and "satisfaction," the study of pride as hubris has until recently received little attention. However, more work now is beginning to appear. Recently, Tracy, Robins, and Lagattuta (2005) have shown that this recognition of pride occurs relatively early (by 4 years of age) and has a set of specific behavioral markers.

Embarrassment and Shyness

From a behavioral as well as a phenomenological point of view, shame and guilt can be differentiated; however, embarrassment and shyness appear to be confused with these as well.

Shyness

Izard and Tyson (1986) consider shyness to be sheepishness, bashfulness, a feeling of uneasiness or psychological discomfort in social situations, and oscillation between fear and interest or between avoidance and approach. In this description, shyness is related to fear and is a nonevaluative emotion centered around the individual's discomfort response to others. Such a description fits Buss's (1980) notion of shyness as an emotional response that is elicited by experiences of novelty or conspicuousness. For Buss, shyness and fear are closely related and represent a fearfulness toward others. A way of distinguishing shyness from shame is that it appears much earlier than either shame or guilt.

Such an approach to shyness seems reasonable because it fits with other notions relating the self to others, or what we might call the "social self." Eysenck (1954) has characterized people as social or asocial by genetic disposition, and Kagan (2003) has pointed out the physiological responses of children he calls "inhibited." These inhibited or shy children are withdrawn, are uncomfortable in social situations, and appear fearful. Shyness may be a dispositional factor not related to self-evaluation (DiBiase & Lewis, 1997; Lewis & Ramsay, 1997). Rather, it may simply be the discomfort of being in the company of other social objects—in other words, the opposite of sociability.

Embarrassment

For Tomkins (1963), embarrassment is closely linked to shame. The most notable difference between embarrassment and shame is the intensity level. Whereas shame appears to be an intense and disruptive emotion, embarrassment is clearly less intense and does not involve the disruption of thought and language that shame does. Second, in terms of body posture, people who are embarrassed do not assume the posture of one wishing to hide, disappear, or die. In fact, their bodies reflect an ambivalent approach-and-avoidance posture. Repeated looking and then looking away, accompanied by smiling behavior, seem to index embarrassment (see Edelman, 1987; Geppert, 1986; Lewis, Stanger, & Sullivan, 1989). Rarely in a shame situation do we see gaze aversion accompanied by smiling behavior. Thus, from a behavioral point of view, these two emotions appear to be different. Finally, whereas shame can occur in the physical absence of another, embarrassment almost always occurs in the company of others.

Phenomenologically, embarrassment is less clearly differentiated from shame than from guilt. People often report that embarrassment is "a less intense experience of shame." Similar situations that invoke shame are found to invoke embarrassment, although its intensity, duration, and disruptive quality are not the same. However, in order to understand embarrassment, I have suggested (Lewis, 1995) that there are two types of embarrassed behavior: (1) embarrassment as exposure, and (2) embarrassment as less intense shame.

EMBARRASSMENT AS EXPOSURE

In certain situations of exposure, people become embarrassed. It is not related to negative evaluation, as is shame. Perhaps the best example is the case of being complimented. One phenomenological experience of those who appear before audiences is that of embarrassment caused by the positive comments of the introduction. Consider the moment when the speaker is introduced: The person introducing the speaker extols his or her virtues. Surprisingly, praise, rather than displeasure or negative evaluation, elicits embarrassment!

Another example of this type of embarrassment can be seen in reactions to public display. When people observe someone looking at them, they are apt to become self-conscious, look away, and touch or adjust their bodies. When an observed person is a woman, she will often adjust or touch her hair; men are less likely to touch their hair, but may adjust their clothes or change their body posture. In few cases do the observed people look sad. If anything, they appear pleased by the attention. This combination—gaze turned away briefly, no frown, and nervous touching—looks like this first type of embarrassment.

A third example of embarrassment as exposure can be seen in this experiment: When I wish to demonstrate that embarrassment can be elicited just by exposure, I announce that I am going to point randomly to a student. I repeatedly mention that my pointing is random and that it does not reflect a judgment about the person. I close my eyes and point. My pointing invariably elicits embarrassment in the student pointed to.

In each of these examples, there is no negative evaluation of the self in regard to SRGs. In these situations, it is difficult to imagine embarrassment as a less intense form of shame. Since praise cannot readily lead to an evaluation of failure, it is likely that embarrassment resulting from compliments, from being looked at, and from being pointed to has more to do with the exposure of the self than with evaluation. Situations other than praise come to mind, in which a negative evaluation can be inferred, although it may not be the case. Take, for example, walking into a room before the speaker has started to talk. It is possible to arrive *on time* only to find people already seated. When you are walking into the room, eyes turn toward you, and you may experience embarrassment. One could say that there is a negative self-evaluation: "I should have been earlier; I should not have made noise (I did not make noise)." I believe, however, that the experience of embarrassment in this case may not be elicited by negative self-evaluation, but simply by public exposure. We (Lewis & Ramsay, 2002) have shown that this type of embarrassment produces less stress (e.g., lower cortisol responses) than does shame.

EMBARRASSMENT AS LESS INTENSE SHAME

The second class of embarrassment, which I call "embarrassment as less intense shame," seems to me to be related to a negative self-evaluation. The difference in intensity can probably be attributed to the nature of the failed SRG. Some SRGs are more or less associated with the core of self; for me, failure at driving a car is less important than is failure at helping a student. Failures associated with less important and central SRGs result in embarrassment rather than shame. If this analysis is correct, then it is possible that each of the four self-conscious emotions has a less intense form.

It may well be that embarrassment is not the same as shame. From a phenomenological stance, they appear very different. On the other hand, there is the possibility that embarrassment and shame are in fact related and that they vary only in intensity. It is safe to say that, as a working definition, there appear to be at least two different types of embarrassment.

SHAME AND PSYCHOPATHOLOGY

Recently my colleagues and I have extended our interest in the development of shame to study its relation to psychopathology. Specifically, we are concerned with how traumatic events influence shame, and how shame then influences psychosocial adjustment.

Figure 46.2 presents our general model. On the far left side of the model is the traumatic event. Trauma leads to shame through the mediation of cognitive attributions about the abuse (a), and shame (b) in turn leads to poor adjustment (d). The model also allows for the trauma to directly influence shame (c) and adjustment (e), although our central hypothesis is that the outcomes of trauma are mediated by how the child thinks about the event(s). The support for this model comes from the research

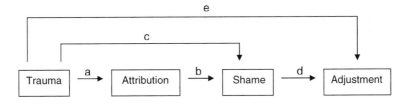

FIGURE 46.2. A model of trauma and adjustment as they relate to shame.

suggesting that individuals who are shame-prone are more likely to evidence poor self-esteem, depression, and dissociation (Lewis, 1992; Tangney, Wagner, & Gramzow, 1990). Consequently, an internal, stable, global attribution style for negative events constitutes a risk factor for shame and subsequent poor adjustment.

Sexual Abuse and Shame

The experience of shame as a consequence of sexual abuse is a central mechanism related to subsequent behavior problems (Lewis, 1992). The theory of the elicitation of shame is particularly relevant to abuse, because attributions as they are related to self-conscious emotions and attributions related to the cause of abuse are connected. If the abuse is attributed to an internal, global cause, the resulting emotion is shame; therefore, how the victim evaluates the sexual abuse event(s) is important. It is likely to mediate subsequent long-lasting effects of the abuse (Janoff-Bulman & Frieze, 1983; Wyatt & Mickey, 1988). Given that making internal, stable, global attributions for negative events is related to poor adjustment, low self-esteem, helplessness, psychological distress, and depression (Metalsky, Abramson, Seligman, Semmel, & Peterson, 1982; Peterson & Seligman, 1983; Tangney et al., 1990), shame as the intervening cause of symptoms following sexual abuse is likely.

The work available on the relation between attribution style and sexual abuse in adults who were victimized in childhood supports the idea that attribution style mediates the long-term outcome of sexual abuse. Gold (1986) compared the current functioning of women who had been sexually abused as children to that of women who did not report being abused, and found a strong relation between a victim's attribution style and her adult functioning. Women who were sexually victimized in childhood, and who reported psychological distress and low self-esteem, were more likely to have an attribution style characterized by internal, stable, global attributions for negative events.

We have been able to show the relations among sexual abuse, shame, and adjustment (Feiring, Taska, & Lewis, 2002). In a longitudinal study of children ages 8–15 years who were known to have been sexually abused, we examined the relations of the severity of sexual abuse, shame, and attribution to adjustment (in this case, depression), using risk and protective factors as covariants.

Figure 46.3 presents these data. Our findings indicate that within 6 months of the reported abuse (left side of the figure), severity of abuse and amount of shame were both related to depression. However, by 1 year after the reported abuse (right side of the figure), only amount of shame was related to depression. Perhaps more importantly, children whose shame decreased over the year showed decreases in depression, while children whose shame stayed the same or increased actually showed increases in depression.

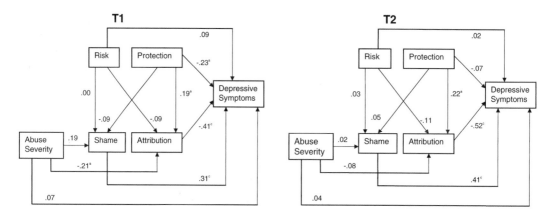

FIGURE 46.3. Depression and shame in sexually abused children. [a]$p < .05$; [b]$p < .01$; [c]$p < .001$. Data from Feiring, Taska, and Lewis (2002).

Maltreatment, Shame, and Attribution

The same model underlying psychopathology in sexually abused children should be evident for maltreated children. Although the literature on maltreatment in children (i.e., physical abuse and neglect) is extensive, there has been relatively little work on the relation between maltreatment and shame. We (Alessandri & Lewis, 1996), for example, have looked at this relation and found that shame and pride in regard to failure and success in learning achievement-like tasks are influenced by shame. Specifically, maltreatment should result in more shame and less pride relative to nonmaltreatment. The results of this study indicate that maltreated children show less pride when they succeed and more shame when they fail, relative to children from the same background who have not been maltreated (see Figure 46.4).

Moreover, important sex differences appear. Maltreated girls show more shame when they fail a task, and less pride when they succeed, than do nonmaltreated girls. Boys, on the other hand, show a suppression of both shame and pride. These sex difference findings are particularly important, since for girls trauma may result in depression (little pride and much shame), while for boys trauma may result in a suppression of emotion in general and there-

fore an increase in the likelihood of aggression, since they are not constrained by feelings of shame, guilt, or regret. Observations of these boys indicate higher amounts of such behaviors as throwing the test materials away, verbally aggressive statements, and (although not common) angry faces. In our more recent work (Sullivan & Lewis, 1999), we have measured these behaviors more carefully and found significant differences for maltreated and nonmaltreated boys' aggressive laboratory behavior. If these findings persist, the sex differences in response to traumas like maltreatment may explain why girls and women show high likelihood of depression, while boys and men show high likelihood of aggressive behavior, as a consequence of similar traumas. It is also interesting to note that children who are physically abused show less shame than those who are neglected (Lewis & Sullivan, 2005).

Abuse, especially in early childhood, is likely to lead to serious forms of pathology through the mediation of shame and attributions. Recently, we (Gold, Sullivan, & Lewis, 2007) studied over 100 adolescents who were incarcerated for antisocial behavior. Examined was how parental punishment, particularly harsh punishment, affected these adolescents' delinquent behavior. The effect of harsh parental punishment was mediated by shame and attributions in regard to responsibility for their ag-

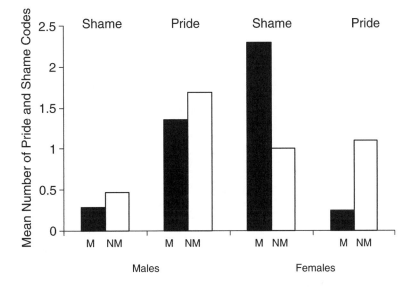

FIGURE 46.4. Shame and pride in maltreated children. M, maltreated; NM, nonmaltreated. Data from Alessandri and Lewis (1996).

gressive behavior. Using data on parental harsh punishment (beating and physical abuse), as well as data from the Test of Self-Conscious Affect–2 (TOSCA-2; Tangney, Ferguson, Wagner, Crowley, & Gramzow, 1996), we were able to examine the adolescents' violent behavior. As seen in Figure 46.5, harsh punishment was directly related to violent delinquent acts. It was also related to not taking responsibility (blaming others), which mediated the effects of punishment on violent delinquent behavior. Interestingly, the more they blamed others (the less responsibility they took), the less shame these adolescents showed. Here again, the connection between attribution and shame is apparent.

CONCLUSION

The study of self-conscious emotions continues to be conducted. The structural model outlined here (see Figure 46.1) provides a model for the self-conscious emotions. Without a more accu-

rate or agreed-upon taxonomy, the harder it will be to study these emotions. Given the interest in emotional life, and in the relation between emotions and health, it seems increasingly necessary to study these complex emotions, rather than only the more "primary" or "basic" ones. Moreover, as others have pointed out and as we are now discovering, these self-conscious emotions are intimately connected with other emotions, such as anger and sadness, as well as with psychopathology. Finally, given the place of self-evaluation in adult life, it seems clear that the self-conscious evaluative emotions are likely to stand in the center of our emotional life.

REFERENCES

Alessandri, S. A., & Lewis, M. (1996). Differences in pride and shame in maltreated and nonmaltreated preschoolers. *Child Development*, 67, 1857–1869.

Barrett, K. C., & Zahn-Waxler, C. (1987, April). *Do toddlers express guilt?* Poster presented at the bien-

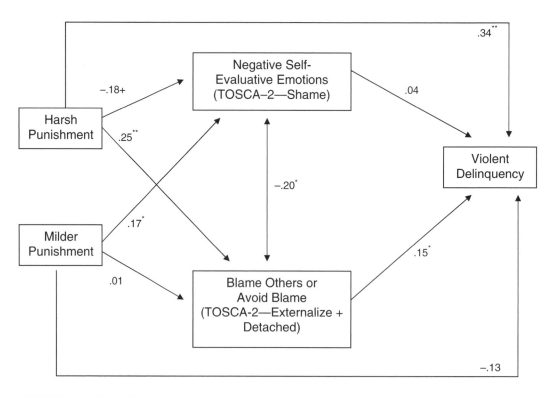

FIGURE 46.5. The effects of harsh parenting on adolescents' emotions, attributions, and delinquent behavior: Model of relations among maltreatment, emotions/attributions, and delinquency. + $p < .10$; *$p < .05$; **$p < .01$. Data from Gold, Sullivan, and Lewis (2007).

nial meeting of the Society for Research in Child Development, Toronto.

Beck, A. T. (1979). *Cognitive therapy and the emotional disorders*. New York: Meridian.

Broucek, F. J. (1991). *Shame and the self*. New York: Guilford Press.

Buss, A. H. (1980). *Self-consciousness and social anxiety*. San Francisco: Freeman.

Darwin, C. R. (1965). *The expression of the emotions in man and animals*. Chicago: University of Chicago Press. (Original work published 1872)

DiBiase, R., & Lewis, M. (1997). The relation between temperament and embarrassment. *Cognition and Emotion, 11,* 259–271.

Dweck, C. S., Hong, Y., & Chiu, C. (1993). Implicit theories: Individual differences in the likelihood and meaning of dispositional inferences. *Personality and Social Psychology Bulletin, 19,* 644–656.

Dweck, C. S., & Leggett, E. L. (1988). A social-cognitive approach to motivation and personality. *Psychological Review, 95,* 256–273.

Edelman, R. J. (1987). *The psychology of embarrassment*. Chichester, UK: Wiley.

Elliot, A. J., & Dweck, C. S. (2005). Competence and motivation: Competence as the core of achievement motivation. In A. J. Elliot & C. S. Dweck (Eds.), *Handbook of competence and motivation* (pp. 3–12). New York: Guilford Press.

Erikson, E. H. (1950). *Childhood and society*. New York: Norton.

Eysenck, H. J. (1954). *The psychology of politics*. London: Routledge & Kegan Paul.

Feiring, C., Taska, L., & Lewis, M. (2002). Adjustment following sexual abuse discovery: The role of shame and attributional style. *Developmental Psychology, 38*(1), 79–92.

Freud, S. (1953). Three essays on the theory of sexuality. In J. Strachey (Ed. & Trans.), *The standard edition of the complete psychological works of Sigmund Freud* (Vol. 7, pp. 123–231). London: Hogarth Press. (Original work published 1905)

Freud, S. (1963). *The problem of anxiety* (H. A. Bunker, Trans.). New York: Norton. (Original work published 1936)

Geppert, U. (1986). *A coding-system for analyzing behavioral expressions of self-evaluative emotions*. Munich: Max-Planck-Institute for Psychological Research.

Gold, E. R. (1986). Long-term effects of sexual victimization in childhood: An attributional approach. *Journal of Consulting and Clinical Psychology, 54,* 471–475.

Gold, J., Sullivan, M., & Lewis, M. (2007). *Emotions and attributions as mediators between harsh and abusive parenting and juvenile delinquency*. Manuscript submitted for publication.

Heckhausen, H. (1984). Emergent achievement behavior: Some early developments. In J. Nicholls (Ed.), *The development of achievement motivation* (pp. 1–32). Greenwich, CT: JAI Press.

Izard, C. E. (1979). *The Maximally Discriminative Facial Movement Coding System (MAX)*. Newark: Instructional Resources Center, University of Delaware.

Izard, C. E., & Tyson, M. C. (1986). Shyness as a discrete emotion. In W. H. Jones, J. M. Cheek, & S. R. Briggs (Eds.), *Shyness: Perspectives on research and treatment* (pp. 147–160). New York: Plenum Press.

Janoff-Bulman, R. (1979). Characterological versus behavioral self-blame: Inquiries into depression and rape. *Journal of Personality and Social Psychology, 37,* 1798–1809.

Janoff-Bulman, R., & Frieze, I. (1983). A theoretical perspective for understanding reactions to victimization. *Journal of Social Issues, 39,* 1–17.

Kagan, J. (2003). Biology, context, and developmental inquiry. *Annual Review of Psychology, 54,* 1–23.

Kochanska, G. (1997). Multiple pathways to conscience for children with different temperaments: From toddlerhood to age 5. *Developmental Psychology, 33,* 597–615.

Lansky, M. R., & Morrison, A. P. (1997). *The widening scope of shame*. Hillsdale, NJ: Analytic Press.

Lewis, H. B. (1971). *Shame and guilt in neurosis*. New York: International Universities Press.

Lewis, M. (1992). *Shame: The exposed self*. New York: Free Press.

Lewis, M. (1995). Embarrassment: The emotion of self-exposure and evaluation. In J. P. Tangney & K. W. Fischer (Eds.), *Self-conscious emotions: The psychology of shame, guilt, embarrassment, and pride* (pp. 198–218). New York: Guilford Press.

Lewis, M. (2003). The emergence of consciousness and its role in human development. *Annals of the New York Academy of Sciences, 1001,* 1–29.

Lewis, M., Alessandri, S. M., & Sullivan, M. W. (1992). Differences in shame and pride as a function of children's gender and task difficulty. *Child Development, 63,* 630–638.

Lewis, M., & Ramsay, D. (1997). Stress reactivity and self-recognition. *Child Development, 68,* 621–629.

Lewis, M., & Ramsay, D. (2002). Cortisol response to embarrassment and shame. *Child Development, 73*(4), 1034–1045.

Lewis, M., Stanger, C., & Sullivan, M. W. (1989). Deception in three-year-olds. *Developmental Psychology, 25,* 439–443.

Lewis, M., & Sullivan, M. W. (2005). The development of self-conscious emotions. In A. J. Elliott & C. S. Dweck (Eds.), *Handbook of competence and motivation* (pp. 185–201). New York: Guilford Press.

Mandler, G. (1975). *Mind and emotion*. New York: Wiley.

Metalsky, G. J., Abramson, L. Y., Seligman, M. E. P., Semmel, A., & Peterson, C. (1982). Attributional styles and life events in the classroom: Vulnerability and invulnerability to depressive mood reactions. *Journal of Personality and Social Psychology, 43,* 612–617.

Morrison, A. P. (1989). *Shame: The underside of narcissism*. Hillsdale, NJ: Analytic Press.

Mueller, C. M., & Dweck, C. S. (1998). Praise for intelligence can undermine children's motivation and performance. *Journal of Personality and Social Psychology, 75*, 33–52.

Oatley, K., & Johnson-Laird, P. N. (1987). Toward a cognitive theory of emotions. *Cognitions and Emotion, 1*, 29–50.

Ortony, A., Clore, G. L., & Collins, A. (1988). *The cognitive structure of emotions*. New York: Cambridge University Press.

Peterson, C., & Seligman, M. E. P. (1983). Learned helplessness and victimization. *Journal of Social Issues, 39*, 105–118.

Plutchik, R. (1980). A general psychoevolutionary theory of emotion. In R. Plutchik & H. Kellerman (Eds.), *Emotion: Theory, research, and experience* (Vol. 1, pp. 3–33). New York: Academic Press.

Schachter, S., & Singer, J. E. (1962). Cognitive, social, and physiological determinants of emotional state. *Psychological Review, 69*, 379–399.

Seligman, M. E. P., Peterson, C., Kaslow, N., Tanenbaum, R., Alloy, L., & Abramson, L. (1984). Attributional style and depressive symptoms among children. *Journal of Abnormal Psychology, 39*, 235–238.

Stipek, D. J. (1983). A developmental analysis of pride and shame. *Human Development, 25*, 42–54.

Stipek, D. J., Recchia, S., & McClintic, S. (1992). Self-evaluation in young children. *Monographs of the Society for Research in Child Development, 57*(1, Serial No. 226).

Sullivan, M. W., & Lewis, M. (1999, April). *The emotions of maltreated children in response to success and failure*. Paper presented at the biennial meeting of the Society for Research in Child Development, Albuquerque, NM.

Tangney, J. P., & Dearing, R. L. (2002). *Shame and guilt*. New York: Guilford Press.

Tangney, J. P., Ferguson, T. J., Wagner, P. E., Crowley, S. L., & Gramzow, R. (1996). *The Test of Self-Conscious Affect–2 (TOSCA-2)*. Fairfax, VA: George Mason University.

Tangney, J. P., Wagner, P., & Gramzow, R. (1990, June). *Shame-proneness, but not guilt-proneness, is linked to psychological maladjustment*. Poster presented at the meeting of the American Psychological Society, Dallas, TX.

Tomkins, S. S. (1963). *Affect, imagery, and consciousness: Vol. 2. The negative affects*. New York: Springer.

Tracy, J. L., & Robins, R. W. (2004). Show your pride: Evidence for a discrete emotion expression. *Psychological Science, 15*(3), 194–197.

Tracy, J. L., Robins, R. W., & Lagattuta, K. H. (2005). Can children recognize pride? *Emotion, 5*(3), 251–257.

Weiner, B. (1986). *An attributional theory of motivation and emotion*. New York: Springer-Verlag.

Wyatt, G. E., & Mickey, M. R. (1988). The support of parents and others as it mediates the effects of child sexual abuse: An exploratory study. In G. E. Wyatt & G. J. Powell (Eds.), *Lasting effects of child sexual abuse* (pp. 211–226). Newbury Park, CA: Sage.

CHAPTER 47

Disgust

PAUL ROZIN, JONATHAN HAIDT, and CLARK R. McCAULEY

For North Americans, elicitors of disgust come from nine domains: food, body products, animals, sexual behaviors, contact with death or corpses, violations of the exterior envelope of the body (including gore and deformity), poor hygiene, interpersonal contamination (contact with unsavory human beings), and certain moral offenses (Haidt, McCauley, & Rozin, 1994; Rozin, Haidt, & McCauley, 1993; Rozin, Haidt, McCauley, & Imada, 1997). What unites these disparate domains? Although all involve negative or unpleasant events, there are many negative events, such as pain and loss, that are not disgusting. The primary goal of this chapter is to make sense of this varied set of elicitors—that is, to describe the meaning of disgust within evolutionary, developmental, and cultural contexts. We argue for a path of development in individuals and cultures that extends from the presumed origin of disgust as a rejection response that protects the body from "bad" foods, to a rejection system that protects the soul from the full range of elicitors listed above.

DEFINING DISGUST

There are two classic papers describing disgust, published some 70 years apart. The first, a chapter in Darwin's *The Expression of the Emotions in Man and Animals* (1872/1965), defined disgust as referring to "something revolting, primarily in relation to the sense of taste, as actually perceived or vividly imagined; and secondarily to anything which causes a similar feeling, through the sense of smell, touch and even of eyesight" (p. 253). Darwin related disgust not only to the experience of revulsion but to a characteristic facial expression. The second paper, by psychoanalyst Andras Angyal (1941), held that disgust is revulsion at the prospect of oral incorporation of an offensive object. He identified body waste products as a focus of disgust, and related the strength of disgust to the degree of intimacy of contact. Our own description of disgust, or what we call "core disgust," follows on Angyal's definition above, adding this sentence: "The offensive objects are contaminants; that is, if they even briefly contact an acceptable food, they tend to render that food unacceptable" (Rozin & Fallon, 1987, p. 23).

Most definitions focus on the mouth and real or imagined ingestion. Tomkins (1963, 1982) held that of all the emotions, disgust has the clearest linkage to a specific motivation (hunger), and functions to oppose this motive. Ekman and Friesen (1975) see disgust as an aversion that centers on oral rejection. Wierzbicka (1986) defines disgust as a bad feeling about another person's action, "similar to what one feels when one has something in one's mouth that tastes bad and when one wants to cause it to come to be out of one's mouth" (p. 590).

Some have proposed systems other than ingestion as the origin of disgust. Freud (1905/1953) predictably linked it to sex, and others (e.g., Renner, 1944; Plutchik, 1980) see its origin as a defense against infection, with the skin playing a central role. Curtis and her colleagues (Curtis & Biran, 2001; Curtis, Aunger, & Rabie, 2004) have presented evidence that the best single account for what is currently disgusting is infection potential, and have suggested that protection from infection provides the adaptive reason for the evolution of disgust. The fact that contamination sensitivity is a basic feature of disgust supports this claim. Kelly (2007) proposes that disgust has a dual origin. His entanglement hypothesis posits a convergence of an orally focused toxin avoidance system (present in nonhumans) and a broader parasite avoidance system that arose during human evolution.

It seems likely that threats of disease and infection shaped the disgust response as humans increased their intake of foods of animal origin and as group densities increased. Both of these major changes increased parasite risk. Still, we find the arguments for a food origin convincing (Rozin & Fallon, 1987). The English term "disgust" itself means "bad taste," and the facial expression of disgust can be seen as functional in rejecting unwanted foods and odors. The most distinct physiological concomitant of disgust—nausea—is a food-related sensation that inhibits ingestion. Finally, the brain region most often activated in studies of disgust (including non-food-related stimuli, such as mutilations and disgust faces) is the anterior insula (Husted, Shapira, & Goodman, 2006), which, among its other functions, is the gustatory cortex in primates (Rolls, 1994).

COMPONENTS OF DISGUST

Almost all of the literature on emotion prior to 1990 focused on fear, anger, happiness, and sadness. However, disgust seems to have "arrived" in the 1990s. Between 1997 and 2006, PsycINFO listed 178 articles with "disgust" in the title (see also Olatunji & Sawchuk, 2005). In the same period, two academically oriented books about disgust were published (W. I. Miller, 1997; S. B. Miller, 2004), and two influential trade books about psychology devoted considerable attention to disgust (Bloom, 2004; Pinker, 1997). One stimulus to the investigation of disgust has probably been the fact that it appears primitive and basic, while at the same time the broad range of elicitors implicates disgust in many uniquely human concerns, including morality and divinity. For this reason, we have described disgust in the title of one publication as "the body and soul emotion" (Rozin, Haidt, & McCauley, 1999), and this contrast has provoked considerable interest (e.g., Bloom, 2004). A related framing of disgust conceives it as the emotion that is the guardian of the borders of both the bodily self and the social self (Fessler & Haley, 2006; S. B. Miller, 2004; Rozin, Nemeroff, Horowitz, Gordon, & Voet, 1995).

Paul Ekman (1992) has provided the clearest articulation of the characteristics of an emotion, and disgust meets all nine of his criteria. We consider here four of Ekman's criteria.

Behavioral Component

Disgust is manifested as a distancing from some object, event, or situation, and can be characterized as a rejection.

Physiological Component

Disgust is associated with a *specific* physiological state—nausea—that is typically measured by self-report. Another specific physiological aspect of disgust has been suggested by Angyal (1941), who pointed to increased salivation, itself associated with nausea, as a concomitant of disgust. We know of no experimental studies of the relation of disgust to nausea or salivation. More conventional psychophysiological investigations of disgust suggest that it is associated with some degree of parasympathetic autonomic response, particularly lowered heart rate, whereas fear and anger are associated with a predominantly sympathetic response (Levenson, Ekman, & Friesen, 1990; Levenson, 1992).

Expressive Component

The expressive component of disgust has been studied almost entirely with reference to the face. The characteristics of the "disgust face" have received particular attention from Darwin (1872/1965), Izard (1971), Ekman (Ekman, 1972; Ekman & Friesen, 1975), and Rozin, Lowery, and Ebert (1994). Scholars are not in complete agreement about a prototypical disgust face, but the three main components seem to be the gape (Action Unit [AU] 25 or 26in the Facial Action Coding System [FACS; Ekman & Friesen, 1978]), retraction of the upper lip (AU 10), and the nose wrinkle (AU 9). Activity centers around the mouth and nose, and the movements tend either to discourage entry into the body (e.g., nose wrinkle) or to encourage discharge (gape with or without tongue extension). Facial electromyographic measurements confirm the observational data, involving some of the same facial muscles, and including some of the muscles around the eyes (Wolf et al., 2005). Laughter is a common response (as opposed to the disgust face) in some disgust-eliciting situations (Hemenover & Schimmack, 2007).

The *Nāṭyaśāstra* (Masson & Patwardhan, 1970), an ancient Hindu treatise on drama (see Shweder, Haidt, Horton, & Joseph, Chapter 25, this volume), treats disgust as one of eight or nine basic emotions. As described by Hejmadi (2000), the multiple portrayals of disgust designated in this document are dynamic (as opposed to the standard "frozen face" used in almost all Western research), and involve actions of the whole body, especially the hands. Americans as well as Indians are able to identify these disgust expressions remarkably well (Hejmadi, Davidson, & Rozin, 2000).

Qualia

Qualia, the mental or feeling component of emotion, may be at once the most central component of disgust and the most difficult to study. The *qualia* of disgust is often described as revulsion. In comparison to other emotions, the experience of disgust appears to be rather short in duration (Scherer & Wallbott, 1994).

CORE DISGUST

We believe that disgust was shaped by evolutionary forces that elaborated upon an older food rejection system based on distaste. In this and subsequent sections, we describe how core disgust differs from distaste, and then how disgust may have expanded to a much wider range of elicitors—including reminders of our animal nature, and certain types of interpersonal contact and moral violations.

Core disgust is one of four categories of food rejection, the others being distaste (rejection motivated by bad sensory properties), danger (rejection motivated by fear of bodily harm), and inappropriateness (rejection of a food culturally classified as not edible) (Fallon & Rozin, 1983; Rozin & Fallon, 1987). Like inappropriateness, disgust is defined by ideational forces: beliefs about the nature or origin of a potential food. Unlike inappropriate entities, disgusting entities are presumed to be both distasteful and dangerous. The appraisal that elicits core disgust requires (1) a sense of potential oral incorporation (and hence a linkage with food or eating), (2) a sense of offensiveness, and (3) contamination potency (Angyal, 1944; Rozin & Fallon, 1987).

Oral Incorporation

Rozin and Fallon (1987) noted that the mouth is the principal route by which material things enter the body, and hence can be thought of as the gateway to the body. Aversion to an offensive entity in the mouth is usually stronger than aversion to the same entity on the body surface near but not inside the mouth, or inside the stomach (Rozin et al., 1995).

The threat of oral incorporation is framed by a widespread belief that one takes on the properties of the food one eats ("You are what you eat"). In *The Golden Bough*, Frazer (1890/1922) noted: "The savage commonly believes that by eating the flesh of an animal or man, he acquires not only the physical but even the moral and intellectual qualities which are characteristic of that animal or man" (p. 573). This belief is consistent with our general experience that when two things combine (in this case, a food and a person), the product resembles both. Nemeroff and Rozin (1989) found, using the Asch impression-listing technique, that American college students attribute boar-like qualities to boar eaters, and turtle-like qualities to turtle eaters.

Offensive Entities: Animals and Their Products

Angyal (1941) held that the center of disgust is animal (including human) waste products, which he saw as debasing. Body products are a focus of disgust, and are central to the related anthropological concept of pollution (Douglas, 1966; Meigs, 1978, 1984). There is widespread historical and cultural evidence for aversion and disgust to virtually all body products, including feces, vomit, urine, and blood (especially menstrual blood). In accord with Angyal's (1941) suggestion of an animal focus for disgust, Rozin and Fallon (1987) proposed that the elicitor category for core disgust consists of all animals and their products as potential foods. Relatedly, Martins and Pliner (2006) report a dimension of livingness/animalness emerging from multidimensional scaling of ratings of the disgustingness of a wide range of novel foods. Almost all cultures eat only a small subset of potential animal foods. Angyal (1941) pointed out that in many cultures some care is taken to disguise the animal origin of animal food by cutting, chopping, and other culinary preparations, as well as by having names for animal foods (e.g., "pork" and "beef" in English) that are distinct from the corresponding animal names.

Animals and their products seem cross-culturally to be both the most favored of foods and the most tabooed. In short, animal foods are emotionally charged (Tambiah, 1969) and tend to give rise to ambivalent responses. Many animal taboos involve disgust. Some animals are disgusting because they bear some resemblance to body products such as mucus (e.g., slugs), or because they are commonly in contact with rotting animal flesh, feces, or other human wastes (e.g., flies, cockroaches, rats, vultures, and other scavengers). Carnivorous land animals eat raw, often decaying animal flesh, and produce putrid feces; they are disgusting at both ends. Herbivores are much less likely to be prohibited cross-culturally. Even the hunter–gatherer !Kung bushmen, who eat a much wider variety of species than most Westerners do, reject rodents, carnivores, and most insects (Howell, 1986).

Two other categories of animal food prohibitions deserve mention. Animals that are close to humans, either in appearance (e.g., other primates) or by virtue of a relationship with humans as pets, are rarely eaten. And finally, there is a group of anomalous animals that seem to produce a mixture of fear (danger) and disgust (e.g., spiders and snakes). These animals are feared, although they are rarely harmful to humans. Davey and his colleagues (Davey, 1993; Matchett & Davey, 1991; Ware, Jain, Burgess, & Davey, 1993; Webb & Davey, 1993) offer evidence that the aversion to these animals is based more on disgust than fear.

Contamination

The contamination response—rejection of a potential food if it even briefly contacted a disgusting entity—appears to be powerful and universal among adults. North American college students reject liked beverages after these have briefly contacted a sterilized cockroach (Rozin, Millman, & Nemeroff, 1986), and virtually all North Americans reject foods that have been handled or bitten by either unsavory or disliked persons (Rozin, Nemeroff, Wane, & Sherrod, 1989). Although this aversion is typically justified as an avoidance of disease, removal of this justification (e.g., by sterilizing the offending dead cockroach) typically has only a small effect. Contamination may have been shaped as an adaptation for disease avoidance, but it operates largely independently of conscious beliefs about disease.

Rozin and his colleagues have suggested that contamination effects may be instances of the sympathetic magical law of contagion (Tylor, 1871/1974; Frazer, 1890/1922; Mauss, 1902/1972), which essentially holds that "once in contact, always in contact" (Rozin & Fallon, 1987; Rozin & Nemeroff, 1990). The law of contagion as applied to disgust is potentially crippling; everything people might eat or touch is potentially contaminated. Humans deal with this problem in a number of ways. First, contamination rules are developed in some cultures, such as the explicit rules establishing a threshold for contamination in the Hebrew dietary system (Grunfeld, 1982). These rules provide ritualistic relief but not necessarily psychological relief of a sense of contamination (Nemeroff & Rozin, 1992).

Most often, framing is the strategy that keeps potential contamination out of consideration—as when we do not think of the people in the kitchen who prepare our food in a restaurant, or the animal that was the source of our meat, or the fact that our body contains a host of disgusting substances. The framing solution fails when the source of contamination is too salient.

A second law of sympathetic magic, the law of similarity, accounts for some other aspects of disgust. The law of similarity, also dating from Tylor, Frazer, and Mauss (for reviews, see Rozin & Nemeroff, 1990; Nemeroff & Rozin, 2000), holds in one form that if things are superficially similar, then they resemble each other in a deep sense as well. In other words, appearance is reality. The law of similarity is evident when objects that look like something disgusting are treated as disgusting. For example, many North Americans are reluctant to consume imitation dog feces that they know are made out of chocolate fudge (Rozin, Millman, & Nemeroff, 1986).

ANIMAL-NATURE DISGUST

Our discussion of disgust up to this point has focused on issues surrounding food and eating. We have presented core disgust as an oral defense against harm from potential foods, or things that can easily contaminate foods such as body products and some animals. However, when we asked North American and Japanese respondents to list the things they thought were disgusting, fewer than 25% of listed examples came from the three core disgust domains of food, animals, and body products (Haidt, Rozin, McCauley, & Imada, 1997). Many of the other examples could be classified into four additional domains: inappropriate sexual acts, poor hygiene, death, and violations of the ideal body "envelope" or exterior form (e.g., gore, deformity, obesity). In the four additional domains, the focus of threat has spread from the mouth to the body in general. This spread is captured in a psychoanalytic treatment of disgust: "In summary, any modality that represents a means of entry into the self or body—the mouth, the nose, the skin, the eyes—seems to play a part in the disgust experience" (S. B. Miller, 1986, p. 300). All four of these domains involve potential sources of biological contagion and infection (e.g., venereal diseases from sex, or skin-to-skin or hair-to-hair infection from parasites on an unclean person); thus core disgust was preadapted and easily expanded to apply contamination sensitivity to these addi-

tional classes of threats. However, we think that something more symbolic was and is going on as well.

Contact with death and corpses is a particularly potent elicitor of disgust. Two of the items in our 32-item Disgust Scale (discussed in more detail later) that correlate most highly with the total score are about contact with dead bodies (Haidt et al., 1994). The prototypical odor of disgust is the odor of decay, which is the odor of death. The centrality of death in disgust suggests a more general construal of disgust within a modified psychoanalytic framework.

Becker (1973) has argued that the most important threat to the psyche is not sexuality and aggression, but the certainty of death. Only human animals know they are to die, and only humans need to repress this threat. In this framework, Becker's "denial of death" is served by disgust, which helps to suppress thoughts or experiences that suggest human mortality. Research on terror management theory has shown a strong connection between disgust and the fear of death: People who are asked to imagine their own death later show an increase in disgust sensitivity, and an increase in liking for an essay that argues for human uniqueness rather than human continuity with other animals (Goldenberg et al., 2001). Conversely, exposure to disgusting stimuli, under some conditions, increases implicit death-related ideation (Cox, Goldenberg, Pyszczynski, & Weise, 2007).

These speculations about death lead to an overarching description of disgust elicitors: Anything that reminds us that we are animals elicits disgust (Rozin & Fallon, 1987). Humans must eat, excrete, and have sex, just like other animals. Each culture prescribes the proper way to perform these actions—for example, by placing most animals off limits as potential foods, and all animals and most people off limits as potential sexual partners. People who ignore these prescriptions are reviled as disgusting and animal-like. Furthermore, humans are like animals in having fragile body envelopes that, when breached, reveal blood and soft viscera that display our commonalities with animals. Human bodies, like animal bodies, die. Envelope violations and death are disgusting because they are uncomfortable reminders of our animal vulnerability. Finally, hygienic rules govern the proper use and maintenance of the human body, and the failure to meet these culturally defined standards places a person below the level of humans. Animals are (often inappropriately) seen as dirty and inattentive to hygiene. Insofar as we humans behave like animals, the distinction between humans and animals is blurred, and we see ourselves as lowered, debased, and mortal.

Elias (1939/1978), in *The History of Manners*, concludes that "people, in the course of the civilizing process, seek to suppress in themselves every characteristic that they feel to be 'animal' " (p. 120). Tambiah (1969) emphasizes the importance of this distinction for humans, and points to the paradox of human fascination with and aversion to animals. Ortner (1973) notes that the one body product that does not reliably elicit disgust is tears, and these are seen as uniquely human. And Leach (1964) has pointed out that animal words are used as insults in many cultures. In general, the ethnographic literature is filled with references to the fact that humans consider themselves better than animals, and work to maintain a clear animal–human boundary. Violations of that boundary—for example, treating an animal as a person in a pet relationship—are rather rare cross-culturally.

W. I. Miller's (1997) broad, historically based conception of disgust comes to a conclusion like ours: "ultimately the basis for all disgust is *us*—that we live and die and that the process is a messy one emitting substances and odors that make us doubt ourselves and fear our neighbors" (p. xiv).

INTERPERSONAL DISGUST

The fact that contact with other people can elicit disgust was noted by Darwin (1872/1965). Furthermore, Angyal (1941) noted that other persons, as containers of waste products, are potentially disgusting. There is widespread evidence in the United States for aversion to contact with possessions, utensils, clothing, cars, and rooms used by unknown or undesirable persons (Rozin et al., 1989; Rozin, Markwith, & McCauley, 1994). Interpersonal aversion can be analyzed into four separately identifiable components: strangeness, disease, misfortune, and moral taint (Rozin, Markwith, & McCauley, 1994). Thus a sweater worn once by a healthy stranger and then laundered is less desirable than an unworn sweater (aversion to strangeness). This negativity is substantially enhanced if the stranger has had a misfortune

(e.g., an amputated leg), a disease (e.g., tuberculosis), or a moral taint (e.g., a conviction for murder). These types of contacts are both offensive and contaminating; thus they seem to be instances of disgust.

Interpersonal disgust clearly discourages contact with other human beings who are not intimates. This is probably adaptive by reducing an infection risk, and can serve the purpose of maintaining social distinctiveness and social hierarchies. In Hindu India, interpersonal contagion, mediated in part by contacts with food, is a major feature of society and a major basis for the maintenance of the caste system (Appadurai, 1981; Marriott, 1968).

MORAL DISGUST

Studies that ask people to recall times they were disgusted elicit stories that often focus on moral violations, and that involve high levels of anger as well (Haidt et al., 1997; Izard, 1977; Nabi, 2002; Scherer, 1997). Some of these stories involve issues of sexuality, gore, or other instances of the misuse or abuse of human bodies, and are thus consistent with animal-nature disgust. However, many of the stories people tell about disgust do not involve the body at all; for North Americans, they often involve such issues as betrayal, hypocrisy, and racism. Do these disembodied moral violations really elicit disgust?

Nabi (2002) has argued that they do not. She found that the phrase "grossed out" did an excellent job of eliciting stories about core disgust, but the words "disgust" and "disgusted" elicited stories that were closer to those elicited by "anger" than those elicited by "grossed out." She suggests that the lay understanding of the word "disgust" is a mixture of disgust and anger, and that researchers should be careful about following ordinary language by assuming that the blend is a single emotion. In short, disgust is really about bodily issues, and the moral part of moral disgust is really anger (see also Royzman & Sabini, 2001).

We agree that the lay use of emotion words can be misleading, particularly in cross-cultural research (Haidt & Keltner, 1999). But there is evidence to suggest that cases of apparent moral disgust are really disgust; they are not just linguistic errors made by English speakers. First, if the broad expansion of the word "disgusting" into the sociomoral domain is a quirk of the English language, it is also a quirk of almost every language we have looked at. French *dégoût*, German *Ekel*, Russian *otvraschenie*, Spanish *asco*, Hebrew *go-al*, Japanese *ken-o*, Chinese *aw-shin*, and Bengali *ghenna* all have a semantic domain covering concerns about the body as well as concerns about other people's social behavior (Haidt et al., 1997). People of diverse cultures and languages apparently *feel* some similarity in their emotional reactions to feces and to sleazy politicians.

Second, research in neuroscience is increasingly focusing on the anterior insula as a crucial site of "somatic marking" (Damasio, 2003), the process by which interoceptive information (gut feelings) meets up with higher-level social cognition to produce motives for social approach or avoidance. In a functional magnetic resonance imaging (fMRI) study of people playing the "ultimatum game," those given a very low "take it or leave it" division of a pool of money usually left it, and their decision was well predicted by a surge of activity in the anterior insula (Sanfey, Rilling, Aronson, Nystrom, & Cohen, 2003)—the brain area most often linked to disgust in neuroimaging studies.

Third, Sherman, Haidt, and Coan (2007) found that in response to a video about American neo-Nazis that elicited very high ratings of disgust and moderately high ratings of anger, heart rates went down—the expected physiological response to disgust, and the opposite of the usual response to anger. Furthermore, the heart rate decrement was much larger in the subset of subjects who reported tightness or clenching in their throats (a marker of core disgust). In other words, Nazis really are disgusting, at least to some people.

These moral offenses on the outer limits of disgust's expansion show not just the property of offensiveness but also the property of contamination. Indirect contact with people who have committed moral offenses (such as murders) is highly aversive, to about the same extent as similar contact with someone with a serious contagious illness (Rozin, Markwith, & McCauley, 1994).

Shweder, Much, Mahapatra, and Park (1997) offer a theory of moral judgment that may help clarify the moral significance of disgust, contempt, and anger (the three other-condemning moral emotions; Izard's [1977] hostility triad). The theory proposes that three codes of ethics underlie the morality of most cultures. One code, called the "ethics of community," focuses on issues of duty, hierarchy, and the proper fulfillment of one's social roles. Violations of this code seem to elicit the emotion of contempt. A second code, the "ethics of autonomy," encompasses issues of rights and justice. This is the most fully elaborated code in Western societies, where violations of this code are usually associated with anger. A third code, the "ethics of divinity," focuses on the self as a spiritual entity and seeks to protect that entity from degrading or polluting acts. We see a rough match between Shweder et al.'s three moral codes and the three other-condemning moral emotions, with disgust as the emotion elicited by violations of the ethics of divinity, the guardian of the sanctity of the soul as well as purity of the body. We call this the "CAD triad" hypothesis (community/contempt, autonomy/anger, divinity/disgust), and provide evidence supporting it from the correspondence between the three moral codes and the three emotions in Japanese and Americans (Rozin, Lowery, Imada, & Haidt, 1999).

Disgust plays a special role in the moral domain as a means of socialization. Insofar as entities viewed as immoral are also disgusting, there is no temptation to have traffic with them. For example, as cigarette smoking has moved from being a preference to a negative moral value in modern North America, there is an accompanying increase in disgust responses to cigarettes, cigarette smoke, cigarette residues (e.g., ashes), and cigarette smokers (Rozin & Singh, 1999). This process of conversion of an entity from a preference into a value has been called "moralization" (Rozin, 1997). It is often associated with the recruitment of a disgust response to the entity or activity in question.

PREADAPTATION AND THE CULTURAL EVOLUTION OF DISGUST

We believe that the output side of disgust (physiology, behavior, expression) has remained relatively constant over human history, and that it still bears noticeable similarities to its animal precursors. However, the input side (elicitors and meanings) has been transformed and greatly expanded.

We have suggested a course of biological and cultural evolution of disgust, summarized in Table 47.1 (Rozin et al., 1993, 1997). The pro-

TABLE 47.1. Proposed Pathway of Expansion of Disgust and Disgust Elicitors

	Disgust stage				
	0. Distaste	1. Core	2. Animal nature	3. Interpersonal	4. Moral
Function	Protect body from poison	Protect body from disease/infection	Protect body and soul; deny mortality	Protect body, soul, and social order	Protect social order
Elicitors	Bad tastes	Food/eating, body products, animals	Sex, death, hygiene, envelope violations	Direct and indirect contact with strangers or undesirables	Certain moral offenses

posed origin is the rejection response to bad-tasting foods, even though taste in the mouth ultimately has little to do with the emotion of disgust. However, oral rejection remains an organizing principle of disgust reactions, in what we have called "core disgust." Core disgust can be thought of as a guardian of the mouth, and therefore as a guardian of the physical body. Food and its potential contaminants (body products and some animals) are the elicitors for core disgust.

Disgust then expanded further to become a guardian of the temple of the body, responding to direct threats of contagion or infection to parts other than the mouth, and also to any evidence that our bodies are really no different from animal bodies (i.e., animal-nature disgust in the domains of sexuality, body envelope violations, death, and hygiene). Driving a desire to distinguish ourselves from animals may be our fear of animal mortality.

Interpersonal disgust and moral disgust are not easily accounted for as reminders of our animal nature. They may both be linked to the prior forms of disgust, because they are extensions of a disease avoidance mechanism to become a broader social avoidance mechanism. This model suggests what might be called an opportunistic accretion of new domains of elicitors to a rejection system that is already in place. A parallel to this model in evolutionary biology is the concept of "preadaptation" (Mayr, 1960). Mayr suggests that the major source of evolutionary "novelties" is the coopting of an existing system for a new function. Preadaptation can operate either to replace an original function, or to accrete new functions to an existing system. A particularly appropriate example is the human mouth, whose teeth and tongue clearly evolved for food handling. However, by a process of preadaptation, they

have come to be shared by the language expression system. Teeth and tongue are critical in pronunciation, but they did not evolve for that purpose. We suggest that in both cultural evolution and individual development, a process like preadaptation occurs; in development, it can be described as the accessing of previously inaccessible systems for a wider range of activities, functions, or elicitors (Rozin, 1976).

We have described the cultural evolution of disgust as a sequence of stages that takes disgust further and further away from its mouth-and-food origins, through a process of preadaptation. But it has not really expanded that far beyond food, because, by a parallel process of preadaptation, food itself has come to serve many functions—aesthetic, social, and moral—besides its original nutritive function (Kass, 1994). In parallel, the food vocabulary has taken on other, metaphorical functions, again by a process of preadaptation. Thus the very words "taste" and "distaste" have come to indicate general aesthetic judgments. In Hindu India, food and eating are quintessentially social and moral activities (Appadurai, 1981).

The latter part of the 19th century included two events with important impact on the evolution of disgust in the Western world: Darwin's theory of evolution (which blurred the human–animal distinction) and the rise of germ theory following on the work of Pasteur and others. Detailed analyses of lay and elite thinking about disgust during the 19th century have been provided in two cultural histories of France (Corbin, 1986; Barnes, 2006). Prior to the development of germ theory, the French had already adapted to serious contagion risks by showing disgust to and avoidance of odors of decay and contact with ill individuals. Quarantine was in practice before germ theory, and odor was believed to be part and parcel of the source of illness, rather than a correlate of it. Germ theory thus provided scientific justification for disgust sensibilities that were already present, and germ theory and disgust were both advanced in what Barnes (2006) has described as the marriage of lay contagion beliefs and germ theory—a "sanitary–bacteriological synthesis."

THE DEVELOPMENT OF DISGUST

For adults, feces seems to be a universal disgust substance (Angyal, 1941; Rozin & Fallon, 1987), with the odor of decay as perhaps the most potent sensory attribute associated with disgust. It is also conceivable that vomit is a primary substance for disgust. Since feces, vomit, and decay are associated with disease vectors, it would be reasonable to suppose that there would be an innate rejection of such things. However, neither one seems to be reliably rejected by nonhuman animals or young children (Rozin, Hammer, Oster, Horowitz, & Marmara, 1986). Rather, it appears that infants may be attracted to feces, and that disgust is a powerful cultural force that turns this attraction into aversion (Freud, 1910/1957; Jones, 1912/1948). The preponderance of evidence suggests that there are no innately negative nonirritant odors, and that a rejection of decay odors (without a referent object present) appears somewhere between 3 and 7 years of age (Petó, 1936; Schmidt & Beauchamp, 1988; Stein, Ottenberg, & Roulet, 1958; but see Steiner, 1979).

As far as we know, there is no sense of offensiveness or rejection outside of the sensory realm in either infants or nonhumans, and hence no gape elicitors other than negative tastes. Disgust seems to require enculturation—a supposition confirmed by Malson's (1964/1972) review of some 50 feral humans, none of whom showed any sign of disgust.

Toilet training is probably the initial disgust-generating experience. For 3-year-olds, feces are rejected, but not contaminating and possibly not offensive. In the period following toilet training, children develop an aversion for substances resembling feces (e.g., mud, dirt, and mushy substances) and sometimes a marked concern for cleanliness (Senn & Solnit, 1968; Ferenczi, 1914/1952).

Further extension of aversion to core disgust elicitors is likely to occur either by generalization from existing disgusting entities (e.g., from feces to mud) or by evaluative conditioning (although attempts to capture this phenomenon in the laboratory have yielded mixed outcomes; see Schienle, Stark, & Vaitl, 2001; Rozin, Wrzesniewski, & Byrnes, 1998). There may be a predisposition or expectancy to associate certain entities, such as certain types of animals, with already disgusting entities (Davey, Cavanagh, & Lamb, 2003). Disgust may be acquired by witnessing facial displays of emotions that elicit the experience of those emotions (Tomkins, 1963), perhaps engaging processes that involve mirror neurons (Gallese, Keysers, & Rizzolatti, 2004).

Locating the onset of true disgust in development depends on subtle measures of "offensiveness" or "ideational rejection" and the appearance of contamination sensitivity. Contamination sensitivity is not present in children under 3–5 years of age (Fallon, Rozin, & Pliner, 1984; Rozin, Fallon, & Augstoni-Ziskind, 1985; Siegal, 1988; Siegal & Share, 1990; Hejmadi, Rozin, & Siegal, 2004). Contamination sensitivity is a sophisticated ability, requiring a separation of appearance and reality. There is no sensory residue of past contamination in a contaminated entity; it is the history of contact that is critical (Rozin & Nemeroff, 1990; Nemeroff & Rozin, 2000). Furthermore, contamination implies some conception of invisible entities (e.g., traces of cockroach) that are the vehicle of contamination. The notion of invisible entities and the notion that appearance is distinct from reality are cognitive achievements of considerable abstraction, and both seem to be absent in young children (Piaget & Inhelder, 1941/1974; Flavell, 1986; Rosen & Rozin, 1993; but see Siegal & Share, 1990). This cognitive limitation may be the principal barrier to a full childhood acquisition of disgust.

Adult contamination sensitivity is a mixture of at least two types of conceptions. One involves transfer of invisible material through contact, and hence is often sensitive to manipulations like washing (material essence). A second is more indelible and involves the passing of some type of "spiritual" force that is not subject to removal by chemical and physical treatments ("spiritual essence"; Nemeroff & Rozin, 1994). There is evidence that at its first appearance in children, the essence producing contamination sensitivity is more like the indelible, "spiritual" than the material form (Hejmadi et al., 2004), and it appears somewhat earlier and in greater intensity in Hindu Indian children than in American children.

A measure of contamination sensitivity that focused on disgust contaminants showed a substantial correlation between young adults and their parents: $r = .52$ for Americans (Rozin, Fallon, & Mandell, 1984); $r = .33$ in Britain (Davey, Forster, & Mayhew, 1991). A study using the broader Disgust Scale (see below) found a more modest correlation ($r = .21$) across three generations of Americans (Rozin & Wolf, 2007).

CULTURAL DIFFERENCES IN DISGUST

Almost the entire literature on disgust comes from the approximately 6% of the world in which English is the native language. We believe that the cultural evolution of disgust has made few changes on the output side, as noted above, but that it has created substantial cultural variation on the input side. The simplest variations can be seen when cultures differ in the particular elicitors of disgust within one of the domains we have described. For example, most cultures value some kind of decayed/fermented food that is disgusting in most other cultures, but such food varies quite a bit (e.g., cheese for Europeans, decayed meat for Inuit, fermented fish sauce for Southeast Asians). Similarly, cultures differ about whether dogs are best friends or dirty scavengers, about whether or not corpses should be touched during mourning, or about whether mouth-to-mouth kissing is erotic or disgusting.

It is primarily in the last two steps of the expansion of disgust—interpersonal and moral disgust—that cultural differences seem to be greatest. Interpersonal and moral disgust appear to be particularly elaborated in Hindu India, compared to Western nations in which people rarely worry about the caste or background of the people cooking their food. Purity is a moral virtue to be protected in India, and in this respect, food is a "biomoral" substance (Appadurai, 1981). Moral disgust in the United States seems to focus on acts that strip others of their basic humanity (of their souls, Bloom [2004] would say; e.g., acts of brutality, cruelty, and racism), as well as to more mundane acts

of sleaziness and insincerity (such as hypocrisy and fawning). In Japan, participants applied the word *ken-o* more to situations in which there had been a failure to achieve a good fit in social relationships, such as when somebody else ignored them or criticized them unfairly. American moral disgust may be guarding against threats to an individualist, rights-based social order, whereas Japanese *ken-o* may be guarding against threats to a more collectivist, interdependent social order (Haidt et al., 1997).

An additional cultural difference is found in the moral significance attached to the activities that disgust regulates. Haidt, Koller, and Dias (1993) asked North Americans and Brazilians of higher and lower socioeconomic status about a number of actions that were disgusting yet harmless, including incestuous kissing, eating one's dead pets, and eating a chicken one has just had sex with. They found that North Americans of high socioeconomic status separated their emotional reactions from their moral judgments, while other groups were more likely to condemn disgusting actions, even when they were harmless. W. I. Miller (1997) suggests that many Westerners may be uncomfortable using disgust as a moral emotion, because it is often at odds with our egalitarian ethos: Disgust puts people down, and it is easily used to condemn people who are obese, are deformed, or have sexual preferences at odds with the majority. It is partly for this reason that Nussbaum (1999) argues that disgust should play little or no role in the legal system or the legislature. She disagrees strongly with Kass's (1997) claim that disgust sometimes embodies "wisdom" about being human that is difficult for us to articulate rationally.

INDIVIDUAL DIFFERENCES IN DISGUST SENSITIVITY

Based on our theorizing about the expansion of disgust, we created a paper-and-pencil measure of individual differences in disgust sensitivity toward seven kinds of elicitors (Haidt et al., 1994). Three were core disgust elicitors (food, animals, and body products), and four were animal-nature disgust elicitors (inappropriate sexuality, envelope violations, death, and poor hygiene). We also included an eighth category of magical thinking across the various kinds of elicitors. The 32-item Disgust Scale (DS) included two true–false and two disgust-rating items for each of these eight categories. The DS has an overall alpha of .84, and it has been shown to predict hands-on disgust-relevant behavior among Americans (Rozin, Haidt, McCauley, Dunlop, & Ashmore, 1999), and Swedes (Björklund & Hursti, 2004), and to predict the behavior of people with obsessive–compulsive symptoms even after other negative affects were controlled for (Olatunji, Lohr, Sawchuck, & Tolin, 2007). It also predicts the degree to which brain regions associated with disgust are activated when subjects look at disgusting pictures in an fMRI scanner (Caseras et al., 2007).

Studies using the DS have consistently found that women score higher than men (Haidt et al., 1994), that disgust sensitivity declines with age in adulthood (Quigley, Sherman, & Sherman, 1996; Fessler & Navarette, 2005), and that it may decline faster for women than for men (Doctoroff & McCauley, 1996). Disgust sensitivity is inversely related to education and socioeconomic status (Doctoroff & McCauley, 1996). Personality correlates of the DS are consistent with disgust's role as an inhibitor of approach and consumption. It correlates positively with scales related to anxiety (e.g., Big Five neuroticism), particularly anxieties related to mortality and bodily concerns (e.g., blood–injection phobia, contamination fears), and it correlates negatively with scales related to sensation seeking and openness to experience. (See Haidt et al., 1994, for a list of articles reporting findings using the DS; see *people.virginia.edu/~jdh6n/disgustscale.html*) for information about the scale itself.

Our goal in creating the DS was not to achieve a high alpha by selecting items that were similar to each other. Rather, it was to create a broad instrument that would allow researchers to look for relationships between subtypes of disgust and various other behaviors and clinical conditions. For example, the sex and death subscales are good predictors of religious obsessions even after fearfulness is controlled (Olatunji, Tolin, Huppert, & Lohr, 2005), as terror management theorists would expect.

It is now clear, however, that our original subscales are not reliably discriminated in psychometric analyses. Rather, the 32 items include just three psychometrically stable factors (Olatunji et al., 2007): core disgust (most of the food, animal, and body product items); animal-reminder disgust (most of the death and envelope violation items), and interpersonal-contamination disgust (items in which the interpersonal nature of the contact is salient). These three subscales have much higher internal consistency (alphas above .70) than the four-item scales of the original DS.

In a series of studies, Olatunji and his collaborators have found that the core and interpersonal-contamination subscales predict clinical conditions, such as the contamination aspects of obsessive–compulsive disorder (OCD) (Olatunji, Williams, Lohr, & Sawchuck, 2005). The animal-reminder scale predicts clinical conditions such as blood–injection–injury fears (Olatunji, Sawchuck, de Jong, & Lohr, 2006).

In recent years, two additional measures of disgust sensitivity have been published. The Disgust Propensity and Sensitivity Scale—Revised (Van Overveld, de Jong, Peters, Cavanagh, & Davey, 2006) offers one subscale that assesses frequency of disgust experiences, and another that assesses the degree to which disgust experiences are upsetting. The Disgust Emotion Scale (Kleinknecht, Kleinknecht, & Thorndike, 1997) offers five subscales to assess disgust toward rotten foods, small animals, injections and blood draws, mutilation and death, and bad smells. The development of these two scales was motivated in part by the low internal reliabilities of the eight DS subscales. A similar concern led to Olatunji et al.'s (2007) modification of the DS to create the 25-item, three-factor DS-R.

DISGUST AND THE BRAIN

Since the early 1990s, there has been a great deal of research on the neural correlates of disgust. A main concern of this research is to identify areas of the brain that are activated by or mediate disgust. An early study (confirmed by some later work) demonstrated that disgust experiences are associated with increased activity in the right frontal cortex, a broad region associated with negative affect (Davidson, 1992). More specific is the finding that people with Huntington's disease, caused by late-onset degeneration of the basal ganglia, show a remarkably specific deficit in identifying disgust facial expressions (Sprengelmeyer et al., 1996; Sprengelmeyer, Rausch, Eysel, & Przuntek, 1998) that may extend to other modalities (e.g., Mitchell, Heims, Neville, & Rickards, 2005). Disgust recognition deficits are also seen in people who have the Huntington genotype, but are still too young to show any of the classical symptoms (Gray, Young, Barker, Curtis, & Gibson, 1997).

A good part of the neuroimaging literature has aimed to establish a link among OCD, disgust, and the basal ganglia or insula (Shapira et al., 2003; Phillips et al., 2000; for a review, see Husted et al., 2006). Dozens of experiments using imaging techniques (principally fMRI), beginning with a study by Phillips et al. (1997; see also Wicker et al., 2003; Wright, He, Shapira, Goodman, & Liu, 2004), have suggested that three interconnected brain areas are characteristically activated when there is exposure to disgust faces, disgust-eliciting images, disgust-related odors, or thoughts about disgusting entities. The areas are the anterior insula, the basal ganglia, and parts of the prefrontal cortex (for a review, see Husted et al., 2006). The evidence for a linkage between the anterior insula and basal ganglia and disgust is confirmed by a demonstration that a patient with damage to both areas showed a selective impairment in both the recognition and experience of disgust (Calder, Keane, Manes, Antoun, & Young, 2000). However, one line of research questions whether insula and basal ganglia activation distinguishes disgust from fear (e.g., Stark et al., 2003; Schienle, Schafer, Stark, Walter, & Vaitl, 2005).

Research on the neural basis of disgust can also provide evidence related to psychological issues. First, the relation between the anterior insula and disgust supports the idea that disgust has particularly strong links to food and eating, since the insula is part of the gustatory cortex and is activated by unpleasant tastes and smells (Rolls, 1994). Second, with regard to the controversy about whether moral disgust is really disgust, Moll et al. (2005) have reported overlap in brain areas activated by core or animal-nature disgust elicitors and by moral disgust elicitors.

DISGUST AND PSYCHOPATHOLOGY

Interest in disgust in relation to psychopathology has increased dramatically since 1990. Davey and his colleagues (Matchett & Davey, 1991; Davey, 1993) provided evidence for a link between disgust and some types of animal phobias, and Power and Dalgleish (1997) proposed links between disgust and many psychopathologies, including depression. A central role for disgust in anxiety disorders (specifically, phobias and OCD; see below) has been described in special issues of the *Journal of Anxiety Disorders* (McKay, 2002) and the *Journal of Behavior Therapy and Experimental Psychiatry* (Olatunji & McKay, 2006), as well as in three review articles (Woody & Teachman, 2000; Berle & Phillips, 2006; Olatunji & Sawchuk, 2005). A plausible linkage between disgust and eating disorders has also been proposed (Quigley et al., 1996; Davey, Buckland, Tantow, & Dallos, 1998; Troop, Treasure, & Serpell, 2002). Furthermore, relations between increased disgust sensitivity and schizophrenia (Schienle et al., 2003) and hypochondriasis (Davey & Bond, 2006) have been reported.

The relations between disgust and two major categories of anxiety disorders—phobias (particularly spider and blood–injury phobia) and OCD—have received most attention. Seven kinds of evidence have been advanced.

First is identification of disgust in the symptoms of the disorder. OCD has an obvious link with disgust, since a common form of OCD involves excessive cleaning and washing based on fears of contamination. Hypersensitivity to disgust (in all or some domains) is one possible account of OCD, as is a potentially separable hypersensitivity to contamination (for reviews, see Berle & Phillips, 2006; Husted et al., 2006; and Olatunji & Sawchuk, 2005). Similarly, phobias often overtly include feelings of disgust (Davey, 1993; Matchett & Davey, 1991; Woody, McLean, & Klassen, 2005; Woody & Teachman, 2000).

Second is correlation of disgust sensitivity with the disorder. For OCD, both the clinically defined disorder and individual differences in OCD tendency have been found to be associated with disgust sensitivity (e.g., Quigley et al., 1996; Rozin, Taylor, Ross, Bennett, & Hejmadi, 2005; Tolin, Woods, & Abramowitz, 2006). Findings are quite consistent, with cleaning OCD more closely related to disgust sensitivity than other forms of OCD (e.g., Mancini, Gragnani, & D'Olimpio, 2001). There are indications that sensitivity to interpersonal contamination and concern with hygiene may be specifically related to cleaning OCD (Olatunji, Williams, Lohr, & Sawchuk, 2005; Tolin et al., 2006). Disgust sensitivity is also generally higher in individuals with small-animal or blood–injury phobias (Tolin, Lohr, Sawchuk, & Lee, 1997; Koch, O'Neill, Sawchuk, & Connolly, 2002), but there is still some question as to whether this is general disgust sensitivity or sensitivity in particular domains (for a review, see Woody & Teachman, 2000). There are also important questions about distinguishing between state and trait disgust (e.g., Woody & Tolin, 2002; Woody et al., 2005) as the principal correlates of phobias.

Third is demonstration that recognition of disgust faces or disgust situations is enhanced or compromised in the disorder. Whereas there are abundant data on disgust face recognition in Huntington's disease (Sprengelmeyer et al., 1996), there are no parallel data for phobias, and there are mixed reports on disgust face recognition in OCD.

Fourth is demonstration of deficits or enhancements in disgust expressions (facial or otherwise). There are no data on this point for OCD, but there is evidence indicating enhanced disgust facial expressions for persons with animal phobias in the presence of phobic elicitors (Lumley & Melamed, 1992; Schienle, Schafer, Walter, Stark, & Vaitl, 2005).

Fifth is demonstration of a parallel psychophysiology in disgust and the disorder in question. The signature physiological sign of disgust, nausea, has not been studied in this context for either phobias or OCD. Fainting, associated with parasympathetic activation, is a frequent feature of blood–injury phobia, and a link between disgust and fainting in blood–injury phobia has been reported (Page, 1994, 2003).

Sixth is demonstration that disgust stimuli activate (or inhibit) brain areas associated with the disorder. Supportive data exist for OCD and disgust: There are signs of an overlap in activated brain areas, with the anterior insula prominently engaged in both (e.g., Shapira et al., 2003; Husted et al., 2006).

Seventh is a more refined analysis that probes whether disgust is a direct cause, a noncausal correlate, an indirect cause, or a consequence of the disorder. In the case of phobias, the issue has largely been whether disgust increases symptoms directly, or increases them indirectly by increasing anxiety. Davey and his colleagues have addressed this issue with normal individuals, showing that while induced anxiety increases disgust, induced disgust does not increase anxiety (Marzillier & Davey, 2005). The same group has shown that experienced disgust causes a negative interpretational bias that may enhance threat perceptions, and that this effect is not fully accounted for by a disgust–anxiety linkage (Davey, Bickerstaffe, & MacDonald, 2006; but see Sawchuk, Meunier, Lohr, & Westendorf, 2002). Davey and Bond (2006) have dissected independent roles for trait anxiety and trait disgust in hypochondriasis and health anxiety. For acquisition of disgust-related phobias, a likely mechanism is evaluative conditioning (Schienle et al., 2001).

The psychopathology literature has understandably focused on above-normal activation of disgust (and other emotions). However, we close this section by noting that very low activation of disgust may generate a highly antisocial person, since disgust is in many respects the emotion of civilization. Scores of nondisordered subjects on the DS correlate negatively with scores on the psychopathy subscale of the Eysenck Personality Questionnaire (Eysenck & Eysenck, 1975); however, it is not known whether persons with true psychopathy score lower than nondisordered individuals on measures of disgust sensitivity (J. Blair, personal communication, February 18, 2007).

THE DELICATE BOUNDARY BETWEEN DISGUST AND PLEASURE

Given that the human body is a repository of disgusting entities, and that we live in a contaminated environment, humans are frequently poised on the edge of potential disgust. While we manage most of the time, by habituation or framing (e.g., Rozin, in press), to ignore the disgust elicitors all around us, there are some situations in which we seek out and enjoy disgust. The powerful negativity of disgust seems perversely to encourage its involvement and enjoyment in at least two domains: humor and romantic attachments.

Disgust plays a significant role in humor, via jokes, cartoons, and casual word play. Disgust stimuli often elicit amusement. Generally, it seems that disgust can be amusing when it is not personally threatening; when a person in formal wear (other than the self) steps in dog feces, it is amusing. Disgust plays a central role in the humor of boys and adolescent males, who use it to tease, to question or confront adult norms, and to establish status within their peer groups (Fine, 1988). Bloom (2004) emphasizes the dignity-destroying aspect of disgust, and sees disgust humor as taking advantage of the fact that the human body is disgusting, at the same time that it abhors disgust and sees itself as at a higher plane of existence. The shift in perspective, from soul to body, is a fertile base for humor.

A number of authors, including S. B. Miller (2004), Fessler and Haley (2006), and ourselves (e.g., Rozin et al., 1995) have emphasized the self-boundary or gateway-guarding function of disgust. A distinct self generally resists mixing of the self's substance with the substance of another. Thus treating the other as self, and enjoying what are usually disgusting interactions such as mouth-to-mouth kissing between lovers, is a way of affirming love and intimacy (W. I. Miller, 1997; Bloom, 2004). As Bloom (2004, p. 180) suggests, "In love, you see the person not as a body, but as a soul."

DISGUST IN INTERGROUP RELATIONS

Recent research in social psychology has given new attention to intergroup emotions in relation to intergroup conflict and intergroup violence, including feelings of disgust toward an enemy or minority group.

Dehumanization is often cited as part of the explanation of particularly horrific forms of intergroup violence, including genocide (Chirot & McCauley, 2006). In a theoretical analysis of dehumanization, Haslam (2006) distinguishes between "animalistic dehumanization," which makes others less human by making them more like animals, and "mechanistic dehumanization," which makes enemies less human by denying them uniquely human emotions and traits and making them more like machines. Haslam suggests that disgust is the emotional reaction associated with animalistic dehumanization, whereas indifference is the reaction to mechanistic dehumanization.

In a related analysis of perception of outgroups, Fiske, Cuddy, Glick, and Xu (2002) followed Brown (1965) in suggesting that social perceptions can be understood in relation to two dimensions: status and solidarity. Groups seen as low in status and dissimilar to one's own group (as welfare mothers were seen by participants in the study by Fiske et al.) tend to be viewed with disgust and contempt. Disgust in relation to low-status and dissimilar outgroups is also implicated in results showing that disgust sensitivity is positively correlated with negative attitudes to foreigners, outgroups, immigrants, and deviant individuals (Faulkner, Schaller, Park, & Duncan, 2004; Hodson & Costello, 2007; Navarette & Fessler, 2006). To some degree, this effect is mediated by fear of infection or contamination (Faulkner et al., 2004; Navarette & Fessler, 2006).

Cottrell and Neuberg (2005) have offered a more complex categorization of perceived threats and associated emotional reactions to these threats. Groups representing physical or moral contaminants (gay men for the participants in this study) elicit disgust, whereas groups representing barriers to desired goals (fundamentalist Christians, for these participants) elicit anger. These studies have in common that group perceptions are analyzed beyond a simple dimension of positive or negative affect to distinguish the different characteristics and different threats associated with different groups. Associated with these different appraisals are different emotional reactions, including feelings of disgust for groups seen as animal-like, low-status, and dissimilar. Disgust may signal a particularly potent threat, the threat of contamination.

CONCLUSION

Darwin and Angyal offered prescient analyses of the emotion of disgust. Despite this early attention to an all-too-common emotional experience, and the accessibility of experimental manipulations of this emotion, empirical investigation of disgust has taken off only since 1990. As a result, there are many unanswered questions. We know little about the evolutionary and ancient history of disgust. It is absent in nonhuman primates, yet extremely frequent and probably universal among contemporary humans. We do not know much about the sequence of events that introduced and expanded disgust over historical time (but see W. I. Miller, 1997, for the most thorough analysis of this expansion for Western cultures). We do not know whether the acceptance of the theory of evolution, and hence of human continuity with animals, played a role in the development or expression of animal nature disgust. We do not know how disgust originates in development;

nor what the principal causes of differences in disgust sensitivity are; nor why it is a focus of humor, especially in children. Many of the fundamental questions posed by Darwin and Angyal remain unanswered.

Our analysis suggests a cultural evolution of disgust that brings it to the heart of what it means to be human. We have suggested that disgust originated as a rejection response to bad tastes, and then evolved into a much more abstract and ideational emotion. In this evolution, the function of disgust shifted: A mechanism for avoiding harm to the body became a mechanism for avoiding harm to the soul. The elicitors of disgust may have expanded to the point where the only thing they have in common is that decent people want nothing to do with them. At this level, disgust becomes a moral emotion and a powerful form of negative socialization. We have presented a skeleton of evidence in support of this analysis, but there are many alternatives and points of difficulty. In our view, because cultures have capitalized on disgust as a way of internalizing some of their particular negative attitudes, there is no overarching abstract definition of the class of disgust elicitors. In the view of Royzman and Sabini (2001), the lack of a single abstract description of disgust elicitors compromises the status of disgust as an emotion. The elicitors of anger and fear, they suggest, are more coherent (i.e., insult and threat appraisals, respectively). Our view is that the appraisal that elicits disgust is indeed more cognitively complex than other emotions. There are multiple appraisals, as we have indicated—some quite abstract, such as reminders of our animal nature. The complexity of disgust reflects the complexity of a species that is both animal and human.

ACKNOWLEDGMENTS

We thank the Whitehall Foundation for supporting some of the research reported in this chapter and the preparation of the original (1993) version of this chapter, and the Edmund J. and Louise W. Kahn Chair for Faculty Excellence Fund for supporting the preparation of this revision.

REFERENCES

Angyal, A. (1941). Disgust and related aversions. *Journal of Abnormal and Social Psychology, 36*, 393–412.

Appadurai, A. (1981). Gastro-politics in Hindu South Asia. *American Ethnologist, 8*, 494–511.

Barnes, D. S. (2006). *The great stink of Paris and the marriage of filth and germs.* Baltimore: Johns Hopkins University Press.

Becker, E. (1973). *The denial of death.* New York: Free Press.

Berle, D., & Phillips, E. S. (2006). Disgust and obsessive–compulsive disorder: An update. *Psychiatry, 69*, 228–238.

Björklund, F., & Hursti, T. (2004). A Swedish translation and validation of the Disgust Scale: A measure of disgust sensitivity. *Scandinavian Journal of Psychology, 45*, 279–284.

Bloom, P. (2004). *Descartes' baby: How the science of child development explains what makes us human.* New York: Basic Books

Brown, R. (1965). *Social psychology.* New York: Free Press.

Calder, A. J., Keane, J., Manes, F., Antoun, N., & Young, A. W. (2000). Impaired recognition and experience of disgust following brain injury. *Nature Neuroscience, 3*, 1077–1088.

Caseras, X., Mataix-Cols, D., An, S. K., Lawrence, N. S., Speckens, A., Giampietro, V., et al. (2007). Sex differences in neural responses to disgusting visual stimuli: Implications for disgust-related psychiatric disorders. *Biological Psychiatry, 62*, 464–471.

Chirot, D., & McCauley, C. (2006). *Why not kill all of them?: The logic and prevention of mass political murder.* Princeton, NJ: Princeton University Press.

Corbin, A. (1986). *The foul and the fragrant: Odor and the French social imagination.* Cambridge, MA: Harvard University Press.

Cottrell, C. A., & Neuberg, S. L. (2005). Different emotional reactions to different groups: A sociofunctional threat-based approach to "prejudice." *Journal of Personality and Social Psychology, 88*, 770–789.

Cox, C. R., Goldenberg, J. L., Pyszczynski, T., & Weise, D. (2007). Disgust, creatureliness and the accessibility of death-related thoughts. *European Journal of Social Psychology, 37*, 494–507.

Curtis, V., Aunger, R., & Rabie, T. (2004). Evidence that disgust evolved to protect from risk of disease. *Proceedings of the Royal Society of London, Series B, 271*(Suppl.), S131–S133.

Curtis, V., & Biran, A. (2001). Dirt, disgust, and disease: Is hygiene in our genes? *Perspectives in Biology and Medicine, 44*, 17–31.

Damasio, A. (2003). *Looking for Spinoza.* Orlando, FL: Harcourt.

Darwin, C. R. (1965). *The expression of the emotions in man and animals.* Chicago: University of Chicago Press. (Original work published 1872)

Davey, G. C. L. (1993). Factors influencing self-rated fear to a novel animal. *Cognition and Emotion, 7*, 461–471.

Davey, G. C. L., Bickerstaffe, S., & MacDonald, B. A. (2006). Experienced disgust causes a negative interpretation bias: A causal role for disgust in anxious psychopathology. *Behaviour Research and Therapy,* *44,* 1375–1384.

Davey, G. C. L., & Bond, N. (2006). Using controlled comparisons in disgust psychopathology research: The case of disgust, hypochondriasis and health anxiety. *Journal of Behavior Therapy and Experimental Psychiatry.* 37, 4–15.

Davey, G. C. L., Buckland, G., Tantow, B., & Dallos, R. (1998). Disgust and eating disorders. *European Eating Disorders Review,* 6, 201–211.

Davey, G. C. L., Cavanagh, K., & Lamb, A. (2003). Differential aversive outcome expectancies for high- and low-predation fear-relevant animals. *Journal of Behavior Therapy and Experimental Psychiatry,* 34, 117–128.

Davey, G. C. L., Forster, L., & Mayhew, G. (1991). Familial resemblance in disgust sensitivity and animal phobias. *Behaviour Research and Therapy,* 31, 41–50.

Davidson, R. J. (1992). Emotion and affective style: Hemispheric substrates. *Psychological Science,* 3, 39–43.

Doctoroff, G., & McCauley, C. (1996, March). *Demographic differences in sensitivity to disgust.* Poster presented at the annual meeting of the Eastern Psychological Association, Philadelphia.

Douglas, M. (1966). *Purity and danger.* London: Routledge & Kegan Paul.

Ekman, P. (1972). Universals and cultural differences in facial expressions of emotion. In J. K. Cole (Ed.), *Nebraska Symposium on Motivation* (Vol. 19, pp. 207–283). Lincoln: University of Nebraska Press.

Ekman, P. (1992). An argument for basic emotions. *Cognition and Emotion,* 6, 169–200.

Ekman, P., & Friesen, W. V. (1975). *Unmasking the face.* Englewood Cliffs, NJ: Prentice Hall.

Ekman, P., & Friesen, W. V. (1978). *Facial Action Coding System: A technique for the measurement of facial movement.* Palo Alto, CA: Consulting Psychologists Press.

Elias, N. (1978). *The history of manners: Vol. 1. The civilizing process* (E. Jephcott, Trans.). New York: Pantheon Books. (Original work published 1939)

Eysenck, H. J., & Eysenck, S. B. G. (1975). *The Eysenck Personality Questionnaire.* London: Hodder & Stoughton.

Fallon, A. E., & Rozin, P. (1983). The psychological bases of food rejections by humans. *Ecology of Food and Nutrition,* 13, 15–26.

Fallon, A. E., Rozin, P., & Pliner, P. (1984). The child's conception of food: The development of food rejections with special reference to disgust and contamination sensitivity. *Child Development,* 55, 566–575.

Faulkner, J., Schaller, M., Park, J. H., & Duncan, L. A. (2004). Evolved disease-avoidance mechanisms and contemporary xenophobic attitudes. *Group Processes and Intergroup Relations,* 7, 333–353.

Ferenczi, S. (1952). The ontogenesis of the interest in money. In S. Ferenczi (Ed.) & E. Jones (Trans.), *First contributions to psychoanalysis* (pp. 319–331). London: Hogarth Press. (Original work published 1914)

Fessler, D. M. T., & Haley, K. J. (2006). Guarding the perimeter: The outside–inside dichotomy in disgust and bodily experience. *Cognition and Emotion,* 20, 3–19.

Fessler, D. M. T., & Navarrete, C. D. (2005). The effect of age on death disgust: A critique of terror management perspectives. *Journal of Evolutionary Psychology,* 3, 279–296.

Fine, G. A. (1988). Good children and dirty play. *Play and Culture,* 1, 43–56.

Fiske, S. T., Cuddy, A. J. C., Glick, P., & Xu, J. (2002). A model of (often mixed) stereotype content: Competence and warmth. *Journal of Personality and Social Psychology,* 82, 878–902.

Flavell, J. (1986). The development of children's knowledge of the appearance–reality distinction. *American Psychologist,* 41, 418–425.

Frazer, J. G. (1922). *The golden bough: A study in magic and religion* (abridged ed., T. H. Gaster, Ed.). New York: Macmillan. (Original work published 1890)

Freud, S. (1953). Three essays on the theory of sexuality. In J. Strachey (Ed. & Trans.), *The standard edition of the complete psychological works of Sigmund Freud* (Vol. 7, pp. 123–231). London: Hogarth Press. (Original work published 1905)

Freud, S. (1957). Five lectures on psychoanalysis. In J. Strachey (Ed. & Trans.), *The standard edition of the complete psychological works of Sigmund Freud* (Vol. 11, pp. 3–56). London: Hogarth Press. (Original work published 1910)

Gallese, V., Keysers, C., & Rizzolatti, G. (2004). A unifying view of the basis of social cognition. *Trends in Cognitive Science,* 8, 398–403.

Goldenberg, J. L., Pyszczynski, T., Greenberg, J., Solomon, S., Kluck, B., & Cornwell, R. (2001). I am not an animal: Mortality salience, disgust, and the denial of human creatureliness. *Journal of Experimental Psychology: General,* 130, 427–435.

Gray, J. M., Young, A. W., Barker, W. A., Curtis, A., & Gibson, D. (1997). Impaired recognition of disgust in Huntington's disease gene carriers. *Brain,* 120, 2029–2038.

Grunfeld, D. I. (1982). *The Jewish dietary laws: Vol. 1. Dietary laws regarding forbidden and permitted foods, with particular reference to meat and meat products* (3rd ed.). London: Soncino Press.

Haidt, J., & Keltner, D. (1999). Culture and facial expression: Open-ended methods find more faces and a gradient of recognition. *Cognition and Emotion,* 13, 225–266.

Haidt, J., Koller, S., & Dias, M. (1993). Affect, culture, and morality, or is it wrong to eat your dog? *Journal of Personality and Social Psychology,* 65, 613–628.

Haidt, J., McCauley, C. R., & Rozin, P. (1994). A scale to measure disgust sensitivity. *Personality and Individual Differences,* 16, 701–713.

Haidt, J., Rozin, P., McCauley, C. R., & Imada, S.

(1997). Body, psyche, and culture: The relationship between disgust and morality. *Psychology and Developing Societies, 9,* 107–131.

Haslam, N. (2006). Dehumanization: An integrative review. *Personality and Social Psychology Review, 10,* 252–264.

Hejmadi, A. (2000). *Rasa or aesthetic emotion: An ancient Hindu perspective.* Unpublished manuscript.

Hejmadi, A., Davidson, R., & Rozin, P. (2000). Exploring Hindu Indian emotion expressions: Evidence for accurate recognition by Americans and Indians. *Psychological Science, 11,* 183–187.

Hejmadi, A., Rozin, P., & Siegal, M. (2004). Once in contact, always in contact: Contagious essence and conceptions of purification in American and Hindu Indian children. *Developmental Psychology, 40,* 467–476.

Hemenover, S. H., & Schimmack, U. (2007). That's disgusting! . . . But very amusing: Mixed feelings of amusement and disgust. *Cognition and Emotion, 21,* 1102–1113.

Hodson, G., & Costello, K. (2007). Interpersonal disgust, ideological orientations and dehumanization as predictors of intergroup attitudes. *Psychological Science, 18,* 691–698.

Howell, N. (1986). Feedbacks and buffers in relation to scarcity and abundance: Studies of hunter–gatherer populations. In R. Scofield (Ed.), *Beyond Malthus* (pp. 156–187). Cambridge, UK: Cambridge University Press.

Husted, D. S., Shapira, N. A., & Goodman, W. K. (2006). The neurocircuitry of obsessive–compulsive disorder and disgust. *Progress in Neuro-Psychopharmacology and Biological Psychiatry, 30,* 389–399.

Izard, C. E. (1971). *The face of emotion.* New York: Appleton-Century-Crofts.

Izard, C. E. (1977). *Human emotions.* New York: Plenum Press.

Jones, E. (1948). Anal–erotic character traits. In E. Jones, *Papers on psychoanalysis* (pp. 413–437). Boston: Beacon Press. (Original work published 1912)

Kass, L. R. (1994). *The hungry soul.* New York: Free Press.

Kass, L. R. (1997, June 2). The wisdom of repugnance. *The New Republic,* pp. 17–26.

Kelly, D. R. (2007). *Towards a cognitive theory of disgust.* Manuscript in preparation.

Kleinknecht, R. A., Kleinknecht, E. A., & Thorndike, R. M. (1997). The role of disgust and fear in blood and injection-related fainting symptoms: A structural equation model. *Behaviour Research and Therapy, 35,* 1075–1087.

Koch, M. D., O'Neill, H. K., Sawchuk, C. N., & Connolly, K. (2002). Domain-specific and generalized disgust sensitivity in blood–injection–injury phobia: The application of behavioral approach/avoidance tasks, *16,* 511–527.

Leach, E. (1964). Anthropological aspects of language: Animal categories and verbal abuse. In E. Lenneberg (Ed.), *New directions in the study of language* (pp. 23–64). Cambridge, MA: MIT Press.

Levenson, R. W. (1992). Autonomic nervous system differences among emotions. *Psychological Science, 3,* 23–27.

Levenson, R. W., Ekman, P., & Friesen, W. V. (1990). Voluntary facial action generates emotion-specific autonomic nervous system activity. *Psychophysiology, 27,* 363–384.

Lumley, M. A., & Melamed, B. G. (1992). Blood phobics and nonphobics: psychological differences and affect during exposure. *Behaviour Research and Therapy, 30,* 425–434.

Malson, L. (1972). *Wolf children* (E. Fawcett, P. Ayrton, & J. White, Trans.). New York: Monthly Review Press. (Original work published 1964)

Mancini, F., Gragnani, A., & D'Olimpio, F. (2001). The connection between disgust and obsessions and compulsions in a non-clinical sample. *Personality and Individual Differences, 31,* 1173–1180.

Marriott, M. (1968). Caste ranking and food transactions: A matrix analysis. In M. Singer & B. S. Cohn (Eds.), *Structure and change in Indian society* (pp. 133–171). Chicago: Aldine.

Martins, Y., & Pliner, P. (2006). "Ugh! That's disgusting!": Identification of the characteristics of foods underlying rejections based on disgust. *Appetite, 46,* 75–85.

Marzillier, S. L., & Davey, G. C. L. (2005). Anxiety and disgust: Evidence for a unidirectional relationship. *Cognition and Emotion, 19,* 729–750.

Masson, J. L., & Patwardhan, M. V. (1970). *Aesthetic rapture: the Rāsadhyāya of the Nāṭyaśāstra.* Poona, India: Deccan College.

Matchett, G., & Davey, G. C. L. (1991). A test of a disease-avoidance model of animal phobias. *Behaviour Research and Therapy, 29,* 91–94.

Mauss, M. (1972). *A general theory of magic* (R. Brain, Trans.). New York: Norton. (Original work published 1902)

Mayr, E. (1960). The emergence of evolutionary novelties. In S. Tax (Ed.), *Evolution after Darwin: Vol. 1. The evolution of life* (pp. 349–380). Chicago: University of Chicago Press.

McKay, D. (2002). Introduction to the special issue: The role of disgust in anxiety disorders. *Journal of Anxiety Disorders, 16,* 475–476.

Meigs, A. S. (1978). A Papuan perspective on pollution. *Man, 13,* 304–318.

Meigs, A. S. (1984). *Food, sex, and pollution: A New Guinea religion.* New Brunswick, NJ: Rutgers University Press.

Miller, S. B. (1986). Disgust: Conceptualization, development, and dynamics. *International Review of Psychoanalysis, 13,* 295–307.

Miller, S. B. (2004). *Disgust: The gatekeeper emotion.* Hillsdale, NJ: Analytic Press.

Miller, W. I. (1997). *The anatomy of disgust.* Cambridge, MA: Harvard University Press.

Mitchell, I. J., Heims, H., Neville, E. A., & Rickards, H. (2005). Huntington's disease patients show impaired perception of disgust in the gustatory and olfactory modalities. *Journal of Neuropsychiatry and Clinical Neurosciences, 17,* 119–121.

Moll, J., deOliveira-Souza, R., Moll, F. T., Ignacio, F. A., Bramati, I. E., Caparelli, D. E. M., et al. (2005). The moral affiliations of disgust: A functional MRI study. *Cognitive and Behavioral Neurology, 8,* 68–78.

Nabi, R. L. (2002). The theoretical versus the lay meaning of disgust: Implications for emotion research. *Cognition and Emotion, 16,* 695–703.

Navarette, C. D., & Fessler, D. M. T. (2006). Disease avoidance and ethnocentrism: The effects of disease vulnerability and disgust sensitivity on intergroup attitudes. *Evolution and Human Behavior, 27,* 270–282.

Nemeroff, C., & Rozin, P. (1989). "You are what you eat": Applying the demand-free "impressions"technique to an unacknowledged belief. *Ethos: The Journal of Psychological Anthropology, 17,* 50–69.

Nemeroff, C., & Rozin, P. (1992). Sympathetic magical beliefs and kosher dietary practice: The interaction of rules and feelings. *Ethos: The Journal of Psychological Anthropology, 20,* 96–115.

Nemeroff, C., & Rozin, P. (1994). The contagion concept in adult thinking in the United States: Transmission of germs and interpersonal influence. *Ethos: The Journal of Psychological Anthropology, 22,* 158–186.

Nemeroff, C., & Rozin, P. (2000). The makings of the magical mind. In K. Rosengren, C. Johnson, & P. Harris (Eds.), *Imagining the impossible: Magical, scientific, and religious thinking in children* (pp. 1–34). New York: Cambridge University Press.

Nussbaum, M. C. (1999). "Secret sewers of vice": Disgust, bodies, and the law. In S. A. Bandes (Ed.), *The passions of law* (pp. 19–62). New York: New York University Press.

Olatunji, B. O., Lohr, J.-M., Sawchuk, C.-N., & Tolin, D.-F. (2007). Multimodal assessment of disgust in contamination-related obsessive–compulsive disorder. *Behaviour Research and Therapy, 45,* 263–276.

Olatunji, B. O., & McKay, D. (2006). Introduction to the special series: Disgust sensitivity in anxiety disorders. *Journal of Behavior Therapy and Experimental Psychiatry, 37,* 1–3.

Olatunji, B. O., & Sawchuk, C. N. (2005). Disgust: Characteristic features, social manifestations, and clinical implications. *Journal of Social and Clinical Psychology, 24,* 932–962.

Olatunji, B. O., Sawchuk, C. N., de Jong, P. J., & Lohr, J. M. (2006). The structural relation between disgust sensitivity and blood–injection–injury fears: A cross-cultural comparison of US and Dutch data. *Journal of Behavior Therapy and Experimental Psychiatry, 37,* 16–29.

Olatunji, B. O., Tolin, D. F., Huppert, J. D., & Lohr, J. M. (2005). The relation between fearfulness, disgust sensitivity and religious obsessions in a non-clinical sample. *Personality and Individual Differences, 38,* 713–722.

Olatunji, B. O., Williams, N. L., Lohr, J. M., & Sawchuk, C. N. (2005). The structure of disgust: Domain specificity in relation to contamination ideation and excessive washing. *Behaviour Research and Therapy, 43,* 1069–1086.

Olatunji, B. O., Williams, N. L., Tolin, D. F., Sawchuck, C. N., Abramowitz, J. S., Lohr, J. M., et al. (2007). The Disgust Scale: Item analysis, factor structure, and suggestions for refinement. *Psychological Assessment, 19,* 281–297.

Ortner, S. B. (1973). Sherpa purity. *American Anthropologist, 75,* 49–63.

Page, A. C. (1994). Blood–injury phobia. *Clinical Psychology Review, 14,* 443–461.

Page, A. C. (2003). The role of disgust in faintness elicited by blood and injection stimuli. *Journal of Anxiety Disorders, 17,* 45–58.

Petó, E. (1936). Contribution to the development of smell feeling. *British Journal of Medical Psychology, 15,* 314–320.

Phillips, M. L., Marks, I. M., Senior, C., Lythgoe, D., O'Dwyer, A. M., Meehan, O., et al. (2000). A differential neural response in obsessive–compulsive disorder patients with washing compared with checking symptoms to disgust. *Psychological Medicine, 30,* 1037–1050.

Phillips, M. L., Young, A. W., Senior, C., Brammer, M., Andrew, C., Williams, S. C. R., et al. (1997). A specific neural substrate for perceiving facial expressions of disgust. *Nature, 389,* 495–498.

Piaget, J., & Inhelder, B. (1974). From conservation to atomism. In J. Piaget & B. Inhelder, *The child's construction of quantities* (pp. 67–116). London: Routledge & Kegan Paul. (Original work published 1941)

Pinker, S. (1997). *How the mind works.* New York: Norton.

Plutchik, R. (1980). *Emotion: A psychoevolutionary synthesis.* New York: Harper & Row.

Power, M., & Dalgleish, T. (1997). *Cognition and emotion: From order to disorder.* Hove, UK: Psychology Press.

Quigley, J. F., Sherman, M., & Sherman, N. (1996, March). *Personality disorder symptoms, gender, and age as predictors of adolescent disgust sensitivity.* Poster presented at the annual meeting of the Eastern Psychological Association, Philadelphia.

Renner, H. D. (1944). *The origin of food habits.* London: Faber & Faber.

Rolls, E. T. (1994). Central taste anatomy and physiology. In R. L. Doty (Ed.), *Handbook of clinical olfaction and gustation* (pp. 549–573). New York: Marcel Dekker.

Rosen, A., & Rozin, P. (1993). Now you see it. . . . Now you don't: The preschool child's conception of invisible particles in the context of dissolving. *Developmental Psychology, 29,* 300–311.

Royzman, E. B., & Sabini, J. (2001). Something it takes to be an emotion: The interesting case of disgust.

Journal for the Theory of Social Behaviour, 31, 29–59.

Rozin, P. (1976). The evolution of intelligence and access to the cognitive unconscious. In J. A. Sprague & A. N. Epstein (Eds.), *Progress in psychobiology and physiological psychology* (Vol. 6, pp. 245–280). New York: Academic Press.

Rozin, P. (1997). Moralization. In A. Brandt & P. Rozin (Eds.), *Morality and health* (pp. 379–401). New York: Routledge.

Rozin, P. (in press). Hedonic "adaptation": Specific adaptation to disgust/death elcicitors as a result of dissecting a cadaver. *Judgment and Decision Making.*

Rozin, P., & Fallon, A. E. (1987). A perspective on disgust. *Psychological Review, 94,* 23–41.

Rozin, P., Fallon, A. E., & Augustoni-Ziskind, M. (1985). The child's conception of food: The development of contamination sensitivity to "disgusting" substances. *Developmental Psychology, 21,* 1075–1079.

Rozin, P., Fallon, A. E., & Mandell, R. (1984). Family resemblance in attitudes to food. *Developmental Psychology, 20,* 309–314.

Rozin, P., Haidt, J., & McCauley, C. R. (1993). Disgust. In M. Lewis & J. M. Haviland (Eds.), *Handbook of emotions* (pp. 575–594). New York: Guilford Press.

Rozin, P., Haidt, J., & McCauley, C. R. (1999). Disgust: The body and soul emotion. In T. Dalgleish & M. Power (Eds.), *Handbook of cognition and emotion* (Pp. 429–445). Chichester, UK: Wiley.

Rozin, P., Haidt, J., & McCauley, C. R. (2000). Disgust. In M. Lewis & J. M. Haviland-Jones (Eds.), *Handbook of emotions* (2nd ed., pp. 637–653). New York: Guilford Press.

Rozin, P., Haidt, J., McCauley, C. R., Dunlop, L., & Ashmore, M. (1999). Individual differences in disgust sensitivity: Comparisons and evaluations of paper-and-pencil versus behavioral measures. *Journal of Research in Personality, 33,* 330–351.

Rozin, P., Haidt, J., McCauley, C. R., & Imada, S. (1997). The cultural evolution of disgust. In H. M. Macbeth (Ed.), *Food preferences and taste: Continuity and change* (pp. 65–82). Oxford: Berghahn.

Rozin, P., Hammer, L., Oster, H., Horowitz, T., & Marmara, V. (1986). The child's conception of food: Differentiation of categories of rejected substances in the 1.4 to 5 year age range. *Appetite, 7,* 141–151.

Rozin, P., Lowery, L., & Ebert, R. (1994). Varieties of disgust faces and the structure of disgust. *Journal of Personality and Social Psychology, 66,* 870–881.

Rozin, P., Lowery, L., Imada, S., & Haidt, J. (1999). The CAD triad hypothesis: A mapping between three moral emotions (contempt, anger, disgust) and three moral codes (community, autonomy, divinity). *Journal of Personality and Social Psychology, 76,* 574–586.

Rozin, P., Markwith, M., & McCauley, C. R. (1994). The nature of aversion to indirect contact with other persons: AIDS aversion as a composite of aversion to strangers, infection, moral taint and misfortune. *Journal of Abnormal Psychology, 103,* 495–504.

Rozin, P., Millman, L., & Nemeroff, C. (1986). Operation of the laws of sympathetic magic in disgust and other domains. *Journal of Personality and Social Psychology, 50,* 703–712.

Rozin, P., & Nemeroff, C. J. (1990). The laws of sympathetic magic: A psychological analysis of similarity and contagion. In J. Stigler, G. Herdt, & R. A. Shweder (Eds.), *Cultural psychology: Essays on comparative human development* (pp. 205–232). Cambridge, UK: Cambridge University Press.

Rozin, P., Nemeroff, C., Horowitz, M., Gordon, B., & Voet, W. (1995). The borders of the self: Contamination sensitivity and potency of the mouth, other apertures and body parts. *Journal of Research in Personality, 29,* 318–340.

Rozin, P., Nemeroff, C., Wane, M., & Sherrod, A. (1989). Operation of the sympathetic magical law of contagion in interpersonal attitudes among Americans. *Bulletin of the Psychonomic Society, 27,* 367–370.

Rozin, P., & Singh, L. (1999). The moralization of cigarette smoking in America. *Journal of Consumer Behavior, 8,* 321–337.

Rozin, P., Taylor, C., Ross, L., Bennett, G., & Hejmadi, A. (2005). General and specific abilities to recognise negative emotions, especially disgust, as portrayed in the face and the body. *Cognition and Emotion, 19,* 397–412.

Rozin, P., & Wolf, S. (2007). *Family resemblance in preferences and values across three generations of Americans.* Manuscript in preparation.

Rozin, P., Wrzesniewski, A., & Byrnes, D. (1998). The elusiveness of evaluative conditioning. *Learning and Motivation, 29,* 397–415.

Sanfey, A. G., Rilling, J. K., Aronson, J. A., Nystrom, L. E., & Cohen, J. D. (2003). The neural basis of economic decision-making in the ultimatum game. *Science, 300,* 1755–1758.

Sawchuk, C. N., Meunier, S. A., Lohr, J. M., & Westendorf, D. H. (2002). Fear, disgust, and information processing in specific phobia: The application of signal detection theory. *Journal of Anxiety Disorders, 16,* 495–510.

Scherer, K. R. (1997). The role of culture in emotion–antecedent appraisal. *Journal of Personality and Social Psychology, 73,* 902–922.

Scherer, K. R., & Wallbott, H. G. (1994). Evidence for universality and cultural variation of differential emotion response patterning. *Journal of Personality and Social Psychology, 66,* 310–328.

Schienle, A., Schafer, A., Stark, R., Walter, B., Franz, M., & Vaitl, D. (2003). Disgust sensitivity in psychiatric disorders: A questionnaire study. *Journal of Nervous and Mental Diseases, 191,* 831–834.

Schienle, A., Schafer, A., Stark, R., Walter, B., & Vaitl, D. (2005). Relationship between disgust sensitivity, trait anxiety and brain activity during disgust induction. *Neuropsychobiology, 51,* 86–92.

Schienle, A., Schafer, A., Walter, B., Stark, R., & Vaitl, D. (2005). Elevated disgust sensitivity in blood phobia. *Cognition and Emotion*, 19, 1229–1241.

Schienle, A., Stark, R., & Vaitl, D. (2001). Evaluative conditioning: A possible explanation for the acquisition of disgust responses? *Learning and Motivation*, 32, 65–83.

Schmidt, H., & Beauchamp, G. (1988). Adult-like odor preferences and aversions in three-year-old children. *Child Development*, 59, 1136–1143.

Senn, M. J. E., & Solnit, A. J. (1968). *Problems in child behavior and development*. Philadelphia: Lea & Febiger.

Shapira, N. A., Liu, Y., He, A. G., Bradley, M. M., Lessig, M. C., James, G. A., et al. (2003). Brain activation by disgust-inducing pictures in obsessive–compulsive disorder. *Biological Psychiatry*, 54, 751–756.

Sherman, G., Haidt, J., & Coan, J. (2007). *Nazis really are disgusting*. Unpublished manuscript, University of Virginia.

Shweder, R. A., Much, N. C., Mahapatra, M., & Park, L. (1997). The "big three" of morality (autonomy, community, divinity), and the "big three" explanations of suffering. In A. Brandt & P. Rozin (Eds.), *Morality and health* (pp. 119–169). New York: Routledge.

Siegal, M. (1988). Children's knowledge of contagion and contamination as causes of illness. *Child Development*, 59, 1353–1359.

Siegal, M., & Share, D. L. (1990). Contamination sensitivity in young children. *Developmental Psychology*, 26, 455–458.

Sprengelmeyer, R., Rausch, M., Eysel, U. T., & Przuntek, H. (1998). Neural structures associated with recognition of facial expressions of basic emotions. *Proceedings of the Royal Society of London, Series B*, 265, 1927–1931.

Sprengelmeyer, R., Young, A. W., Calder, A. J., Karnat, A., Lange, H., Homberg, V., et al. (1996). Loss of disgust: perception of faces and emotions in Huntington's disease. *Brain*, 119, 1647–1665.

Stark, R., Schienle, A., Walter, B., Kirsch, P., Sammer, G., Ott, U., et al. (2003). Hemodynamic responses to fear and disgust-inducing pictures: An fMRI study. *International Journal of Psychophysiology*, 50, 225–234.

Stein, M., Ottenberg, P., & Roulet, N. (1958). A study of the development of olfactory preferences. *Archives of Neurology and Psychiatry*, 80, 264–266.

Steiner, J. E. (1979). Human facial expressions in response to taste and smell stimulation. In H. W. Reese & L. P. Lipsitt (Eds.), *Advances in child development and behavior* (Vol. 13, pp. 257–295). New York: Academic Press.

Tambiah, S. J. (1969). Animals are good to think and good to prohibit. *Ethnology*, 8, 423–459.

Tolin, D. F., Lohr, J. M., Sawchuk, C. M., & Lee, T. C. (1997). Disgust and disgust sensitivity in blood–injection–injury and spider phobia. *Behaviour Research and Therapy*, 35, 949–953.

Tolin, D. F., Woods, C. M., & Abramowitz, J. S. (2006). Disgust sensitivity and obsessive–compulsive symptoms in a non-clinical sample. *Journal of Behavior Therapy and Experimental Psychiatry*, 37, 30–40.

Tomkins, S. S. (1963). *Affect, imagery, consciousness: Vol. 2. The negative affects*. New York: Springer.

Tomkins, S. S. (1982). Affect theory. In P. Ekman (Ed.), *Emotion in the human face* (2nd ed., pp. 353–395). Cambridge, UK: Cambridge University Press.

Troop, N. A., Treasure, J. L., & Serpell, L. (2002). A further exploration of disgust in eating disorders. *European Eating Disorders Review*, 10, 218–226.

Tylor, E. B. (1974). *Primitive culture: Researches into the development of mythology, philosophy, religion, art and custom*. New York: Gordon Press. (Original work published 1871)

Van Overveld, W. J. M., de Jong, P. J., Peters, M. L., Cavanagh, K., & Davey, G. C. L. (2006). Disgust propensity and disgust sensitivity: Separate constructs that are differentially related to specific fears. *Personality and Individual Differences*, 41, 1241–1252.

Ware, J., Jain, K., Burgess, L., & Davey, G. C. L. (1994). Disease-avoidance model: Factor analysis of common animal fears. *Behaviour Research and Therapy*, 32, 57–63.

Webb, K., & Davey, G. C. L. (1993). Disgust sensitivity and fear of animals: effect of exposure to violent or repulsive material. *Anxiety, Coping, and Stress*, 5, 329–335.

Wicker, B., Keysers, C., Plailly, J., Royet, J. P., Gallese, V., & Rizzolatti, G. (2003). Both of us disgusted in my insula: The common neural basis of seeing and feeling disgust. *Neuron*, 40, 655–664.

Wierzbicka, A. (1986). Emotions: Universal or culture-specific? *American Anthropologist*, 88, 584–594.

Wolf, K., Mass, R., Ingenbleek, T., Kiefer, F., Naber, D., & Wiedemann, K. (2005). The facial pattern of disgust, appetence, excited joy and relaxed joy: An improved facial EMG study. *Scandinavian Journal of Psychology*, 46, 403–409.

Woody, S. R., McLean, C., & Klassen, T. (2005). Disgust as a motivator of avoidance of spiders. *Journal of Anxiety Disorders*, 19, 461–475.

Woody, S. R., & Teachman, B. A. (2000). Intersection of disgust and fear: Normative and pathological views. *Clinical Psychology: Science and Practice*, 7, 291–311.

Woody, S. R., & Tolin, D. F. (2002). The relationship between disgust sensitivity and avoidant behavior: Studies of clinical and nonclinical samples. *Journal of Anxiety Disorders*, 16, 543–559.

Wright, P., He, G., Shapira, N. A., Goodman, W. K., & Liu, Y. (2004). Disgust and the insula: fMRI responses to pictures of mutilation and contamination. *NeuroReport*, 15, 2347–2351.

CHAPTER 48

Positive Emotions

BARBARA L. FREDRICKSON and MICHAEL A. COHN

Positive emotions have attracted increased scientific attention in the past decade. They have long been studied as markers of people's overall well-being or happiness (Diener & Seligman, 2004; Kahneman, Kreuger, & Schkade, 2004), but looking at positive emotions as outcomes is just the beginning. In large, well-controlled studies, positive emotions and experiences have been found to predict or contribute to many different life outcomes (Lyubomirsky, King, & Diener, 2005), as well as increased longevity (Danner, Snowdon, & Friesen, 2001; Levy, Slade, & Kunkel, 2002; Moskowitz, 2003; Ostir, Markides, & Black, 2000); improved immune function (Cohen, Doyle, & Turner, 2003); and less pain, impairment, and mortality in people with chronic disease (Gil et al., 2004; Cohen & Pressman, 2006). The "broaden-and-build" theory of positive emotions (Fredrickson, 1998, 2001) encompasses this great variety of empirical results, and this chapter uses this theory as a framework for organizing and interrelating past findings and current questions about positive emotions. Through this synthesis, we hope to explain the central paradox of positive emotions: How is it that fleeting experiences of joy, interest, or love—which can be so easily squelched or dismissed—produce lasting gains in strengths and well-being?

OUTLINE OF THE CHAPTER

We begin the chapter with a general definition of positive emotions and discuss some of the issues involved in studying them. We then briefly lay out our broaden-and-build theory, which we use as a framework for organizing research on positive emotions throughout the chapter. The broaden-and-build theory begins with the immediate effects of positive emotions, which serve to broaden attention, cognition, and behavioral repertoires. These lead to the long-term effects of frequent positive emotions, which serve to build resources that make lasting contributions to survival, health, and happiness. Finally, we take stock of what is known about positive emotions, what questions remain, and how the study of positive emotions can contribute to the field of positive psychology more generally.

DEFINING POSITIVE EMOTIONS

The theories of emotions that dominated psychology for most of its history proved fruitful for studying negative emotions, but were often unsuitable for the study of positive emotions (Fredrickson, 1998). In the past 10 years, positive emotions have come into their own. The renaissance in positive emotions research stems from two sources: a growing interest in the psychology of the "good life" (Ryff & Singer, 1998; Fredrickson, 1998; Csikszentmihalyi & Csikszentmihalyi, 2006); and several research programs that have sought to build an empirical, bottom-up model of positive emotions, rather than shoehorning them into older models that were constructed primarily for the negative emotions. Below we review these findings—refining what makes an emotion or other state "positive," determining what differentiates a positive emotion from other pleasant affective states, and investigating some of the challenges unique to the study of positive emotions.

Positive Emotions versus Other Positive Affective States

The distinctions between positive emotions and other closely related affective states, such as sensory pleasure and positive mood, have often been blurry. Although working definitions of emotions vary somewhat across researchers, a consensus is emerging that emotions (both positive and negative) are best conceptualized as multicomponent response tendencies—incorporating muscle tension, hormone release, cardiovascular changes, facial expression, attention, and cognition, among other changes—that unfold over a relatively short time span. Typically, emotions begin with an individual's assessment of the personal meaning of some antecedent event—what Lazarus (1991) called the "person–environment relationship" or "adaptational encounter." Either conscious or unconscious, this appraisal process triggers a cascade of responses incorporating mental, physical, and subjective changes.

Sensory pleasure includes such experiences as sexual gratification, satiation of hunger or thirst, and the remedying of unpleasant states (e.g., cold, pain, or excessive noise). Cabanac (1971) suggested that sensory pleasure arises whenever a stimulus "corrects an internal trouble" (e.g., cooling down when overheated, eating when hungry). Sensory pleasure shares with positive emotions a pleasant subjective feel and may include physiological changes, but an emotion also requires an appraisal of some stimulus or an assessment of its meaning. Emotion and sensation often co-occur: A good meal satisfies hunger, and can also lead to feelings of contentment; sex provides pleasant sensations, and may also lead to gratitude or love toward one's partner. Positive emotions can also occur without a physical stimulus (e.g., joy at receiving good news, or interest in a new idea). Berridge (Berridge & Robinson, 2003, Peciña, Smith, & Berridge, 2006) finds evidence for perhaps a similar distinction at the neurological level: Positive affect includes a passive "liking" component, mediated by opioid receptors, and a motivational "wanting" component, mediated by dopamine.

Positive emotions also resemble positive moods. Yet emotions differ from moods, in that emotions are *about* some personally meaningful circumstance (i.e., they have an object), are typically short-lived, and occupy the foreground of consciousness. In contrast, moods are typically free-floating or objectless, are more long-lasting, and occupy the background of consciousness (Oatley & Jenkins, 1996; Rosenberg, 1998). These distinctions between emotions and moods, however, are made more often at theoretical than at empirical levels. In research practice, virtually identical techniques are used for inducing positive moods and positive emotions (e.g., giving gifts, viewing comedies). Many experimental techniques involve presenting a positive stimulus in order to lead a participant to respond to an unrelated task with a generally positive mindset. In this case, multiple forms of positive mood or emotion may lead to the same results. However, research on the tendencies linked to specific emotions (e.g., gratitude, pride, awe), or on positive states with more specific meaning (e.g., optimism, confidence, enjoyment), requires a more careful distinction between mood and emotion.

Links to Urges to Approach or Continue

Most commonly, the function common to all positive emotions has been conceptualized as facilitating approach behavior (Cacioppo,

Priester, & Berntson, 1993; Davidson, 1993; Frijda, 1994) or continued action (Carver & Scheier, 1990; Clore, 1994). From this perspective, experiences of positive emotions prompt individuals to engage with their environments and take part in activities, many of which are evolutionarily adaptive for the individuals, their species, or both. This link between positive emotions and activity engagement provides an explanation for the often-documented "positivity offset," or the tendency for individuals to experience mild positive affect frequently, even in neutral contexts (Diener & Diener, 1996; Ito & Cacioppo, 1999). Without such an offset, individuals most often would be unmotivated to engage with their environments. Yet with such an offset, individuals exhibit the adaptive bias to approach and explore novel objects, people, or situations.

However, other positive affective states share these effects. Sensory pleasure, for instance, motivates people to approach and continue consuming whatever stimulus is (or appears) biologically useful at the moment (Cabanac, 1971). Free-floating positive moods motivate people to continue along any line of thinking or action that they have initiated (Clore, 1994). Thus the approach model can be seen as a lowest common denominator underlying subjectively pleasant states, but it is not sufficient to define or capture the effects of the class of positive emotions. Furthermore, positive emotions such as relief can be conceptualized as approaching a desired state by avoiding an undesired one, but "approach" is by itself a poor description of the associated elicitors or behavioral tendencies. Clearly, positive emotions can arise from a variety of approach- and avoidance-related situations.

Core Appraisal Dimensions

Theorists differ as to whether emotions are best modeled as points on a two-dimensional plane (Russell, Weiss, & Mendelson, 1989), points in a higher-dimensional space (Smith & Ellsworth, 1985), or separately evolved modules (Tooby & Cosmides, Chapter 8, this volume). However, there is general agreement that a primary characteristic of every emotion is valence on a bipolar continuum from highly unpleasant to highly pleasant (reviewed in Smith & Ellsworth, 1985). Indeed, this pleasantness rating may be one of the earliest determinations we make when processing sensory input

from our environment (Chen & Bargh, 1999). An appraisal of pleasantness can arise when a stimulus fulfills a biological need (e.g., Cabanac, 1971), when it contributes to a personally relevant goal, or when it remedies a noxious or goal-inconsistent state. Others have argued that an appraisal of pleasantness is based on a favorable comparison between our actual rate of goal attainment and our expected rate (Carver, 2003). This distinction may relate to the distinction between sensations and emotions: Anything that we recognize as progress toward a goal should elicit an immediately pleasant response, but when appraised in the context of our expectations or other considerations, it may or may not give rise to a pleasant (positive) emotion.

The pleasantness dimension of emotions is separate from and orthogonal to other aspects of emotional experience. Consider, for example, the emotions of joy (high arousal) versus contentment (low arousal), or gratitude (low personal control) versus pride (high control). Past emotion measures have often conflated pleasantness with either high arousal or high personal control, even though pleasant emotions can span the range of these dimensions. For example, one prominent scale, the Positive and Negative Activation Schedule[1] (PANAS; Watson, Wiese, Vaidya, & Tellegen, 1999), deliberately focuses on high-arousal positive emotions for psychometric reasons. This PANAS has been effective in the past, perhaps because different positive emotions tend to correlate, or because Americans tend to value high-arousal positive emotions more highly than low-arousal ones (Tsai, Knutson, & Fung, 2006). There are two reasons to favor measures with greater distinction between positive emotions. First, the fact that different positive emotions co-occur does not mean that do not have distinct effects. Low-arousal positive emotions are likely to have different thought–action tendencies from high-arousal ones, and ignoring these emotions impedes our ability to make specific predictions about emotions and behavior. Second, looking at only a subset of positive emotions can tell us whether a person is generally having a positive experience, but it is less helpful in quantitatively measuring the person's level of positive emotion. Increasing evidence suggests that a person's ratio of positive to negative emotions is an important predictor of psychological and social outcomes (Fredrickson & Losada, 2005; Gottman, 1994).

These quantitative measures are best assembled when the participant rates a more inclusive set of positive emotions. Therefore, positive emotion measures perhaps work best when they cast the widest possible net.

Additional Appraisal Dimensions

Appraisal-based emotion theories have generally found that positive emotions are less cognitively distinct than negative ones (Smith & Ellsworth, 1985; Ellsworth & Smith, 1988; Fredrickson & Branigan, 2001). This dovetails with experience-sampling research showing that experiences of various positive emotions covary more strongly than experiences of negative emotions (i.e., people are more likely to feel multiple positive emotions at one time than multiple negative ones; Barrett, Gross, Christensen, & Benvenuto, 2001). Because negative emotions are adapted for specific, survival-critical situations (see the description of the broaden-and-build theory later in this chapter), it is plausible that negative situations would evoke only one emotion, or a closely related cluster. Positive emotions initiate a broader range of thoughts and actions, so it is more likely that—for example—an experience of contentment could lead to thoughts about new challenges to take on, leading quickly to experiences of pride or excitement.

However, there is also evidence that our past research methods have been restrictive. Tong (2007) proposed new appraisal dimensions based on research on individual positive emotions, and found evidence of several higher-order dimensions—each associated with several discrete positive emotions—that made the positive emotions appear just as distinct from one another as the negative emotions. Whereas the negative emotions seem to be differentiated from each other by appraisals of threat, personal responsibility, and self-efficacy, the positive emotions require additional dimensions, such as interpersonal relationship, mastery, and spiritual experience. Similarly, Shiota, Keltner, and John (2006) found that the Big Five personality traits predict dispositions toward different positive emotions, beyond the well-documented association between extraversion and positive affect more generally. Thus recent results suggest that the antecedents, effects, and subjective dimensions of such emotions as contentment, compassion, and amusement are just as different as those of any negative emotions. Finally, individuals show different levels of

ability in noting fine distinctions between emotions (lexithymia), with higher levels predicting lower correlations among the experiences of different positive emotions (Tugade, Fredrickson, & Barrett, 2004).

ISSUES IN THE STUDY OF POSITIVE EMOTIONS

Qualitatively Distinct from Negative Emotions

Historically, emotion research has focused on negative emotions. The most general reason is that psychology as a whole tends to focus on understanding and ameliorating psychological problems (Seligman & Csikszentmihalyi, 2000). Negative emotions—when extreme, prolonged, or contextually inappropriate—are implicated in many grave problems, including anxiety disorders, aggression and violence, eating disorders and self-injury, and depression and suicide. Medicine and health psychology have also focused on negative emotions, which contribute to problems ranging from sexual dysfunction to life-threatening immune disorders (Kiecolt-Glaser, McGuire, Robles, & Glaser, 2002). Although positive emotions can contribute to problems (e.g., mania, drug addiction), negative emotions are more prominent in psychopathology and thus have captured the majority of research attention. Studies of positive functioning and strengths have only recently begun to catch up, concomitantly raising interest in the contributions of positive emotions. We also argue later in the chapter that even the study of pathology has been hindered by overlooking positive emotions, which play a critical role in recovering from adversity and developing compensatory strengths.

The study of positive emotions has also suffered from the long-running effort to create a single, general theory of emotion. Such models are typically built with the more attention-grabbing negative emotions (e.g., fear and anger) as prototypes, with positive emotions squeezed in later. For instance, many theories of emotions associate each emotion with a *specific action tendency* (Frijda, 1986; Frijda, Kuipers, & Schure, 1989; Lazarus, 1991; Levenson, 1994; Oatley & Jenkins, 1996; Tooby & Cosmides, 1990). Fear, for example, is linked with the urge to escape, anger with the urge to attack, disgust with the urge to expel, and so on. No theorist argues that these are irresistible compulsions, but rather that people's ideas about possible courses of action narrow in on a specific set of behavioral options. Often the specific action tendency is linked to the emotion's evolutionary adaptive value. Its action tendencies are presumed to incline people toward behaviors that helped get early humans out of life-or-death situations. Another key idea is that specific action tendencies and physiological changes go hand in hand: For example, when you feel fear your thoughts will tend toward escape, and your autonomic nervous system will change in ways that would help you run or climb.

Although specific action tendencies were invoked to describe the form and function of positive emotions as well, these tendencies were notably vague and underspecified (Fredrickson & Levenson, 1998). Joy, for instance, was linked with aimless activation, interest with attending, and contentment with inactivity (Frijda, 1986). These tendencies seem far too general to be called specific; nor do they present the same obvious adaptive value as negative emotions' action tendencies (Fredrickson, 1998). Although a few theorists noted that fitting positive emotions into emotion-general models posed problems (Ekman, 1992; Lazarus, 1991), this acknowledgment was not accompanied by any new or revised models to better accommodate the positive emotions. Instead, the difficulty of shoehorning the positive emotions into emotion-general models merely tended to marginalize them further. The prevailing models were successful for studying the negative emotions, so researchers pursued that work and often neglected the positive emotions—either because it was more difficult to make progress, or because the positive emotions challenged the validity of the model.

Challenging to Measure and Evoke

Another reason why positive emotions may have been featured in less past research is simply that they are harder to study. Negative emotions, as we have discussed, lead to a focus on a single, clear action tendency. In the lab, this translates into clear, reliable results. The results of positive emotions are more diffuse and generally less urgent, making them more difficult to operationalize or observe.

Empirical evidence from many areas of psychology (Baumeister, Bratslavsky, Finkenauer, & Vohs, 2001; Rozin & Royzman, 2001; Cacioppo, Gardner, & Berntson, 1999) and

economics (Tversky & Kahneman, 1981) suggests that negative emotions command more attention than positive ones, and that negative events evoke a stronger response than positive events of the same magnitude. The observed health effects of prolonged negative emotions also contribute to the impression that negative emotions are more significant. In addition, psychologists have a wide range of established protocols for evoking fear, disgust, and anger, but fewer for evoking joy, contentment, or love.

Thus scientists who wish to study positive emotions face procedural difficulties, less obvious dependent variables, and smaller effect sizes. However, this should not be taken to mean that positive emotions are less important! Negative emotions appear strongly in the moment because they were sculpted by evolution to mobilize immediate action; positive emotions exert their power over the long term, and are critical to building a healthy and fruitful life (Fredrickson & Losada, 2005; Lyubomirsky et al., 2005). We will return to this asymmetry repeatedly: Negative emotions help us respond to a single, immediate threat; positive emotions help us take advantage of life's numerous opportunities.

Widely, but Not Universally, Appropriate

Some critics have suggested that researchers who study the benefits of positive emotions pathologize negative emotions, ignore situations where feeling good is inappropriate, or tacitly endorse an unsophisticated hedonism or a Pollyanna-like disregard for life's difficulties (Lazarus, 2003; see also Fineman, 2006). We recognize the critical role of negative emotions and their associated physiological responses in dealing with threatening situations, as well as in appropriately marking the emotional importance of serious losses. We also acknowledge that extremes of positive emotion can be disruptive, especially in high-performance states, which are often marked by an overall lack of self-focus (Csikszentmihalyi, 1990).

The emerging picture is not that people should experience high levels of positive emotion at all times and in all situations, or that positive emotions are a panacea for all of life's challenges. Rather, it appears beneficial for people to cultivate positive emotions as a general backdrop to their emotional lives, while still responding positively or negatively to emotionally meaningful events as they occur. It may also be natural: Recall the evidence for a pervasive and cross-cultural "positivity offset" (Diener & Diener, 1996; Ito & Cacioppo, 1999), suggesting that people usually feel a little better than neutral. This is appropriate if they are usually in a position to amass resources, rather than responding to an immediate threat. Negative emotions help people achieve survival and short-term material ends, while positive emotions help them build toward a more widely construed "good life" (Ryff & Singer, 1998; Keyes & Haidt, 2003).

THE BROADEN-AND-BUILD THEORY OF POSITIVE EMOTIONS

The broaden-and-build theory (Fredrickson, 1998) arose from a desire to move beyond negative-emotion-based models of emotion, and capture the unique effects of positive emotions. Fredrickson's broaden-and-build theory of positive emotions holds that positive emotions *broaden* people's momentary thought–action repertoires and lead to actions that *build* enduring personal resources (Fredrickson, 1998, 2001).

The specific action tendencies described by traditional models are appropriate descriptions of the function of negative emotions: They are the outcomes of thought–action repertoires that *narrow* individuals' urges and perceived affordances so that they are likely to act in a specific way (e.g., escape, attack, expel). In a life-threatening situation, a narrowed thought–action repertoire promotes quick and decisive action that carries direct and immediate benefit.[2] The various negative emotions available to humans comprise the thought–action repertoires that worked best to save their ancestors' lives and limbs (or genes) in similar situations.

Positive emotions, in contrast, seldom occur in response to life-threatening situations. Thus there is less need for them to evoke specific, focused response tendencies. Instead, positive emotions lead to *broadened* and *more flexible* response tendencies, widening the array of the thoughts and actions that come to mind (Fredrickson, 1998). Joy, for instance, creates the urge to play, push the limits, and be creative—urges evident not only in social and physical behavior, but also in intellectual and artistic behavior. Interest, a phenomenologically distinct positive emotion, creates the urge to explore, take in new information and experi-

ences, and expand the self in the process. Contentment, a third distinct positive emotion, creates the urge to sit back and savor current life circumstances, and to integrate these circumstances into new views of self and of the world. And love—which we view as an amalgam of distinct positive emotions (e.g., joy, interest, and contentment) experienced within contexts of safe, close relationships—creates recurring cycles of urges to play with, explore, and savor loved ones. The appraisal dimensions that are unique to positive emotions, such as interpersonal relationship, mastery, and spirituality (Tong, 2007), can also be seen as different domains in which various thought–action tendencies (to play, to explore, or to savor and integrate) broaden habitual modes of thinking or acting.

In contrast to negative emotions, which were shaped by evolution to provide direct and immediate adaptive benefits when survival is threatened, the broadened thought–action repertoires triggered by positive emotions evolved because of their indirect and long-term adaptive benefits. Broadening *builds* enduring personal resources.

Take play as an example. Specific forms of chasing play evident in juveniles of a species—such as running into a flexible sapling or branch and catapulting oneself in an unexpected direction—are reenacted in adults of that species exclusively during predator avoidance (Dolhinow, 1987). Such correspondences between juvenile play maneuvers and adult survival maneuvers suggest that juvenile play builds enduring physical resources (Boulton & Smith, 1992; Caro, 1988). Social play also builds enduring social resources. Laughter appears to function as a social signal of openness to new, friendly interactions (broadening), which can lead to lasting social bonds and attachments (building; Gervais & Wilson, 2005). Shared amusement and smiles have many of the same effects (Lee, 1983; Simons, McCluskey-Fawcett, & Papini, 1986; Keltner & Bonanno, 1997). Childhood play also builds enduring intellectual resources, by increasing levels of creativity (Sherrod & Singer, 1989) and fueling brain development (Panksepp, 1998). Similarly, the exploration prompted by the positive emotion of interest creates knowledge and intellectual complexity, and the savoring prompted by contentment produces self-insight and alters world views. So these phenomenologically distinct positive emotions all share the feature of augmenting individuals' personal resources, ranging from physical and social resources to intellectual and psychological ones (for more detailed reviews, see Fredrickson, 1998, 2001; Fredrickson & Branigan, 2001).

Importantly, the personal resources accrued during states of positive emotions are durable. They outlast the transient emotional states that led to their acquisition. These resources can be drawn on in subsequent moments and in different emotional states. So through experiences of positive emotions, people *transform* themselves—becoming more creative, knowledgeable, resilient, socially integrated, and healthy individuals. Figure 48.1 represents these three sequential effects of positive emotions (broadening, building, transforming). It also suggests that initial experiences of positive emotions produce upward spirals toward further experiences of positive emotions—a point we have begun to investigate empirically (Fredrickson & Joiner, 2002; see the following section for more details).

In short, the broaden-and-build theory describes the form of positive emotions in terms of broadened thought–action repertoires, and describes their function in terms of building enduring personal resources. The theory explains the evolved adaptive significance of

positive emotions. Those of our ancestors who succumbed to the urges sparked by positive emotions—to play, explore, and so on—would have by consequence accrued more personal resources. When these same ancestors later faced inevitable threats to life and limb, their greater personal resources would have translated into greater odds of survival, and in turn greater odds of living long enough to reproduce. To the extent that the capacity to experience positive emotions is innate and heritable, natural selection would have driven it to become a basic trait shared by our entire species (for early evidence that the broaden effect of positive emotions is indeed cross-cultural, see Waugh, Hejmadi, Otake, & Fredrickson, 2006).

SHORT-TERM AND LONG-TERM EFFECTS OF POSITIVE EMOTIONS

Our empirical investigation of the broaden-and-build theory has rested on two hypotheses: the "broaden hypothesis," which targets the ways people change while experiencing a positive emotion, and the "build hypothesis," which targets the lasting changes that follow repeated positive emotional experiences over time.

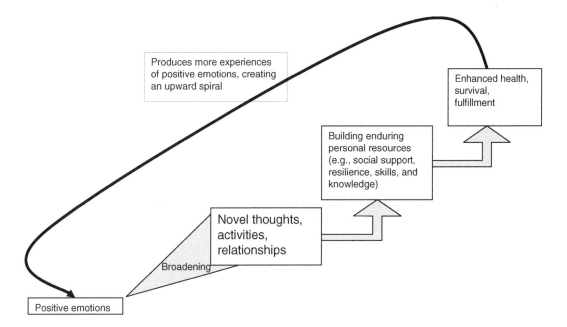

FIGURE 48.1. The broaden-and-build theory of positive emotions.

The Broaden Hypothesis

The first central claim of the broaden-and-build theory is that experiences of positive emotions broaden a person's momentary thought–action repertoire. We call this the "broaden hypothesis," and have found evidence for it across a range of domains, from visual attention to self-construal and social group perception.

Visual Attention

The most cognitively basic form of broadening we have examined appears in global–local visual processing tasks. Participants are asked to make a choice about a figure that can be judged on the basis of either its global, overall shape or its local detail elements (see Figure 48.2a for an example). Positive emotions, with their broadened focus, produce a preference for the global level, whereas negative emotions often produce a preference for the details. This pattern holds both for emotionally relevant traits like optimism and anxiety (Basso, Schefft, Ris, & Dember, 1996), and for emotional states induced through a variety of means (Brandt, Derryberry, & Reed, 1992, cited in Derryberry & Tucker, 1994; Fredrickson & Branigan, 2005; Johnson & Fredrickson, 2005). Wadlinger and Isacowitz (2006) tracked participants' eye movements, and found that induced positive emotion broadened visual search patterns, leading to increased attention to peripheral stimuli.

Our lab's work with the global–local visual processing paradigm was the first to introduce a neutral control condition, and to demonstrate that positive emotions broaden attention relative to a nonemotional baseline (Fredrickson & Branigan, 2005). We also tested distinct emotions in each valence type (e.g., contentment and joy; anxiety and anger), to build the case that the broaden effect was linked to positive emotions in general, and not to arousal level or another specific property of the emotions tested.

Cognition and Behavior

Emotions affect both the focus and the process of cognition, and many long-standing findings on the effects of positive affect on cognition and behavior are consistent with the broaden hypothesis. For instance, Isen and colleagues tested the effects of positive states on a wide range of cognitive outcomes, ranging from creativity puzzles to simulations of complex, life-or-death work situations (Estrada, Isen, & Young, 1997). Their work demonstrates that positive emotions produce patterns of thought that are notably unusual (Isen, Johnson, Mertz, & Robinson, 1985), flexible and inclusive (Isen & Daubman, 1984), creative (Isen, Daubman, & Nowicki, 1987), and receptive to new information (Estrada et al., 1997). Confirming an interpretation of these results in terms of the broaden effect, Rowe, Hirsch, and Anderson (2007) replicated Isen et al.'s (1987) findings of improved performance on the verbal Remote Associates Test (Figure 48.2b), and found that this improvement was correlated with *decreased* performance on a visual task that required participants to ignore peripheral cues (i.e., a task that required attentional narrowing).

In the domain of more personally relevant behavior, we (Fredrickson & Branigan, 2005) induced positive, negative, or no emotions, and asked participants to step away from the specifics of the induction and list all the things they felt like doing. Participants induced to feel positive emotions listed *more* and *more varied* potential actions, relative to the neutral group; participants induced to feel negative emotions listed fewer potential actions than the neutral group. Similar research has shown that positive emotions produce more creative (Isen et al., 1987) and variable (Kahn & Isen, 1993) actions. (See also Isen, Chapter 34, this volume.)

Another perspective on positive affect and cognition comes from the mood-as-information theorists. Their view resembles the broaden hypothesis in suggesting that positive emotions lead to creative, unusual, or integrative thinking, but it differs in predicting a concomitant reduction in attention to detail and negative feedback, sometimes leading to an overreliance on heuristics or stereotypes. There is substantial empirical support for this view (for a review, see the volume by Martin & Clore, 2001). However, other work suggests that people in positive emotional states are *more* likely to incorporate challenging evidence (Trope & Pomerantz, 1998) and carefully consider difficult problems (for reviews, see Aspinwall, 1998, and Abele, 1992; see also the work by Isen et al. cited above).

It is unlikely that either of these bodies of evidence is entirely spurious, or that either the mood-as-information or the mood-as-resource model will be entirely disproven by future evi-

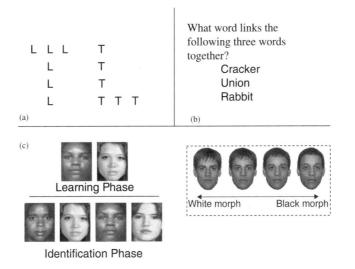

FIGURE 48.2. Three forms of broadened attention. (a) The participant is instructed to find the letter T as quickly as possible. It is present in both figures, but finding the first is facilitated by a broadened visual focus, while finding the second is facilitated by a narrowed (detail-oriented) focus (Johnson, 2005; Fredrickson & Branigan, 2005). (b) In this item from the Remote Associates Test, the participant is asked to find a word that ties the three stimulus words together. Participants are more likely to find the answer ("jack") when experiencing a positive emotion (Isen, Daubman, & Nowicki, 1987). (c) White individuals are typically *poor* at distinguishing one black face from another (solid box) and *good* at determining where a morphed series crosses from "more white" to "more black." Positive emotions improve face recognition (Johnson & Fredrickson, 2005) and impair racial categorization (Johnson, 2005).

dence. The broaden-and-build model as it currently stands is not specific enough to offer a priori guidance: The general term "broadening" could apply to either vague, heuristic thinking or thorough, nondefensive exploration, and little has been done to reconcile these opposing interpretations. What work there is suggests that *flexibility* and *openness* are important attributes of positive emotions' cognitive effects (Dreisbach & Goschke, 2004; Bless et al., 1996). Properties of the particular situation may well determine whether these attributes are beneficial or harmful. We are continuing this work, considering variables such as method of emotion induction, level of intrinsic motivation, social and personal relevance, and amount of mental set switching involved, to determine when the thought–action tendencies associated with positive emotions are beneficial to problem solving and when they are detrimental.

Social Cognition

Broadening in the social domain takes the form of enhanced attention to others and reduced distinctions between self and other, or between different groups. Participants experiencing pos-

itive emotions report more overlap between their concept of themselves and their concept of their best friend (Waugh & Fredrickson, 2006; Waugh et al., 2006), and they become more imaginative and attentive regarding things they could do for friends, relative to things friends could do for them (Otake, Waugh, & Fredrickson, 2007). When a close relationship does not yet exist, induced positive emotions can increase trust (Dunn & Schweitzer, 2005), and may underlie the creation of a wide variety of bonds and interdependence opportunities (Cohn & Fredrickson, 2006; Gable, Reis, Impett, & Asher, 2004).

Positive emotions also broaden social group concepts and break down an essentialized sense of "us versus them" (Dovidio, Gaertner, Isen, Rust, & Guerra, 1995). We have discovered the same result in a racial context: When we induce positive emotions in participants, people become better at remembering the faces of individuals of other races,[3] and simultaneously *worse* at perceiving physical differences between races (Figure 48.2c) (Johnson, 2005; Johnson & Fredrickson, 2005).

The studies we have discussed demonstrate variety in the broaden effect, but more importantly, the outcomes they involve can make a substantive difference in how people act. These changes can then lead to differences in their circumstances, abilities, resources, and relationships in the future. In other words, these *broadened* mindsets can lead people to *build* enduring resources.

The Build Hypothesis

The second central claim of the broaden-and-build theory is that *temporary and transient* experiences of positive emotions, by encouraging a broadened range of actions, over time build *enduring* personal resources. It is now established that positive emotions function as causes, results, and concomitants of success in life. A large meta-analysis by Lyubomirsky et al. (2005) reviews the links between positive affect and outcomes ranging from satisfaction at work and in relationships, to physical health and effective problem solving. We refer interested readers to their excellent review for specifics. In this section we review a selection of research that helps fill in the missing pieces necessary to test our overarching model: that positive emotions lead to broader thought–action repertoires, and that these broadened mindsets enable people to build resources over time.

Correlational and experimental studies of humans and animals help us link positive traits, positive states, and behaviors linked with positive states (e.g., play) to increases in physical, intellectual, and social resources. As previously mentioned, ethologists who have observed nonhuman mammals have associated juvenile play with the development of specific survival maneuvers evident in both predator avoidance and aggressive fighting (Boulton & Smith, 1992; Caro, 1988), suggesting that play builds enduring physical resources. In laboratory experiments, rats deprived of juvenile social play were slower to learn a complex motor task than nondeprived controls were (Einon, Morgan, & Kibbler, 1978).

Evidence suggesting that positive emotions build intellectual resources can be drawn from studies on individual differences in attachment styles. Securely attached children—those who experience the most consistent caregiver love—are more persistent, flexible, and resourceful problem solvers than their peers (Arend, Gove, & Sroufe, 1979; Matas, Arend, & Sroufe, 1978). They also engage in more independent exploration of novel places, and, as a consequence, develop superior cognitive maps of those spaces (Hazen & Durrett, 1982). The intellectual resources associated with secure attachment also appear to last into adulthood. Securely attached adults are more curious and open to information than their insecurely attached peers (Mikulincer, 1997). Experiments with children ranging from preschool to high school age reinforce the claim that positive emotions build intellectual resources by showing that induced positive states—in comparison to neutral and negative states—produce faster learning and improved intellectual performance (Bryan & Bryan, 1991; Bryan, Mathur, & Sullivan, 1996; Masters, Barden, & Ford, 1979). Finally, correlational studies with both humans and nonhuman mammals suggest that social play builds enduring social relationships (Boulton & Smith, 1992; Lee, 1983; Martineau, 1972). Research from our lab has shown that positive emotions, experienced over the course of a month, predict whether a new acquaintance becomes a friend (Waugh & Fredrickson, 2006). Mutually supportive social relationships in turn predict longevity (Brown, Nesse, & Vinokur, 2003), and in times of need they can directly influence survival.

In a direct test of the build hypothesis, we randomly assigned working adults to an intervention to increase daily experiences of positive emotions over the course of 8 weeks. Participants in the experimental group were trained in loving-kindness meditation—a practice that is similar to mindfulness meditation (Davidson et al., 2003; Kabat-Zinn, 2005), but that focuses on deliberately generating broadened mindsets and the positive emotions of compassion and love. They were compared to those assigned to a wait list for the same meditation workshop. All participants in this study reported daily on their experience of several discrete positive and negative emotions, and filled out pre- and postintervention batteries to assess psychological, social, mental, and physical resources, plus their life satisfaction.

After 3 weeks of practice, participants in the meditation group began experiencing higher daily levels of various positive emotions than those in the wait-list control group. After 8 weeks, these participants also showed increases in a number of personal resources, including physical wellness, agency for achieving important goals, ability to savor positive experiences, and quality of close relationships. These gains were mediated by increased positive emotion.

Finally, meditators showed an increase relative to the control group in life satisfaction, and this gain was mediated by the increase in resources (see Figure 48.3). These results provide strong and specific evidence for the build hypothesis: Positive emotions led people to build a variety of important resources, and these resources proved valuable in increasing their life satisfaction and functioning in general (Fredrickson, Cohn, Coffey, Pek, & Finkel, 2008).

Positive Emotions and Stress

Researchers have also examined the ways in which positive emotions affect coping with chronic stressors. Prolonged negative situations such as bereavement or joblessness evoke negative emotions, but cannot be solved by the kind of immediate, narrowly defined action that negative emotions encourage. Consistent with this view, studies have shown that people who experienced some level of positive emotions during bereavement (alongside their negative emotions) showed greater psychological well-being a year or more later, and that this occurred partly because positive emotions were associated with the ability to take a longer view and develop plans and goals for the future (Stein, Folkman, Trabasso, & Richards, 1997; Moskowitz, Folkman, & Acree, 2003). Similarly, we performed a longitudinal assessment of college students' emotions and mental health before and after the terrorists attacks of September 11, 2001 (Fredrickson, Tugade, Waugh, & Larkin, 2003). We found that precrisis trait resilience predicted psychological growth and reduced risk of depression, but that this difference was fully mediated by experiences of positive emotion in the wake of the attacks. Resilient participants fared better, and this was because they were more likely than nonresilient participants to experience positive emotions. Resilient participants were not devoid of negative emotions—they felt fear and grief, much as their less resilient peers did—but finding occasional opportunities to feel positive emotions seems to have alleviated some of the negative effects of a prolonged narrowed mindset. It may be difficult to find positive emotions that are fully appropriate while in a prolonged negative situation; perhaps this is why people who can feel a wider variety of finely differentiated positive emotions show greater psychological resilience (Tugade, Fredrickson, & Barrett, 2004).

These results contradict common-sense criticisms that positive emotions are unhelpful or inappropriate for people in negative circumstances: Even adults dealing with suicidal thoughts (Joiner, Pettit, Perez, & Burns, 2001) or disclosure of childhood sexual abuse (Bonanno et al., 2002) showed better coping when some degree of positivity accompanied their painful feelings. In a longitudinal study of college students coping with ordinary life problems (Fredrickson & Joiner, 2002), we found that state positive emotions correlated with the use of creative and broad-minded coping strategies, and that use of these strategies in turn predicted increased positive emotions 5 weeks

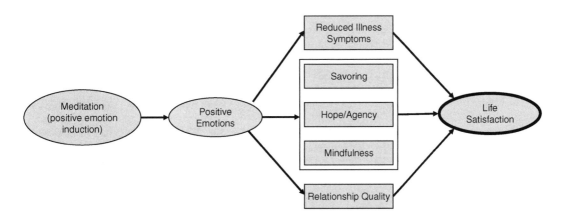

FIGURE 48.3. Results from a positive emotions intervention study. The intervention increased daily positive emotions, which led to building physical resources (top box), psychological resources (middle box), and social resources (bottom box). Resource building, in turn, led to increased life satisfaction.

later (above and beyond initial level of positive emotion).

The literature on depression has long documented a downward spiral in which depressed mood and the narrowed, pessimistic thinking it engenders feed into one another, leading to ever-worsening moods and even clinical levels of depression (Peterson & Seligman, 1984). The findings we have reviewed suggest that positive emotions can disrupt the spiral, and in some cases even initiate a comparable upward spiral: Positive emotions make people feel good in the present moment, which broadens their mindsets, which allows them to build resources that increase their likelihood of feeling good in the future. The upward spiral effect is represented by the feedback loop in Figure 48.1.

Positive Emotions and Health

One of the newest frontiers in positive emotions research is evidence linking positive emotions to physiology. People who experience high levels of positive emotions tend to experience less pain and disability related to chronic health conditions (Gil et al., 2004), to fight off illness and disease more successfully (Cohen & Pressman, 2006; Ong & Allaire, 2005), and even to live longer (Danner et al., 2001; Levy et al., 2002; Moskowitz, 2003; Ostir et al., 2000). We believe that these findings may be explained by the ability of positive emotions to lift people out of stressed, narrowed states. It is already established that the physiological changes accompanying negative emotions are beneficial for decisive, short-term action, but detrimental to long-term health. If biochemicals such as cortisol and epinephrine remain elevated for too long, they can lead to physical deterioration and immune dysregulation (Sapolsky, 1999). In line with this, individuals whose biological stress markers take longer to return to baseline following a stressor show poorer health than those who return to baseline quickly (McEwen & Seeman, 1999). Thus we have explored whether positive emotions play a role in physiological as well as psychological well-being.

The basic observation that positive and negative emotions (or key components of them) are to some extent incompatible has a long lineage in work on anxiety disorders (e.g., systematic desensitization—Wolpe, 1958), motivation (e.g., opponent-process theory; Solomon & Corbit, 1974), and aggression (e.g., the princi-

ple of incompatible responses; Baron, 1976).[4] Even so, the mechanism ultimately responsible for this incompatibility has not been adequately identified. The broaden effect may turn out to be the mechanism. Negative emotions are linked to preparation for a specific action, and if a positive emotion dissipates that focus, then the negative emotion loses its hold.

Because negative emotions were shaped by evolution to deal with pressing threats, we would not expect them to be easily neutralized; this may be the basis for the "bad-is-stronger-than-good" effect referenced earlier (Baumeister et al., 2001; Rozin & Royzman, 2001; Tversky & Kahneman, 1981). Instead, we have hypothesized that the "undo effect" may function when the threat is no longer apparent, but the narrowed focus and biochemical response to threat nonetheless linger.

Our laboratory has tested this by first inducing a high-arousal negative emotion in all participants, removing the negative stimulus, and then immediately inducing a randomly assigned emotion by showing a short, emotionally evocative film clip. Participants in the two positive emotion conditions (mild joy and contentment) exhibited faster cardiovascular recovery than those in the neutral control condition, who recovered more quickly than those in the sadness condition (Fredrickson, Mancuso, Branigan, & Tugade, 2000, Study 1; see also Fredrickson & Levenson, 1998). When participants viewed the positive films without a preceding stressor, they had no cardiovascular effects of any kind (Fredrickson et al., 2000, Study 2). In other words, the positive and neutral films did not differ in what they *did* to the cardiovascular system, but they differed in what they could *undo* within this system.

In subsequent work, we discovered that self-reported levels of psychological resilience (Block & Kremen, 1996) correlate with speed of cardiovascular recovery, and that this relationship is mediated by self-generated levels of positive emotions during recovery (Tugade & Fredrickson, 2004). Resilient individuals seem to be experts at harnessing the undo effect of positive emotions on their own.

We take these laboratory experiments as a microcosm for the influence of emotions on coping, and of coping on health. Imagine that some individuals typically seek positive emotions to help them bounce back quickly from life's stressors, while others spend more time remaining physiologically activated and prepared to react, even after the threat is gone. Over time, the latter group will accumulate more physiological wear and tear, and will be more vulnerable to a wide range of stress-related illnesses (McEwen & Seeman, 1999; Kiecolt-Glaser et al., 2002). Whether the undo effect of positive emotions factors into long-term health in this way is a challenging but deeply important question for future research.

DIRECTIONS FOR FUTURE RESEARCH

There is growing evidence that the broaden-and-build theory describes the most basic form and function of positive emotions, but there is also much yet to learn. In this section, we describe some critical directions for future research.

Physiological and Neurological Connections

We are eager to see empirical findings on positive emotions embedded in a broader physiological context. We know that positive emotions such as liking and intimacy can lead to closer relationships (Waugh & Fredrickson, 2006; Aron, Normal, Aron, McKenna, & Heyman, 2000). Recent work suggests that these emotions are linked to heightened levels of the hormones oxytocin (Zak, Kurzban, & Matzner, 2005; Gonzaga, Turner, Keltner, Campos, & Altemus, 2006) and progesterone (Schultheiss, Wirth, & Stanton, 2004), and that exogenous oxytocin can induce positive social feelings (Kosfelt, Heinrichs, & Zak, 2005). Further research on this relationship will allow us to bring the human research on relationship formation and the predominantly nonhuman research on hormone release and behavior to bear on each other, and to expand our understanding of the antecedents and consequences of relationship-relevant emotions.

The broaden effect is also amenable to physiological exploration. A review by Ashby, Isen, and Turken (1999) suggests that the broaden effect may be associated with release of meso-limbic dopamine, which enhances cognitive flexibility, set switching, and proactive curiosity. Notably, this is the same neurological system Berridge and Robinson (2003) associate with the motivational component of positive affect. It is also the mesolimbic dopamine sys-

tem that is impaired by older antipsychotic drugs, which lead to notable cognitive narrowing and rigidity (Berger et al., 1989). There is no doubt that the neurological substrate of the broaden effect will turn out to be more complex than a single neurotransmitter or neuronal system, but Ashby et al.'s observations help pave the way for future investigation.

Scattered results linking neurology and positive emotional effects are emerging in other areas. Haidt (2005) has early but suggestive evidence linking elevation and other moral emotions to changes in vagal tone. Results from neuroimaging studies demonstrate heightened left-hemispheric activation both in persons experiencing short-term positive emotions, and tonically in individuals with higher trait positive emotionality (Davidson, 2004). Our work on the undo effect (Fredrickson & Levenson, 1998; Fredrickson et al., 2000) demonstrates that positive emotions can reduce the duration of cardiovascular response evoked by a stressor. We are currently undertaking work to examine relationships between psychophysiological measures and meditation outcomes, and among positive emotions, affiliation-related hormones, and relationship formation.

Interventions

Our loving-kindness meditation intervention was the first to investigate the effects of positive emotions in light of the broaden-and-build theory, but other investigators have also found ways to create relatively lasting increases in positive emotions. Emmons and McCullough (2003) designed an intervention based on counting blessings; Sheldon and Lyubomirsky (2006) combined counting blessings with visualizing one's best possible self; and Seligman, Steen, and Park (2005) had participants count blessings, express gratitude, and practice using their signature strengths. Practitioners of cognitive-behavioral therapy also have a stable of techniques for generating positive emotions (Beck, 1995), although these are usually tested only among depressed individuals.

These early efforts might best be seen as proof of the concepts that positive emotions can be reliably evoked and that they have significant effects beyond momentary hedonic satisfaction. Next, positive emotion interventions need to become more mature: We can determine how best to deliver them, which interventions function for different populations, and how to maximize their effectiveness while minimizing their cost and time commitment. Also, larger studies could test long-term health outcomes, relationships with others, and school or work outcomes, in addition to the personal outcomes already investigated. Unlike interventions that focus on specific problems and therefore address only a specific group of people (e.g., those with depression, drug dependence, or extreme aggression), interventions that teach how to generate positive emotions could be of value to nearly anyone, in any situation. Therefore, they pose a wider variety of theoretical challenges, and possibly offer greater potential benefits as well.

Properties of Specific Emotions

So far, the empirical evidence suggests that the broaden effect is common to many positive emotions, and may describe their most general shared effect on cognition and attention. However, different positive emotions should also have distinct thought–action repertoires, subjective components, and physiological effects. For example, Tiedens and Linton (2001) compared the cognitive effects of contentment and pleasant surprise along a certainty–uncertainty continuum, and Gonzaga et al. (2006) studied cognitive, behavioral, and biological distinctions among romantic love, friendship, and sexual desire. Tong (2007) found that distinguishing different positive emotions may require attention to dimensions of experience that we have not previously thought of as inherent to emotion, such as social connection and spiritual experience.

However, most work on discrete positive emotions remains inconclusive (Barrett, 2006). We have suggested, for example, that joy is designed to encourage physical play and exploration, and so has a physiological arousal component (Fredrickson, 1998). Gratitude seems to encourage reflection and reconceptualization of one's experiences, targeted toward encouraging reciprocal behavior in the future (McCullough, Kilpatrick, Emmons, & Larson, 2001; Bartlett & DeSteno, 2006), and may differ from the related negative emotion of indebtedness by involving more insight into the perspective and desires of the benefactor (F. Flynn, personal communication, April 2006; Fredrickson, 2004). Keltner and Haidt (2003) suggest that awe functions to facilitate a Piagetian process of "accommodation," in which our mental structures enlarge to incorporate an important and wholly new experience; Haidt (2003) has suggested that there is a phenomenologically distinct and generally recognized emotion called "elevation," which causes people to attend to and emulate other people who show skillful or morally excellent behavior (i.e., people broaden their self-concept to incorporate the others' good example). Empirical tests of these proposals are not difficult to imagine, and at present the field is wide open for exploration.

Models

The broaden-and-build theory provides a description of the short-term effects of positive emotions and a plausible mechanism for long-term growth, but at a very general level. There is much more to learn about how the broaden effect works and what it does in specific situations. How does a broad mindset affect perceived familiarity with and interest in a new relationship partner? In a learning situation, is it likely to increase interest in the topic at hand, or increase the tendency to switch between topics? In what situations does it lead to use of heuristics versus careful processing?

Similarly, the build effect is difficult to observe directly. We have demonstrated that positive emotions lead people to build personal resources, but what specific actions lead to this growth? What situational or personal characteristics beyond positive emotions encourage behavior that leads to new resources? Because positive emotions encourage novel, divergent behavior that leads to long-term benefits, we may find that traditional methods based on a single manipulation and a single, clear outcome are inadequate to capture all their effects. Instead, we may need analytical methods that take into account individuals' specific resources, their adaptation to their situation, and the opportunities they can detect in their environment. Our lab has collaborated with Marcial Losada, who has used nonlinear dynamic models (similar to those used to analyze highly complex systems, such as weather and stock market fluctuations) to represent moment-by-moment interactions within high- and low-performing business teams. People experiencing positive emotions and teams achieving high performance show patterns characteristic of complex, multiply determined systems, whereas people experiencing fewer positive emotions and teams with lower performance are characterized by less complex, more predictable patterns (Schuldberg & Gottlieb, 2002; Losada & Heaphy, 2004). Our analysis suggests that the shift to novel behavior and resource building may begin precipitously when the ratio between positive and negative emotions exceeds a critical threshold of about 3:1 (Fredrickson & Losada, 2005), and early evidence supports this view (Cohn et al., 2007; Waugh & Fredrickson, 2006). Using these methods, we may be able to look more closely at the dynamics of resource building within a single observation session, or to recognize the course that the build effect takes over time, even when we are limited to a few discrete assessments within a longitudinal study.

Limitations of Positive Emotions

Most of the research we have surveyed discusses benefits of positive emotions, but a full scientific understanding should include pitfalls and boundary conditions of these benefits. For example, although more securely attached infants show faster cognitive development, insecure attachment may be an appropriate response to threatening or unreliable family circumstances. Positive emotions help undo the lingering cardiovascular effects of stressors, but people in particularly dangerous circumstances may have good reason to remain ready to act, even when a threat appears to be gone. Additionally, there is some suggestion that extremely high levels of positive emotions, untempered by sufficient negative emotions, can degrade performance (Diener, 2004; Fredrickson & Losada, 2005). We would like to develop a nuanced understanding of when positive emotions can help resolve a negative situation (as in Stein et al., 1997; Moskowitz et al., 2003; Fredrickson et al., 2003), and when they might be dangerous, excessive, or unacceptably costly.

Regardless of these caveats, we believe that there is good reason to celebrate and encourage positive emotions. Research on critical ratios of positivity to negativity (Fredrickson & Losada, 2005; Gottman, 1994) suggests that nearly all individuals and groups have low ratios. There are important questions about when and how to experience positive emotions, and which emotions are appropriate in different situations—but few of us are fortunate enough to have the problem of simply experiencing too much joy, interest, contentment, and love.

CONCLUSION

At the most general level, the broaden-and-build theory offers three new avenues for exploration:

1. For researchers on positive emotions, it provides an empirical framework for investigating the dynamics of such emotions and more clearly specifying their effects. Whether the theory is corroborated "as is" or whether it undergoes substantial changes, it is currently the best starting point for learning more.

2. For emotion theorists, the broaden-and-build theory suggests that the action tendencies model be expanded to include not just the narrowed repertoires associated with negative emotions, but also the broadened, less predictable repertoires associated with positive emotions. Psychology's understanding of emotion will be hampered if we deal exclusively with resource-consuming emotions that operate in a short time frame, and not with resource-building emotions that show their adaptive effects over longer periods.

3. Finally, the broaden-and-build theory suggests that positive emotions are fruitful targets for basic and applied research in any field that deals with personal growth, change, learning, social coordination, or physical health. As we have seen, positive emotions are more than just desirable endpoints; they also affect a wide variety of cognitive, social, and biological processes, and can help people to build a variety of personal resources. Right now we have a basic scheme for learning more about how positive emotions work and how they affect other areas of life; we look forward to broadening and building on it as research continues.

ACKNOWLEDGMENTS

Barbara L. Fredrickson's research on positive emotions is supported by the National Institute of Mental Health (Grant No. MH59615).

NOTES

1. The PANAS was formerly the Positive and Negative *Affect* Schedule. The authors renamed it to indicate that it actually measures valence mostly for high-activation states (Watson et al., 1999).

2. Note that a life-saving response need not involve action per se. For example, evolutionary research sug-

gests that sadness may be adaptive because it *prevents* action, thus conserving resources at times when prospects are so poor that no available action would be worth the risk and/or calories it requires (Keller & Nesse, 2005).

3. There is strong evidence that face recognition typically relies on a holistic (broad) representation of the face, and that impaired other-race face recognition results partly from a focus on narrowly construed racial features (Johnson & Fredrickson, 2005).

4. We previously reviewed studies in which frightened or grieving individuals reported both positive and negative emotions. The incompatibility of positive and negative emotions relates to feelings in a single moment, whereas the participants in bereavement studies were surveyed about their emotions over a long period of time, which can encompass many individual episodes of different emotions.

REFERENCES

Abele, A. (1992). Positive versus negative mood influences on problem solving. *Polish Psychological Bulletin, 23,* 187–202.

Arend, R., Gove, F. L., & Sroufe, L. A. (1979). Continuity of individual adaptation from infancy to kindergarten: A predictive study of ego-resiliency and curiosity in preschoolers. *Child Development, 50,* 950–959.

Aron, A., Norman, C. C., Aron, E. N., McKenna, C., & Heyman, R. (2000). Couples shared participation in novel and arousing activities and experienced relationship quality. *Journal of Personality and Social Psychology, 78,* 273–283.

Ashby, F. G., Isen, A. M., & Turken, U. (1999). A neuropsychological theory of positive affect and its influence on cognition. *Psychological Review, 106,* 529–550.

Aspinwall, L. (1998). Rethinking the role of positive affect in self-regulation. *Motivation and Emotion, 22*(1), 1–32.

Baron, R. A. (1976). The reduction of human aggression: A field study of the influence of incompatible reactions. *Journal of Applied Social Psychology, 6,* 260–274.

Barrett, L. F. (2006). Emotions as natural kinds? *Perspectives on Psychological Science, 1,* 28–58.

Barrett, L. F., Gross, J., Christensen, T. C., & Benvenuto, M. (2001). Knowing what you're feeling and knowing what to do about it: Mapping the relation between emotion differentiation and emotion regulation. *Cognition and Emotion, 15,* 713–724.

Bartlett, M. Y., & Desteno, D. (2006). Gratitude and prosocial behavior: Helping when it costs you. *Psychological Science, 17,* 319–325.

Basso, M. R., Schefft, B. K., Ris, M. D., & Dember, W. N. (1996). Mood and global–local visual processing. *Journal of the International Neuropsychological Society, 2,* 249–255.

Baumeister, R. F., Bratslavsky, E., Finkenauer, C., & Vohs, K. D. (2001). Bad is stronger than good. *Review of General Psychology, 5,* 323–370.

Beck, J. S. (1995). *Cognitive therapy: Basics and beyond.* New York: Guilford Press.

Berger, H. J. C., van Hoof J. J. M., van Spaendonck, K. P. M., Horstink, M. W. I., van den Bercken, J. H. L., Jaspers, R., et al. (1989). Haloperidol and cognitive shifting. *Neuropsychologia, 27,* 629–639.

Berridge, K. C., & Robinson, T. E. (2003). Parsing reward. *Trends in Neuroscience, 26,* 507–513.

Bless, H., Clore, G., Schwarz, N., Golisano, V., Rabe, C., & Wölk, M. (1996). Mood and the use of scripts: Does a happy mood really lead to mindlessness? *Journal of Personality and Social Psychology, 71*(4), 665–679.

Block, J., & Kremen, A. M. (1996). IQ and ego-resilience: Conceptual and empirical connections and separateness. *Journal of Personality and Social Psychology, 70,* 349–361.

Bonanno, G. A., Keltner, D., Noll, J. G., Putnam, F. W., Trickett, P. K., LeJune, J., et al. (2002). When the face reveals what words do not: Facial expressions of emotion, smiling, and the willingness to disclose childhood sexual abuse. *Journal of Personality and Social Psychology, 83,* 94–110.

Boulton, M. J., & Smith, P. K. (1992). The social nature of play fighting and play chasing: Mechanisms and strategies underlying cooperation and compromise. In J. H. Barkow, L. Cosmides, & J. Tooby (Eds.), *The adapted mind: Evolutionary psychology and the generation of culture* (pp. 429–444). New York: Oxford University Press.

Brown, S. L., Nesse, R. M., Vinokur, A. D., & Smith, D. M. (2003). Providing social support may be more beneficial than receiving it: Results from a prospective study of mortality. *Psychological Science, 14,* 320–327.

Bryan, T., & Bryan, J. (1991). Positive mood and math performance. *Journal of Learning Disabilities, 24,* 490–494.

Bryan, T., Mathur, S., & Sullivan, K. (1996). The impact of positive mood on learning. *Learning Disabilities Quarterly, 19,* 153–162.

Cabanac, M. (1971). Physiological role of pleasure. *Science, 173,* 1103–1107.

Cacioppo, J. T., Gardner, W. L., & Berntson, G. G. (1999). The affect system has parallel and integrative processing components: Form follows function. *Journal of Personality and Social Psychology, 76,* 839–855.

Cacioppo, J. T., Priester, J. R., & Berntson, G. G. (1993). Rudimentary determinants of attitudes: II. Arm flexion and extension have differential effects on attitudes. *Journal of Personality and Social Psychology, 65,* 5–17.

Caro, T. M. (1988). Adaptive significance of play: Are we getting closer? *Tree, 3,* 50–54.

Carver, C. S. (2003). Pleasure as a sign you can attend to

something else: Placing positive feelings within a general model of affect. *Cognition and Emotion*, *17*, 241–261.

Carver, C. S., & Scheier, M. F. (1990). Origins and functions of positive and negative affect: A control-process view. *Psychological Review*, *97*, 19–35.

Chen, M., & Bargh, J. (1999). Consequences of automatic evaluation: Immediate behavioral dispositions to approach or avoid the stimulus. *Personality and Social Psychology Bulletin*, *25*(2) 215–224.

Clore, G. L. (1994). Why emotions are felt. In P. Ekman & R. Davidson (Eds.), *The nature of emotion: Fundamental questions* (pp. 103–111). New York: Oxford University Press.

Cohen, S., Doyle, W. J., & Turner, R. B. (2003). Emotional style and susceptibility to the common cold. *Psychosomatic Medicine*, *65*, 652–657.

Cohen, S., & Pressman, S. D. (2006). Positive affect and health. *Current Directions in Psychological Science*, *15*, 122–125.

Cohn, M. A., & Fredrickson, B. L. (2006). Beyond the moment, beyond the self: Shared ground between selective investment theory and the broaden-and-build theory of positive emotion. *Psychological Inquiry*, *17*, 39–44.

Cohn, M. A., Fredrickson, B. L., Brown, S. L., Mikels, J. A., & Conway, A. (2007). *Happiness unpacked: Positive emotions increase life satisfaction by building resilience.* Manuscript in preparation.

Csikszentmihalyi, M. (1990). *Flow: The psychology of optimal experience.* New York: Harper & Row.

Csikszentmihalyi, M., & Csikszentmihalyi, I. (2006). *A life worth living: Contributions to positive psychology.* New York: Oxford University Press.

Danner, D., Snowdon, D. A., & Friesen, W. V. (2001). Positive emotions in early life and longevity: Findings from the nun study. *Journal of Personality and Social Psychology*, *80*, 804–813.

Davidson, R. J. (1993). The neuropsychology of emotion and affective style. In M. Lewis & J. M. Haviland (Eds.), *Handbook of emotions* (pp. 143–154). New York: Guilford Press.

Davidson, R. J. (2004). What does the prefrontal cortex 'do' in affect?: Perspectives on frontal EEG asymmetry research. *Biological Psychiatry*, *67*, 219–233.

Davidson, R. J., Kabat-Zinn, J., Schumacher, J., Rosenkrantz, M., Muller, D., Santorelli, S. F., et al. (2003). Alterations in brain and immune function produced by mindfulness meditation. *Psychosomatic Medicine*, *65*, 564–570.

Derryberry, D., & Tucker, D. M. (1994). Motivating the focus of attention. In P. M. Niedenthal & S. Kitayama (Eds.), *The heart's eye: Emotional influences in perception and attention* (pp. 167–196). San Diego, CA: Academic Press.

Diener, E. (2004, February). "Was Pollyanna right? Determining when positive affect will be beneficial." Talk presented at the meeting of the Society for Personality and Social Psychology, Austin TX.

Diener, E., & Diener, C. (1996). Most people are happy. *Psychological Science*, *7*, 181–185.

Diener, E., & Seligman, M. E. P. (2004). Beyond money: Toward an economy of well-being. *Psychological Science in the Public Interest*, *5*, 1–31.

Dolhinow, P. J. (1987). At play in the fields. In H. Topoff (Ed.), *The natural history reader in animal behavior* (pp. 229–237). New York: Columbia University Press.

Dovidio, J., Gaertner, S., Isen, A., Rust, M., & Guerra, P. (1995). Positive affect and the reduction of intergroup bias. In C. Sedikides, J. Schopler, & C. A. Insko (Eds.), *Intergroup cognition and intergroup behavior* (pp. 337–366). Mahwah, NJ: Erlbaum.

Dreisbach, G., & Goschke, T. (2004). How positive affect modulates cognitive control: Reduced perseveration at the cost of increased distractibility. *Journal of Experimental Psychology: Memory and Cognition*, *30*, 343–353.

Dunn, J. R., & Schweitzer, M. E. (2005). Feeling and Believing: The influence of emotion on trust. *Journal of Personality and Social Psychology*, *88*, 736–748.

Einon, D. F., Morgan, M. J., & Kibbler, C. C. (1978). Brief periods of socialization and later behavior in the rat. *Developmental Psychobiology*, *11*, 213–225.

Ekman, P. (1992). An argument for basic emotions. *Cognition and Emotion*, *6*, 169–200.

Ellsworth, P. C., & Smith, C. A. (1988). Shades of joy: Patterns of appraisal differentiating pleasant emotions. *Cognition and Emotion*, *2*, 301–331.

Emmons, R. A., & McCullough, M. E. (2003). Counting blessings vs. burdens: An experimental investigation of gratitude and subjective well-being in daily life. *Journal of Personality and Social Psychology*, *84*, 377–389.

Estrada, C. A., Isen, A. M., & Young, M. J. (1997). Positive affect facilitates integration of information and decreases anchoring in reasoning among physicians. *Organizational Behavior and Human Decision Processes*, *72*, 117–135.

Fineman, S. (2006). On being positive: Concerns and counterpoints. *Academy of Management Review*, *31*, 270–91.

Fredrickson, B. L. (1998). What good are positive emotions? *Review of General Psychology*, *2*, 300–319.

Fredrickson, B. L. (2000). Cultivating positive emotions to optimize health and well-being. *Prevention and Treatment*, *3*. Article 0001a. Retrieved from *content.apa.org/journals/pre/3/1/1a.html*

Fredrickson, B. L. (2001). The role of positive emotions in positive psychology: The broaden-and-build theory of positive emotions. *American Psychologist*, *56*, 218–226.

Fredrickson, B. L. (2004). Gratitude, like other positive emotions, broadens and builds. In R. A. Emmons & M. E. McCullough (Eds.), *The psychology of gratitude* (pp. 145–166). New York: Oxford University Press.

Fredrickson, B. L., & Branigan, C. (2001) Positive emotions. In T. J. Mayne & G. A. Bonnano (Eds.), *Emo-

tions: Current issues and future directions. New York: Guilford Press.

Fredrickson, B. L., & Branigan, C. (2005). Positive emotions broaden thought–action repertoires: Evidence for the broaden-and-build model. *Cognition and Emotion, 19,* 313–332.

Fredrickson, B. L., Cohn, M. A., Coffey, K. A., Pek, J., & Finkel, S. M. (2008). *Open hearts build lives: Positive emotions, induced through loving-kindness meditation, meditation, build consequential personal resources.* Manuscript under review.

Fredrickson, B. L., & Joiner, T. (2000). Positive emotions trigger upward spirals toward emotional well-being. *Psychological Science, 13,* 172–175.

Fredrickson, B. L., & Levenson, R. W. (1998). Positive emotions speed recovery from the cardiovascular sequelae of negative emotions. *Cognition and Emotion, 12,* 191–220.

Fredrickson, B. L., & Losada, M. F. (2005). Positive affect and the complex dynamics of human flourishing. *American Psychologist, 60,* 678–686.

Fredrickson, B. L., Mancuso, R. A., Branigan, C., & Tugade, M. (2000). The undoing effect of positive emotions. *Motivation and Emotion, 24*(4), 237–258.

Fredrickson, B. L., Tugade, M. M., Waugh, C. E., & Larkin, G. (2003). What good are positive emotions in crises? A prospective study of resilience and emotions following the terrorist attacks on the United States on September 11, 2001. *Journal of Personality and Social Psychology, 84,* 365–376.

Frijda, N. H. (1986). *The emotions.* Cambridge, UK: Cambridge University Press.

Frijda, N. H. (1994). Emotions are functional, most of the time. In P. Ekman & R. Davidson (Eds.), *The nature of emotion: Fundamental questions* (pp. 112–122). New York: Oxford University Press.

Frijda, N. H., Kuipers, P., & Schure, E. (1989). Relations among emotion, appraisal, and emotional action readiness. *Journal of Personality and Social Psychology, 57,* 212–228.

Gable, S. L., Reis, H. T., Impett, E. A., & Asher, E. R. (2004). What do you do when things go right?: The intrapersonal and interpersonal benefits of sharing positive events. *Journal of Personality and Social Psychology, 87,* 228–245.

Gervais, M., & Wilson, D. S. (2005). The evolution and functions of laughter and humor: A synthetic approach. *Quarterly Review of Biology, 80,* 395–451.

Gil, K. M., Carson, J. W., Porter, L. S., Scipio, C., Bediako, S. M., & Orringer, E. (2004). Daily mood and stress predict pain, health care use, and work activity in African American adults with sickle-cell disease. *Health Psychology, 23,* 267–274.

Gonzaga, G. C., Turner, R. A., Keltner, D., Campos, B., & Altemus, M. (2006). Romantic love and sexual desire in close relationships. *Emotion, 6,* 163–179.

Gottman, J. M. (1994). *What predicts divorce?: The relationship between marital processes and marital outcomes.* Hillsdale, NJ: Erlbaum.

Haidt, J. (2003). Elevation and the positive psychology of morality. In C. L. M. Keyes & J. Haidt (Eds.), *Flourishing: Positive psychology and the life well-lived* (pp. 275–289). Washington, DC: American Psychological Association.

Haidt, J. (2005). *The happiness hypothesis: Finding the modern truth in ancient wisdom.* New York: Basic Books.

Hazen, N. L., & Durrett, M. E. (1982). Relationship of security of attachment and cognitive mapping abilities in 2-year-olds. *Developmental Psychology, 18,* 751–759.

Isen, A. M., & Daubman, K. A. (1984). The influence of affect on categorization. *Journal of Personality and Social Psychology, 47,* 1206–1217.

Isen, A. M., Daubman, K. A., & Nowicki, G. P. (1987). Positive affect facilitates creative problem solving. *Journal of Personality and Social Psychology, 52,* 1122–1131.

Isen, A. M., Johnson, M. M. S., Mertz, E., & Robinson, G. F. (1985). The influence of positive affect on the unusualness of word associations. *Journal of Personality and Social Psychology, 48,* 1413–1426.

Ito, T. A., & Cacioppo, J. T. (1999). The psychophysiology of utility appraisals. In D. Kahneman, E. Diener, & N. Schwartz (Eds.), *Well-being: Foundations of hedonic psychology* (pp. 470–488). New York: Russell Sage Foundation.

Johnson, K. J. (2005). *We all look the same to me: Positive emotions eliminate the own-race bias in face recognition.* Unpublished doctoral dissertation, University of Michigan.

Johnson, K. J., & Fredrickson, B. L. (2005). "We all look the same to me:" Positive emotions eliminate the own-race bias in face recognition. *Psychological Science, 16,* 875–881.

Joiner, T. E., Pettit, J. W., Perez, M., & Burns, A. B. (2001). Can positive emotion influence problem-solving among suicidal adults? *Professional Psychology: Research and Practice, 32,* 507–512.

Kabat-Zinn, J. (2005). *Full catastrophe living: Using the wisdom of your body and mind to face stress, pain, and illness* (15th anniversary ed.). New York: Bantam.

Kahn, B. E., & Isen, A. M. (1993). The influence of positive affect on variety seeking among safe, enjoyable products. *Journal of Consumer Research, 20,* 257–270.

Kahneman, D., Kreuger, A. B., & Schkade, D. A. (2004). A survey method for characterizing daily life experience: The day reconstruction method. *Science, 306,* 1776–1780.

Keller, M. C., & Nesse, R. M. (2005). Is low mood an adaptation?: Evidence for subtypes with symptoms that match precipitants. *Journal of Affective Disorders, 86,* 27–35.

Keltner, D., & Bonanno, G. A. (1997). A study of laughter and dissociation: Distinct correlates of laughter and smiling during bereavement. *Journal of Personality and Social Psychology, 73,* 687–702.

Keltner, D., & Haidt, J. (2003). Approaching awe, a moral, spiritual, and aesthetic emotion. *Cognition and Emotion, 17,* 297–314.

Keyes, C. L. M., & Haidt, J. (Eds.). (2003). *Flourishing: Positive psychology and the life well-lived.* Washington, DC: American Psychological Association.

Kiecolt-Glaser, J. K., McGuire, L., Robles, T. F., & Glaser, R. (2002). Emotions, morbidity, and mortality. *Annual Review of Psychology, 53,* 83–107.

Kosfelt, M., Heinrichs, M., & Zak, P. J. (2005). Oxytocin increases trust in humans. *Nature, 435,* 673–676.

Lazarus, R. S. (1991). *Emotion and adaptation.* New York: Oxford University Press.

Lazarus, R. S. (2003). Does the positive psychology movement have legs? *Psychological Inquiry, 14,* 93–109.

Lee, P. C. (1983). Play as a means for developing relationships. In R. A. Hinde (Ed.), *Primate social relationships* (pp. 82–89). Oxford, UK: Blackwell.

Levenson, R. W. (1994). Human emotions: A functional view. In P. Ekman & R. Davidson (Eds.), *The nature of emotion: Fundamental questions* (pp. 123–126). New York: Oxford University Press.

Levy, B. R., Slade, M. D., & Kunkel, S. R. (2002). Longevity increased by positive self-perceptions of aging. *Journal of Personality and Social Psychology, 83,* 261–270.

Losada, M., & Heaphy, E. (2004). The role of positivity and connectivity in the performance of business teams: A nonlinear dynamics model. *American Behavioral Scientist, 47*(6), 740–765.

Lyubomirsky, S. L., King, L., & Diener, E. (2005). The benefits of frequent positive affect: Does happiness lead to success? *Psychological Bulletin, 131,* 803–855.

Martin, L. L., & Clore, G. (Eds.). (2001). *Theories of mood and cognition: A user's guidebook.* Mahwah, NJ: Erlbaum.

Martineau, W. H. (1972). A model of the social functions of humor. In J. H. Goldstein & P. E. McGee (Eds.), *The psychology of humor: Theoretical perspectives and empirical issues* (pp. 101–128). New York: Academic Press.

Masters, J. C., Barden, R. C., & Ford, M. E. (1979). Affective states, expressive behavior, and learning in children. *Journal of Personality and Social Psychology, 37,* 380–390.

Matas, L., Arend, R. A., & Sroufe, L. A. (1978). Continuity of adaptation in the second year: The relationship between quality of attachment and later competence. *Child Development, 49,* 547–556.

McCullough, M. E., Kirkpatrick, S. D., Emmons, R. A., & Larson, D. B. (2001). Is gratitude a moral affect? *Psychological Bulletin, 127,* 249–266.

McEwen, B. S., & Seeman, T. (1999). Protective and damaging effects of mediators of stress: Concepts of allostasis and allostatic load. *Annals of the New York Academy of Sciences, 896,* 30–47.

Mikulincer, M. (1997). Adult attachment style and information processing: Individual differences in curiosity and cognitive closure. *Journal of Personality and Social Psychology, 72,* 1217–1230.

Moskowitz, J. T. (2003). Positive affect predicts lower risk of AIDS mortality. *Psychosomatic Medicine, 65,* 620–626.

Moskowitz, J. T., Folkman, S., & Acree, M. (2003). Do positive psychological states shed light on recovery from bereavement?: Findings from a 3-year longitudinal study. *Death Studies, 27,* 471–500.

Oatley, K., & Jenkins, J. M. (1996). *Understanding emotions.* Cambridge, MA: Blackwell.

Ong, A. D., & Allaire, J. C. (2005). Cardiovascular intraindividual variability in later life: The influence of social connectedness and positive emotions. *Psychology and Aging, 20,* 476–485.

Ostir, G. V., Markides, K. S., & Black, S. A. (2000). Emotional well-being predicts subsequent functional independence and survival. *Journal of the American Geriatrics Society, 48,* 473–78.

Otake, K., Waugh, C. E., & Fredrickson, B. L. (2007). *Positive emotions unlock other-focused thinking.* Manuscript in preparation.

Panksepp, J. (1998). Attention deficit hyperactivity disorders, psychostimulants, and intolerance of childhood playfulness: A tragedy in the making? *Current Directions in Psychological Science, 7,* 91–98.

Peciña, S., Smith, K. S., & Berridge, K. C. (2006). Hedonic hot spots in the brain. *Neuroscientist, 12,* 500–511.

Peterson, C., & Seligman, M. E. P. (1984). Causal explanations as a risk factor for depression: Theory and evidence. *Psychological Review, 91,* 347–374.

Rosenberg, E. L. (1998). Levels of analysis and the organization of affect. *Review of General Psychology, 2,* 247–270.

Rowe, G., Hirsch, J., & Anderson, A. K. (2007). Positive affect increases the "breadth" of attentional selection. *Proceedings of the National Academy of Sciences of the USA, 104,* 338–383.

Rozin, P., & Royzman, E. B. (2001). Negativity bias, negativity dominance, and contagion. *Personality and Social Psychology Review, 5,* 296–320.

Russell, J. A., Weiss, A., & Mendelsohn, G. A. (1989). Affect Grid: A single-item scale of pleasure and arousal. *Journal of Personality and Social Psychology, 57,* 493–502.

Ryff, C. D., & Singer, B. (1998). The contours of positive human health. *Psychological Inquiry, 9,* 1–28.

Sapolsky, R. M. (1999). The physiology and pathophysiology of unhappiness. In D. Kahneman, E. Diener, & N. Schwarz (Eds.), *Well-being: The foundations of hedonic psychology* (pp. 453–469). New York: Russell Sage Foundation.

Schuldberg, D., & Gottlieb, J. (2002). Dynamics and correlates of microscopic changes in affect. *Nonlin-*

ear Dynamics, Psychology, and Life Sciences, 6, 231–257.

Schultheiss, O. C., Wirth, M. M., & Stanton, S. J. (2004). Effects of affiliation and power motivation arousal on salivary progesterone and testosterone. *Hormones and Behavior, 46*, 592–599.

Seligman, M. E. P., & Csikszentmihalyi, M. (2000). Positive psychology: An introduction. *American Psychologist, 55*, 5–14.

Seligman, M. E. P., Steen, T. A., & Park, N. (2005). Positive psychology progress: Empirical validation of interventions. *American Psychologist, 60*, 410–421.

Sheldon, K. M., & Lyubomirsky, S. (2006). How to increase and sustain positive emotion: The effects of expressing gratitude and visualizing best possible selves. *Journal of Positive Psychology, 1*, 73–82.

Sherrod, L. R., & Singer, J. L. (1989). The development of make-believe play. In J. Goldstein (Ed.), *Sports, games and play* (pp. 1–38). Hillsdale, NJ: Erlbaum.

Shiota, M. N., Keltner, D., & John, O. P. (2006). Positive emotion dispositions differentially associated with Big Five personality and attachment style. *Journal of Positive Psychology, 1*, 61–71.

Simons, C. J. R., McCluskey-Fawcett, K. A., & Papini, D. R. (1986). Theoretical and functional perspective on the development of humor during infancy, childhood, and adolescence. In L. Nahemow, K. A. McCluskey-Fawcett, & P. E. McGhee (Eds.), *Humor and aging* (pp. 53–77). Orlando, FL: Academic Press.

Smith, C. A., & Ellsworth, P. C. (1985). Patterns of cognitive appraisal in emotion. *Journal of Personality and Social Psychology, 48*, 813–838.

Solomon, R. L., & Corbit, J. D. (1974). An opponent-process theory of motivation: I. Temporal dynamics of affect. *Psychological Review, 81*, 119–145.

Stein, N. L., Folkman, S., Trabasso, T., & Richards, T. A. (1997). Appraisal and goal processes as predictors of psychological well-being in bereaved caregivers. *Journal of Personality and Social Psychology, 72*, 872–884.

Tiedens, L. Z., & Linton, S. (2001). Judgment under emotional certainty and uncertainty: The effects of specific emotions on information processing. *Journal of Personality and Social Psychology, 81*, 973–988.

Tong, E. M. W. (2007). Appraisal processes in emotional experiences. *Dissertation Abstracts International: Section B: The Sciences and Engineering, 67*, 4161.

Tooby, J., & Cosmides, L. (1990). The past explains the present: Emotional adaptations and the structure of ancestral environments. *Ethology and Sociobiology, 11*, 375–424.

Trope, Y., & Pomerantz, E. (1998). Resolving conflicts among self-evaluative motives: Positive experiences as a resource for overcoming defensiveness. *Motivation and Emotion, 22*(1), 53–72.

Tsai, J. L., Knutson, B., & Fung, H. H. (2006). Cultural variation in affect valuation. *Journal of Personality and Social Psychology, 90*, 288–307.

Tugade, M. M., & Fredrickson, B. L. (2004). Resilient individuals use positive emotions to bounce back from negative emotional experiences. *Journal of Personality and Social Psychology, 86*, 320–333.

Tugade, M. M., Fredrickson, B. L., & Barrett, L. F. (2004). Psychological resilience and positive emotional granularity: Examining the benefits of positive emotions on coping and health. *Journal of Personality, 72*, 1161–1190.

Tversky, A., & Kahneman, D. (1981). The framing of decisions and the psychology of choice. *Science, 211*, 453–458.

Wadlinger, H. A., & Isaacowitz, D. M. (2006). Positive mood broadens visual attention to positive stimuli. *Motivation and Emotion.*

Watson, D., Wiese, D., Vaidya, J., & Tellegen, A. (1999). The two general activation systems of affect: Structural findings, evolutionary considerations, and psychobiological evidence. *Journal of Personality and Social Psychology, 76*, 820–838.

Waugh, C. E., & Fredrickson, B. L. (2006). Nice to know you: Positive emotions, self–other overlap, and complex understanding in the formation of a new relationship. *Journal of Positive Psychology, 1*, 93–106.

Waugh, C. E., Hejmadi, A., Otake, K., & Fredrickson, B. L. (2006). Cross-cultural evidence that positive emotions broaden views of self to include close others. Unpublished raw data.

Wolpe, J. (1958). *Psychotherapy by reciprocal inhibition.* Stanford, CA: Stanford University Press.

Zak, P. J., Kurzban, R., & Matzner, W. T. (2005). Oxytocin is associated with human trustworthiness. *Hormones and Behavior, 48*, 522–527.

CHAPTER 49

Sadness and Grief

GEORGE A. BONANNO, LAURA GOORIN, and KARIN G. COIFMAN

Sadness and grief are universal and inevitable aspects of the human experience. They are conceptually and phenomenally similar—so similar, in fact, that sometimes the terms are used interchangeably. But it is important to underscore that sadness and grief are not the same, and that their distinction helps illuminate unique and important aspects of human behavior. We begin this chapter by detailing four crucial ways in which sadness and grief differ. We next review the functional role played by sadness in normal human experience, and we describe how, when those functions go awry, sadness can become depression. We then consider how similar patterns may characterize the normative experience of sadness in response to the death of a loved one, and how bereavement-related sadness can sometimes deteriorate into complicated grief reactions. To this end, we speculate about the possible role played by sadness and grief in our ancestral past, and also in the social life of nonhuman primates. Finally, we consider the role of positive emotional experiences after loss, as well as the growing

body of evidence regarding the oscillation of positive and negative affect and its role in normal self-regulatory processes.

FOUR CRUCIAL DIFFERENCES BETWEEN SADNESS AND GRIEF

We begin our chapter with the question of how sadness and grief differ from each other. We argue that sadness is a basic emotion, but that grief represents a broader and more elaborate construct similar to (though not identical with) depression (Bonanno, 2001; Lazarus, 1991). Grief and emotion each involve complex behavioral responses whose respective operational definitions have been subject to considerable debate. (For reviews of some of the key definitional issues regarding emotion, see Barrett, 2006a, 2006b; Ekman, 1992; Ekman & Davidson, 1994; Izard, 1994; Oatley & Jenkins, 1996; and Russell, 1994. Regarding grief, see Bonanno, 2001; Bonanno & Kaltman, 1999; Hansson, Carpenter, & Fairchild,

1993; M. S. Stroebe, Hansson, Stroebe, & Schut, 2001; W. Stroebe, Schut, & Stroebe, 2005.)

Grief is typically a highly emotionally distressing experience, and at a superficial level it appears to share features with specific emotions, most notably sadness (Lazarus, 1991). Perhaps for this reason, some investigators have preferred to blur the distinction between the concepts, and have viewed grief as a form of emotion (Averill & Nunley, 1993; Stearns & Knapp, 1996; Panksepp, 2005). However, a careful analysis reveals that grief is most appropriately conceptualized as a complex and enduring molar experience that generates various molecular components, including a range of specific emotions (Bonanno, 2001; Lazarus, 1991). Most prominent among the emotions experienced during grief is sadness.

There are at least four ways in which the emotion of sadness differs from the molar experience of grief (Bonanno, 2001). First, sadness and grief each encompass dramatically different temporal intervals. Emotions, such as sadness, are commonly defined as ephemeral phenomena, generally lasting a few seconds but sometimes up to several hours (Ekman, 1984; Ekman & Davidson, 1994; Izard, 1993; Chow, Ram, Boker, Fujita, & Clore, 2005). In contrast, grief is an enduring state that for most bereaved individuals persists for several weeks and up to several years (Bonanno, 2004; Bonanno & Kaltman, 2001). In some cases, aspects of grief have been found to endure 7 to 8 years or longer after the loss (Lehman, Wortman, & Williams, 1987; Lundin, 1984).

Second, myriad different emotions typically occur within the course of a single period of grief. Although the death of a loved one is most commonly associated with sadness, grieving is far from a one-dimensional emotional phenomenon. In addition to sadness, grief has been associated with a wide range of negative emotions, such as anger, contempt, hostility, fear, and guilt (Abraham, 1924; Belitsky & Jacobs, 1986; Bonanno & Keltner, 1997; Bonanno, Mihalecz, & LeJeune, 1998; Bowlby, 1980; Cerney & Buskirk, 1991; Kavanagh, 1990; Lazare, 1989; Osterweis, Solomon, & Green, 1984; Raphael, 1983)—and, as we discuss in greater detail below, genuinely positive emotional experiences related to amusement, affection, happiness, and pride (see Bonanno & Kaltman, 1999, 2001).

Third, grief and emotions are associated with different types of underlying meaning structures. Emotions are typically linked to relatively simple, proximal appraisals related to the immediate situational context. Emotion-related appraisals often encompass, for example, issues of personal danger or benefit, coping potential, or their interaction with motivational states (Frijda, 1993; Lazarus, 1991; Roseman, Antoniou, & Jose, 1996). In many cases, emotional responses occur without the benefit of even these simple cognitive appraisals. For instance, the chemical and physical responses associated with basic emotions, such as fear, can be triggered solely on the basis of rapid, automated, subcortical processing of crude perceptual information (LeDoux, 1989, 1996; Phelps, 2006). Moreover, there is emerging evidence that the amygdala also responds to sadness-related stimuli (Wang, McCarthy, Song, & LaBar, 2005).

The emotion of sadness in particular is generally associated with the appraisal of permanent loss. Grief is, of course, also associated with the cognitive understanding of loss. However, in contrast to the relatively simple way this appraisal manifests itself in sadness, the sense of loss that informs grief is typically far more profound and all-encompassing. When the loss involves the death of someone of importance in a person's life, the impact on meaning structures includes a dramatic impact on that person's identity and cognitive understanding of the world (Schwartzberg & Janoff-Bulman, 1991) and the future (Horowitz et al., 1997; Lehman et al., 1987; Shuchter & Zisook, 1993). Indeed, bereaved people commonly report that they feel as if "a piece of me is missing" (Kastenbaum, 1995; Shuchter & Zisook, 1993). These longer-term appraisals typically encompass a bereaved person's evaluation and understanding of the entire course of bereavement, as well as major portions of his or her own life (Bonanno & Kaltman, 1999, 2001).

Fourth, grief and emotions evoke different types of coping responses. Emotions are proximal, and thus are generally implicated in proximal, short-term coping responses aimed at either changing or maintaining the immediate psychological or physical state (Gross & John, 2003; Mauss, Levenson, McCarter, Wilhelm, & Gross, 2005). Indeed, emotion and proximal coping are so intimately related that Folkman and Lazarus (1988, 1990) described coping as a mediator of emotion. Grieving, on the other hand, typically evokes longer-term coping efforts aimed at ameliorating the enduring emotional upsets as well as myriad concrete disruptions wrought by the loss, such as changes in social roles, economic situation, or familial configuration (Bonanno & Keltner, 1997; Lazarus, 1991; Neimeyer, 2006; Neimeyer, Prigerson, & Davies, 2002; Shuchter & Zisook, 1993; W. Stroebe & Stroebe, 1987).

THE FUNCTIONS OF SADNESS

In this section, we consider the functional role played by the everyday experience and expression of sadness. A key adaptive function of sadness is to promote personal reflection following the irrevocable loss of a person or object of importance to the self (Lazarus, 1991). The experience of sadness turns our attention inward, promoting resignation and acceptance (Izard, 1977, 1993; Lazarus, 1991; Stearns, 1993). Physiological arousal is decreased, allowing for a "time out" to update cognitive structures and to accommodate lost objects (Welling, 2003). The reflective function of sadness, therefore, opportunely affords us a pause, allowing us to take stock and to revise our goals and plans (Bonanno & Keltner, 1997; Oatley & Johnson-Laird, 1996).

An extensive body of experimental data has associated sadness with more detail-oriented information processing, more accurate performance appraisals, and less overall reliance on heuristics and stereotyping for decision making (see Bodenhausen, Gabriel, & Lineberger, 2000; Schwarz, 1998). Overskeid (2000) has argued that the decreased arousal associated with sadness facilitates problem solving by allowing for the deployment of more time-consuming analytic strategies. Alternatively, Schwarz (1990) has suggested that sadness tends to be accompanied by a decrease in people's confidence in their first impressions. In an attempt to compensate for this insecurity, an individual experiencing sadness may engage in a more extensive deliberation during decision making. Based on their research showing that induction of a sad emotional state decreases the likelihood of false-memory bias, Storbeck and Clore (2005) similarly concluded that "with sadness comes accuracy" (p. 785).

In addition to the reflective function associated with the experience of sadness, the non-verbal expression of sadness is thought to serve an important interpersonal function. From a social-functional perspective, expressions of emotion in mammals are evolutionary adaptations to social environments related to the creation and maintenance of social relationships and the organization of interindividual interactions (Darwin, 1872/1998; Keltner & Kring, 1998). Facial displays of emotion evoke and shape the responses of others by inducing specific emotional responses and reinforcing or discouraging social behaviors (Keltner & Kring, 1998). The facial expression of sadness is thought to support group social behavior by evoking sympathy and helping responses in others (Keltner & Kring, 1998; Izard, 1977, 1993; Lazarus, 1991; Stearns, 1993).

Research on distress eliciting sympathy suggests that sadness functions in a reciprocal manner (Batson & Shaw, 1991; Keltner & Kring, 1998). Sad images evoke both sad affect (Gross & Levenson, 1995) and increased amygdala activation in observers (Wang et al., 2005). Moreover, experimental research reveals that newborn infants are capable of distinguishing between an audiotape recording of their own cry and another neonate's cry, and that the sound of another newborn's cry provokes distress in the infants, evidenced through consistent facial grimaces, turning red-faced, and showing visible signs of agitation (Dondi, Simion, & Caltran, 1999). Physiological responses accompanying sympathy in adults, including concerned gaze and reduced heart rate, are predictive of altruistic or helping behaviors. Such reciprocal responses increase the probability that individuals expressing sadness will receive needed attention and/or assistance from others (Keltner & Kring, 1998).

It is important to note, however, that the functional benefits of sadness are not entirely free of cost. For example, Gray (2001) showed that experimentally induced sadness enhanced some aspects of working memory while reducing others. In particular, sadness induction enhanced spatial memory while reducing verbal memory. Notably, the opposite pattern was evident in a condition that involved a happiness induction (Gray, 2001). Similarly, despite the fact that sadness is generally linked to decreased susceptibility to judgmental bias, Bodenhausen et al. (2000) found that a sadness induction resulted in greater vulnerability to an anchoring bias wherein final judgments were altered toward a provided starting point, even if the particular starting point was arbitrary.

There are also social consequences associated with sadness. Ambady and Gray (2002) found that a sadness induction led to reduced accuracy in participants' social judgments of brief video clips. In one of their studies, for example, sadness reduced participants' ability to accurately gauge teacher effectiveness. In another study, sadness reduced participants' ability to correctly categorize the type of relationship enacted in brief video clips of dyadic interactions.

WHEN SADNESS BECOMES DEPRESSION

Sadness can sometimes deteriorate into more chronic dysphoric mood states, or, in extreme cases, depressogenic states. In contrast to the cognitive and social benefits associated with brief sadness episodes, more prolonged dysphoric states have been associated with withdrawal and despair, as well as with the elicitation of rejection from others (Bonanno & Keltner, 1997; Lazarus, 1991; Smith & Ellsworth, 1985).

One of the mechanisms that probably mediates the transition from the brief, episodic experience of sadness to a more elaborate and dysfunctional depressive state is rumination. Considerable research indicates that transient dysphoric mood is most likely to develop into a more prolonged depressive state when people engage in ruminative responses, such as "repetitively and passively focusing on symptoms of distress and the possible causes and consequences of these symptoms" (Nolen-Hoeksema, Wisco & Lyubomirsky, in press). Moreover, the tendency to ruminate appears to be a relatively stable response style—one linked to increased vulnerability not only for depression, but also for negative thinking, decreased problem solving abilities, disruption in the execution of instrumental behaviors, and the dissolution of social relationships (see Nolen-Hoeksema, 1991; Nolen-Hoeksema et al., in press). And rumination has been shown to mediate other risk factors for depression, such as negative cognitive styles, self-criticism, neediness, and a history of depression (Spasojevic & Alloy, 2001).

The potentially dysfunctional influence of depressive rumination is perhaps most pro-

nounced in situations where psychological threat is acute, as in the case of a serious interpersonal loss. For example, Nolen-Hoeksema, Morrow, and Frederickson (1993) found that in a longitudinal study of bereaved men, initial rumination levels were uniquely predictive of depression 12 months later, even after initial depressive symptomatology was controlled for. Recent evidence indicates that rumination predicts the onset of depression, and is moderated by negative cognitive styles in predicting the duration of depression (Nolen-Hoeksema et al., in press).

There also appear to be genetic vulnerabilities to depression that emerge when people are exposed to loss or other extremely aversive events, suggesting a gene × environment interaction (Moffitt, Caspi, & Rutter, 2006). Convincing prospective evidence has shown, for example, that a functional polymorphism in the promoter region of the serotonin transporter gene (5-HTT) moderates the impact of stressful life events on depression (Caspi et al., 2003). Such findings suggest the compelling possibility that ruminative responses to sad states may be at least partially informed by a person's genetic makeup.

But is the transition from sadness to depression always maladaptive? This pivotal question becomes especially important in the context of loss, where bereavement scholars have traditionally assigned functional significance to grief reactions (e.g., Bowlby, 1980). Nesse (2000) has argued, for example, that the cognitive and behavioral manifestations of depression—specifically, pessimism and lack of motivation—help to inhibit potentially dangerous actions that might lead to further loss, thus conserving necessary resources for survival. In their situation–symptom congruence hypothesis, Keller and Nesse (2006) theorize that because of the distinct adaptive functions of various depressive symptoms, different contexts (including failure and social loss) are likely to evoke discrete depressive symptoms, which will in turn enhance survival capacities in these diversely challenging situations.

However, other fundamental social and cognitive survival skills may be lost at the expense of these inhibited behaviors. Whereas transient sadness may boost some forms of problem solving, when sadness becomes depression, the concomitant lack of motivation and pessimism will tend to interrupt problem-solving efforts (Overskeid, 2000). Similarly, whereas brief displays of sadness evoke sympathy and helping responses from others, more prolonged dysphoric expressions tend to extract a serious toll on personal relationships and to threaten overall social adjustment. Several studies have suggested that intense and prolonged expressions of negative emotions, such as sadness, tend to drive away people who might otherwise offer support (Coyne, 1976; Gottlieb, 1991; Harber & Pennebaker, 1992; Pennebaker, 1993). In his interpersonal theory of depression, for instance, Coyne (1976) argued that depression is transmitted between people through excessive reassurance seeking. However, reassurance seeking in turn tends to lead to social rejection (Joiner, 1999; Joiner, Alfano, & Metalsky, 1992).

The type of negative social exchange fueled by excessive dysphoric expressions creates a downward spiral of social rejection. For example, Strack and Coyne (1983) found that participants who had engaged in 15 minutes of conversation with depressed partners endorsed greater anxiety, depression, and hostile mood following the interaction, compared to those who conversed with nondepressed partners. Participants who conversed with a depressed partner also endorsed less willingness to interact with the partner in the future and a greater willingness to share negative social perceptions with the depressed partner. The depressed partners, in turn, had accurately anticipated their partners' rejection, and acted reciprocally by rejecting their nondepressed counterparts.

WHEN SADNESS BECOMES GRIEF

The phenomenology of sadness as it moves into more depressed states is mirrored, to some extent, by the ways in which sadness appears to give way to more complicated grief reactions during bereavement. From a comparative and historical perspective, it is easy to envision how the functional relevance of sadness would facilitate human survival of loss. However, it is more difficult to fathom that there would be much usefulness to prolonged dysphoric states. In this section, we briefly consider what the experience of loss might have been like in our ancestral past, and how it may still operate among our nonhuman primate relatives.

One salient feature of virtually our entire ancestral past is that humans and protohumans were constantly faced with the death of genetic relatives or others within the broader social group. It was only recently, for example, with the advent of modern medicine, that humans began to exceed a normal life expectancy of 20–35 years (Galor & Moav, 2005). For all but a relatively brief period of the time humans have lived on earth, daily life has been beset with disease, poor nutrition, predation, and other threats to survival. Moreover, because humans and protohumans were until only recently nomadic, any psychological mechanisms that might have evolved to deal with these continual losses would have by necessity been a mechanism commensurate to group life on the move.

In this context, grief-related sadness in response to the loss would clearly be most adaptive as an ephemeral reaction that ran its course in relatively short order. Each of the intrapersonal functional characteristics we have discussed above—the turning of attention inward, the temporary decrease in arousal, the promotion of resignation and acceptance, the facilitation of problem solving, and the updating of cognitive structures—offer obvious mechanisms that would help a person adjust to the social and personal changes wrought by the death of an important relative or group member. Likewise, the expressive functions of sadness—the evocation of sympathy and helping responses in others—would also facilitate bereavement in the context of the broader social group.

By the same token, it seems obvious that more prolonged sadness reactions, or more elaborate grief or depressive states, would be incompatible with nomadic life and would put a bereaved nomad in this context at considerable risk. The withdrawal and despair associated with longer-term sadness and depressive states would make it difficult to keep up with the moving tribe or group, and would be likely to increase susceptibility to disease or predation. Similarly, the association of prolonged sadness and depression with rejection from others would mean that the bereaved nomad would receive less support or perhaps even elicit treachery from other members of the group or tribe.

We can no longer directly observe the pressing demands of nomadic group living as these would have manifested themselves in our own ancestral past, when easy-communication, mass produced goods or foods, and effective medical care were nonexistent. However, it is still possible to observe nomadic group living in our closest primate relatives. Here Jane Goodall's famously patient observations of wild chimpanzees in Gombe National Park, Tanzania, provide compelling examples.

In her field observations, Goodall (1986) repeatedly described apparent instances of sadness, depression, and grief in young chimpanzees following the death of their mothers. Chimps younger than 3 years of age are still dependent on mothers' milk, and thus cannot survive unless adopted by another female. Yet all of the orphaned chimps Goodall observed in this age group eventually died following their mothers' deaths, regardless of whether or not they were adopted by another female. Most of the older orphans survived, even though some exhibited ostensible developmental deficits (e.g., unusual levels of violence, poor coordination) that may have been occasioned by the loss. For younger orphans, however, prolonged sadness or depression-like behaviors were almost always lethal. In fact, each of the chimps that failed to survive following its mother's death, regardless of age, had been observed as listless and lethargic. By stark contrast, none of the surviving orphans exhibited lethargy; moreover, the orphans that were oldest (i.e., 7–9 years) at the time of their mothers' deaths showed no noticeable adverse reactions.

It is simply not possible to ascribe emotional states to animals with full confidence. However, laboratory studies have shown that interruption of the mother–child bond in nonhuman primates tends to produce significant behavioral disturbances, depression-like reactions (e.g., lethargy, slouched posture), and what appear to be sad facial expressions (e.g., Reite, Short, Seiler, & Pauley, 1981). Nonhuman primates also appear to recognize (or at least to attend to) sad facial expressions, even in humans. For example, Japanese monkeys have been found to engage in longer search time when presented with sad than with neutral human faces (Kanazawa, 1996). Because monkeys do not have the same capacity for eyebrow movement as humans, they tend to devote greater attention in differentiating sadness to the cheek muscles (Kanazawa, 1998).

Goodall (1986) consistently observed proto-emotional expressions in the orphaned chimps that were similar to human sadness expressions. We could speculate that these expressions would play some role in restructuring social relations following the loss. A key element

of chimpanzee survival with particular relevance to bereavement is social bonding with siblings and other adults. All of the orphaned chimps in Goodall's sample, even those that did not survive, had either been adopted by another adult or sibling, or traveled with another chimp when the group was on the move. Survival would no doubt depend, at least in part, on the success of these bonds (Trivers, 1972). The orphans that did not survive appeared to have somewhat troubled and ambivalent relations with their newly adopted partners, and it seems that these difficulties might be attributed at least in part to the social friction caused by their lethargic expressions and neediness. For example, one 4- to 5-year-old orphan, given the name Merlin, was adopted by an older female sibling. Merlin was described as lethargic, with sunken eyes; as engaging in minimal play; and as socially unresponsive. The sibling allowed Merlin to sleep with her, but rejected him when he attempted to ride her dorsally, as young chimps often do with their mothers. He died 18 months later (Goodall, 1986, p. 102).

Together, these data suggest that the experience and expressions of sadness are functionally useful following an important loss, but also that more prolonged and extreme sadness will be less functionally relevant; as sadness gives way to depressive expressions and lethargy, it begins to compromise functioning and to undermine potentially crucial avenues for interpersonal bonding and support.

POSITIVE EMOTION AND OSCILLATION IN GRIEF REACTIONS

As noted earlier, although sadness is the prototypical emotion of bereavement, it is not the only emotion evoked by the death of a loved one. Somewhat counterintuitively, loss experiences also commonly involve positive memories and reflections, as well as positive emotional expressions (Bonanno & Kaltman, 1999; Bonanno, Moskowitz, Papa, & Folkman, 2005; Moskowitz, Folkman, & Acree, 2003; Shuchter & Zisook, 1993; Stein et al., 1997). Facial coding from videotaped interviews conducted within months after the death of a spouse showed, for example, that most bereaved people exhibited at least one genuine laugh or smile, even as they discussed their recent loss (Bonanno & Keltner, 1997). Moreover, consistent with the adaptive value of positive emotions observed in other contexts (Fredrickson, 1998, 2001; Fredrickson & Joiner, 2002), bereaved people who expressed positive emotions early in bereavement had better long-term adjustment (Bonanno & Keltner, 1997) and also evoked more favorable reactions from untrained observers who viewed videotapes of the interviews (Keltner & Bonanno, 1997).

How can grief involve sadness, longing, withdrawal, and disorientation on the one hand, and laughter and positive emotional experiences on the other? The answer seems to be that bereavement, like other stress reactions, has a kind of wave-like periodicity characterized by oscillation between a focus inward (on the stressor event and its implications and meanings) and a focus outward (toward the external world and other people). Grief reactions are not uniform or static. Rather, as many bereavement investigators have noted, grief seems to occur in waves. The wave-like nature of grief has been observed, for example, in studies of 19th-century American diaries (e.g., Rosenblatt, 1983). Robert Kastenbaum (1995), one of the first social scientists to consider how humans adapt to death and loss, noted that "distress does not end with the first wave of shock and grief. After the realization that a loved one is dead often comes the realization that life is supposed to go on" (p. 316).

The oscillatory nature of these reactions has been documented in many theories about severe or pathological reactions to loss and trauma. The key point is that a moderate level of oscillation is an adaptive feature of normal, short-lived stress reactions. The inability to self-regulate sadness and other emotions during bereavement, however, tends to be associated with more extreme and unregulated forms of oscillation, with more enduring and extreme negative affective reactions, and consequently with more chronic or complicated grief reactions.

The oscillating quality of grief reactions is not unlike similar wave-like or oscillatory reactions observed in response to other stressor events. Litz (quoted in Greer, 2005) has noted, for example, "We tend to think of [posttraumatic stress disorder] as this discrete disorder that is a steady state. But research suggests it's much more dynamic . . . the symptoms can wax and wane over time" (p. 39). Similarly, in a widely cited book about trauma, Herman (1992) describes the "dialectic of trauma . . . In

the aftermath of an experience of overwhelming danger, the two contradictory responses of intrusion and constriction establish an oscillating rhythm" (p. 47).

In an attempt to move beyond the traditional emphasis in bereavement theory on grief work, M. S. Stroebe and Schut (1999) have incorporated the wave-like nature of grief into a broader model of bereavement coping behaviors: the dual-process model of bereavement. The dual-process model specifies that adaptive coping with bereavement requires two types of processes or coping orientations: a "loss orientation" and a "restoration orientation." A loss orientation is described as dealing with "processing of some aspect of the loss experience itself, most particularly, with respect to the deceased person" (M. S. Stroebe & Schut, 1999, p. 212). By contrast, a restoration orientation involves processes that deal with the secondary sources of stress associated with the loss—the indirect consequences of a loss that must be dealt with in order to move beyond the loss.

The crucial theoretical advance of the dual-process model is that it emphasizes the alternating quality or *oscillation* of the two orientations. Not only are both loss-oriented and restoration-oriented processes deemed necessary for successful recovery from loss; according to the model, "optimal adjustment" (M. S. Stroebe & Schut, 1999, p. 216) over time also requires a relatively constant switching back and forth, or oscillation, between the processes. As we discuss below, however, because the Stroebe and Schut dual-process model focuses primarily on coping rather than emotion during bereavement, it may overestimate the duration and extent of oscillation required for healthy adjustment.

Oscillation in Emotion Regulation

Under normal conditions, we can conceptualize self-regulation as the relatively simple and straightforward task of maintaining an optimal psychological and emotional equilibrium (Bonanno, 2001; Carver, 1998; Carver & Scheier, 1982, 1990; Westphal & Bonanno, 2004). One key issue to consider when we think of oscillation is how positive and negative states may function in relation to each other. There has been quite a bit of debate in psychology about this issue. Some theorists have argued that positive and negative states represent two ends of a bipolar continuum (e.g., Barrett & Russell, 1998). One of the primary sources of evidence for this position comes from factor-analytic studies of the way people describe their affective states; it seems that when people say they are feeling good, they don't say they are feeling bad, and vice versa. Other theorists have argued, however, that positive and negative states are relatively independent, and thus represent distinct and uncorrelated dimensions of experience. Evidence for the independence of emotional states comes from studies of biological markers of emotion, such as brain functions (Cacioppo, Gardner, & Berntson, 1997, 1999) and facial expressions (Bonanno & Keltner, 1997).

One way to think about this controversy is that under typical conditions, when self-regulation demands are considerably mild, positive and negative states will appear to function relatively independently. By contrast, however, when there is a serious disturbance or aversive threat to the system, we should see extremes of these behaviors as individuals tend to experience more bipolar affective reactions. Stressful situations tend naturally to evoke negative emotions, and these emotions should serve their functional purpose. For example, getting angry helps people to mobilize their resources and communicate their readiness to defend themselves. However, people also tend to experience positive emotions and even moments of calm in the aftermath of extreme adversity. The presence of positive emotion in the context of adversity is supported by evidence suggesting that positive emotions may play a crucial role in undoing or regulating the physiological effects of negative emotions (Bonanno & Keltner, 1997; Fredrickson & Levenson, 1998; Fredrickson, 1998, 2001; Tugade & Fredrickson, 2004). Because it is rather difficult, if not impossible, to experience negative and positive emotions simultaneously, and because the experience of positive emotions may minimize or undo negative emotions, it is reasonable to expect that such experiences will tend to alternate.

This is precisely what is predicted by Zautra and colleagues' dynamic model of affect (Reich, Zautra, & Davis, 2003; Zautra, Reich, Davis, Potter, & Nicolson, 2000; Zautra, Berkhof, & Nicolson, 2002). They argue that when there is low stress, it is relatively easy for people to engage in complex, differentiated, and multidimensional processing of the surrounding environment and of their own affec-

tive reactions in response to that environment. During an ordinary social gathering with friends, for instance, one may have different perceptions and attributions about one's own behavior or the behavior of the various people in the room, and these perceptions and attributions will probably result in a range of affective experiences as the gathering progresses. In such a casual situation, there is relatively little demand on attention, and the mind is ostensibly free to roam among, monitor, and catalogue these affective states. However, in more demanding and stressful situations—say, for example, a heated interpersonal conflict or a rush to catch a plane—one's attention becomes more clearly concentrated on the most immediate and necessary behaviors and information in the environment. Thus perceptions and attributions become more narrowly focused, and the experience of positive or negative states seems to "collapse into a single bipolar dimension with highly inversely coupled affect" (Reich et al., 2003, p. 70). It is important to note that stress does not necessarily change the *functions* of positive and negative emotions, and indeed the biological and behavioral data suggest that positive and negative emotions are functionally independent (Bonanno & Keltner 1997; Cacioppo et al., 1999). What does change in stressful situations is the subjective *experience* of affect; one's perception is shifted toward experiencing affect more as a bipolar, or one-or-the-other, phenomenon.

The inverse relationship between positive and negative affect in times of stress suggests a direct relationship among the severity of the stress, the strength of the bipolarity, and the strength of the regulatory oscillation (Bisconti, Bergeman, & Boker, 2004). For example, in longitudinal studies of people suffering from chronic pain syndromes, Zautra and Smith (2001) found that across a number of weeks, positive and negative affect tended to show a mild correlation—and, not surprisingly, that pain tended to increase negative affect and decrease positive affect. More interestingly, however, they also found that when pain was more pronounced, the presence of positive affect was predictive of a weaker relationship between pain and negative affect. In other words, "as pain escalates, positive affect appears to play an increasing role in the regulation of negative affect" (Zautra & Smith, 2001, p. 690).

Recently, Bisconti, Bergeman, Boker, and Ong (Bisconti et al., 2004; Bisconti, Bergeman,

& Boker, 2006; Ong, Bergeman, & Bisconti, 2004) replicated these findings, using daily ratings of positive and negative affect across several different samples, including a recently bereaved sample. They obtained reports of emotional well-being and depression from a small sample of widows each day during the first 1–4 months of bereavement. The explicit goal of this study was to test the idea, central to this chapter, that "a stressful life event, such as the death of a spouse, perturbs the emotional well-being state of the individual away from equilibrium, contributing to emotional shifts that vacillate between negative and positive affect" (Bisconti et al., 2004, p. 164). Thus they predicted that the widows' daily well-being ratings would conform to a linear oscillator model (Bisconti et al., 2004; Chow et al., 2005) that looks something like a "pendulum with friction" (Bisconti et al., 2004, p. 159). The most obvious features of this type of model are its gradual decrease in oscillation and the slope of change over time. For example, well-being is more variable and swings to its lowest point early in bereavement, and then gradually becomes more stable and increases on average across time. Essentially, these types of dynamics indicate that change in reaction to stress is not static, but rather a product of different self-regulation processes and behaviors over time. Thus the change is best characterized as an oscillation.

It goes without saying that immediately following the death of someone of personal importance, people are likely to feel deep and painful despair. However, even in the early days of bereavement, people can also temporarily forget about the loss and laugh, or experience moments of normal or even heightened pleasure. Because of the severity of the disturbance to normal equilibrium, and the volatility of the system, the oscillations tend to be more frequent and extreme—to have a greater amplitude—and then gradually to lessen or "dampen" across time.

Oscillation and Resilience after Loss

Bisconti et al.'s (2004) data on the first 4 months of bereavement conform nicely to the linear oscillator model. What's more, although these findings generally seem to support M. S. Stroebe and Schut's (1999) dual-process model, Bisconti et al. (2004) conclude that the regulatory oscillations "occur more rapidly" (p. 165) and earlier in bereavement, and also seem to dampen more quickly than the dual-process model would imply.

Stroebe and Schut's dual-process model also predicts that because oscillation has an adaptive regulatory function, the strength of the oscillation can be taken as a marker of adjustment to bereavement. This idea leads to the compatible assumption that "people who show little or no oscillation will adapt less well to loss" (M. S. Stroebe, Schut, & Stroebe, 2005, p. 52). However, both the dynamic model of affect and the work of Bisconti and colleagues (e.g., Bisconti et al., 2004, 2006) suggest the opposite hypothesis: that people who show healthy adaptation or resilience after loss will be *less* dysregulated by the loss, and thus will evidence *less* and not more oscillation.

Support for this idea was further evidenced in a recent study of recently bereaved adults who participated in a series of brief laboratory interviews (Coifman, Bonanno, & Rafaeli, 2007). The most resilient bereaved individuals in this study ("resilience" was defined as having relatively minimal disruption in functioning across the first 18 months of bereavement; see Bonanno et al., 2005) showed less oscillation in affect across interview topics. More specifically, when current levels of distress were statistically controlled for, resilient bereaved individuals had weaker correlations between self-reported negative and positive affect, suggesting relatively greater independence in affect, less bipolarity, and therefore less oscillation. In contrast, for those individuals who had chronically elevated symptom levels similar to complicated grief reactions, positive and negative affect were more strongly inversely correlated, suggesting less independence between affects, greater bipolarity, and therefore more oscillation.

In another recent study, Bisconti et al. (2006) also suggested a relationship between resilience after loss and individual differences in the oscillatory pattern during bereavement. They concluded that bereaved individuals whose outcome trajectory was similar to that observed among resilient individuals in previous bereavement studies (e.g., Bonanno et al., 2002) showed "a temporary influx of lability in emotional well-being, followed by a high level of positive and stable functioning" (Bisconti et al., 2006, p. 596). They further contrast this resilient pattern of oscillation with another trajectory more clearly suggestive of the chronic or complicated grief reactions, in which the widow was "exhibiting a continued amount of oscillation across the duration of the study" (p. 596).

CONCLUSION

The results of these investigations not only support our understanding of oscillatory processes during bereavement; they also illuminate the crucial distinction between the emotion of sadness and the more enduring and complex experiences captured under the broader construct of grief. As we have described earlier, sadness exists within the experience of grief but is not exclusive to grief. By the same token, the experience of grief is dominated by, but not limited to, sadness; the process of grieving encompasses a variety of other negative emotions (such as anger or guilt), as well as positive emotions (such as happiness, amusement, and affection). Moreover, the periodic experience of positive emotion while grieving appears to serve the valuable function of helping to regulate sadness and other negative emotional experiences over the course of bereavement. Although this model is somewhat at odds with modern conceptualizations of grief as an exclusively painful and somber experience, the oscillatory nature of positive and negative affect during bereavement makes sense from the perspective of our nomadic ancestral heritage. Because long-term grief would almost certainly have led to isolation, abandonment, and predation, the utility of experiencing episodes of sadness punctuated with positive emotional experiences would have been favored over more ruminative and depressogenic responses, and would have evolved as an adaptive means to achieve both necessary respite and resources from within the broader social group.

REFERENCES

Abraham, K. (1953). A short study of the development of the libido, viewed in the light of mental disorders. In D. Bryan & J. A. Strachey (Eds.), *Selected papers of Karl Abraham* (pp. 418–501). New York: Basic Books.

Ambady, N., & Gray, H. M. (2002). On being sad and mistaken: Mood effects on the accuracy of thin-slice judgments. *Journal of Personality and Social Psychology, 83,* 947–961.

Averill, J. R., & Nunley, E. P. (1993). Grief as an emotion and as a disease: A social-constructionist perspective. In M. S. Stroebe, W. Stroebe, & R. O. Hansson (Eds.), *Handbook of bereavement: Theory, research, and intervention* (pp. 77–90). New York: Cambridge University Press.

Barrett, L. F. (2006a). Solving the emotion paradox: Categorization and the experience of emotion. *Personality and Social Psychology Review, 10,* 20–46.

Barrett, L. F. (2006b). Are emotions natural kinds? *Current Directions in Psychological Science, 1,* 28–58.

Barrett, L. F., & Russell, J. A. (1998). Independence and bipolarity in the structure of current affect. *Journal of Personality and Social Psychology, 74*(4), 967–984.

Batson, C. D., & Shaw, L. L. (1991). Evidence for altruism: Toward a pluralism of prosocial motives. *Psychological Inquiry, 2,* 107–122.

Belitsky, R., & Jacobs, S. (1986). Bereavement, attachment theory, and mental disorders. *Psychiatric Annals, 16*(5), 276–280.

Bisconti, T. L., Bergeman, C. S., & Boker, S. M. (2004). Emotional well-being in recently bereaved widows: A dynamic systems approach. *Journals of Gerontology: Series B. Psychological Sciences and Social Sciences, 59B,* 158–168.

Bisconti, T. L., Bergeman, C. S., & Boker, S. M. (2006). Social support as a predictor of variability: An examination of recent widows' adjustment trajectories. *Psychology and Aging, 21,* 590–599.

Bodenhausen, G. V., Gabriel, S., & Lineberger, M. (2000). Sadness and susceptibility to judgmental bias: The case of anchoring. *Psychological Science, 11*(4), 320–323.

Bonanno, G. A. (2001). Grief and emotion: A sociofunctional perspective. In M. Stroebe, R. O. Hansson, W. Stroebe, & H. Schut (Eds.), *Handbook of bereavement research: Consequences, coping, and care* (pp. 493–516). Washington, DC: American Psychological Association.

Bonanno, G. A. (2004). Loss, trauma, and human resilience: Have we underestimated the human capacity to thrive after extremely aversive events? *American Psychologist, 59,* 20–28.

Bonanno, G. A., & Kaltman, S. (1999). Toward an integrative perspective on bereavement. *Psychological Bulletin, 125*(6), 760–776.

Bonanno, G. A., & Kaltman, S. (2001). The varieties of grief experience. *Clinical Psychology Review, 21*(5), 705–734.

Bonanno, G. A., & Keltner, D. (1997). Facial expressions of emotion and the course of conjugal bereavement. *Journal of Abnormal Psychology, 106*(1), 126–137.

Bonanno, G. A., & Keltner, D. (2004). The coherence of emotion systems: Comparing "on-line" measures of appraisal and facial expression, and self-report. *Cognition and Emotion, 18,* 431–444.

Bonanno, G. A., Mihalecz, M. C., & LeJeune, J. T.

(1999). The core emotion themes of conjugal bereavement. *Motivation and Emotion*, 23, 175–201.

Bonanno, G. A., Moskowitz, J. T., Papa, A., & Folkman, S. (2005). Resilience to loss in bereaved spouses, bereaved parents, and bereaved gay men. *Journal of Personality and Social Psychology*, 88, 827–843.

Bonanno, G. A., Wortman, C. B., Lehman, D. R., Tweed, R. G., Haring, M., Sonnega, J., et al. (2002). Resilience to loss and chronic grief: A prospective study from pre-loss to 18 months post-loss. *Journal of Personality and Social Psychology*, 83, 1150–1164.

Bowlby, J. (1980). *Attachment and loss: Vol. 3. Loss: Sadness and depression.* New York: Basic Books.

Cacioppo, J. T., Gardner, W. L., & Berntson, G. G. (1997). Beyond bipolar conceptualizations and measures: The case of attitudes and evaluative space. *Personality and Social Psychology Review*, 1(1), 3–25.

Cacioppo, J. T., Gardner, W. L., & Berntson, G. G. (1999). The affect system has parallel and integrative processing components: Form follows function. *Journal of Personality and Social Psychology*, 76(5), 839–855.

Carver, C. S. (1998). Resilience and thriving: Issues, models, and linkages. *Journal of Social Issues*, 54, 245–268.

Carver, C. S., & Scheier, M. F. (1982). Control theory: A useful conceptual framework for personality–social, clinical and health psychology. *Psychological Bulletin*, 92, 111–135.

Carver, C. S., & Scheier, M. F. (1990). Origins and functions of positive and negative affect: A control-process view. *Psychological Review*, 97, 19–35.

Caspi, A., Sugden, K., Moffitt, T., Taylor, T., Craig, I. W., Harrington, H., et al. (2003). Influence of life stress on depression: Moderation by a polymorphism in the 5-HTT gene. *Science*, 301, 386–389.

Cerney, M. S., & Buskirk, J. R. (1991). Anger: The hidden part of grief. *Bulletin of the Menninger Clinic*, 55(2), 228–237.

Chow, S.-Y., Ram, N., Boker, S. M., Fujita, F., & Clore, G. (2005). Emotion as a thermostat: Representing emotion regulation using a damped oscillator model. *Emotion*, 5, 208–225.

Coifman, K. G., Bonanno, G. A., & Rafaeli, E. (2007). Affective dynamics, bereavement, and resilience to loss. *Journal of Happiness Studies*, 8, 371–392.

Coyne, J. C. (1976). Depression and the response of others. *Journal of Abnormal Psychology*, 85, 186–193.

Darwin, C. (1998). *The expression of the emotions in man and animals* (3rd ed.). New York: Oxford University Press. (Original work published 1872)

Dondi, M., Simion, F., & Caltran, G. (1999). Can newborns discriminate between their own cry and the cry of another newborn infant? *Developmental Psychology*, 35(2), 418–426.

Ekman, P. (1984). Expression and the nature of emotion. In K. Scherer & P. Ekman (Eds.), *Approaches to emotion* (pp. 319–344). Hillsdale, NJ: Erlbaum.

Ekman, P. (1992). Are there basic emotions? *Psychological Review*, 99(3), 550–553.

Ekman, P., & Davidson, R. J. (Eds.). (1994). *The nature of emotion: Fundamental questions.* New York: Oxford University Press.

Folkman, S., & Lazarus, R. S. (1988). Coping as a mediator of emotion. *Journal of Personality and Social Psychology*, 54(3), 466–475.

Folkman, S., & Lazarus, R. S. (1990). Coping and emotion. From N. L. Stein, B. Leventhal, & T. Trabasso (Eds.), *Psychological and biological approaches to emotion* (pp. 313–332). Hillsdale, NJ: Erlbaum.

Fredrickson, B. L. (1998). What good are positive emotions? *Review of General Psychology*, 2, 300–319.

Fredrickson, B. L. (2001). The role of positive emotions in positive psychology: The broaden-and-build theory of positive emotions. *American Psychologist*, 56, 218–226.

Fredrickson, B. L., & Joiner, T. (2002). Positive emotions trigger upward spirals toward emotional well-being . *Psychological Science*, 13, 172–175.

Fredrickson, B. L., & Levenson, R. W. (1998). Positive emotions speed recovery from the cardiovascular sequelae of negative emotions. *Cognition and Emotion*, 12(2), 191–220.

Frijda, N. H. (1993). Moods, emotion episodes, and emotions. In M. Lewis & J. M. Haviland (Eds.), *Handbook of emotions* (pp. 381–403). New York: Guilford Press.

Galor, O., & Moav, O. (2005). *Natural selection and the evolution of life expectancy* (Minerva Center for Economic Growth, Paper No. 02-05). Retrieved from *ssrn.com/abstract=563741*

Goodall, J. (1986). *The chimpanzees of Gombe.* Cambridge, MA: Belknap Press of Harvard University Press.

Gottlieb, B. H. (1991). Advances in research on social support and issues applying to adolescents at risk. In G. Albrecht, H.-W. Otto, S. Karstedt-Henke, K. Bollert, & F. Deutsche (Eds.), *Social prevention and the social sciences: Theoretical controversies, research problems, and evaluation strategies* (pp. 199–216). Berlin: de Gruyter.

Gray, J. R. (2001). Emotional modulation of cognitive control: Approach–withdrawal states double-dissociate spatial from verbal two-back task performance. *Journal of Experimental Psychology: General*, 130(3), 436–452.

Greer, M. (2005). A new kind of war. *American Psychological Association Monitor on Psychology*, 36, 40.

Gross, J. J., & John, O. P. (2003). Individual differences in two emotion regulation processes: Implications for affect, relationships, and well-being. *Journal of Personality and Social Psychology*, 85(2), 348–362.

Gross, J. J., & Levenson, R. W. (1995). Emotion elicitation using films. *Cognition and Emotion*, 9, 87–108.

Hansson, R. O., Carpenter, B. N., & Fairchild, S. K.

(1993). Measurement issues in bereavement. In M. S. Stroebe, W. Stroebe, & R. O. Hansson (Eds.), *Handbook of bereavement: Theory, research, and intervention* (pp. 62–74). New York: Cambridge University Press.

Harber, K. D., & Pennebaker, J. W. (1992). Overcoming traumatic memories. In S.-A. Christianson (Ed.), *The handbook of emotion and memory: Research and theory* (pp. 359–387). Hillsdale, NJ: Erlbaum.

Herman, J. L. (1992). *Trauma and recovery*. New York: Basic Books.

Horowitz, M. J., Siegel, B., Holen, A., Bonanno, G. A., Milbrath, C., & Stinson, C. (1997). Diagnostic criteria for complicated grief disorder. *American Journal of Psychiatry, 154*(7), 904–910.

Izard, C. (1977). *Human emotions*. New York: Plenum Press.

Izard, C. E. (1993). Four systems for emotion activation: Cognitive and noncognitive processes. *Psychological Review, 100*(1), 68–90.

Izard, C. E. (1994). Innate and universal facial expressions: Evidence from developmental and cross-cultural research. *Psychological Bulletin, 115*(2), 288–299.

Jenkins, J. M., & Oatley, K. (1996). Emotional episodes and emotionality through the life span. In C. Magai & S. H. McFadden (Eds.), *Handbook of emotion, adult development, and aging* (pp. 421–441). San Diego, CA: Academic Press.

Joiner, T. E. (1999). A test of interpersonal theory of depression in youth psychiatric inpatients. *Journal of Abnormal Child Psychology, 27*, 77–85.

Joiner, T. E., Alfano, M. S., & Metalsky, G. I. (1992). When depression breeds contempt: Reassurance seeking, self-esteem, and rejection of depressed college students by their roommates. *Journal of Abnormal Psychology, 101*(1), 165–173.

Kanazawa, S. (1996). Recognition of facial expressions in a Japanese monkey (*Macaca fuscata*) and humans (*Homo sapiens*). *Primates, 37*, 25–38.

Kanazawa, S. (1998). What facial part is important for Japanese monkeys (*Macaca fuscata*) in recognition of smiling and sad faces of humans (*Homo sapiens*)? *Journal of Comparative Psychology, 112*, 363–370.

Kastenbaum, R. J. (1995). *Death, society, and human experience* (5th ed.). Boston: Allyn & Bacon.

Kavanagh, D. J. (1990). Towards a cognitive-behavioural intervention for adult grief reactions. *British Journal of Psychiatry, 157*, 373–383.

Keller, M. C., & Nesse, R. M. (2006). The evolutionary significance of depressive symptoms: Different adverse situations lead to different depressive symptom patterns. *Journal of Personality and Social Psychology, 91*(2), 316–330.

Keltner, D., & Bonanno, G. A. (1997). A study of laughter and dissociation: Distinct correlates of laughter and smiling during bereavement. *Journal of Personality and Social Psychology, 73*, 687–702.

Keltner, D., & Kring, A. (1998). Emotion, social func-

tion, and psychopathology. *Review of General Psychology, 2*(3), 320–342.

Lazare, A. (1989). Bereavement and unresolved grief. In A. Lazare (Ed.), *Outpatient psychiatry: Diagnosis and treatment* (2nd ed., pp. 381–397). Baltimore: Williams & Wilkins.

Lazarus, R. S. (1991). *Emotion and adaptation*. New York: Oxford University Press.

LeDoux, J. E. (1989). Central pathways of emotional plasticity. In H. Weiner, I. Florin, R. Murison, & D. Hellhammer (Eds.), *Frontiers of stress research* (pp. 122–136). Lewiston, NY: Huber.

LeDoux, J. E. (1996). *The emotional brain: The mysterious underpinnings of emotional life*. New York: Simon & Schuster.

Lehman, D. R., Wortman, C. B., & Williams, A. F. (1987). Long-term effects of losing a spouse or child in a motor vehicle crash. *Journal of Personality and Social Psychology, 52*(1), 218–231.

Litz, B. T. (2005). Has resilience to severe trauma been underestimated? *American Psychologist, 60*(3), 262.

Lundin, T. (1984). Long-term outcome of bereavement. *British Journal of Psychiatry, 145*, 424–428.

Mauss, I. B., Levenson, R. W., McCarter, L., Wilhelm, F. H., & Gross, J. J. (2005). The tie that binds?: Coherence among emotion experience, behavior, and physiology. *Emotion, 5*(2), 175–190.

Moffitt, T. E., Caspi, A., & Rutter, M. (2006). Measures of gene–environment interactions in psychopathology: Concepts, research strategies, and implications for research, intervention, and public understanding of genetics. *Perspectives on Psychological Science, 1*, 5–27.

Moskowitz, J., Folkman, S., & Acree, M. (2003). Do positive psychological states shed light on recovery from bereavement?: Findings from a 3-year longitudinal study. *Death Studies, 27*(6), 471–500.

Neimeyer, R. A. (2006). Widowhood, grief, and the quest for meaning: A narrative perspective on resilience. In D. Carr, R. M. Nesse, & C. B. Wortman (Eds.), *Late life widowhood: New directions in research, theory, and practice* (pp. 227–246). New York: Springer.

Neimeyer, R. A., Prigerson, H. G., & Davies, B. (2002). Mourning and meaning. *American Behavioral Scientist, 46*(2), 235–251.

Nesse, R. (2001). Is depression an adaptation? *Archives of General Psychiatry, 57*, 14–20.

Nolen-Hoeksema, S. (1991). Responses to depression and their effects on the duration of depressive episodes. *Journal of Abnormal Psychology, 100*(4), 569–582.

Nolen-Hoeksema, S., Morrow, J., & Fredrickson, B. L. (1993). Response styles and the duration of episodes of depressed mood. *Journal of Abnormal Psychology, 102*(1), 20–28.

Nolen-Hoeksema, S., Wisco, B., & Lyubomirsky, S. (in press). Rethinking rumination. *Perspectives in Psychological Science*.

Oatley, K., & Jenkins, J. M. (1996). *Understanding emotions.* Cambridge, MA: Blackwell.

Oatley, K., & Johnson-Laird, P. N. (1996). The communicative theory of emotions: Empirical tests, mental models, and implications for social interaction. In L. L. Martin & A. Tesser (Eds.), *Goals and affect* (pp. 363–393). Hillsdale, NJ: Erlbaum.

Ong, A. D., Bergeman, C. S., & Bisconti, T. L. (2004). The role of daily positive emotions during conjugal bereavement. *Journals of Gerontology: Series B. Psychological Sciences and Social Sciences, 59B*(4), P168–P176.

Osterweis, M., Solomon, F., & Green, F. (Eds.). (1984). *Bereavement: Reactions, consequences, and care.* Washington, DC: National Academy Press.

Overskeid, G. (2000). The slave of the passions: Experiencing problems and selecting solutions. *Review of General Psychology, 4*(3), 284–309.

Panksepp, J. (2005). Why does separation distress hurt?: Comment on MacDonald and Leary (2005). *Psychological Bulletin, 131,* 224–230.

Pennebaker, J. W. (1993). Social mechanisms of constraint. In D. M. Wegner & J. W. Pennebaker (Eds.), *Handbook of mental control* (pp. 200–219). Englewood Cliffs, NJ: Prentice-Hall.

Phelps, E. A. (2006). Emotion and cognition: Insights from the study of the human amygdala. *Annual Review of Psychology, 57,* 27–53.

Raphael, B. (1983). *The anatomy of bereavement.* New York: Basic Books.

Reich, J. W., Zautra, A. J., & Davis, M. (2003). Dimensions of affect relationships: Models and their integrative implications. *Review of General Psychology, 7*(1) 66–83.

Reite, M., Short, R., Seiler, C., & Pauley, J. D. (1981). Attachment, loss, and depression. *Journal of Child Psychology and Psychiatry, 22,* 141–169.

Roseman, I. J., Antoniou, A. A., & Jose, P. E. (1996). Appraisal determinants of emotions: Constructing a more accurate and comprehensive theory. *Cognition and Emotion, 10*(3), 241–277.

Rosenblatt, P. C. (1993). Grief: The social context of private feelings. In. M. S. Stroebe, W. Stroebe, & R. O. Hansson (Eds.), *Handbook of bereavement: Theory, research, and intervention* (pp. 102–111). New York: Cambridge University Press.

Russell, J. A. (1994). Is there universal recognition of emotion from facial expression?: A review of cross-cultural studies. *Psychological Bulletin, 115,* 102–141.

Schwartzberg, S. S., & Janoff-Bulman, R. (1991). Grief and the search for meaning: Exploring the assumptive worlds of bereaved college students. *Journal of Social and Clinical Psychology, 10*(3), 270–288.

Schwarz, N. (1990). Feelings as information: Informational and motivational functions of affective states. In E. T. Higgins & R. M. Sorrentino (Eds.), *Handbook of motivation and cognition: Foundations of social behavior* (Vol. 2, pp. 527–561). New York: Guilford Press.

Schwarz, N. (1998). Warmer and more social: Recent developments in cognitive social psychology. *Annual Review of Sociology, 24,* 239–264.

Shuchter, S. R., & Zisook, S. (1993). The course of normal grief. In M. S. Stroebe, W. Stroebe, & R. O. Hansson (Eds.), *Handbook of bereavement: Theory, research, and intervention* (pp. 23–43). New York: Cambridge University Press.

Smith, C. A., & Ellsworth, P. C. (1985). Patterns of cognitive appraisal in emotion. *Journal of Personality and Social Psychology, 48*(4), 813–838.

Spasojevic, J., & Alloy, L. B. (2001). Rumination as a common mechanism relating depressive risk factors to depression. *Emotion, 1*(1), 25–37.

Stearns, C. Z. (1993). Sadness. In M. Lewis & J. M. Haviland (Eds.), *Handbook of emotions* (pp. 547–561). New York: Guilford Press.

Stearns, P. N., & Knapp, M. (1996). Historical perspectives on grief. In R. Harr & W. G. Parrott (Eds.), *The emotions: Social, cultural, and biological dimensions* (pp. 132–150). Thousand Oaks, CA: Sage.

Stein, N., Folkman, S., Trabasso, T., & Richards, T. (1997). Appraisal and goal processes as predictors of psychological well-being in bereaved caregivers. *Journal of Personality and Social Psychology, 72*(4), 872–884.

Strack, S., & Coyne, J. C. (1983). Social confirmation of dysphoria: Shared and private reactions to depression. *Journal of Personality and Social Psychology, 44,* 798–806.

Storbeck, J., & Clore, G. (2005). With sadness comes accuracy; With happiness, false memory: Mood and the false memory effect. *Psychological Science, 16*(10), 785–791.

Stroebe, M., Schut, H., & Stroebe, W. (2005). Attachment in coping with bereavement: A theoretical integration. *Review of General Psychology, 9,* 48–66.

Stroebe, M. S., Hansson, R. O., Stroebe, W., & Schut, H. (2001). Concepts and issues in contemporary research on bereavement. In M. S. Stroebe, R. O. Hansson, W. Stroebe, & H. Schut (Eds.), *Handbook of bereavement research: Consequences, coping, and care* (pp. 3–22). Washington, DC: American Psychological Association.

Stroebe, M. S., & Schut, H. (1999). The dual process model of coping with bereavement: Rationale and description. *Death Studies, 23*(3), 197–224.

Stroebe, W., Schut, H., & Stroebe, M. S. (2005). Grief work, disclosure and counseling: Do they help the bereaved? *Clinical Psychology Review, 25*(4), 395–414.

Stroebe, W., & Stroebe, M. S. (1987). *Bereavement and health: The psychological and physical consequences of partner loss.* New York: Cambridge University Press.

Trivers, R. L. (1972). Parental investment and sexual selection. In B. Campbell (Ed.), *Sexual selection and the descent of man* (pp. 136–179). Chicago: Aldine-Atherton.

Tugade, M. M., & Fredrickson, B. L. (2004). Resilient individuals use positive emotions to bounce back from negative emotional experiences. *Journal of Personality and Social Psychology, 86*, 320–333.

Wang, L., McCarthy, G., Song, A. W., & LaBar, K. S. (2005). Amygdala activation to sad pictures during high-field (4 tesla) functional magnetic resonance imaging. *Emotion, 5*, 12–22.

Welling, H. (2003). An evolutionary function of the depressive reaction: The cognitive map hypothesis. *New Ideas in Psychology, 21*(2), 147–156.

Westphal, M., & Bonanno, G. A. (2004). Emotion self-regulation. In M. Beauregard (Ed.), *Consciousness,* *emotional self-regulation and the brain* (pp. 1–33). Amsterdam: Benjamins.

Zautra, A. J., Berkhof, J., & Nicolson, N. A. (2002). Changes in affect interrelations as a function of stressful events. *Cognition and Emotion, 16*, 309–318.

Zautra, A. J., Reich, J. W., Davis, M. C., Potter, P., & Nicolson, N. A. (2000). The role of stressful events in the relationship between positive and negative affects: Evidence from field and experimental studies. *Journal of Personality, 68*, 927–951.

Zautra, A. J., & Smith, B. W. (2001). Depression and reactivity to stress in older women with rheumatoid arthritis and osteoarthritis. *Psychosomatic Medicine, 63*, 687–696.

Author Index

Subject Index

Page numbers followed by an *n, f,* or *t* indicate notes, figures, or tables.